Stedman's

MEDICAL & SURGICAL
EQUIPMENT WORDS

FOURTH EDITION

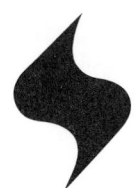

Stedman's
MEDICAL & SURGICAL
EQUIPMENT WORDS

FOURTH EDITION

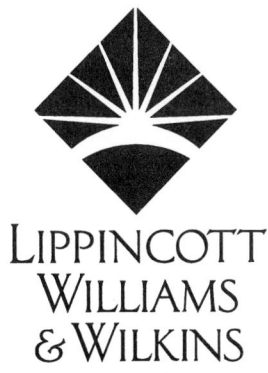

LIPPINCOTT
WILLIAMS
& WILKINS

Publisher: Julie K. Stegman
Series Managing Editor: Trista A. DiPaula
Production Coordinator: Jason Delaney
Typesetter: Peirce Graphic Services, LLC.
Printer & Binder: Malloy Litho, Inc.

Copyright © 2004 Lippincott Williams & Wilkins
351 West Camden Street
Baltimore, Maryland 21201-2436

Printed in the United States of America

2004

Library of Congress Cataloging-in-Publication Data

Stedman's medical & surgical equipment words.— 4th ed.
    p. ; cm.— (Stedman's word books)
Rev. ed. of: Stedman's equipment words. 3rd ed. 2001.
Includes bibliographical references.
  ISBN 0–7817-5440–2
  1. Medical instruments and apparatus—Terminology. 2. Medical technology—
Terminology. I. Title: Stedman's medical and surgical equipment words. II. Title:
Medical & surgical equipment words. III. Stedman, Thomas Lathrop, 1853–1938. IV.
Lippincott Williams & Wilkins. V. Stedman's equipment words. VI. Series.
  [DNLM: 1. Equipment and Supplies—Terminology—English. W 15 S8126 2004]
R123.S698 2004
610′.1′4—dc22

2003024518
01
1 2 3 4 5 6 7 8 9 10

Contents

Acknowledgments

An important part of our editorial process is the involvement of medical transcriptionists—as advisors, reviewers, and/or editors.

We extend special thanks to Catherine S. Baxter and R. Jo-Ann Clarke, for editing the manuscript, helping resolve many difficult questions, and reviewing material for the appendix sections. We are grateful to those who spent numerous hours doing research: Jeanne Bock, CSR, MT; Jo-Ann Clarke; Darcy Johnson; Andrea Linderman; and Nicole Peck, CMT who were instrumental in the refinement and development of this reference. They recommended sources and shared their valuable judgment, insight, and perspective. Additional thanks to Jeanne Bock for performing the final prepublication review. Other important contributors to this edition include Susan Caldwell, Cheryl A. Letner, CMT, and Beverly S. Oberline, CMT.

And, as always, Barb Ferretti played an integral role in the process by reviewing the content files for format, updating the content, and providing a final quality check. Special thanks also goes to Lisa Fahnestock for her assistance with this work.

As with all our *Stedman's* word references, this resource incorporates the suggestions and expertise of our many contacts in the medical transcriptionist community. Thanks to all of our advisory board participants, reviewers, and editors; AAMT meeting attendees; and others who have written us with requests and comments—keep talking, and we'll keep listening.

Editor's Preface

Alas, the call has come from my editorial team. It's time once again to prepare the *Editor's Preface*. This is the fourth such request that I have received over the past dozen years for this very special title, *Stedman's Medical & Surgical Equipment Words*. Ah, the name of the book has been changed over time, but the content and intent have not deviated from our original scope of purpose.

In preparing to write a preface, I always begin by re-reading the prefaces of the previous editions. I'm sure the obvious comment would be that she doesn't want to say something that she has already said in a previous edition. But, in truth, I relish walking back in time and rekindling those feelings of excitement, and at times exhaustion, I felt during the year of work that went into each of the first three editions. As I re-read the preface to that first edition and recall how, ". . . it all started with the Veress needle," I also recall that my youngest child, Erin, was a skinny little horse-crazy 12 year old at the time. A few weeks ago, I watched as a beautiful young woman of 24 walked down the aisle on her wedding day. By the way, she's still horse crazy, but someone else is paying the feed bills.

Now, I sit before my Dell Pentium IV with Zip drive, sound system, scanner, color printer, and fax—all online at lightening fast connection speeds through a cable modem. Twelve years ago, I sat in the archives of the Texas Medical Center Library in Houston, Texas, fighting off dust allergies as I researched one term at a time, one book at a time, and one journal at a time, dutifully recording each term in writing with the proper reference cited. Then, those terms were typed in Word Perfect and stored on floppies, and I do mean the real floppy disks of old . . . you know, the ones that were about 5 inches across and could be bent and destroyed with one good fold.

By the second edition, we at least had the beginnings of a database. Certainly nothing like what Lippincott Williams & Wilkins currently maintains on behalf of the *Stedman's Word Books,* but a significant improvement none the less. And, the icing on the cake for me was that I didn't have to manually alphabetize the majority of the terms, as I did with the first edition.

And then came the third edition and the new millennium. Truly, I felt that we had reached the brave new world of publishing. For the very first time in preparing this title, I did not have to set foot in a medical library to do my research. The database was rich and robust, though it did stumble at one point, which I've since learned databases do from time to time just to keep us honest and humble and indebted to the database managers who seem to belong to some secret society that has all the answers, password protected, encrypted, and guarded under threat of permanent loss of access privileges.

So, after this walk down memory lane, I can say that I'm pleased to announce the release of the best edition yet thanks to the patient efforts of the very capable LWW editorial team and the guidance provided by the editorial advisory board comprised of some of the most respected medical transcription experts and educators in the world.

The technology available to us in 2004 has made the creative and review processes much more streamlined and efficient. Our beloved databases have allowed us to dice, slice, reorganize, and refine thousands of words and phrases into a very consistently presented reference book.

As always, LWW and I continue to share the vision of providing all types of medical language specialists with a text that simply has no equal in quality and quantity of content with respect to medical and surgical equipment. We know that this book has become the reference of choice for medical transcriptionists, medical editors, as well as medical translators and interpreters throughout the world. Our commitment to each of you is to continue to provide the most up-to-date, accurate, and complete resource possible to assist you in your daily work.

To this day, nothing gives me more pleasure, nothing repays me more fairly than when a person tells me, "*Stedman's Medical & Surgical Equipment Words* made my job easier today. I found a word in there, I couldn't find anywhere else."

This edition, more than any other, was prepared with many helping hands. For the first time, I was assisted by a second editor, Jo-Ann Clarke. I would like to thank Jo-Ann for the countless hours of work she has contributed to reviewing both the first and second pass edits. There is absolutely no doubt that two sets of eyes are far better than one, especially when dealing with so many terms.

In addition, I'd like to thank my friends and colleagues at Scott & White Memorial Hospital and Clinic in Temple, Texas, for gathering new terms and keeping me on my toes with challenging QA questions. It takes the combined efforts of over 225 MTs to support all the documentation for this sprawling Central Texas integrated healthcare delivery system. We rely on the *Stedman's Word Books Series* to provide our organization with the quality they demand and deserve.

Special thanks go to my "handlers" at Lippincott Williams & Wilkins, Trista DiPaula and Julie Stegman. Both ladies displayed the patience of Job in working with me, an individual who is not known to take "no" for an answer. My grandmother once told my mother that being hardheaded was a good character trait for me to have. I'm not so certain my mother ever bought that line, and I'm quite sure that Trista and Julie would beg to differ with Big Mama at this point in time.

But, in the end, we have prepared for you a thorough reference book that will meet your needs for the next three years . . . augmented, of course, by the wonderful *Stedman's Online* resources.

So, as we put to bed the fourth edition, let the fifth edition begin!

Catherine S. Baxter

Publisher's Preface

Stedman's Medical & Surgical Equipment Words, Fourth Edition, offers an authoritative assurance of quality and exactness to the wordsmiths of the healthcare professions—medical transcriptionists, medical editors and copyeditors, health information management personnel, court reporters, and the many other users and producers of medical documentation.

Users will find an extensive array of medical and surgical equipment terminology. The appendix sections, substantially enhanced over the previous edition include illustrations with useful captions and labels; sample reports and dictation; common terms by procedure; and common manufacturers and websites.

This new edition, including more than 70,000 entries, includes the Stedman's Word Book Series trademarks: fully cross-indexed by first and last word, A-Z format with main entries and subentries, and appendix material for additional comprehension and application of the terminology.

We at Lippincott Williams & Wilkins strive to provide you with the most up-to-date and accurate word references available. Your use of this Word Book will prompt new editions, which we will publish as often as updates and revisions justify. We welcome your suggestions for improvements, changes, corrections, and additions—whatever will make this *Stedman's* product more useful to you. Please complete the postage-paid card in this book for future suggestions and recommendations, or visit us online at www.stedmans.com.

Explanatory Notes

Medical transcription is an art as well as a science. Both approaches are needed to correctly interpret the dictation of a physician, whose language is a product of education, training, and experience. This variety in medical language means that there are several acceptable ways to express certain terms, including jargon. *Stedman's Medical & Surgical Equipment Words, Fourth Edition,* provides variant spellings and phrasings for many terms. These elements, in addition to complete cross-indexing, make *Stedman's Medical & Surgical Equipment Words, Fourth Edition,* a valuable resource for determining the validity of terms as they are encountered.

Alphabetical Organization

Alphabetization of main entries is letter by letter as spelled, ignoring punctuation, spaces, prefixed numbers, or other characters. For example:

VSG 2/3F graphic card
V-slit lamp
VSR

Terms beginning or ending with Greek letters show the Greek letters spelled out and listed alphabetically. For example:

alpha, α
- a. angle
- b. crystallin

In subentry alphabetization, the abbreviated singular form or the spelled-out plural form of the noun main entry word is ignored.

Format and Style

All main entries are in **boldface** to expedite locating a sought-after term, to enhance distinction between main entries and subentries, and to relieve the textual density of the pages.

Irregular plurals and variant spellings are shown on the same line as the singular or preferred form of the word. For example:

ampulla, pl. ampullae
disc, disk

Capitalization

Trade/brand names (proprietary) and proper names (eponyms) begin with a capital letter.

Axiom thoracic trocar
Equinox occlusion balloon system
Kjelland blade

Product names that are represented in all upper case by the manufacturer are represented with an initial upper case in this book as shown in bold below.

INTERCEED absorbable adhesion barrier = **Interceed absorbable adhesion barrier**
ENDOCAM digital camera = **Endocam digital camera**

Irregular capitalization used by the manufacturer is maintained as shown below.

IsoMed implantable drug pump
MAGneedle

Hyphenation

As a rule of style, multiple eponyms (e.g., Smith-Fisher knife) are hyphenated. Also, hyphens have been added between a manufacturer and one or more eponyms (e.g., Storz-Duredge steel cataract knife). Please note that in many cases, hyphenation is a question of style, not of accuracy, and thus is a matter of choice.

Possessives

Possessive forms have been dropped in this reference for the sake of consistency and conformance with the guidelines of the American Association for Medical Transcription (AAMT) and other groups. Please note, however, that in many cases, retaining the possessive, like hyphenating, is a question of style, not of accuracy, and thus is a matter of choice. To form the possessive of a word, simply add the apostrophe or apostrophe "s" to the end of the word.

Cross-indexing

The word list is in an index-like main entry-subentry format that contains two combined alphabetical listings:

(1) A *noun* main entry-subentry organization, which is typical of the A-Z section of medical dictionaries like *Stedman's:*

Smith	**bed**
S. expressor	air b.
S. expressor hook	hyperbaric b.
S. eyelid operation	Lumex shower b.

(2) An *adjective* main entry-subentry organization, which lists words and phrases as you hear them. The main entries are the adjectives or modifiers in a multiword term. The subentries are the nouns around which the terms are constructed and to which the adjectives or modifiers pertain:

long	**round**
l. arm splint	r. cutting bur
l. needle	r. dissector
l. tissue forceps	r. speculum

This format provides the user with more than one way to locate and identify a multiword term. For example:

curved   **scissors**
  c. scissors   curved s.

epithelial   **cyst**
  e. inclusion cyst   epithelial inclusion c.

It also allows the user to see together all terms that contain a particular descriptor, as well as all types, kinds, or variations of a noun entity. For example:

ocular   **multifocal**
  o. adnexa   m. chorioretinal disease
  o. adnexal tumor   m. choroiditis
  o. albinism   m. choroiditis with panuveitis

Wherever possible, abbreviations are separately defined and cross-referenced. For example:

IMT
  integrated massage therapy

integrated
  i. massage therapy (IMT)

therapy
  integrated massage t. (IMT)

References

In addition to the manufacturers' literature we gather at various medical meetings, scientific reports from hospitals, and the lists of our MT Editorial Advisory Board members (from their daily transcription work), we used the following sources for new terms in *Stedman's Medical & Surgical Equipment Words, Fourth Edition.*

Books

The AAMT Book of Style, 2nd Edition. Modesto, CA: AAMT, 2002.

Dorland's Medical Equipment Word Book for Medical Transcriptionists. Philadelphia: Elsevier, 2002.

Lance LL. Quick Look Drug Book. Baltimore: Lippincott Williams & Wilkins, 2003.

Pyle V. Current Medical Terminology, 9th Edition. Modesto, CA: Health Professions Institute, 2003.

Stedman's Abbreviations, Acronyms & Symbols, 3rd Edition. Baltimore: Lippincott Williams & Wilkins, 2003.

Stedman's Alternative Medicine Words. Baltimore: Lippincott Williams & Wilkins, 2000.

Stedman's Anatomy & Physiology Words, 2nd Edition. Baltimore: Lippincott Williams & Wilkins, 2002.

Stedman's Cardiovascular & Pulmonary Words, 3rd Edition. Baltimore: Lippincott Williams & Wilkins, 2001.

Stedman's Dermatology & Immunology Words, 2nd Edition. Baltimore: Lippincott Williams & Wilkins, 2002.

Stedman's Emergency Medicine Words. Baltimore: Lippincott Williams & Wilkins, 2004.

Stedman's Endocrinology Words. Baltimore: Lippincott Williams & Wilkins, 2001.

Stedman's Equipment Words, 3rd Edition. Baltimore: Lippincott Williams & Wilkins, 2001.

Stedman's GI & GU Words, 3rd Edition. Baltimore: Lippincott Williams & Wilkins, 2002.

Stedman's Internal Medicine & Geriatric Words. Baltimore: Lippincott Williams & Wilkins, 2002.

Stedman's Medical Dictionary, 27th Edition. Baltimore: Lippincott Williams & Wilkins, 2000.

Stedman's Neurology & Neurosurgery Words, 3rd Edition. Baltimore: Lippincott Williams & Wilkins, 2003.

Stedman's OB/GYN & Genetics Words, 3rd Edition. Baltimore: Lippincott Williams & Wilkins, 2001.

Stedman's Oncology Words, 4th Edition. Baltimore: Lippincott Williams & Wilkins, 2004.

Stedman's Ophthalmology Words, 3rd Edition. Baltimore: Lippincott Williams & Wilkins, 2004.

Stedman's Organisms & Infectious Disease Words. Baltimore: Lippincott Williams & Wilkins, 2002.

Stedman's Orthopaedic & Rehab Words, 4th Edition. Baltimore: Lippincott Williams & Wilkins, 2003.

Stedman's Pathology & Lab Medicine Words, 3rd Edition. Baltimore: Lippincott Williams & Wilkins, 2002.

Stedman's Pediatric Words. Baltimore: Lippincott Williams & Wilkins, 2001.

Stedman's Plastic Surgery/ENT/Dentistry Words, 3rd Edition. Baltimore: Lippincott Williams & Wilkins, 2003.

Stedman's Psychiatry Words, 3rd Edition. Baltimore: Lippincott Williams & Wilkins, 2003.

Stedman's Radiology Words, 4th Edition. Baltimore: Lippincott Williams & Wilkins, 2004.

Stedman's Surgery Words, 2nd Edition. Baltimore: Lippincott Williams & Wilkins, 2002.

Journals

American Journal of Audiology. Rockville, MD: American Speech-Language-Hearing Association, 2000–2003.

Alternative Therapies in Health and Medicine. Aliso Viejo, CA: Innovision Communications, 2000–2003.

American Journal of Cardiology. New York: Excerpta Medica, 2000–2003.

American Journal of Clinical Pathology. Chicago: American Society for Clinical Pathology, 2000–2003.

American Journal of Gastroenterology. New York: Elsevier, 2000–2003.

American Journal of Ophthalmology. New York: Elsevier, 2000–2003.

American Journal of Surgical Pathology. Philadelphia: Lippincott Williams & Wilkins, 2000–2003.

Archives of Otolaryngology—Head & Neck Surgery. Chicago: American Medical Association, 2000–2003.

AUA News. Baltimore: Lippincott Williams & Wilkins, 2000–2003.

CA-A Cancer Journal for Clinicians. Atlanta: American Cancer Society. 2000–2003.

Cancer. New York: John Wiley & Sons, 2000–2003.

Cardiology in Review. Baltimore: Lippincott Williams & Wilkins, 2000–2003.

Chiropractic Products. Los Angeles: Novicom, 2000–2003.

Clinical Pulmonary Medicine. Baltimore: Lippincott Williams & Wilkins, 2000–2003.

Computer-Aided Surgery. New York: Wiley, 2000–2003.

Contemporary OB/GYN. Montvale, NJ: Medical Economics, 2000–2003.

Cornea. Philadelphia: Lippincott Williams & Wilkins, 2000–2003.

The Endocrinologist. Baltimore: Lippincott Williams & Wilkins, 2000–2003.

Extended Care Product News. Malvern, PA: HMP Communications, 2000–2003.

Foot & Ankle International. Seattle: American Orthopaedic Foot & Ankle Society, 2000–2003.

Gastrointestinal Endoscopy. St. Louis: Mosby, 2000–2003.

Hypertension. Philadelphia: Lippincott Williams & Wilkins, 2000–2003.

Implant Dentistry. Philadelphia: Lippincott Williams & Wilkins, 2000–2003.

Infectious Diseases in Clinical Practice. Baltimore: Lippincott Williams & Wilkins, 2000–2003.

The Integrative Medicine Consult. Newton, MA: Integrative Medicine Communications, 2000–2003.

Journal of Alternative and Complementary Medicine. Larchmont, NY: Mary Ann Liebert Publishers, Inc. 2000–2003.

Journal of the American Association for Medical Transcriptionists. Modesto, CA: AAMT, 2000–2003.

Journal of the American College of Cardiology. Orlando: Elsevier, 2000–2003.

Journal of the American College of Surgeons. New York: Elsevier, 2000–2003.

Journal of the American Society of Nephrology. Baltimore: Lippincott Williams & Wilkins, 2000–2003.

Journal of Bone and Joint Surgery. Needham, MA: The Journal of Bone and Joint Surgery, Incorporated, 2000–2003.

Journal of Clinical Rheumatology. Baltimore: Lippincott Williams & Wilkins, 2000–2003.

Journal of Oral and Maxillofacial Surgery. Philadelphia: Saunders, 2000–2003.

Journal of the National Cancer Institute. Bethesda, MD: Oxford University Press, 2000–2003.

Journal of Neuro-Ophthalmology. Philadelphia: Lippincott Williams & Wilkins, 2000–2003.

The Latest Word. Philadelphia: Saunders, 2000–2003.

Neurosurgery. Baltimore: Lippincott Williams & Wilkins, 2000–2003.

O & P Almanac. Alexandria, VA: American Orthotic and Prosthetic Association, 2000–2003.

OB/GYN Clinical Alert. Atlanta: American Health Consultants, 2000–2003.

OB/GYN News. Rockville, MD: International Medical News Group, 2000–2003.

Obstetrical & Gynecological Survey. Philadelphia: Lippincott Williams & Wilkins, 2000–2003.

Obstetrics & Gynecology. New York: Elsevier. 2000–2003.

Ophthalmology. Philadelphia: Lippincott Williams & Wilkins, 2000–2003.

Ophthalmology Times. New York: Advanstar Communications, 2000–2003.

Ostomy Wound Management. Malvern, PA: HMP Communications, 2000–2003.

Physical Therapy Products. Los Angeles: Novicom, 2000–2003.

Plastic and Reconstructive Surgery. Philadelphia: Lippincott Williams & Wilkins, 2000–2003.

Plastic Surgery Products. Los Angeles: Novicom, 2000–2003.

Podiatric Products. Los Angeles: Novicom, 2000–2003.

Radiology. Oak Brook, IL: Radiological Society of North America: 2000–2003.

Retina. Baltimore: Lippincott Williams & Wilkins, 2000–2003.

Images

Blackbourne LH, MD. Advanced Surgical Recall, 2nd Edition. Baltimore: Lippincott Williams & Wilkins, 2004.

Hardy NO, Westport, CT. From Stedman's Medical Dictionary, 27th Edition. Baltimore: Lippincott Williams & Wilkins, 2000.

LifeART Emergency Collection 2, CD-ROM. Baltimore: Lippincott Williams & Wilkins.

LifeART Emergency Collection 4, CD-ROM. Baltimore: Lippincott Williams & Wilkins.

LifeART Emergency Collection 5, CD-ROM. Baltimore: Lippincott Williams & Wilkins.

LifeART Health Care 1, CD-ROM. Baltimore: Lippincott Williams & Wilkins.

LifeART Nursing Collection 1, CD-ROM. Baltimore: Lippincott Williams & Wilkins.

LifeART Nursing Collection 2, CD-ROM. Baltimore: Lippincott Williams & Wilkins.

LifeART Nursing Collection 3, CD-ROM. Baltimore: Lippincott Williams & Wilkins.

LifeART Pediatrics Collection 1, CD-ROM. Baltimore: Lippincott Williams & Wilkins.

LifeART Super Anatomy Collection 3, CD-ROM. Baltimore: Lippincott Williams & Wilkins.

LifeART Super Anatomy Collection 8, CD-ROM. Baltimore: Lippincott Williams & Wilkins.

LifeART Super Anatomy Collection 9, CD-ROM. Baltimore: Lippincott Williams & Wilkins.

MediClip Clinical Cardiopulmonary, CD-ROM. Baltimore: Lippincott, Williams & Wilkins.

MediClip Clinical OB/GYN, CD-ROM. Baltimore: Lippincott, Williams & Wilkins.

Websites

http://www.fda.gov/cdrh

http://www.hpisum.com

http://www.mdrweb.com

http://www.mtdaily.com

http://www.mtdesk.com

http://www.mtmonthly.com

http://www.stedmans.com/section.cfm/36

A13 Sequel programmable behind-the-ear hearing aid
A1-Askari needle holder
A1cNow glucose monitoring device
A675 Sequel Audio Vision hearing aid
A-6S wheelchair
AAI single-chamber pacemaker
Aaron cautery
AART
    Aesthetic and Reconstructive
    Technologies
    AART calf implant
    AART chin implant
    AART gluteal implant
    AART malar implant
    AART pectoralis implant
    AART silicone carving block
AAT pacemaker
Abacus Concepts StatView 4.02 statistical analyzer
Abadie
    A. intestinal clamp
    A. self-retaining intestinal retractor
ABaer newborn hearing screening system
Abanda drape sheet
Abbe
    A. condenser
    A. refractometer
Abbey needle holder
ABBI
    Advanced Breast Biopsy Instrumentation
    ABBI breast biopsy system
Abbokinase catheter
Abbott
    A. elevator
    A. infusion pump
    A. LifeCare PCA Plus II infuser
    A. LifeCare PCA Plus II infusion system
    A. Lifeshield needleless system
    A. Plum infusion system
    A. scoop
    A. tube
Abbott-Mayfield forceps
Abbott-Rawson gastrointestinal double-lumen tube
abdominal
    a. aortic counterpulsation device
    a. bandage
    a. belt
    a. binder
    a. brace
    a. compression cylinder

    A. Left Ventricular Assist Device (ALVAD)
    a. patch electrode
    a. scissors
    a. scoop
    a. trocar
    a. vascular retractor
abduction
    a. finger splint
    a. pillow
    a. splint
Abel-Aesculap-Pratt tenaculum
Abelson
    A. adenotome
    A. cricothyrotomy cannula
    A. cricothyrotomy trocar
Aberhart
    A. disposable urinal bag
    A. hemostatic bag
Abernaz strut forceps
aberrometer
    Shack-Hartmann a.
ABG cement-free hip system
ABI
    ABI fluorescence dye
    ABI Prism dye terminator cycle sequencing ready reaction kit
    ABI Vest airway clearance system
AbioCor replacement heart
Abiomed
    A. biventricular support system
    A. BVAD 5000 left ventricular assist device
    A. BVS 5000 biventricular support system
ABL520 blood gas measurement system
Ablaser laser delivery catheter
Ablatherm
    A. HIFU system
    A. high-intensity focused ultrasound system
ablation
    a. catheter
    outpatient endometrial resection and a. (OPERA)
    radiofrequency interstitial tissue a. (RITA)
    ThermaChoice thermal balloon a.
    transurethral needle a. (TUNA)
ablative device
ablator
    cautery a.
    Concept a.
    endometrial a.
    Hydro TherAblator a.

ablator *(continued)*
    NovaSure a.
    radiofrequency a.
    Trident resection arthroscopic a.
Ablatr temperature control device
Ablaza
    A. aortic wall retractor
    A. patent ductus clamp
Ablaza-Blanco cardiac valve retractor
Ablaza-Morse rib approximator
Ableware Bath+Safe deluxe tub safety rail
AbMap
    A. electrophysiologic imaging system
    A. imaging system
abortion scoop
above-knee suction enhancement system
Abradabloc dermabrasion instrument
abrader
    a. bur
    cartilage a.
    corneal a.
    Dingman a.
    Haverhill dermal a.
    Howard corneal a.
    Lieberman a.
    Montague a.
Abraham
    A. contact lens
    A. elevator
    A. iridectomy laser lens
    A. iridectomy YAG laser lens
    A. laryngeal cannula
    A. peripheral button iridotomy lens
    A. rectal curette
    A. tonsillar knife
Abrams
    A. biopsy needle
    A. pleural biopsy punch
Abrams-Lucas mitral valve prosthesis
Abramson
    A. catheter
    A. hook
    A. retractor
    A. sump drain
Abramson-Allis breast clamp
Abramson-Dedo microlaryngoscope
abrasive
    micromesh cushioned a.
abscess
    a. drainage catheter
    a. forceps
Abscession fluid drainage catheter
abscission needle
Absolok
    A. endoscopic clip applicator
    A. forceps
    A. ligating clip

Absolute absorbable screw
absorbable
    a. gelatin film
    a. gelatin sponge
    a. plate
    a. stent
    a. suture
absorbent cover dressing (ACD)
absorber
    Hollister wound exudate a.
    laser fume a.
absorptiometer
    Hologic 1000 QDR dual-energy a.
    Lunar DPX dual-energy a.
    single-energy x-ray a.
absorptiometry
    dual-energy x-ray a. (DEXA)
absorption spectrophotometer
A/B switch box
abutment
    CerAdapt a.
    CeraOne a.
    Dalla Bona ball and socket a.
    dovetail stress broken a.
    Hex-Lock a.
    Impac PDQ a.
    ProTect a.
    ThreadLoc non-cast-to a.
    tooth-colored a.
AC
    anterior chamber
    AC intraocular lens
    AC IOL
Acapella chest physical therapy device
ACAT
    Arrow Cardiac Assist Technology
    ACAT 1 Plus intraaortic balloon pump
accelerator
    alpha particle a.
    Becker a.
    dual-energy digital linear a.
    electron linear a.
    high-energy bent-beam linear a.
    A. II aspirator
    linear a. (LINAC)
    Mevatron 74 linear a.
    Microtron a.
    Mobetron mobile, self-shielded electron a.
    Philips linear a.
    plasma prothrombin conversion a.
    racetrack Microtron a.
    Siemens Mevatron 74 linear a.
    University of Florida linear a.
    Varian linear a.
accelerometer
    Caltrac a.
    intracardiac a.

piezoelectric a.
triaxial a.
TriTrac a.
uniaxial a.
Accellon Combi cervical biosampler
Accel stopcock
Accent DG balloon catheter
Accents
A. micropigmentation system
A. permanent lash liner
Access
Advanced Venous A. (AVA)
A. immunoassay system
A. MV coronary stabilizer
A. MV stabilizer system
A. needle stiffening cannula
accessor
Auto Glide walker a.
accessory
BabyFace 3-D surface rendering a.
ScanLite Computer Pattern
Generator laser a.
Wegenke stent exchange a.
AccESS wand
ACCO
ACCO cotton roll
ACCO impression material
ACCO orthodontic appliance
Accolade hip prosthesis
accommodative IOL
Accorde bur
Accor dental matrix
accordion
a. drain
a. graft
AccuAngle indicator
AccuBrush dental system
Accucap CO₂/O₂ monitor
Accucare TENS unit
Accu-Chek
A.-C. blood glucose monitor
A.-C. Easy blood glucose monitor
A.-C. II Freedom blood glucose
monitor
A.-C. II, III glucometer
A.-C. InstantPlus blood glucose
monitor
A.-C. InstantPlus glucometer
Accucom cardiac output monitor
AccuCore biopsy needle
Accu-Cut osteotomy guide

accuDEXA
a. bone densitometer
a. bone mineral density assessment
system
AccuFilm articulating film
Accufix
A. pacemaker
A. pacemaker lead
AccuFlex dynamic elbow orthosis
Accuflex intraocular lens
Accu-Flo
A.-F. button
A.-F. connector
A.-F. CSF reservoir
A.-F. dural film
A.-F. pressure valve
A.-F. spring catheter
A.-F. U-channel stripping cannula
A.-F. ventricular cannula
A.-F. ventricular catheter
Accuform nasal splint
AccuGage vessel calipers
AccuGel
A. impression material
A. lens
AccuGuide injection monitor
Accuguide syringe
Accuject dental needle
AccuLase excimer laser
**AccuLength arthroplasty measuring
system**
Accu-line surgical marker
Acculink self-expanding stent
Acculith pacemaker
**AccuMark calibrated infant feeding
tube**
AccuMax
A. bed
A. self-adjusting pressure
management mattress
Accu-Measure personal body fat tester
AccuMeter
ChemTrak A.
A. cholesterol test system
Choles Trak A.
Accu-Mix
A.-M. amalgamator
A.-M. impression material
Accunet embolic protection system
Accu-o-Matic TENS unit
AccuPoint targeting sphere
AccuPort seal

NOTES

AccuPressure heel cup
AccuProbe
    A. 450 cryosurgical system
    A. 600 cryotherapy probe
    A. thermometer
Accura hydrocephalus shunt
Accurate
    A. catheter
    A. Surgical and Scientific Instruments (ASSI)
Accuratome precurved papillotome
Accuray Neurotron 1000 machine
Accurette
    A. endometrial suction curette
    A. microcurette
Accur hemofiltration system
Accurox mask
AccurRx constant flow implantable pump
Accurus vitrectomy system
Accusat pulse oximeter
AccuScan
    A. CO$_2$ laser scanner
    A. transducer
Accu-Scope
    A.-S. colposcope
    A.-S. microscope
AccuSharp instrument
Accu-Sorb gauze sponge
Accu-Space plain gut seeding spacer
AccuSpan tissue expander
AccuStick II introducer system
AccuSway balance measurement system
Accu-Temp cautery
Accutome low-speed diamond saw
Accutorr
    A. A1 blood pressure monitor
    A. oscillometric device
    A. Plus blood pressure monitor
Accutracker
    A. ambulatory blood pressure monitor
    A. ambulatory blood pressure recorder
    A. ambulatory BP recorder
    A. II ambulatory blood pressure monitor
    A. II ambulatory blood pressure recorder
AccuTrack eye-tracking system
AccuVac smoke evacuation attachment
Accu-Vu sizing angiographic catheter
ACD
    absorbent cover dressing
    active compression-decompression
    alternative communication device
    CombiDerm ACD
    ACD resuscitator

ACE
    Aerosol Cloud Enhancer
Ace
    A. adherent bandage
    A. autografter bone filter
    A. balloon
    A. bone screw tack
    A. brace
    A. fixed-wire balloon catheter
    A. halo-cast assembly
    A. halo pelvic girdle
    A. inhaler
    A. intramedullary femoral nail system
    A. longitudinal strips dressing
    A. low-profile MR halo
    A. Mark III halo
    A. OsteoGenic distractor
    A. spica bandage
    A. Trippi-Wells tongs cervical traction device
    A. Universal tongs cervical traction device
    A. wrap
Ace-Colles half ring
Ace-Fischer
    A.-F. external fixator
    A.-F. frame
Ace-Hershey halo jig
Ace-Hesive dressing
Ace/Normed
    A./N. bidirectional distractor
    A./N. osteodistractor
acetabular
    a. allograft
    a. component
    a. cup
    a. cup positioner
    a. grater
    a. reamer
    a. reconstruction plate
    a. shell guide
    a. skid
    a. trial cup
ACFS
    anterior cervical plate fixation system
    Dogbone ACFS
achalasia dilator
Achieva portable ventilator
Achieve off-pump system
Achiever
    A. balloon dilatation catheter
    A. balloon dilator
Achilles densitometer
Achilles+ ultrasonometer
Achillotrain active Achilles tendon support
acid
    hyaluronic a. (HA)

A

Acier stainless steel suture
ACIST
 Angiographic Contrast Injection System Technology
 ACIST injection system
Ackerman
 A. clip
 A. lingual bar
 A. needle
Ackrad
 A. balloon-bearing catheter
 A. Bronchitrac L^2 suction catheter
 A. Cervicet dilator
 A. esophageal balloon catheter
 A. H/S Elliptosphere catheter
 A. Tampa catheter set
ACL
 anterior cruciate ligament
 ACL drill
 ACL drill guide
 ACL graft knife
Aclaim nasal mask
Acland
 A. clasp
 A. clip
 A. microvascular clamp
 A. needle
Acland-Banis arteriotomy set
Acland-Bunke counterpressor
Aclec resin
Acme articulator
ACMI
 American Cystoscope Makers, Inc.
 ACMI ACN-2 flexible cystonephroscope
 ACMI Alcock catheter
 ACMI antroscope
 ACMI bag
 ACMI biopsy loop electrode
 ACMI Bunts catheter
 ACMI cannula
 ACMI coated Foley catheter
 ACMI cutting loop electrode
 ACMI cystourethroscope
 ACMI Dolphin pump
 ACMI duodenoscope
 ACMI Emmett hemostatic catheter
 ACMI endoscope
 ACMI fiberoptic colonoscope
 ACMI fiberoptic esophagoscope
 ACMI fiberoptic proctosigmoidoscope

ACMI flexible sigmoidoscope
ACMI gastroscope
ACMI hysteroscope
ACMI laparoscope
ACMI Marici bronchoscope
ACMI Martin endoscopic forceps
ACMI Micro-H hysteroscope
ACMI microlens foroblique telescope
ACMI monopolar electrode
ACMI operating colonoscope
ACMI Owens catheter
ACMI Pezzer drain
ACMI positive pressure catheter
ACMI proctoscope
ACMI resectoscope
ACMI retrograde electrode
ACMI severance catheter
ACMI Thackston catheter
ACMI transvaginal hydro laparoscope
ACMI transvaginal hydro laparoscopy
ACMI ulcer-measuring device
ACMI ureteral catheter
ACMI ureteral stent
ACMI Word Bartholin gland catheter
Acmix Foley catheter
Acolysis
 A. coronary probe
 A. ultrasound thrombolysis system
Acoma
 A. portable x-ray machine
 A. scanner
acorn
 a. cannula
 A. CorCap cardiac support device
 A. II nebulizer
 a. reamer
acorn-shaped eye implant
acorn-tipped
 a.-t. bougie
 a.-t. catheter
Acoustascope esophageal stethoscope
acoustic
 a. impedance probe
 a. microscope
 a. otoscope
AC-powered euthyscope
ACP plating system
AcQSIM CT simulator

NOTES

5

Acquacel Hydrofiber dressing
Acra-clip system
Acra-Cut spiral craniotome blade
Acragun system
AcroFlex artificial disc
AcroMed Isola device
acromionizer bur
acromioplasty
    a. electrode
    a. rasp
Acrotorque
    A. bur
    A. hand engine
AcryDerm
    A. border island dressing
    A. sheet wound dressing
    A. Strands
    A. Strands absorbent wound
    dressing
Acry Island border dressing
acrylic
    a. bar prosthesis
    a. bite block
    a. cap splint
    a. cement
    a. conformer eye implant
    Dentex a.
    Durabase soft rebase a.
    Duralay a.
    Dura-Liner a.
    fast-setting a.
    Flexacryl hard rebase a.
    a. implant material
    a. lens
    a. mold
    a. ocular implant
    a. resin dressing
    Setacure denture repair a.
    a. splint
    Splintline a.
    Vitacrilic dental a.
    Vita-Gel a.
    a. wafer TMJ splint
Acryl-X-II bone cement removal system
Acryl-X orthopaedic cement removal
system
AcrySof
    A. foldable intraocular lens
    A. single-piece intraocular lens
ACS
    Advanced Cardiovascular System
    ACS Amplatz guidewire
    ACS Anchor exchange device
    ACS angioplasty catheter
    ACS angioplasty Y connector
    ACS balloon catheter
    ACS Concorde
    ACS Concorde coronary dilatation
    catheter

ACS Concorde over-the-wire
    catheter system
ACS Eclipse catheter
ACS Endura coronary dilatation
    catheter
ACS exchange guiding catheter
ACS Flowtrack-40 catheter
ACS Hi-Torque Balance
    middleweight guidewire
ACS Hi-Torque Iron Man
    guidewire
ACS LIMA guidewire
ACS Monorail perfusion balloon
    catheter
ACS Multi-Link Duet coronary
    stent
ACS Multi-Link OTW Duet stent
ACS Multi-Link RX Duet stent
ACS Multi-Link RX Ultra
    coronary stent
ACS Multi-Link Tristar coronary
    stent
ACS Multi-Link Ultra coronary
    stent
ACS OTW Lifestream coronary
    dilatation catheter
ACS OTW Photon coronary
    dilatation catheter
ACS OTW Solaris coronary
    dilatation catheter
ACS percutaneous introducer
ACS RSX Multi-Link stent
ACS RX Comet VP coronary
    dilatation catheter
ACS RX Ellipse angioplasty
    catheter
ACS RX Gemini coronary
    dilatation catheter
ACS RX Rocket coronary
    dilatation catheter
ACS RX Solaris coronary
    dilatation catheter
ACS RX Streak angioplasty
    catheter
ACS Torquemaster catheter
ACS Tourguide II guiding catheter
ACS Tx2000 VP catheter
ACS Viking catheter
ACT
    Advanced Coronary Technology
    ACT MicroCoil delivery system
Actaeon probe
Actalyke activated clotting time test
system
Acticoat
    A. composite dressing
    A. foam dressing
    A. silver-based burn dressing

Acticon
- A. neosphincter
- A. neosphincter implant

Acti-Fit incontinence brief
Actifoam collagen sponge
Actigraph
- Mini-Motionlogger A.

Action
- A. elbow wrap
- A. Jr pediatric wheelchair
- A. OR pad
- A. Ranger II power chair
- A. ThumSling
- A. traction system
- A. wrist wrap
- A. 4XP tilt system wheelchair

Actis
- A. venous flow controller
- A. venous flow device
- A. VFC

Activa
- A. Parkinson control system
- A. tremor control system

activator
- Andresen a.
- Andresen-Haupl a.
- Bimler a.
- Karwetsky U-bow a.
- Klammt elastic open a.
- Metzelder modification a.
- Nuva-Lite ultraviolet a.
- palate-free a.
- Pfeiffer-Grobety a.
- Schmuth modification a.
- Schwarz bow a.
- Wunderer modification a.

Activator adjusting instrument
active
- A. Can defibrillator lead system
- A. Can-RV defibrillator lead system
- A. Cath catheter
- a. compression-decompression (ACD)
- a. electrode monitoring (AEM)
- a. fixation lead
- a. fixation pacemaker lead
- A. Free beta-hCG ELISA test kit
- A. Life 1-piece opqaue stoma cap
- A. Life urostomy pouch
- A. Response Catheter (ARC)

Activent ear tube

ActiveTrac traction treatment table
Activitrax
- A. II pacemaker
- A. variable-rate pacemaker

activity-guided pacemaker
activity-sensing pacemaker
Act joint support
actocardiotocograph fetal monitor
ACT-one coronary stent
Actros pacemaker
actuator
- linear a.
- NYU-Hosmer electric elbow and prehension a.

AcuBlade
- A. robotic laser
- A. robotic laser microsurgery system

Acucair continuous airflow system
Acucare bed
Acucise
- A. balloon
- A. cutting balloon device
- A. RP35 retrograde endopyelotomy catheter
- A. ureteral cutting cautery

AcuClip endoscopic multiple-clip applier
Acu-Derm
- A.-D. IV/TPN dressing
- A.-D. wound dressing

Acu-Dispo-Curette disposable dermal curette
Acufex
- A. alignment drill guide
- A. arthroscope
- A. arthroscopic instrument
- A. basket
- A. bioabsorbable Suretac suture
- A. bioabsorbable suture anchor
- A. curved basket forceps
- A. drill
- A. MosaicPlasty comprehensive system
- A. MosaicPlasty instrument
- A. rotary basket forceps
- A. rotary punch
- A. straight basket forceps
- A. Suretac fixation device

AcuFix anterior cervical plate system
Acuflex
- A. impression material
- A. intraocular lens

NOTES

Acuforce 7.0 massage therapy tool
acuity
    a. card
    a. visual projector
AcuMaster acupuncture needle
AcuMatch M Series modular femoral hip prosthesis
Acumed
    A. bone graft system
    A. suture anchor
AcuNav diagnostic ultrasound catheter
Acupoint finder
AcuPressor myotherapy tool
acupuncture laser
Acu-Ray x-ray unit
Acuscope microcurrent stimulator
AcuSeal cardiovascular patch
AcuSnare
    A. polypectomy device
    A. snare
Acuson
    A. cardiovascular ultrasound system
    A. color Doppler
    A. computed sonography
    A. echocardiograph
    A. model 128XP ultrasound scanner
    A. transvaginal sonogram
    A. ultrasound
    A. ultrasound scanner
    A. V510B biplane TEE transducer
    A. V5M ultrasound transducer
    A. 128XP/10 Doppler ultrasound
    A. XP10 scanner
    A. 128XP transducer
Acuspot
    Sharplan Laser 710 A.
AcuSyst-Xcell cell culturing system
Acutome 2000 Reich-Hasson laparoscopic CO_2 laser coupler
AcuTouch tissue forceps
AcuTrainer
    A. bladder retraining device
    A. bladder trainer
Acutrak
    A. bone fixation system
    A. bone replacement system
    A. fusion system
    A. Mini screw
    A. Plus screw
    A. screw
Acutrol suture
Acuvance catheter
Acuvue
    A. bifocal lens
    A. disposable contact lens
    A. Etafilcon A lens
ADAC
    ADAC Forte gamma camera
    ADAC SPECT camera
    ADAC Vertex Plus MCD/AC gamma camera
Adair
    A. adenotome
    A. breast clamp
    A. breast tenaculum forceps
    A. screw compressor
    A. tissue forceps
    A. tissue-holding forceps
    A. uterine forceps
Adair-Allis tissue forceps
Adair-Veress needle
Adam and Eve rib belt splint
Adams
    A. aspirator
    A. clasp
    A. kidney stone filter
    A. modification of Bethune tourniquet
    A. orthodontic clip
    A. retractor
    A. rib contractor
    A. saw
Adams-DeWeese vena caval serrated clip
Adamson retractor
Adante Monorail catheter shaft
Adapta
    A. massage table
    A. MC-100 massage chair
adapter
    Air-Lon a.
    Alcock catheter a.
    Amsco Hall a.
    Bard-Tuohy-Borst a.
    BD a.
    Bernaco a.
    BioLase laser a.
    Bodai a.
    Brown-Roberts-Wells ring a.
    butterfly a.
    catheter a.
    Christmas tree a.
    chuck a.
    collet screwdriver a.
    Cook plastic Luer-Lok a.
    Cooper laser a.
    Cordis-Dow shunt a.
    Freestyle CAPD catheter a.
    friction-fit a.
    Grace plate 4-hole a.
    Greenberg Maxi-Vise a.
    halo-ring a.
    House a.
    Hudson a.
    Jacobs chuck a.
    Kaufman a.
    King connector a.

A

KleenSpec otoscope a.
laser a.
LifePort endotracheal tube a.
Lloyd a.
Luer-Lok a.
Luer suction cannula a.
Mayfield skull clamp a.
Medi-Jector a.
Merrimack laser a.
metal a.
Morch swivel a.
Neuroguide suction-irrigation a.
Nickell cystoscope a.
peripheral interface a.
PMV O_2 a.
power a.
Rosenblum rotating a.
rotating a.
SafeTrak epidural catheter a.
Sanders ventilation a.
Sheehy-Urban sliding lens a.
Shiley pressure-relief a.
side-arm a.
sleeve a.
suction a.
swivel a.
Telestill photo a.
terminal electrode a.
Trinkle chuck a.
tubing a.
Tuohy-Borst sideport a.
venous Y a.
ventilation a.
Venturi ventilation a.
Volk Minus power noncontact a.
Volk Plus power noncontact a.
Volk retinal scale a.
Volk UltraField contact lens a.
Volk yellow filter a.
Wullstein chuck a.
Xanar laser a.
Y a.
Zeiss cine a.
Adapteur
A. multifunctional drill guide
A. power system
Adaptic
A. gauze
A. gauze dressing
A. II dental restorative material
A. nonadhering dressing
A. petroleum gauze dressing

A. PG gauze dressing
A. X Xeroform gauze nonadhering dressing
adaptometer
color a.
Feldman a.
Ada scissors
ADC Medicut shears
Add-A-Cath
A.-A.-C. catheter
Lawrence A.-A.-C.
Add-A-Clamp
Hex-Fix A.-A.-C.
Additions multifocal soft progressive lens
Addix needle
AddOn-Bucky
A.-B. direct x-ray detector
A.-B. image acquisition system
ADDStat laser
adductus/varus
metatarsus a./v. (MTA)
AddVent atrioventricular pacemaker
A-Dec
A-D. amalgamator
A-D. handpiece
adenoid
a. curette
a. cutter
a. forceps
a. punch
adenotome
Abelson a.
Adair a.
a. blade
Box a.
Box-DeJager a.
Breitman a.
Cullom-Mueller a.
Daniels a.
direct-vision a.
guillotine a.
Kelly direct-vision a.
LaForce a.
LaForce-Grieshaber a.
LaForce-Stevenson a.
LaForce-Storz a.
Mueller-LaForce a.
Myles guillotine a.
reverse a.
Shambaugh reverse a.
Shulec a.

NOTES

9

adenotome *(continued)*
   Sluder a.
   St. Clair-Thompson a.
   Stevenson-LaForce a.
   Storz-LaForce a.
   Storz-LaForce-Stevenson a.
   V. Mueller-LaForce a.
Aderer alloy
Adeza TLi system
adherent
   Tuf-Skin tape a.
Ad-Hese-Away dressing
adhesive
   a. absorbent dressing
   Aron Alpha a.
   autologous fibrin tissue a.
   a. band
   a. bandage
   bioactive bone cement a.
   Biobond tissue a.
   BioGlue protein-based surgical a.
   Bond-Eze a.
   bone cement a.
   Brown sterile a.
   Cel Touch a.
   Coe-Pak paste a.
   Cover-Roll gauze a.
   cyanoacrylate tissue a.
   Dermabond topical skin a.
   fibrin glue a.
   fibrin sealant a.
   a. flange
   gelatin-resorcin-formalin tissue
    glue a.
   HA a.
   Hollister a.
   hydroxyapatite a.
   Indermil tissue a.
   Klutch denture a.
   LiquiBand topical skin tissue a.
   Liquiderm liquid a.
   LPPS hydroxyapatite a.
   Mammopatch gel self a.
   Mastisol liquid a.
   Medipatch Gel Z self a.
   methyl methacrylate cement a.
   Nexacryl tissue a.
   Nu-Hope a.
   Orthomite II a.
   Orthoset radiopaque bone
    cement a.
   Palacos cement a.
   a. plastic drape
   Plastodent dental impression a.
   Scanpor acrylate a.
   Silastic medical a.
   silicone a.
   Simplex cement a.
   Superglue a.

   Surfit a.
   Surgical Simplex P radiopaque a.
   a. tape remover
   Technovit 7210 VLC a.
   Tisseel biologic fibrogen a.
   tissue a.
   T-Stick a.
   Urihesive expandable a.
   Uro-Bond II brush-on silicone a.
   VersaBond structural a.
   Zimmer low-viscosity a.
Adjustaback wheelchair backrest system
adjustable
   a. advanced reciprocating gait
    orthosis
   a. breast implant
   a. headrest
   a. leg and ankle repositioning
    mechanism (ALARM)
   A. OA Defiance knee brace
   a. ostomy appliance belt
   a. pedicle connector
   A. Postoperative Protective and
    Preparatory Systems (APOPPS)
   a. skull traction tongs
   a. thigh antiembolism stocking
   a. vaginal stent
Adjust-A-Flow colostomy irrigation kit
Adjust-A-Lift heel lift
Adjusta-Rak hanger
Adjusta-Wrist splint
adjuster
   Seibel ophthalmic paracentesis
    valve a.
   Serdarevic suture a.
Adkins strut
Adler
   A. attic ear punch
   A. bone forceps
   A. punch forceps
   A. tripronged lens loop
Adlerkreutz forceps
adnexal forceps
adolescent vaginal speculum
Adolph Gasser camera system
"adoptable" baby cholangioscope
ADR Ultramark 4 ultrasound
Adson
   A. aneurysm needle
   A. angular hook
   A. arterial forceps
   A. aspirating tube
   A. bayonet dressing forceps
   A. bipolar forceps
   A. blunt dissecting hook
   A. bone rongeur
   A. brain cannula
   A. brain clip
   A. brain forceps

A. brain hook
A. brain retractor
A. brain suction tip
A. brain suction tube
A. bur
A. cerebellar retractor
A. clamp
A. clip-applying forceps
A. conductor
A. cranial rongeur
A. dissecting hook
A. dissector
A. drainage cannula
A. dressing forceps
A. drill guide
A. dural hook
A. dural knife
A. dural needle holder
A. dural protector
A. forceps
A. ganglion scissors
A. Gigli saw
A. Gigli-saw guide
A. headrest
A. hemostat
A. hemostatic forceps
A. hypophyseal forceps
A. laminectomy chisel
A. microbipolar forceps
A. microdressing forceps
A. microforceps
A. microtissue forceps
A. monopolar forceps
A. neurosurgical suction tube
A. perforating bur
A. periosteal elevator
A. pickups
A. scalp clip
A. scalp clip-applying forceps
A. scalp needle
A. sharp hook
A. speculum
A. spiral drill
A. splanchnic retractor
A. suture needle
A. thumb forceps
A. tissue forceps
A. tooth forceps
A. twist drill
Adson-Beckman retractor
Adson-Biemer forceps

Adson-Brown
    A.-B. clamp
    A.-B. tissue forceps
Adson-Callison tissue forceps
Adson-Love periosteal elevator
Adson-Mixter neurosurgical forceps
Adson-Murphy trocar point needle
Adson-Rogers
    A.-R. cranial bur
    A.-R. perforating drill
Adson-Vital tissue forceps
Adsorba hemoperfusion cartridge
adult
    a. laryngoscope
    a. reverse-bevel laryngoscope
    a. sigmoidoscope
    A. Star 2000 ventilator
    a. ventilation bronchoscope
Advance
    A. Dynamic ROM orthosis
    A. EX self-adhesive urinary
    external catheter
    A. Zoneaire sleep surface
Advanced
    A. Beta 200 otoscope
    A. Breast Biopsy Instrumentation
    (ABBI)
    A. Breast Biopsy Instrumentation
    system
    A. Cardiovascular System (ACS)
    A. Collection breast pump
    A. Coronary Technology (ACT)
    A. Medical Systems fetal
    monitoring system
    A. NMR Systems scanner
    A. Real-Time Motion Analysis
    (ARTMA)
    A. Reciprocating Gait Orthosis
    (ARGO)
    A. Surgical Intervention, Inc. (ASI)
    A. Surgical suture applier
    A. Technology Laboratories (ATL)
    A. Venous Access (AVA)
advancement
    a. forceps
    a. needle
Advancer
    Arrow A.
Advancit guidewire system
Advanta
    A. bed
    A. facial implant

NOTES

Advantage
- A. 1000 CBA-RCA gas mask
- A. DP artificial leg prosthesis
- A. glucometer
- A. ultrasound
- A. ultrasound system

AdvanTeq II TENS unit
Advantim revision knee system
Advantx-E Legacy system
Advantx LC+ cardiovascular imaging system
Advent
- A. Flurofocon contact lens
- A. pachymeter

AdVent implant
Advia 1650 chemistry analyzer
Advocate electric flexion distraction table
AdzorbStar
EndoDynamics A.
AE-7277 Rubenstein LASIK cannula
Aebli
- A. corneal scissors
- A. tenotomy scissors

Aebli-Manson scissors
AECD
automatic external cardioverter-defibrillator
PowerHeart AECD
AED
automatic external defibrillator
AED automatic external defibrillator
FirstSave AED
Aegis
- A. ICD system
- A. implantable cardioverter-defibrillator system
- A. sonography management system

AEM
active electrode monitoring
AEM current flow monitoring system
Aequalis
- A. humeral head implant
- A. shoulder prosthesis

Aequitron
- A. apnea monitor
- A. pacemaker
- A. ventilator

AER+ automated endoscope reprocessing system
Aeris 590 concentrator
Aerobicycle
- A. exercise bicycle
Universal A.
AeroChamber
- A. bronchial inhaler
- A. face mask

- A. metered-dose inhaler
- A. Plus valved holding chamber
- A. spacer
- A. spacing device
- A. VHC

AeroDose inhaler
Aerodyne bicycle
AeroEclipse breath-actuated nebulizer
AeroGear asthma action kit
Aero-Kromayer lamp
Aeroneb portable nebulizer
AeroNOx nitric oxide delivery and analysis system
AeroPEP
- A. Plus valve holding chamber
- A. Plus VHC

aeroplane splint
Aeroplast dressing
aerosol
- A. Cloud Enhancer (ACE)
- A. Cloud Enhancer inhaler
- a. inhalation monitor
- a. respiratory therapy

aerosol-barrier pipette tip
AeroSonic ultrasonic nebulizer
AeroStat cholangiography catheter
AeroTech II nebulizer
AeroTrach Plus valve holding chamber
AeroVent
- A. CHC
- A. collapsible holding chamber

AeroView optical intubation system
AERx
AERx diabetes management system
AERx electronic inhaler
AERx pain management system
AERx pulmonary drug delivery system
Aescula left ventricular lead
Aesculap
- A. alpha vessel clip
- A. argon ophthalmic laser
- A. drill
- A. forceps
- A. Meditec excimer laser
- A. needle holder
- A. ScalpFix scalp clip system
- A. skull perforator
- A. traction bow
- A. Unitrac retraction and retention system
- A. Vascu Cut punch system
- A. Verio wound hook system

Aesculap-Pratt tenaculum
Aesculap-Spiegelberg brain pressure monitor
AE-series implantable pronged unipolar electrode

Aesop
>A. 2000, 3000 endoscopic
>stabilizer robot
>A. robotic arm

Aesthetic and Reconstructive
Technologies (AART)
Aestiva/5 MRI anesthesia machine
AF
>aortofemoral

Affinity
>A. arterial filter
>A. bed
>A. blood pump
>A. NT oxygenator
>A. pacemaker

Affirm VP microbial identification
system
Affymetrix GeneChip system
a-fiX cannula seal
AFO
>ankle-foot orthosis
>AFO brace
>AFO brace sock

AFocus steerable diagnostic catheter
A-Force dorsal night splint
A-frame orthosis
aftercataract bur
afterload
>a. applicator
>a. colpostat

afterloader
>Fletcher a.
>Henschke a.

afterloading
>a. catheter
>a. implant
>a. probe

AFx
>AFx DR AutoCapture pacing
>system
>AFx pacemaker

Ag/AgCl electrode
Agarloid impression material
Agarwal irrigating phaco chopper
agate burnisher
AGC
>Anatomical Graduated Components
>AGC dual-pivot resection guide
>AGC knee prosthesis
>AGC unicondylar knee component

Agee
>A. carpal tunnel release system

>A. endoscope
>A. 4-pin fixation device
>A. WristJack fracture reduction
>system

Agfa
>A. CR system
>A. PACS system
>A. scanner

aggregate
>bone a.

aggregometer
>Alivi a.
>electronic a.
>fully automatic erythrocyte a.
>platelet a.
>whole blood a.

Aggressor
>A. blade
>A. meniscal shaver

Agiltrac peripheral dilatation catheter
Agnew
>A. canaliculus knife
>A. keratome
>A. splint
>A. tattooing needle

agraffe clamp
Agricola
>A. eye speculum
>A. lacrimal sac retractor
>A. tattooing needle

Agris-Dingman submammary dissector
Agris rasp
AgX antimicrobial Foley catheter
Ahlquist-Durham embolism clamp
Ahmed
>A. glaucoma valve
>A. glaucoma valve tube extender

Ahn thrombectomy catheter
AICD
>automatic implantable cardioverter-
>defibrillator
>Cadence AICD
>CPI Ventak AICD
>Guardian AICD
>AICD pacemaker
>Ventak AICD
>Ventak Mini IV AICD
>Ventak P AICD

AICD-B pacemaker
AICD-BR pacemaker
aid
>air-conduction hearing a.

NOTES

13

aid *(continued)*

Amplitone-3 hearing a.
Argosy Cameo CIC hearing a.
Argosy in-the-ear hearing a.
A675 Sequel Audio Vision
hearing a.
A13 Sequel programmable behind-
the-ear hearing a.
Audibel hearing a.
Audicraft hearing a.
Audionics PB Max hearing a.
AudioTone hearing a.
Audivisette hearing a.
Auriculina hearing a.
Bansaton behind-the-ear hearing a.
BD Sensability breast self-
examination a.
behind-the-ear hearing a.
bone-anchored hearing a.
bone-conduction hearing a.
Canal-Mate hearing a.
Carex ambulatory a.
CIC hearing a.
completely-in-the-canal hearing a.
compression hearing a.
cryostat frozen sectioning a.
Crystal Tone hearing a.
CunMeter accupuncture a.
Dahlberg hearing a.
Ear-Tronics hearing a.
eyeglass hearing a.
Fonix hearing a.
hearing a.
Highlighter low-vision a.
in-the-ear hearing a.
Jade Audio-Starr hearing a.
linear hearing a.
Lion hearing a.
Listening Glass hearing a.
lower extremity mobility a.
(LEMA)
low-vision a.
Magnatone hearing a.
Maico Gamma hearing a.
MasterCraft hearing a.
Mecon-I hearing a.
Metavox hearing a.
Microson hearing a.
Nuway in-the-ear hearing a.
Omnitone hearing a.
Ortho-Turn transfer a.
Ovation in-the-ear hearing a.
Pacific Coast hearing a.
Panasonic hearing a.
postauricular hearing a.
Prescriptor hearing a.
PrimoFocus hearing a.
Prisma digital hearing a.
Quantum hearing a.

ReSound CC4 hearing a.
ReSound digital hearing a.
Rexton hearing a.
Rionet hearing a.
Servox electronic speech a.
Servox Inton speech a.
SmartLine low vision a.
sock a.
SolarEar hearing a.
Songbird disposable hearing a.
Soundtec hearing a.
Starkey hearing a.
Star Optica hearing a.
Tactaid hearing a.
Tactaid VII vibrotactile a.
Trilogy I hearing a.
Turn-Easy transfer a.
Ultra Voice speech a.
Unitron Esteem CIC hearing a.
Widex hearing a.

AID-B pacemaker
AI 5200 diagnostic ultrasound
Ailee needle
aimer

Arthrotek femoral a.
Puddu tibial a.

Aim titanium femoral nail system
Ainslie acrylic splint
Ainsworth

A. arch
A. punch

air

a. aspirator needle
a. bag
a. bed
A. Cam boot
a. chamber
a. compressor
a. cystotome
a. dermatome
a. drill
a. inflatable vessel occluder clamp
a. injection cannula
a. pillow
a. plethysmograph
A. Plus low-air-loss bed
a. saw
a. splint
A. Supply
A. Supply air purifier
A. Temp Advantage back support
belt

Air-3787 static air mattress overlay
AirBack spinal system
air-brace

PP knee a.-b.

Aircast

A. Air-Stirrup leg brace
A. Cryo/Cuff

A. fracture brace
A. knee system
A. patellar brace
A. pneumatic brace
A. Swivel-Strap brace
A. Swive-Strap
A. walking brace
air-conduction hearing aid
air-core magnet
Airdance pressure-reducing mattress
overlay
air-driven
  a.-d. artificial heart
  a.-d. saw
Air-Drop chiropractic table
Aire-Cuf
  A.-C. endotracheal tube
  A.-C. tracheostomy tube
Airex balance pad
AirFlex carpal tunnel splint
Air-Flex chiropractic table
AirFlo alternating pressure system
air-flow enclosure
air-fluidized bed
airfoam splint
airfuge
  Beckman a.
AirGel ankle brace
airgun retractor
Airis II MRI system
AirKair seat cushion
AirLife
  A. heated wire circuit
  A. MediSpacer
  A. nasal cannula
Airlift balloon retractor
Air-Limb
  A.-L. amputation protector
  A.-L. edema control system
Airlite
  A. alignable ankle block
  A. monolithic prosthesis
AirLITE wheelchair support pad
Air-Lon
  A.-L. adapter
  A.-L. decannulation plug
  A.-L. inhalation cannula
  A.-L. inhalation catheter
  A.-L. laryngectomy tube
  A.-L. tracheal tube
Air-O-Ease static air flotation mattress
Air-O-Pad air mattress

AirPacks backpack
airplane splint
air-powered
  a.-p. drill
  a.-p. nebulizer
Airprene
  A. hinged knee prosthesis
  A. hinged knee support
air-puff tonometer
AirSep ultimate nasal mask
Airshields isolette
Air-Shield-Vickers syringe tip
Airsoft replacement mattress
air-spaced electrode
Air-Stirrup ankle brace
Airstrip composite dressing
Air-1517 vacuum-formed static air
wheelchair cushion
airway
  Beck mouth tube a.
  Berman intubating pharyngeal a.
  binasal pharyngeal a.
  Coburg-Connell a.
  Combitube a.
  Connell a.
  double-lumen gastric laryngeal
    mask a.
  esophageal obturator a.
  Guedel a.
  LMA-Unique disposable laryngeal
    mask a.
  Lumbard a.
  Luomanen oral a.
  oral pharyngeal a.
  pharyngeal a.
  Portex nasopharyngeal a.
  Robertazzi nasopharyngeal a.
  rubber a.
  Safar-S a.
AirZone flowmeter
AIS CELLector device
AK-10 dialysis machine
Akahoshi
  A. hydrodissection cannula
  A. nucleus manipulator
  A. nucleus sustainer
  A. ophthalmic hydrodissection
  A. phaco prechopper forceps
AK diamond knife
Aker lens pusher
Akins valve re-do forceps
Akorn Pak

NOTES

Akron tilt table
Akros
    A. DFD wheelchair wedge cushion
    A. extended-care mattress
AkroTech mattress
Akton
    A. pad
    A. positioning roll
Akura partial-depth astigmatic keratotomy marker
Akutsu III total artificial heart
AL-1 catheter
Alabama
    A. needle holder
    A. University forceps
Alabama-Green eye needle holder
Aladdin
    A. II nasal CPAP
    A. II nasal CPAP system
    A. infant flow system
    A. mixer/blender
    A. nasal CPAP system
Alamo alternating low-air-loss mattress overlay
alar
    a. cinch
    a. cinch suture
    a. protector
    a. retractor
    a. screw
Alara
    A. DenOptix filmless dental imaging system
    A. MetriScan bone density system
alar-columellar implant
ALARM
    adjustable leg and ankle repositioning mechanism
alarm
    Bárány a.
    bedwetting a.
    enuresis a.
    Nite Train'r bedwetting a.
    Nite Train'r DVC bedwetting a.
    Nytone enuretic a.
    Silent Nite a.
    Wet-Stop enuresis a.
AlaStat allergy immunoassay system
A-Lastic module
Albany eye guard
Albarran
    A. bridge
    A. deflector
    A. laser
    A. laser cystoscope
    A. lens
    A. urethroscope
Albarran-Reverdin needle

Albee
    A. bone graft calipers
    A. bone saw
    A. drill
    A. olive-shaped bur
    A. orthopaedic fracture table
    A. osteotome
Albert
    A. Grass Heritage digital EEG system
    A. Grass Heritage polysomnograph
    A. Grass Heritage PSG system
    A. slotted bronchoscope
Albert-Andrews laryngoscope
Albert-Smith pessary
Albin-Bunegin pressure sensor
Albizzia nail
albumin-coated vascular graft
albuminized woven Dacron tube graft
Alcatel pacemaker
Alcock
    A. bladder syringe
    A. catheter adapter
    A. catheter plug
    A. hemostatic bag
    A. lithotrite
    A. obturator
    A. return-flow hemostatic catheter
Alcock-Timberlake obturator
Alcon
    A. A-OK phacoemulsification slit knife
    A. A-OK ShortCut knife
    A. aspirator
    A. closure system
    A. crescent blade
    A. crescent knife
    A. cryoextractor
    A. cryophake
    A. cryosurgical unit
    A. cystotome
    A. Digital B 2000 ultrasound
    A. disposable drape
    A. handheld cautery
    A. I-knife
    A. indirect ophthalmoscope
    A. intraocular lens
    A. irrigating needle
    A. MA 60 BM lens
    A. microsponge
    A. nylon suture
    A. Phaco-Emulsifier phacoemulsification unit
    A. pocket blade
    A. reverse-cutting needle
    A. spatula needle
    A. sponge
    A. taper-cut needle
    A. taper-point needle

A. tonometer
A. vitrectomy probe
A. vitrector
Alcon-Biophysic Ophthascan
Alden retractor
Alden-Senturia specimen collector
Alderkreutz tissue forceps
Aldrete needle
Aldridge rectus fascia sling
Aleman meniscotomy knife
Aleo meter
Alert
A. cardioversion catheter
A. Companion II defibrillator
Sears Wee A.
Alert-TD catheter
Alesen tube
Alexa 1000 breast diagnostic system
Alexander
A. antrostomy punch
A. approximator
A. bone chisel
A. bone lever
A. dressing forceps
A. elevator
A. mastoid chisel
A. mastoid gouge
A. otoplasty knife
A. perforating osteotome
A. retractor
A. rib raspatory
A. tonsillar needle
Alexander-Ballen orbital retractor
Alexander-Farabeuf
A.-F. costal periosteotome
A.-F. elevator
A.-F. forceps
Alexander-Matson retractor
Alexander-Reiner ear syringe
alexandrite DP laser
Alexian
A. Brothers overhead fracture
frame
A. Hospital retractor
AlexLAZR
Candela A.
A. laser
Alfa II electrode
Alfonso
A. eyelid speculum
A. guarded bur
A. nucleus ophthalmic trisector

Alfreck retractor
Alfred
A. Becht temporary crown
A. M. Large vena caval clamp
A. snare
Algee impression material
Alger brush
algesimeter
coiled pressure a.
AlgiDerm wound dressing
alginate
a. impression material
a. wound dressing
AlgiSite alginate wound dressing
Algisorb wound dressing
Algitec impression material
Algometer
Commander A.
Algo newborn hearing screener
algorithm
Artek colony counting a.
Algosteril alginate dressing
Alice 4 sleep diagnostic system
Alien WildEyes lens
aligner
Charnley femoral inlay a.
femoral a.
Geo-Matt 30-degree body a.
orthodontic a.
patellar a.
tibial a.
alignment catheter
AL II guiding catheter
AliMed
A. diabetic night splint
A. Freedom arthritis support
A. Freedom thumb spica splint
A. PF night splint
A. QualCraft neoprene thigh
support
A. QualCraft wrist support
A. surgical drape
alimentation catheter
Alio
A. MICS capsulorrhexis forceps
A. MICS knife
A. MICS scissors
Aliplast custom molded foot orthosis
Alivi aggregometer
Alivium prosthesis cup
alkaline battery cautery

NOTES

alkaliner
> Masterpiece Jupiter ionizer a.

Alkare adhesive remover wipe

Alken set

All Access laser system

Alladin Infant Flow nasal continuous positive air pressure

Alldress multilayer wound dressing

Allegretto unicompartmental knee prosthesis

Allen
- A. arm surgery table
- A. cecostomy trocar
- A. ePTFE ocular implant
- A. fetal stethoscope
- A. finger trap
- A. hand positioner
- A. hex key
- A. intestinal anastomosis clamp
- A. intestinal forceps
- A. laparoscopic stirrups
- A. preschool card
- A. retractor
- A. root pliers
- A. spherical eye introducer
- A. splint
- A. stereo separator
- A. Supramid implant
- A. tenaculum forceps
- A. traction system
- A. Universal stirrup system
- A. uterine forceps
- A. well leg holder
- A. wire threader

Allen-Barkan
- A.-B. forceps
- A.-B. knife

Allen-Braley
- A.-B. forceps
- A.-B. intraocular lens
- A.-B. lens implant

Allen-Brown
- A.-B. cannula
- A.-B. prosthesis
- A.-B. vascular access shunt

Allen-Burian trabeculotome

Allen-Hanbury knife

Allen-headed screwdriver

Allen-Heffernan nasal speculum

Allen-Kocher clamp

Allen-Schiotz tonometer

Allen-Thorpe
- A.-T. goniolens
- A.-T. gonioprism

Allerdyce
- A. approximator
- A. dissector
- A. elevator

Allergan-Humphrey
- A.-H. lensometer
- A.-H. photokeratoscope

Allergan Medical Optics (AMO)

Allergan-Simcoe C-loop intraocular lens

Allevyn
- A. adhesive hydrocellular dressing
- A. cavity wound dressing
- A. hydrophilic polyurethane dressing
- A. island dressing
- A. polyurethane foam dressing
- A. tracheostomy dressing

Allgower stitch

Alliance
- A. cable system table
- A. catheter
- A. integrated inflation system
- A. rehabilitation system

alligator
- a. clip
- a. crimper forceps
- a. cup forceps
- a. ear forceps
- a. forceps
- a. jaw forceps
- a. MacCarty scissors
- a. nasal forceps
- a. scissors

Allingham rectal speculum

all-in-one laparoscopic electrode

all-in-the-bag intraocular lens

Allis
- A. catheter
- A. clamp
- A. dry dissector
- A. forceps
- A. hemostat
- A. intestinal forceps
- A. lung retractor
- A. Micro-Line pediatric forceps
- A. periosteal elevator
- A. thoracic forceps
- A. tissue clamp
- A. tissue forceps

Allis-Abramson breast biopsy forceps

Allis-Adair
- A.-A. intestinal forceps
- A.-A. tissue forceps

Allis-Coakley
- A.-C. tonsillar forceps
- A.-C. tonsil-seizing forceps

Allis-Duval forceps

Allis-Ochsner
- A.-O. tissue forceps
- A.-O. tonsillar forceps

Allison lung retractor

Allis-Willauer
   A.-W. thoracic forceps
   A.-W. tissue forceps
AllKare protective barrier wipe
AlloAnchor RC anchor
Alloclassic hip system
AlloDerm
   A. dermal tissue graft
   A. processed tissue graft
Allofit acetabular cup system
Allofix cortical bone pin
allogeneic
   a. cellular immune therapy system
   a. lyophilized bone graft implant
      material
allograft
   acetabular a.
   AlloGro freeze-dried bone a.
   Bi-Metric impaction a.
   a. bone vise
   bovine a.
   CryoVein saphenous vein a.
   decalcified freeze-dried bone a.
   Dermaplant dermal a.
   Endius MiCOR precision bone a.
   fresh frozen a.
   HTO wedge tissue a.
   intercalary a.
   MD-111 bone a.
   napkin ring calcar a.
   osteoarticular a.
   OsteoStim traditional a.
   Repliform dermal a.
   Triad lumbar interbody a.
   Tutoplast processed a.
AlloGrip bone vise
AlloGro
   A. demineralized bone matrix
   A. freeze-dried bone allograft
AlloMatrix
   A. injectable putty
   A. injectable putty bone graft
      substitute
AlloMune system
Allon thermoregulation system
alloplastic graft material
Allo-Pro hip system
all-optical frequency shifter
alloy
   Aderer a.
   amalgam a.
   Arjalloy amalgam a.

Ceradelta a.
Ceramalloy a.
Cerapall a.
Cer-Mate a.
Cer-On R a.
cobalt-chromium-molybdenum a.
Co-Cr-Mo a.
Co-Cr-W-Ni a.
Coltene a.
Coronet a.
Co-Span a.
d'Arcet metal a.
Degucast a.
Degudent a.
Densilay a.
Dentsply a.
GFH a.
Hammond a.
Imperial a.
Leff a.
Lumi a.
Ostalloy 202 a.
Phase-A-Caps a.
Primallor a.
Remanium star a.
Safco a.
shape-memory a. (SMA)
Shasta a.
Sierra a.
Stabilor a.
Steldent a.
Summar a.
Summit a.
Thriftcast a.
tivanium a.
Ultracast a.
Vera bond a.
Victory a.
Vitallium a.
Wilgnath a.
Wilkadium a.
Wilkoro a.
Wil-Tex a.
Zimaloy cobalt-chromium-
   molybdenum a.
all-PMMA one-piece C-loop intraocular
lens
Allport
   A. cutting bur
   A. gauze packer
   A. hook
   A. mastoid bayonet retractor

NOTES

Allport *(continued)*
    A. mastoid searcher
    A. mastoid sound
Allport-Babcock
    A.-B. mastoid searcher
    A.-B. retractor
Allport-Gifford retractor
All-Tronics scanner
Allurion foot prosthesis
Alm
    A. clip applier
    A. dilator
    A. microsurgery retractor
    A. retractor
    A. self-retaining retractor
Almeida forceps
Alnico Magneprobe magnet
Aloka
    A. 650CL ultrasound
    A. 2000 color Doppler
    A. echocardiograph machine
    A. linear ultrasound
    A. MP-PN ultrasound probe
    A. OB/GYN ultrasound
    A. SD, SSD ultrasound system
    A. sector ultrasound
    A. SSD-720 real-time scanner
    A. SSD1700 transducer
    A. SSD-500 ultrasound system
    A. ultrasound linear scanner
    A. ultrasound sector scanner
Alpar intraocular lens implant
Alpern cortex aspirator
alpha
    A. Active pressure-relieving support
      surface
    a. cradle
    A. fiberoptic pocket otoscope
    A. I penile implant
    a. particle accelerator
Alphabed bed
AlphaCare monitor
alpha-chymotrypsin cannula
AlphaCor synthetic cornea
alpha-particle emitter
AlphaStar operating room table
Alphatec
    A. large cannulated screw system
    A. small fragment system
Alpine reusable leg bag
ALPS
    anterior locking plate system
    Amset ALPS
Alta
    A. cancellous screw
    A. CFX reconstruction rod
    A. channel bone plate
    A. condylar buttress plate
    A. cortical screw

    A. cross-locking screw
    A. distal fracture plate
    A. femoral intramedullary rod
    A. femoral plate
    A. lag screw
    A. modular trauma system
    A. supracondylar bone plate
    A. supracondylar screw
    A. tibial-humeral rod
    A. transverse screw
Altaire open MRI system
Altchek vaginal mold
Alter lip retractor
alternative communication device (ACD)
alternator
    film a.
Alterns therapeutic seating system
Altmann needle
Altona finger extension device
Alton and Dean blood/fluid warmer
Altra Flux hemodialyzer
Alukart hemoperfusion cartridge
Alumafoam nasal splint
alumina cemented total hip prosthesis
aluminum
    a. cortex retractor
    a. eye shield
    a. fence splint
    a. oxygen regulator
aluminum-bronze wire suture
aluminum/foam cot splint
Aluwax bite and impression wax
ALVAD
    Abdominal Left Ventricular Assist
    Device
    ALVAD partial artificial heart
Alvarado
    A. Orthopedic Research (AOR)
    A. surgical knee holder
Alvarez-Rodriguez cardiac catheter
Alvis
    A. fixation forceps
    A. foreign body eye curette
    A. foreign body spud
Alvis-Lancaster sclerotome
Alway groover
Alyea vas clamp
Alzate catheter
Alzer osmotic minipump
Alzet continuous-infusion osmotic pump
Alzheimer lamp
AM1 asthma monitor
Amadeus
    A. microkeratome
    A. ventilator
amalgam
    a. alloy
    a. burnisher
    a. carrier

A

a. carver
a. condenser
Dispersalloy dental a.
a. packer
Paragon a.
Phasealloy dental a.
a. plugger
a. plugger elevator
a. scraper
amalgamator
Accu-Mix a.
A-Dec a.
Bantex a.
CapMix a.
crown a.
Dentomat a.
McShirley a.
Vari-Mix II a.
Amazr 6-pole linear lesion catheter
AMBI
AMBI compression hip screw system
AMBI reamer
Ambicor inflatable penile prosthesis
Ambler dilator
amblyoscope
Major a.
Orthoptic Therapy a.
Worth a.
Ambroise dynamic wrist orthosis
Ambrose
A. eye forceps
A. suture forceps
Ambu
A. bag
A. CardioPump
A. infant resuscitator
A. MediBag
A. NAJO Pedi-Air-Align backboard
A. ResCue key
A. respirator
A. SPUR disposable resuscitator
Ambu-E valve
Ambulator
A. biomechanical footwear
A. H1200 healing shoe
ambulatory
a. electrocardiographic recorder
a. volumetric infusion pump
AmbulMate walker
Amcath catheter
Amdent ultrasonic scaler

Amdur lid forceps
AME
American Medical Electronics
AME bone growth stimulator
AME PinSite shield
Ameda Egnell breast pump
A-Med A-Syst right heart support system
Amelogen
A. dental implant
A. Lite kit
A. UltraLite kit
A. Universal kit
Amenabar
A. capsular forceps
A. discission hook
A. iris retractor
A. lens loop
Amercal intraocular lens
Amercal-Shepard intraocular lens
American
A. artificial larynx
A. circle nephrostomy tube
A. Cystoscope Makers, Inc. (ACMI)
A. Endoscopy dilator
A. Hanks uterine dilator
A. Heyer-Schulte brain retractor
A. Heyer-Schulte chin prosthesis
A. Heyer-Schulte elastomer
A. Heyer-Schulte-Hinderer malar prosthesis
A. Heyer-Schulte mammary prosthesis
A. Heyer-Schulte-Radovan tissue expander prosthesis
A. Heyer-Schulte rhinoplasty prosthesis
A. Heyer-Schulte-Robertson suprapubic trocar
A. Heyer-Schulte sphere
A. Heyer-Schulte stent
A. Heyer-Schulte testicular prosthesis
A. Heyer-Schulte T-tube
A. Hydron instrument
A. Lapidus bed
A. Medical Electronics (AME)
A. Medical Electronics PinSite shield
A. Medical Optics (AMO)
A. Medical Optics Baron lens

NOTES

21

American *(continued)*
 A. Medical Source laparoscope
 A. Medical Systems (AMS)
 A. Optical (AO)
 A. Optical Cardiocare pacemaker
 A. Optical coagulator
 A. Optical ophthalmometer
 A. Optical oximeter
 A. Optical photocoagulator
 A. Safety Razor (ASR)
 A. Shared CuraCare scanner
 A. silk suture
 A. Sterilizer operating table
 A. Surgical Instruments Corp.
 (ASICO)
 A. umbilical scissors
 A. vascular stapler
 A. wire gauge
Amersham
 A. CDCS A-type needle
 A. J tube
Amerson bone elevator
Ames ventriculoperitoneal shunt
Amfit orthotic
Amico
 A. chisel
 A. drill
Amicon
 A. arteriovenous blood tubing set
 A. D-20 filter
Amicus blood collection separator
Amigo mechanical wheelchair
Ami infant apnea monitor
amino acid analyzer
**Amis 2000 respiratory mass
 spectrometer**
AMK
 Anatomic Modular Knee
 AMK total knee system
Amko vaginal speculum
AML
 Anatomic Medullary Locking
 AML total hip prosthesis
 AML total hip system
**AmniHook amniotic membrane
 perforator**
amnioscope
 Erosa a.
 Saling a.
amniotome
 Baylor a.
 Beacham a.
 Glove-n-Gel a.
AMO
 Allergan Medical Optics
 American Medical Optics
 AMO Advent contact lens
 AMO Array foldable intraocular
 lens

AMO Diplomax phacoemulsification
 system
AMO lensometer
AMO phacoemulsification lens-
 folder forceps
AMO Phacoflex II foldable
 intraocular lens
AMO photokeratoscope
AMO Prestige advanced cataract
 extraction system
AMO refractometer
AMO scleral implant
AMO Sensar intraocular lens
AMO Ultraviolet-Absorbing lens
AMO ultraviolet-absorbing lens
AMO vitreous aspiration cutter
AMO YAG 100 laser
Amoena breast form
Amoils
 A. cryoextractor
 A. cryopencil
 A. cryophake
 A. cryoprobe
 A. cryosurgical unit
 A. iris retractor
 A. probe
 A. refractor
Amoils-Keeler cryo unit
AMO-PhacoFlex lens inserter
AmpErase electrocautery
amperemeter
Amplatz
 A. anchor system
 A. angiography needle
 A. aortography catheter
 A. cardiac catheter
 A. Clot Buster
 A. clot buster catheter
 A. coronary catheter
 A. dilator set
 A. fascial dilator
 A. femoral catheter
 A. gooseneck microsnare
 A. gooseneck snare
 A. guidewire
 A. Hi-Flo torque-control catheter
 A. injector
 A. left I, II coronary catheter
 A. retinal snare
 A. right coronary catheter
 A. sheath
 A. Super Stiff guidewire
 A. thrombectomy device
 A. torque wire
 A. TractMaster system
 A. tube guide
 A. ureteral stent
 A. ventricular septal defect device

Amplatzer
- A. duct occluder
- A. occluder
- A. septal occluder
- A. VSD occluder device

Amplex guide wire

Amplicor
- A. automated PCR system
- A. HIV-1 test kit
- A. PCR kit
- A. tissue typing kit

amplifier
- Botox injection a.
- Cona-Tone office-use hearing a.
- gradient a.
- hearing aid a.
- lock-in a.
- power a.
- pulse a.
- Servox a.
- triode tube a.
- voltage a.

Amplitone-3 hearing aid

Ampoxen sling

amputation
- a. knife
- a. retractor
- a. saw
- a. screw

amputator
- Smith intraocular capsular a.

AMS
- American Medical Systems
- AMS Ambicor penile prosthesis
- AMS 800 artificial urethral sphincter
- AMS autoclavable laparoscope
- AMS Coaguloop resection electrode
- AMS CX penile prosthesis cylinder
- AMS 700CX-series penile prosthesis
- AMS disposable trocar
- AMS Endoview camera
- AMS Hydroflex penile prosthesis
- AMS malleable penile prosthesis
- AMS M-series malleable penile prosthesis
- AMS penile prosthesis
- AMS SPARC sling system
- AMS Sphincter 800 urinary prosthesis
- AMS Ultrex penile prosthesis
- AMS urethral stent

Amsco
- A. Hall adapter
- A. headholder
- A. hysteroscope
- A. light
- A. Orthairtome drill

Amset
- A. ALPS
- A. anterior locking plate system
- A. R-F reduction fixation system
- A. R-F rod
- A. R-F screw

Amsler
- A. aqueous transplant needle
- A. chart
- A. grid
- A. scleral marker

Amsoft lens

Amsterdam
- A. biliary stent
- A. ventilator

Amsterdam-type prosthesis

Amstutz
- A. cemented hip prosthesis
- A. femoral component
- A. total hip replacement

Amstutz-Wilson osteotomy

Amtech-Killeen pacemaker

AM-UP-75WET dialyzer

Amussat probe

AN69 membrane dialyzer

anal
- a. dilator
- a. retractor
- a. speculum

analgizer
- Penthrane a.

analmoscope
- Pickford-Nicholson a.

analog
- a. electronic inclinometer
- a. rate meter

Analogic Anatom 2000 mobile CT scanner

analysis
- Advanced Real-Time Motion A. (ARTMA)
- Fourier harmonic a.
- Immediate Response Mobile A. (IRMA)

NOTES

analysis *(continued)*
    Mass Isotopomer Distribution A.
      (MIDA)
    multidimensional a.
    Multidimensional Scalogram a.
    point-of-care a.
    Topcon noncontact specular
      morphometric a.
analytical electron microscope
analyzer
    Abacus Concepts StatView 4.02
      statistical a.
    Advia 1650 chemistry a.
    amino acid a.
    arterial blood gas a.
    Aution Max AX-4280 automated
      urine a.
    automated biochemical a.
    automated cerebral blood flow a.
    automatic chemical a.
    automatic clinical a.
    AVL Medical Instruments model
      995-Hb arterial blood gas a.
    AVL Omni 1, 2 blood gas a.
    AVL Opti 1 portable blood gas a.
    AVL 9110 pH a.
    BacT/Alert a.
    Beckman O_2 a.
    BiliCheck bilirubin a.
    bioimpedance a.
    Bio-Optics cell a.
    blood color a.
    blood gas a.
    840 blood gas a.
    BRACAnalyzer gene a.
    Capnomac multiple gas a.
    Capnomac Ultima gas a.
    CA-6000 spine motion a.
    Cat-a-Kit a.
    Cell Soft 2000 semen a.
    Cell Trak/DMS semen a.
    Cell Trak 11 semen a.
    Cell Trak/S semen a.
    Chiroslide leg discrepancy a.
    ChromaVision digital a.
    Clinitek 50 urine chemistry a.
    Cobas Fara H centrifugal a.
    Cobas Helios differential a.
    Corning 170 pH/blood gas a.
    CO Sleuth handheld carbon
      monoxide a.
    Coulter Channelyser cell a.
    Coulter STKS hematology a.
    C-Trak a.
    Dantec Menuet urodynamic a.
    Dicon ocular blood flow a.
    Dow Corning hollow-fiber a.
    Ela Medical Elatec V 3.03A
      arrhythmia a.

Electra 1000C coagulation a.
E-Spart a.
ESRA-10 erythrocyte sedimentation
    rate a.
ESR-Auto Plus erythrocyte
    sedimentation rate a.
Fast Fourier Transform spectrum a.
Fourier transformation spectrum a.
Friedman visual field a.
Futrex a.
Gas Check blood a.
GastrograpH Mark III pH a.
GDx nerve fiber a.
Gem Premier Plus whole blood a.
halothane a.
Hamilton-Thorn motility a.
HemoCue blood glucose a.
HemoCue blood hemoglobin a.
Hitachi automated chemistry a.
Hosokawa E-Spart a.
Humphrey lens a.
Humphrey visual field a.
Immulite Dynamic Duo a.
immunoturbidimetry a.
i-STAT handheld a.
IVEC-10 neurotransmitter a.
Jayco H2 lactose breath a.
KC1 Delta coagulation a.
Keystone PF a.
Leadcare handheld blood lead a.
Malvern a.
MedGraphics diffusion a.
medical gas a.
Menuet Compact primary
    urodynamic nerve fiber a.
Microlyzer Gas a.
miniature centrifugal fast a.
MiniOX IA oxygen a.
MMS-10 tympanic displacement a.
multichannel a.
Myograph 2000 neuromuscular
    function a.
nerve fiber a.
New Glucorder a.
nitric oxide a.
Nova Celltrak 12 hematology a.
Olympus SP-series image a.
Omni 1, 2 blood gas a.
Opti 1 portable pH/blood gas a.
Orion model AE-940 ion a.
Osteomeasure computer-assisted
    image a.
Oxisensor oxygen a.
oxygen a.
Pachymetric a.
Packard Auto-Gamma 5650 a.
Paradigm Dicon ocular blood
    flow a.
platelet function a.

portable blood gas a.
pulse-height a.
Radiometer ABL 500 blood gas a.
Rapidlab 800 a.
reflectance TS-200 spectrum a.
retinal thickness a. (RTA)
Reynolds Pathfinder 3 a.
scanning retinal thickness a.
Serono SR1 FSH a.
Shimadzu DAR-2400 coronary
  arteriographic a.
Sievers model 280 nitric oxide a.
single-channel a.
Sole Primeur 33D a.
Sonoclot coagulation a.
SRI automated immunoassay a.
Stat Profile pHOx blood
  gas/critical care a.
STKS hematology a.
Stride a.
Sweat-Chek a.
Synchron CX-series automated a.
Synchron LX20 Pro chemical a.
Syntheses critical care a.
Sysmex NE-8000 CBC a.
Tanita Professional body
  composition a.
thermal energy a.
ultrasound bone a.
ULT-Svi calibrated end-tidal gas a.
Urisys 2400 urine a.
Vitalab Flexor clinical chemistry a.
Vitalab ViVa clinical chemistry a.
Anastaflo
A. intravascular shunt
A. stent
Anastasia bougie
anastigmatic aural magnifier
**Anastomark coronary artery bypass
  graft marker**
anastomosis
a. apparatus
a. clamp
a. forceps
gastrointestinal a. (GIA)
anastomotic button
anatomic
a. hip prosthesis
A. hip system
A. Medullary Locking (AML)
A. Medullary Locking total hip
  system

A. Modular Knee (AMK)
porous-coated a. (PCA)
a. porous revision (APR)
A. Precoat hip prosthesis
Anatomical
A. Graduated Components (AGC)
A. Vertebral Body Replacement
  (AVR)
Anatomic/Intracone reamer
Anatomotor traction/massage table
Ancap braided silk suture
anchor
Acufex bioabsorbable suture a.
Acumed suture a.
AlloAnchor RC a.
AnchorLok soft tissue a.
Arthrex Bio-FASTak suture a.
Arthrex FASTak suture a.
Arthrotek suture a.
AxyaWeld bone a.
Bio-Anchor suture a.
Bio-Corkscrew suture a.
Bio-FASTak suture a.
BioKnotless suture a.
Biologically Quiet mini-screw
  suture a.
Bionx suture a.
Bio-Phase suture a.
BioROC EZ suture a.
BioSphere suture a.
Bio-Statak suture a.
Bone Bullet suture a.
Bone Button orthopaedic suture a.
Catera suture a.
ConTack labral a.
Corkscrew suture a.
Cuff Tack a.
DRG Sherlock threaded suture a.
EndoAnchor a.
FASTak suture a.
FastIn threaded a.
Hall sacral a.
Harpoon suture a.
a. hook
A. IIa osseointegrated titanium
  implant system
Innovasive Devices ROC XS
  suture a.
Kurer a.
Lemoine-Searcy a.
Mainstay soft tissue a.
Mainstay urologic soft tissue a.

NOTES

25

anchor *(continued)*
    Mitek absorbable bone a.
    Mitek bone a.
    Mitek Fastin threaded a.
    Mitek GII Easy a.
    Mitek GII suture a.
    Mitek GL a.
    Mitek Knotless a.
    Mitek Ligament a.
    Mitek Micro a.
    Mitek Mini GII a.
    Mitek Mini GLS a.
    Mitek Panalok a.
    Mitek rotator cuff a.
    Mitek Tacit threaded a.
    A. needle holder
    Ogden soft tissue to bone a.
    Panalok absorbable a.
    Panalok RC QuickAnchor Plus
      suture a.
    PeBA a.
    a. plate
    Precision SpeedTac transvaginal a.
    Precision Twist transvaginal a.
    Radix a.
    Revo suture a.
    Roc EZ a.
    Roc hXS bone a.
    Roc XS suture a.
    a. screw
    SD Sorb E-Z TAC suture a.
    Searcy fixation a.
    Sherlock threaded suture a.
    SmartAnchor-D suture a.
    SmartAnchor-L suture a.
    SmartTack absorbable bone a.
    Snap-Pak a.
    A. soft tissue biopsy device
    a. splint
    Statak suture a.
    A. sterilizer box
    Stryker wedge suture a.
    Super Revo suture a.
    A. surgical needle
    suture a.
    Tacit threaded a.
    TAG Rod II suture a.
    Therap-Loop door a.
    traction a.
    TwinFix AB absorbable suture a.
    UltraFix a.
    UltraSorb suture a.
    Zest dental bone a.
anchored catheter
anchoring peg
AnchorLok
    A. soft tissue anchor
    A. system
Ancor imaging system

Ancrofil clasp wire
Ancure
    A. balloon catheterization system
    A. bifurcated system
    A. endograft system
    A. stent-graft
Andersen mercury-weighted tube
Anderson
    A. acetabular prosthesis
    A. biopsy punch
    A. clamp
    A. columellar prosthesis
    A. converse iris scissors
    A. curette
    A. distractor
    A. double ball
    A. double-end knife
    A. double-end retractor
    A. elevator
    A. flexible suction tube
    A. nasal strut
    A. splint
    A. suture pusher and double hook
    A. traction bow
Anderson-Adson self-retaining retractor
Anderson-Neivert osteotome
Ando
    A. aortic clamp
    A. motor-driven probe
Andre hook
Andresen
    A. activator
    A. monoblock appliance
    A. removable orthodontic appliance
Andresen-Haupl activator
Andrews
    A. applicator
    A. chisel
    A. comedo extractor
    A. gouge
    A. infant laryngoscope
    A. mastoid gouge
    A. osteotome
    A. rigid chest support holder
    A. spinal frame
    A. spinal surgery table
    A. suction tip
    A. tongue depressor
    A. tonsillar forceps
    A. tonsil-seizing forceps
    A. tracheal retractor
Andrews-Hartmann
    A.-H. forceps
    A.-H. rongeur
Andrews-Pynchon
    A.-P. suction tip
    A.-P. suction tube
    A.-P. tongue depressor
Andries stethoscope

AnEber probe
Anel
  A. lacrimal probe
  A. syringe
anemometer
  hot wire a.
  mass flow a.
aneroid
  a. chest bellows
  a. manometer
anesthesiometer
  Semmes-Weinstein pressure a.
Aneuroplast acrylic material
AneuRx
  A. AAA stent graft system
  A. aortic aneurysm stent-graft
  A. bifurcated stent graft system
  A. DTA stent graft system
  A. endograft system
  A. stent endograft
  A. stent graft system
aneurysm, aneurysmal
  a. clamp
  a. clip
  a. clip applier
  a. forceps
  a. neck dissector
  a. needle
AngeCool RF catheter ablation system
AngeFix lead
AngeFlex defibrillation lead
Angeion 2000 ICD generator
AngeLase combined mapping-laser probe
Angelchik antireflux prosthesis
Angeles
  University of California Los A.
  (UCLA)
Angell
  A. curette
  A. gauze packer
Angell-James
  A.-J. dissector
  A.-J. hypophysectomy forceps
  A.-J. punch forceps
Angell-Shiley
  A.-S. bioprosthetic heart valve
  A.-S. porcine xenograft
  A.-S. xenograft prosthetic valve
AngelWings device
Ange-Med Sentinel ICD device

AngePass
  A. defibrillation lead
  A. lead system
Anger
  A. gamma camera system
  A. scintillation camera
Angestat introducer with hemostasis valve
Angetear tear-away introducer sheath
Angiocath
  A. autoguard shielded IV catheter
  A. flexible catheter
  A. PRN catheter
angiocatheter
  Brockenbrough a.
  Corlon a.
  Deseret a.
  Eppendorf a.
  large-bore a.
  Mikro-Tip a.
Angiocor
  A. prosthetic valve
  A. rotational thrombolizer
Angioflow high-flow catheter
angiogram
  Epistar subtraction a.
  FluoroPlus a.
  helical computed tomographic a.
  indocyanine green a.
  Medis off-line quantitative
    coronary a.
angiograph
  Heidelberg retinal a.
angiographic
  a. catheter
  A. Contrast Injection System
    Technology (ACIST)
  a. portacaval shunt
angiography
  a. catheter
  a. needle
Angioguard guidewire filter device
AngioJet
  A. catheter
  A. e-Train 110 catheter
  A. rapid thrombectomy system
  A. Rheolytic thrombectomy system
  A. thrombectomy catheter
  A. thrombectomy device
  A. Xpeedior catheter
Angio-Kit catheter

NOTES

angiolaser
    pulsed a.
AngioLink vascular closure device
Angiomat
    A. angiographic injector
    A. 6000 contrast delivery system
    A. Illumena injector system
Angiomedics catheter
AngioOPTIC catheter
angiopigtail catheter
angioplasty
    a. balloon
    a. balloon catheter
    a. guiding catheter
    percutaneous transluminal a. (PTA)
    percutaneous transluminal
      coronary a. (PTCA)
    a. sheath
AngioRad radiation system
angioscope
    Baxter a.
    Coronary Imagecath a.
    flexible a.
    Imagecath a.
    Imagecath rapid exchange a.
    Masy a.
    Mitsubishi a.
    Olympus a.
    Optiscope a.
angioscopic valvulotome
Angio-Seal
    A.-S. catheter
    A.-S. hemostasis system
    A.-S. hemostatic puncture closure
      device
    A.-S. puncture closure device
AngioStent balloon-expandable coronary
   stent
AngioSurf scan system
angiotribe
    Ferguson a.
    a. forceps
    Zweifel a.
AngioVista angiographic system
angle
    intermetatarsal a. (IMA)
    a. splint
Anglebasic E arch appliance
angled
    a. Glidewire
    a. guidewire
    a. high-flow aortic cannula
    a. pigtail catheter
    a. probe
    a. scissors
2-angled polypropylene loop
angled-tip ureteral catheter
Angle-Iron skull immobilizer

AngleLoop curette
Angle-Pezzer drain
angle-tip
    a.-t. Glidewire
    a.-t. guidewire
Angstrom
    A. II ICD system
    A. II implantable cardioverter-
      defibrillator system
    A. MD implantable cardioverter-
      defibrillator
angular
    a. bolster
    a. elevator
    a. needle
    a. scissors
angulator
    Heidelberg a.
    incisor-mandibular plane a.
    integral spinal a.
    orthodontic a.
Anis
    A. aspirating cannula
    A. ball reverse-curvature capsular
      polisher
    A. capsulotomy forceps
    A. corneal forceps
    A. corneoscleral forceps
    A. disc capsular polisher
    A. intraocular lens forceps
    A. irrigating vectis
    A. microforceps
    A. microsurgical tying forceps
    A. needle holder
    A. staple lens
    A. straight corneal forceps
    A. tying forceps
Anis-Barraquer needle holder
Ankeney sternal retractor
Ank-L-Aid brace
ankle
    a. hitch
    a. isolator
    a. orthosis (AO)
    a. weight
AnkleCiser exerciser
ankle-foot
    a.-f. orthosis (AFO)
    a.-f. orthotic
    a.-f. orthotic splint
AnkleTough ankle rehabilitation system
Ann Arbor
    A. A. phrenic retractor
    A. A. towel clamp
Anne anesthesia infuser
AnnuloFlex
    A. annuloplasty system
    A. flexible annuloplasty ring

AnnuloFlo
  A. annuloplasty ring
  A. annuloplasty ring system
anode
  molybdenum a.
  rhodium a.
  a. tube
  tungsten a.
anomaloscope
  Kamppeter a.
  Nagel a.
  Pickford-Nicholson a.
anoscope
  Bacon a.
  Bensaude a.
  Bodenheimer a.
  Boehm a.
  Brinkerhoff a.
  Buie-Hirschman a.
  Burnett a.
  Fansler a.
  fiberoptic a.
  Goldbacher a.
  Hirschman a.
  Ives a.
  Ives-Fansler a.
  KleenSpec disposable a.
  Muer a.
  Munich-Crosstreet a.
  Otis a.
  Pratt a.
  Proscope a.
  Pruitt a.
  rotating speculum a.
  Sims a.
  Sklar a.
  slotted a.
  Smith a.
  speculum a.
  Welch Allyn a.
anosigmoidoscope
Anprolene sterilizer
Ansaldo AU560 ultrasound
Anspach
  A. cranial perforator
  A. craniotome
  A. diamond dissecting cutter
  A. 65K drill
  A. 65K instrument system
  A. leg holder
antegrade
  a. cardioplegia catheter

  a. compression nail
  a. internal stent
  a. ureteral stent
  a. valvulotome
Antense antitension device
antepartum monitor
anterior
  a. capsule forceps
  a. cervical fusion kit
  a. cervical plate fixation system (ACFS)
  a. cervical plate system
  a. chamber (AC)
  a. chamber acrylic implant
  a. chamber intraocular lens
  a. chamber irrigating cannula
  a. chamber irrigating vectis
  a. chamber irrigator
  a. chamber maintainer
  a. chamber synechia scissors
  a. commissure laryngoscope
  a. commissure microlaryngoscope
  a. cruciate ligament (ACL)
  a. cruciate ligament guide
  a. crurotomy knife
  a. crurotomy nipper
  a. distraction instrumentation
  a. footplate pick
  a. internal fixation device
  a. locking plate system (ALPS)
  a. plate system
  a. prostatic retractor
  a. quadrilateral triplane frame
  a. resection clamp
  a. segment forceps
anterior-posterior (AP)
  a.-p. cutting block
  a.-p. cystoresectoscope
Anthony
  A. aspirating tube
  A. cast boot
  A. elevator
  A. enucleation compressor
  A. gorget
  A. mastoid suction tube
  A. orbital compressor
  A. pillar retractor
  A. Products, Inc. (API)
  A. quadrisected dilator
  A. suction tube

NOTES

Anthony-Fisher
    A.-F. antral balloon
    A.-F. forceps
Anthron
    A. heparinized catheter
    A. II catheter
anthropometric total hip
antibiotic-coated stent
antibiotic-loaded
    a.-l. acrylic cement
    a.-l. acrylic cement total joint
      prosthesis
anticavitation drill
anticoagulator
    argon gas a.
anticomplementary
antiembolic stocking
antiembolism stocking
antifog tube
antigravity suit
anti-G suit
antimicrobial
    a. catheter
    a. catheter cuff
antimony pH electrode
antiprotrusio cage
antireflux prosthesis
antirotation guide
antiseptic dressing
antishock suit
Anti-Shox gel insole
antisiphon valve
antitachycardia pacemaker
Antlantis ACP plating system
Antoni-Hook lumbar puncture cannula
antral
    a. balloon
    a. bur
    a. chisel
    a. curette
    a. forceps
    a. gouge
    a. irrigator
    a. perforator
    a. punch
    a. rasp
    a. retractor
    a. sinus cannula
    a. trocar
    a. trocar needle
Antron catheter
antroscope
    ACMI a.
    Nagashima right-angle a.
    Reichert a.
anular
    a. detector
    a. gouge
anular-array transducer

Anustim electronic neuromuscular
    stimulator
anvil
    Bunnell a.
Anywear shoe
Anzio catheter
A-O
    A-O minus cylinder Phoroptor
    A-O plus cylinder Phoroptor
AO
    American Optical
    ankle orthosis
    AO blade plate
    AO brace
    AO cancellous screw
    AO coagulator
    AO compression plate
    AO condylar blade plate
    AO contoured T plate
    AO cortex screw
    AO drill bit
    AO dynamic compression plate
    AO dynamic compression plate
      construct
    AO femoral distractor
    AO fixateur interne
    AO fixateur interne instrumentation
    AO gouge
    AO guidepin
    AO hook plate
    AO indirect ophthalmoscope
    AO internal fixator
    AO lag screw
    AO mandibular system
    AO notched instrumentation
    AO ophthalmometer
    AO oximeter
    AO photocoagulator
    AO plate bender
    AO reconstruction plate
    AO reduction forceps
    AO semitubular plate
    AO slotted medullary nail
    AO small fragment plate
    AO spinal internal fixation
    AO spongiosa screw
    AO spoon plate
    AO stopped-drill guide
    AO tap
    AO tension band
AOA cervical immobilization brace
AOA/Chick ambulatory halo system
AO/ASIF
    AO/ASIF orthopaedic implant
    AO/ASIF titanium craniofacial
      system
AOO pacemaker
AOR
    Alvarado Orthopedic Research

AOR check traction device
AOR collateral ligament retractor
aortic
  a. air aspirator needle
  a. aneurysm clamp
  a. aneurysm forceps
  a. arch cannula
  a. balloon pump
  a. bifurcation graft
  a. bioprosthetic valve
  a. catheter
  a. clamp
  a. connector system
  a. cross-clamp
  a. direct ellipse cannula
  a. occluder
  a. occlusion clamp
  a. occlusion forceps
  a. perfusion cannula
  a. punch
  a. root cannula
  a. root perfusion needle
  a. sump tube
  a. tube graft
aortofemoral (AF)
  a. prosthesis
aortography
  a. catheter
  a. needle
aortopulmonary shunt
AP
  anterior-posterior
  AP cutting block
  AP portal
APC
  Arthroplasty Products Consultants
  APC foot and leg holder
APC-3, -4 collimator
Apdyne phenol applicator kit
Apex
  A. irrigation system
  A. MiniTENS TS-1701 TENS unit
  A. pin
  A. Plus excimer laser
  A. Universal driver
Apexo elevator
ApexPro telemetry system
Apfelbaum
  A. bipolar forceps
  A. cerebellar retractor
  A. mirror
Apgar timer

apheresis catheter
API
  Anthony Products, Inc.
  API Universal foam chin strap
  API V-notched osteotome
apicitis curette
apicoaortic
  a. conduit heart valve
  a. shunt heart valve
apicolysis retractor
Aplicap
  Espe Ketac-Bond A.
  Espe Photac-Bond A.
Apligraf
  A. graft
  A. Graftskin
  A. skin graft material
  A. venous ulcer graft material
APM-2000 vital signs monitor
apnea
  a. alarm mattress
  a. monitor
Apogee
  A. 9300/6200 alexandrite laser
  A. CX-series echocardiography system
  A. hair removal laser
  A. 100 long pulse diode
  A. RX-series diagnostic ultrasound system
Apollo
  A. DXA bone densitometry system
  A. 95E tooth-whitening and curing system
  A. hip prosthesis
  A. hip system
  A. knee prosthesis
  A. knee system
  A. Light Systems
  A. Pak hot/cold knee pack
  A. 3 triple-lumen papillotome
APOPPS
  Adjustable Postoperative Protective and Preparatory Systems
  APOPPS transtibial prosthetic socket
A-Port implantable port
apparatus
  anastomosis a.
  aspiration a.
  Barcroft a.
  Barcroft-Warburg a.

NOTES

apparatus *(continued)*
>Benedict-Roth a.
>biphase Morris fixation a.
>Brawley suction a.
>Buck convoluted traction a.
>Buck extension a.
>C-arm fluoroscopic a.
>cryosurgical a.
>Davidson pneumothorax a.
>dental a.
>Desault a.
>Dewald halo hoop a.
>Deyerle a.
>electro-oculogram a.
>extension a.
>eye movement measuring a.
>Fell-O'Dwyer a.
>fixation a.
>FracSure a.
>Frigitronics nitrous oxide cryosurgery a.
>Gibson-Cooke sweat test a.
>Golgi a.
>Guthrie-Smith a.
>Heyns abdominal decompression a.
>Hilal embolization a.
>Hodgen a.
>Holman flushing a.
>Jackson-Rees a.
>Jaquet a.
>Kanavel a.
>Kandel stereotactic a.
>Kinetron muscle strengthening a.
>Kirschner traction a.
>lacrimal a.
>Lewy suspension a.
>Lynch suspension a.
>Malgaigne a.
>Manifold II slot-blot a.
>Marstock a.
>masticatory a.
>Mayfield-Kees skull fixation a.
>McAtee a.
>McKesson pneumothorax a.
>mechanical joint a.
>mobile electroconvulsive therapy a.
>Morris biphase a.
>Morwel silhouette suction a.
>Naugh os calcis a.
>optoelectric measuring a.
>OsteoStim a.
>Parham-Martin fracture a.
>Pearson flexed-knee a.
>pneumothoracic a.
>portable insulin dosage-regulating a.
>R&B portable pneumothorax a.
>Reichert stereotaxic brain a.
>Riechert-Mundinger a.
>Robinson artificial pneumothorax a.
>Roger Anderson a.
>Roughton-Scholander a.
>Ruth-Hedwig pneumothorax a.
>Sayre suspension a.
>Scholander a.
>Seldinger a.
>self-contained underwater breathing a.
>Semm pneumoperitoneum a.
>Singer portable pneumothorax a.
>Skatron a.
>Spiegel-Wycis stereotactic a.
>Stader extraoral a.
>stereotactic a.
>suction a.
>surgical exhaust a.
>suspension a.
>Swenko gastric-cooling a.
>Tallerman a.
>Taylor spinal support a.
>Tobold laryngoscopic a.
>traction a.
>Vactro perilimbal suction a.
>vacuum a.
>van Slyke a.
>Venturi a.
>Volutrol control a.
>von Petz a.
>Wagner a.
>Waldenberg a.
>Wangensteen a.
>Warburg a.
>Watanabe a.
>Wells stereotaxic a.
>Zander a.
>Zavod aneroid pneumothorax a.
>Zund-Burguet a.

AP-PA skull immobilizer
Appel-Bercie sheath
appendage clamp
appendectomy retractor
appendiceal retractor
applanation tonometer
applanator
>Goldmann a.
>Johnston LASIK flap a.
>Posner-Inglima a.

applanometer
Applause Super-Hemi wheelchair
Apple
>A. laparoscopic stone grabber
>A. Medical bipolar forceps
>A. trocar

Applebaum prosthesis
appliance
>ACCO orthodontic a.
>Andresen monoblock a.
>Andresen removable orthodontic a.
>Anglebasic E arch a.

arch bar facial fracture a.
Balters a.
Begg a.
Bimler a.
Bipro orthodontic a.
Bradford fracture a.
Brooks a.
Buck fracture a.
craniofacial fracture a.
Crozat removable orthodontic a.
dental arch bar facial fracture a.
extraoral fracture a.
Fairdale orthodontic a.
Fränkel a.
Gentle Touch colostomy a.
Gerster fracture a.
Goldthwait fracture a.
Graber a.
Hasund a.
Hibbs fracture a.
Hyrax a.
ileostomy a.
intraoral fracture a.
Janes fracture a.
Jelenko facial fracture a.
Jewett fracture a.
Jobst a.
Johnson twin-wire a.
Joseph septal fracture a.
Karaya adhesive ileostomy a.
Kesling a.
Klearway a.
Latham a.
light wire a.
mandibular advancement a.
mandibular orthopaedic
  repositioning a.
Margolis a.
Marlen colostomy a.
microstomia prevention a.
Mitek anchor a.
Nu-Comfort colostomy a.
obturator a.
oral a.
Ormco a.
orthodontic a.
ostomy a.
prosthetic a.
Proxi-Floss cleaning a.
Remedy colostomy a.
Remedy ileostomy a.
Rest Assured oral a.

ribbon arch a.
Roger Anderson pin fixation a.
SACH orthopaedic a.
Schacht colostomy a.
Seep-Pruf ileostomy a.
"stick-and-carrot" a.
Stockfisch a.
surgical a.
TheraSnore oral a.
Unitek a.
vasocillator fracture a.
Whip a.
Whitman fracture a.
Wilson fracture a.
Winter facial fracture a.
wire a.

applicator
Absolok endoscopic clip a.
afterload a.
Andrews a.
balloon a.
Barth double-end a.
Betadine PrepStick a.
Betadine PrepStick Plus a.
beta irradiation a.
beta ray a.
Bloedorn a.
brachytherapy balloon a.
Brown a.
Brown-Dean cotton a.
Buck ear a.
Buck nasal a.
Burnett a.
Campbell-type Heyman fundus a.
cesium a.
Chaoul a.
Cohen suture a.
colpostat a.
cotton a.
cotton-tipped a.
Dean a.
Delrin a.
ear a.
EndoAvitene disposable a.
endocavitary a.
Falope-ring a.
Farrior suction a.
Filshie clip minilaparotomy a.
Fletcher-Suit a.
Fletcher-Suit-Delclos
  brachytherapy a.
a. forceps

NOTES

applicator *(continued)*
Gass dye a.
Gifford corneal a.
GliaSite RTS balloon
  brachytherapy a.
global force a.
Grafco cotton tip a.
Henschke seed a.
Hex heat a.
Holinger a.
Huzly a.
infrared a.
intracavitary afterloading a.
iontophoretic a.
Ivan laryngeal a.
Ivan nasopharyngeal a.
Jackson laryngeal a.
Jobson-Horne cotton a.
Kevorkian-Younge uterine a.
Kyle a.
laryngeal a.
laser-induced thermotherapy a.
Lathbury cotton a.
Lejeune cotton a.
LITT a.
Ludwig middle ear a.
Ludwig sinus a.
Mayfield clip a.
Mick seed a.
Mick TP-200 a.
Milex Jel-Jector vaginal a.
Miralva a.
Montrose dressing a.
multifire clip a.
NeuroAvitene a.
Nucletron a.
Playfair uterine caustic a.
Plummer-Vinson radium
  esophageal a.
Pynchon a.
Ralks sinus a.
ring a.
Roberts a.
Sawtell laryngeal a.
Sr-90 eye a.
Stille laryngeal a.
strontium-90 ophthalmic beta ray a.
suture a.
Syed-Puthawala-Hedger
  esophageal a.
tandem a.
tandem and ovoid a.
Ter-Pogossian cervical radium a.
Turnbull a.
Uckermann cotton a.
Uebe a.
University of Iowa cotton a.
Wang a.

Wolf-Yoon a.
Yoon-ring a.
Applied
A. Biosystems 340A nucleic acid
  extractor
A. Medical mini ureteroscope
applier
AcuClip endoscopic multiple-clip a.
Advanced Surgical suture a.
Alm clip a.
aneurysm clip a.
Autoclip a.
Auto Suture Clip-A-Matic clip a.
bayonet clip a.
clip a.
Endo Clip a.
Ethicon clip a.
Gam-Mer clip a.
Hamby right-angle clip a.
Heifitz clip a.
Hulka clip a.
Kaufman clip a.
Kees clip a.
Kerr clip a.
LDS clip a.
Ligaclip MCA multiple-clip a.
Malis clip a.
Mayfield miniature clip a.
Mayfield temporary aneurysm
  clip a.
McFadden Vari-Angle clip a.
mini a.
Mount-Olivecrona clip a.
Mt. Clemens Hospital clip a.
Multifire Endo hernia clip a.
Olivecrona clip a.
pivot clip a.
Raney scalp clip a.
Right Clip a.
Sano clip a.
Schwartz clip a.
Scoville clip a.
Scoville-Drew clip a.
Sugita jaws clip a.
surgical clip a.
Surgiclip clip a.
TiGold clip a.
Vari-Angle McFadden clip a.
vascular clip a.
Weck clip a.
Yasargil aneurysm clip a.
Zmurkiewicz clip a.
Applipak
IntraSite gel A.
Appolionio eye lens implant
Appose skin stapler
approximation forceps
approximator
Ablaza-Morse rib a.

Alexander a.
Allerdyce a.
Bailey rib a.
Biemer a.
Bruni-Wayne clamp a.
Brunswick-Mack a.
Bunke-Schulz clamp a.
Christoudias a.
Henderson clamp a.
hook a.
Ikuta clamp a.
Iwashi clamp a.
Kleinert-Kutz clamp a.
Lalonde tendon a.
Leksell sternal a.
Lemmon sternal a.
Link a.
Microspike a.
Neuromeet nerve a.
Neuromeet Universal soft tissue a.
Nunez sternal a.
Pilling-Wolvek sternal a.
pivot microanastomosis a.
rib a.
sternal a.
Tamai clamp a.
Vari-Angle temporary clip a.
Wolvek sternal a.

APR
anatomic porous revision
APR acetabular cup
APR I femoral stem
APR total hip system
Aprema II device
A-Probe
Soft-Touch A.-P.
apron
Grafco x-ray a.
Hottentot a.
lead a.
lead-rubber a.
perineal surgical a.
APS
AutoCapture Pacing System
Pacesetter APS
Aptima Combo 2 assay kit
Aqua
A. Spray debridement system
A. Thermassage table
Aquacel
A. Ag Hydrofiber wound dressing
A. Hydrofiber wound dressing

Aqua-Cel Aqua-Relief heating pad system
Aquaciser underwater treadmill
AquaFlate balloon catheter
Aquaflex
A. contact lens
A. ultrasound gel pad
Aquaflo hydrogel wound dressing
Aqua-Flow collagen glaucoma drainage device
AquaGaiter treadmill
Aqualase cataract removal system
Aqualogger buoyancy belt
AquaMED hydrotherapy device
AquaMotion therapy pool
Aquanex hydrodynamic measurement system
Aquaphor
A. gauze
A. gauze dressing
Aquaplast
A. cast
A. mask
A. mold
A. splint
A. tie-down dressing
Aqua-Purator suction device
AquariusBLUE 2D/3D imaging workstation
AquariusNET streaming 2D/3D medical imaging server
Aqua-Seal system
AquaSens FMS 1000 fluid monitoring system
AquaShield
A. bandage protector
A. cast protector
A. reusable orthopaedic cast cover
Aquasight lens
Aquasil Smart Wetting impression material
Aquasorb
A. Border gel matrix
A. Border hydrogel dressing
A. hydrogel dressing
A. transparent hydrogel dressing
AquaTack hydrocolloid barrier
Aquatic Bike aquatic therapy machine
AquaTrek device
aqueous
a. scintillator

NOTES

aqueous *(continued)*
    a. transplant needle
    a. tube shunt
Aquilion CT scanner
AR-1, AR-2 diagnostic guiding catheter
arachnoid
    a. Beaver blade
    a. knife
arachnoid-shaped blade
arachnophlebectomy needle
Aramis laser
Arani double-loop guiding catheter
Arans pulley passer
Arbuckle-Shea trocar
Arbuckle sinus probe
ARC
    Active Response Catheter
    ARC reciprocating cannula
arc
    Leksell a.
    shoulder ROM a.
    xenon a.
arch
    Ainsworth a.
    a. bar
    a. bar cutter
    a. bar facial fracture appliance
    Bimler a.
    FemoStop femoral artery
      compression a.
    lingual a.
    LockJaw dental bonding a.
    a. rake retractor
    Simon expansion a.
    a. support
    Wilson bimetric distalizing a.
Archer splinter forceps
arch-expander
    Ormco orthodontic a.-e.
Archimedean drill
archwire
    Jarabak-type a.
arcitumomab diagnostic imaging system
Arclite light source
Arco
    A. atomic pacemaker
    A. lithium pacemaker
ArCom
    A. compression-molded polyethylene
    A. processed polyethylene
ARC-22 PTCA catheter
arc-quadrant stereotactic system
arcuate skin staple
Ardee denture liner
Arem-Madden retractor
Arem retractor
Arenberg
    A. dural palpator elevator
    A. endolymphatic sac knife

Arenberg-Denver inner-ear valve implant
AREx inhaler
ArF
    argon fluoride
    ArF excimer laser
Argen dental attachment
Arglaes wound dressing
ARGO
    Advanced Reciprocating Gait Orthosis
argon
    a. beam coagulator
    a. blue laser
    a. fluoride (ArF)
    a. fluoride laser
    a. gas anticoagulator
    a. green laser
    a. guidewire
    a. ion laser
    a. krypton laser
    a. laser
    a. laser photocoagulator
    a. plasma coagulator
    a. pump dye laser
    a. vessel dilator
argon-pumped
    a.-p. dye laser
    a.-p. tunable dye laser
Argosy
    A. Cameo CIC hearing aid
    A. in-the-ear hearing aid
Argyle
    A. anti-reflux valve
    A. arterial catheter
    A. chest tube
    A. CPAP nasal cannula
    A. endotracheal tube
    A. esophageal stethoscope
    A. feeding tube
    A. Medicut R catheter
    A. oxygen catheter
    A. Penrose tubing
    A. Salem sump tube
    A. Sentinel Seal chest tube
    A. silicone Salem sump
    A. sump tube
    A. trocar
    A. trocar catheter
    A. Turkel safety thoracentesis system
    A. umbilical vessel catheter
Argyle-Dennis tube
Argyle-Salem sump anti-reflux valve
Argyle-Turkel safety thoracentesis system
Aria
    A. CABG
    A. LX CPAP system

Arion
    A. implant
    A. rod eye prosthesis
Arizona AFO brace
Arjalloy amalgam alloy
Arjo sling
Arkan sharpening-stone needle
Arlt
    A. fenestrated lens scoop
    A. lens loupe
arm
    Aesop robotic a.
    a. board
    a. elevator sling
    Heidelberg a.
    Leyla flexible a.
    mechanical articulated a.
    pediatric retractor adjustable a.
    Pinpoint stereotactic a.
    a. retractor
    scanning a.
    a. and shoulder immobilizer
    Utah artificial a.
    Wittmoser optical a.
armed bougie
2-arm goniometer
Armstrong
    A. beveled grommet drain tube
    A. beveled grommet myringotomy
    tube
    A. beveled grommet ventilation
    tube
    A. CPR mask
    A. handheld pulse oximeter
    A. V-Vent tube
Army
    A. bone gouge
    A. chisel
    A. osteotome
Army-Navy retractor
Arndorfer
    A. esophageal motility probe
    A. infusion system
    A. pneumohydraulic capillary
    infusion system
Arndt endobronchial blocker
Arnett Lefort implant
Arnett-TMP system
Arnoff external fixation device
Arnold brace

Arnold-Bruening
    A.-B. intracordal injection set
    A.-B. syringe
Arnott
    A. bed
    A. dilator
    A. 1-piece all-PMMA intraocular
    lens
AromaScan aroma analysis device
Aron Alpha adhesive
Aronson
    A. esophageal retractor
    A. lateral sternomastoid retractor
Aronson-Fletcher antrum cannula
AR+ portable heart monitor
array
    A. foldable intraocular lens
    a. processor
    a. ultrasound transducer
AR 1000 refractor
Arrequi
    A. KPL laparoscopic knot pusher
    A. laparoscopic knot pusher ligator
arrhythmia
    a. control device
    a. mapping system
    A. Net monitor
    A. Research 1200 EPX
    electrocardiograph
arrow
    A. Advancer
    A. articulation paper forceps
    A. AutoCAT intraaortic balloon
    pump
    A. balloon wedge pressure catheter
    Biofix a.
    A. Blue FlexTip catheter
    A. Cardiac Assist Technology
    (ACAT)
    A. catheter
    A. EID catheter
    A. emergency infusion device
    A. FlexTip Plus catheter
    A. Hands-Off thermodilution
    catheter
    A. LionHeart left ventricular assist
    system
    A. Multi-Lumen Access catheter
    A. PICC
    A. PICC catheter
    A. PICC line
    A. pneumothorax kit

NOTES

arrow *(continued)*
    polylactic acid a.
    A. pullback atherectomy catheter
    A. pulmonary artery catheter
    A. QuadPolar electrode catheter
    A. QuickFlash arterial catheter
    A. Raulerson spring-wire
      introduction syringe
    A. sheath obturator
    A. TheraCath epidural catheter
    A. TransAct intraaortic balloon
      pump console
    A. true torque wire guide
    A. tube
    A. Twin Cath
    A. TwinCath 2-lumen peripheral
      catheter
    A. TwinCath multilumen peripheral
      catheter
    A. UserGard injection cap system
Arrow-Berman
    A.-B. angiographic balloon
    A.-B. angiographic catheter
    A.-B. balloon catheter
Arrow-Clarke thoracentesis catheter
Arrow-Fischell
    A.-F. EVAN needle
    A.-F. pullback atherectomy catheter
Arrow-Flex
    A.-F. intraaortic balloon catheter
    A.-F. sheath
Arrowgard
    A. Blue antiseptic-coated catheter
    A. Blue central venous catheter
Arrow-Howes
    A.-H. multilumen catheter
    A.-H. quad-lumen catheter
Arrowsmith
    A. corneal marker
    A. electrode
    A. fixation forceps
Arrow-Trerotola
    A.-T. percutaneous thrombectomy
      device
    A.-T. PTD
    A.-T. PTD catheter
    A.-T. PTD rotator drive unit
Arroyo
    A. expressor
    A. forceps
    A. implant
    A. protector
    A. trephine
Arruga
    A. curved capsular forceps
    A. extraction hook
    A. eye expressor
    A. eye holder
    A. eye implant

    A. eye retractor
    A. eye speculum
    A. eye trephine
    A. globe retractor
    A. globe speculum
    A. lacrimal trephine
    A. lens expressor
    A. needle holder
    A. protector
    A. surface electrode
Arruga-Gill forceps
Arruga-McCool capsular forceps
Arruga-Moura-Brazil orbital implant
ArtAssist
    A. arterial assist device
    A. compression dressing
    A. pneumatic compression device
    A. wrap
Artec balloon catheter
Artecoll injectable microimplant
Artegraft
    A. bovine graft
    A. natural collagen vascular graft
Artek colony counting algorithm
arterial
    a. blood gas analyzer
    a. cannula
    a. clamp
    a. embolectomy catheter
    a. filter
    a. forceps
    a. graft prosthesis
    a. line
    a. needle
    a. oscillator endarterectomy
      instrument
    a. port catheter system
    a. portography
    A. Vascular Engineering (AVE)
arteriography needle
arteriotomy scissors
arteriovenous (AV)
    a. catheter
    a. malformation (AVM)
artery
    inferior mesenteric a. (IMA)
    internal mammary a. (IMA)
    left internal mammary a. (LIMA)
Arthopor acetabular cup
Arthrex
    A. AR-6400 Continuous Wave II
      arthroscopy pump
    A. arthroscope
    A. Bio-Corkscrew suture
    A. Bio-FASTak suture anchor
    A. biointerference drill
    A. Bio-Transfix cross pin fixation
    A. coring reamer
    A. drill guide

A. FASTak suture anchor
A. FiberWire suture
A. meniscal dart
A. meniscal dart gun
A. OATS bone plug
A. sheathed interference screw
A. suture anchor guide
A. tibial tunnel cannula
A. Transfix II cross pin fixation
A. zebra pin
ArthroCare
   A. arthroscopic system
   A. Coblation-based cosmetic
     surgery system
   A. plasma scalpel wand
   A. Rubo-Vac device
arthrodesis clamp
ArthroDistractor distractor
Arthrofile orthopaedic rasp
Arthro-Flo powered irrigation system
ArthroForce
   A. basket cutting forceps
   A. hook scissors
ArthroGuide carbon dioxide laser
Arthro-Lok
   A.-L. knife
   A.-L. system
arthrometer
   Genucom a.
   KT1000, 2000 knee ligament a.
   KT1000/S knee ligament a.
   Medmetric KT1000/S knee
     laxity a.
   Robinson pocket a.
   Stryker a.
ArthroPlastics ankle instrumentation
arthroplasty
   Global total shoulder a.
   Gustilo-Kyle cementless total hip a.
   A. Products Consultants (APC)
   Stanmore shoulder a.
   total articular replacement a.
     (TARA)
ArthroProbe laser
Arthroscan imaging system
arthroscope
   Acufex a.
   Arthrex a.
   Baxter angled a.
   Circon a.
   CitScope a.
   Codman a.

Concept Intravision a.
Dyonics a.
Dyonics rod lens a.
Eagle straight-ahead a.
examining a.
fiberoptic a.
Hopkins a.
Lumina rod lens a.
Medical Dynamics 5990 needle a.
O'Connor operating a.
PanoView a.
Richard Wolf a.
Sapphire View a.
spinal a.
Storz a.
Stryker a.
Takagi a.
Watanabe a.
Wolf a.
Zimmer a.
arthroscopic
   a. ankle holder
   a. banana blade
   a. cannula
   a. knife
   a. leg holder
   a. osteotome
   a. probe
   a. punch
   a. scissors
   a. shaver
   a. sheath
   a. synovector
arthroscopy
   Electrosurgical A. (ESA)
   a. knife
**Arthroscrew arthroscopic suturing
   device**
ArthroSew
   A. arthroscopic suturing device
   A. suturing system
Arthrotek
   A. calibrated cylinder
   A. Ellipticut hand instrument
   A. femoral aimer
   A. meniscus staple
   A. suture anchor
   A. tibial fixation device
arthrotome
   Hall a.
ArthroWands
   CAPSure A.

NOTES

ArthroWands *(continued)*
    Caps X A.
    CoVac 50, 70 A.
    Eliminator A.
    Microblator A.
    RazorVac A.
    right angle A.
    Saber A.
    Saber Bisector A.
Arthur splinter forceps
articular insert
Articu-Lase
    A.-L. laser
    A.-L. laser mirror
articulated
    a. chin implant
    a. chin prosthesis
    a. external fixator
articulating paper forceps
articulator
    Acme a.
    Balkwell a.
    Bonwill a.
    Christensen a.
    Denar a.
    Dentatus a.
    Galetti a.
    Granger a.
    Gysi a.
    Hanau 130-21 a.
    Handy II a.
    hinge a.
    hinged a.
    KSK a.
    Ney a.
    non-arcon a.
    Oliair a.
    Olyco a.
    Olympia a.
    plain-line a.
    semiadjustable a.
    Steele a.
    Stuart a.
    Walker a.
    Whip-Mix a.
Articulator injection needle
Articul/eze femoral ball
artificial
    a. breast prosthesis
    a. bur
    a. eye
    a. heart
    a. hip joint
    a. joint implant
    a. larynx
    a. lung
    a. pacemaker
    a. sphincter
Arti-holder tweezers

Artilk forceps
Artisan
    A. phakic intraocular lens
    A. wide-angle vaginal speculum
ARTMA
    Advanced Real-Time Motion Analysis
    ARTMA virtual patient technology
Artmann
    A. disarticulation chisel
    A. elevator
    A. raspatory
Artoscan
    A. MRI scanner
    A. MRI system
Artus power system
Arvee model 2400 infant apnea monitor
Arzbaecher pill electrode
Arzco
    A. pacemaker
    A. preamplifier
    A. Tapsul pill electrode
    A. transesophageal cardiac stimulator
AS-800 artificial sphincter
Asahi
    A. Biomembrane hollow-fiber dialyzer
    A. blood plasma pump
    A. hollow fiber dialyzer
    A. Plasmaflo plasma separator
    A. pressure controller
ASAP
    ASAP automated biopsy system
    ASAP channel-cut automated biopsy needle
    ASAP PinPoint guiding introducer needle
    ASAP prostate biopsy needle
    ASAP Stacker automated multisample biopsy system
A-scan
    Contact A.-s.
    A.-s. scanner
    A.-s. ultrasonogram
Ascension
    A. Bird position tracker
    A. MCP total joint
    A. PIP total joint
Ascent
    A. guiding catheter
    A. total knee system
Asch
    A. clamp
    A. nasal splint
    A. septal forceps
    A. septal straightener
    A. septum-straightening forceps
    A. uterine secretion scoop

ASDOS
atrial septal defect occlusion system
ASDOS double umbrella
ASDOS double umbrella system
ASDOS umbrella occluder
aseptic saw
Asepto
A. bulb irrigation syringe
A. suction tube
Ash
A. dental forceps
A. septum-straightening forceps
A. Split Cath catheter
A. Split Cath II catheter
Ashbell hook
Ashby fluoroscopic foreign body forceps
Asher high-pull facebow
Asherman chest seal
Ashhurst leg splint
Ashley
A. cleft palate elevator
A. natural-Y breast prosthesis
A. retractor
Ashworth-Blatt implant
ASI
Advanced Surgical Intervention, Inc.
ASI uroplasty balloon
ASI uroplasty prostatic dilatation
catheter
ASI uroplasty TCU dilatation
catheter
asia-med acupuncture needle
ASICO
American Surgical Instruments Corp.
ASICO capsulorrhexis forceps
ASICO diamond knife
Asid Bonz PP infusion pump
ASIF
Association for the Study of Internal
Fixation
ASIF broad dynamic compression
bone plate
ASIF plate
ASIF screw pin
ASIF T plate
Asissto-Seat
Maddapult A.-S.
Ask-Upmark kidney
Aslan
A. endoscopic scissors
A. laparoscope
A. needle holder

Asmalert Lo-Range peak flowmeter
Asnis
A. guided screw
A. 2 guided screw
A. III cannulated screw
A. pin
Aspect computer
Aspen
A. cervical thoracic orthosis
A. CTO system
A. digital ultrasound
A. digital ultrasound system
A. echocardiography system
A. electrocautery
A. Excaliber electrosurgical unit
A. laparoscopic electrode
A. ultrasound platform
A. ultrasound system
AspenVAC smoke evacuation system
aspheric
a. cataract lens
a. lens
aspherical ophthalmoscopic lens
Aspiradeps dissector
aspirating
a. cannula
a. curette
a. dissector
a. needle
a. syringe
a. tube
aspiration
a. apparatus
irrigation and a. (I&A)
a. tube
aspirator
Accelerator II a.
Adams a.
Alcon a.
Alpern cortex a.
Aspirette endocervical a.
blue-tip a.
Bovie ultrasonic a.
Bovie ultrasound a.
bronchoscopic a.
Broyles a.
Carabelli a.
Care-E-Vac portable a.
Carmody a.
Castroviejo orbital a.
cataract a.
Cavi-Pulse ultrasonic a.

NOTES

aspirator *(continued)*
Cavitron a.
Cavitron Ultrasonic Surgical A. (CUSA)
Cogswell tip a.
Cook County Hospital a.
Cooper a.
CPI 6260 a.
CUSA Excel ultrasonic surgical a.
DeLee meconium a.
DeVilbiss Vacu-Aide a.
Dia pump a.
Dieulafoy a.
Dissectron ultrasonic a.
Egnell uterine a.
Endo-Assist sponge a.
endocervical a.
endometrial a.
faucet a.
Fibra Sonics phaco a.
Fink cataract a.
Fluvog a.
Frazier suction tip a.
Fritz a.
gallbladder a.
Gesco a.
Gomco uterine a.
Gottschalk middle ear a.
GynoSampler endometrial a.
Hahnenkratt a.
Hu-Friedy suction tip a.
Huzly a.
Hydrojette a.
InDuct breast a.
Junior Tompkins portable a.
Kelman a.
Leasure a.
Lukens a.
LySonix 250 a.
meconium a.
Monoject bone marrow a.
nasal a.
Nugent soft cataract a.
Penberthy double-action a.
Pilling-Negus clamp-on a.
portable suction a.
Potain a.
Printz a.
red-tip a.
Selector ultrasonic a.
Senoran a.
Sharplan Ultra ultrasonic a.
Sklar-Junior Tompkins a.
soft cataract a.
Sonocut ultrasonic a.
Sonop ultrasonic a.
Sorensen uterine a.
Stat a.
Stedman suction pump a.
suction a.
surgical a.
Taylor a.
Thorek gallbladder a.
Tompkins a.
Ultra ultrasonic a.
Universal a.
uterine a.
Vabra a.
Vabra cervical a.
vacuum a.
Vent-O-Vac a.
walker a.
yellow-tip a.

Aspire continuous imaging system
Aspirette endocervical aspirator
Aspir-Vac probe
Aspisafe nasogastric tube
A-splint dental splint
ASR
American Safety Razor
ASR blade
ASR scalpel
assembly
Ace halo-cast a.
Brown-Roberts-Wells arc-ring a.
Dosick bellows a.
emergency oxygen mask a.
Endoscopic Carpal Tunnel Release A. (ECTRA)
Feild retractable blade a.
infant nasal cannula a.
infant nasal CPAP a. (INCA)
linear array hydrophone a.
malleus-footplate a.
malleus-stapes a.
Massie nail a.
Vabra a.
Assess peak flowmeter
ASSI
Accurate Surgical and Scientific Instruments
ASSI air-injection cannula
ASSI bipolar coagulating forceps
ASSI breast dissector
ASSI cranial blade
ASSI forceps
ASSI METE-series Microspike approximator clamp
ASSI METS-series Microspike approximator clamp
ASSI MKCV-series Microspike approximator clamp
ASSI MSPK-series Microspike approximator clamp
ASSI no-scalpel vasectomy fixator ring clamp
ASSI no-scalpel vasectomy forceps
ASSI S&T microsurgical instrument

assist
Thera-Band A.
Assistant
A. Free calibrated femoral-tibial spreader
A. Free coated femoral-tibial spreader
A. Free retractor
A. Free self-retaining hip surgery retractor system
A. Free Stulberg leg positioner
Suture A.
Association for the Study of Internal Fixation (ASIF)
Assura
A. EasiClose ostomy pouch
A. 1-piece post-op drainable pouch
Assurant
Bridge A.
ASSureBite hot polypectomy snare
Assure blood glucose monitoring system 600 Asta air support therapy
Asta-Cath
A.-C. catheter device
A.-C. female catheter guide
Astech
A. peak flow meter
A. peak flowmeter
Asteion computed tomography system
AsthmaCheck peak flow meter
AsthmaMentor peak flowmeter
Asthmastik
Bird A.
astigmatic marker
astigmatome
Terry a.
Aston
A. cartilage reduction system
A. facelift scissors
A. nasal retractor
A. submental retractor
Aston-Daniel EndoForehead cannula
Astra
A. pacemaker
A. Tech dental implant system
AstraZeneca dental cartridge
Astro-Med Albert Grass Heritage digital EEG system
Astron
A. dental resin
A. denture

A. investment material
A. resin
Astropulse cuff
Astro-Trace Universal adapter clip
Asuka PTCA catheter
asynchronous
a. mode pacemaker
a. ventricular VOO pacemaker
AT
MemoryTrace AT
A-T
Auto-Tie
A-T antiembolism stocking
AT-10 spirometer
AT-2 ECG
Atad
A. cervical ripening device
A. ripener device
Atakr RF ablation system
Atavi
A. atraumatic spine fusion system
A. MDS system
A. microdebrider system
A. TiTLE top-loading rod fixation system
AT-1 3-channel resting ECG system
Aten olecranon screw
Athena high frequency mammography system
Athens
A. forceps
A. suture spreader
atherectomy catheter
atheroblation laser
AtheroCath
A. Bantam coronary atherectomy catheter
A. GTO catheter
Simpson coronary A.
Simpson peripheral A.
A. spinning blade catheter
atherotome
balloon a.
Athlete coronary guidewire
Athos laser
Atkins
A. esophagoscopic telescope
A. nasal splint
A. tonsillar knife
Atkins-Cannard tracheotomy tube
Atkinson
A. corneal scissors

NOTES

Atkinson *(continued)*
    A. endoprosthesis
    A. G-series short curved cystotome
    A. introducer
    A. keratome
    A. prosthesis
    A. retrobulbar needle
    A. sclerotome
    A. single-bevel blunt-tip needle
    A. tip peribulbar needle
    A. tube
    A. tube stent
Atkinson-Walker scissors
Atkins-Tucker
    A.-T. antiembolism stocking
    A.-T. shadow-free laryngoscope
    A.-T. surgical shield
ATL
    Advanced Technology Laboratories
    ATL duplex scanner
    ATL HDI-series cardiovascular
    ultrasound system
    ATL high definition imaging
    systems
    ATL Mark 600 real-time sector
    scanner
    ATL Neurosector real-time scanner
    ATL Ultramark-series real-time
    ultrasound
    ATL ultrasound scanner
Atlanta-Scottish Rite hip brace
Atlantic
    A. ileostomy catheter
    A. "O-Dor-Less" pouch
Atlantis
    A. anterior cervical plating system
    A. SR coronary intravascular
    ultrasound catheter
    A. SR IVUS catheter
atlas
    A. 2.0 diagnostic ultrasound system
    A. LP PTCA balloon dilatation
    catheter
    A. orthogonal percussion instrument
    Schaltenbrand-Wahren stereotactic a.
    A. shoulder prosthesis
    stereotactic a.
    A. ULP PTCA balloon dilatation
    catheter
Atlas-Storz eye magnet
AtLast blood glucose system
Atlee
    A. bronchus clamp
    A. uterine dilator
Atmolit suction unit
atomic absorption spectrophotometer
atomizer
    DeVilbiss a.
    Jackson laryngeal a.

    laryngeal a.
    Ono laryngobronchoscope a.
A-Trac
    A-T. atraumatic clamping system
    A-T. clamp
    A-T. insert
ATRAC multipurpose balloon catheter
Atraloc needle
Atrauclip
    A. ligating clip
    A. ligating clip system
AtrauGrip
    A. clamp
    A. dissecting forceps
    A. Weck scissors
atraumatic
    a. braided silk suture
    a. chromic suture
    a. clamp
    a. curved grasper
    a. forceps
    a. grasper
    a. intestinal clamp
    a. needle
    a. suture needle
    a. tissue forceps
    a. visceral forceps
Atraumax
    A. peripheral vascular clamp
    A. SofTrac bulldog spring clip
atrial
    a. cannula
    a. clamp
    a. demand-inhibited pacemaker
    a. demand-triggered pacemaker
    a. electrode
    a. endocardial electrode
    a. pacing wire
    a. septal defect occluder system
    umbrella
    a. septal defect occlusion system
    (ASDOS)
    a. synchronous ventricular-inhibited
    pacemaker
    a. tracking pacemaker
    a. triggered ventricular-inhibited
    pacemaker
atrial-based pacemaker
atrial-synchronous ventricular-inhibited
    pacemaker
Atricor pacemaker
AtriCure ablation and sensing unit
Atridox drug system
Atrigel drug delivery system
atrioseptostomy catheter
atrioventricular
    a. junctional pacemaker
    a. sequential demand pacemaker
    a. valve ring

atrioverter
    a. implantable defibrillator
    Metrix implantable a.
Atri-pace I bipolar flared pacing catheter
Atrisorb
    A. FreeFlow GTR barrier
    A. FreeFlow tissue regeneration barrier
Atrium
    A. blood recovery System
    A. hemodialysis graft
Atrostim phrenic nerve stimulator
ATS
    ATS Open Pivot bileaflet heart valve
    ATS 500/1500 tourniquet system
attachment
    AccuVac smoke evacuation a.
    Argen dental a.
    bar-clip a.
    Distaflex dental a.
    Hader dental a.
    HepaCoat end-point a.
    Hudson cerebellar a.
    Mayfield-Kees table a.
    O-ring a.
    pathometer a.
    PRAFO KAFO a.
    Preci-Slot dental a.
    pyramid a.
    Roach ball precision a.
    Specular reflectance a.
    Stern dental a.
    Tach-EZ dental a.
    Tasserit shoulder a.
    Thomas splint with Pearson a.
Attenborough total knee prosthesis
Attends
    A. beltless undergarment
    A. brief
    A. pad
    A. underpad
attic
    a. cannula
    a. dissector
    a. hook
Atwood
    A. bridge/crown remover
    A. loop
    A. orthodontic cement
A-type dental implant

Audibel hearing aid
Audicraft hearing aid
audiometer
    AudioScope 3 a.
    Crib-O-Gram neonatal screening a.
    GSI 16 a.
    MA 53 2-channel a.
    Madsen OB822 clinical a.
    Maico-MA 20 a.
    Pilot a.
Audionics PB Max hearing aid
AudioScope 3 audiometer
AudioTone hearing aid
AudiSil silicone ear mold material
Audivisette hearing aid
Aufranc
    A. arthroplasty gouge
    A. cup
    A. dissector
    A. femoral neck retractor
    A. finishing ball reamer
    A. finishing cup reamer
    A. hip retractor
    A. hook
    A. offset reamer
    A. periosteal elevator
    A. psoas retractor
    A. push retractor
    A. trochanteric awl
Aufranc-Turner hip prosthesis
Aufricht
    A. diamond nasal rasp
    A. facelift scissors
    A. glabellar rasp
    A. nasal elevator
    A. nasal retractor
    A. septal speculum
Aufricht-Lipsett nasal rasp
auger
    A. electron spectroscope
    Hough stapedial footplate a.
    a. wire
Auger-electron emitter
Augmen bone-grafting material
augmentative communication device
August automatic gauze packer
Augustine
    A. boat nail
    A. guide
    A. scope
Ault intestinal clamp

NOTES

Aura
    A. desktop laser
    A. laser system
AuRA cemented total hip system
aural
    a. forceps
    a. magnifier
    a. speculum
Aureomycin
    A. gauze dressing
    A. suture
auricular
    a. appendage catheter
    a. appendage clamp
    a. appendage forceps
    a. prosthesis
Auriculina hearing aid
Aurora
    A. dedicated breast MRI system
    A. diode-based dental laser system
    A. diode laser
    A. dual-chamber pacemaker
    A. HL laser
    A. MR breast imaging scanner
    A. pulse generator
Aurovest investment material
Ausculscope carotid bruit detector
Aus-Jena-Gullstrand lens loop
Austin
    A. attic dissector
    A. awl
    A. clip
    A. dental knife
    A. dental retractor
    A. dissection knife
    A. duckbill elevator
    A. endolymph dispersement shunt
    A. excavator
    A. footplate elevator
    A. forceps
    A. measuring gauge
    A. middle ear instrument
    A. Moore bone reamer
    A. Moore corkscrew
    A. Moore curved endoprosthesis
    A. Moore endoprosthesis
    A. Moore extractor
    A. Moore head
    A. Moore hip prosthesis
    A. Moore inside-outside calipers
    A. Moore mortising chisel
    A. Moore-Murphy bone skid
    A. Moore pin
    A. Moore rasp
    A. Moore standard stem
    A. Moore straight-stem
    endoprosthesis
    A. needle
    A. oval curette

    A. pick
    A. piston
    A. right-angle elevator
    A. sickle knife
    A. strut calipers
Australian
    A. orthodontic wire
    A. Special Plus wire
Auth
    A. atherectomy catheter
    A. knife
Autima II dual-chamber cardiac pacemaker
Aution Max AX-4280 automated urine analyzer
Auto
    A. D-dimer assay kit
    A. Glide walker accessor
    A. Ref-keratometer instrument
    A. Suture ABBI system
    A. Suture clip
    A. Suture Clip-A-Matic clip applier
    A. Suture curette
    A. Suture device
    A. Suture endoscopic suction-
    irrigation device
    A. Suture forceps
    A. Suture Mini-CABG occlusion
    clamp
    A. Suture Multifire Endo GIA 30
    stapler
    A. Suture One-Shot anastomotic
    device
    A. Suture Premium CEEA stapler
    A. Suture Soft Thoracoport
    A. Suture surgical mesh
    A. Suture SurgiStitch
    A. Suture SurgiStitch device
    A. Syringe AS50 infusion pump
AutoAdjust CPAP device
autoanalyzer
    Beckman a.
    Kodak Ektachem a.
Auto-Band Steri-Drape drape
Autoblock safety syringe
AutoCapture
    Integrity AFx A.
    A. Pacing System (APS)
AutoCat intraaortic balloon pump
autoclave sterilizer
Autoclip
    A. applier
    Totco A.
Autoclix fingerstick lancet device
Autocon electrosurgical unit
AutoCorr digital pulse oximeter
AutoCyte image analysis system
Autoflex II continuous passive motion unit

autofluoroscope
digital a.
autofunduscope
autogenic graft
autogenous graft
autograft
AutoGuard shielded IV catheter
Autohaler
Maxair A.
autoinfuser
Gish a.
auto-injector
Lido-Pen a.-i.
Simple-Ject a.-i.
autokeratometer
Canon K1 a.
AutoLensmeter
Tomey Trooper A.
Autolet fingerstick device
AuTolo cure process
autoLog autotransfusion system
autologous
a. fibrin tissue adhesive
a. stem
automated
a. biochemical analyzer
a. biopsy gun
a. biopsy needle
a. brainstem auditory evoked
response
a. cellular imaging system
a. cerebral blood flow analyzer
a. corneal shaper
a. endoscope reprocessor
a. gamma counter
a. laser fluorescence sequencer
a. refractor
a. trephine
automatic
a. catheter
a. chemical analyzer
a. clinical analyzer
a. collimator
a. external cardioverter-defibrillator
(AECD)
a. external defibrillator (AED)
a. implantable cardioverter-
defibrillator (AICD)
a. implantable defibrillator
a. reprocessor
a. screwdriver
a. skin retractor

a. stapling device
a. suction device
a. tourniquet
**Automator computerized distraction
device**
AutoPap
A. automated screening device
A. Pap smear system
A. 300 QC automatic Pap screener
A. reader
autoperfusion
a. balloon
a. balloon catheter
autopsy
a. blade
a. handle
autoradiographic film
Autoread centrifuge hematology system
Autoref keratometer
autorefractor
Hoya AR-570 a.
Nikon Retinomax K-Plus a.
Retinomax cordless handheld a.
AutoSet
A. portable riveting system
A. T titration system
AutoSPECT processing module
autostainer
Biotek a.
autostapling device
Autostat
A. hemostatic clip
A. ligating clip
Autosyringe pump
Autotechnicon tissue processor
Auto-Tie (A-T)
autotitration device
autotitrator
Radiometer a.
autotome drill
autotopographer
Tomey a.
autotransfuser
Biosurge synchronous a.
autotransfusion system
Autovac
A. autotransfusion system
A. LF autotransfusion system
A. needle
Autraugrip tissue forceps
Auvard
A. Britetrac speculum

NOTES

Auvard *(continued)*
  A. clamp
  A. cranioclast
  A. weighted vaginal retractor
Auvard-Remine vaginal speculum
Auvard-Zweifel
  A.-Z. basiotribe
  A.-Z. forceps
auxiliary lens
AV
  arteriovenous
    AV DeClot catheter
    AV fistula needle
    AV Gore-Tex graft
    AV Impulse foot pump
    AV junctional pacemaker
    AV Paceport thermodilution
      catheter
    AV sequential demand pacemaker
    AV sequential pacemaker
    AV synchronous pacemaker
AVA
  Advanced Venous Access
    AVA 3Xi triple-lumen venous
      access device
Avanar F/X IVUS imaging catheter
Avanta soft skeletal implant
Avanti introducer
Avant nonwoven gauze
Avco intraaortic balloon pump
AVE
  Arterial Vascular Engineering
    AVE bridge biliary stent
    AVE GFX coronary stent
    AVE Microstent II coronary stent
    AVE S-series coronary stent
    AVE stent system
Avea ventilator
Avenida dilator
Avenida-Torres dilator
Avenue insertion tool
Avera breast imaging system
averager
  multichannel signal a.
Averett total hip endoprosthesis
Avesta procedure kit
Avian transport ventilator
Avi lens system
Avina female urethral plug
Avitene
  A. collagen hemostatic material
  A. hemostatic material
  A. microfibrillar collagen hemostat
  A. Ultrafoam collagen hemostat
  A. Ultrafoam collagen sponge
Avit handpiece
Avius sequential pacemaker
Aviva mammography system

AVL
  AVL Medical Instruments model
    995-Hb arterial blood gas
    analyzer
  AVL Omni 1, 2 blood gas
    analyzer
  AVL Opti 1 portable blood gas
    analyzer
  AVL 9110 pH analyzer
AVM
  arteriovenous malformation
**AvocetPT rapid prothrombin time
  meter**
AVR
  Anatomical Vertebral Body Replacement
    AVR spinal reconstruction system
Aware breast self-examination pad
awl
  Aufranc trochanteric a.
  Austin a.
  bone a.
  Carroll a.
  Carter-Rowe a.
  DePuy a.
  Ferran a.
  Kelsey-Fry bone a.
  Kirklin sternal a.
  lacrimal a.
  Mark II Kodros radiolucent a.
  Mustarde a.
  Obwegeser a.
  pointed a.
  reamer a.
  reaming a.
  rectangular a.
  rib brad a.
  Rochester a.
  Rush pin reamer a.
  starter a.
  Stedman a.
  Swanson scaphoid a.
  T-handle bone a.
  trochanteric a.
  Uniflex distal targeting a.
  Wangensteen a.
  Wilson a.
  wire-passing a.
  Zelicof orthopaedic a.
  Zuelzer a.
Axcis
  A. laser catheter
  A. percutaneous myocardial
    revascularization laser
  A. percutaneous myocardial
    revascularization laser system
Axenfeld nerve loop
Axhausen needle holder

axial
 a. gradiometer
 a. tractor
Axiom
 A. DG balloon angioplasty catheter
 A. double sump pump
 A. drain
 A. knee component
 A. modular knee system
 A. thoracic trocar
Axios pacemaker
3-axis gradient coil
Axisonic II computerized biometer
axis-traction forceps
Axius Vacuum 2 stabilizer
Axostim nerve stimulator
Axxess spinal cord stimulator
Axya bone anchor system
AxyaWeld
 A. bone anchor
 A. bone anchor system
 A. instrument
 A. J-tip suture welding system
 A. laparoscopic sonic J system
Ayers
 A. chalazion forceps
 A. spatula

Ayerst instrument
Aylesbury
 A. cervical spatula
 A. spatula
Ayre
 A. brush
 A. cervical spatula
 A. cone knife
 A. spatula
 A. tube
Ayre-Scott cervical cone knife
Azar
 A. corneal scissors
 A. cystotome
 A. intraocular forceps
 A. iris retractor
 A. lens forceps
 A. lens hook
 A. lid speculum
 A. Mark II intraocular lens
 A. needle holder
 A. Tripod eye implant
 A. tying forceps

NOTES

Babbington nebulizer
Babcock
   B. clamp
   B. empyema trocar
   B. Endo Grasp
   B. grasper
   B. intestinal forceps
   B. jointed vein stripper
   B. lung-grasping forceps
   B. needle
   B. plate
   B. raspatory
   B. retractor
   B. stainless steel suture wire
   B. thoracic tissue-holding forceps
   B. tissue clamp
   B. tissue forceps
Babcock-Beasley forceps
Babcock-Vital
   B.-V. atraumatic tissue forceps
   B.-V. intestinal forceps
Babe OB ultrasound reporting system
Babinski percussion hammer
BA bone cement
baby
   b. Adson brain retractor
   b. Adson forceps
   b. Allis forceps
   b. Babcock forceps
   b. Balfour retractor
   b. Barraquer needle holder
   b. Bishop clamp
   b. Collin abdominal retractor
   b. Crile forceps
   b. Crile needle holder
   b. Crile-Wood needle holder
   B. Dopplex 3000 antepartum fetal
     monitor
   b. dressing forceps
   b. hemostatic forceps
   b. Inge bone spreader
   b. Inge laminar spreader
   b. intestinal tissue forceps
   b. Kocher clamp
   b. Lane bone-holding forceps
   b. Metzenbaum scissors
   b. Mikulicz forceps
   b. Miller blade
   b. Miller laryngoscope
   b. Mixter forceps
   b. mosquito forceps
   b. Overholt forceps
   b. Payr pylorus clamp
   b. rib contractor
   b. Roux retractor

   b. Satinsky clamp
   b. scope
   b. Senn-Miller retractor
   b. spur crusher
   b. Tischler biopsy punch
   b. Weitlaner retractor
BabyBeat ultrasound instrument
Babybird
   B. II respirator
   B. II ventilator
BabyFace 3-D surface rendering
accessory
Babyflex
   B. heated ventilation system
   B. ventilator
Babyhaler spacer device
BabyHugger prenatal back and
abdominal support
Babytherm IC gel mattress
BacFix system
back
   B. atYa rebounder for plyometric
     exercise
   b. board
   b. brace
   B. Bubble gravity traction unit
   B. Bull lumbar support cushion
   b. range-of-motion device
   B. Seat back brace
   B. Specialist table
backbiter
   MicroFrance pediatric b.
BackBiter forceps
backbiting
   b. bone punch
   b. forceps
backboard
   Ambu NAJO Pedi-Air-Align b.
BackCycler continuous passive motion
device
Back-Ease aromatherapy hot/cold pack
Backhaus
   B. cervical knife
   B. dilator
   B. forceps
   B. towel clamp
   B. towel clip
Backhaus-Jones towel clamp
Backhaus-Kocher towel clamp
Backhaus-Roeder forceps
Back-Huggar
   Bodyline B.-H.
   B.-H. lumbar support
   B.-H. lumbar support cushion
Backjoy spine repositioning cushion

B

back-leg-chest dynamometer
Backlund
    B. spiral biopsy needle
    B. stereotactic instrument
Backmann thyroid retractor
BackMaster device
Backnobber II massage tool
backpack
    AirPacks b.
back-stop laser probe
BackThing lumbar support
backward-cutting knife
Bacon
    B. anoscope
    B. bone rongeur
    B. cranial forceps
    B. cranial retractor
    B. periosteal raspatory
    B. proctoscope
    B. shears
Bac-Stat
    B.-S. drainage ring
    B.-S. LASIK spear
BacStop anti-retraction checkvalve
BacT/Alert
    BacT/Alert analyzer
    BacT/Alert automated blood culture
     system
    BacT/Alert glass bottle
Bactec automated blood culture system
bacterial filter
Bactigras dressing
Bacti-Swab
    B.-S. II collection and transport
     system
    B.-S. NPG collection and transport
     system
Bactron 1.5 anaerobic chamber
Badal stimulus system
Badgley
    B. laminectomy retractor
    B. plate
Baer
    B. bone-cutting forceps
    B. bone rongeur
    B. rib shears
Baerveldt
    B. glaucoma drainage implant
    B. glaucoma implant tube
    B. seton implant
    B. shunt
    B. shunt tube
baffle
    Gore-Tex b.
    Senning intraatrial b.
bag
    Aberhart disposable urinal b.
    Aberhart hemostatic b.
    ACMI b.

air b.
Alcock hemostatic b.
Alpine reusable leg b.
Ambu b.
Bard Dispoz-A-Bag leg b.
Bardex drainage b.
Barnes b.
B. Bath
bedside drainage b.
Belly Bag urine storage b.
bile b.
biohazard b.
Bogota b.
bowel b.
Brake hemostatic b.
breathing b.
Brodney hemostatic b.
Bunyan b.
Cardiff resuscitation b.
b. catheter
Champetier de Ribes obstetrical b.
Coloplast colostomy b.
Coloplast contoured urine leg b.
colostomy b.
Conveen bedside drainage b.
Conveen Security+ deluxe
  contoured leg b.
coudé b.
Curity ureteral drainage b.
Curity urine leg b.
Davol b.
dialysate b.
Diamed leg b.
Douglas b.
drainage b.
Duval b.
Dynacor leg b.
Emmet hemostatic b.
Endobag specimen b.
Endocatch II b.
Endopouch Pro specimen
  retrieval b.
Endosac specimen b.
Endo-Sock specimen retrieval b.
exudate disposal b.
Foley-Alcock b.
Foley hemostatic b.
Freedom T-tap leg b.
Frenta enteral feeding b.
Gambro freezing b.
GaSampler multilaminate b.
gauze tissue b.
Grafco colostomy b.
Grafco ileostomy b.
Hagner hemostatic b.
Hagner urethral b.
Hemofreeze blood b.
hemostatic b.
Hendrickson b.

Heyer-Schulte disposal b.
Heyer-Schulte Pour-Safe exudate b.
Higgins b.
Hofmeister drainage b.
Hollister colostomy b.
Hollister drainage b.
Hollister urostomy b.
Hope resuscitation b.
hydrostatic b.
ice b.
ileostomy b.
Incono b.
Infu-Surg pressure infuser b.
intestinal b.
intracervical b.
isolation b.
Karaya seal ileostomy stomal b.
Lahey b.
Lapides collecting b.
Lapides ileostomy b.
latex b.
Lyster water b.
Mac-Lee enema b.
manual resuscitation b.
Marlen ileostomy b.
Marlen leg b.
Melmed blood freezing b.
micturition b.
millinery b.
3M limb isolation b.
Mosher b.
Nesbit hemostatic b.
night drainage b.
ostomy b.
Owen hemostatic b.
Paul condom b.
Paul hemostatic b.
Pearman transurethral hemostatic b.
pear-shaped fluted b.
Peel Pak b.
Pennine leg b.
Perry ileostomy b.
Petersen rectal b.
Pilcher suprapubic hemostatic b.
Plummer b.
pneumatic b.
3-point spreader b.
4-point spreader b.
Politzer air b.
Ponsky Endo-Sock specimen
  retrieval b.
prostatectomy b.

ProSys leg b.
Rainy Day playground b.
rebreathing b.
replacement collection b.
Robinson b.
Rusch leg b.
Rutzen ileostomy b.
severance transurethral b.
Shea-Anthony b.
short-tip hemostatic b.
sleeve b.
Soft Guard XL fecal
  incontinence b.
Sones hemostatic b.
sterile isolation b.
stomal b.
suprapubic hemostatic b.
SureGrip resuscitation b.
Sur-Fit colostomy b.
Sur-Fit urinary drainage b.
Surgi-Flo leg b.
Swenko b.
Tassett vaginal cup b.
Tedlar b.
Teflo-Kapton freezing b.
Thackston retropubic b.
Trach-Mist aerosol drainage b.
Travenol heart b.
Uri-Drain leg b.
urinary drainage b.
urinary leg b.
Urocare latex reusable leg b.
Uro-Safe vinyl disposable leg b.
vaginal b.
Van Hove b.
Versi-Splint carry b.
Vi-Drape bowel b.
Void-Ease urine collection b.
Voorhees b.
VPI urinary leg b.
Wheelchair Buddy b.
Whitmore b.
Wolf hemostatic b.
Bagby
  B. compression plate
  B. and Kuslich (BAK)
  B. and Kuslich cable
  B. and Kuslich cage
  B. and Kuslich interbody fusion
    system
BagEasy disposable manual resuscitator
bag-fixated intraocular lens

NOTES

Baggish hysteroscope
Bagley helical basket
Bagley-Wilmer lens expressor
Bagolini lens
bag-valve-mask (BVM)
    b.-v.-m. resuscitator
Bahama suture scissors
Bahler
    Gschwend, Scheier, B. (GSB)
Bahnson
    B. aortic aneurysm clamp
    B. aortic cannula
    B. appendage clamp
    B. sternal retractor
Bahnson-Brown forceps
Bahn spud
Baikoff lens
Bailey
    B. aortic clamp
    B. aortic valve-cutting forceps
    B. aortic valve rongeur
    B. chalazion forceps
    B. dilator
    B. drill
    B. duckbill clamp
    B. fontonal needle
    B. foreign body remover
    B. Gigli-saw guide
    B. lacrimal cannula
    B. leukotome
    B. punch
    B. rib approximator
    B. rib contractor
    B. rib spreader
    B. round knife
    B. saw conductor
    B. skull bur
    B. transthoracic catheter
    B. wire saw
Bailey-Cowley clamp
Bailey-Gibbon rib contractor
Bailey-Glover-O'Neill commissurotomy
  knife
Bailey-Morse
    B.-M. clamp
    B.-M. mitral knife
Bailey-Williamson obstetrical forceps
Bailliart
    B. goniometer
    B. ophthalmodynamometer
    B. ophthalmoscope
    B. tonometer
bail-lock brace
bailout
    b. autoperfusion balloon catheter
    b. stent
Baim pacing catheter

Baim-Turi
    B.-T. cardiac device
    B.-T. monitoring/pacing catheter
Bainbridge
    B. anastomosis clamp
    B. hemostatic forceps
    B. intestinal clamp
    B. intestinal forceps
    B. resection forceps
    B. thyroid forceps
    B. vessel clamp
Bair
    B. Hugger forced-air warmer
    B. Hugger patient warming blanket
    B. Hugger patient warming system
Baird
    B. chalazion forceps
    B. Electric System 5000 Power
      Plus electrosurgical unit
BAK
  Bagby and Kuslich
    BAK cage
    BAK interbody fusion system
BAK/C
    BAK/C cervical interbody fusion
     cage
    BAK/C cervical interbody fusion
     implant
    BAK/C interbody fusion system
Bakelite
    B. cystoscopy sheath
    B. dental chisel
    B. mallet
    B. rectoscope sheath
    B. retractor
    B. spatula
Baker
    B. amniocentesis needle set
    B. continuous flow capillary drain
    B. jejunostomy tube
    B. punch
    B. self-sumping tube
    B. tissue forceps
    B. velum
Bakes
    B. bile duct dilator
    B. common duct dilator
    B. probe
Bakes-Pearce dilator
BAK/Proximity interbody fusion implant
Bakst
    B. cardiac scissors
    B. valvulotome
BAK/T interbody fusion system
Baladi inverter
balance
    b. beam scale
    b. board
    b. bridge

B

B. hip prosthesis
Humphriss binocular b.
B. Master rocker board
B. Master training and assessment
  system
b. pad
b. padding orthosis
balanced forearm orthosis (BFO)
Baldwin
  B. butterfly ventilation tube
  B. perineum needle
Balfour
  B. bladder blade
  B. center blade
  B. center-blade abdominal retractor
  B. clamp
  B. lateral blade
  B. pediatric abdominal retractor
  B. self-retaining abdominal retractor
Balkan
  B. bed
  B. femoral splint
  B. fracture frame
Balkin Up & Over introducer
Balkwell articulator
ball
  Anderson double b.
  Articul/eze femoral b.
  birthing b.
  Body B.
  b. burnisher
  Cajal axonal retraction b.
  cauterizing b.
  b. coagulator
  cold-weld femoral b.
  cotton b.
  b. dissector
  Exertools gym b.
  b. extractor
  b. fastener
  Finger Fitness spring b.
  B. forceps
  Gertie b.
  Gripp squeeze b.
  gym b.
  Gymnastik b.
  Gymnic b.
  Gymnic Plus b.
  hand exercise b.
  HeavyMed b.
  b. joint block
  Jurgan pin b.

Ledraplastic exercise b.
b. nerve hook
PhysioGymnic exercise b.
Physio-Roll VisuaLiser exercise b.
Pinky b.
Plyoback Rebounder medicine b.
Plyoball medicine b.
b. poppet
Silastic b.
Slo-Mo b.
Spondex sponge b.
squeeze b.
Stycar graded b.
Super Pinky b.
Swiss b.
Thera-Band exercise b.
Thera-Band Slow Deflate System
  exercise b.
Theragym b.
therapy b.
TissueLink monopolar floating b.
b. valve prosthesis
b. wedge
Ballade needle
Ballance mastoid spoon
ball-and-cage prosthesis
ball-and-socket prosthesis
Ballantine
  B. clamp
  B. hemilaminectomy retractor
  B. hysterectomy forceps
  B. uterine curette
Ballantine-Drew coagulator
Ballantine-Peterson hysterectomy forceps
Ballen-Alexander
  B.-A. forceps
  B.-A. orbital retractor
ball-end elevator
Ballenger
  B. cartilage knife
  B. chisel
  B. ethmoidal curette
  B. follicle electrode
  B. gouge
  B. hysterectomy forceps
  B. mastoid bur
  B. mucosal knife
  B. nasal swivel knife
  B. periosteotome
  B. raspatory
  B. septal elevator
  B. septal knife

NOTES

Ballenger *(continued)*
    B. sponge forceps
    B. tonsillar forceps
Ballenger-Foerster forceps
Ballenger-Hajek
    B.-H. chisel
    B.-H. elevator
Ballenger-Lillie mastoid bur
Ballenger-Sluder
    B.-S. guillotine
    B.-S. tonsillectome
ballistic energy generator
ballistocardiograph
Ballobes gastric balloon
ball-occluder valve
balloon
    Ace b.
    Acucise b.
    angioplasty b.
    b. angioplasty catheter
    Anthony-Fisher antral b.
    antral b.
    b. applicator
    Arrow-Berman angiographic b.
    ASI uroplasty b.
    b. atherotome
    autoperfusion b.
    Ballobes gastric b.
    banana-shaped b.
    Bandit low-profile over-the-wire b.
    Bardex Lubricath red latex
      double b.
    barium enema retention b.
    barostat b.
    Baxter Intrepid b.
    Baylor cervical b.
    bifoil b.
    b. biliary catheter
    Bilisystem stone-removal b.
    Blue Max high-pressure b.
    Brandt cytology b.
    Brighton epistaxis b.
    catheter b.
    b. catheter
    b. catheter sealing device
    centering b.
    b. cervical cannula
    compliant b.
    Cook b.
    Cordis Powerflex PTA b.
    counterpulsation b.
    Cribier-Letac aortic valvuloplasty b.
    cutting b.
    cylindrical b.
    Datascope b.
    delivery b.
    b. dilatation catheter
    b. dilating catheter
    b. dilator

Dispatch b.
b. dissector
Distaflex b.
doughnut-shaped b.
DURAglide^3 stone removal b.
electrode b.
Eliminator dilatation b.
b. embolectomy catheter
endocapsular b.
Epistat double b.
epistaxis b.
esophageal b.
extraction b.
Extractor XL triple-lumen
  retrieval b.
ExtraView b.
fixed-wire b.
b. flotation catheter
Fogarty b.
Foley b.
Force b.
Fox postnasal b.
French Swan-Ganz b.
Garren-Edwards gastric b.
gastric b.
Grüntzig b.
Guidant b.
b. guide catheter
Hadow b.
helix b.
Helmstein b.
high-pressure Blue Max b.
Honan b.
Hunter b.
Hunter-Sessions b.
hydrostatic b.
b. imaging catheter
inflated b.
Inoue self-guiding b.
Integra II b.
intraaortic b. (IAB)
intraaortic counterpulsation b.
intragastric b.
intraocular b.
Katzin-Long b.
Kaye tamponade b.
kissing b.
Knead-A-Ball therapy b.
laser b.
latex b.
LEAP b.
low-compliance b.
low-profile angioplasty b.
Mansfield b.
metrizamide-filled b.
Micross SL b.
Microvasive retrieval b.
Microvasive Rigiflex through-the-
  scope b.

Microvasive Rigiflex TTS b.
Monorail Speedy b.
Multi-Link Duet coronary stent b.
Multi-Link Penta coronary stent b.
Multi-Link Zeta coronary stent b.
NC Cobra b.
noncompliant b.
nondetachable endovascular b.
nondetachable occlusive b.
NoProfile b.
NuMED single b.
occlusion b.
occlusive b.
Olbert b.
Omega-NV b.
Omni SST b.
Origin PDB 1000 b.
Orion b.
Owen b.
Passage exchange b.
PDB preperitoneal distention b.
Percival gastric b.
Percor-Stat intraaortic b.
percutaneous transluminal
  angioplasty b.
PET b.
Piccolino b.
pillow-shaped b.
polyethylene terephthalate b.
polyolefin copolymer b.
polyvinyl chloride b.
positron emission tomography b.
postnasal b.
Powerflex PTA b.
preperitoneal distention b.
Prime b.
ProCross Rely b.
Provocative sensitivity b.
pulmonary b.
b. pump
QuickFurl double-lumen b.
QuickFurl single-lumen b.
QuickTrack coronary stent b.
radiofrequency hot b.
Raptor PTCA b.
Rashkind b.
rectal b.
RediFurl double-lumen b.
RediFurl single-lumen b.
retrieval b.
Riepe-Bard gastric b.
Rigiflex achalasia b.

Rushkin b.
Schneider-Shiley b.
Schwarten Microglide LP b.
scintigraphic b.
self-sealing latex b.
Seloris b.
Sengstaken b.
Sengstaken-Blakemore esophageal b.
b. septostomy catheter
Shadow b.
Shea-Anthony b.
Short Speedy b.
b. shunt
Simpson epistaxis b.
sinus b.
sizing b.
Slalom b.
Slider b.
Slinky b.
Soft-Wand atraumatic tissue
  manipulator b.
Soto USCI b.
Spacemaker II b.
Spears USCI laser b.
Stack autoperfusion b.
Stealth catheter b.
b. stone extractor
stone-retrieval b.
Stretch b.
b. tamponade
Taylor gastric b.
TEGwire b.
ThermaChoice uterine b.
thigh b.
through-the-scope b.
Thruflex b.
transluminal b.
Triad PET b.
Tri-Ex triple-lumen extraction b.
Tru-Trac high-pressure PTA b.
Tyshak b.
ultra-thin b.
Ultrathin Diamond b.
b. valvuloplasty catheter
VasoView b.
b. wedge pressure catheter
Wilson-Cook dilating b.
Wilson-Cook gastric b.
windowed esophageal b.
wire-guided hydrostatic b.
balloon-centered argon laser

NOTES

57

balloon-expandable
  b.-e. flexible coil stent
  b.-e. intravascular stent
balloon-flotation pacing catheter
ballooning esophagoscope
balloon-on-a-wire
  b.-o.-a.-w. device
  b.-o.-a.-w. dilatation catheter
balloon-tipped
  b.-t. angiographic catheter
  b.-t. catheter
  b.-t. flow-directed catheter
  b.-t. thermodilution catheter
ball-peen splint
ball-tipped seeker
ball-type retractor
ball-wedge catheter
Balmer tongue depressor
Balmoral shoe
Balnetar implant
Baloser hysteroscope
Balser hook plate
Balshi packer
Balters appliance
Baltherm thermal dilution catheter
Baltimore
  B. nasal scissors
  B. Therapeutic Equipment work
    stimulator
Bambi cell analysis system
Banaji
  B. LASIK cannula
  B. LASIK flap spatula
banana
  b. Beaver blade
  b. catheter
  b. split splint
banana-shaped balloon
band
  adhesive b.
  AO tension b.
  BB b.
  belly b.
  Can-Do exercise b.
  coffer b.
  Colvin-Galloway Future
    annuloplasty b.
  copper b.
  Cosgrove-Edwards annuloplasty b.
  Dentaform b.
  DOC b.
  dynamic orthotic cranioplasty b.
  encircling b.
  ExerBand therapy b.
  exercise b.
  EZ band hemostasis b.
  Falope-ring tubal occlusion b.
  Fit-Lastic therapy b.
  fracture b.

Fränkel head b.
GelBand arm b.
Hahnenkratt matrix b.
Harris b.
hemostasis b.
Jobst air b.
Johnson dental b.
latex O b.
b. ligator device
Lukens orthodontic b.
Magill orthodontic b.
Marlex b.
Matas vessel b.
matrix b.
Mersilene b.
Ormco preformed b.
Orthoband traction b.
orthodontic b.
Parham b.
Parham-Martin b.
Parma b.
patellar b.
PD copper b.
PD SS matrix b.
Ray-Tec b.
Remak b.
Resist-A-Band exercise b.
scultetus binder b.
Silastic b.
silicone elastomer b.
Simonart b.
table b.
Thera-Band exercise b.
Thera-Band Max b.
Tofflemire matrix b.
tooth b.
tourniquet b.
True Blue exercise b.
vessel b.
Vistnes rubber b.
Watzke b.
Xercise b.
Xertube resistance b.
Zipper Medical hypoallergenic
  tracheostomy tube neck b.
bandage
  abdominal b.
  Ace adherent b.
  Ace spica b.
  adhesive b.
  Band-Aid b.
  barrel b.
  Barton b.
  Bennell b.
  binocular b.
  Borsch b.
  Bulkee II gauze b.
  Buller b.
  butterfly b.

capeline b.
Cellamin resin plaster-of-Paris b.
Cellona resin plaster-of-Paris b.
Champ elastic b.
CircAid compression b.
circular b.
ClearSite b.
Coban b.
Coflex b.
cohesive b.
collodion-treated self-adhesive b.
Comperm tubular elastic b.
compression b.
Comprilan b.
Conco elastic b.
Conform stretch b.
b. contact lens
cotton crepe b.
cotton elastic b.
cotton-wool b.
Cover-Roll stretch b.
cravat b.
crepe b.
Curad b.
demigauntlet b.
Desault wrist b.
Dressinet tubular b.
DuoDERM SCB sustained
  compression b.
Dynaflex elastic b.
E-cotton b.
elastic foam-backed b.
Elastikon b.
Elastomull b.
Elastoplast b.
Equiflex b.
Esmarch b.
eye b.
Fabco gauze b.
fiberglass b.
figure-of-8 b.
fixation b.
flat eye b.
flexible b.
Flexicon gauze b.
Flexilite conforming elastic b.
FoaMTrac traction b.
Fractura Flex b.
Fricke b.
Galen b.
Garretson b.
gauntlet b.

gauze b.
Gauztape b.
Gauztex b.
Gibney fixation b.
Gibson b.
Guibor bubble b.
Guibor Expo flat eye b.
Haftelast self-adhering b.
Hamilton b.
hammock b.
Heliodorus b.
Hermitex b.
Hippocrates b.
Hollister medical adhesive b.
Hueter b.
Hydron burn b.
Hypertie b.
immobilizing b.
Kerlix gauze b.
Kiwisch b.
Kling gauze b.
Kold Wrap cold compression b.
Larrey b.
4-layer b.
Liquiderm liquid healing b.
Lister b.
Maisonneuve b.
many-tailed b.
Marlex b.
Martin b.
3M Clean Seals waterproof b.
Medi-Band b.
Medicopaste b.
moleskin b.
monocular b.
Morton b.
oblique b.
Orthoflex elastic plaster b.
Ortho-Vent b.
Pearlcast polymer plaster b.
perineal b.
plaster b.
plaster-of-Paris b.
Plast-O-Fit thermoplastic b.
polyurethane b.
pressure b.
Priessnitz b.
Profore four-layer b.
protective b.
QuikStrip adhesive b.
recurrent b.
Rep Bands exercise b.

NOTES

bandage *(continued)*

Ribble b.
Richet b.
Robert Jones b.
roller b.
rubber-reinforced b.
Sayre b.
scarf b.
b. scissors
Scultetus b.
Setopress high-compression b.
Seutin b.
b. shears
short-stretch b.
Shur-Band self-closure elastic b.
Silesian b.
sling-and-swathe b.
Sof-Band bulky b.
Sof-Kling conforming b.
b. soft contact lens
Spandage b.
spica b.
spiral reverse b.
spray b.
starch b.
Stereocrepe crepe b.
Steri-Band b.
stockinette amputation b.
SurePress high compression b.
Sureseal cellulose sponge b.
Sureseal pressure b.
Surgiflex b.
suspensory b.
T b.
4-tailed b.
Telfa 4 x 4 b.
Theden b.
Thera-Boot compression b.
Thillaye b.
triangular b.
Tricodur Epi compression
support b.
Tricodur Omos compression
support b.
Tricodur Talus compression
support b.
Tru-Support EW b.
Tru-Support SA b.
T-Spica b.
Tubegauz seamless tubular knitted
cotton b.
TubiFast b.
Tubigrip elastic support b.
Tubipad b.
Tubiton b.
Tuffnell b.
Unna-Flex paste b.
Velpeau b.
Watson-Jones b.

Webril b.
wet b.
woven elastic b.
wrist b.
zinc oxide b.

BandageGuard half-leg guard

Band-Aid

B.-A. bandage
B.-A. sterile adhesive surgical
dressing

Bandeloux bed

banding

Lap-Band adjustable gastric b.
(LAGB)

Bandit

B. low-profile over-the-wire balloon
B. PTCA catheter

Band-It tennis elbow strap

bandpass filter

Bane

B. hook
B. mastoid rongeur
B. rongeur
B. rongeur forceps

Bane-Hartmann bone rongeur

Bangerter

B. muscle forceps
B. spatula

Bangs bougie

banjo

b. curette
b. splint
b. tractor

Bankart

B. rasp
B. retractor
B. shoulder prosthesis
B. shoulder repair set
B. shoulder retractor

Banks bone graft

Banno catheter

Bannon-Klein implant

Bansal LASIK forceps

Bansaton behind-the-ear hearing aid

Bantam

B. Bovie coagulator
B. irrigation set
B. wire cutter
B. wire-cutting scissors

Bantex amalgamator

BAR

biofragmentable anastomotic ring
Valtrac BAR

bar

Ackerman lingual b.
arch b.
Bendick dental arch b.
Berens prism b.
Bill b.

Bookwalter horizontal b.
Bose b.
Brookdale b.
Buck extension b.
Burns prism b.
calcaneonavicular b.
clasp b.
cross b.
Denis Browne b.
dental arch b.
distraction b.
b. drill
Erich malleable dental arch b.
EZ-Guide SL light b.
facial fracture appliance dental
arch b.
Fillauer b.
fixed arch b.
fracture b.
Gerster traction b.
Goldman b.
Goldthwait b.
grab b.
Greenberg b.
Hader implant b.
Hahnenkratt lingual b.
hex b.
intramedullary b.
Jelenko arch b.
Jewett b.
Joseph septal b.
Kangoo Thera-P b.
Kennedy b.
Leyla self-retaining tractor b.
lingual b.
Livingston intramedullary b.
LockJaw arch b.
lumbrical b.
mandibular arch b.
maxillary arch b.
Niro arch b.
occlusal rest b.
palatal b.
Passavant b.
Posey b.
posterior thigh b.
b. prism
retainer arch b.
retention b.
screw alignment b.
Simonart b.
skiascopy b.

spondylitic b.
spreader b.
stabilizing b.
stall b.
strut b.
T b.
tarsal b.
Thera-Band FlexBar b.
Thera-P b.
Tommy hip b.
Tommy trapeze b.
traction b.
trapeze b.
b. T-tube
valgus b.
Vistnes applier b.
Zielke derotator b.
4-bar
4-b. linkage prosthetic knee
mechanism
4-b. polycentric knee prosthesis
Bara-Med
B.-M. clinical acrylic monoplace
hyperbaric chamber
B.-M. clinical multiplace hyperbaric
chamber
bar-and-shoe orthosis
Bárány
B. alarm
B. box
B. noise apparatus whistle
B. speculum
Barbara needle
barbed
b. broach
b. epicardial pacing lead
b. myringotome
b. Richards staple
bar-clip attachment
Barcroft apparatus
Barcroft-Warburg apparatus
Bard
B. absorption drape
B. absorption dressing
B. adhesive and barrier film
remover
B. AlgiDerm dressing
B. AlgiDerm rope
B. alligator cup
B. ambulatory PCA device
B. arterial cannula
B. automatic endoscope reprocessor

NOTES

61

Bard *(continued)*
- B. balloon-directed pacing catheter
- B. biopsy needle
- B. Biopty cut needle
- B. Biopty gun
- B. BladderScan bladder volume instrument
- B. button feeding tube
- B. cardiopulmonary support pump
- B. cardiopulmonary support system
- B. catheter
- B. catheter sterile insertion tray
- B. catheter strap
- B. cervical cannula
- B. clamshell septal occluder
- B. clamshell septal umbrella
- B. closed-end pouch
- B. coil stent
- B. collagen Contigent implant
- B. Commander PTCA guidewire
- B. Companion papillotome
- B. Composix Kugel hernia patch
- B. Composix mesh
- B. Composix mesh graft
- B. CPS system
- B. Cunningham urinary incontinence clamp
- B. Dispoz-A-Bag leg bag
- B. drainage adhesive pouch
- B. electrode
- B. electrophysiology catheter
- B. EndoCinch suturing system
- B. endoscopic suture system
- B. evacuator
- B. extension tubing
- B. FCD fecal containment device
- B. Federal containment device
- B. forceps
- B. gastrostomy catheter
- B. gastrostomy feeding tube
- B. guiding catheter
- B. helical catheter
- B. Infus-OR syringe-type infusion pump
- B. irrigation sleeve
- B. leg bag holder
- B. male external catheter
- B. malleable tip catheter stylet
- B. Marlex mesh
- B. Medi-aire
- B. Memotherm
- B. Memotherm colorectal stent
- B. nonsteerable bipolar electrode
- B. oval cup
- B. PCA pump
- B. PDA umbrella
- B. PEG tube
- B. probe
- B. protective barrier film

- B. PTFE graft
- B. regular one-piece stoma
- B. resectoscope
- B. rotary atherectomy system
- B. Safety Excalibur
- B. security pouch
- B. Sequence II Plus incontinent skin care kit
- B. soft double-pigtail ureteral stent
- B. Sperma-Tex preshaped mesh
- B. sterile infection control tray
- B. sterile red rubber catheter
- B. sterilizer
- B. Stinger S ablation catheter
- B. Touchless intermittent catheter
- B. TransAct IABP
- B. TransAct intraaortic balloon pump
- B. ureteroscopic cytology brush
- B. urethral dilator
- B. urinary sterile collection system
- B. Urolase fiber
- B. Urolase fiber laser system
- B. Visilex mesh
- B. wide leg bag strap
- B. x-ray ureteral catheter
- B. XT coronary stent

Bardam red rubber catheter
Bardco-Matic catheter
Bardeleben
- B. bone-holding forceps
- B. rasp

Bardex
- B. drain
- B. drainage bag
- B. IC silver-coated latex Foley catheter
- B. Lubricath latex Foley catheter
- B. Lubricath red latex double balloon
- B. Lubricath sterile Foley tray
- B. stent

Bardex-Bellini drain
Bardex-Foley
- B.-F. balloon catheter
- B.-F. return-flow retention catheter

Bard-Hamm fulgurating electrode
Bardic
- B. cannula
- B. curette
- B. cutdown catheter
- B. translucent catheter
- B. tube
- B. Uro Sheath reusable male external catheter

Bardic-Deseret Intracath catheter
Bard-Parker
- B.-P. dermatome
- B.-P. handle

B.-P. keratome
B.-P. knife
B.-P. razor
B.-P. scalpel
B.-P. surgical blade
B.-P. transfer forceps
B.-P. trephine
B.-P. U-Mid/Lo humidifier
BardPort implanted port
Bard-Steigmann-Goff variceal ligation kit
Bard-Tuohy-Borst adapter
Bard-U-Cath self-adhering male external catheter
bare-metal stent
Bareskin knee positioner
Bare-Tip fiber
Bari-800i system bariatric bed
bariatric mat platform
BariKare advanced power system
barium enema retention balloon
barium-impregnated poppet
Barkan
B. bident retractor
B. goniolens
B. gonioscope
B. gonioscopic lens
B. goniotomy knife
B. illuminator
B. infant lens
B. infant lens implant
B. iris forceps
B. light
B. operating lens
B. scissors
Barker
B. calipers
B. spinal anesthesia needle
B. Vacu-tome dermatome
B. Vacu-tome suction knife
Barlow forceps
Barnard mitral valve prosthesis
Barnes
B. bag
B. cervical dilator
B. common duct dilator
B. compressor
B. perineorrhaphy scissors
B. spirometer
B. suction tube
B. vessel scissors
Barnes-Crile hemostatic forceps

Barnes-Dormia stone basket
Barnes-Hill forceps
Barnes-Hind ophthalmic dressing
Barnes-Simpson obstetrical forceps
Barnhill adenoid curette
Barnhill-Jones curette
baromacrometer
Baron
B. ear knife
B. ear tube
B. forceps
B. intraocular lens
B. retractor
B. suction tube
B. suction tube-cleaning wire
Baron-Frazier suction tube
baroreceptor
cardiac b.
barospirator
barostat balloon
Barouk
B. button
B. button spacer
B. cannulated bone screw
B. microscrew
B. microstaple
B. spacer
Barr
B. anal speculum
B. bolt
B. crypt hook
B. fistula probe
B. pin
B. rectal fistular hook
B. rectal probe
B. rectal retractor
B. rectal speculum
B. self-retaining rectal retractor
Barraquer
B. blade
B. cannula
B. ciliary forceps
B. conjunctival forceps
B. corneal dissector
B. corneal forceps
B. corneal knife
B. corneal section scissors
B. corneal trephine
B. curved holder
B. cyclodialysis spatula
B. erysiphake
B. eye shield

B

NOTES

Barraquer *(continued)*
- B. eye speculum
- B. fixation forceps
- B. hemostatic mosquito forceps
- B. implant
- B. iris scissors
- B. iris spatula
- B. irrigator
- B. irrigator spatula
- B. J-loop intraocular lens
- B. keratoplasty knife
- B. lid retractor
- B. microkeratome
- B. needle carrier
- B. needle holder
- B. needle holder clamp
- B. operating room tonometer
- B. razor bladebreaker
- B. sable brush
- B. silk suture
- B. speculum
- B. sweep
- B. tonometer
- B. vitreous strand scissors
- B. wire guide
- B. wire speculum

Barraquer-Carriazo microkeratome
Barraquer-Colibri
- B.-C. eye speculum
- B.-C. forceps

Barraquer-DeWecker iris scissors
Barraquer-Douvas eye speculum
Barraquer-Floyd speculum
Barraquer-Karakashian scissors
Barraquer-Katzin forceps
Barraquer-Krumeich-Swinger (BKS)
- B.-K.-S. microkeratome
- B.-K.-S. refractor
- B.-K.-S. retractor

Barraquer-Troutman
- B.-T. corneal forceps
- B.-T. needle holder

Barraquer-Vogt needle
Barraquer-von Mandach
- B.-v. M. capsular forceps
- B.-v. M. clot forceps

Barraya tissue forceps
barrel
- b. bandage
- b. bur
- b. cutting bur
- b. dressing
- b. guide
- Opti-Vue plastic b.

Barrett
- B. appendix inverter
- B. flange lens manipulator
- B. hebosteotomy needle
- B. hydrodelineation cannula

- B. hydrogel intraocular lens
- B. intestinal forceps
- B. lens forceps
- B. placental forceps
- B. tenacular forceps
- B. uterine knife
- B. uterine tenaculum forceps

Barrett-Adson cerebellum retractor
Barrett-Allen
- B.-A. placental forceps
- B.-A. uterine forceps

Barrett-Murphy intestinal forceps
Barrie-Jones angled crocodile forceps
barrier
- AquaTack hydrocolloid b.
- Atrisorb FreeFlow GTR b.
- Atrisorb FreeFlow tissue regeneration b.
- Capset bone graft b.
- DermaMend b.
- Durahesive moldable convex skin b.
- external urethral b.
- b. gown
- Hollister Flextend skin b.
- Interceed absorbable adhesion b.
- Kraylex odor b.
- B. laparoscopy drape
- B. laparoscopy/LAVH pack
- B. lower extremity sheet
- Marlen SkinShield adhesive skin b.
- b. membrane
- Nu-Hope adhesive waterproof skin b.
- Oxiplex/AP adhesion b.
- Seprafilm adhesion b.
- Sil-K OB b.
- space-maintaining b.
- sterile field b.
- TC-7 adhesion b.
- VitaCuff tissue-interface b.

Barron
- B. corneal punch
- B. epikeratophakia trephine
- B. hemorrhoidal ligator
- B. pump
- B. radial vacuum trephine
- B. retractor
- B. scalpel handle
- B. vacuum trephine

Barron-Hessburg corneal trephine
Barr-Shuford speculum
Barsky
- B. cleft palate raspatory
- B. elevator
- B. forceps
- B. nasal osteotome
- B. nasal rasp

B. nasal retractor
B. nasal scissors
bar-supported overdenture
Bart abdominoperipheral angiography unit
Barth double-end applicator
Bartholdson-Stenstrom rasp
Bartholin gland catheter
Bartkiewicz two-sided drain
Bartlett fascial stripper
Bartley
B. anastomosis clamp
B. partial-occlusion clamp
bar-to-bar clamp
Barton
B. bandage
B. blade
B. double hook
B. dressing
B. obstetrical forceps
B. skull traction tongs
B. sling
B. suction
B. traction device
B. traction handle
B. wrench
Barton-Cone tongs
Baruch circumcision scissors
BAS-300 transurethral thermotherapy device
basal body thermometer
Baschui pigtail catheter
base
Brown-Roberts-Wells phantom b.
Getz rubber b.
Lok-Mesh bonding b.
Profix nonporous tibial b.
Vibram walking b.
baseball finger splint
base-down prism
Basek chisel
Baseline dynamometer
Basic
One Touch B.
B. Sequences ColorCards
Basile hip screw
basin
catch b.
urological soaking b.
basiotribe
Auvard-Zweifel b.
Tarnier b.

Basis breast pump
Basix pacemaker
basket
Acufex b.
Bagley helical b.
Barnes-Dormia stone b.
Browne stone b.
b. catheter
Dormia biliary stone b.
Dormia gallstone b.
Dormia ureteral stone b.
Duette b.
Eliminator stone extraction b.
Ellik kidney stone b.
Ferguson stone b.
b. forceps
gallstone b.
Gemini helical wire b.
Glassman b.
Hobbs stone b.
Howard stone b.
InSurg common bile duct b.
Johns Hopkins stone b.
Johnson ureteral stone b.
kidney stone b.
lithotripter b.
Medi-Tech stone b.
Memory b.
Mill-Rose spiral stone b.
Mitchell stone b.
Moss-Harms b.
Olympus stone retrieval b.
Pfister-Schwartz stone b.
Pfister stone b.
Positrap mini-retrieval b.
Pursuer CBD helical b.
b. retriever
Robinson stone b.
rotary b.
Rutner stone b.
Schutte shovel-nose b.
Segura CBD b.
Segura-Dretler stone b.
Segura Hemisphere stone retrieval b.
Segura stone b.
sphincterotomy b.
sterilizing b.
stone b.
b. stone extractor catheter
stone-holding b.
stone-retrieval b.

NOTES

basket *(continued)*
    Sur-Catch paired-wire b.
    ultrasonic cleaner b.
    ureteral stone b.
    Vantec stone b.
    VPI stone b.
    Wilson-Cook stone b.
    6-wire spiral-tip Segura b.
    ZeroTip nitinol stone retrieval b.
basket-cutting forceps
basket-punch forceps
basket-type crushing forceps
Bassett electrical stimulation device
Basswood splint
bastard suture
basting suture
Bastow raspatory
Batchelor plate
Bateman
    B. endoprosthesis
    B. finger prosthesis
    B. UPF II bipolar endoprosthesis
    B. UPF II bipolar knee system
    B. UPF II shoulder prosthesis
Bates-Jensen pressure ulcer status tool
bath
    Bag B.
    Charcot b.
    Dickson paraffin b.
    Finsen b.
    HydraClense sitz b.
    B. respirator
    Therabath paraffin therapy b.
    ThermaSplint heating b.
    Travel B.
Bathlifter
    Leo B.
Baton laser pointer
Batson-Carmody elevator
batten graft
battery
    Duracell Activair hearing aid b.
    external pacemaker b.
    lithium iodine b.
    Renata b.
battery-assisted heart assist device
battery-operated breast pump
battery-powered endoscope
batting
    cotton b.
Batt tip
bat-wing
    b.-w. catheter
    b.-w. dissector
Batzdorf
    B. cervical wire passer
    B. cervical wire twister
Baudelocque pelvimeter

Bauer
    B. dissecting forceps
    B. hernia belt
    B. kidney pedicle clamp
    B. retractor
    B. sponge forceps
    B. Temno biopsy needle
Bauerfeind
    B. Achillotrain Achilles tendon
    brace
    B. ankle brace
    B. Champion Powersox sock
    B. Comprifix knee brace
    B. Malleolic ankle orthosis
    B. silicone heel pad
    B. ViscoSpot heel cushion
Baumanometer sphygmomanometer
Baumberger forceps
Baumer locking nail
Baumgarten wire twister
Baumgartner
    B. forceps
    B. needle holder
    B. punch
Baum-Hecht tarsorrhaphy forceps
Baum-Metzenbaum sternal needle holder
Baum needle holder
Baumrucker
    B. clamp irrigator
    B. electrode
    B. post-TUR irrigation clamp
    B. resectoscope
    B. urinary incontinence clamp
Bausch
    B. articulation paper forceps
    B. & Lomb Duoloupe lens loupe
    B. & Lomb manual keratometer
    B. & Lomb Optima lens
    B. & Lomb Softlens 66 contact
    lens
    B. & Lomb Surgical L161U lens
    B. & Lomb-Thorpe slit lamp
Bausch-Lomb-Thorpe slit lamp
Bavarian splint
Baxa oral dispenser
Baxter
    B. ambulatory PCA device
    B. ambulatory PCA pump
    B. ambulatory volumetric infusion
    pump
    B. angioplasty catheter
    B. angioscope
    B. angled arthroscope
    B. CA-series filter
    B. dialyzer
    B. dilatation catheter
    B. fiberoptic spectrophotometry
    catheter

B. Flo-Gard 8200 volumetric infusion pump
B. hemodialyzer
B. infuser
B. InterLink needle system
B. INtermate
B. Intrepid balloon
B. mechanical valve
B. mechanical valve prosthesis
B. personal Von-Loc ice pack
B. PSN dialyzer
B. surgical clipper
B. V. Mueller laparoscopic instrumentation
Baxter-V. Mueller catheter
Bayer/Technicon H1 automated flow cytometer
Bay external fixator
Bayless neurosurgical headholder
Baylis Medical Company (BMC)
Baylor
B. adjustable cross splint
B. amniotic perforator
B. amniotome
B. cervical balloon
B. intracardiac sump tube
B. metatarsal splint
B. pelvic traction belt
B. rapid autologous transfusion system
B. total artificial heart
Bayne Pap brush
Baynton dressing
bayonet
b. aneurysm clip
b. bipolar forceps
b. clip applier
b. curette
b. forceps
b. handle
b. knife
Lucae b.
b. monopolar forceps
b. needle holder
b. osteotome
b. root tip forceps
b. scissors
b. separator
b. transsphenoidal mirror
Bazooka support surface bed

BB
BB band
BB shot forceps
B&B Trachguard
BCD Plus cardioplegic unit
BCell-HDM filtering system
BCI
BCI FingerPrint handheld pulse oximeter
BCI 3301 handheld pulse oximeter
BCNU-impregnated polymer wafer
BCO$_2$
Cardiac Stimulator B.
BD
BD adapter
BD bone marrow biopsy needle
BD butterfly swab dressing
BD gun
BD Insyte Autoguard shielded intravenous catheter
BD K-3000 microkeratome
BD Luer syringe
BD Potain thoracic trocar
BD Safety-Gard needle
BD SafetyGlide shielding hypodermic needle
BD Sensability breast self-examination aid
BD Vacutainer system
B-D
B-D Sensability breast self-examination pad
B-D spinal needle
BDProbeTec ET system
beach
b. bum rocker-bottom cast sandal shoe
b. chair positioner
Beacham amniotome
beachchair shoulder positioning system
Beachcomber prosthetic foot
Beacon
B. radiopaque tip
B. Tip Royal Flush pigtail catheter
bead
b. bed
carbon particle b.
Cida-Gel absorbent b.'s
B. ethmoidal forceps
gentamicin-impregnated Biodel b.
glass b.
hydroxyapatite b.

NOTES

67

bead *(continued)*
    immunomagnetic b.
    magnetic b.
    methyl methacrylate b.
    Percoll b.
    Sephadex b.
    Septobal b.
beaded
    b. cerclage wire
    b. guidewire
    b. hip pin
    b. pin wrench
beaked
    b. cowhorn forceps
    b. sheath
Beall
    B. bulldog clamp
    B. circumflex artery scissors
    B. disc heart valve
    B. mitral valve
    B. mitral valve prosthesis
Beall-Feldman-Cooley sump tube
Beall-Morris ascending aortic clamp
Beall-Surgitool disc prosthetic valve
beam
    pencil electron b.
    b. splitter
Beamer
    B. injection stent system
    B. stent
4-beam laser Doppler probe
beam-splitter optimal element
bean forceps
Bear
    B. 1, 2, 3 adult-volume ventilator
    B. Cub infant ventilator
    B. NUM-1 tidal volume monitor
    B. 5 respirator
Beard
    B. cystotome
    B. eye speculum
    B. lid knife
Beardsley
    B. aortic dilator
    B. cecostomy trocar
    B. empyema tube
    B. esophageal retractor
    B. forceps
    B. intestinal clamp
bearing
    patellar tendon b. (PTB)
    pretibial b. (PTB)
bearing-seating forceps
Beasley-Babcock tissue forceps
BeasyTrans transfer device
Beath
    B. guidewire
    B. needle
    B. pin

Beatty
    B. pillar retractor
    B. tongue depressor
Beaufort seating orthosis
Beaulieu camera
Beaupre
    B. ciliary forceps
    B. epilation forceps
Beaver
    B. bent blade
    B. blade
    B. blade cataract knife
    B. blade discission knife
    B. blade keratome
    B. cataract blade
    B. cataract cryoextractor
    B. cataract knife
    B. clear cornea incision system
    B. curette
    B. discission blade
    B. dissector
    B. ear knife
    B. goniotomy needle knife
    B. handle
    B. keratome blade
    B. knife
    B. lamellar blade
    B. limbus blade
    B. microblade
    B. Microsharp blade
    B. miniblade
    B. myringotomy blade
    B. Ocu-1 curved cystotome
    B. Optimum blade
    B. phacokeratome blade
    B. rhinoplasty blade
    B. ring cutter
    B. scleral Lundsgaard blade
    B. tail-tip electrode
    B. tonsillar knife
    B. tonsillectomy blade
    B. Xstar knife
Beaver-DeBakey blade
Beaver-Lundsgaard blade
Beaver-Okamura blade
beaver-tail
    b.-t. burnisher
    b.-t. retractor
Beaver-Ziegler blade
Bebax
    B. Bootie
    B. orthosis
Bechert
    B. capsular polisher
    B. intraocular lens cannula
    B. intraocular lens implant
    B. lens-holding forceps
    B. nucleus rotator

B. 1-piece all-PMMA intraocular
lens
B. spatula
Bechert-Hoffer nucleus rotator
Bechert-Kratz nucleus rotator
Bechert-McPherson tying forceps
Bechert-Sinskey needle holder
Bechtol prosthesis
Beck
B. abdominal scoop
B. aortic clamp
B. forceps
B. gastrostomy
B. gastrostomy scoop
B. mouth tube airway
B. pericardial raspatory
B. pliers
B. tonsillar knife
B. twisted wire snare loop
B. vascular clamp
B. vessel clamp
Becker
B. accelerator
B. accelerator cannula
B. aspiration cannula
B. brace
B. breast prosthesis
B. corneal section spatulated
scissors
B. cranial remolding orthosis
B. dissector liposuction cannula
B. expandable implant
B. gonioscopic prism
B. Greater dissecting cannula
B. hand prosthesis
B. 655 motion control limiter
B. orthopaedic spinal system
(BOSS)
B. orthotic device
B. probe
B. retractor
B. round dissector tip
B. screwdriver
B. septum scissors
B. skull trephine
B. spatulated corneal section
scissors
B. thermoformable ankle system
B. tissue expander
B. tissue expander prosthesis
B. twist dissector tip
B. vibrating cannula system

Becker-Joseph saw
Becker-Parkin pliers
Becker-Park speculum
Becker-Rojas Sub-Sonic surgical system
Beckerscope binocular microscope
Beckman
B. airfuge
B. autoanalyzer
B. distractor
B. goiter retractor
B. ICS Nephelometer system
B. J5.0 elutriation rotor
B. JE10X elutriation rotor
B. J6M centrifuge
B. nasal scissors
B. nasal speculum
B. O_2 analyzer
B. probe
B. self-retaining retractor
B. Silastic bulb
B. stomach electrode
B. thyroid retractor
B. UV spectrophotometer
Beckman-Adson
B.-A. laminectomy blade
B.-A. laminectomy retractor
Beckman-Colver nasal speculum
Beckman-Eaton
B.-E. laminectomy blade
B.-E. laminectomy retractor
Beckmann adenoid curette
Beckman-Weitlaner retractor
Beck-Mueller tonsillectome
Beck-Potts
B.-P. aortic clamp
B.-P. pulmonic clamp
Beck-Satinsky clamp
Beck-Schenck
B.-S. tonsillectome
B.-S. tonsil snare
Beck-Steffee total ankle prosthesis
Beck-Storz tonsillar snare
Becton
B. Colles fracture plate
B. Dickinson
B. Dickinson Teflon-sheathed
catheter
bed
AccuMax b.
Acucare b.
Advanta b.
Affinity b.

NOTES

B

bed *(continued)*
  air b.
  air-fluidized b.
  Air Plus low-air-loss b.
  Alphabed b.
  American Lapidus b.
  Arnott b.
  Balkan b.
  Bandeloux b.
  Bari-800i system bariatric b.
  Bazooka support surface b.
  bead b.
  BioDyne II kinetic therapy low-air-loss b.
  Biologics Airlift b.
  Burke bariatric treatment system powered bariatric b.
  Burke plus low-air-loss b.
  Cardiopulmonary Paragon 8500 b.
  Chick-Foster orthopaedic b.
  CircOlectric b.
  Clensicair low-air-loss hydrotherapy b.
  Clini-Care low-air-loss b.
  Clini-Dyne low-air-loss b.
  Clinitron air-fluidized b.
  Comfort Care b.
  dynamic b.
  electric b.
  Excel electric hospital b.
  EZ Flex b.
  Fisher b.
  Flexicair II low-air-loss therapy unit b.
  Flexicair MC3 low-air-loss therapy unit b.
  Fluid-Air Plus b.
  Foster b.
  fracture b.
  Gatch b.
  Gelastic b.
  GellyComb b.
  Guthrie-Smith b.
  HomeKair b.
  hospital b.
  Hough b.
  Hoverbed b.
  hydrostatic b.
  hyperbaric b.
  IC b.
  Isoflex b.
  Keane Mobility b.
  KinAir II, TC low-air-loss b.
  Klondike b.
  low-air-loss b.
  Lumex shower b.
  Magnum bariatric b.
  Medicus b.
  Medline Alpha subacute care b.
  Mega-Air b.
  Mega Tilt and Turn b.
  Ohio b.
  Orthoderm consummate air therapy b.
  PediKair pediatric low-air-loss b.
  Plastazote foot b.
  Pneu Care ICU dynamic low-air-loss b.
  Pneu Care Pedibed dynamic pediatric low-air-loss b.
  Pulmonair 40 b.
  pulsating low-air-loss b.
  Restcue CC dynamic air therapy b.
  Roho b.
  rotational dynamic air therapy b.
  Roto Kinetic b.
  Roto-Rest b.
  Sanders oscillating b.
  sawdust b.
  Skytron air-fluidized b.
  stress echo b.
  Stryker CircOlectric b.
  Swinger car b.
  TheraPulse pulsating air suspension b.
  Tilt and Turn Paragon b.
  TriaDyne b.
  Ultra Dream Ride infant car b.
  water b.

BedBath
  Centurion B.

Bedfont carbon monoxide monitor

Bedge
  B. antireflux mattress
  B. pillow

Bedrossian eye speculum

bedside
  b. air chair
  b. drainage bag
  b. monitor
  b. scale
  b. spirometer

bedwetting alarm

Beebe
  B. hemostatic forceps
  B. lens loop
  B. wire-cutting forceps
  B. wire-cutting scissors

Beehler irrigating pupil expander

Beekhuis-Supramid mentoplasty augmentation implant

Beekley
  B. breast bolster
  B. skin marking system

Beer
  B. blade
  B. canaliculus knife

B

B. cataract knife
B. ciliary forceps
Beeson cast spreader
Begg
B. appliance
B. straight-wire combination bracket
Behen ear forceps
behind-the-ear (BTE)
b.-t.-e. hearing aid
b.-t.-e. listening device
Behrend
B. cystic duct forceps
B. periosteal elevator
Beimer-Clip aneurysm clip
Beird eye catheter
Belcher clamp
bell
B. erysiphake
Gomco circumcision b.
b. rasp
b. stethoscope
Bellavar support stocking
Bellfield wire retractor
bellied bougie
Bellman retractor
Bellocq
B. cannula
B. sound
B. tube
bellows
aneroid chest b.
B. cryoextractor
B. cryoextractor extractor
B. cryophake
Bellucci
B. alligator scissors
B. cannula
B. curette
B. ear forceps
B. elevator
B. hook
B. lancet knife
B. middle ear scissors
B. pick
B. suction tube
Bellucci-Wullstein retractor
belly
B. Bag urine storage bag
b. band
BellyBeats fetal Doppler monitor
Belmont collar
Bel-O-Pak suction tube

Belos compression pin
below-elbow
medium b.-e. (MBE)
below-knee (BK)
b.-k. prosthesis
b.-k. walking cast
b.-k. walking plaster
Belscope laryngoscope blade
Belsey perfusor
belt
abdominal b.
adjustable ostomy appliance b.
Air Temp Advantage back
support b.
Aqualogger buoyancy b.
Bauer hernia b.
Baylor pelvic traction b.
Bili Button abdominal b.
Black hernia b.
body b.
Carabelt therapeutic b.
Coloplast ostomy b.
compression b.
Conco abdominal b.
Cool-Flex A/K suspension b.
Dover abdominal b.
gait b.
Grafco pelvic traction b.
Grotena abdominal b.
Grotena lumbar b.
Hackett sacroiliac cinch b.
Little Ones Sur-Fit pediatric b.
Loc-Light lumbar support b.
magnetic support b.
Marsupial b.
Meek pelvic traction b.
MicroTeq portable b.
pelvic traction b.
Posey b.
Pouchkins pediatric ostomy b.
PowerBelt lower back and
abdominal support b.
Pro-Comelastic abdominal b.
Reed cast b.
sacroiliac cinch b.
safety b.
Serola sacroiliac b.
SI-LOC sacroiliac b.
Soma sacroiliac stabilization b.
Spine Power pelvic stabilizer b.
Sports Plus II back b.
traction b.

NOTES

belt *(continued)*
 Tri-Flex auxiliary suspension b.
 Vera-Lift back b.
 waist b.
Belz lacrimal rongeur
BEMA
 bioerodible mucoadhesive
Bemis
 B. air humidifier
 B. air purifier
 B. suction cannister
 B. Vac-U-Port
Benaron scalp-rotating forceps
bench
 Champion TE-II total exercise b.
 Invacare vinyl transfer b.
 meditation b.
 pelvic b.
 b. scale calorimeter
Benchekroun ileal valve
Bend-A-Boot foot splint
Benda finger vise
bender
 AO plate b.
 Bunnell knuckle b.
 French rod b.
 plate b.
 rod b.
 Tessier rib b.
Bendick dental arch bar
bending pliers
Bendixen-Kirschner traction bow
Benedict
 B. operating gastroscope
 B. retractor
Benedict-Roth
 B.-R. apparatus
 B.-R. calorimeter
 B.-R. spirometer
Benestent I, II stent
Beneventi self-retaining retractor
Beneys tonsillar compressor
Bengash needle
Benger probe
Bengolea arterial forceps
Béniqué
 B. catheter
 B. dilator
 B. sound
Benjamin
 B. binocular slimline laryngoscope
 B. pediatric operating laryngoscope
 B. tube
Benjamin-Havas fiberoptic light clip
Benjamin-Lindholm microsuspension laryngoscope
Ben-Jet tube

Bennell
 B. bandage
 B. forceps
Bennett
 B. bone elevator
 B. bone lever
 B. bone retractor
 B. Cascade II Servo controlled heated humidifier
 B. ciliary forceps
 B. common duct dilator
 B. contour mammography system
 B. epilation forceps
 B. foreign body spud
 B. MA-1 ventilator
 B. monitoring spirometer
 B. pressure-cycled ventilator
 B. PR-2 ventilator
 B. raspatory
 B. respirator
 B. seal
 B. self-retaining retractor blade
 B. tibial retractor
Benoist penetrometer
Bensaude anoscope
Benson
 B. baby pyloric separator
 B. pyloric clamp
 B. pylorus spreader
Bentall cardiovascular prosthesis
Bentley
 B. button
 B. Duraflo II extracorporeal perfusion circuit
 B. oxygenator
 B. transducer
Bentson
 B. floppy-tip guidewire
 B. Glidewire guidewire
 B. guidewire
 B. straight guidewire
Bentson-Hanafee-Wilson catheter
Bentson-type Glidewire guidewire
Benzaquen-Chajchir extraction/reinjection system
benzene scintillator
Berbecker
 B. needle
 B. pliers
Berchtold cautery
Berci-Schore choledochoscope-nephroscope
Berci-Ward
 B.-W. laryngonasopharyngoscope
 B.-W. laryngopharyngoscope
Bercovici wire lid speculum
Berens
 B. bident electrode
 B. blade

B. capsular forceps
B. cataract knife
B. common duct scoop
B. conical eye implant
B. corneal dissector
B. corneal transplant forceps
B. corneal transplant scissors
B. corneoscleral punch
B. enucleation compressor
B. esophageal retractor
B. eye speculum
B. glaucoma knife
B. graft
B. iridocapsulotomy scissors
B. iris knife
B. keratoplasty knife
B. lens expressor
B. lens loop
B. lens scoop
B. lid everter
B. lid retractor
B. marking calipers
B. mastectomy skin flap retractor
B. muscle clamp
B. muscle recession forceps
B. orbital compressor
B. orbital implant
B. partial keratome
B. prism
B. prism bar
B. ptosis forceps
B. ptosis knife
B. punctum dilator
B. pyramidal eye implant
B. recession forceps
B. refractor
B. scleral hook
B. sclerotomy knife
B. spatula
B. sphere eye implant
B. sterilizing case
B. suturing forceps
B. thyroid retractor
B. tonometer
Berens-Rosa scleral implant
Berenstein
B. guiding catheter
B. occlusion balloon catheter
Berens-Tolman ocular hypertension indicator
Bergen retractor

Berger
B. biopsy forceps
B. loop
B. spur crusher
Bergeret-Reverdin needle
Bergeron pillar forceps
Berges-Reverdin needle
Berget lens loop
Bergh ciliary forceps
Berghmann-Foerster sponge forceps
Bergland-Warshawski phaco/cortex adapter kit
Bergman
B. mallet
B. plaster saw
B. plaster scissors
B. scalpel
B. tissue forceps
B. tracheal retractor
B. wound retractor
Bergmann Optical laser scanner
Bergström muscle cannula
Beriplast P fibrin tissue glue
Berke
B. chalazion forceps
B. ciliary forceps
B. clamp
B. double-end lid everter
B. ptosis clamp
B. ptosis forceps
Berkefeld filter
Berke-Jaeger lid plate
Berkeley
B. Bioengineering bipolar cautery
B. Bioengineering brass scleral plug
B. Bioengineering infusion terminal port
B. Bioengineering mechanized scissors
B. Bioengineering ocutome
B. Bioengineering ptosis forceps
B. Bioengineering stiletto
B. cannula
B. clamp
B. optic zone marker
B. retractor
B. scarifier
B. suction cup
B. suction machine
B. Vacurette
B. Vacurette curettage system

B

NOTES

Berkeley-Bonney
    B.-B. hysterectomy forceps
    B.-B. self-retaining abdominal
      retractor
    B.-B. vaginal clamp
Berkovits-Castellanos hexapolar electrode
Berlin curette
Berlind-Auvard
    B.-A. retractor
    B.-A. weighted vaginal speculum
Berliner neurological percussion
  hammer
Berman
    B. angiographic catheter
    B. aortic clamp
    B. balloon flotation catheter
    B. cardiac catheter
    B. foreign body locator
    B. intubating pharyngeal airway
    B. localizer
    B. locator
    B. magnet
    B. vascular clamp
Bermen-Werner probe
Bernaco adapter
Berna infant abdominal retractor
Bernard uterine forceps
Bernay
    B. sponge
    B. tracheal retractor
    B. uterine gauze packer
Berndt hip ruler
Berne
    B. nasal forceps
    B. nasal rasp
Bernell
    B. grid
    B. tangent screen
Bernhard
    B. clamp
    B. towel forceps
Bernstein
    B. catheter
    B. gastroscope
    B. nasal retractor
Berry
    B. pile clamp
    B. rib raspatory
    B. rotating inlet
    B. sternal needle holder
    B. uterine-elevating forceps
Berry-Lambert periosteal elevator
Bertillon
    B. calipers
    B. cephalometer
Bertin hip retractor
Best
    B. bite block
    B. common duct stone forceps

    B. direct forward-vision telescope
    B. gallstone forceps
    B. intestinal clamp
    B. right-angle colon clamp
BeStent
    B. balloon-expandable stent
    B. 2 coronary stent
    B. Rival coronary stent system
    B. Rival stent
Bestneb nebulizer
beta
    b. irradiation applicator
    B. Pile II, III splint strap
    b. ray applicator
    b. scintillation counter
Betabed alternating pressure pump
Beta-Cap II catheter closure
Beta-Cath
    B.-C. catheter
    B.-C. delivery system
Betaclassic surgical table
Betadine
    B. PrepStick applicator
    B. PrepStick Plus applicator
Beta-Rail catheter
Betaseron needle-free delivery system
BetaSorb hemodialysis device
Bethea sheet holder
Bethune
    B. clamp
    B. lobectomy tourniquet
    B. lung tourniquet
    B. nerve hook
    B. periosteal elevator
    B. phrenic retractor
    B. rib shears
Bethune-Coryllos rib shears
Better Than Another Pair of Hands
  retractor system
Bettman empyema tube
Bettman-Noyes fixation forceps
Beurrier connector
Bevalac system
Bevan
    B. gallbladder forceps
    B. hemostatic forceps
bevel
    Menghini-type coring b.
beveled
    b. chisel
    b. needle
bevel-point Rush pin
Bevel wand
Beverly referential valve
Beyer
    B. bone rongeur
    B. endaural rongeur
    B. forceps
    B. laminectomy rongeur

B

B. paracentesis needle
B. pigtail probe
Beyer-Lempert rongeur
Beyer-Stille bone rongeur
BFO
balanced forearm orthosis
BGC Matrix dressing
BHTU microscope
Biacore system
Biad
B. camera
B. SPECT imaging system
Bianchi valve
Bi-Angular shoulder prosthesis
BIAS
Biologic Ingrowth Anatomic System
BIAS prosthesis
BIAS slaphammer
BIAS total hip system
bias
b. stockinette
b. wrap
bias-cut stockinette dressing
Biatain foam dressing
bibeveled cutting instrument
bicanalicular silicone tube
BICAP
Bipolar Circumactive Probe
BICAP bipolar hemostasis probe
BICAP cautery
BICAP II cautery
BICAP monopolar electrode
BICAP unit
Bicek vaginal retractor
Bicer-val
B.-v. mitral heart valve prosthesis
B.-v. prosthetic valve
Bickel
B. intramedullary nail
B. intramedullary rod
B. legholder
B. ring
Bickle microsurgical knife
BiCoag bipolar laparoscopic forceps
Bicol collagen sponge
Bicomatic bipolar cable
biconcave
b. contact lens
b. washer
Bicon dental implant
bicondylar knee prosthesis
Bicon-Plus cup

biconvex intraocular lens
Bicor catheter
bicortical
b. screw
b. superior border screw
bicurved needle
bicycle
Aerobicycle exercise b.
Aerodyne b.
b. dynamometer
b. ergometer
MedGraphics CPE 2000
electronically braked b.
Monark b.
Schwinn Air-Dyne b.
Tredex b.
bicylindrical lens
bidet toilet
bidirectional
b. Butterworth digital filter
b. cavopulmonary shunt
b. shunt
b. telescopic distractor
Biegeleisen needle
Bielawski heart clamp
Biemer
B. approximator
B. vessel clip
Bier
B. amputation saw
B. lumbar puncture needle
Bierer ovum forceps
Bierman needle
Biestek thyroid retractor
Bietti
B. eye implant
B. lens
bifid
b. gallbladder retractor
b. hook
bifocal
b. demand pacemaker
executive b.
b. glasses
b. intracorneal lens
b. lens implant
b. multiplane transducer
bifoil
b. balloon
b. balloon catheter
bifurcated
b. drain extension

NOTES

75

bifurcated *(continued)*
    b. stent
    b. vascular graft
bifurcation prosthesis
Bigelow
    B. calvaria clamp
    B. evacuator
    B. forceps
    B. lithotrite
Biggs retractor
Bihrle
    B. dorsal clamp
    B. dorsal clamp-T-C needle holder
    B. T-C needle holder
BiLAP
    BiLAP bipolar probe
    BiLAP cautery
bilateral
    b. breast coil
    b. breast pump
    b. variable screw placement system
    b. ventricular assist device
      (BIVAD)
Bilbao-Dotter hypotonic duodenography
  tube
bileaflet
    b. prosthesis
    b. tilting-disc prosthetic valve
bile bag
bilevel positive pressure device
Bili
    B. Button abdominal belt
    B. mask
    B. mask phototherapy eye cover
biliary
    b. balloon catheter
    b. balloon probe
    b. drainage catheter
    b. duct balloon dilator
    b. endoprosthesis
    b. stent
BiliBed phototherapy unit
BiliBlanket Plus high-output
  phototherapy system
BiliBottoms light-permeable phototherapy
  diaper
BiliCheck bilirubin analyzer
BiliLight
    Olympic B.
    B. phototherapy system
bilirubin blanket
bilirubinometer
    transcutaneous b.
    Unistat b.
Bilisystem
    B. ERCP cannula
    B. stone-removal balloon
    B. wire-guided papillotome
Bili-Timer timer

Bill
    B. bar
    B. traction handle forceps
Billeau
    B. ear hook
    B. ear loop
    B. ear wax curette
Billeau-House ear loop
Billingham-Bookwalter rectal fenestrated
  blade
Billroth
    B. curette
    B. ovarian retractor
    B. tube
    B. tumor forceps
Billroth-Stille retractor
Bilos pin extractor
Bilson fixable-removable cross arch bar
  splint
Biltzer laryngeal blade
bilumen mammary implant
Bi-Metric
    B.-M. hip prosthesis
    B.-M. hip system
    B.-M. impaction allograft
    B.-M. Interlok femoral prosthesis
    B.-M. porous primary femoral
      prosthesis
Bimler
    B. activator
    B. appliance
    B. arch
    B. elastic plate
binasal
    b. cannula
    b. pharyngeal airway
Bindazyme ELISA kit
binder
    abdominal b.
    breast b.
    cesarean b.
    compression b.
    Dale abdominal b.
    Dale surgical b.
    Fuller perineal b.
    HK b.
    Orthomatrix b.
    OsteoGraf b.
    postpartum b.
    Scultetus b.
    surgical b.
    Texal-Muller chest b.
Binder Submalar facial implant
Bingham knee prosthesis
Bing stylet
Binkhorst
    B. capsular forceps
    B. collar stud intraocular lens
    B. collar stud lens implant

B. eye implant
B. hooked cannula
B. irrigating cannula
B. lens
B. lens forceps
B. lens implant
B. 2-loop intraocular lens
B. 4-loop iris-fixated implant
B. mustache lens intraocular lens
Binkhorst-Fyodorov lens
Binner
B. diaphanoscope
B. head lamp
binocular
b. bandage
b. eye dressing
b. fixation forceps
B. Infrared Oculography (BIRO)
b. loupe
b. shield
Zeiss MD b.
binophthalmoscope
binoscope
Bio
B. Core therapeutic mattress
B. Flote air flotation system
B. Gard Plus mattress
bioabsorbable
b. closure device
b. double-spiral stent
b. interference screw
b. staple
b. stent
bioaccumulator
bioactive
b. bone cement
b. bone cement adhesive
Bio-Anchor suture anchor
bioartificial liver support device
BioBands bracelet
BioBarrier membrane
Biobond tissue adhesive
Biobrane
B. biosynthetic dressing
B. glove
B. graft
B. sheet
B. skin substitute
B. transparent film
Biobrane/HF
B. experimental skin substitute

B. graft material
B. wound dressing
BioCardia Universal deflectable guide catheter
Biocare
B. dental implant
B. portable handheld irrigation device
BioCare thread
biocavity laser
Biocell
B. anatomical reconstructive mammary implant
B. breast implant
B. breast implant system
B. RTV saline-filled mammary implant
B. textured breast implant
B. textured silicone
B. wrap
bioceramic implant material
Bioceram 2-stage series II endosteal dental implant
Bio-Chromatic hand prosthesis
Bio-Clad acetabular prosthesis
Bioclusive
B. drape
B. MVP Select transparent dressing
Biocol dressing
BioComFold foldable intraocular lens
biocompatible
b. spacing material
b. stent
Biocompression pneumatic sleeve
Biocon impedance plethysmography cardiac output monitor
Biocor
B. 200 high-performance oxygenator
B. porcine stented mitral valve
B. prosthetic valve
B. stentless porcine aortic valve
Biocoral
B. graft
B. implant
BioCore collagen dressing
Bio-Corkscrew suture anchor
BioCuff
B. screw
B. washer
BioCurve Gold toric contact lens

NOTES

biodegradable
- b. plate
- b. polymer scaffold
- b. screw
- b. stent
- b. surgical tack

Biodel implant

BioDerm external continence device

Biodex
- B. balance system
- B. isokinetic dynamometer
- B. isokinetic testing machine
- B. Unweighing system
- B. XYZ imaging table

BioDiamond
- B. bare stent
- B. coronary stent
- B. F stent
- B. Micro F12 stent

BioDimensional
- B. breast reconstruction system
- B. saline-filled implant

BiodivYsio
- B. AS stent
- B. OC stent
- B. PC coated coronary stent
- B. SV stent

Biodrape dressing

Biodynamic
- B. acetabular component
- B. molding system

BioDyne II kinetic therapy low-air-loss bed

BioEnterics gastric balloon suction catheter

bioerodible mucoadhesive (BEMA)

Bio-Esthetic abutment system

Bio-eye hydroxyapatite ocular implant

Bio-FASTak suture anchor

biofeedback
- b. electroencephalograph
- b. electromyometer
- b. galvanic skin response device
- b. instrumentation

Biofil
- Trio-Temp X B.

Biofilter cardiovascular hemoconcentrator

Bio-Fit total hip system

Biofix
- B. absorbable screw
- B. arrow
- B. arrow gun
- B. biodegradable fixation rod
- B. biodegradable implant
- B. system pin

BIOflex
- B. magnetic orthotic
- B. magnet lumbar back support

Biofoot orthotic

biofragmentable anastomotic ring (BAR)

Biogel
- B. Indicator underglove
- B. orthopaedic surgical glove
- B. Reveal puncture indication system
- B. Reveal surgical glove
- B. Sensor surgical glove
- B. Surgeons glove

BioGen nonporous barrier membrane

Bio-Gide bilayer membrane

Bioglass
- B. bone substitute material
- B. middle ear device
- B. prosthesis
- B. synthetic bone graft

BioGlide catheter

BioGlue
- B. protein-based surgical adhesive
- B. surgical sealant

Biograft
- B. bovine heterograft material
- Dakin B.
- Dardik B.
- B. graft
- Meadox Dardik B.

BioGran resorbable synthetic bone graft

Biographer
- GlucoWatch B.

Bio-Groove
- B.-G. acetabular prosthesis
- B.-G. HA hip system
- B.-G. Macrobond HA femoral prosthesis
- B.-G. stem

Bio-Guard Spectrum antimicrobial-bonded catheter

BioGun automated biopsy system

biohazard bag

BioHorizon
- B. implant
- B. thread

bioimpedance analyzer

bioimplant
- DynaGraft b.

biointerference screw

Bioject jet injector

Biojector 2000 needle-free injection management system

Biokinetics pedobarograph

BioKnit garment electrode

BioKnotless suture anchor

BioLab modular motility system

BioLase laser adapter

Biolex
- B. wound cleanser dressing
- B. wound glue

Biolite ventilation tube

B

Biologically
- B. Quiet interference screw
- B. Quiet mini-screw suture anchor
- B. Quiet reconstruction screw
- B. Quiet staple

BioLogic-DT system
BioLogic-HT system
Biologic Ingrowth Anatomic System (BIAS)
Biologics Airlift bed
Biolox
- B. ball head
- B. ball head prosthesis
- B. ceramic ball head for hip replacement

biomagnetometer
- Magnes b.

BioMask mask
biomaterial
- Delrin joint replacement b.
- DualMesh b.
- DualMesh Plus b.
- Gore-Tex DualMesh Plus b.
- Gore-Tex MycroMesh Plus b.
- MycroMesh b.
- MycroMesh Plus b.
- polymeric b.
- Thoralon b.

Biomatrix ocular implant
Biomedical
- Continuum B. (CB)

BioMedic microdelivery peel pump
Bio-Medicus
- B.-M. centrifugal pump
- B.-M. percutaneous cannula set
- B.-M. 1-piece femoral arterial catheter

Bio-Med MVP-10 neotal/pediatric transport ventilator
BioMed TENS unit
BioMedx portable air flotation system
biomembrane
BioMend
- B. absorbable collagen membrane
- B. periodontal material

Biomer microsuturing instrument
Biomet
- B. AGC knee component
- B. AGC knee prosthesis
- B. AGC knee system
- B. ankle arthrodesis nail
- B. Ascent total knee system
- B. cement removal hand chisel
- B. Discovery elbow prosthesis
- B. Finn salvage/oncology knee reconstruction system
- B. Liverpool radial head replacement
- B. MARS acetabular reconstructive system
- B. M2a-taper metal-on-metal hip system prosthesis
- B. Maxim revision knee system
- B. Repicci II unicompartment implant
- B. shoulder joint resurfacing component
- B. total toe prosthesis
- B. tripolar acetabular system
- B. Ultra-Drive cement remover
- B. Ultra-Drive ultrasonic revision system

biometer
- Axisonic II computerized b.
- Contact A-scan b.
- Ophthasonic Ultrasonic b.

Biometric prosthesis
biometry probe
biomicroscope
- high-frequency ultrasound b.
- Nikon FS-3 photo slit lamp b.
- ultrasonic b.

biomicroscopic indirect lens
Bio-Modular
- B.-M. humeral rasp
- B.-M. shoulder component
- B.-M. total shoulder system

Bio-Moore
- B.-M. II instrumentation
- B.-M. II provisional neck spacer
- B.-M. II stem impactor
- B.-M. rasp

Bionicare
- B. stimulator
- B. stimulator system

Bionic Ear prosthesis
Bionit
- B. vascular graft
- B. vascular prosthesis

Bionix nasal speculum
Bionx
- B. BioCuff screw
- B. SmartNail bioresorbable implant
- B. suture anchor

NOTES

79

Bio-Optics
> B.-O. Bambi image analysis system
> B.-O. camera
> B.-O. cell analyzer
> B.-O. specular microscope

Bio-Oss
> B.-O. bone graft material
> B.-O. collagen
> B.-O. collagen hemostatic material
> B.-O. freeze-dried demineralized bone
> B.-O. maxillofacial bone filler

Biopac gingival retraction cord
Biopatch antimicrobial dressing
Bio-Pen biometric ruler
Biopharm leeches
Bio-Phase suture anchor
Biophysic
> B. Medical YAG laser
> B. Ophthascan S instrument

Bioplant hard tissue replacement synthetic bone
Bioplastique
> B. injectable microimplant
> B. nasal augmentation material
> B. polymer

Bioplate rigid fixation system
Bio-Plug
> B.-P. canal plug
> B.-P. component

Bioplus dispersive electrode
BioPolyMeric
> B. femoropopliteal bypass graft
> B. vascular graft

Biopore membrane
Bioport collection and transport system
biopotential skin electrode
bioprosthesis
> Carpentier-Edwards Perimount RSR pericardial b.
> Carpentier-Edwards porcine b.
> Freestyle aortic root b.
> Freestyle stentless b.
> Hancock II aortic b.
> Hancock II mitral b.
> Hancock II porcine b.
> Hancock MO II aortic b.
> Hancock MO II porcine b.
> Intact porcine b.
> Medtronic Hancock II b.
> Medtronic Intact porcine b.
> Mitroflow Synergy PC stented pericardial b.
> Mosaic cardiac b.
> pericarbon b.
> Perimount RSR pericardial b.
> PhotoFix alpha pericardial b.
> porcine b.

> SJM X-Cell cardiac b.
> Toronto SPV b.

bioprosthetic heart valve
biopsy
> b. cannula
> b. forceps
> b. gun
> b. loop electrode
> minimally invasive breast b. (MIBB)
> b. needle
> b. probe
> b. punch
> b. punch forceps
> b. specimen forceps
> b. suction curette
> b. telescope

Biopsys Mammotome vacuum biopsy system
bioptic
> b. amorphic lens system
> b. telescope

bioptome
> Bycep PC Jr b.
> cardiac b.
> Caves b.
> Cordis b.
> King cardiac b.
> Mansfield b.
> Scholten endomyocardial b.
> Stanford b.
> Stanford-Caves b.

Biopty biopsy gun
Biopty-Cut biopsy needle
Biopulse stimulator
Bio-Pump
> B.-P. centrifugal blood pump
> Medtronic B.-P.

BioRad 5000 titanium system
Biorate pacemaker
BioRCI screw
bioresorbable
> b. drug delivery system
> b. orbital implant

Biorigid Nail unreamed tibial nailing system
BioROC EZ suture anchor
Bio-R-Sorb resorbable poly-L-lactic acid ministaple
biosampler
> Accellon Combi cervical b.

BioScrew
> B. bio-absorbable interference screw
> B. XtraLok tibial fixation device

Biosearch
> B. anorectal biofeedback system
> B. enteroclysis catheter

B. female/male intermittent urinary catheter
B. jejunostomy kit
Biosense
B. DMR system
B. intracardiac mapping system
B. NOGA catheter-based endocardial mapping system
Bio-sentry telemeter
BioSkin support
Biosling urethral sling
BioSole-GEL orthotic
BioSorb
B. endoscopic browlift screw
B. FX dental implant
B. FX tack system
B. resorbable urology stent
Biosound
B. AU-series echocardiography system
B. 2000 II ultrasound unit
B. Phase 2 ultrasound system
B. Surgiscan echocardiograph
B. wide-angle monoplane ultrasound scanner
Biospal
B. filter
B. hemodialyzer
Biospan
B. anatomical tissue expander
B. breast tissue expander
BioSpec
B. MR imaging system
B. MRI/MRS system
BioSphere suture anchor
Bio-Statak suture anchor
Biostent stent
Biostil blood transfusion set
BioStim digital NMS muscle stimulator
BioStinger
B. fixation device
B. gun
B. Hornet meniscal fixation inserter
B. meniscal repair system
BioStinger-V bioabsorbable meniscal repair device
BioStop G cement restrictor
Biosurge synchronous autotransfuser
BioSymMetRic PIP fixator
Biosyn suture
Biosystems feeding tube

BioTac
B. biopsy cannula
B. ECG electrode
Biotek autostainer
biotelemetry system
Bio-Tenodesis screw
BioTENS neurostimulator
Bioteque vaginal pessary
Bio-Thesiometer
penile B.-T.
Biothotic
B. foot orthotic
B. orthotic mold
Biotrack coagulation monitor
BioTrainer exercise monitor
Biotronik
B. demand pacemaker
B. lead
B. pacemaker electrode
BioTwist soft tissue anchor system
Bio-Vascular prosthetic valve
Bio-Vent implant
Biovert
B. ceramic implant
B. implant material
Biovue catheter
Bio-Wick sock
BioWrap support
Biox III ear oximeter
BioZtect sensor system
BiPAP
biphasic positive airway pressure
BiPAP Duet LX system
BiPAP Pro system
BiPAP S/T-D ventilatory support system
BiPAP unit
BiPAP Vision system
BIP breast implant protector
biphase Morris fixation apparatus
biphasic
b. pin
b. positive airway pressure (BiPAP)
b. system
bipivotal hinge knee brace
biplanar fixator
bipolar
b. bayonet forceps
b. catheter
b. cautery
B. Circumactive Probe (BICAP)

NOTES

81

bipolar *(continued)*
    b. clip electrode
    b. coagulating forceps
    b. coagulator
    b. coaptation forceps
    b. cutting forceps
    b. cutting loop
    b. diathermy forceps
    b. electrocautery
    b. electrocautery forceps
    b. electrode
    b. electrosurgical unit
    B. EndoStasis probe
    b. eye forceps
    b. forceps
    b. generator
    b. glass electrode
    b. hemostasis probe
    b. laparoscopic forceps
    b. needle
    b. needle electrode
    b. pacemaker
    b. pacemaker electrode
    b. pacing catheter
    b. pacing lead
    b. scissors
    b. sphincterotome
    b. temporary pacemaker catheter
    b. transsphenoidal forceps
    b. urological loop
Bi-Pol endoscopic cutter
BiPort hemostasis introducer sheath kit
BIPP
    bismuth iodoform parafin paste
    BIPP ribbon gauze
biprong muscle marker
Bipro orthodontic appliance
Bi-Rads breast imaging and reporting system
Birch
    B. lamp
    B. trocar
Bircher
    B. bone-holding clamp
    B. cartilage clamp
    B. cartilage knife
Bircher-Ganske cartilage forceps
Birch-Hirschfeld lamp
bird
    B. Asthmastik
    b. eye catheter
    b. low-flow blender
    B. Mark 8 respirator
    B. micronebulizer
    B. MK VIII pressure-cycled ventilator
    B. neonatal CPAP generator
    b. nest IVC filter
    B. OP cup

    B. pressure-cycled ventilator
    B. 8400STi ventilator
    B. vacuum extractor
BirdBeak orthopaedic grasper instrument
birdcage
    b. coil
    b. head coil
    b. resonator
    b. splint
Birdseye quilted underpad
Birkenstock
    B. blue footbed arch support
    B. high-flange arch support
Birkett hemostatic forceps
Birkhauser eye testing chart
Birks
    B. Mark II grooved forceps
    B. Mark II hook
    B. Mark II micro cross-action holder
    B. Mark II micro push/pull spatula
    B. Mark II needle holder
    B. Mark II needle-holder forceps
    B. Mark II suture-tying forceps
    B. Mark II toothed forceps
    B. Mark II trabeculectomy scissors
    B. suture-tying forceps
Birks-Mathelone microforceps
BIRO
    Binocular Infrared Oculography
    BIRO system
Birtcher
    B. cautery
    B. defibrillator
    B. electrocautery probe
    B. electrode
    B. electrosurgical generator
    B. electrosurgical needle
    B. endoscopic forceps
    B. Hyfrecator
    B. Hyfrecator cautery wire
    B. Hyfrecator coagulator
    B. Hyfrecator electrosurgical unit
    B. laparoscopic coagulator
birth cushion
birthing
    b. ball
    b. chair
bisected minigraft dilator
Bi-Set catheter
Bishop
    B. antral perforator
    B. bone clamp
    B. mastoid chisel
    B. mastoid gouge
    B. oscillatory bone saw
    B. putty

B. retractor
B. sphygmoscope
B. tendon tucker
Bishop-Black tendon tucker
Bishop-DeWitt tendon tucker
Bishop-Harman
   B.-H. anterior chamber irrigator
   B.-H. bladebreaker
   B.-H. dressing
   B.-H. dressing forceps
   B.-H. foreign body forceps
   B.-H. iris forceps
   B.-H. irrigating cannula
   B.-H. knife
   B.-H. mules
   B.-H. spud
   B.-H. Superblade
   B.-H. tissue forceps
Bishop-Peter tendon tucker
bismuth iodoform parafin paste (BIPP)
BiSNARE bipolar polypectomy snare
Bi-Soft lens
bispherical lens
Bisping electrode
bisque-baked prosthesis
BIS Sensor electrode
Bistite II DC resin cement
bistoury
   b. blade
   Brophy b.
   Converse button-end b.
   Jackson tracheal b.
   Jackson tracheotomic b.
   b. knife
   straight b.
Biswas Silastic vaginal pessary
bit
   AO drill b.
   cannulated drill b.
   cone bur b.
   Howmedica Microfixation System
     drill b.
   Leibinger Micro System drill b.
   Luhr microfixation system drill b.
bite
   b. block
   b. force transducer
   b. protector
   b. stick
   B. wafer denture bite wax
Bi-tec forceps

biter
   suction b.
biterminal electrode
biting
   b. forceps
   b. rongeur
Bitome
   B. bipolar sphincterotome
   B. bipolar system
   B. catheter
BitPad digitizer
Bitumi monobjective microscope
BIVAD
   bilateral ventricular assist device
bivalve
   b. nasal splint
   b. splint
bivalved
   b. anal speculum
   b. cannula
   b. cast
   b. retractor
biventricular
   b. assist device
   b. implantable cardioverter-
     defibrillator
Bivona
   B. cuff maintenance device
   B. duckbill voice prosthesis
   B. epistaxis catheter
   B. Fome-Cuf tracheostomy tube
   B. Medical Technologies
     customized tracheostomy tube
   B. Optivox artificial electronic
     larynx
   B. sleep apnea tracheostomy tube
   B. TTS tracheostomy tube
   B. Ultra Low voice prosthesis
Bivona-Colorado
   B.-C. button
   B.-C. dummy prosthesis
   B.-C. sizing device
   B.-C. template
   B.-C. voice prosthesis
Bi-Wave
   B.-W. mattress overlay
   B.-W. plus mattress replacement
Bizzarri-Giuffrida laryngoscope
Bjerrum
   B. scotometer
   B. screen
Björk rib drill

NOTES

Björk-Shiley
- B.-S. convexoconcave 60-degree valve prosthesis
- B.-S. floating-disc prosthesis
- B.-S. graft
- B.-S. heart valve holder
- B.-S. heart valve sizer
- B.-S. mitral valve

Björk-Stille diathermy forceps

BK
- below-knee
- BK prosthesis

BKS
- Barraquer-Krumeich-Swinger
- BKS microkeratome

black
- B. Beauty ureteral stent
- b. braided nylon suture
- b. braided silk suture
- b. hatchet
- B. hernia belt
- b. light lamp
- B. Max mid size knee component
- B. meatal clamp
- B. rasp
- B. retractor
- B. spanner stent
- b. twisted suture

Blackburn
- B. skull traction tractor
- B. trephine

Black-Decker needle

blackened
- b. hemostat
- b. speculum

Blackmon needle

Blackstone
- B. anterior cervical plate
- B. spinal fixation system

black/white occluder

Black-Wylie obstetric dilator

bladder
- b. blade
- b. catheter
- b. dilator
- b. evacuator
- b. flap tube
- gel-filled b.
- b. neck support pessary
- b. neck support prosthesis
- b. pacemaker
- PyMaH nylon balanced b.
- b. replacement urinary pouch
- b. retractor
- b. scan
- b. sound
- b. specimen forceps

BladderManager
- B. portable ultrasound scanner
- B. ultrasound

BladderScan
- B. BVI2500 diagnostic ultrasound
- B. monitor
- B. scanner

blade
- Acra-Cut spiral craniotome b.
- adenotome b.
- Aggressor b.
- Alcon crescent b.
- Alcon pocket b.
- arachnoid Beaver b.
- arachnoid-shaped b.
- arthroscopic banana b.
- ASR b.
- ASSI cranial b.
- autopsy b.
- baby Miller b.
- Balfour bladder b.
- Balfour center b.
- Balfour lateral b.
- banana Beaver b.
- Bard-Parker surgical b.
- Barraquer b.
- Barton b.
- Beaver b.
- Beaver bent b.
- Beaver cataract b.
- Beaver-DeBakey b.
- Beaver discission b.
- Beaver keratome b.
- Beaver lamellar b.
- Beaver limbus b.
- Beaver-Lundsgaard b.
- Beaver Microsharp b.
- Beaver myringotomy b.
- Beaver-Okamura b.
- Beaver Optimum b.
- Beaver phacokeratome b.
- Beaver rhinoplasty b.
- Beaver scleral Lundsgaard b.
- Beaver tonsillectomy b.
- Beaver-Ziegler b.
- Beckman-Adson laminectomy b.
- Beckman-Eaton laminectomy b.
- Beer b.
- Belscope laryngoscope b.
- Bennett self-retaining retractor b.
- Berens b.
- Billingham-Bookwalter rectal fenestrated b.
- Biltzer laryngeal b.
- bistoury b.
- bladder b.
- Blitzer laryngeal b.
- Blount bent b.
- bone saw b.

Bookwalter-Cook anal rectal b.
Bookwalter-Gelpi point retractor b.
Bookwalter-Kelly retractor b.
Bookwalter malleable retractor b.
Bookwalter-Mayo b.
Bookwalter-Parks anal sphincter b.
Bookwalter rectal b.
Bookwalter retractor b.
Bookwalter vaginal Deaver b.
Bovie b.
Bowen BAS-30 b.
breakable b.
Brown dermatome b.
capsulotomy b.
carbolized knife b.
carbon steel b.
Caspar b.
cast b.
Castroviejo razor b.
cataract b.
cervical biopsy b.
Chang Quick Chop combo
  ophthalmic b.
chisel b.
chondroplasty Beaver b.
circular b.
CLM McCoy articulating
  laryngoscope b.
Cloward single-tooth retractor b.
Collin radiopaque sternal b.
conization instrument b.
Converse retractor b.
Cooley-Pontius sternal b.
CooperVision Surgeon-Plus
  Ultrathin b.
copper b.
Cranwall laryngoscope b.
crescent b.
crescentic b.
Crile b.
Crockard small-tongue retractor b.
Curdy b.
Curdy-Hebra b.
Davidoff b.
Davis b.
Davis-Crowe tongue b.
Dean b.
Deaver b.
DeBakey b.
DeBakey-Beaver b.
deep spreader b.

Denis Browne abdominal
  retractor b.
Denis Browne-Hendren pediatric
  retractor b.
Denis Browne malleable copper
  retractor b.
Denis Browne mastoid pediatric
  retractor b.
Dennis b.
dermatome b.
diamond saw b.
Dingman cheek b.
discission b.
Dixon b.
double-angled b.
double-vector b.
Duotrak b.
Dyonics arthroscopic b.
Edge b.
b. electrode
electrodermatome sterile b.
electrosurgical b.
electrosurgical spatula b.
Elliot trephine b.
E-Mac laryngoscope b.
Emir razor b.
Endo-Assist retractable b.
b. endosteal implant
English MacIntosh fiberoptic
  laryngoscope b.
English profile laryngoscope b.
Epstein hemilaminectomy b.
Eschmann b.
expandable b.
eye b.
Feather carbon breakable b.
Field b.
folding b.
Franceschetti-type b.
Fugo b.
Genesis diamond b.
Gigli-saw b.
Gill b.
Gillette Blue b.
Gill-Hess b.
Goulian b.
Grandview laryngoscope b.
Grieshaber b.
GS-9 b.
Guedel laryngoscope b.
Hammond winged retractor b.
Hebra b.

B

NOTES

blade *(continued)*
hemilaminectomy b.
Hendren pediatric retractor b.
Henley retractor b.
Hibbs spinal retractor b.
Hopp anterior commissure
  laryngoscope b.
Horgan center b.
Hoskins razor fragment b.
House detachable b.
House knife b.
House ophthalmic b.
Incisor arthroscopic b.
infant urethrotome b.
jigsaw b.
K b.
Katena double-edged sapphire b.
K-Blade microsurgical b.
Keeler retractable b.
Kellan sutureless incision b.
keratome b.
Kjelland b.
Knapp b.
knife b.
b. knife
K-2000 surgical saw b.
LaForce adenotome b.
lamellar b.
laminectomy b.
lancet b.
Lange b.
laryngoscope b.
Leivers b.
Lemmon b.
limbal relaxing incision diamond b.
Lite b.
LRI diamond b.
Lundsgaard b.
MacIntosh fiberoptic
  laryngoscope b.
Magrina-Bookwalter vaginal
  Deaver b.
Mako shaver b.
malleable b.
malleable retractor b.
Martin b.
Martinez corneal trephine b.
Mastel trifaceted diamond b.
McCoy laryngoscope b.
McPherson-Wheeler b.
meniscectomy b.
meniscotome b.
Merlin arthroscopy b.
Merlin bendable b.
Meyerding laminectomy b.
Meyerding retractor b.
Microplaner b.
Micro-Sharp b.
microvitreoretinal b.

Miller fiberoptic laryngoscope b.
miniature b.
Morse b.
Mueller tongue b.
Mullins b.
multi-incision 10-facet diamond b.
Murphy-Balfour center b.
MVR b.
Myocure b.
myringotomy b.
myringotomy knife b.
New Skimmer b.
notchplasty b.
Nounton b.
nubular b.
ocutome vitreous b.
ophthalmic b.
Optimum b.
Orbit b.
Orca surgical b.
Organdi b.
Otocap myringotomy b.
Oxford laryngoscope b.
Oxiport b.
Padgett dermatome b.
Park b.
Parker-Bard b.
Paufique b.
pediatric mastoid retractor b.
Penlon Crystal laryngoscope b.
Personna surgical prep b.
planar b.
b. plate
b. plate fixation device
PowerCut drill b.
3-pronged rake b.
5-prong rake b.
Rad airway laryngeal b.
RADenoid b.
RAD40 sinus b.
Rad 60 X-Treme curved b.
ramus b.
razor b.
rectangular b.
Reese dermatome b.
replaceable b.
b. retractor
retractor b.
retrograde meniscal b.
Rew-Wyly b.
Rhein 3-D trapezoid diamond b.
Rhinotec b.
Rhinotec shaver b.
ribbon b.
ring retractor b.
ring tongue b.
Robertshaw pediatric
  laryngoscope b.
Rubin b.

Rusch laryngoscope b.
Satterlee bone saw b.
b. scalpel
ScalpelTec keratome slit b.
Schanz b.
Scheie b.
scimitar b.
scleral b.
sclerotome b.
Scoville retractor b.
Security b.
self-retaining retractor b.
semilunar-tip b.
b. septostomy catheter
serrated b.
Sharpoint spoon b.
Sharpoint V-lance b.
Sharptome crescent b.
shoulder b.
sickle b.
sickle-shaped Beaver b.
side b.
side-cutting b.
Silver Bullet b.
single-tooth retractor b.
Skimmer b.
slimcut b.
slit b.
Sofield retractor b.
spear b.
spinal retractor b.
Sputnik Russian razor b.
stainless steel b.
Stealth DBO diamond b.
sterile electrodermatome b.
Sterling arthroscopy b.
sternal b.
sternal retractor b.
Stryker b.
Supercut b.
surgical saw b.
Surgistar ophthalmic b.
Swann-Morton surgical b.
Swiss b.
Synovator arthroscopic b.
synovectomy b.
tapered b.
Taylor laminectomy b.
Taylor spinal b.
Temperlite saw b.
The Edge coated b.
Thornton arcuate triple-edged b.

Thornton tri-square b.
throw-away manual dermatome b.
Tiger b.
tongue b.
tongue depressor b.
Tooke b.
Torpin vectis b.
trephine b.
Tricut b.
tri-radial resector b.
Troutman b.
Tucker-Luikart b.
Turner-Warwick b.
Typhoon cutter b.
Typhoon microdebrider b.
UltraEdge keratome b.
ultra-thin surgical b.
Universal nasal saw b.
urethrotome b.
Vascutech circular b.
vectis b.
V-lance b.
V. Mueller myringotomy b.
Weck Prep b.
Welch Allyn laryngoscope b.
Wheeler b.
Wilkinson-Deaver b.
winged retractor b.
wire side b.
Wisconsin laryngoscope b.
Wis-Hipple laryngoscope b.
wood tongue b.
Yu-Holtgrewe b.
Zalkind-Balfour b.
Ziegler b.
Zimmer saw b.
bladebreaker
  Barraquer razor b.
  Bishop-Harman b.
  b. holder
  I-tech-Castroviejo b.
  Jarit b.
  b. knife
  Swiss b.
  Vari b.
3-bladed clamp
2-bladed dilator
blade-form implant
Blade-Safe case
Blade-Vent implant system
Blade-Wilde ear forceps

NOTES

Blair
- B. cleft palate clamp
- B. cleft palate elevator
- B. cleft palate knife
- B. Gigli-saw guide
- B. head drape
- B. modification of Gellhorn pessary
- B. nasal chisel
- B. palate hook
- B. 4-prong retractor
- B. serrefine
- B. silicone drain
- B. stiletto
- B. talar body fusion blade plate
- B. tibiotalar arthrodesis blade plate

Blair-Brown
- B.-B. graft
- B.-B. implant
- B.-B. needle
- B.-B. needle holder
- B.-B. skin graft knife
- B.-B. vacuum retractor

Blair-Ivy loop

Blajwas-Schwartz-Marcinko irrigation/drainage system

Blake
- B. ear forceps
- B. embolus forceps
- B. gallstone forceps
- B. gingivectomy knife
- B. silicone drain
- B. uterine curette

Blakemore
- B. esophageal tube
- B. nasogastric tube

Blakemore-Sengstaken tube

Blakesley
- B. ethmoid forceps
- B. grasper
- B. lacrimal trephine
- B. laminectomy rongeur
- B. nasal forceps
- B. septal bone forceps
- B. septal compression forceps
- B. tongue depressor
- B. uvular retractor

Blakesley-Weil upturned ethmoidal forceps

Blakesley-Wilde
- B.-W. ear forceps
- B.-W. ethmoidal forceps
- B.-W. nasal forceps

Blalock
- B. forceps
- B. pulmonary stenosis clamp
- B. shunt
- B. suture

Blalock-Kleinert forceps

Blalock-Niedner pulmonic stenosis clamp

Blalock-Taussig shunt

Blanchard
- B. cryptotome
- B. hemorrhoidal forceps
- B. pile clamp
- B. traction device
- B. traction device blade plate

Blanco
- B. retractor
- B. scissors
- B. valve spreader

Bland
- B. cervical traction forceps
- B. perineal retractor
- B. vulsellum
- B. vulsellum forceps

blank
- implant b.
- Nickelplast b.

blanket
- Bair Hugger patient warming b.
- bilirubin b.
- CareDrape b.
- circulating water b.
- cooling b.
- EBI Temptek b.
- Gaymar water-circulating b.
- Hollister Hot/Ice knee b.
- Hot/Ice System III knee b.
- hypothermia b.
- Mediwrap b.
- Rowe b.
- b. suture
- thermal space b.

Blasucci
- B. clamp
- B. pigtail ureteral catheter

Blauth knee prosthesis

Blaydes
- B. angled lens
- B. angled lens forceps
- B. corneal forceps
- B. lens-holding forceps

Bledsoe
- B. adjustable brace
- B. cast brace
- B. knee brace

bleeding needle

Bleier clip

blender
- Bird low-flow b.

Blenderm
- B. surgical tape
- B. surgical tape dressing
- B. tape

blepharochalasis forceps

blepharoplasty clip

blepharostat
b. clamp
Goldman-McNeill b.
McNeill-Goldmann b.
b. ring
Schachar b.
blind
b. endosonography probe
b. medullary nail
Bliskunov implantable femoral distractor
BlisterFilm transparent wound dressing
Blitzer laryngeal blade
block
AART silicone carving b.
acrylic bite b.
Airlite alignable ankle b.
anterior-posterior cutting b.
AP cutting b.
ball joint b.
Best bite b.
bite b.
Brightbill corneal cutting b.
Bunnell b.
calipers b.
B. cardiac device
Cerrobend trim b.
cervical b.
Constructa foam b.
corneal b.
4-in-1 cutting b.
Delrin cutting b.
Dembone demineralized cortical
   dental b.
disposable Styrofoam b.
ENT bite b.
ESI bite b.
Ethox bite b.
Fine folding b.
Guilford-Wright cutting b.
hand b.
House-Delrin cutting b.
House Teflon cutting b.
Jackson bite b.
lateral skull b.
lead b.
Lell bite b.
MaxBloc bite b.
methyl methacrylate b.
Neumann calipers b.
New Orleans corneal cutting b.
OB-10 Comfort bite b.
Omni Bloc bite b.

Ora-Gard disposable intraoral
   bite b.
Oxyguard mouth b.
paraffin b.
pelvic b.
Plexiglas tissue equivalency b.
punch b.
push-up b.
B. right coronary guiding catheter
Shepard calipers b.
Shepard-Kramer calipers b.
shielding b.
shock b.
silicone b.
skull b.
Speed-E-Rim denture bite b.
Stahl calipers b.
Tanne corneal cutting b.
Teflon cutting b.
tibial augmentation b.
tibial cutting b.
Ultima Bloc bite b.
Wright-Guilford cutting b.
blocker
Arndt endobronchial b.
hook b.
MacIntosh b.
Wallach cryosurgical pain b.
Block-Potts intestinal forceps
Bloedorn applicator
Blohmka
B. tonsillar forceps
B. tonsillar hemostat
Blomqvist external tissue extender
Blom-Singer
B.-S. esophagoscope
B.-S. indwelling low-pressure voice
   prosthesis
B.-S. tracheoesophageal prosthesis
B.-S. valve
blood
b. agar plate
b. cell separator
b. color analyzer
b. flow imaging
b. flowmeter
b. gas analyzer
840 b. gas analyzer
b. glucose reagent strip
b. perfusion monitor (BPM)
b. pressure cuff
b. pressure recorder

B

NOTES

blood *(continued)*
    b. pump
    b. warmer cuff
blood-contacting catheter
blood-flow probe
bloodless circumcision clamp
Bloodshot WildEyes lens
Bloodwell
    B. tissue forceps
    B. vascular forceps
Bloodwell-Brown forceps
Bloomberg
    B. lens forceps
    B. lens ophthalmic ring
    B. SuperNumb anesthetic ring
    B. trabeculotome set
bloomer
    KINS pull-on waterproof b.
Bloom programmable stimulator
Blount
    B. bent blade
    B. blade plate
    B. bone spreader
    B. brace
    B. double-prong retractor
    B. epiphyseal staple
    B. fracture staple
    B. hip retractor
    B. knee retractor
    B. knife
    B. laminar spreader
    B. nylon mallet
    B. scoliosis osteotome
    B. single-prong retractor
    B. splint
    B. V-blade
Blount-Schmidt-Milwaukee brace
blow bottle
blow-by ventilator
blower
    DeVilbiss plastic powder b.
    powder b.
    Rica powder b.
    SMIC powder b.
Blucher low-quarter shoe
blue
    B. Brand therapy putty
    Daimas B.
    B. Dolphin denture instrument
    B. FlexTip catheter
    B. Line cuffed endotracheal tube
    B. Line orthotic
    B. Max balloon dilation catheter
    B. Max cannula
    B. Max high-pressure balloon
    B. Max triple-lumen catheter
    B. multi-vector external distraction
      system
    b. ring pessary

    b. sponge dressing
    b. twisted cotton suture
blue-black monofilament suture
Bluemle pump
blue-tip aspirator
Blum
    B. arterial scissors
    B. forceps
Blumenthal
    B. anterior chamber maintainer
    B. bone rongeur
    B. intraocular lens
    B. irrigating cystotome
    B. uterine dressing forceps
blunt
    b. dissecting hook
    b. elevator
    b. forceps
    b. needle
    b. nerve hook
    b. obturator
    b. probe
    b. trocar
blunt-end needle
blunt-nose
    b.-n. hemostat
    b.-n. scissors
Bluntport trocar
blunt-ring curette
blunt-tip
    b.-t. obturator
    b.-t. probe
BMC
    Baylis Medical Company
    BMC coaxial injectable catheter
    BMC radiofrequency perforation
      system
B-mode ultrasound machine
BMSI 5000 electroencephalograph
BNA-100-Behring Diagnostics
   immunonephelometer
board
    arm b.
    back b.
    balance b.
    Balance Master rocker b.
    cartilage cutting b.
    competitive ankle b. (CAB)
    cutting b.
    Fisher tape b.
    Flexisplint arm b.
    full spine b.
    Gabarro b.
    graft b.
    Hadfield hand b.
    J b.
    manipulation b.
    Massageboard b.
    memory b.

papoose b.
pivoting surgical arm b.
powder b.
rocker b.
Rock & Roller exercise b.
Slippery Slider transport b.
b. splint
Spri Xercise b.
Steffensmeier b.
string drawing b.
SummaSketch III digitizing b.
tape b.
Targa+ image capture b.
Tegtmeier hand b.
Wooden Wobble balance b.
Boari button
boat
    b. hook
    b. nail
bobbin myringotomy tube
bobbin-type laryngectomy button
Bobechko
    B. sliding barrel hook
    B. spreader
Boberg-Ans
    B.-A. intraocular lens
    B.-A. lens implant
Boberg lens
Bock
    B. knee prosthesis
    B. knife
Bodai adapter
Bodenham
    B. dermabrasion cylinder
    B. saw
Bodenham-Blair skin graft knife
Bodenham-Humby knife
Bodenheimer
    B. anoscope
    B. rectal speculum
Bodenstab tourniquet
Bodi
    B. Dynamic orthosis
    B. knee extension orthosis
Bodian
    B. discission knife
    B. lacrimal probe
    B. minilacrimal probe
Bodkin thread holder
Bodnar knee retractor
BodPod body composition system

body
    B. Armor short leg walker
    B. Armor walker
    B. Ball
    b. belt
    B. Belt body massager
    B. buddy-body pillow
    Cloward lumbar retractor b.
    b. coil
    Crockard transoral retractor b.
    B. Gard neoprene support
    B. glue
    b. jacket
    B. Logic rehabilitation system
    B. Masters MD 510 hi-lo pulley system
    b. oscillation integrates neuromuscular gain
    b. positioner
    B. prop positioning splint
    B. Response system
    B. Solid exercise equipment
    B. Wrap foam positioner
BodyBilt chair
Bodyblade exercise equipment
The Bodyguard emboli containment system
BodyIce
    B. cold pack
    B. cold pack wrap
Bodyline
    B. Back-Huggar
    B. sleeper mattress overlay
BodyTable
    HiLo B.
    TouchAmerica B.
BodyWrap premium overlay
Boebinger tongue depressor
Boehler-Braun fracture frame
Boehm
    B. anoscope
    B. drop syringe
    B. proctoscope
    B. resectoscope
    B. sigmoidoscope
Boehringer
    B. Autovac autotransfusion system
    B. kit
    B. suction regulator
Boer craniotomy forceps
Boerma obstetrical forceps

NOTES

Boettcher
- B. antral trocar
- B. arterial forceps
- B. hemostat
- B. pulmonary artery clamp
- B. pulmonary artery forceps
- B. tonsillar artery forceps
- B. tonsillar hook
- B. tonsil scissors

Boettcher-Farlow snare
Boettcher-Jennings mouthgag
Boettcher-Schnidt
- B.-S. antral trocar
- B.-S. forceps

Bogle rongeur
Bogota bag
Böhler
- B. exerciser
- B. extension bow
- B. guideline
- B. hip nail
- B. iron
- B. os calcis clamp
- B. pin
- B. plaster cast breaker
- B. reducing fracture frame
- B. rongeur
- B. tongs
- B. traction bow
- B. tractor
- B. wire splint

Böhler-Braun
- B.-B. fracture frame
- B.-B. leg sling
- B.-B. splint

Böhler-Knowles hip pin
Bohlman pin
Bohm dropper sponge
Boiler septal trephine
Boilo retinoscope
Boing exercise device
Boise
- B. cutting forceps
- B. nasal fracture elevator

Boise-Lombard mastoid rongeur
Boldrey brace
Bolero lift bath trolley
Bolex
- B. cine camera
- B. gastrocamera

Boley
- B. dental gouge
- B. gauge
- B. retractor

Bolin x-ray filter system
Bollinger knee brace
bolster
- angular b.
- Beekley breast b.

breast b.
- b. buddy
- Hollister bridge suture b.
- knee b.
- knee arthrography b.
- retention suture b.
- roll control b.
- b. suture
- Telfa b.
- tie-over b.

bolt
- Barr b.
- Camino microventricular b.
- cannulated b.
- DePuy b.
- Fenton tibial b.
- Herzenberg b.
- hexhead b.
- Hubbard b.
- Hubbard-Nylok b.
- Norman tibial b.
- Nylok b.
- Philly b.
- Richmond b.
- tibial b.
- transfixion b.
- trochanteric b.
- Webb b.
- Webb stove b.
- wire fixation b.

Bolton forceps
bolus dressing
Bonaccolto
- B. cup-jaw forceps
- B. eye implant
- B. fragment forceps
- B. jeweler's forceps
- B. magnet
- B. magnet tip forceps
- B. monoplex orbital implant material
- B. orbital implant
- B. scleral ring
- B. splinter forceps
- B. strabismus forceps
- B. trephine
- B. utility forceps

Bonaccolto-Flieringa scleral ring
Bonchek-Shiley
- B.-S. cardiac jacket
- B.-S. vein distention system

Bond
- B. arm splint
- B. placental forceps

Bondek absorbable suture
Bond-Eze adhesive
Bondeze resin
bonding
- In-Ceram Alumina b.

In-Ceram Cerestore b.
In-Ceram Dicor b.
In-Ceram Empress b.
In-Ceram Fortress b.
In-Ceram Optec b.
In-Ceram Spinell b.
Poly-Lock b.

bone

b. abduction instrument
b. aggregate
b. awl
Bio-Oss freeze-dried
 demineralized b.
Bioplant hard tissue replacement
 synthetic b.
B. Bullet suture anchor
b. bur
B. Button orthopaedic suture
 anchor
b. calipers
b. cement
b. cement adhesive
b. chisel
b. clamp
b. clasp
b. collector
b. crusher
b. curette
b. cutter
Dembone demineralized freeze-dried
 cortical b.
demineralized b.
b. densitometer
b. elevator
b. extension clamp
b. femoral plug
b. file
b. fixation device
b. fixation wire
b. flap fixation plate
b. gouge
B. Grafter instrument
b. graft impactor
b. growth stimulator
b. guide
b. hand drill
b. hole punch
b. hook
b. implant material
b. injection gun
Lambone demineralized laminar b.

b. lever
b. mallet
b. marrow biopsy needle
B. Mulch screw
Osteomin demineralized b.
Osteomin freeze dried b.
b. punch
b. punch forceps
b. punch rongeur
b. rasp
b. reamer
b. retractor
b. rongeur
b. rongeur forceps
b. saw
b. saw blade
b. scalpel
b. screw
b. screw depth gauge
b. screw targeter
b. skid
b. substitute material (BSM)
b. tack system
b. tunnel plug
Tutoplast b.
Vitoss synthetic b.
b. wax
b. wax suture
bone-anchored hearing aid
bone-biting
 b.-b. forceps
 b.-b. rongeur
BoneCollector device
bone-conduction hearing aid
bone-cutting
 b.-c. double-action forceps
 b.-c. rongeur
Bone-Dri femoral surgical wick
bone-graft holder
bone-holding
 b.-h. clamp
 b.-h. forceps
Boneloc cement
Bone-Lok bone fixation system
bone-measuring calipers
BonePlast
 B. bone void filler
 B. graft
bone-plate
 TiMesh b.-p.
bone-reduction forceps

NOTES

BoneSource
 B. hydroxyapatite cement
 B. implant
bone-splitting forceps
Bonfiglio bone graft
Bongort
 B. Max-E-Pouch pouch
 B. urinary diversion pouch
Bonn
 B. European suturing forceps
 B. iris forceps
 B. iris scissors
 B. microhook
 B. micro iris hook
 B. microiris hook
 B. peripheral iridectomy forceps
 B. suturing forceps
Bonnano catheter
Bonnet
 Hydro B.
Bonney
 B. blue ink
 B. cervical dilator
 B. clamp
 B. clip
 B. insufflator
 B. needle
 B. retrograde inflator
 B. tissue forceps
 B. uterine tube
Bonnie balloon catheter
Bonta mastectomy knife
Bonwill articulator
Bookler swivel-ball laparoscopic instrument holder
Bookwalter
 B. horizontal bar
 B. malleable retractor blade
 B. rectal blade
 B. retractor
 B. retractor blade
 B. retractor ring
 B. ring retractor
 B. segmented ring
 B. vaginal Deaver blade
 B. vaginal retractor ring
Bookwalter-Balfour retractor
Bookwalter-Cook anal rectal blade
Bookwalter-Gelpi point retractor blade
Bookwalter-Goulet retractor
Bookwalter-Harrington retractor
Bookwalter-Hill-Ferguson rectal retractor
Bookwalter-Kelly
 B.-K. retractor
 B.-K. retractor blade
Bookwalter-Magrina vaginal retractor
Bookwalter-Mayo blade
Bookwalter-Parks anal sphincter blade

Bookwalter-St. Mark deep pelvic retractor
boomerang
 b. bladder needle
 b. needle holder
Booster clip
boot
 Air Cam b.
 Anthony cast b.
 b. brace
 CAM Walker II b.
 cast b.
 Castaway II CAM Walker b.
 Chukka b.
 Circulator b.
 compression b.
 Conformer diabetic b.
 ConvaTec Unna-Flex elastic Unna b.
 cradle b.
 Cryo/Cuff pressure b.
 Darkos b.
 DeLorme b.
 derotation b.
 Duke b.
 DuraBoot b.
 Elasto-Gel heel/ankle b.
 external sequential pneumatic compression b.
 fracture b.
 gelatin compression b.
 Gelocast Unna b.
 Gibney b.
 Heelift suspension b.
 Hi-Top II CAM Walker b.
 hyperbaric b.
 intermittent pneumatic compression b.
 Jobst postoperative air b.
 Junod b.
 Kangoo Jumps exercise b.
 L'Nard b.
 Lunax b.
 Markell brace b.
 Moon B.
 MPO Active walking Multi Podus b.
 MultiBoot Basic flexion b.
 pneumatic compression b.
 PNS Unna b.
 Primer flexible Unna b.
 Primer modified Unna b.
 quadriceps b.
 Rik FootHugger fluid heel b.
 rocker b.
 rocker-bottom cast b.
 Rooke perioperative b.
 Scotch b.
 sheepskin b.

SlimLine cast b.
Spenco b.
Tenderwrap Unna b.
Unna b.
Unna-Flex elastic Unna b.
Unna paste b.
Unna zinc b.
Venodyne b.
weight b.
Wilke b.

Bootie
Bebax B.
Boplant graft
Borazon blade cutting machine
Borchard
B. Gigli-saw guide
B. wire threader
Borchardt olive-shaped bur
Bores
B. corneal fixation forceps
B. incision spreader
B. optic zone marker
B. radial marker
B. twist fixation ring
B. U-shaped fixation forceps
Borge
B. bile duct clamp
B. catheter
boron counter
Boros esophagoscope
Borsch
B. bandage
B. dressing
Borst-Tuohy side-arm introducer set
Bortone shears
Bortz clamp
Boruchoff forceps
Bosch ERG 501 ergometer
Bose
B. bar
B. retractor
B. tracheostomy hook
Bosher commissurotomy knife
Bosker
B. TMI Reconstruction system
B. TMI surgery
B. transmandibular implant
B. transmandibular reconstructive
surgical system
BosPac cardiopulmonary bypass system

BOSS
Becker orthopaedic spinal system
BOSS surgical instrument
Bossi cervical dilator
Bostick staple
Boston
B. bivalve brace
B. brace
B. Children's frame
B. Dynamics surgical simulator
B. elbow system
B. Envision lens
B. gauze sponge
B. hip orthosis
B. Lying-In cervical forceps
B. neurosurgical couch
B. overlap brace
B. Scientific Sonicath imaging
catheter
B. scleral lens
B. scoliosis brace
B. soft body jacket
B. soft corset
B. stethoscope
B. trephine
Bosu balance trainer
Bosworth
B. coracoclavicular screw
B. crown drill
B. headband
B. nasal snare
B. nasal wire speculum
B. nerve root retractor
B. osteotomy spline
B. saw
B. screwdriver
B. spline plate
B. temporary crown
B. tongue depressor
Bosworth-Joseph nasal saw
Botox injection amplifier
bottle
BacT/Alert glass b.
blow b.
Castaneda b.
hot water b.
McGaw plastic b.
night drain b.
Nu-Hope urine collection b.
Ohio safety trap overflow b.
PlasmaPlex b.

NOTES

B

bottle *(continued)*
  urinary night drainage b.
  Ziegler wash b.
Bottoms-Up posture system
Botvin
  B. iris forceps
  B. vulsellum forceps
Botvin-Bradford enucleator
Bouchayer grasping forceps
Boucheron ear speculum
Bouchut laryngeal tube
bougie
  acorn-tipped b.
  Anastasia b.
  armed b.
  Bangs b.
  bellied b.
  bronchoscopic b.
  Buerger dilating b.
  bulbous b.
  Celestin b.
  Chevalier Jackson b.
  conic b.
  cylindrical b.
  dilating b.
  b. dilator
  Dittel dilating urethral b.
  Dourmashkin tunneled b.
  ear b.
  elastic b.
  elbowed b.
  EndoLumina b.
  eustachian b.
  filiform b.
  fusiform b.
  Gabriel Tucker b.
  Garceau b.
  Gruber b.
  b. guide
  Guyon dilating b.
  Guyon exploratory b.
  Harold Hayes eustachian b.
  Hegar b.
  Holinger-Hurst b.
  Holinger infant b.
  Hurst mercury-filled esophageal b.
  Jackson radiopaque b.
  Jackson steel-stem woven
   filiform b.
  Jackson tracheal b.
  Klebanoff b.
  LeFort filiform b.
  Maloney tapered mercury-filled
   esophageal b.
  Maloney-type b.
  mercury-filled esophageal b.
  mercury-weighted rubber b.
  Miller b.
  olive-tipped b.

  Phillips urethral whip b.
  Plummer modified b.
  polyvinyl b.
  Ravich b.
  retrograde b.
  rosary b.
  Rusch b.
  Ruschelit urethral b.
  Savary-Gilliard Silastic flexible b.
  Savary-Gilliard wire-guided b.
  spiral-tipped b.
  Szuler eustachian b.
  through-the-scope b.
  Trousseau esophageal b.
  Tucker retrograde b.
  Urbantschitsch eustachian b.
  b. urethrotome
  Wales rectal b.
  Waltham-Street b.
  wax b.
  whalebone filiform b.
  whip b.
  Whistler b.
  wire-guided polyvinyl b.
  yellow-eyed dilating b.
boule
  Friedman-Otis bougie à b.
  Otis bougie à b.
Bourassa catheter
Bourdon
  B. tube
  B. tube pressure gauge
Bourns
  B. electronic adult respirator
  B. infant pressure ventilator
  B. infant respirator
Bourns-Bear ventilator
Boutin
  B. optics
  B. thoracoscope
boutonniere splint
Bovie
  B. blade
  B. cautery
  B. coagulating forceps
  B. conization electrode
  B. CSV coagulator
  B. electrocautery
  B. electrocautery device
  B. electrocautery unit
  B. grounding pad
  B. holder
  B. needle
  B. suction device
  B. ultrasonic aspirator
  B. ultrasound aspirator
  B. wet-field cautery
bovine
  b. allograft

b. biodegradable collagen
b. collagen implant
b. collagen material prosthesis
b. heterograft
b. pericardial heart valve xenograft
b. pericardial valve
b. pericardium dural graft
b. pericardium strip
b. xenograft
Bovino scleral-spreading forceps
Bovin-Stille vaginal speculum
Bovin vaginal speculum
bow
Aesculap traction b.
Anderson traction b.
B. & Arrow cannulated drill guide
Bendixen-Kirschner traction b.
Böhler extension b.
Böhler traction b.
Crego-McCarroll traction b.
Crutchfield traction b.
extension b.
Framer finger extension b.
Granberry finger traction b.
harelip traction b.
Keys-Kirschner traction b.
Kirschner extension b.
Kirschner wire traction b.
lip traction b.
Logan lip traction b.
Pease-Thomson traction b.
Peterson skeletal traction b.
Schwarz finger extension b.
Schwarz traction b.
Steinmann extension b.
traction b.
bowel
b. bag
b. forceps
b. grasper
b. retractor
Bowen
B. BAS-30 blade
B. double-bladed scalpel
B. gooseneck chisel
B. gouge
B. osteotome
B. periosteal elevator
B. rasp
B. resin
B. suction
B. suction loose body forceps

B. suture drill
B. wire tightener
Bowen-Grover meniscotome
Bower PEG tube
Bowers cannula
bowl
b. curette
Latham b.
rubber spa b.
Bowlby arm splint
bowleg brace
Bowling lens
Bowls septal gouge
Bowman
B. cataract needle
B. discission knife
B. discission needle
B. eye knife
B. eye speculum
B. iris needle
B. iris scissors
B. lacrimal dilator
B. lacrimal probe
B. needle stop
B. speculum
B. stop needle
B. strabismus scissors
B. tube
box
A/B switch b.
B. adenotome
Anchor sterilizer b.
Bárány b.
Brite Lite III light b.
BTE Bolt B.
b. curette
digital constant-current pacing b.
Elecath switch b.
FootPrinter b.
Hogness b.
b. joint forceps
mammographic view b.
Mammo-Lume view b.
b. osteotome
steam b.
sterilizer b.
SunBox light therapy b.
switch b.
Box-DeJager adenotome
boxing strip
Boxwood mallet
Boyce needle holder

NOTES

B

97

Boyd
B. bone graft
B. bone scoop
B. dissecting scissors
B. orbital implant
B. perforator
B. retractor
B. tonsillar scissors
Boyden
B. chamber
B. chamber assay device
Boyd-Stille tonsillar scissors
Boyes-Goodfellow
B.-G. hook
B.-G. hook retractor
Boyes muscle clamp
Boyle-Davis mouthgag
Boyle-Rosin clip
Boyle uterine elevator
Boynton needle holder
Boys-Allis tissue forceps
Boys-Smith laser lens
Bozeman
B. catheter
B. clamp
B. curette
B. dilator
B. forceps
B. hook
B. Lorenz-Barmesh holding forceps
B. LR packing forceps
B. LR uterine-dressing forceps
B. needle holder
B. scissors
B. speculum
B. suture
B. uterine dressing forceps
B. uterine packing forceps
Bozeman-Douglas forceps
Bozeman-Finochietto needle holder
Bozeman-Fritsch catheter
Bozeman-Wertheim needle holder
B-P
B-P surgical handle
B-P transfer forceps
BPM
blood perfusion monitor
BPS spinal angiographic catheter
BQ 900 slit lamp
bra
Circumpress compression b.
lead b.
Woods Surgitek b.
Braasch
B. bladder specimen forceps
B. bulb
B. bulb ureteral catheter
B. direct catheterization cystoscope
B. ureteral dilator

Braasch-Kaplan direct vision cystoscope
Braastad costal arch retractor
BRACAnalyzer gene analyzer
Bracco system
brace
abdominal b.
Ace b.
Adjustable OA Defiance knee b.
AFO b.
Aircast Air-Stirrup leg b.
Aircast fracture b.
Aircast patellar b.
Aircast pneumatic b.
Aircast Swivel-Strap b.
Aircast walking b.
AirGel ankle b.
Air-Stirrup ankle b.
Ank-L-Aid b.
AO b.
AOA cervical immobilization b.
Arizona AFO b.
Arnold b.
Atlanta-Scottish Rite hip b.
back b.
Back Seat back b.
bail-lock b.
Bauerfeind Achillotrain Achilles
  tendon b.
Bauerfeind ankle b.
Bauerfeind Comprifix knee b.
Becker b.
bipivotal hinge knee b.
Bledsoe adjustable b.
Bledsoe cast b.
Bledsoe knee b.
Blount b.
Blount-Schmidt-Milwaukee b.
Boldrey b.
Bollinger knee b.
boot b.
Boston b.
Boston bivalve b.
Boston overlap b.
Boston scoliosis b.
bowleg b.
Buck knee b.
Caligamed b.
Callender derotational b.
CAM lock knee b.
Camp b.
CAM Walker leg b.
Can-Am b.
canvas b.
Capener b.
carpal lock wrist b.
Cash back b.
cast b.
Castaway leg b.
cervical b.

B

Chairback b.
Charleston bending b.
Charleston scoliosis b.
Chopart b.
Cincinnati ACL b.
clamshell b.
CM-Band 505N rubber b.
contraflexion b.
Cook walking b.
Cotrel-Dubousset orthopaedic b.
CounterForce osteoarthritis knee b.
Count'R-Force arch b.
CRS b.
Cruiser hip abduction b.
CTEV b.
C.Ti.2 b.
Cunningham b.
cutout patellar b.
DarcoGel ankle b.
derotation b.
DonJoy ALP ankle b.
DonJoy Defiance CI b.
DonJoy Goldpoint hinged knee b.
DonJoy Legend ACL knee b.
DonJoy 4-point ACL Super Sport
  knee b.
drop foot b.
Duncan shoulder b.
Easy Lok ankle b.
Easy-On elbow b.
Eclipse gel ankle b.
Edge knee b.
elastic-hinge knee b.
Elite knee b.
English b.
Exotec b.
Extreme Select ligament b.
figure-of-8 b.
Fillauer Tiny Titans pediatric
  knee b.
Fisher b.
Flex Foam b.
flexor hinge hand splint b.
Floam ankle stirrup b.
Florida back b.
Florida cervical b.
Florida contraflexion b.
Florida extension b.
Florida hyperextension b.
Florida J-series b.
Florida postfusion b.
Florida spinal b.

foot-ankle b.
footdrop b.
Forrester cervical collar b.
fracture b.
Friedman splint b.
functional electronic peroneal b.
functional fracture b.
Futuro wrist b.
gait lock splint b.
Galveston metacarpal b.
Generation II Matrix knee b.
Genutrain knee b.
G II Unloader ADJ knee b.
Gillette b.
Goldthwait b.
Guilford b.
halo b.
hand b.
head b.
Hessing b.
Hilgenreiner b.
Hi-Top foot/ankle b.
Hoke lumbar b.
Hudson-Jones knee cage b.
Hudson TLSO b.
hyperextension b.
Ilfeld b.
InCare b.
Industrial Work b.
Inner Lok ankle b.
internal tibial torsion b.
I-Plus humeral b.
ischial weightbearing b.
Jace knee b.
Jewett-Benjamin cervical b.
Jewett contraflexion b.
Jewett hyperextension b.
Jewett postfusion b.
Jones b.
Joseph nasal b.
Juzo Patellaligner b.
Kallassy ankle b.
Kicker Pavlik harness b.
King cervical b.
Klenzak b.
knee cage b.
knee MD b.
Knight b.
Knight-Taylor b.
Korn Cage knee b.
Kuhlman cervical b.
Küntscher-Hudson b.

NOTES

brace *(continued)*
Kydex b.
kyphosis b.
lace-on b.
leaf-spring b.
LeCocq b.
left long leg b.
leg b.
Lenox Hill Spectralite knee b.
Lerman hinge b.
Liberty thumb b.
Lofstrand b.
long double upright b.
long leg b.
Lorenz b.
Lovitt-Uhler postfusion b.
Lyman-Smith toe drop b.
Maliniac nasal b.
Masterbrace 3 functional ACL knee b.
McCollough internal tibial torsion b.
McDavid knee b.
McKee b.
Medical Design b.
Metcalf spring drop b.
Miami cervical fracture b.
Miami TLSO scoliosis b.
Milwaukee scoliosis b.
MKS II knee b.
Monarch knee b.
Moon Boot b.
MTA b.
Mueller Ultralite b.
Murphy b.
Nakamura b.
neoprene hinged-knee b.
neoprene Osgood-Schlatter knee b.
neoprene wrist b.
New England scoliosis b.
Nextep knee b.
nonweightbearing b.
Northville b.
OAdjuster knee b.
OAsys b.
Omni knee b.
Opiela b.
Oppenheim b.
Orbital shoulder stabilizer b.
Orthomedics b.
Ortho-Mold spinal b.
Orthoplast fracture b.
Orthotech Performer knee b.
OS-5/Plus 2 knee b.
OsteoArthritic knee b.
Pacesetter knee b.
Palumbo dynamic patellar b.
Palumbo knee b.
Palumbo stabilizing knee b.

pantaloon b.
Patellaligner knee b.
patellar b.
Patten-Bottom-Perthes b.
performer ultralight knee b.
Perlstein b.
Phelps b.
Phemister b.
piano-wire dorsiflexion b.
PMT halo b.
PneuGel postop knee b.
Pneu Knee b.
4-point cervical b.
6-point knee b.
postoperative flexor tendon traction b.
Power Play knee b.
PPT gel stirrup ankle b.
Pro-8 ankle b.
Pro 50 KS 5 ACL b.
Propoint multifunction knee b.
ProShifter ACL sports b.
PTB b.
Push medical b.
Quadrant shoulder b.
QualCare knee b.
Quick-Tie ankle b.
Raney flexion jacket b.
range-of-motion b.
ratchet-type b.
Rhino Triangle hip abduction b.
Richie b.
Rolyan Firm D-Ring wrist b.
Rolyan tibial fracture b.
ROM knee b.
Sarmiento b.
SAS II b.
Schanz collar b.
Scoi b.
scoliosis b.
Scottish Rite b.
seton hip b.
short leg caliper b.
shoulder b.
shoulder subluxation inhibitor b.
SmartBrace b.
SmartWrap elbow b.
Smedberg b.
snap-lock b.
SofTec genu knee b.
SOMI b.
SOMI Jr. b.
Speed b.
Spinal Technology bivalve TLSO b.
Sports-Caster I, II knee b.
sterno-occipital-mandibular immobilizer b.
Stille b.

Stimprene electrotherapy b.
stirrup b.
straight walker b.
Strap Lok ankle b.
Stromgren ankle b.
Sully shoulder stabilizer b.
Sure Step b.
Swede-O ankle b.
Swede-O Arch Lok b.
Swede-O Inner Lok 8 ankle b.
Swede-O-Universal b.
Swivel-Strap ankle b.
Taylor-Knight b.
Taylor spine b.
telescoping b.
Teufel cervical b.
Teurlings wrist b.
Thermoskin b.
Thomas-type cervical collar b.
Thomas walking b.
tibial fracture b.
toedrop b.
Townsend knee b.
Tracker knee b.
triangle shoulder abduction b.
Trinkle b.
turnbuckle ankle b.
turnbuckle knee b.
UBC b.
UCLA functional long leg b.
Ultrabrace b.
University of British Columbia b.
Unloader Bi-ComPF b.
Unloader Express knee b.
ValueWalker b.
Verlow b.
VertaBrace b.
walking b.
Warm Springs b.
weightbearing b.
Wheaton b.
Wilke boot b.
Williams back b.
Women's Tradition b.
Wright Universal b.
Wrist Restore b.
Yale b.
Zinco Hyperex thoracolumbar b.
bracelet
BioBands b.
Nussbaum b.
Q-Ray b.

braceRAP wrap
brachial artery catheter
BrachySeed brachytherapy seed
brachytherapy
b. balloon applicator
Genetra seedless b.
BrachyVision brachytherapy planning system
Bracken
B. anterior chamber cannula
B. fixation forceps
B. iris forceps
B. irrigating cannula
B. scleral fixation forceps
Bracken-Forkas corneal forceps
bracket
Begg straight-wire combination b.
Broussard b.
Cusp-Lok b.
Hanson speed b.
Lee b.
Lee-Fischer plastic b.
Lewis vertical slot b.
ligatureless b.
molar b.
Ormco wire b.
orthodontic b.
plastic b.
Siamese twin b.
steel-slotted plastic b.
Steiner b.
torqued slot b.
bracketed splint
Brackett dental probe
Brackmann
B. facial nerve monitor
B. II EMG system
B. suction-irrigator
Braden
B. flushing reservoir
B. scale
Bradford
B. enucleation neurotome
B. fracture appliance
B. fracture frame
B. snare enucleator
B. thyroid forceps
Bradley femoral canal preparation scraper
Bradshaw-O'Neill aortic clamp
Brady balanced suspension splint
Bragg-Paul respirator

NOTES

Brahler ultrasonic dental scaler
braided
- b. diagnostic catheter
- b. Ethibond suture
- b. Mersilene suture
- b. Nurolon suture
- b. nylon suture
- b. occlusion device
- b. polyamide suture
- b. polyester fiber
- b. polyester suture
- b. silk suture
- b. Spectra UHMWPE surgical cable
- b. titanium cable
- b. Vicryl suture
- b. wire
- b. wire suture

brain
- b. biopsy cannula
- b. biopsy needle
- b. clip
- b. clip carrier
- b. clip forceps
- b. depressor
- b. dressing forceps
- b. lead
- b. probe
- b. retractor
- b. silicone-coated retractor
- b. spatula
- b. spatula forceps
- b. tissue forceps
- b. trocar
- b. tumor forceps

BrainLab VectorVision neuronavigational system
BrainSCAN
- B. Linac radiosurgery system
- B. stereotactic system

Braithwaite
- B. clip remover
- B. forceps
- B. nasal chisel
- B. skin graft knife

Brake hemostatic bag
Bralon suture
Brand
- B. passing forceps
- B. shunt-introducing forceps
- B. tendon-holding forceps
- B. tendon passer
- B. tendon-passing forceps
- B. tendon stripper

Brandel cell harvester
Brandt
- B. brassiere
- B. cytology balloon

Brandy
- B. front closure scalp stretcher
- B. scalp stretcher I, II, front closure
- B. scalp stretcher I, II, rear closure

Brånemark
- B. endosteal implant
- B. implant system

Brannock
- B. device shoe sizer
- B. foot measuring device

Brannon
- B. extracapsular cleaving forceps
- B. extracapsular removal forceps

Bransford-Lewis ureteral dilator
Brant aluminum splint
Brantley-Turner vaginal retractor
Branula cannula
brass
- b. mallet
- b. scleral plug
- b. wire

Brasseler Optipost root post
brassiere
- Brandt b.
- Foerster surgical support b.

brassiere-type dressing
Brauer chisel
Braun
- B. cranioclast
- B. decapitation hook
- B. episiotomy scissors
- B. forceps
- B. frame
- B. graft
- B. implant
- B. ligature carrier
- B. needle
- B. obstetrical hook
- B. speculum
- B. stent
- B. uterine depressor
- B. uterine tenaculum

Braun-Schroeder single-tooth tenaculum
Braun-Stadler
- B.-S. episiotomy scissors
- B.-S. sternal shears

Braunstein fixed calipers
Braunwald-Cutter ball prosthetic valve
Braunwald heart valve
Braun-Wangensteen graft
Braun-Yasargil right-angle clip
Brava breast enhancement and shaping system
Brawley
- B. nasal suction tube
- B. refractor
- B. scleral wound retractor

B

B. sinus rasp
B. suction apparatus
Brawner orbital implant
bread knife valvulotome
breakable blade
breakaway
  b. lap cushion
  b. pin
  b. splice
BreakAway wound dressing
breaker
  Böhler plaster cast b.
  cast b.
  Castroviejo blade b.
  Jarit-Mason cast b.
  Troutman-Barraquer mini blade b.
  Troutman blade b.
  Wölfe-Böhler cast b.
Breakstone lithotripter
Breas PV10 CPAP device
breast
  b. binder
  b. bolster
  b. calipers
  b. form
  b. implant
  b. keyhole template
  b. localization needle
  b. plate
  b. prosthesis
  b. pump
  b. reduction pattern
  b. tenaculum
  B. Vest Exu-Dry one-piece wound
    dressing
BreastAlert
  B. differential temperature sensor
  B. DTS breast cancer screening
    device
Breathables air-permeable underpad
BreathCO breathe carbon monoxide
  monitor
Breathe Right nasal strip
breathing
  b. bag
  b. pacemaker
breath-operated inhaler
Brecht feeder
Breck
  B. pin
  B. pin cutter
Bredall amalgam plugger

breeder reactor
Breen retractor
Breeze
  B. E150 ventilator
  B. infant ventilator
  B. respirator
Breg slingshot arm and shoulder
  immobilizer
Breinin suction cup
Breisky
  B. vaginal retractor
  B. vaginal speculum
Breisky-Navratil
  B.-N. straight retractor
  B.-N. vaginal speculum
Breisky-Stille speculum
Breitman adenotome
Bremer
  B. AirFlo thoracic stabilization vest
  B. halo
  B. halo cervical traction
  B. halo Crown system
  B. halo vest
  B. torque-limiting cap
Brems astigmatism marker
Brenman camera
Brennen biosynthetic surgical mesh
Brenner
  B. carotid bypass shunt
  B. forceps
  B. mesher
  B. rectal probe
Brent pressure earring
brephoplastic graft
Brescia-Cimino
  B.-C. AV fistula
  B.-C. shunt
Bresgen
  B. cannula
  B. catheter
  B. frontal sinus probe
Brett bone graft
Brevi-Kath epidural catheter
Brewer vaginal speculum
Brewster retractor
bridge
  Albarran b.
  B. Assurant
  balance b.
  Burns converting b.
  catheter deflecting b.
  B. clamp

NOTES

bridge *(continued)*
B. deep surgery forceps
B. hemostatic forceps
B. hip system
1-horn b.
B. intestinal forceps
Maryland b.
pediatric b.
retention suture b.
Rochette b.
Short b.
b. splint
B. telescope
Wappler b.
3-way b.
B. X3 renal stent system
bridged loop-gap resonator
bridgeless mask
Bridgemaster nasal splint
bridle
control b.
b. suture
brief
Acti-Fit incontinence b.
Attends b.
Conveen disposable stretch b.
Harmonie Classic Plus b.
KINS all-in-1 cotton b.
PrimeTime Plus adult disposable b.
Shamp AK casting b.
SlimLine disposable b.
Slim and Trim b.
Sofnit 300 fitted b.
Ultra-Fit b.
Brierley nucleus splitter
Briesky pelvimeter
Briggs
B. laryngoscope
B. retractor
B. transilluminator
Brigham
B. brain tumor forceps
B. dressing forceps
B. tissue forceps
B. 1x2 teeth forceps
Brightbill corneal cutting block
Brighton epistaxis balloon
Brilliant light-cured resin
Brimfield
B. cannulated grasping hook
B. magnetic retriever
Brimms
B. denture reliner
B. Quik-Fix denture repair kit
Brinkerhoff
B. anoscope
B. rectal speculum
Brinker hygienic tissue retractor
Brink PeriPyriform implant

Brisman-Nova carotid endarterectomy shunt
Bristow
B. lever
B. periosteal elevator
B. rasp
Bristow-Bankart
B.-B. humeral retractor
B.-B. soft tissue retractor
Brite
B. Lite III light box
B. Tip guiding catheter
BriteSmile laser tooth whitening system
Britetrac
B. fiberoptic instrument
B. illuminator
B. retractor
B. speculum
B. Taylor retractor
Britt
B. argon pulsed ion laser
B. BL-12 laser
B. krypton laser
B. pulsed argon laser
BRK-series transseptal needle
broach
barbed b.
Charnley femoral b.
crescent b.
endodontic b.
b. extractor
femoral b.
glenoid fin b.
Harris b.
intramedullary b.
Koenig metatarsal b.
metacarpal b.
metatarsal stem b.
Monaco b.
orthopaedic b.
phalangeal b.
root canal b.
square-hole b.
starter b.
Swanson intramedullary b.
Swanson metatarsal b.
tibial b.
broadbill hemostat with push fork
Brock
B. auricular clamp
B. biopsy forceps
B. cardiac dilator
B. cardiovascular forceps
B. infundibular punch
B. mitral valve knife
B. probe
B. pulmonary valve knife
B. valvulotome

Brockenbrough
  B. angiocatheter
  B. cardiac device
  B. curved-tip occluder
  B. mapping catheter
  B. modified bipolar catheter
  B. transseptal catheter
  B. transseptal needle
Brockington pile clamp
Brodie
  B. director
  B. fistula director
  B. fistular probe
Brodmerkel colon decompression set
Brodney
  B. catheter
  B. hemostatic bag
  B. urethrographic cannula
  B. urethrographic clamp
Broggi-Kelman dipstick gauge
Brombach perimeter
Bromley uterine curette
Brompton Hospital retractor
bronchial
  b. biopsy forceps
  b. catheter
  b. clamp
  b. dilator
  b. grasping forceps
  b. tube
Bronchitrac-L suction catheter
Broncho-Cath double-lumen endotracheal tube
bronchocele
  b. sound
  b. sound raspatory
bronchofiberscope
  Pentax b.
bronchoscope
  ACMI Marici b.
  adult ventilation b.
  Albert slotted b.
  Broyles b.
  Broyles-Negus b.
  Bruening b.
  Bryan-Dumon rigid b.
  Chevalier Jackson b.
  Davis b.
  Doesel-Huzly b.
  double-channel irrigating b.
  Dumon-Harrell b.
  Dumon rigid b.

Efer-Dumon b.
Emerson b.
fiberoptic b.
flexible fiberoptic b.
Foregger b.
foroblique b.
Fujinon flexible b.
Haslinger b.
Holinger infant b.
Holinger-Jackson b.
Holinger ventilating fiberoptic b.
Jackson costophrenic b.
Jackson full-lumen b.
Jesberg infant b.
Kernan-Jackson coagulating b.
Life White Light b.
Marici b.
Michelson infant b.
Moersch b.
Negus b.
Negus-Broyles b.
Olympus BF-series b.
Olympus fiberoptic b.
Overholt-Jackson b.
Pentax b.
Pilling b.
respiration b.
Riecker respiration b.
rigid ventilation b.
Safar ventilation b.
Savary b.
SFB-I right-angled b.
Shapshay laser b.
single-channel fiberoptic b.
Storz b.
Storz-Hopkins b.
Storz infant b.
Tucker b.
ventilation b.
Waterman folding b.
Xanar laser b.
Yankauer b.
bronchoscopic
  b. aspirator
  b. biopsy forceps
  b. bougie
  b. brush
  b. disposable suction tube
  b. forceps
  b. magnet
  b. probe
  b. ruler

NOTES

B

bronchoscopic *(continued)*
    b. sponge
    b. sponge carrier
bronchospirometric catheter
Bronkhorst Hi-Tec controller
Bronkometer
Bronner clamp
Bronson
    B. magnet
    B. speculum
    B. ultrasonoscope
Bronson-Magnion
    B.-M. eye magnet
    B.-M. forceps
Bronson-Park speculum
Bronson-Ray pituitary curette
Bronson-Turner foreign body locator
Bronson-Turtz
    B.-T. iris retractor
    B.-T. refractor
    B.-T. speculum
bronze wire suture
Brookdale bar
Brooke Army Hospital splint
Brooker
    B. double-locking unreamed tibial nail
    B. wire
Brooker-Wills nail
Brookfield viscometer
Brooks
    B. adenoidal punch
    B. appliance
    B. gallbladder scissors
broomstick cast
Brophy
    B. bistoury
    B. bistoury knife
    B. cleft palate knife
    B. dressing forceps
    B. gag
    B. mouthgag
    B. needle
    B. periosteal elevator
    B. periosteotome
    B. plate
    B. retractor
    B. scissors
    B. tenaculum
    B. tissue forceps
    B. tooth elevator
Brophy-Deschamps needle
Broselow
    B. chart
    B. tape
Broselow/Hinkle pediatric resuscitation system
Broussard bracket
Broviac catheter

Browlift Bone Bridge system
Brown
    B. air dermatome
    B. applicator
    B. chisel
    B. cleft palate knife
    B. cleft palate needle
    B. dermatome blade
    B. dissecting scissors
    B. ear speculum
    B. electrodermatome
    B. hook
    B. lip clamp
    B. mallet
    B. nasal splint
    B. ophthalmic insertion forceps
    B. periosteotome
    B. rasp
    B. saw
    B. and Sharp digital electronic calipers
    B. side-grasping forceps
    B. sphenoidal cannula
    B. staphylorrhaphy needle
    B. sterile adhesive
    B. thoracic forceps
    B. tissue forceps
    B. tonsillar snare
    B. tonsillectome
    B. tooth elevator
    B. uvular retractor
Brown-Adson
    B.-A. side-grasping forceps
    B.-A. tissue forceps
Brown-Bahnson bayonet forceps
Brown-Blair
    B.-B. dermatome
    B.-B. skin graft knife
Brown-Bovari machine
Brown-Buerger
    B.-B. cystoscope
    B.-B. dilator
    B.-B. forceps
Brown-Burr modified Gillies retractor
Brown-Cushing forceps
Brown-Davis mouthgag
Brown-Dean cotton applicator
Brown-Dohlman Silastic corneal implant
Browne
    B. stone basket
    B. UroBreeze urodynamics monitor
Brown-Fillebrown-Whitehead mouthgag
Brown-Grabow capsulorrhexis forceps
Brown-Joseph saw
Brown-McHardy pneumatic dilator
Brown-Mueller
    B.-M. T-bar fastener
    B.-M. T-fastener set

Brown-Pusey corneal trephine
Brown-Roberts-Wells (BRW)
    B.-R.-W. arc-ring assembly
    B.-R.-W. base ring
    B.-R.-W. computerized tomography
        stereotaxic guidance system
    B.-R.-W. floor stand
    B.-R.-W. head frame
    B.-R.-W. headrest
    B.-R.-W. head ring halo
    B.-R.-W. phantom base
    B.-R.-W. ring adapter
    B.-R.-W. stereotactic frame
    B.-R.-W. stereotactic guide
Brown-Sanders fascial needle
Brown-Sharp gauge suture
Brown-Swan forceps
Brown-Whitehead mouthgag
Broyles
    B. anterior commissure
        laryngoscope
    B. aspirator
    B. bronchoscope
    B. esophageal dilator
    B. esophagoscope
    B. nasopharyngoscope
    B. optical forceps
    B. optical laryngoscope
    B. retrograde cystoscope
    B. telescope
    B. wasp-waist laryngoscope
Broyles-Negus bronchoscope
Bruch mastoid retractor
Bruecke tube
Brueckmann lead hand
Bruel
    B. & Kjaer axial transducer
    B. & Kjaer transvaginal ultrasound
        probe
Bruening
    B. biting tip
    B. bronchoscope
    B. cannula
    B. chisel
    B. cutting-tip forceps
    B. ear snare
    B. electroscope
    B. esophagoscope
    B. ethmoid exenteration forceps
    B. forceps stylet
    B. intracordal injection set

    B. Japanese anastigmatic aural
        magnifier
    B. nasal-cutting septal forceps
    B. nasal snare
    B. otoscope set
    B. pneumatic otoscope
    B. pressure syringe
    B. punch
    B. retractor
    B. septal forceps
    B. speculum
    B. tongue depressor
**Bruening-Arnold intracordal injection
set**
Bruening-Citelli
    B.-C. forceps
    B.-C. rongeur
Bruening-Storz
    B.-S. anastigmatic aural magnifier
    B.-S. diagnostic head
Bruening-Work diagnostic head
Brughleman needle
Bruker
    B. AMX 300 NMR spectrometer
    B. Avance spectrometer
    B. BioSpec system
    B. console
    B. CSI MR system
    B. PC-10 relaxometer
    B. scanner
Bruker/GE CSI Omega MR system
Brun
    B. ear curette
    B. guarded chisel
    B. mastoid bone curette
    B. plaster scissors
    B. plaster shears
Bruner vaginal speculum
Brunetti chisel
Bruni counterpressor
Bruni-Wayne clamp approximator
Brunner
    B. chisel
    B. colon clamp
    B. goiter dissector
    B. intestinal clamp
    B. intestinal forceps
    B. ligature needle
    B. probe
    B. raspatory
    B. retractor
    B. rib shears

NOTES

Brunner *(continued)*
    B. sigmoid anastomosis forceps
    B. tissue forceps
Brunschwig
    B. arterial forceps
    B. visceral forceps
    B. visceral retractor
Brunswick-Mack
    B.-M. approximator
    B.-M. bur
    B.-M. chisel
    B.-M. rotating drill
Brunswick serrefine
Brunton otoscope
brush
    Alger b.
    Ayre b.
    Bard ureteroscopic cytology b.
    Barraquer sable b.
    Bayne Pap b.
    bronchoscopic b.
    bur b.
    Castaneda over-the-wire
      thrombolytic b.
    Cohort bone b.
    Combo Cath wire-guided
      cytology b.
    Cox cytology b.
    Cragg thrombolytic b.
    Cytobrush Plus b.
    cytological b.
    cytology b.
    DexTBrush b.
    Diaflex cytology b.
    disposable cytology b.
    endotracheal tube b.
    Endovations disposable cytology b.
    Geenan biliary cytology b.
    Gill biopsy b.
    Glassman b.
    Grafco tracheal tube b.
    Haidinger b.
    Hobbs sheath b.
    Howell biliary introducer b.
    intramedullary b.
    Kurtin planing dermabrasion b.
    Kurtin wire b.
    manual dermatome b.
    Marten hair eye b.
    Medscand cytology b.
    Medscand endometrial b.
    Mill-Rose cytology b.
    ophthalmic sable b.
    Oral-B soft foam interdental b.
    Plak-Vac oral suction b.
    polishing b.
    polypropylene hand b.
    protected bronchoscopic b.
    protected specimen b.

    protected specimen microbiology b.
    Rusch cleaning b.
    sable b.
    SafeClean instrument cleaning b.
    scraping b.
    scrub b.
    Sklar b.
    soft scrub b.
    specimen b.
    stomach b.
    Stormby b.
    Storz cleaning b.
    Sulcabrush b.
    Superfine Microbrush b.
    Surgi-Prep sponge b.
    Thomas b.
    thrombolytic b.
    tracheal tube b.
    Unimar Cervex b.
    Viba-Brush endocervical b.
    Wagner laryngeal b.
    Wilson-Cook cytology b.
Bruus scoop
BRW
    Brown-Roberts-Wells
      BRW CT stereotaxic guide
      BRW stereotactic system
Bryan-Dumon rigid bronchoscope
Bryant
    B. mitral hook
    B. nasal forceps
    B. traction
    B. tractor
Brymill cryosurgical probe
B-scan
    Contact B-s.
    Humphrey B-s.
    B-s. ultrasonogram
BSM
    bone substitute material
BTA S-2000 biofeedback system
BTE
    behind-the-ear
      BTE Assembly Tree
      BTE Bolt Box
      BTE dynamic lift
      BTE listening device
      BTE Work simulator
bubble
    b. chamber equipment
    b. humidifier
    b. jar
    b. oxygenator
buccal cortical plate
Buchbinder
    B. Omniflex catheter
    B. Thruflex over-the-wire catheter
Buch-Gramcko gouge

Buchholz
    B. acetabular cup
    B. hip prosthesis
Bucholz bipolar cauterizer
Buchwald tongue depressor
Buck
    B. bone curette
    B. convoluted traction apparatus
    B. ear applicator
    B. ear curette
    B. ear probe
    B. extension
    B. extension apparatus
    B. extension bar
    B. extension frame
    B. extension splint
    B. femoral cement restrictor
    B. foreign body forceps
    B. fracture appliance
    B. hook
    B. knee brace
    B. mastoid curette
    B. myringotome
    B. myringotomy knife
    B. nasal applicator
    B. neurological percussion hammer
    B. osteotome
    B. periosteal elevator
    B. plug
    B. traction
    B. traction splint
    B. tractor
    B. Universal convoluted traction
        unit
    B. wax curette
bucket
    Denis Browne b.
    kick b.
    Lenox b.
Buck-Gramcko
    B.-G. bone lever
    B.-G. retractor
Buck-House curette
Buckingham
    B. drill
    B. mirror
buckle
    wire-fixation b.
Buckley chisel
Buckstein colonic insufflator
Bucky
    B. diaphragm

    B. digital x-ray device
    B. hand drill
    B. high-contrast imaging
    B. view tray
bucrylate collagen hemostatic material
Bucy
    B. cordotomy knife
    B. laminectomy rongeur
    B. spinal cord retractor
    B. suction tube
Bucy-Frazier
    B.-F. coagulation cannula
    B.-F. suction cannula
    B.-F. suction tube
Bud bur
Budde
    B. halo neurosurgical retractor
    B. halo ring
**Budde-Greenberg-Sugita stereotactic
    head frame**
buddy
    bolster b.
    Ostomy Shadow B.
    b. strap
Budin
    B. hammertoe splint
    B. toe splint
Buechel-Pappas total ankle prosthesis
**Buedding squeegee cortex extractor and
    polisher**
Bueleau empyema trocar
Buerger
    B. dilating bougie
    B. prostatic needle
    B. punch
    B. snare
Buerger-McCarthy
    B.-M. bladder forceps
    B.-M. scissors
Buettner-Parel vitreous cutter
Buffalo
    B. dental cement
    B. ultrasonic scaler
Bugbee
    B. electrocautery
    B. fulgurating electrode
buggy
    Maclaren mobile b.
Buhl spirometer
Buie
    B. biopsy forceps
    B. cannula

B

NOTES

Buie *(continued)*
B. fistula probe
B. fulgurating electrode
B. pile clamp
B. rectal forceps
B. rectal scissors
B. rectal suction tube
B. retractor
B. sigmoidoscope
B. specimen forceps
Buie-Hirschman
B.-H. anoscope
B.-H. pile clamp
Buie-Smith
B.-S. anal retractor
B.-S. rectal speculum
Builder Grip hand exerciser
build-up eye implant
Bülau trocar
bulb
Beckman Silastic b.
Braasch b.
dilating b.
b. dynamometer
b. grenade
nasal suction b.
nystagmus b.
b. retractor
self-inflating b.
Selrodo b.
b. syringe
b. and thumb screw valve
b. ureteral catheter
bulb-operated nebulizer
bulbous
b. bougie
b. catheter
bulbous-tip ear syringe
Bulkee
B. II gauze bandage
B. super fluff sponge
bulky
b. compressive dressing
b. hand dressing
b. pressure dressing
Bullard intubating laryngoscope
bulldog
b. clamp
b. clamp-applying forceps
b. scissors
Buller
B. bandage
B. eye shield
bullet
b. forceps
b. probe
b. tip catheter
bullet-shaped cannula
Bullseye femoral guide

Bulnes-Sanchez retractor
Bumgardner dental holder
Bumm
B. placental curette
B. uterine curette
bumper
PEG b.
b. wedge
Bumpus specimen forceps
Buncke quartz needle
Bunegin-Albin pressure catheter
Bunge
B. curette
B. evisceration spoon
B. exenteration spoon
B. scissors
B. ureteral meatotome
Bunim urethral forceps
bunion
b. last
b. shield
Bunke clamp
Bunker
B. implant
B. modification of Jackson
laryngeal forceps
Bunke-Schulz clamp approximator
Bunnell
B. active hand splint
B. anvil
B. block
B. bone drill
B. digital exertion measurer
B. dissecting probe
B. dressing
B. finger extension splint
B. finger loop
B. forwarding probe
B. gutter splint
B. hand drill
B. knuckle bender
B. knuckle-bender splint
B. outrigger splint
B. pull-out wire
B. reverse knuckle bender splint
B. safety-pin splint
B. tendon needle
B. tendon passer
B. tendon stripper
B. wire pull-out suture
Bunnell-Howard arthrodesis clamp
Bunnell-Littler dressing
Bunny Boot foot splint
Bunsen burner
Bunt
B. catheter
B. forceps holder
B. tendon stripper
Bunyan bag

B

bur

abrader b.
Accorde b.
acromionizer b.
Acrotorque b.
Adson b.
Adson perforating b.
Adson-Rogers cranial b.
aftercataract b.
Albee olive-shaped b.
Alfonso guarded b.
Allport cutting b.
antral b.
artificial b.
Bailey skull b.
Ballenger-Lillie mastoid b.
Ballenger mastoid b.
barrel b.
barrel cutting b.
bone b.
Borchardt olive-shaped b.
Brunswick-Mack b.
b. brush
Bud b.
Caparosa cutting b.
carbide finishing b.
cataract b.
Cavanaugh-Israel b.
Cavanaugh sphenoid b.
choanal b.
coarse carbide cone b.
coarse-olive b.
cone b.
conical b.
corneal foreign body b.
countersink b.
cranial b.
Cross corneal b.
Cushing cranial b.
cutting b.
cylindrical b.
Davidson b.
decortication b.
Densco b.
dental b.
dentate b.
denture vulcanite b.
dermabrasion b.
D'Errico perforating b.
diamond b.
diamond-coated b.
diamond-dust b.

diamond finishing b.
Doyen cylindrical b.
Doyen spherical b.
b. drill
Dyonics arthroplasty b.
endodontic b.
enlarging b.
eustachian b.
excavating b.
Farrior b.
Feldman b.
fenestration b.
Ferris-Smith-Halle sinus b.
FG diamond b.
fine olive b.
finishing b.
Fisch cutting b.
fissure b.
flame b.
fluted finishing b.
foreign body b.
friction grip diamond b.
Gam-Mer b.
Gates-Glidden b.
gold b.
guarded b.
Guilford-Wright b.
Hall bone b.
Hall mastoid b.
Hannahan b.
Happy podiatric b.
high-speed diamond wheel b.
high-speed tungsten carbide b.
high-speed two-grit b.
high-torque b.
b. hole cover
b. hole transducer
Hough-Wullstein crurotomy saw b.
House b.
House-Wullstein perforating b.
Hudson brace b.
Hudson conical b.
Hudson cranial b.
Hu-Friedy dental b.
inverted cone b.
Jordan-Day cutting b.
Jordan-Day fenestration b.
Jordan-Day polishing b.
Jordan perforating b.
Kopetzky sinus b.
lacrimal sac b.
large nail spicule b.

NOTES

bur *(continued)*
Le Blond R diamond dental b.
Lee diamond b.
Lempert diamond-dust polishing b.
Lempert fenestration b.
Light-Veley b.
Lindemann b.
low-speed Christmas tree
diamond b.
low-speed tapered carbide b.
Martin b.
Masseran trepan b.
mastoid b.
McKenzie enlarging b.
Micro-Aire b.
MTM 2 b.
Mueller b.
neurosurgical b.
Old Smoothie b.
orthopaedic b.
Osteon b.
oval cutting b.
Parapost b.
paronychia b.
Patton b.
pear-shaped b.
perforating b.
pilot b.
pineapple b.
plug-finishing b.
pointed cone b.
polishing b.
primary trimming b.
Redi B.
Red Witch b.
RhinoBur rhinoplasty b.
rhinoplasty diamond b.
rosehead b.
Rosen b.
Rotablator rotating b.
rotary b.
round cutting b.
round diamond b.
Sachs skull b.
Scheer-Wullstein cutting b.
Shannon b.
Shea b.
side-cutting Swanson b.
sinus b.
skull b.
slotting b.
small nail spicule b.
Smoothie Junior b.
Somerset b.
sphenoidal b.
spherical b.
spiral fluted tungsten carbide b.
Starlite Omni-AT b.
Stille b.
Storz corneal b.
straight fissure crosscut b.
straight shank b.
Stryker b.
Stumer perforating b.
Supercut diamond b.
surgical b.
Surgitome b.
tapered fissure b.
Thomas b.
tungsten carbide b.
Turbo-Jet dental b.
vulcanite b.
Wachsberger b.
wheel b.
Wilkerson choanal b.
Worst corneal b.
Wullstein diamond b.
Wullstein high-speed b.
Yazujian cataract b.
Zimmer b.

Buratto
B. flap forceps
B. flap protector
B. irrigating cannula
B. LASIK forceps
B. LASIK irrigating cannula
B. ophthalmic forceps

bur-bearing catheter

Burch
B. biopsy forceps
B. eye calipers
B. fixation fork
B. fixation pick
B. hook
B. ophthalmic pick
B. tendon tucker

Burch-Greenwood tendon tucker

Burch-Schneider antiprotrusio cage

Burdick
B. cautery
B. Eclipse ECG machine
B. microwave diathermy
electrosurgical unit

Buretrol solution set

Burette multiple patient delivery system

Burford
B. clamp
B. coarctation forceps
B. rib retractor
B. rib spreader

Burford-Finochietto infant rib spreader

Burford-Lebsche sternal knife

Burgess Vibro-Graver

Burget nasal splint

Burge vagotometer

Burhenne steerable catheter

Burian-Allen
    B.-A. contact lens
    B.-A. contact lens electrode
Burkard spore trap
Burke
    B. bariatric treatment system powered bariatric bed
    B. Plus frameless air support therapy
    B. plus low-air-loss bed
burlisher clamp
burner
    Bunsen b.
Burnett
    B. anoscope
    B. applicator
    B. bidirectional TMJ device
    B. cylinder
    B. mouth positioning device
    B. Pap smear kit
    B. Sani-Spec disposable speculum
Burnham
    B. bandage scissors
    B. biopsy forceps
burnisher
    agate b.
    amalgam b.
    ball b.
    beaver-tail b.
    fishtail b.
    fissure b.
    flat b.
    gold b.
    Nordent b.
    SMIC b.
    straight b.
Burn Jel dressing
Burns
    B. bone forceps
    B. bridge telescope
    B. chisel
    B. converting bridge
    B. prism bar
burr
    B. butterfly needle
    B. corneal ring
    B. silicone button
Burron stopcock
burst pacemaker
Burton
    B. Electricator electrosurgical unit

    B. laryngoscope
    B. osteotome
Busch umbilical cord scissors
Buselmeier shunt
B.U.S. Endotron-Lipectron ultrasonic liposuction
Busenkell posterior hip retractor
Bushey compression clamp
bushing
    patellar planer b.
    reamer b.
    Uniflex drill b.
Bush intervertebral curette
Buster
    Amplatz Clot B.
Butcher saw
Butler
    B. bayonet forceps
    B. dental retractor
    B. pillar retractor
    B. stimulator
    B. tonsillar suction tube
Butte dissector
Butterfield cystoscope
butterfly
    b. adapter
    b. bandage
    b. catheter
    b. clip
    B. cushion
    b. drain
    b. dressing
    b. needle
    b. needle infusion port
butterfly-shaped monoblock vertebral plate
Butterworth bidirectional four-pole high-pass digital filter
button
    Accu-Flo b.
    anastomotic b.
    Barouk b.
    Bentley b.
    Bivona-Colorado b.
    Boari b.
    bobbin-type laryngectomy b.
    Burr silicone b.
    Charnley suture b.
    Chlumsky b.
    collar b.
    Converse fracture-wiring b.
    coronary artery b.

NOTES

button *(continued)*
    DiaTap vascular access b.
    Drummond b.
    b. electrode
    Emesay suture b.
    Endobutton 6 b.
    fixation b.
    gastrostomy b.
    b. gastrostomy device
    Groningen b.
    Helsper laryngectomy b.
    b. hook
    Husen b.
    Jaboulay b.
    Kazanjian tooth b.
    Kistner tracheal b.
    Lardennois b.
    Lee lingual b.
    ligament b.
    Moore tracheostomy b.
    Murphy-Johnson anastomosis b.
    Norris b.
    B. One-Step gastrostomy device
    Panje voice b.
    patellar b.
    peritoneal b.
    Perspex b.
    polyethylene collar b.
    polypropylene b.
    pull-out b.
    Reuter bobbin collar b.
    Sheehy collar b.
    Silastic suture b.
    silicone b.
    Smithwick buttonhook b.
    b. spacer
    stoma b.
    Surgitek b.
    suture b.
    Teflon collar b.
    tracheal b.
    tracheostomy b.
    Villard b.
    voice b.
buttoned device

button-end knife
buttonhook
    b. nerve retractor
    Smithwick b.
button-tip manipulator
button-type G-tube
buttress
    Omni pretibial b.
    b. pad
    b. plate
    pretibial b. (PTB)
    Rotator Cuff B. (RCB)
    Teflon pledget suture b.
buttressed hook
buttress-type plate
butyl cyanoacrylate glue
Buxton
    B. clamp
    B. uterine clamp
Buzard-Barraquer Diamond
   Microkeratome system
Buzard-Thornton fixation ring
BVI neurosurgical dissection kit
BVM
    bag-valve-mask
    BVM device
BVS-5000 biventricular support system
BVS pump
BWM spine system
Bx
    Bx IsoStent stent
    Bx Sonic coronary stent
    Bx Velocity coronary artery stent
Byars mandibular prosthesis
Bycep PC Jr bioptome
Bycroft-Brunswick thyroid retractor
Byford retractor
bypass
    b. connector
    b. graft catheter
    b. machine
    b. Speedy balloon catheter
Byrel SX/Versatrax pacemaker
Byrne expulsive hemorrhage lens

C.
C. B. T. bumper wedge
C. L. Jackson head-holding forceps
C. L. Jackson pin-bending
   costophrenic forceps
C. R. Bard catheter
C. R. Bard Urolase fiber
C-2 OsteoCap hip prosthesis
CA-6000 spine motion analyzer
CAAS
Cardiovascular Angiography Analysis
   System
CAB
competitive ankle board
CABG
coronary artery bypass graft
Aria CABG
cabin
magnetic shielded c.
cabinet
grid c.
c. respirator
cable
Bagby and Kuslich c.
Bicomatic bipolar c.
braided Spectra UHMWPE
   surgical c.
braided titanium c.
chrome-cobalt c.
coaxial c.
Dall-Miles c.
ESI Lite-Pipe fiberoptic c.
European bipolar c.
fiberoptic light c.
FlexStrand c.
Gallie fusion-using c.
c. graft
internal fiberoptic c.
interspinous c.
Oklahoma City c.
OxyLead interconnect c.
SecureStrand c.
Songer c.
Sullivan variable stiffness c.
c. system
c. tie
titanium c.
c. wire suture
world standard Olsen bipolar c.
cable-twister orthosis
Cabot
C. cannula
C. leg splint
C. Medical Corporation
   diagnostic/operating laparoscope

C. nephroscope
C. Optima laparoscopic Roticulator
C. trocar
CADD
continuous ambulatory drug delivery
caddie
Cath C.
SwingAlong walker c.
CADD-Plus intravenous infusion pump
CADD-Prizm pain control system
CADD-TPN
CADD-TPN ambulatory infusion
   system
CADD-TPN pump
Cadence
C. AICD
C. biphasic ICD
C. defibrillator
C. implantable cardioverter-
   defibrillator
C. tiered therapy defibrillator
   system
C. TVL nonthoracotomy lead
Cadet
C. defibrillator
C. V-115 implantable cardioverter-
   defibrillator
Cadlow shoulder stabilizer
cadmium
c. iodide detector
c. selenide Vidicon video camera
**Cadogan-Hough footpedal suction
   control**
**Cadwell 5200A somatosensory evoked
   potential unit**
**CADx SecondLook computer-aided
   detection system**
CAFET
Computer-Aided Fluency Establishment
   Training
CAFET speech therapy system
Caffinière prosthesis
cage
antiprotrusio c.
Bagby and Kuslich c.
BAK c.
BAK/C cervical interbody fusion c.
Burch-Schneider antiprotrusio c.
carbon fiber composite c.
DePuy Lumbar I/V c.
derotation knee c.
Faraday c.
fusion c.
Harm c.
Inter Fix threaded spinal fusion c.

cage *(continued)*
    Link acetabular c.
    lumbar interbody fusion c.
    lumbar intersomatic fusion
      expandable c.
    metallic c.
    Moss c.
    Motech c.
    nonmetallic c.
    Novus LC threaded interbody
      fusion c.
    Polaris c.
    protrusio c.
    Pyramesh c.
    Ray threaded fusion c.
    stereolithography c.
    Swedish knee c.
    thoracic c.
    threaded interbody fusion c.
    titanium c.
    VariLift spinal c.
caged-ball
    c.-b. heart valve
    c.-b. valve prosthesis
CAH
    Camber axis hinge
Caire Breeze oxygen concentrator
Cairns
    C. clamp
    C. dissection forceps
    C. hemostatic forceps
    C. rongeur
    C. scalp retractor
Cairns-Dandy hemostasis forceps
Cairpad incontinence pad
Cajal axonal retraction ball
"cake mix" kit
Calandruccio
    C. clamp
    C. II compression device
    C. triangular compression fixation
      device
Calasept delivery system
calcaneal
    c. spreader
    c. spur cookie orthosis
calcaneonavicular bar
calcar
    c. planer
    c. reamer
    c. replacement implant
    c. stem
    c. trimmer
Cal-Chek CD Plus hematology
    calibrator
calcified tissue scissors
Calcigen-S calcium sulfate bone
    substitute
Calcipulpe calcium hydroxide paste

Calcitek
    C. drill
    C. implant
    C. implant system
    C. retaining screw
    C. spline
Calcitite
    C. bone graft
    C. bone replacement
calcium
    c. alginate swab
    c. phosphate ceramic implant
    c. sodium alginate wound dressing
Calculair spirometer
Calcusplit pneumatic lithotripter
Calcutript electrohydraulic lithotripter
Caldwell
    C. guide
    C. hanging cast
Calgiswab calcium alginate swab
Calgitrol dressing
Calhoun-Hagler lens needle
Calhoun-Merz needle
Calhoun needle
calibrated
    c. clubfoot splint
    c. depth gauge
    c. grasping tube
    c. pin
    c. probe
    c. V-Lok cuff
calibrator
    Cal-Chek CD Plus hematology c.
    Fogarty c.
    isotope c.
    radioisotope c.
    screw depth c.
Calibri forceps
California hatchet
Caligamed
    C. ankle orthosis
    C. brace
calipers
    AccuGage vessel c.
    Albee bone graft c.
    Austin Moore inside-outside c.
    Austin strut c.
    Barker c.
    Berens marking c.
    Bertillon c.
    c. block
    bone c.
    bone-measuring c.
    Braunstein fixed c.
    breast c.
    Brown and Sharp digital
      electronic c.
    Burch eye c.
    Castroviejo marking c.

Castroviejo-Schacher angled c.
Cone ice-tong c.
Cottle c.
digital c.
EKG c.
electronic c.
eye c.
Fat-O-Meter skinfold c.
Green eye c.
Harpenden skinfold c.
House strut c.
ice-tong c.
Jameson eye c.
John Green c.
Kapp Surgical Instrument total
   hip c.
Ladd c.
Lafayette skinfold c.
Lange skinfold c.
Machemer c.
McGaw skinfold c.
Mendez degree c.
Mipron digital computer-assisted c.
Mitutoyo Digimatic c.
Miyajima LASIK c.
ophthalmic c.
Osher internal c.
Paparella rasp c.
restraint c.
Ruddy stapes c.
ruler c.
Sentalloy digital c.
skinfold c.
Stahl ophthalmic c.
Storz c.
strut c.
Tenzel c.
Tesa S.A. handheld electronic
   digital c.
Thomas c.
Thorpe c.
Thorpe-Castroviejo c.
tibial c.
Townley c.
Vernier c.
V. Mueller ruler c.
x-ray c.
Cali-Press graft press
Callahan
   C. flange
   C. lacrimal rongeur
   C. lens loop

C. lens loupe
   C. modification speculum
   C. retractor
   C. scleral fixation forceps
Callender
   C. clip
   C. derotational brace
   C. technique hip prosthesis
Callison-Adson tissue forceps
Calman
   C. carotid clamp
   C. ring clamp
Calnan-Nicolle synthetic digital joint
   prosthesis
calomel electrode
calorimeter
   bench scale c.
   Benedict-Roth c.
   differential scanning c.
   MedGem c.
   Scientech c.
Calot jacket
Caltagirone
   C. chisel
   C. skin graft knife
Caltrac accelerometer
Caluso PEG gastrostomy tube
calvarial clamp
Calve cannula
Calvitron hair replacement system
Calypso Rely catheter
CAM
   controlled ankle motion
   CAM lock knee brace
   CAM stimulator
   CAM Walker
   CAM Walker II boot
   CAM Walker leg brace
Camber axis hinge (CAH)
Cambridge
   C. acuity card
   C. defibrillator
   C. electrocardiograph
   C. jelly electrode
Cameco syringe pistol aspiration device
CA membrane hollow-fiber dialyzer
camera
   ADAC Forte gamma c.
   ADAC SPECT c.
   ADAC Vertex Plus MCD/AC
      gamma c.
   AMS Endoview c.

C

NOTES

camera *(continued)*
Anger scintillation c.
Beaulieu c.
Biad c.
Bio-Optics c.
Bolex cine c.
Brenman c.
cadmium selenide Vidicon video c.
Canon CF-60U fundus c.
Carl Zeiss Jena fundus c.
CeraSPECT c.
CFA digital c.
charge-coupled device video c.
CIDtech c.
cine c.
Circon ACMI MicroDigital-I c.
Circon video c.
Coburn c.
CompuCam digital intraoral c.
CooperVision c.
Cr6-45NMf retinal c.
crystal gamma c.
CTI-Siemens 933/08-12 PET c.
Dental Pro II c.
DentCAM dental c.
Digirad gamma c.
DigiScope c.
Dine SLR digital c.
Docustar fundus c.
Donaldson fundus c.
DSX Sopha c.
dual-head coincidence c.
dual-head gamma c.
DyoCam 550 arthroscopic video c.
E.CAM photon emission c.
electron diffraction c.
Elmo c.
Elscint dual-detector cardiac c.
Endius spinal c.
Endocam digital c.
EndoVideo-Five endoscopic c.
EndoView c.
Endo zoom lens c.
Eyecor c.
field-of-view c.
Fujica c.
fundus c.
gamma c.
gamma scintillation c.
gantry-free gamma c.
GE Maxicamera gamma c.
Genesys Vertex variable angle
  gamma c.
GE single-detector SPECT-
  capable c.
GE Starcam single-crystal
  tomographic scintillation c.
Haifa c.
handheld fundus c.
Handy non-mydriatic video
  fundus c.
4-head c.
HealthCam 2 c.
Helix c.
Hitachi SPECT 2000H-40
  gamma c.
Holofax Oxford retroillumination
  cataract c.
House-Urban microsurgery cine c.
House-Urban-Pentax c.
House-Urban-Stille c.
House-Urban UEM-100 cine c.
hybrid PET/SPECT c.
Icarex 25 Med mirror reflex
  lens c.
immersible video c.
infrared c.
integral uniformity scintillation c.
Isocon c.
Israel c.
Keeler c.
Kowa angiographic c.
Kowa fundus c.
Kowa hand c.
Kowa-Optimed c.
Kowa PRO II retinal c.
Kowa RC-XV fundus c.
large field-of-view gamma c.
Leicaflex c.
Lester A. Dine c.
Macro-5 c.
MedCam Pro Plus video c.
Medicam c.
MedX c.
Micro-Imager high-resolution
  digital c.
MLR+ c.
multicrystal gamma c.
multiwire gamma c.
MyoSIGHT nuclear cardiology c.
Neitz CT-R cataract c.
Nidek 3Dx c.
Nikon microprocessor-controlled c.
Nikon Retinopan fundus c.
nuclear medicine c.
Odelca c.
Olympus OM-1 endoscopic c.
Olympus operating c.
Olympus OTV-S-series miniature c.
ophthalmoscope c.
Orthicon c.
Pentax Spotmatic c.
PET/SPECT c.
Picker c.
pinhole c.
Pixsys FlashPoint c.
Polaroid CB-100 c.
positron scintillation c.

Prism 2000XP gamma c.
radioisotope c.
radionuclide c.
RC-2 fundus c.
Reflec UV instant c.
Reichert c.
Release-NF c.
Retcam 120 digital c.
Retinopan 45 c.
Reveal MLR+ c.
Reveal single lens reflex c.
Robot Starr II c.
Rotacamera c.
rotating gamma c.
Scheimpflug c.
Schepens binocular indirect c.
Scinticore multicrystal
    scintillation c.
scintillation c.
Siemens Orbiter gamma c.
single-crystal gamma c.
single-head rotating gamma c.
single-head SPECT c.
Skylight gantry-free nuclear
    medicine gamma c.
slip-ring c.
Sony CCD/RGB DXC-151 color
    video c.
Sopha Medical gamma c.
SPECT c.
StarCam c.
SteriCam Endoscopic c.
Storz c.
Strichman SME-810 c.
Stryker chip c.
Syn-optics c.
Technicare c.
Technicare Omega 500 gamma c.
telecentric fundus c.
TeliCam intraoral c.
time-of-flight positron emission
    tomographic c.
Topcon stereoscopic TRC-series
    fundus c.
Trionix c.
triple-head gamma c.
TroCam endoscopic c.
Urocam video c.
variable-angle gamma c.
Vertex c.
Vertex Plus MCD/AC gamma c.
video display c.

Virtuoso shape c.
Vision c.
Yashica Dental Eye II c.
Zeiss FF450 fundus c.
Zeiss-Nordenson fundus c.
Zeiss operating c.
Zeiss-Scheimpflug c.
Cameron
    C. cautery
    C. elevator
    C. fracture device
    C. omni-angle gastroscope
    C. periosteal elevator
Cameron-Haight periosteal elevator
Cameron-Miller
    C.-M. electrode
    C.-M. monopolar forceps
Camey reservoir
Camino
    C. catheter-tip transducer
    C. fiberoptic ICP monitor
    C. intracranial catheter
    C. intracranial pressure monitor
    C. intracranial pressure probe
    C. intraparenchymal fiberoptic
        device
    C. micromanometer catheter
    C. microventricular bolt
    C. OLM intracranial pressure
        monitor
    C. postcraniotomy subdural pressure
        monitor
    C. subdural screw
    C. transducer catheter
Cammann stethoscope
Camo disposable dental splint
camouflage prosthesis
Campbell
    C. airplane splint
    C. arthroplasty gouge
    C. graft
    C. infant catheter
    C. lacrimal sac retractor
    C. laminectomy rongeur
    C. ligature-carrier forceps
    C. miniature urethral sound
    C. nerve rongeur
    C. nerve root retractor
    C. osteotome
    C. periosteal elevator
    C. refractor
    C. self-retaining retractor

NOTES

Campbell *(continued)*
- C. slit lamp
- C. suprapubic cannula
- C. suprapubic retractor
- C. suprapubic trocar
- C. traction splint
- C. ureteral forceps
- C. ureterotome
- C. ventricular needle

Campbell-Boyd
- C.-B. pneumatic tourniquet
- C.-B. tourniquet

Campbell-French sound
Campbell-type Heyman fundus applicator
Camp brace
campimeter
- Damato c.
- Goldman c.
- Gringnolo-Tagliasco-Zingirian projection c.
- stereo c.

Camp-Sigvaris stocking
CamStar
- C. power leg press
- C. rotary twist
- C. 8-way cervical exercise machine

Cam tent
Canadian
- C. chest retractor
- C. hip disarticulation prosthesis
- C. Ibex quilted underpad
- C. serial knee orthosis

Canad meniscal knife
Canakis
- C. beaded hip pin
- C. wrench

canal
- c. chisel
- completely in c. (CIC)
- c. finder system
- c. knife
- C. Master drill
- c. reamer

canalicular scissors
canaliculus
- c. dilator
- c. knife
- c. probe

Canal-Mate hearing aid
Can-Am brace
cancellous
- c. bone screw
- c. pin

Cancer and Blood Institute (CBI)
Candela
- C. AlexLAZR
- C. C-beam laser
- C. dynamic cooling device

- C. laser
- C. laser lithotripter
- C. miniscope
- C. MOL Lasertripter laser
- C. pulsed dye laser
- C. ScleroLaser laser
- C. videoimaging system

candle
- cesium c.
- vaginal c.
- c. vaginal cesium implant

Can-Do exercise band
candy
- C. Cane cannula
- c. cane stirrups

cane
- C. bone-holding forceps
- large-base quad c.
- MAFO c.
- molded ankle-foot orthosis c.
- narrow-base quad c.
- offset c.
- SBQC c.
- single-base c.
- small-based quad c.
- wide-base quad c.

Canfield
- C. facial plastics garment
- C. tonsillar knife

cannister, canister
- Bemis suction c.
- Lipovacutainer c.
- Sep-T-Vac suction c.
- Sorensen reusable c.

Cannon
- C. Bio-Flek nasal splint
- C. endarterectomy loop

Cannon-Rochester lamina elevator
CannuFlex guidewire
cannula
- Abelson cricothyrotomy c.
- Abraham laryngeal c.
- Access needle stiffening c.
- Accu-Flo U-channel stripping c.
- Accu-Flo ventricular c.
- ACMI c.
- acorn c.
- Adson brain c.
- Adson drainage c.
- AE-7277 Rubenstein LASIK c.
- air injection c.
- AirLife nasal c.
- Air-Lon inhalation c.
- Akahoshi hydrodissection c.
- Allen-Brown c.
- alpha-chymotrypsin c.
- angled high-flow aortic c.
- Anis aspirating c.
- anterior chamber irrigating c.

Antoni-Hook lumbar puncture c.
antral sinus c.
aortic arch c.
aortic direct ellipse c.
aortic perfusion c.
aortic root c.
ARC reciprocating c.
Argyle CPAP nasal c.
Aronson-Fletcher antrum c.
arterial c.
Arthrex tibial tunnel c.
arthroscopic c.
aspirating c.
ASSI air-injection c.
Aston-Daniel EndoForehead c.
atrial c.
attic c.
Bahnson aortic c.
Bailey lacrimal c.
balloon cervical c.
Banaji LASIK c.
Bard arterial c.
Bard cervical c.
Bardic c.
Barraquer c.
Barrett hydrodelineation c.
Bechert intraocular lens c.
Becker accelerator c.
Becker aspiration c.
Becker dissector liposuction c.
Becker Greater dissecting c.
Bellocq c.
Bellucci c.
Bergström muscle c.
Berkeley c.
Bilisystem ERCP c.
binasal c.
Binkhorst hooked c.
Binkhorst irrigating c.
biopsy c.
BioTac biopsy c.
Bishop-Harman irrigating c.
bivalved c.
Blue Max c.
Bowers c.
Bracken anterior chamber c.
Bracken irrigating c.
brain biopsy c.
Branula c.
Bresgen c.
Brodney urethrographic c.
Brown sphenoidal c.

Bruening c.
Bucy-Frazier coagulation c.
Bucy-Frazier suction c.
Buie c.
bullet-shaped c.
Buratto irrigating c.
Buratto LASIK irrigating c.
Cabot c.
Calve c.
Campbell suprapubic c.
Candy Cane c.
Cantlie c.
Carabelli mirror c.
cardiovascular c.
Casselberry sphenoid c.
Castaneda c.
Castroviejo cyclodialysis c.
cataract-aspirating c.
caval c.
cerebral c.
cervical c.
Charlton c.
Chilcott venoclysis c.
Christmas tree c.
Churchill cardiac suction c.
Cimochowski cardiac c.
Circon ACMI c.
c. clamp
clysis c.
Coakley frontal sinus c.
coaxial c.
Cobe small vessel c.
Cobra K+ c.
Cobra LASIK irrigating c.
Codman c.
Cohen-Eder uterine c.
Cohen intrauterine c.
Cohen tubal insufflation c.
Cohen uterine c.
Coleman aspiration c.
Coleman infiltration c.
Coleman V-dissector infiltration c.
Colt c.
Concept c.
Concorde disposable c.
Cone-Bucy c.
Cone cerebral c.
Connor silicone oil removal c.
Continental c.
Contour ERCP c.
Cook balloon cervical c.
Cooper chemopallidectomy c.

NOTES

cannula *(continued)*
    Cooper double-lumen c.
    Cope needle introducer c.
    Core Dynamics disposable c.
    coronary artery c.
    coronary perfusion c.
    coronary sinus c.
    cortex-aspirating c.
    cortical cleaving hydrodissector c.
    Corydon HydroExpression c.
    cricothyrotomy c.
    Crystal c.
    cyclodialysis c.
    dacryocystorhinostomy c.
    Dankner Panariello cortex c.
    Day attic c.
    de la Vega vitreous-aspirating c.
    DeRoyal c.
    Devonshire-Mack c.
    DeWecker syringe c.
    Dexide disposable c.
    Digiflex c.
    DirectFlow arterial c.
    disposable c.
    disposable cystotome c.
    disposable inner c. (DIC)
    DLP aortic root c.
    Dorsey ventricular c.
    double-barreled irrigating-
      aspirating c.
    double-lumen c.
    double-lumen irrigation c.
    Dougherty anterior chamber c.
    Douglas c.
    Dow Corning c.
    Drews irrigating c.
    Duke c.
    Dulaney antral c.
    duodenoscope c.
    Dwellcath c.
    ear c.
    ECMO c.
    egress c.
    Elecath ECMO c.
    Elsberg ventricular c.
    Embol-X arterial c.
    endometrial c.
    Endo-Pool suction c.
    EndoTIP access c.
    Endotrac c.
    Entree II c.
    Entree Plus c.
    ERCP c.
    Eriksson muscle biopsy c.
    esophagoscopic c.
    Ethicon disposable c.
    Everett fallopian c.
    exploring c.
    fallopian c.

    Fasanella lacrimal c.
    Feaster K7-5460 hydrodissecting c.
    Fein c.
    femoral artery c.
    femoral perfusion c.
    Fink cul-de-sac c.
    Fish infusion c.
    flattened irrigating c.
    Flexi-Cath silicone subclavian c.
    Floyd loop c.
    Fluoro Tip ERCP c.
    flute c.
    Ford Hospital ventricular c.
    Franklin-Silverman biopsy c.
    Frazier brain-exploring c.
    Frazier suction c.
    Frazier ventricular c.
    Freeman Blue-Max c.
    Freeman positioning c.
    frontal sinus c.
    frontal sinus wash c.
    Fujita suction c.
    gallbladder c.
    Galt aspirating c.
    Gans cyclodialysis c.
    Gass cataract-aspirating c.
    Gass retinal detachment c.
    Gass vitreous-aspirating c.
    Gesco c.
    Gill double I&A c.
    Gill double Luer-Lok c.
    Gill sinus c.
    Gill-Welsh double c.
    Gill-Welsh irrigation-aspiration c.
    Gill-Welsh olive-tip c.
    Gimbel fountain c.
    Girard irrigating c.
    Goldstein anterior chamber c.
    Goldstein irrigating c.
    Goldstein lacrimal c.
    golf tee hollow titanium c.
    goniotomy knife c.
    Gott c.
    Grafco c.
    gravity infusion c.
    Gregg c.
    Grinfeld c.
    Grizzard subretinal c.
    Grüntzig femoral stiffening c.
    guiding c.
    Gulani triple function laser-assisted
      intrastromal keratomileusis c.
    Gulani triple function LASIK c.
    Gundry c.
    Hahn c.
    Hajek c.
    Hanscom transscleral c.
    Harvard c.
    Hasson c.

Hasson balloon uterine elevator c.
Hasson blunt-end c.
Hasson-Eder laparoscopy c.
Hasson open-laparoscopy c.
Hasson stable access c.
Haverfield brain c.
Havlicek spiral c.
Haynes brain c.
Healon injection c.
Heartport-Endoclamp balloon c.
Heartport endovenous drainage c.
Hendon venoclysis c.
Hepacon c.
Heyer-Schulte-Fischer ventricular c.
Heyner c.
high-flow coaxial c.
Hilton self-retaining sutureless
  infusion c.
Hirschman hooked c.
Hoen ventricular c.
Hoffer forward-cutting knife c.
3-hole aspiration c.
Holinger c.
Holman-Mathieu salpingography c.
Hudgins salpingography c.
Hudson All-Clear nasal c.
Hulka uterine c.
Hulten-Stille c.
HUMI c.
Hunt-Reich secondary c.
Huse c.
Hyde irrigating-aspirating c.
hydrodelineation c.
hydrodissection c.
I&A coaxial c.
Illouz suction c.
indwelling c.
infiltration c.
inflow c.
infusion c.
Ingals antral c.
Ingals flexible silver c.
Ingals rectal injection c.
ingress/egress c.
inhalation c.
injection c.
Interlink lever lock c.
Interlink threaded lock c.
Interlink vial access c.
intraarterial c.
intracardiac c.
Intraducer peritoneal c.

intragastric c.
intraocular lens c.
intrauterine balloon c.
intrauterine insemination c.
Ipas flexible c.
iris hook c.
irrigating c.
irrigating-aspirating c.
irrigation c.
I-tech c.
IUI disposable c.
Jarcho self-retaining uterine c.
Jarit air injection c.
Jarit lacrimal c.
Jensen-Thomas I&A c.
Jensen-Thomas irrigating-
  aspirating c.
Jetco spray c.
Johnson double c.
J-shaped I&A c.
Judd c.
Kahn uterine trigger c.
Kanavel brain-exploring c.
Kara cataract-aspirating c.
Karickhoff double c.
Karman c.
Katena c.
Katzenstein rectal c.
KDF-2.3 intrauterine
  insemination c.
Keeler-Keislar lacrimal c.
Keisler lacrimal c.
Kellan hydrodissection c.
Kelman cyclodialysis c.
Kesilar c.
Keyes-Ultzmann-Luer c.
Khouri hydrodissection c.
Kidde uterine c.
Killian antral c.
Killian antrum c.
Killian-Eichen c.
Killian nasal c.
Kleegman c.
Klein curved c.
Knolle anterior chamber
  irrigating c.
Knolle-Pearce c.
Kos attic c.
Kraff cortex c.
Krause nasal snare c.
Kreutzmann c.
lacrimal irrigating c.

C

NOTES

cannula *(continued)*
    Lamb c.
    Landolt c.
    laparoscopic c.
    large antral c.
    large-bore c.
    laryngeal c.
    laser-assisted intrastromal
      keratomileusis c.
    LASIK Lindstrom irrigating c.
    Leon cobra c.
    Lewicky threaded infusion c.
    Lichtwicz antral c.
    Lifemed c.
    ligature c.
    Lillie attic c.
    Lindemann self-retaining uterine
      vacuum c.
    Linvatec c.
    liquid vitreous-aspirating c.
    Littell c.
    Litwak c.
    Look I&A coaxial c.
    Lübke uterine vacuum c.
    Luer tracheal c.
    Lukens c.
    lumen c.
    Luongo sphenoid irrigating c.
    LV apex c.
    Makler c.
    Malette-Spencer coronary c.
    Malstrm-Westman c.
    Mandelbaum c.
    Marlow disposable c.
    Maumenee goniotomy c.
    maxillary sinus c.
    Mayo coronary perfusion c.
    Mayo-Ochsner c.
    McCain TMJ c.
    McCaskey sphenoid c.
    McGoon c.
    McIntyre anterior chamber c.
    McIntyre-Binkhorst irrigating c.
    McIntyre coaxial c.
    McIntyre lacrimal c.
    mediastinal c.
    Medicut c.
    Medi-Tech flexible stiffening c.
    Menghini c.
    Mercedes tip c.
    metal c.
    metal-ball tip c.
    mirror c.
    Mladick concave c.
    Mladick convex c.
    Moehle c.
    Moncrieff anterior chamber
      irrigating c.
    Montgomery tracheal c.

Morris c.
Morwel c.
Mueller coronary perfusion c.
MultAport c.
MVS c.
Myerson-Moncrieff c.
Myles sinus c.
nasal c.
nasal snare c.
Neal fallopian c.
Neubauer lancet c.
New York Eye and Ear c.
Nichamin hydrodissection c.
Nichamin LASIK irrigating c.
nucleus delivery c.
Oaks double straight c.
O'Gawa cataract-aspirating c.
O'Gawa irrigating c.
O'Gawa two-way I&A c.
olive-tipped c.
Olympus disposable c.
O'Malley-Heintz infusion c.
Osher air-bubble removal c.
Osher lens-vacuuming c.
outflow c.
outlet c.
Pacifico c.
Packo pars plana c.
Padgett-Concorde suction c.
Padgett shark-mouth c.
Park irrigating c.
Paterson laryngeal c.
Patton c.
Pautler infusion c.
Peacekeeper c.
Pearce coaxial I&A c.
Peczon I&A c.
Pemco c.
Pereyra ligature c.
perfusion c.
Pierce attic c.
Pinto superficial dissection c.
plastic c.
polyethylene c.
Polystan perfusion c.
portal c.
Portex nylon c.
Portnoy ventricular c.
Power c.
Pritchard c.
ProForma c.
Pye c.
Pynchon c.
pyramid c.
quad-ported LASIK irrigating c.
QuickDraw venous c.
Rabinov c.
Ramirez Silastic c.
Ramirez telescoping c.

Randolph cyclodialysis c.
Ranfac stiffening c.
RAP c.
Reddick-Saye c.
reel aspiration c.
Reipen c.
remote access perfusion c.
Research Medical straight multiple-
holed aortic c.
return-flow c.
Rica tracheostomy c.
Rigg c.
Riordan flexible silver c.
Robb antral c.
Robles cutting point c.
Rockey mediastinal c.
Rockey tracheal c.
Rohrschneider c.
Rolf-Jackson c.
Roper alpha-chymotrypsin c.
Rosenberg dissecting c.
Rowsey fixation c.
Rubin fallopian tube c.
Rycroft c.
Sachs brain-exploring c.
saphenous vein c.
Sarns aortic arch c.
Sarns soft-flow aortic c.
Sarns 2-stage c.
Sarns venous drainage c.
Schanz c.
Scheie anterior chamber c.
Scheie cataract-aspirating c.
c. scissors
Scott attic c.
Scott rubber ventricular c.
Sedan-Nashold biopsy c.
Seibel LASIK flap irrigator and
squeegee c.
Seletz ventricular c.
self-retaining infusion c.
self-retaining irrigating c.
self-sealing c.
Semm uterine vacuum c.
Sewall antral c.
Shahinian lacrimal c.
shark-mouth c.
Sheets irrigating vectis c.
Shepard incision irrigating c.
Shepard radial keratotomy
irrigating c.
side-cutting c.

sideport c.
sidewall infusion c.
Silastic coronary artery c.
silicone c.
silicone oil removal c.
Silverman-Boeker c.
Silver trachea c.
Simcoe cortex c.
Simcoe double-barreled c.
Simcoe II PC double c.
Simcoe nucleus delivery c.
Simcoe reverse-aperture c.
Simcoe reverse I&A c.
Sims c.
single-lumen c.
sinoscopy c.
sinus antral c.
sinus irrigating c.
Skillern sphenoid c.
Slade c.
Sluijter-Mehta SMK-C10 c.
small-bore c.
soft-tipped c.
soft tissue shaving c.
Soresi c.
Southey c.
SpaceSEAL balloon tip c.
spatula c.
Spencer c.
sphenoid c.
sphenoidal c.
Spielberg sinus c.
Spizziri-Simcoe c.
stable access c.
2-stage c.
2-stage Sarns c.
Stangel fallopian tube c.
step-down c.
Steriseal disposable c.
Storz c.
straightening c.
straight lacrimal c.
StraightShot arterial c.
Strauss c.
subclavian c.
subretinal fluid c.
sub-tenon anesthesia c.
suction c.
suprapubic c.
surgical c.
Swets goniotomy c.
Sylva irrigating c.

NOTES

cannula *(continued)*

TAC2 atrial caval c.
Tandem XL triple-lumen ERCP c.
Teflon ERCP c.
Tenner lacrimal c.
Ternamian EndoTIP access c.
Texas c.
Thomas I&A c.
Thora-Port c.
Thurmond nucleus-irrigating c.
Tibbs arterial c.
Toledo V-dissector c.
Tomey angled c.
Tomey G-bevel c.
Topper c.
Torchia nucleus-aspirating c.
tracheal c.
tracheostomy c.
tracheotomy c.
transseptal c.
Tremble sphenoid c.
Trendelenburg c.
Trevisani c.
TriEye c.
trigeminus c.
trigger c.
Tri-Port sub-Tenon anesthesia c.
Trocan disposable CO_2 trocar
  and c.
Troutman alpha-chymotrypsin c.
trumpet valve c.
TruPro c.
tubal insufflation c.
Tulevech lacrimal c.
Turnbull c.
Ulanday double c.
Uldall subclavian hemodialysis c.
Ultra-Sil c.
Unitech Toomey c.
Unitri c.
Universal c.
urethral instillation c.
urethrographic c.
USCI c.
U-shaped c.
uterine c.
uterine self-retaining c.
uterine vacuum c.
Vabra c.
vacuum c.
vacuum intrauterine c.
Van Alyea antral c.
Van Alyea frontal sinus c.
Van Alyea sphenoid c.
Vancaillie uterine c.
Vance prostatic aspiration c.
Van Osdel irrigating c.
vein graft c.
Veirs c.

vena caval c.
Venflon c.
venoclysis c.
venous c.
ventricular c.
Veress laparoscopic c.
Veress peritoneum c.
Vidaurri c.
Viking c.
Viscoflow angled c.
Visitec anterior chamber c.
Visitec I&A c.
Vitalcor cardioplegia infusion c.
vitreous aspirating c.
von Eichen antral c.
Wallace Flexihub central venous
  pressure c.
washout c.
Webb c.
Webster infusion c.
Weck disposable c.
Weil lacrimal c.
Weiner c.
Weisman c.
Wells Johnson c.
Welsh cortex-stripper c.
Welsh flat olive-tipped double c.
Wergeland double c.
West lacrimal c.
Wisap disposable c.
Wolf disposable c.
Wolf drainage c.
Wolf return-flow c.
Ximed disposable c.
Yamagishi viscocanalostomy c.
Yankauer middle meatus c.
Zinn endoillumination infusion c.
Zylik c.

cannulated

c. bolt
c. bone tunnel plug
c. cancellous lag screw
c. drill bit
c. nail
c. obturator
c. pin cutter
C. Plus screw system
c. reamer
c. screw system

cannulation catheter
cannulatome

Cotton c.

Canon

C. autorefraction keratometer
C. auto refractometer
C. CF-60U fundus camera
C. K1 autokeratometer
C. perimeter

C. refractor
C. scanner
Can-Opt
    C.-O. dual-lumen ERCP system
    C.-O. stand-alone dual lumen ERCP catheter
canted finger hook
Cantlie cannula
Cantor intestinal tube
canvas brace
Canyons wound irrigation system
cap
    Active Life 1-piece opaque stoma c.
    Bremer torque-limiting c.
    Dansac Colo F mini c.
    Dansac Combi micro c.
    Dansac Contour I mini c.
    Gelfilm c.
    Interlink injection c.
    Lehnhardt Universal c.
    Multiseal c.
    Oneseal reducer c.
    Oves cervical c.
    Oves fertility c.
    Prentif cavity-rim cervical c.
    Silipos mesh c.
    c. splint
    Sur-Fit flange c.
    syringe c.
    Universal reducer c.
    Zang metatarsal c.
    Zimmer tibial nail c.
capacitive sensor
capacitor
Caparosa
    C. cutting bur
    C. wire crimper
Capasee diagnostic ultrasound system
CAPD
    continuous ambulatory peritoneal dialysis
capeline bandage
Capello slim-line abduction pillow
Capener
    C. brace
    C. coil splint
    C. finger splint
    C. nail
    C. nail plate
Capes clamp

Capetown
    C. aortic prosthetic valve
    C. aortic valve prosthesis
cap-fitted
    c.-f. endoscope
    c.-f. panendoscope
capillary
    c. flow dialyzer
    c. tube
    c. tube plasma viscosimeter
Capintec
    C. gamma counter
    C. Generation II Vest monitor
    C. VEST system
Capio
    C. CL suture-capturing device
    C. suture passer
    C. transvaginal suture-capturing device
Capiox
    C. hollow flow oxygenator
    C. SX gas and heat exchange oxygenation system
Capiox-E bypass oxygenator system
CAPIS
    Computer-Aided Patient Information System
    CAPIS bone plate system
capitonnage suture
Caplan
    C. angular scissors
    C. dorsal scissors
    C. nasal scissors
    C. septal scissors
CapMix amalgamator
Capner gouge
Capnocheck
    C. handheld capnometer
    C. II handheld CO_2/SpO_2 monitor
    C. Sleep capnograph
Capno-Flo resuscitator
Capnogard capnograph monitor
capnograph
    Capnocheck Sleep c.
    Microcap handheld c.
    Tidal Wave handheld c.
Capnomac
    C. multiple gas analyzer
    C. Ultima gas analyzer
    C. Ultima sidestream spirometer
capnometer
    Capnocheck handheld c.

C

NOTES

capnometer *(continued)*
 Cardiocap c.
 MicroSpan c.
Capnostat
 C. Mainstream carbon dioxide
  module
 C. Mainstream CO_2 sensor
capped lead
Caprolactam suture
Caprosyn suture
Capset bone graft barrier
Capsitome cystotome
capsular
 c. forceps
 c. fragment forceps
 c. knife
 c. scraper
 c. scrubber
capsule
 c. coupeur
 Crosby-Kugler biopsy c.
 dental c.
 Entero-Test c.
 Entero-Test Hp c.
 Gastro-Test c.
 Heyman-Simon c.
 pH-sensitive radiotelemetry c.
 c. polisher
 pyxigraphic sampling c.
 radioisotope c.
 Saf-T-Fit amalgamator c.
 Watson c.
capsule-grasping forceps
Capsulform lens
capsulorrhexis forceps
capsulotome
 Darling c.
capsulotomy
 c. blade
 c. forceps
 c. knife
 c. scissors
CAPSure
 C. ArthroWands
 C. electrode
 C. EPI pacing lead
 C. Fix pacing lead
 C. SP Novus pacing lead
 C. SP pacing lead
 C. steroid-eluting electrode
 C. VDD pacing lead
 C. Z Novus pacing lead
Caps X ArthroWands
Captiflex polypectomy snare
Captivator polypectomy snare
caput forceps
Carabelli
 C. aspirator
 C. cancer cell collector

 C. endobronchial tube
 C. irrigator
 C. lumen finder
 C. mirror cannula
Carabelt
 C. lower back support
 C. lumbar support
 C. therapeutic belt
Carapace face shield
Carasyn hydrogel wound dressing
Carb-Bite
 C.-B. needle holder
 C.-B. tissue forceps
Carb-Edge scissors
carbide finishing bur
carbide-jaw forceps
CarboFlex odor-control dressing
CarboJet lavage system
carbolized knife blade
CarboMedics
 C. bileaflet prosthetic heart valve
 C. cardiac valve prosthesis
 C. Orbis prosthetic heart valve
 C. Top Hat supraannular valve
 C. valve device
carbon
 c. arc lamp
 C. Copy HP foot prosthesis
 C. Copy II lightweight foot
  prosthesis
 c. dioxide generator
 c. dioxide laser
 c. dioxide laser scalpel
 c. fiber
 c. fiber composite cage
 c. fiber-reinforced polyethylene
 c. implant
 c. monoxide monitor
 c. particle bead
 c. steel blade
Carboplast
 C. II sheeting
 C. II thermoplastic composite sheet
  material
Carborundum grinding wheel
Carbo-Seal
 C.-S. cardiovascular composite graft
 C.-S. Valsalva ascending aortic
  prosthesis
Carbostent coronary stent
Carbo-Zinc skin barrier material
Carcon stent
card
 acuity c.
 Allen preschool c.
 Cambridge acuity c.
 CardioCard optical memory c.
 CloneSaver c.
 digital acuity c.

Guthrie c.
Jaeger acuity c.
memory exercise c.
microendoscopic test c.
Novus Medical image c.
pace c.
pattern matching c.
reduced Snellen c.
Teller acuity c.
Wound Stick Photo Facts C.

Cardak percutaneous catheter introducer

Carden
C. bronchoscopy tube
C. jetting device
C. laryngoscopy tube

cardiac
C. Assessment System for Exercise (CASE)
C. Assist intraaortic balloon catheter
c. baroreceptor
c. bioptome
c. monitor
c. output recorder
c. pacemaker
c. patch
c. probe
C. Protect scan
c. pulse duplicator
c. sling
C. Stimulator BCO_2
c. thermodilution catheter
c. transplant monitoring (CTM)

cardiac/apnea monitor
Cardiff resuscitation bag
Cardifix EZ endocardial pacing lead
Cardillo retractor
Cardima
C. Pathfinder microcatheter
C. Revelation Tx microcatheter

cardinal suture
Cardio3DScope imaging system
CardioBeat vascular Doppler
CardioBeeper CB-12L cardiac monitor
Cardioblate
C. BP surgical handle
C. surgical ablation system

CardioCamera imaging system
Cardiocap capnometer

CardioCard
C. optical memory card
C. system

Cardiocare stethoscope
CardioCoil coronary stent
Cardio-Control pacemaker
CardioCOOL myocardial cooling system
Cardio-Cuff
Childs C.-C.

CardioData
C. Mark IV computer
C. MK-3 Holter scanner

CardioDiary heart monitor
cardiodilator
cardioesophageal junction dilator
CardioFix
C. patch
C. pericardium cardiovascular patch
C. pericardium patch
C. pericardium with PhotoFix technology

Cardioflon suture
CardioFocus Lightstic
Cardiofreezer cryosurgical system
CardioGenesis PMR system
cardiograph
Minnesota impedance c.

Cardio-Grip
C.-G. anastomosis clamp
C.-G. aortic clamp
C.-G. bronchus clamp
C.-G. iliac forceps
C.-G. ligature carrier
C.-G. pediatric clamp
C.-G. renal artery clamp
C.-G. tangential occlusion clamp
C.-G. tissue forceps
C.-G. vascular clamp

CardioGrip exercise device
Cardioguard 4000 electrocardiographic monitor
cardiokymograph
CardioLab 7000 electrophysiology monitoring system
Cardiology II stethoscope
Cardiomarker catheter
CardioMatic electrocardiograph
Cardiomed
C. Bodysoft epidural catheter
C. endotracheal ventilation catheter
C. flow-directed thermodilution catheter

NOTES

C

Cardiomemo device
Cardiometrics
    C. cardiotomy reservoir
    C. FloWire Doppler echo crystal
    C. Flowire guidewire
cardiomyostimulator
    Transform c.
CardioNet mobile outpatient cardiac
    telemetry unit
Cardionyl suture
Cardio-Pace Medical Durapulse
    pacemaker
cardioplegic needle
Cardiopoint cardiac surgery needle
cardiopulmonary
    c. bypass machine
    c. bypass pump
    C. Paragon 8500 bed
    c. resuscitation (CPR)
CardioPump
    Ambu C.
Cardioscint nuclear probe
cardioscope
    Carlens Universal c.
    Siemens BICOR c.
    Siemens Hicor c.
CardioSeal septal occlusion device
CardioSearch sensor
CardioServ defibrillator
cardiospasm dilator
CardioSync cardiac synchronizer
Cardiotach heart rate monitor
cardiotachometer
    CT-1000 c.
    digital c.
    portable c.
Cardio Tactilaze peripheral angioplasty
    laser catheter
CardioTec scan
Cardiotest portable electrocardiograph
cardiotomy reservoir
cardiovascular
    c. anastomotic clamp
    C. Angiography Analysis System
    (CAAS)
    c. cannula
    C. Imaging Systems (CVIS)
    c. monitor
    c. Prolene suture
    c. scissors
    c. silk suture
    c. stylet
    c. tissue forceps
cardioverter
    Lown c.
cardioverter-defibrillator
    Angstrom MD implantable c.-d.
    automatic external c.-d. (AECD)
    automatic implantable c.-d. (AICD)

    biventricular implantable c.-d.
    Cadence implantable c.-d.
    Cadet V-115 implantable c.-d.
    Contour implantable c.-d.
    Contour LTV135D implantable c.-d.
    Contour MD implantable single-
    lead c.-d.
    CPI Ventak PRx c.-d.
    Endotak nonthoracotomy
    implantable c.-d.
    external c.-d.
    Gem II DR/VR implantable c.-d.
    Gem III AT implantable c.-d.
    implantable c.-d. (ICD)
    implantable automatic c.-d.
    Intermedics RES-Q implantable c.-
    d.
    Jewel AF implantable c.-d.
    Jewel programmable c.-d.
    Lyra implantable c.-d.
    Medtronic external c.-d.
    Medtronic Gem III implantable c.-
    d.
    Medtronic Jewel AF
    implantable c.-d.
    Medtronic Micro Jewel II
    implantable c.-d.
    Micro Jewel II implantable c.-d.
    Micron Res-Q implantable c.-d.
    nonthoracotomy lead implantable c.-
    d.
    PCD Transvene implantable c.-d.
    Photon DR dual-chamber
    implantable c.-d.
    Phylax AV implantable c.-d.
    programmable c.-d. (PCD)
    PRx implantable c.-d.
    Res-Q ACD implantable c.-d.
    Sentinel implantable c.-d.
    Siemens Siecure implantable c.-d.
    Telectronics Guardian ATP
    implantable c.-d.
    tiered-therapy implantable c.-d.
    Transvene nonthoracotomy
    implantable c.-d.
    Ventak AV III DR automatic
    implantable c.-d.
    Ventak Prizm 2 automatic
    implantable c.-d.
    Ventak PRx implantable c.-d.
    Ventritex Angstrom MD
    implantable c.-d.
    Ventritex Cadence implantable c.-d.
    Ventritex Contour c.-d.
Cardiovit
    C. AT-series ECG system
    C. CS-series ECG system
    C. spirometer
Cardizem Lyo-Ject syringe

Cardona
- C. corneal prosthesis forceps
- C. corneal prosthesis trephine
- C. fiberoptic diagnostic lens
- C. focalizing fundus lens implant
- C. focalizing goniolens
- C. goniofocalizing implant
- C. keratoprosthesis prosthesis
- C. laser
- C. threading lens forceps

care
- intensive c. (IC)

CareDrape blanket
Care electrode
Care-E-Vac portable aspirator
CareLink cardiac monitor
CareTone I, II telephonic stethoscope
Carex ambulatory aid
Carey-Coons
- C.-C. biliary endoprosthesis kit
- C.-C. soft stent

Carl
- C. Zeiss instrument
- C. Zeiss Jena fundus camera
- C. Zeiss lens
- C. Zeiss lensometer
- C. Zeiss myringotomy tube
- C. Zeiss tonometer
- C. Zeiss YAG laser

Carle analytic gas chromatograph
Carlens
- C. bronchospirometric catheter
- C. curette
- C. double-lumen endotracheal tube
- C. forceps
- C. mediastinoscope
- C. needle
- C. tracheotomy retractor
- C. Universal cardioscope

Carlens-Stille tracheal retractor
Carlesta ointment
C-arm
- C-a. fluoroscope
- C-a. fluoroscopic apparatus
- C-a. image intensifier
- C-a. portable x-ray unit

Carmack ear curette
Carmalt
- C. arterial forceps
- C. clamp
- C. hemostat
- C. hemostatic forceps
- C. hysterectomy forceps
- C. splinter forceps
- C. thoracic forceps

Carman rectal tube
Carmeda BioActive surface
Carmel clamp
Carmody
- C. aspirator
- C. perforator drill
- C. thumb tissue forceps
- C. valvulotome

Carmody-Batson elevator
Carmody-Brody retractor
carmustine wafer
Carolina
- C. color spectrum CW Doppler
- C. rocker

Caroline finger retractor
Carolon
- C. AFO sock
- C. antiembolism stocking

Caromed surgical garment
Carones
- C. LASEK pump
- C. LASEK spatula

carotid
- c. angiogram needle
- c. artery clamp
- c. artery forceps
- c. stent

CarotidCoil stent
carpal
- c. care exerciser
- c. lock cockup wrist splint
- c. lock wrist brace
- c. lock wrist splint
- c. lunate implant
- c. scaphoid screw
- c. tunnel release relief kit
- c. tunnel syndrome (CTS)
- c. tunnel syndrome gauge

Carpel
- C. One-Step trabeculectomy punch
- C. speculum

Carpenter dissector
Carpentier
- C. annuloplasty ring prosthesis
- C. pericardial valve
- C. ring
- C. ring heart valve
- C. stent

NOTES

Carpentier-Edwards
- C.-E. aortic valve prosthesis
- C.-E. bioprosthetic valve
- C.-E. glutaraldehyde-preserved porcine xenograft prosthesis
- C.-E. mitral annuloplasty valve
- C.-E. pericardial valve
- C.-E. Perimount mitral valve
- C.-E. Perimount RSR pericardial bioprosthesis
- C.-E. Physio annuloplasty ring
- C.-E. porcine bioprosthesis
- C.-E. porcine supraannular valve
- C.-E. xenograft

Carpentier-Rhone-Poulenc mitral ring prosthesis
carposcope
carpular needle
CarraFilm transparent film dressing
CarraGauze
- C. dressing
- C. hydrogel wound dressing pad
- C. packing strip

CarraSmart foam
CarraSorb H wound dressing
Carrasyn V viscous hydrogel wound dressing
Carrel
- C. clamp
- C. hemostatic forceps
- C. mosquito forceps
- C. patch
- C. suture
- C. tube

Carrel-Girard screw
Carrel-Lindbergh pump
Carriazo-Barraquer microkeratome
Carrie car seat
carrier
- amalgam c.
- Barraquer needle c.
- brain clip c.
- Braun ligature c.
- bronchoscopic sponge c.
- Cardio-Grip ligature c.
- Cave-Rowe ligature c.
- Converta-Litter c.
- Cooley ligature c.
- cotton c.
- DeBakey ligature c.
- DeBakey-Semb ligature c.
- deep ligature c.
- Deschamps ligature c.
- double-headed stereotactic c.
- double-pronged ligature c.
- ear snare wire c.
- Endo-Assist endoscopic ligature c.
- Endoclose suture c.
- Favaloro ligature c.
- fiberoptic light c.
- Finochietto clamp c.
- Fitzwater ligature c.
- foil c.
- Fragen c.
- gauze pad c.
- goiter ligature c.
- Jackson sponge c.
- Kilner suture c.
- Kwapis ligature c.
- Lahey ligature c.
- ligature c.
- light c.
- linear inline ligature c.
- London College foil c.
- Macey tendon c.
- Madden ligature c.
- Mayo goiter ligature c.
- Miya hook ligature c.
- Pereyra ligature c.
- Pereyra-Raz ligature c.
- proctological cotton c.
- Rica cotton c.
- sigmoidoscope light c.
- sponge c.
- Storz cotton c.
- suture c.
- Tauber ligature c.
- Thermafil plastic c.
- c. tube
- Wangensteen deep ligature c.
- Yasargil ligature c.
- Young ligature c.

Carrion penile prosthesis
Carrion-Small penile implant
Carr lobectomy tourniquet
Carroll
- C. aluminum mallet
- C. awl
- C. bone holding forceps
- C. bone hook
- C. dressing forceps
- C. finger goniometer
- C. forearm tendon stripper
- C. hook curette
- C. needle
- C. offset hand retractor
- C. osteotome
- C. periosteal elevator
- C. rongeur
- C. self-retaining spring retractor
- C. skin hook
- C. tendon passer
- C. tendon-passing forceps
- C. tendon-pulling forceps
- C. tendon retriever
- C. tissue forceps

Carroll-Adson dural forceps
Carroll-Bennett finger retractor

Carroll-Bunnell drill
Carroll-Legg
C.-L. osteotome
C.-L. periosteal elevator
Carroll-Smith-Petersen osteotome
Carson
C. internal/external endopyelotomy
stent
C. Zero Tip balloon dilatation
catheter
Carson-Bush internal/external
endopyelotomy stent
cart
Datel endoscopy travel c.
Harloff c.
MedGraphics CPX/D metabolic c.
metabolic c.
MetroFlex endoscopic c.
resuscitation c.
Carter
C. clamp
C. immobilization cushion
C. intranasal splint
C. pillow
C. retractor
C. septal knife
C. septal speculum
C. sphere
C. spherical eye introducer
C. submucous elevator
C. submucous elevator curette
C. Tubal Assistant surgical
instrument
Carter-Glassman resection clamp
Carter-Rowe awl
Carter-Thomason
C.-T. suture passer
C.-T. Uplift
cartesian reference coordinate system
cartilage
c. abrader
c. chisel
c. clamp
c. crusher
c. cutting board
c. forceps
c. graft
c. guide
c. implant
c. knife
c. scissors
cartilage-holding forceps

Carti-Loid syringe
Cartman lens insertion forceps
Cartmill feeding tube kit
Carto
C. electrophysiology navigation
system
C. EP navigation system
cartridge
Adsorba hemoperfusion c.
Alukart hemoperfusion c.
AstraZeneca dental c.
ELAD c.
Genotropin 2-chamber c.
Hemocal hemoperfusion c.
Hemokart hemoperfusion c.
Heparinase test c.
Cartwright valve prosthesis
caruncle
c. clamp
c. forceps
carver
amalgam c.
Cooley wax c.
dental wax c.
C. dental wax
Frahm c.
G-C wax c.
Hollenback c.
modeling c.
Nordent c.
SMIC c.
wax c.
CAS-200 image cytometer
CAS-8000V angiography positioner
Cascadeflo plasma component separator
Cascade Up and About system
CASE
Cardiac Assessment System for Exercise
CASE computerized exercise EKG
system
CASE Marquette 16-exercise
system
case
Berens sterilizing c.
Blade-Safe c.
Fine corneal carrying c.
Mazzariello-Caprini stone forceps
sterilizing c.
Casebeer capsulorrhexis forceps
Casebeer-Lindstrom nomogram
CA-series dialyzer
Casey pelvic clamp

C

NOTES

CASH
> cruciform anterior spinal hyperextension
> CASH orthosis

Cash back brace

Caspar
> C. alligator forceps
> C. anterior cervical plate
> C. anterior instrumentation
> C. blade
> C. cervical retractor
> C. cervical screw
> C. disc space spreader
> C. distraction pin
> C. distractor
> C. drill
> C. hook
> C. plating
> C. retraction post
> C. rongeur
> C. speculum
> C. trapezoidal plate
> C. vertebral body spreader

Caspari
> C. shuttle
> C. suture punch

CASS
> computer-assisted stereotactic surgery
> CASS TrueTaper collimator
> CASS whole-brain mapping system

Casselberry
> C. sphenoid cannula
> C. sphenoid tube

Cassidy-Brophy dressing forceps

cast
> Aquaplast c.
> below-knee walking c.
> bivalved c.
> c. blade
> c. boot
> c. brace
> c. breaker
> broomstick c.
> Caldwell hanging c.
> Cerrobend c.
> Comfort C.
> Cotton-Loader position c.
> c. cutter protector
> dermoplasty c.
> Fractura Flex c.
> Freedom memory thumb spica c.
> Freedom Thumb spica c.
> Frejka c.
> C. Gard cast protector
> Gypsona c.
> Hexcelite c.
> hinged c.
> hip spica c.
> c. knife
> LAE c.

> c. liner
> c. lingual splint
> long above-elbow c.
> long arm navicular c.
> long below-elbow c.
> long leg cylinder c.
> long leg plaster c.
> long leg walking c.
> MaxCast c.
> MBE c.
> Minerva c.
> Muenster c.
> Neufeld c.
> Orfizip knee c.
> Orthoplast slipper c.
> c. padding
> plaster-of-Paris c.
> PlastiCast adjustable joint c.
> pontoon spica c.
> Risser-Cotrel body c.
> Risser localizer scoliosis c.
> Risser turnbuckle c.
> SAE c.
> Sarmiento c.
> SBE c.
> semirigid fiberglass c.
> c. shoe
> short above-elbow c.
> short arm cylinder c.
> short arm navicular c.
> short below-elbow c.
> short leg cylinder c.
> short leg nonwalking c.
> short leg nonweightbearing c.
> short leg plaster c.
> short leg walking c.
> spica c.
> c. spreader
> standard above-elbow c.
> sugar-tong c.
> thumb spica c.
> total contact c.
> Velpeau c.
> walking heel c.

CastAlert cast pressure sensing system

Castallo
> C. eyelid retractor
> C. eye speculum
> C. refractor

Castanares facelift scissors

Castaneda
> C. anastomosis clamp
> C. bottle
> C. cannula
> C. IMM vascular clamp
> C. infant sternal retractor
> C. over-the-wire thrombolytic brush
> C. partial-occlusion clamp
> C. vascular forceps

Castaneda-Malecot catheter
Castaneda-Mixter
    C.-M. forceps
    C.-M. thoracic clamp
Castaway
    C. II CAM Walker boot
    C. II fixed ankle walker
    C. leg brace
    C. leg walker
    C. orthotic
    C. surgical shoe
Castech extremity support
Castelli-Paparella collar button tube
Castens
    C. ascites trocar
    C. hydrocele trocar
Castex rigid dressing
Casteyer prostatic punch
CastGuard foot protector
Castillo catheter
casting wax sheet
Castle
    C. Daystar surgical television
      system
    C. surgical light
cast-molded PMMA intraocular lens
Castorit investment material
Castro-Martinez keratome
Castroviejo
    C. acrylic eye implant
    C. adjustable retractor
    C. angled keratome
    C. anterior synechia scissors
    C. blade breaker
    C. blade holder
    C. capsular forceps
    C. clip-applying forceps
    C. compressor
    C. cornea-holding forceps
    C. corneal dissector
    C. corneal scissors
    C. corneal transplant marker
    C. corneal transplant scissors
    C. corneal transplant trephine
    C. corneoscleral forceps
    C. corneoscleral punch
    C. cross-action capsular forceps
    C. cyclodialysis cannula
    C. cyclodialysis spatula
    C. dermatome
    C. discission knife
    C. double-end spatula

    C. electrokeratotome
    C. electromucotome
    C. enucleation snare
    C. erysiphake
    C. eye speculum
    C. fixation forceps
    C. iridocapsulotomy scissors
    C. iris scissors
    C. keratoplasty scissors
    C. lacrimal dilator
    C. lacrimal sac probe
    C. lens clamp
    C. lens loop
    C. lens loupe
    C. lens spoon
    C. lid forceps
    C. lid retractor
    C. marking calipers
    C. microcorneal scissors
    C. mosquito lid clamp
    C. needle holder
    C. needle holder clamp
    C. ophthalmic knife
    C. orbital aspirator
    C. oscillating razor
    C. razor blade
    C. razor holder
    C. refractor
    C. scleral fold forceps
    C. scleral marker
    C. scleral shortening clip
    C. sclerotome
    C. snare enucleator
    C. straight tying forceps
    C. surface electrode
    C. suture forceps
    C. synechia spatula
    C. tenotomy scissors
    C. transplant forceps
    C. twin knife
    C. Universal corneal scissors
    C. vitreous-aspirating needle
    C. wide-grip handle forceps
Castroviejo-Arruga capsular forceps
Castroviejo-Barraquer needle holder
Castroviejo-Colibri corneal forceps
Castroviejo-Furness cornea-holding
    forceps
Castroviejo-Galezowski dilator
Castroviejo-Kalt needle holder
Castroviejo-McPherson keratectomy
    scissors

NOTES

Castroviejo-Schacher angled calipers
Castroviejo-Scheie cyclodiathermy
Castroviejo-Simpson forceps
Castroviejo-Steinhauser mucotome
Castroviejo-Troutman scissors
Castroviejo-Vannas capsulotomy scissors
Castroviejo-Wheeler discission knife
catadioptric lens
Cat-a-Kit analyzer
Catalano
    C. capsular forceps
    C. corneoscleral forceps
    C. dilator
    C. lacrimal intubation set
    C. muscle hook
    C. needle holder
    C. tying forceps
Catalyst microsurgical system
Catamaran swim plug
cataract
    c. aspirating needle
    c. aspirator
    c. blade
    c. bur
    c. knife
    c. knife guard
    c. mask ring
    c. needle
    c. pencil
    c. probe
    c. rotoextractor extractor
    c. scissors
    c. spoon
cataract-aspirating cannula
Catarex cataract removal system
catch basin
Catera suture anchor
Cateye
    C. Ergociser
    C. T-220 treadmill
catgut
    c. needle
    Rica surgical c.
    SMIC surgical c.
    c. suture
Cath
    Arrow Twin C.
    C. Caddie
    Freedom C.
    Microdose C.
    Uni-Gard Quik C.
Cathcart orthocentric hip prosthesis
cathematic catheter
catheter
    Abbokinase c.
    Ablaser laser delivery c.
    ablation c.
    Abramson c.
    abscess drainage c.

Abscession fluid drainage c.
Accent DG balloon c.
Accu-Flo spring c.
Accu-Flo ventricular c.
Accurate c.
Accu-Vu sizing angiographic c.
Ace fixed-wire balloon c.
Achiever balloon dilatation c.
Ackrad balloon-bearing c.
Ackrad Bronchitrac L^2 suction c.
Ackrad esophageal balloon c.
Ackrad H/S Elliptosphere c.
ACMI Alcock c.
ACMI Bunts c.
ACMI coated Foley c.
ACMI Emmett hemostatic c.
ACMI Owens c.
ACMI positive pressure c.
ACMI severance c.
ACMI Thackston c.
ACMI ureteral c.
ACMI Word Bartholin gland c.
Acmix Foley c.
acorn-tipped c.
ACS angioplasty c.
ACS balloon c.
ACS Concorde coronary
    dilatation c.
ACS Eclipse c.
ACS Endura coronary dilatation c.
ACS exchange guiding c.
ACS Flowtrack-40 c.
ACS Monorail perfusion balloon c.
ACS OTW Lifestream coronary
    dilatation c.
ACS OTW Photon coronary
    dilatation c.
ACS OTW Solaris coronary
    dilatation c.
ACS RX Comet VP coronary
    dilatation c.
ACS RX Ellipse angioplasty c.
ACS RX Gemini coronary
    dilatation c.
ACS RX Rocket coronary
    dilatation c.
ACS RX Solaris coronary
    dilatation c.
ACS RX Streak angioplasty c.
ACS Torquemaster c.
ACS Tourguide II guiding c.
ACS Tx2000 VP c.
ACS Viking c.
Active Cath c.
Active Response C. (ARC)
Acucise RP35 retrograde
    endopyelotomy c.
AcuNav diagnostic ultrasound c.
Acuvance c.

c. adapter
Add-A-Cath c.
Advance EX self-adhesive urinary external c.
AeroStat cholangiography c.
AFocus steerable diagnostic c.
afterloading c.
Agiltrac peripheral dilatation c.
AgX antimicrobial Foley c.
Ahn thrombectomy c.
Air-Lon inhalation c.
AL-1 c.
Alcock return-flow hemostatic c.
Alert cardioversion c.
Alert-TD c.
alignment c.
AL II guiding c.
alimentation c.
Alliance c.
Allis c.
Alvarez-Rodriguez cardiac c.
Alzate c.
Amazr 6-pole linear lesion c.
Amcath c.
Amplatz aortography c.
Amplatz cardiac c.
Amplatz clot buster c.
Amplatz coronary c.
Amplatz femoral c.
Amplatz Hi-Flo torque-control c.
Amplatz left I, II coronary c.
Amplatz right coronary c.
anchored c.
Angiocath autoguard shielded IV c.
Angiocath flexible c.
Angiocath PRN c.
Angioflow high-flow c.
angiographic c.
angiography c.
AngioJet c.
AngioJet e-Train 110 c.
AngioJet thrombectomy c.
AngioJet Xpeedior c.
Angio-Kit c.
Angiomedics c.
AngioOPTIC c.
angiopigtail c.
angioplasty balloon c.
angioplasty guiding c.
Angio-Seal c.
angled pigtail c.
angled-tip ureteral c.

antegrade cardioplegia c.
Anthron heparinized c.
Anthron II c.
antimicrobial c.
Antron c.
Anzio c.
aortic c.
aortography c.
apheresis c.
AquaFlate balloon c.
Arani double-loop guiding c.
AR-1, AR-2 diagnostic guiding c.
ARC-22 PTCA c.
Argyle arterial c.
Argyle Medicut R c.
Argyle oxygen c.
Argyle trocar c.
Argyle umbilical vessel c.
Arrow c.
Arrow balloon wedge pressure c.
Arrow-Berman angiographic c.
Arrow-Berman balloon c.
Arrow Blue FlexTip c.
Arrow-Clarke thoracentesis c.
Arrow EID c.
Arrow-Fischell pullback atherectomy c.
Arrow-Flex intraaortic balloon c.
Arrow FlexTip Plus c.
Arrowgard Blue antiseptic-coated c.
Arrowgard Blue central venous c.
Arrow Hands-Off thermodilution c.
Arrow-Howes multilumen c.
Arrow-Howes quad-lumen c.
Arrow Multi-Lumen Access c.
Arrow PICC c.
Arrow pullback atherectomy c.
Arrow pulmonary artery c.
Arrow QuadPolar electrode c.
Arrow QuickFlash arterial c.
Arrow TheraCath epidural c.
Arrow-Trerotola PTD c.
Arrow TwinCath 2-lumen peripheral c.
Arrow TwinCath multilumen peripheral c.
Artec balloon c.
arterial embolectomy c.
arteriovenous c.
Ascent guiding c.
Ash Split Cath c.
Ash Split Cath II c.

NOTES

C

catheter *(continued)*

ASI uroplasty prostatic dilatation c.
ASI uroplasty TCU dilatation c.
Asuka PTCA c.
atherectomy c.
AtheroCath Bantam coronary
  atherectomy c.
AtheroCath GTO c.
AtheroCath spinning blade c.
Atlantic ileostomy c.
Atlantis SR coronary intravascular
  ultrasound c.
Atlantis SR IVUS c.
Atlas LP PTCA balloon
  dilatation c.
Atlas ULP PTCA balloon
  dilatation c.
ATRAC multipurpose balloon c.
atrioseptostomy c.
Atri-pace I bipolar flared pacing c.
auricular appendage c.
Auth atherectomy c.
AutoGuard shielded IV c.
automatic c.
autoperfusion balloon c.
Avanar F/X IVUS imaging c.
AV DeClot c.
AV Paceport thermodilution c.
Axcis laser c.
Axiom DG balloon angioplasty c.
bag c.
Bailey transthoracic c.
bailout autoperfusion balloon c.
Baim pacing c.
Baim-Turi monitoring/pacing c.
balloon c.
c. balloon
balloon angioplasty c.
balloon biliary c.
balloon dilatation c.
balloon dilating c.
balloon embolectomy c.
balloon flotation c.
balloon-flotation pacing c.
balloon guide c.
balloon imaging c.
balloon-on-a-wire dilatation c.
balloon septostomy c.
balloon-tipped c.
balloon-tipped angiographic c.
balloon-tipped flow-directed c.
balloon-tipped thermodilution c.
balloon valvuloplasty c.
balloon wedge pressure c.
ball-wedge c.
Baltherm thermal dilution c.
banana c.
Bandit PTCA c.
Banno c.

Bard c.
Bardam red rubber c.
Bard balloon-directed pacing c.
Bardco-Matic c.
Bard electrophysiology c.
Bardex-Foley balloon c.
Bardex-Foley return-flow
  retention c.
Bardex IC silver-coated latex
  Foley c.
Bardex Lubricath latex Foley c.
Bard gastrostomy c.
Bard guiding c.
Bard helical c.
Bardic cutdown c.
Bardic-Deseret Intracath c.
Bardic translucent c.
Bardic Uro Sheath reusable male
  external c.
Bard male external c.
Bard sterile red rubber c.
Bard Stinger S ablation c.
Bard Touchless intermittent c.
Bard-U-Cath self-adhering male
  external c.
Bard x-ray ureteral c.
Bartholin gland c.
Baschui pigtail c.
basket c.
basket stone extractor c.
bat-wing c.
Baxter angioplasty c.
Baxter dilatation c.
Baxter fiberoptic
  spectrophotometry c.
Baxter-V. Mueller c.
BD Insyte Autoguard shielded
  intravenous c.
Beacon Tip Royal Flush pigtail c.
Becton Dickinson Teflon-
  sheathed c.
Beird eye c.
Béniqué c.
Bentson-Hanafee-Wilson c.
Berenstein guiding c.
Berenstein occlusion balloon c.
Berman angiographic c.
Berman balloon flotation c.
Berman cardiac c.
Bernstein c.
Beta-Cath c.
Beta-Rail c.
Bicor c.
bifoil balloon c.
biliary balloon c.
biliary drainage c.
BioCardia Universal deflectable
  guide c.

BioEnterics gastric balloon suction c.
BioGlide c.
Bio-Guard Spectrum antimicrobial-bonded c.
Bio-Medicus 1-piece femoral arterial c.
Biosearch enteroclysis c.
Biosearch female/male intermittent urinary c.
Biovue c.
bipolar c.
bipolar pacing c.
bipolar temporary pacemaker c.
bird's eye c.
Bi-Set c.
Bitome c.
Bivona epistaxis c.
bladder c.
blade septostomy c.
Blasucci pigtail ureteral c.
Block right coronary guiding c.
blood-contacting c.
Blue FlexTip c.
Blue Max balloon dilation c.
Blue Max triple-lumen c.
BMC coaxial injectable c.
Bonnano c.
Bonnie balloon c.
Borge c.
Boston Scientific Sonicath imaging c.
Bourassa c.
Bozeman c.
Bozeman-Fritsch c.
BPS spinal angiographic c.
Braasch bulb ureteral c.
brachial artery c.
braided diagnostic c.
Bresgen c.
Brevi-Kath epidural c.
Brite Tip guiding c.
Brockenbrough mapping c.
Brockenbrough modified bipolar c.
Brockenbrough transseptal c.
Brodney c.
bronchial c.
Bronchitrac-L suction c.
bronchospirometric c.
Broviac c.
Buchbinder Omniflex c.

Buchbinder Thruflex over-the-wire c.
bulbous c.
bulb ureteral c.
bullet tip c.
Bunegin-Albin pressure c.
Bunt c.
bur-bearing c.
Burhenne steerable c.
butterfly c.
bypass graft c.
bypass Speedy balloon c.
Calypso Rely c.
Camino intracranial c.
Camino micromanometer c.
Camino transducer c.
Campbell infant c.
cannulation c.
Can-Opt stand-alone dual lumen ERCP c.
Cardiac Assist intraaortic balloon c.
cardiac thermodilution c.
Cardiomarker c.
Cardiomed Bodysoft epidural c.
Cardiomed endotracheal ventilation c.
Cardiomed flow-directed thermodilution c.
Cardio Tactilaze peripheral angioplasty laser c.
Carlens bronchospirometric c.
Carson Zero Tip balloon dilatation c.
Castaneda-Malecot c.
Castillo c.
cathematic c.
Cath-Finder c.
Cath-Guide closed suction c.
CathLink 20 c.
Cathlon IV c.
Cathmark suction c.
Caud-A-Kath epidural c.
caval c.
cavity drainage c.
cecostomy c.
central venous pressure c.
cephalad c.
Cerablate Plus Flutter ablation c.
Cereblate c.
cerebral c.
C-Flex c.
Chaffin c.

NOTES

catheter *(continued)*
    Cheetah angioplasty c.
    Chemo-Port c.
    Chilli cooled ablation c.
    Cholangiocath c.
    cholangiographic c.
    cholangiography c.
    CholangioLAPcath c.
    cholecystotomy c.
    chorionic villus sampling c.
    ChronoFlex c.
    Chubby balloon c.
    Cinemagic diagnostic c.
    circular mapping c.
    Cisco covered needle c.
    cisterna magna c.
    Clarke expanding mesh c.
    Clarke helical c.
    Clay Adams PE-series c.
    Clear Advantage latex-free male
      external c.
    CliniCath peripherally inserted c.
    cloverleaf radiofrequency ablation c.
    coaxial c.
    Cobe-Tenckhoff peritoneal
      dialysis c.
    Codman-Holter c.
    Codman ventricular silicone c.
    coiled c.
    coil-tipped c.
    Combicath telescope c.
    Comet VP coronary dilation c.
    Comfort Cath c.
    Compli soft-tip c.
    Concentric balloon guide c.
    Conceptus Soft Seal cervical c.
    Conceptus Soft Torque uterine c.
    Conceptus VS c.
    Concorde c.
    Concord/Portex suction c.
    condom c.
    conductance c.
    conical c.
    Conquest PTA balloon dilatation c.
    Constantine flexible metal c.
    ConstaVac c.
    Constellation mapping c.
    continuous irrigation c.
    Contour balloon dilatation c.
    contrast-filled c.
    Conveen Security+ self-sealing male
      external c.
    Conveen tapered intermittent c.
    Cook arterial c.
    Cook-Cope loop nephrostomy c.
    Cook Enforcer balloon dilatation c.
    Cook Flexi-Tip ureteral c.
    Cook infusion c.
    Cook pressure monitoring c.

    Cook Spectrum c.
    Cook TPN c.
    Cook yellow pigtail c.
    Cooley vena caval c.
    cool-tip c.
    Cope loop nephrostomy c.
    Cordis Brite Tip guiding c.
    Cordis Ducor I, II, III coronary
      pigtail c.
    Cordis Lumelec c.
    Cordis Powerflex balloon c.
    Cordis Predator balloon c.
    Cordis Son-II c.
    Cordis Trakstar PTCA balloon c.
    Cordis TransTaper tip c.
    Cordis-Webster diagnostic/ablation
      deflectable tip c.
    Cordis-Webster mapping c.
    Corlon c.
    coronary angiographic c.
    coronary dilatation c.
    coronary guiding c.
    coronary perfusion c.
    coronary seeking c.
    coronary sinus c.
    corset balloon c.
    Cotton graduated dilation c.
    coudé c.
    coudé-tip demeure c.
    Councill retention c.
    counterpulsation c.
    Cournand quadpolar electrode c.
    Coxeter urologic c.
    Coyote OTW balloon c.
    C. R. Bard c.
    Cribier-Letac c.
    CritiCath flow-directed
      thermodilution c.
    CritiCath pulmonary artery c.
    Critikon balloon thermodilution c.
    Critikon balloon wedge pressure c.
    Critikon-Berman angiographic
      balloon c.
    Critikon Optiva IV c.
    CrossPoint TransAccess c.
    CrossSail coronary dilatation c.
    cryoablation c.
    CryoCath c.
    CryoCor cardiac cryoablation c.
    CUI c.
    Cummings four-wing Malecot
      retention c.
    Cummings nephrostomy c.
    Cummings-Pezzer c.
    cup c.
    Curl Cath peritoneal c.
    cutdown c.
    cutting balloon c.
    CVIS intravascular US imaging c.

CVP c.
CVS c.
cylindrical diffusing balloon c.
Cynosar c.
Cystocath c.
Dacron c.
Dakin c.
Damato curved c.
Datascope DL-II percutaneous translucent balloon c.
Datascope intraaortic balloon pump c.
Davis c.
Davol sterile intermittent red rubber c.
Dawson-Mueller drainage c.
decapolar electrode c.
decapolar pacing c.
decompression c.
decompressive enteroclysis c.
deflectable quadripolar c.
c. deflecting bridge
Delcath double-balloon c.
DeLee infant c.
DeLee suction c.
Dent sleeve c.
de Pezzer mushroom-tipped c.
de Pezzer self-retaining c.
Derek-Harwood-Nash c.
Desai VectorCath mapping c.
Deseret flow-directed thermodilution c.
Desilets c.
Desilets-Hoffman c.
Devonshire c.
Devonshire-Mack c.
DeWeese caval c.
Diaflex ureteral dilatation c.
diagnostic ultrasound c.
Dialy-Nate c.
dialysis c.
Diasonics c.
Digiflex high-flow c.
dilatation c.
dilating pressure balloon c.
dilator c.
directional atherectomy c.
Dispatch balloon c.
Dispatch infusion c.
DLP cardioplegic c.
DLP infant ventricular c.

DLP left atrial pressure monitoring c.
Doppler coronary c.
Dormia stone basket c.
Dorros brachial internal mammary guiding c.
Dorros infusion/probing c.
Dotter c.
Dotter coaxial c.
double-balloon perfusion c.
double-current c.
double-J indwelling c.
double-J ureteral c.
double-lumen c.
double-lumen balloon stone extractor c.
double-lumen central venous c.
double-lumen injection c.
double-lumen Silastic c.
double-lumen subclavian c.
double-lumen Swan-Ganz c.
Dover Premium teflon-coated latex Foley c.
Dover Texas disposable male c.
Dow Corning ileal pouch c.
drainage c.
Drew-Smythe c.
dual-lumen c.
dual-lumen hemodialysis c.
Dualtherm dual-thermistor thermodilution c.
Ducor angiographic c.
Ducor balloon c.
Ducor cardiac c.
Ducor HF c.
Duett c.
duodecapolar c.
Duo-Flow c.
Du Pen long-term epidural c.
DuraGlide3 c.
DVI Simpson coronary AtheroCath c.
Dynacor Foley c.
Dynacor suction c.
dynamic angioplasty c.
Easy Rider c.
E-cath c.
echo c.
EchoMark salpingography c.
EchoMark SSG c.
echo transponder electrode c.
Edge dilatation c.

C

NOTES

catheter *(continued)*

EDM infusion c.
Edslab cholangiography c.
Edwards diagnostic c.
Efficere embryo transfer c.
Eichelter-Schenk vena cava c.
EID percutaneous central venous large-bore c.
elbowed c.
Elecath thermodilution c.
electrode c.
electrohemostasis c.
electrothermal c.
El Gamal coronary bypass c.
Eliminator nasal biliary c.
Elite guide c.
embolectomy c.
Embryon GIFT transfer c.
Embryon HSG c.
Encapsulon epidural c.
Endeavor nondetachable silicone balloon c.
EndoClamp ST aortic c.
EndoCPB c.
endoscopic retrograde cholangiopancreatography c.
EndoSonics IVUS/balloon dilatation c.
EndoSonics ultrasound-guided c.
EndoSound endoscopic ultrasound c.
endotracheal c.
Endura coronary dilation c.
Enhanced Torque guiding c.
EnSite cardiac c.
Entract dilation and occlusion c.
Eppendorf c.
Eppendorf cardiac c.
EPT Dx steerable diagnostic c.
ePTFE ventricular shunt c.
Equinox balloon occlusion balloon c.
ERCP c.
ERCPeel Away c.
esophageal balloon c.
esophageal manometry c.
esophageal motility c.
esophagoscopic c.
eustachian c.
Everett eustachian c.
Everett fallopian c.
Evermed c.
Evert-O-Cath drug delivery c.
Everyday self-adhering urinary external c.
eXamine cholangiography c.
expandable access c.
Explorer coronary dilatation c.
Explorer 360-degree rotational diagnostic c.
Explorer precurved diagnostic EP c.
Explorer ST fixed-curve diagnostic c.
Expo diagnostic c.
Export aspiration c.
Express 2 balloon c.
Express over-the-wire balloon c.
Express Plus PTCA c.
external biliary drainage c.
external ureteral c.
Extreme laser c.
Extreme peripheral c.
extrusion balloon c.
6-eye c.
EZ Cath c.
FACT-22 coronary balloon angioplasty c.
Falcon coronary c.
Falcon single-operator exchange balloon c.
FAST balloon flotation c.
Fast-Cath c.
FasTracker-18 infusion c.
FAST right heart cardiovascular c.
Feldman aortic stenosis c.
femoral cerebral c.
femoral guiding c.
femoral hemodialysis c.
fenestrated c.
FHT Reform coronary c.
fiberoptic oximeter c.
fiberoptic pressure c.
Fidelity intraaortic balloon c.
filiform c.
filiform-tipped c.
Finesse large-lumen guiding c.
Fino vascular c.
fixed-wire c.
Flex-Cath double-lumen intraaortic balloon c.
Flexi-Cath double-lumen intraaortic balloon c.
Flexi-Cath straight dual-lumen c.
FlexiCut coronary c.
Flexima biliary drainage c.
Flexima nephrostomy c.
Flexima ureteral c.
Flexi-Tip ureteral c.
Flexxicon Blue dialysis c.
Flexxicon II PC internal jugular c.
flotation c.
flow-assisted short-term balloon c.
flow-directed balloon cardiovascular c.
flow-directed balloon-tipped c.
flow-directed thermodilution c.

FloWire Doppler c.
flow-oximetry c.
Flow Rider neurovascular c.
fluid-filled balloon-tipped flow-
directed c.
fluid-filled pigtail c.
Fogarty adherent clot c.
Fogarty arterial embolectomy c.
Fogarty arterial irrigation c.
Fogarty balloon biliary c.
Fogarty balloon embolectomy c.
Fogarty-Chin extrusion balloon c.
Fogarty-Chin peripheral dilatation c.
Fogarty dilation c.
Fogarty embolectomy c.
Fogarty gallstone c.
Fogarty graft thrombectomy c.
Fogarty occlusion c.
Fogarty Thru-Lumen c.
Fogarty venous irrigation c.
Fogarty venous thrombectomy c.
Folatex c.
Foley c.
Foley acorn-bulb c.
Foley-Alcock c.
Foley balloon c.
Foley cone-tip c.
Foley 3-way c.
Foltz c.
ForeRunner coronary sinus
guiding c.
Fountain infusion c.
Franz monophasic action
potential c.
Freedom Clear external c.
Freedom external c.
Freedom Pak seven c.
Freeway PTCA balloon c.
French angiographic c.
French Cope loop nephrostomy c.
French curve out-of-plane c.
French double-lumen c.
French Foley c.
French Gesco c.
French in-plane guiding c.
French JR4 Schneider c.
French MBIH c.
French mushroom-tip c.
French pigtail nephrostomy c.
French red rubber Robinson c.
French Robinson c.
French SAL c.

French shaft c.
French Silastic Foley c.
French sizing of c.
French Teflon c.
French Teflon pyeloureteral c.
Fritsch c.
Frontrunner coronary c.
Frydman c.
FullFlow perfusion dilation c.
Furness c.
fused-tip c.
Gambro c.
Garceau ureteral c.
gastroenterostomy c.
gastrojejunostomy c.
gastrostomy c.
Gazelle balloon dilatation c.
Geenan graduated dilation c.
Gensini coronary arteriography c.
Gensini Teflon c.
Gentle-Flo suction c.
Gesco c.
Gesco Umbili-Cath c.
Gibbon urethral c.
Gilbert pediatric balloon c.
Gilbert plug-sealing c.
Gizmo c.
Glidecath hydrophilic coated c.
Glidewire c.
Glo-Tip ERCP c.
Gold probe bipolar hemostasis c.
Goodale-Lubin cardiac c.
Gore-Tex peritoneal c.
Gorlin pacing c.
Gould PentaCath thermodilution c.
Gouley whalebone filiform c.
graduated c.
Graft ACE fixed-wire balloon c.
Graham c.
Greenfield caval c.
Greer Seroma-Cath c.
Grollman pigtail c.
Grollman pulmonary artery-
seeking c.
Groshong double-lumen c.
Grüntzig arterial balloon c.
Grüntzig balloon angiography c.
Grüntzig G, S dilating c.
Grüntzig steerable c.
Guidant guiding c.
c. guide
guide c.

NOTES

catheter *(continued)*
Guidefather c.
c. guide holder
c. guidewire
guiding c.
Günther c.
Guyon ureteral c.
GyneSys Dx diagnostic c.
Hagner bag c.
Hakim c.
Hakko Dwellcath c.
Halo c.
Halocath c.
Hamilton-Steward c.
Hanafee c.
Hancock coronary perfusion c.
Hancock embolectomy c.
Hancock fiberoptic c.
Hancock hydrogen detection c.
Hancock luminal electrophysiologic
  recording c.
Hancock thermodilution c.
Hancock wedge-pressure c.
Hands-Off thermodilution cardiac c.
Harris c.
Hartmann eustachian c.
Hartzler ACS coronary dilatation c.
Hartzler ACX II c.
Hartzler dilatation c.
Hartzler Excel c.
Hartzler LPS dilatation c.
Hartzler Micro-600 c.
Hartzler Micro II angioplasty
  balloon c.
Hartzler Micro XT c.
Hartzler RX-14 balloon c.
Hatch c.
Headhunter visceral angiography c.
HealthShield antimicrobial
  mediastinal wound drainage c.
Heartport endocoronary sinus c.
HeatProbe c.
helical PTCA dilatation c.
helical-tip Halo c.
helium-filled balloon c.
Helixcision cardiovascular c.
Helix PTCA dilatation c.
Hemo-Cath c.
hemodialysis c.
Hemoject injection c.
HemoSplit dialysis c.
hemostatic c.
Hepacon c.
heparin-coated c.
hexapolar c.
Heyer-Schulte c.
Heyer-Schulte-Pudenz cardiac c.
H-H open-end alimentation c.
Hickman c.

Hickman tunneled c.
Hidalgo c.
Hieshima coaxial c.
Higgins c.
high-fidelity micromanometer c.
high-flow c.
high-speed rotation dynamic
  angioplasty c.
Hilal modified headhunter c.
His bundle c.
Hi5 Torq Flow c.
Hi-Torque Floppy guide c.
Hobbs dilatation balloon c.
hockey-stick c.
Hohn c.
Hollister external c.
Hollister self-adhesive c.
Holter distal atrial c.
Holter distal peritoneal c.
Holter-Hausner c.
Holter lumboperitoneal c.
Holter ventricular c.
Holt self-retaining c.
hooked c.
Hopkins Percuflex drainage c.
hot-tipped c.
Hryntschak c.
HSG c.
HUI c.
Huibregtse-Katon ERCP c.
Hunter-Sessions vena cava-occluding
  balloon c.
Hurwitt c.
Hurwitz dialysis c.
HyCoSy c.
HydraCross TLC PTCA c.
HydroCath central venous c.
Hydrogel-coated PTCA balloon c.
Hydrolyser thrombectomy c.
Hydromer grafted c.
hydrophilic-coated guiding c.
hydrostatic balloon c.
Hymes double-lumen c.
hyperalimentation c.
hysterosalpingography c.
IAB c.
ICP c.
ICP-T fiberoptic ICP monitoring c.
Illumen guiding c.
ILUS c.
Imager II angiographic c.
Imager Torque selective c.
imaging-angioplasty balloon c.
Impact balloon dilatation c.
Imperson c.
implantable access c.
implantable cardioverter-
  defibrillator c.
Impra peritoneal c.

indwelling c.
indwelling Foley c.
indwelling subclavian c.
infant female/male c.
inferior vena caval c.
Infiniti c.
inflatable Foley bag c.
Infusaid c.
InfusaSleeve II c.
Infuse-A-Cath c.
Infuse-a-Port c.
infusion c.
Ingram c.
injection c.
injection electrode c.
Inmed whistle tip urethral c.
Innervision ventricular c.
Inoue balloon c.
inside-the-needle infusion c.
Insyte AutoGuard c.
Intact c.
Integra c.
IntelliCath pulmonary artery c.
intercostal c.
internal/external c.
internal mammary artery c.
Interpret ultrasound c.
interventional c.
Intimax arterial embolectomy c.
Intimax biliary c.
Intimax cholangiography c.
Intimax occlusion c.
Intimax vascular c.
intraaortic balloon c.
intracardiac c.
Intracath c.
intracoronary guiding c.
intracoronary perfusion c.
intracranial pressure c.
Intraducer peritoneal c.
intraductal imaging c.
IntraEAR Round Window E C.
intramedullary c.
Intran intrauterine pressure
  measurement c.
Intran Plus c.
intrapleural c.
Intrasil c.
intraurethral prostatic bridge c.
intrauterine c. (IUC)
intrauterine insemination c.
intrauterine pressure c.

intravascular ultrasound c.
intravenous pacing c.
intravenous ultrasound c.
intraventricular pressure
  monitoring c.
Intrepid balloon c.
Intrepid percutaneous transluminal
  coronary angioplasty c.
Intrepid PTCA c.
Introcan Safety IV c.
c. introducer
c. introducing forceps
irrigating c.
irrigation c.
Itard c.
ITC radiopaque balloon c.
IUI c.
IV c.
IVUS c.
Jackman coronary sinus
  electrode c.
Jackman orthogonal c.
Jackson-Pratt c.
Jacques c.
Jaeger-Whiteley c.
James lumbar peritoneal c.
Jansen-Anderson intrauterine c.
Javid c.
Jehle coronary perfusion c.
jejunostomy c.
Jelco intravenous c.
Jelm 2-way c.
Jinotti dual-purpose c.
JL c.
JL4 c.
JL5 c.
Jocath Maestro coronary balloon c.
Jography angiographic c.
Joguide coronary guiding c.
Joguide guiding c.
Jo-Kath c.
Josephson quadripolar c.
Jostra c.
JR c.
JR4 c.
JR5 c.
Judkins coronary c.
Judkins curve LAD c.
Judkins curve LCX c.
Judkins curve STD c.
Judkins 4 diagnostic c.
Judkins guiding c.

C

NOTES

catheter *(continued)*

Judkins left 4 c.
Judkins left coronary c.
Judkins pigtail c.
Judkins right c.
Judkins right coronary c.
Judkins torque-control c.
Judkins USCI c.
jugular venous c.
J-Vac c.
Kaminsky c.
Karmen c.
Katon c.
Katzen long balloon dilatation c.
Kaufman c.
KDF-2.3 intrauterine
  insemination c.
Kearns bag c.
Kensey atherectomy c.
Kensey dynamic angioplasty c.
Kifa green, grey, red, yellow c.
Kimball c.
King guiding c.
King multipurpose coronary
  graft c.
kink-resistant peritoneal c.
Kinsey atherectomy c.
Kish urethral c.
Koala intrauterine pressure c.
Konigsberg 5-channel solid-state c.
Kontron intraaortic balloon c.
Kumpe c.
Labotech embryo transfer c.
LacriCath lacrimal duct c.
lacrimal balloon c.
Lahey c.
LAIS laser energy percutaneous
  coronary c.
Landmark midline c.
Lane rectal c.
laparoscopic cholangiography c.
Lapides c.
LAP-13 Ranfac cholangiographic c.
Lapras c.
large-bore c.
large-lumen c.
Lasso circular mapping c.
latex c.
Latis c.
Latson multipurpose c.
L-Cath peripherally inserted
  neonatal c.
Ledor pigtail c.
LeFort male urethral c.
left coronary c.
left heart c.
left Judkins c.
left ventricular sump c.
c. leg strap

c. leg tube holder
Lehman aortographic c.
Lehman pancreatic manometry c.
Lehman ventriculography c.
LeMaitre biliary c.
lensed fiber-tip laser delivery c.
Leonard c.
LeRoy ventricular c.
LeVeen c.
Levin tube c.
Leycom volume conductance c.
Lifecath c.
LifeJet high-flow chronic
  dialysis c.
Lifemed c.
Lifestream coronary dilation c.
LightRing balloon c.
Lillehei-Warden c.
Lincoff design of Storz scleral
  buckling balloon c.
Lionheart c.
Livewire Duo-Decapolar c.
Livewire TC ablation c.
Livewire TC Compass ablation c.
Lloyd bronchial c.
Lloyd double c.
Lloyd esophagoscopic c.
lobster-tail c.
Lofric disposable urethral c.
Long Brite Tip guiding c.
Longdwel Teflon c.
Long Skinny over-the-wire
  balloon c.
long-term internal jugular c.
Lo-Profile II steerable dilatation c.
low-profile balloon-positioning c.
low-speed rotation angioplasty c.
LTX PTCA c.
Lucae eustachian c.
Lumaguide infusion c.
Lumelec pacing c.
LuMend Frontrunner CTO c.
4-lumen polyvinyl manometric c.
Lunderquist c.
Lynx OTW c.
Magill endotracheal c.
Maglinte enteroclysis c.
magnet-tipped flexible c.
Mahurkar dual-lumen femoral
  dialysis c.
Malecot nephrostomy c.
Malecot self-retaining urethral c.
Malecot Silastic c.
Malecot suprapubic cystostomy c.
Malecot 2-wing c.
Malecot 4-wing c.
Mallinckrodt angiographic c.
Mallinckrodt vertebral c.
Maloney c.

Manashil sialography c.
Mandelbaum c.
Mani cerebral c.
manometer-tipped c.
manometric c.
Mansfield Atri-Pace 1 c.
Mansfield balloon dilatation c.
Mansfield orthogonal electrode c.
Mansfield Scientific dilatation
  balloon c.
Mansfield-Webster deflectable
  curved c.
mapping c.
Marathon guiding c.
marker c.
Mark IV Moss decompression-
  feeding c.
Marlin thoracic c.
Marrs intrauterine c.
mastoid c.
Maverick balloon dilatation c.
Maverick Monorail balloon c.
Max Force balloon dilatation c.
Max Force TTS biliary balloon
  dilatation c.
Maxi LD PTA dilatation c.
Maxxum balloon c.
McCarthy c.
McCaskey antral c.
McGoon coronary perfusion c.
McIntosh double-lumen
  hemodialysis c.
McIver nephrostomy c.
Meadox Surgimed c.
Med-Co flexible c.
Medcomp c.
mediastinal c.
Medicut c.
Medi-Tech arterial dilatation c.
Medi-Tech-Mansfield dilating c.
Medi-Tech occlusion balloon c.
Medi-Tech steerable c.
Medrad angiographic c.
Medtronic balloon c.
Medtronic Zuma guiding c.
MegaSonics PTCA c.
Melker emergency
  cricothyrotomy c.
Memokath c.
memory c.
Menlo Care c.
Mentor continent urinary coudé c.

Mentor Foley c.
Mentor Self-Cath soft c.
Mentor Tele-Cath ileal conduit
  sampling c.
Mentor-UroSan external c.
Mercator atrial high-density
  array c.
Mercier c.
metal ball-tip c.
metallic-tip c.
Metaport c.
Metras bronchial c.
Mewi-5 side-hole infusion c.
Mewissen infusion c.
Micor c.
microdialysis c.
Micro-Guide c.
micromanometer c.
micromanometer-tipped c.
MicroMewi multiple side-hole
  infusion c.
Microsoftrac c.
Micro-Soft Stream side-hole
  infusion c.
Micross dilatation c.
microtransducer c.
MicroVac c.
Microvasive balloon retrieval c.
Microvasive Rigiflex balloon c.
MicroView sheath-based IVUS c.
Mikaelsson c.
Mikro-Tip micromanometer-tipped c.
Mikro-Tip pressure transducer c.
Millar Doppler c.
Millar micromanometer c.
Millar pigtail angiographic c.
Millar urodynamic c.
Millenia balloon c.
Millenia balloon dilatation c.
Millenia percutaneous transluminal
  coronary angioplasty c.
Miller septostomy c.
Mills operative peripheral
  angioplasty c.
Mini-Profile dilatation c.
Minispace IUI c.
Mirage over-the-wire balloon c.
Missouri c.
Mitsubishi angioscopic c.
Mixtner c.
MMG Easycath c.
MMG Ready Cath c.

NOTES

catheter *(continued)*

Molina needle c.
MoniTorr ICP lumbar c.
MoniTorr ICP ventricular c.
monofoil c.
Monorail angioplasty c.
Monorail imaging c.
Monorail Piccolino c.
More-Flow c.
Morris thoracic c.
Moss decompression feeding c.
Moss Suction Buster c.
MPR drain c.
MS Classique balloon dilatation c.
MTC Ventcontrol ventricular c.
Mueller c.
Mullins transseptal c.
multiaccess c. (MAC)
multielectrode basket c.
multielectrode impedance c.
multiflanged Portnoy c.
multilumen manometric c.
Multi-Med triple-lumen infusion c.
multipolar c.
multipolar electrode c.
multipolar impedance c.
Multipurpose-SM c.
multisensor c.
multi-sideport c.
Multistim electrode c.
mushroom c.
Mylar c.
Mystic balloon c.
Namic c.
NarrowFlex intraaortic balloon c.
NarrowFlex Universal IAB c.
nasal c.
nasobiliary c.
nasocystic c.
nasopancreatic c.
nasotracheal c.
nasovesicular c.
NavAblator c.
Navarre Universal drainage c.
Naviport deflectable-tip guiding c.
Naviport hollow-lumen guiding c.
Navi-Star ablation c.
Navi-Star Biosense Webster
  mapping c.
Navi-Star electrophysiology c.
NC Bandit PTCA c.
NC Big Ranger OTW balloon c.
NDSB occlusion balloon c.
Nd:YAG laser c.
Neal c.
Nélaton urethral c.
Neonatal Y TrachCare c.
Neoplex c.
Neo-Sert umbilical vessel c.

NephroMax nephrostomy balloon c.
nephrostomy c.
Nestor guiding c.
Neuroguide Visicath viewing c.
Nexus 2 linear ablation c.
Niagara temporary dialysis c.
Nichols-Jehle coronary multihead c.
NIH left ventriculography c.
nonflotation c.
nontraumatizing c.
NoProfile balloon c.
Norfolk intrauterine aspiration c.
Norton flow-directed Swan-Ganz
  thermodilution c.
NovaCath multilumen infusion c.
Nova thermodilution c.
Novoste c.
NuMED intracoronary Doppler c.
Nutricath silicone elastomer c.
Nycore angiography pigtail c.
Nykanen RF perforation c.
nylon c.
Oasis guiding/pushing c.
Oasis thrombectomy c.
occlusion c.
octapolar c.
Odman-Ledin c.
Olbert balloon c.
Olbert NoProfile balloon
  dilatation c.
olivary c.
olive-tipped c.
Olympus II PTCA dilatation c.
Olympus PW-1L wash c.
Omni c.
OmniCath atherectomy c.
Omniflex balloon c.
Omni flush c.
Omni selective c.
On-Command c.
Onik-Cohen percutaneous access c.
Opaca-Garcea ureteral c.
OpenSail coronary dilatation c.
Opta 5 c.
Optical c.
Opticath c.
Opticon c.
Opti-Flow permanent dialysis c.
Opti-Plast XT balloon c.
OptiQue sensing c.
Optiscope c.
Optiva IV c.
Oracle Focus PTCA c.
Oracle Focus ultrasound imaging c.
Oracle Megasonics c.
Oracle Micro intravascular
  ultrasound c.
Oracle Micro Plus PTCA c.
Oral-Cath c.

ORC-B Ranfac cholangiographic c.
Oreopoulos-Zellerman c.
OriGen Biomedical dual-lumen c.
OTW Lifestream coronary
dilation c.
OTW Photon coronary dilation c.
over-the-needle infusion c.
over-the-wire PTCA balloon c.
Owatusi double c.
Owen Lo-Profile dilation c.
oximetric c.
oximetry c.
Pacel bipolar pacing c.
pacemaker c.
Paceport c.
Pacewedge dual-pressure bipolar
pacing c.
Pacifico c.
pacing c.
Panther c.
Paparella c.
Parahisian EP c.
ParCA c.
Park blade septostomy c.
Parodi c.
partially-implantable c.
P.A.S. Port Fluoro-Free c.
Passage balloon dilation c.
Pathfinder c.
PA Watch position-monitoring c.
PBN hysterosalpingography c.
PE c.
pectoral c.
pediatric balloon c.
pediatric Foley c.
pediatric pigtail c.
peel-away banana c.
peel-off c.
pennate suction c.
Pennine Nélaton c.
PentaCath c.
Pentalumen c.
PentaPace QRS c.
PE Plus II balloon dilatation c.
Per-C-Cath c.
Percor dual-lumen intraaortic
balloon c.
Percor-Stat-DL c.
Percuflex nephrostomy c.
percutaneous central venous c.
percutaneous drainage c.

percutaneous intraaortic balloon
counterpulsation c.
percutaneous nephrostomy
Malecot c.
percutaneous radiofrequency c.
percutaneous rotational
thrombectomy c.
percutaneous transhepatic biliary
drainage c.
percutaneous transhepatic pigtail c.
percutaneous transluminal coronary
angioplasty c.
perfusion c.
perfusion balloon c.
Periflow peripheral balloon
angioplasty-infusion c.
peripheral long-line c.
peripherally inserted central c.
(PICC)
peripherally inserted central
venous c. (PICVC)
peritoneal dialysis c.
peritoneal reflux control c.
PermCath dual-lumen
hemodialysis c.
Per-Q-Cath CVP c.
Perry-Foley c.
Perry pediatric Foley latex c.
Personal Catheter 100% silicone
intermittent c.
Per-Stat-DL c.
pervenous c.
Pezzer mushroom-tipped c.
Pezzer self-retaining urethral c.
Pezzer suprapubic cystostomy c.
Pfeifer c.
Phantom V Plus balloon
dilatation c.
Pharmaseal c.
Pharmex disposable c.
phased-array ultrasound-tipped c.
phase-shifted multielectrode c.
Phillips urethral c.
Phillips urologic c.
Phoenix Anti-Blok ventricular c.
PIBC c.
Piccolino Monorail balloon c.
Pico-ST II low-profile balloon c.
Pico-T II PTCA balloon c.
pigtail c.
pigtail rotation c.
Pilcher c.

C

NOTES

catheter *(continued)*
    Pilotip c.
    Pinkerton balloon c.
    Pipelle c.
    Pivot fixed-wire balloon c.
    plastic Tiemann c.
    Pleur-evac chest c.
    Pleurx indwelling pleural c.
    c. plug
    plugged telescoping c.
    pneumatic balloon c.
    POC Bandit c.
    Polaris-Dx steerable diagnostic c.
    Polaris LE c.
    Polaris steerable diagnostic c.
    20-pole deflectable halo c.
    20-pole deflectable mapping c.
    Pollock c.
    Poly-Cath balloon c.
    polyethylene c.
    PolyFlo peripherally inserted c.
    polypropylene c.
    Polysil-Foley c.
    Polystan venous return c.
    polyurethane c.
    polyurethane nasoenteric c.
    polyvinyl chloride c.
    pop-on self-adhering male
      external c.
    Port-A-Cath implantable c.
    portal c.
    Porterfield c.
    Portex chorionic villus sampling c.
    Portex-Gibbon c.
    Portnoy multiflanged c.
    Portnoy ventricular c.
    Porto-Vac c.
    position-sensing c.
    Positrol II Bernstein c.
    Positrol USCI c.
    Pousson pigtail c.
    Powerflex balloon c.
    Powerflex Extreme PTA
      dilatation c.
    Predator balloon c.
    preformed Cordis c.
    preshaped c.
    Priestly c.
    Pro-Bal protected balloon-tipped c.
    probe balloon c.
    c. probe ultrasound
    probing sheath exchange c.
    Procath electrophysiology c.
    Pro-Cell balloon c.
    ProCross Rely over-the-wire
      balloon c.
    Profile Plus balloon dilatation c.
    Proflex dilatation c.
    Pro-Flo XT c.

    Pro infusion c.
    Prostaprobe c.
    prostatic bridge c.
    ProSys silicone sterile 2-way, 3-
      way Foley c.
    proximal occlusion c. (POC)
    Pruitt-Inahara balloon-tipped
      perfusion c.
    Pruitt irrigation c.
    Pruitt occlusion c.
    PTA balloon c.
    PTBD c.
    PTCA c.
    PTCA rapid exchange c.
    PU c.
    Pudenz barium cardiac c.
    Pudenz-Heyer vascular c.
    Pudenz infant cardiac c.
    Pudenz peritoneal c.
    Pudenz ventricular c.
    pulmonary artery c.
    pulmonary flotation c.
    pulmonary triple-lumen c.
    pulse spray c.
    Pursuit c.
    pusher c.
    push-pull c.
    Putnam evacuator c.
    PVC c.
    pyeloureteral c.
    PythonEC c.
    Quad-Lumen c.
    Quadra-Flo infusion c.
    quadripolar diagnostic c.
    quadripolar electrode c.
    quadripolar 6-French diagnostic
      electrophysiology c.
    quadripolar pacing c.
    quadripolar steerable electrode c.
    Quanticor c.
    Quantum Maverick c.
    Quantum Monorail balloon c.
    Quantum Ranger OTW balloon c.
    QuickFlash arterial c.
    Quinton biopsy c.
    Quinton central venous c.
    Quinton dual-lumen c.
    Quinton-Mahurkar dual-lumen
      peritoneal c.
    Quinton peritoneal c.
    Quinton PermCath c.
    Quinton Q-Port c.
    Raaf Cath vascular c.
    Raaf dual-lumen c.
    Racz c.
    radial artery c.
    Radiofocus Glidewire
      angiography c.
    radiofrequency c.

radiofrequency-generated thermal balloon c.
radiofrequency thermal balloon c.
radiopaque calibrated c.
radiopaque ERCP c.
radiopaque silastic c.
railway c.
Raimondi peritoneal c.
Raimondi ventricular c.
Ramirez winged c.
Ranfac cholangiographic c.
Ranger OTW balloon c.
rapid exchange balloon c.
rapid exchange PTCA c.
Rashkind atrial septostomy balloon c.
rat-tail c.
RC1 c.
recessed balloon septostomy c.
rectal c.
Reddick cystic duct cholangiogram c.
Reddick-Saye screw c.
RediFurl TaperSeal IAB c.
RediGuard IAB c.
red Robinson c.
red rubber c.
reference c.
Reif c.
Release-NF c.
Reliance urinary control insert c.
Rentrop infusion c.
reperfusion c.
Replogle suction c.
Response electrophysiology c.
retention c.
retrograde femoral c.
retrograde occlusion balloon c.
retroperfusion c.
return-flow hemostatic c.
return-flow retention c.
Revivac c.
Reynolds infusion c.
RF Ablatr ablation c.
RF balloon c.
RF Mariner c.
RF Performer c.
rheolytic thrombectomy c.
Rhyder diagnostic c.
Rica eustachian c.
right coronary c.
right heart c.

right Judkins c.
Rigiflex ABD balloon dilatation c.
Rigiflex biliary balloon dilatation c.
Rigiflex OTW balloon dilatation c.
Rigiflex TTS balloon dilatation c.
RIJ c.
Ring-McLean c.
RI Rapid Exchange balloon c.
Rivas vascular c.
Robinson urethral c.
Rochester Medical self-adhering male external c.
Rocket coronary dilatation c.
Rockey-Thompson c.
Rodriguez c.
Rodriguez-Alvarez c.
Rolnel c.
Rosch c.
Rosch-Thurmond fallopian tube c.
Ross c.
Rotablator c.
Rotacs motorized c.
rotatable pigtail c.
rotating cutter c.
Rothene c.
Roubin LuMax flexible guiding c.
Royal Flush angiographic flush c.
R1 rapid exchange balloon dilatation c.
rubber c.
Rumel c.
Rusch bronchial c.
Rusch coudé c.
Ruschelit c.
Rusch external c.
Rusch-Foley c.
Rutner nephrostomy balloon c.
Rutner Universal wedge ureteral c.
RX Comet VP coronary dilatation c.
RX CrossSail coronary dilatation c.
RX Rocket coronary dilatation c.
RX Solaris coronary dilatation c.
RX Streak balloon c.
RX Viatrac 14 peripheral dilatation c.
Sable balloon c.
Sable PTCA balloon c.
Sacks QuickStick c.
Sacks Single-Step c.
Safe-Dwel Plus c.

C

NOTES

catheter *(continued)*

Safe-T-Coat heparin-coated thermodilution c.
SafTouch c.
Salvage c.
Saratoga sump c.
Sarns wire-reinforced c.
Savvy PTA dilatation c.
SCA-Ex ShortCutter c.
Schneider c.
Schneider-Shiley dilatation c.
Schneider trefoil balloon c.
SchonCath long-term c.
Schon hemodialysis c.
SchonXL temporary c.
Schoonmaker femoral c.
Schrotter c.
Schwarten balloon dilatation c.
Schwarten LP balloon c.
Science-Med balloon c.
Scimed angioplasty c.
Scimed guiding c.
Scimed rTRA-GC guiding c.
Scimed SSC Skinny c.
scleral buckling c.
Scoop transtracheal c.
Seidel c.
Seldinger cardiac c.
Selecon coronary angiography c.
Selective-HI c.
Seletz c.
Self-Cath coudé tipped c.
self-guiding c.
self-retaining c.
Sellheim uterine c.
semirigid c.
Semm uterine vacuum c.
Sensation intraaortic balloon c.
sensing c.
Sentron pigtail angiographic micromanometer c.
septostomy balloon c.
Seroma-Cath wound drainage c.
serrated c.
SetPoint coronary c.
SG c.
Shadow over-the-wire balloon c.
Shadow-Stripe c.
Shaldon c.
shaver c.
Shaw c.
c. sheath
shellac-covered c.
shepherd's hook c.
Sherpa guiding c.
Shiley guiding c.
Shiley-Ionescu c.
Shiley irrigation c.
Shiley MultiPro c.

Shiley soft-tip guiding c.
Shone c.
short-arm Grollman c.
ShortCutter c.
Shulitz c.
side-hole c.
side-hole pigtail c.
sidewinder percutaneous intraaortic balloon c.
Siegel-Cohen dilating c.
Silastic c.
Silastic elastomer infusion c.
Silastic ileal reservoir c.
Silastic mushroom c.
Silcath subclavian c.
silicone elastomer infusion c.
silicone epistaxis c.
silicone Robinson c.
silicone rubber Dacron-cuffed c.
Silicore c.
Silitek c.
silk-and-wax c.
Sil-Med c.
silver c.
silver-coated c.
Simmons c.
Simmons sidewinder c.
Simplastic c.
Simplus PE/t dilatation c.
Simpson atherectomy c.
Simpson coronary AtheroCath c.
Simpson-Robert ACS dilatation c.
Simpson suction c.
Simpson Ultra Lo-Profile II balloon c.
single-lumen balloon stone extractor c.
single-lumen infusion c.
single-stage c.
Skene c.
Skinny over-the-wire balloon c.
Sleek c.
Slider c.
sliding-rail c.
Slinky balloon c.
Slinky PTCA c.
Slip-Sheen c.
SMIC eustachian c.
snare c.
Soaker c.
Soehendra Universal dilating c.
Soft-Cell permanent dual-lumen c.
Sof-T guiding c.
Softip arteriography c.
Softip diagnostic c.
Softouch angiography c.
Softouch Cobra 1, 2 c.
Softouch Headhunter 1 c.
Softouch Multipurpose B2 c.

Softouch Simmons 1, 2 c.
Softouch UHF cardiac pigtail c.
Softrac-PTA c.
Soft Seal cervical c.
soft-tip c.
Soft Torque uterine c.
Soft-Vu angiographic c.
Soft-Vu Omni flush c.
Solaris coronary dilatation c.
Solera thrombectomy c.
solid-state esophageal manometry c.
solid-tip c.
SoloCath c.
Sones Cardio-Marker c.
Sones coronary c.
Sones Hi-Flow c.
Sones Positrol c.
Sones vent c.
Sones woven Dacron c.
Sonicath endoluminal ultrasound c.
Sonicath intravascular ultrasound c.
Sorenson thermodilution c.
SOS Omni c.
Soules intrauterine insemination c.
Spectra-Cath STP c.
Spectranetics Extreme peripheral c.
Spectranetics support c.
Spectrum antibiotic-impregnated
  central venous c.
Speedy balloon c.
Spetzler subarachnoid c.
SPI-Argent II peritoneal dialysis c.
spinal c.
SpineCATH intradiscal c.
spiral-tipped c.
split-sheath c.
Spring c.
Sprint c.
Spyglass angiography c.
Squibb c.
Squire c.
Stack perfusion coronary
  dilatation c.
Stamey open-tip ureteral c.
Stanford end-hole pigtail c.
Stargate falloposcopy c.
StatLock-Foley c.
StatLock hemodyalysis c.
St. Bartholomew barium c.
Stealth angioplasty balloon c.
steerable c.
steerable DecaPolar electrode c.

steerable electrode c.
steerable guidewire c.
steering c.
Steerocath-A, -T ablation c.
Steerocath-Dx valve mapping c.
stenting c.
Steri-Cath c.
Stertzer brachial guiding c.
StimuCath nerve block c.
stimulating c.
Stinger M, S ablation c.
Stitt c.
Stormer balloon c.
Storz bronchial c.
Storz-DeKock 2-way bronchial c.
Storz scleral buckling balloon c.
straight flush percutaneous c.
straight-tipped c.
Streamline peripheral c.
StressCath c.
Stretta c.
Stretzer bent-tip USCI c.
Stringer tracheal c.
Stripseal c.
subclavian apheresis c.
subclavian dialysis c.
subclavian hemodialysis c.
subclavian vein access c.
submicroinfusion c.
suction c.
Suction Buster c.
Suggs c.
Sugita c.
SULP II balloon c.
sump drainage c.
Superflow guiding c.
Super-9 guiding c.
Superior suction c.
Supertorque MB 5F marker band
  flush c.
Super Torque Plus c.
SupraFoley suprapubic c.
suprapubic c. (SC)
Supreme electrophysiology c.
SureCath port access c.
Sure Seal Golden Drain c.
Surflo IV c.
Surgimedics cholangiography c.
Surgitek Double-J ureteral c.
Surpass c.
Swan-Ganz balloon flotation c.
Swan-Ganz bipolar pacing c.

NOTES

catheter *(continued)*

Swan-Ganz flow-directed c.
Swan-Ganz pacing TD c.
Swan-Ganz pulmonary artery c.
Swan-Ganz thermodilution c.
swan-neck Missouri c.
swan-neck pediatric Coil-Cath c.
Switzerland dilatation c.
Syntel embolectomy c.
Syntel graft cleaning c.
Syntel latex-free embolectomy c.
systemic arterial c.
TAC atherectomy c.
Tactilaze angioplasty laser c.
Taheri-Leonhardt c.
Takumi PTCA c.
Talon balloon dilatation c.
Tandem thin-shaft transureteroscopic
  balloon dilatation c.
Tant cystic duct c.
tapered c.
tapered-tip hydrophilic-coated
  guiding c.
Tauber male urethrographic c.
Taut cholangiographic c.
Taut cystic duct c.
Taut M-series c.
TEC c.
Tefcat intrauterine insemination c.
Teflon ERCP c.
Teflon guiding c.
Teflon injection c.
Teflon-tipped c.
TEGwire balloon dilatation c.
telescoping plugged c.
temporary pacing c.
Tenckhoff 2-cuff c.
Tenckhoff peritoneal dialysis c.
Tennis Racquet angiographic c.
Ten system balloon c.
Terumo SP coaxial c.
Terumo Surflo intravenous c.
Tesio c.
tetrapolar esophageal c.
Texas condom c.
ThermaChoice c.
thermistor c.
thermistor thermodilution c.
thermodilution balloon c.
thermodilution pacing c.
thermodilution Swan-Ganz c.
thin-walled c.
thin-walled introducer c.
Thompson bronchial c.
ThoraCath c.
thrombectomy c.
thrombosuction c.
through-the-scope c.
Thruflex PTCA balloon c.

Tiemann coudé c.
Tiemann-Foley c.
Tiemann Neoflex c.
Timberlake c.
tip-deflecting c.
c. tip occluder
Tis-U-Trap endometrial suction c.
Titan balloon c.
Tolantins bone marrow infusion c.
Tomac c.
Tomac-Nélaton c.
toposcopic c.
Torcon blue c.
Torcon NB selective
  angiographic c.
Torktherm torque control c.
Toronto-Western Hospital c.
torque-control balloon c.
total parenteral nutrition c.
Tourguide guiding c.
TPN c.
Trabucco double balloon c.
TrachCare multi-access c.
tracheal c.
Trach-Eze closed suction c.
Tracker-18 Soft Stream c.
Tracker-18 Unibody c.
Trac Plus c.
Trakstar balloon c.
transcervical tubal access c.
transcutaneous extraction c.
transducer-tipped c.
transfemoral c.
transfemoral endoaortic occlusion c.
translumbar inferior vena caval c.
transluminal angioplasty c.
transluminal endarterectomy c.
transluminal extraction c. (TEC)
transoral c.
transport c.
transseptal c.
transthoracic c.
transtracheal oxygen c.
transurethral c.
transvenous pacemaker c.
Trattner urethrographic c.
trefoil balloon c.
Trellis infusion c.
Trestle transurethral prostatic c.
Trifecta multipurpose balloon c.
Triguide c.
Trilogy low-profile balloon
  dilatation c.
triple-balloon perfusion c.
triple-lumen c.
triple-lumen Arrow c.
triple-lumen biliary manometry c.
triple-lumen central c.
triple-lumen manometry c.

triple-thermistor coronary sinus c.
tripolar Damato curve c.
tripolar electrode c.
Trocath peritoneal dialysis c.
Troeltsch eustachian c.
True Sheathless c.
T-TAC c.
T-tube c.
c. tube holder
Tun-L-Kath epidural c.
tunnelable ventricular ICP c.
tunneled c.
Tuohy c.
twist drill c.
Tygon c.
Tyshak balloon valvuloplasty c.
Uldall subclavian hemodialysis c.
UltraCross c.
Ultraflex self-adhering male
  external c.
Ultra-Flow double-lumen high-
  flow c.
Ultrafuse c.
Ultra 8 intraaortic balloon c.
Ultramer c.
ultrasound ablation c.
ultrasound-tipped c.
umbilical artery c.
umbilical vein c.
umbilical venous c.
UMI Cath-Seal c.
Unicath all-purpose c.
UniFuse infusion c.
Uni-Sem intrauterine c.
Unisensor unitip pressure sensor c.
UNI shunt c.
Universal drainage c.
Uniweave c.
Ureflex ureteral c.
UreSil biliary c.
UreSil
  embolectomy/thrombectomy c.
UreSil irrigation c.
UreSil occlusion balloon c.
ureteral dilatation c.
ureteral occlusion balloon c.
urethral c.
UrethraMax urethral c.
urethrographic c.
Uridome c.
Uridrop c.
urinary c.

Urocare Foley c.
Uro-Cath external c.
Uro-Con Texas style male
  external c.
urodynamic c.
urological c.
UroMax II high-pressure balloon c.
Uro-San Plus external c.
USCI Bard c.
USCI Finesse guiding c.
USCI Mini-Profile PTCA balloon
  dilatation c.
USCI Positrol coronary c.
uterine cornual access c.
uterine ostial access c.
Vabra c.
Vacurette c.
vacuum aspiration c.
vacuum cup c.
valve-ended c.
valvuloplasty balloon c.
Van Aman pigtail c.
Van Aman pulmonary pigtail c.
Van Andel dilation c.
Van Buren c.
Vance-Kish urethral illuminated c.
Vance percutaneous Malecot
  nephrostomy c.
van Sonnenberg gallbladder c.
van Sonnenberg sump c.
van Sonnenberg-Wittich c.
Van Tassel pigtail c.
Vantec occlusion balloon c.
Vantec ureteral balloon dilatation c.
Vantex central venous c.
Variflex c.
Varisource remote afterloading c.
Vas-Cath dialysis c.
Vas-Cath Opti-Plast peripheral
  angioplasty c.
Vas-Cath Soft-Cell c.
vascular access c.
Vascu-Sheath c.
Vaso-Cath peritoneal dialysis c.
Vaxcel peripherally inserted
  central c.
V-Cath c.
Vector large-lumen guiding c.
Venaport guiding c.
venous c.
venous irrigation c.
venous thrombectomy c.

NOTES

catheter *(continued)*
 venting c.
 Ventra c.
 ventricular c.
 ventriculography c.
 Ventrix True Tech ICP c.
 Ventureyra ventricular c.
 Verbatim balloon c.
 Veripath peripheral guiding c.
 Versaflex steerable c.
 vertebrated c.
 vessel-sizing c.
 Viking Optima guiding c.
 Viper PTA c.
 Virden rectal c.
 Visa II PTCA c.
 Visicath viewing c.
 Vision PTCA c.
 Visi-Tube c.
 Vista Brite Tip guiding c.
 Vitalcor venous return c.
 Vitatron E c.
 Vitax female c.
 Vitesse Cos laser c.
 Vitesse E-II coronary c.
 c. vitrector
 Vivonex jejunostomy c.
 V. Mueller embolectomy c.
 Vnus Closure c.
 Vnus Restore c.
 Voda c.
 von Andel biliary dilation c.
 vonSonnenberg-Wittich c.
 VPI nonadhesive condom c.
 Vueport balloon occlusion
  guiding c.
 Vuport balloon-occlusion c.
 Vygon Nutricath S c.
 c. waist tube holder
 Walrus Advancit c.
 Walrus Angioflus c.
 Walther female c.
 Was-Catheter c.
 washing c.
 Watanabe c.
 water-infusion esophageal
  manometry c.
 water-perfused c.
 waveguide c.
 2-way c.
 3-way Foley c.
 3-way irrigating c.
 Weber rectal c.
 Weber winged c.
 Webster coronary sinus c.
 Webster orthogonal electrode c.
 wedge pressure balloon c.
 Western external urinary c.
 Wexler c.

 whalebone filiform c.
 whistle-tip Foley c.
 whistle-tip ureteral c.
 Wholey balloon occlusion c.
 Wholey-Edwards c.
 wick c.
 Wideband urinary c.
 Williams L-R guiding c.
 Wilson-Cook fine-needle
  aspiration c.
 Wilton-Webster coronary sinus
  thermodilution c.
 Wilton-Webster thermodilution
  pacing c.
 Winer c.
 winged c.
 4-wing Malecot retention c.
 Winston SD c.
 Wishard c.
 Wishard ureteral c.
 Witzel enterostomy c.
 Wolf nephrostomy c.
 Woodruff ureteropyelographic c.
 Word Bartholin gland c.
 Workhorse percutaneous
  transuluminal angioplasty
  balloon c.
 woven Dacron c.
 woven silk c.
 Wurd c.
 Xemex pulmonary artery c.
 XL-11 Ranfac percutaneous
  cholangiographic c.
 Xpeedior series c.
 X-Sizer c.
 X-Trode electrode c.
 XXL balloon dilatation c.
 Yankauer eustachian c.
 Y-trough c.
 Yumiko-Lita c.
 Zavod bronchospirometry c.
 Zimmon c.
 Zinnanti uterine manipulator-
  injector c.
 Z-Med balloon c.
 Zucker multipurpose bipolar c.
 Zuma coronary guiding c.
 Zuma guiding c.
 ZUMI c.
 Zurich dilatation c.
CatheterPump
 Reitan C.
Catheter-Secure tape
catheter-tipped manometer
Cath-Finder
 C.-F. catheter
 C.-F. catheter tracking system
Cath-Guide closed suction catheter

CathLink
    C. 20 catheter
    C. implantable vascular access
        device
    C. 20 implanted port
Cath-Lok catheter locking device
Cathlon IV catheter
Cathmark suction catheter
cathode
    c. ray oscilloscope
    c. ray tube
Cath-Secure
    C.-S. catheter holder
    C.-S. dual-tab holder
    C.-S. tape
Cath-Strip recloseable catheter fastener
CathTrack catheter locator system
Catlin amputation knife
cat paw retractor
Catrix
    C. ointment
    C. wound dressing
CatsEye digital camera system
Cat's Paw exerciser
Cattell
    C. forked-type T- tube
    C. gallbladder tube
Caud-A-Kath epidural catheter
caudal
    c. hook
    c. needle
caulking gun
Cault punch
Causse
    C. piston
    C. stapes sheet
cauterizer
    Bucholz bipolar c.
cauterizing ball
cautery
    Aaron c.
    c. ablator
    Accu-Temp c.
    Acucise ureteral cutting c.
    Alcon handheld c.
    alkaline battery c.
    Berchtold c.
    Berkeley Bioengineering bipolar c.
    BICAP c.
    BICAP II c.
    BiLAP c.
    bipolar c.

Birtcher c.
Bovie c.
Bovie wet-field c.
Burdick c.
Cameron c.
c. clamp
Codman-Mentor Wet-Field c.
cold c.
Concept disposable c.
Concept handheld c.
Corrigan c.
cutting c.
Denis bipolar c.
disposable c.
Downes c.
c. electrode
eraser c.
Eraser-tip c.
Fine micropoint c.
Geiger c.
Gonin c.
Goodhill c.
hand-control c.
handheld c.
Hildreth ocular c.
c. hook
Hotsy high-temperature c.
Ishihara I-Temp c.
Khosia c.
c. knife electrode
L-shaped c.
Magielski coagulation c.
MegaDyne c.
Mentor Wet-Field c.
Mira c.
monopolar c.
Mueller alkaline battery c.
Mueller Currentrol c.
National c.
needlepoint c.
NeoKnife c.
ocular c.
Paquelin c.
Parker-Heath c.
pencil c.
pencil-tip c.
phacoemulsification c.
Prince eye c.
Ritter Bovie c.
Rommel c.
Rommel-Hildreth c.
Schanz c.

C

NOTES

cautery *(continued)*
    Scheie ophthalmic c.
    Schepens eye c.
    c. scissors
    c. snare
    Souttar c.
    Statham c.
    stepped-down c.
    suction c.
    Ultrafyn thermal c.
    unipolar c.
    c. unit
    Valleylab c.
    von Graefe c.
    Wadsworth-Todd c.
    walker c.
    Wappler cold c.
    Wepsic fiberoptic c.
    wet-field c.
    Wills Eye Hospital c.
    Ziegler c.
cava
    inferior vena c. (IVC)
caval
    c. cannula
    c. catheter
    c. occlusion clamp
Cavanaugh-Israel bur
Cavanaugh sphenoid bur
Cavanaugh-Wells tonsillar forceps
Cave
    C. cartilage knife
    C. knee retractor
    C. scaphoid gouge
    C. scaphoid spatula
CaverMap surgical device
cavernospongiosum shunt
Cave-Rowe ligature carrier
Caves bioptome
Cavi-Endo ultrasonic system
Cavi-Jet dental prophylaxis device
Cavi-Pulse ultrasonic aspirator
Cavitat ultrasonograph bone densitometer
Cavitec cavity liner
Cavitron
    C. aspirator
    C. cautery unit
    C. dissector
    C. I&A handpiece
    C. I&A system
    C. laser
    C. machine
    C. phacoemulsification unit
    C. phacoemulsifier
    C. scalpel
    C. SPS ultrasonic scaler
    C. Ultrasonic Surgical Aspirator (CUSA)

Cavitron-Kelman
    C.-K. I&A system
    C.-K. phacoemulsification machine
cavity drainage catheter
Cavoline cavity liner
C-AVR spinal reconstruction system
Cawood nasal splint
Caylor scissors
CB
    Continuum Biomedical
    CB Diode/532 laser
    CB Erbium/2.94 laser
C-bar web-spacer
CBCS
    cord blood collection system
C-beam laser
C-beveled chisel
CBI
    Cancer and Blood Institute
    CBI stereotactic head holder
    CBI stereotactic ring
CC Rider closed-chain rehabilitation system
C-D
    C-D hook
    C-D instrumentation device
CD
    CD Horizon Eclipse spinal system
    CD Horizon Sextant spinal system
    CD instrumentation
C-Dak dialyzer
CD-Chex
    CD-C. CD4 LOW flow cytometer
    CD-C. Plus flow cytometry control
CDH
    CDH Precoat Plus hip prosthesis
    CDH stapler
cDNA probe
CDRPan digital x-ray system
CDX Spiro 850 portable spirometer
Cebotome drill
Cecar electrode
Cecil dressing
cecostomy
    c. catheter
    c. retractor
Cedar anesthesia face rest
Ceegraph 128 EEG system
CeeOn
    C. Edge foldable lens
    C. heparinized intraocular lens
Celay
    C. milling unit
    C. Tech light curing resin
Celestin
    C. bougie
    C. endoesophageal prosthesis
    C. endoesophageal tube
    C. endoprosthesis

C. graduated dilator
C. graft material
C. implant
C. latex rubber tube
Celita
C. Elite knife
C. Sapphire knife
cell
c. analysis system
c. recovery System
C. Saver 4 cardiopulmonary bypass blood centrifuge
C. Saver Haemolite autotransfusion system
C. Saver Haemonetics autotransfusion system
C. Soft 2000 semen analyzer
C. Sweep cervical cytology device
C. Trak/DMS semen analyzer
C. Trak 11 semen analyzer
C. Trak/S semen analyzer
Cellamin resin plaster-of-Paris bandage
Cell-Chex body fluid control
CellFIT acquisition system
Cellolite
C. material
C. patty
Cellona resin plaster-of-Paris bandage
cellophane dressing
cell-seeded stent
Cellugel ophthalmologic viscosurgical device
celluloid
c. implant
c. linen suture
cellulose surgical sponge
Celluron dental roll
Cell-VU disposable semen analysis chamber
Celsite
C. brachial port
C. pediatric port
Cel Touch adhesive
CEM
CUSA electrosurgical module
Cemax/Icon scanner
Cemax PACS platform
cement
acrylic c.
antibiotic-loaded acrylic c.
Atwood orthodontic c.
BA bone c.

bioactive bone c.
Bistite II DC resin c.
bone c.
Boneloc c.
BoneSource hydroxyapatite c.
Buffalo dental c.
Cemex bone c.
c. centralizer
Ceramco dental c.
Ceramlin dental c.
Ceramsave dental c.
Compacement dental c.
composite dental c.
Concert bone c.
Conclude dental c.
Copal bone c.
copper phosphate c.
dental c.
DePuy 1 bone c.
dermatome c.
Diaket root canal c.
Duall 88 c.
Durelon dental c.
Eastman dental c.
c. eater
c. eater drill
Endurance bone c.
Epoxylite CBA dental resin c.
Freegenol c.
Fuji dental c.
Generation 4 bone c.
glass ionomer c.
Howmedica Osteonics bone c.
Howmedica Simplex P c.
Implast bone c.
IMProv c.
inorganic dental c.
Ketac Fil c.
Ketac Silver c.
Kirkland c.
low-viscosity bone c.
master c.
modified zinc oxide-eugenol c.
Mynol endodontic c.
Neutrocim dental c.
Nobetec dental c.
Nogenol dental c.
Norian SRS c.
organic dental c.
Orthocomp c.
orthodontic c.
Orthoset c.

C

NOTES

cement *(continued)*
　　Osteobond copolymer bone c.
　　Osteopal G low-viscosity c.
　　Osteopal V vertebroplasty bone c.
　　Palacos Radiopaque bone c.
　　Palamed bone c.
　　Palamed G bone c.
　　Petralit dental c.
　　polycarboxylate c.
　　polymethyl methacrylate bone c.
　　Pronto c.
　　prosthetic antibiotic-loaded
　　　acrylic c.
　　Pulpdent Ortho Band c.
　　Refobacin Palacos R c.
　　resin c.
　　Restore X dental c.
　　c. restrictor
　　Roth dental c.
　　Selfast dental c.
　　Shofu dental c.
　　silicate c.
　　Simplex P bone c.
　　Skin-Bond skin c.
　　c. spatula
　　Sulfix-6 c.
　　Super-Dent orthodontic c.
　　SuperEBA c.
　　Surgical Simplex P radiopaque
　　　bone c.
　　Tempbond dental c.
　　Temrex dental c.
　　tooth c.
　　Torbot bonding c.
　　VersaBond c.
　　Wacker Sil-Gel 604 silicone c.
　　Zimmer bone c.
**Cementless Sportorno hip arthroplasty
stem**
cement-removal hand tool
Cemex bone cement
Cencit
　　C. facial scanner
　　C. imaging system
　　C. surface scanner
Cenflex central station monitor
CenSlide 2000 urinalysis centrifuge
Centauri Er:YAG laser
Centaur trial cup
center-action forceps
centering
　　c. balloon
　　c. drill
　　c. ring
Centermark vascular access device
CenterPointLock 2-piece ostomy system
centimeter subtraction ruler
Centimist nebulizer
Centra-Flex lens

central
　　c. extensor mechanism
　　c. terminal electrode
　　c. venous pressure (CVP)
　　c. venous pressure catheter
Centralign precoat hip prosthesis
centralizer
　　cement c.
　　Integral distal c.
　　PMMA c.
Centrax
　　C. bipolar endoprosthesis
　　C. bipolar system
Centrica rotational core biopsy system
Centricon-10 filter
CentriFlow mass flow meter
centrifugal pump
centrifuge
　　Beckman J6M c.
　　Cell Saver 4 cardiopulmonary
　　　bypass blood c.
　　CenSlide 2000 urinalysis c.
　　CritSpin c.
　　Eppendorf c.
　　Ficoll-Hypaque gradient c.
　　HemataSTAT portable
　　　microhematocrit c.
　　MicroMax c.
　　Polyprep c.
　　StatSpin Express c.
Centrix
　　C. PDQ ligator
　　C. syringe
**Centronic 200 MGA respiratory mass
spectrometer**
Centurion
　　C. BedBath
　　C. gel moisturizer saliva substitute
Century
　　C. BC-65 birthing chair
　　C. bicarbonate dialysis control unit
　　C. heart lung machine
cephalad catheter
cephalic blade forceps
cephalometer
　　Bertillon c.
　　Plasticeph c.
　　Wehmer c.
cephalometric protractor
cephalostat
　　DuoCeph c.
　　EC Proline c.
　　Orthoceph OC100 c.
　　Wehmer c.
cephalotribe
　　Tarnier c.
**Ceprate SC Instrument II cell-
separation device**
Cerablate Plus Flutter ablation catheter

CerAdapt abutment
Ceradelta alloy
Ceramalloy alloy
Ceramco
    C. dental cement
    C. porcelain kit
ceramic
    c. endosteal implant
    c. ossicular prosthesis
    titanate c.
    c. vertebral spacer
Ceramion prosthesis
Ceramlin dental cement
ceramometal implant
Ceramsave dental cement
CeraOne
    C. abutment
    C. abutment/implant screw
    C. implant system
Cerapall alloy
CeraSPECT camera
CeraSpoon curette
Ceravital incus replacement prosthesis
cerclage
    Howmedica c.
    McDonald c.
    Tylok c.
    c. wire
    c. wire twister
cerebellar retractor
Cereblate catheter
cerebral
    c. cannula
    c. catheter
    c. function monitor
    c. retractor
    c. spinal fluid reservoir
    c. spinal fluid valve
cerebrograph
cerebrospinal
    c. fluid (CSF)
    c. fluid shunt
Cer-Mate alloy
Cer-On R alloy
Cerrobend
    C. cast
    C. trim block
Cerva crane halter
Cervex-Brush
    C.-B. cervical cell collector
    C.-B. cervical cell sampler

cervical
    c. AOA halo traction
    c. biopsy blade
    c. biopsy curette
    c. biopsy forceps
    c. block
    c. brace
    c. cannula
    c. clamp
    c. collar
    c. cone knife
    c. conization electrode
    c. dilator
    c. disc retractor
    c. dislocation reducer
    c. drill guide
    c. fusion plate
    c. grasping forceps
    c. hemostatic forceps
    c. mallet
    c. orthosis
    c. plate
    c. punch
    c. punch forceps
    c. range-of-motion (CROM)
    c. range-of-motion instrument
    c. rest
    c. retractor
    c. roll
    c. rongeur
    c. saddle
    c. skull pillow
    c. sleep pillow
    c. tenaculum
    c. traction forceps
    c. vulsellum
cervicothoracic
    c. jacket
    c. orthosis
Cer-View lateral wall retractor
CerviFix system
Cervi-Lok cervical fixation system
CerviSoft cytology collection device
Cervitrak device
cesarean
    c. binder
    c. forceps
cesium
    c. applicator
    c. candle
    c. fluoride scintillation detector
    c. needle

NOTES

CF-200Z Olympus colonoscope
CFA digital camera
CFC BioScanner system
CFix cable fixation system
C-Flex
C-F. Amsterdam stent
C-F. catheter
C-F. II cervical traction
C-F. supine cervical traction
C-F. ureteral stent
CFS hip prosthesis
CF-UM3 echocolonoscope
CFV wrist component
CGI-1 contact lens
CGR biplane angiographic system
Chadwick scissors
Chaffin catheter
Chaffin-Pratt drain
Chailey go-cart
chain saw
chair
Action Ranger II power c.
Adapta MC-100 massage c.
bedside air c.
birthing c.
BodyBilt c.
Century BC-65 birthing c.
CombiSit surgeon c.
computerized rotary c.
DuraTilt wheeled
shower/commode c.
dynamic integrated stabilization c.
(DISC)
EasyChair massage c.
EZ Rider support c.
fluoroscopic imaging c.
Gardner c.
geriatric c.
Hi-seat Artherapedic hip c.
Invacare padded shower c.
invalid c.
Kaleidoscope c.
Kaye Kinder c.
Kinder c.
Midmark 413 power female
procedure c.
mobile air c.
Orthokinetics travel c.
Pigg-O-Stat x-ray c.
Pogon c.
Portal Pro 3 treatment c.
Portazam portable exam c.
reclining air c.
Relax SLH Deluxe massage c.
seated hamstring curl exercise c.
shower c.
sit/stand c.
SPECTurn c.
STC 900-series travel c.

urodynamics c.
Vancare shower/commode
transfer c.
Vess c.
Chairback brace
ChairCiser exerciser
Chair-Mate system
chalazion
c. clamp
c. curette
c. forceps
c. knife
c. retractor
c. trephine
Challenger digital applanation tonometer
Chalnot valvulotome
chamber
AeroChamber Plus valved
holding c.
AeroPEP Plus valve holding c.
AeroTrach Plus valve holding c.
AeroVent collapsible holding c.
air c.
anterior c. (AC)
Bactron 1.5 anaerobic c.
Bara-Med clinical acrylic
monoplace hyperbaric c.
Bara-Med clinical multiplace
hyperbaric c.
Boyden c.
Cell-VU disposable semen
analysis c.
collapsible holding c. (CHC)
drill c.
drip c.
Finn c.
Fisher-Paykel MR290 water-feed c.
flush c.
hydraulic c.
hyperbaric c.
Hyper-Oxy portable hyperbaric c.
LiteAire disposable dual-valved
holding c.
Makler reusable semen analysis c.
MicroCell c.
MoistAir humidifying c.
moisture c.
monoplace c.
MR 290 humidification c.
multiwire proportional c.
OptiChamber valved holding c.
parallel-plate flow c.
Pari Vortex holding c.
plasma clot diffusion c.
Sechrist monoplace hyperbaric c.
Shandon cytospin c.
Storm Von Leeuwen c.
Ussing c.

valved holding c.
valve holding c. (VHC)
Chamberlain-Fries atraumatic retractor
Chamberlain tongue depressor
Chamberlen obstetrical forceps
ChamberLift 2000 patient lift system
Chambers
    C. doughnut pessary
    C. intrauterine cup
    C. intrauterine pessary
chamfer
    c. guide
    c. jig
    c. reamer
chamois
    c. swab
    c. underpad
Champ
    C. arthritis Hotmitt
    C. cardiac device
    C. elastic bandage
Champetier de Ribes obstetrical bag
Champion
    C. drug eluding stent
    C. TE-II total exercise bench
Championnière
    C. bone drill
    C. forceps
Champy miniplate rigid fixation system
Chandler
    C. bone elevator
    C. felt collar splint
    C. iris forceps
    C. knee retractor
    C. laminectomy retractor
    C. mallet
    C. spinal-perforating forceps
    C. table
    C. transluminal V-pacing probe
    C. unreamed interlocking tibial nail
Chang
    C. bone-cutting forceps
    C. Quick Chop combo ophthalmic
    blade
changer
    film c.
    Littmann galilean magnification c.
    Puck film c.
    Sanchez-Perez automatic film
    cassette c.
    Schonander film c.
    tracheal tube c.

channel
    c. dissector
    c. retractor
4-channel Aesculap ventriculoscope
Chan wrist rest
Chaoul
    C. applicator
    C. voltage x-ray tube
Chaput tissue forceps
charcoal filter
Charcot bath
Charcot-Bottcher filament
Chardack-Greatbatch
    C.-G. implantable cardiac pulse
    generator
    C.-G. Medtronic pacemaker
Charest head frame
char-free carbon dioxide laser
charge-coupled
    c.-c. device scanner
    c.-c. device video camera
Charles
    C. anterior segment sleeve
    C. contact lens
    C. flute needle
    C. infusion sleeve
    C. intraocular lens
    C. irrigating lens
    C. vacuuming needle
    C. vitrector with sleeve
Charleston
    C. bending brace
    C. scoliosis brace
Charlton
    C. antral needle
    C. antral trocar
    C. cannula
Charnley
    C. acetabular cup
    C. acetabular cup prosthesis
    C. acetabular scraper
    C. arthrodesis clamp
    C. bone clamp
    C. bone clasp
    C. brace handle
    C. cemented hip prosthesis
    C. cement restrictor
    C. centering drill
    C. centering ring
    C. compressor
    C. cup-trimming scissors
    C. deepening reamer

C

NOTES

163

Charnley *(continued)*
- C. double-ended bone curette
- C. drain tube
- C. expanding reamer
- C. external fixation clamp
- C. femoral broach
- C. femoral condyle drill
- C. femoral condyle radius gauge
- C. femoral inlay aligner
- C. femoral inlay guillotine
- C. femoral lever
- C. femoral prosthesis neck punch
- C. femoral prosthesis pusher
- C. flat-back femoral component
- C. foam suture pad
- C. gouge
- C. hip prosthesis
- C. horizontal retractor
- C. Howorth ExFlow system
- C. implant
- C. knee prosthesis
- C. narrow stem component
- C. offset-bore cup
- C. pilot drill
- C. pin
- C. pin clamp
- C. pin retractor
- C. rasp
- C. saw
- C. self-retaining retractor
- C. socket gauge
- C. standard stem retractor
- C. starting drill
- C. suction drain
- C. suture button
- C. suture forceps
- C. taper reamer
- C. template
- C. tibial onlay jig
- C. total hip prosthesis
- C. towel
- C. trochanter file
- C. trochanter reamer
- C. trochanter wire
- C. wire-holding forceps
- C. wire passer

Charnley-Hastings bipolar prosthesis
Charnley-Mueller hip prosthesis
Charnley-Riches arterial forceps
Charnow notched ruler
Charriére
- C. amputation saw
- C. aseptic metacarpal saw
- C. bone saw

chart
- Amsler c.
- Birkhauser eye testing c.
- Broselow c.
- contemporary near-point c.

- cross-Polaroid projection c.
- Ferris c.
- Hawley c.
- Illiterate E c.
- Ishihara test c.
- Jaeger eye c.
- Jaeger reading c.
- Konig bar c.
- Landolt C acuity c.
- Lea Symbol c.
- Lebensohn c.
- Lighthouse ETDRS acuity c.
- logMAR c.
- Mentor B-VAT visual acuity c.
- Pelli-Robson letter c.
- Pomard anthropomorphic measurement reference c.
- Regan low-contrast acuity c.
- sclerotome pain c.
- Snellen c.
- Turtle c.
- Vistech wall c.

Chase cardiovascular patch
Chaston eye pad
Chatfield-Girdlestone splint
Chatillon dolorimeter
Chattanooga
- C. balance system
- C. exerciser

Chatzidakis implant
Chauffin-Pratt tube
Chaussier tube
Chavantes-Zamorano neuroendoscope
Chavasse
- C. squint hook
- C. strabismus hook

Chayes handpiece
Chayet corneal marker
CHC
- collapsible holding chamber
- AeroVent CHC

Cheanvechai-Favaloro retractor
Cheatle sterilizing forceps
Checkerboard wheelchair cushion
Check-Flo
- C.-F. introducer
- C.-F. introducer sheath

Checkmate intravascular brachytherapy system
checkvalve
- BacStop anti-retraction c.

cheek retractor
Cheetah angioplasty catheter
cheiroscope
- Maddox c.
- Wolff standup c.

Chelex ionic bead resin
Chelsea-Eaton anal speculum
ChemoBloc vial venting system

chemonucleolysis table
Chemo-Port
> C.-P. catheter
> C.-P. implantable vascular access system
> C.-P. perivena catheter system

Chemstrip MatchMaker blood glucose meter
ChemTrak AccuMeter
Chen-Smith image coder
Cherf
> C. cast stand
> C. leg holder

Chermel
> C. bone chisel
> C. bone gouge
> C. osteotome

Chernov tracheostomy hook
Cheron uterine dressing forceps
cherry
> C. brain probe
> C. drill
> C. forceps
> C. laminectomy self-retaining retractor
> C. osteotome
> C. screw extractor
> C. Secto dissector
> c. sponge
> C. S-shaped brain retractor
> C. S-shape scissors
> C. traction tongs

Cherry-Adson forceps
Cherry-Austin drill
Cherry-Kerrison
> C.-K. forceps
> C.-K. laminectomy rongeur

Cheshire electrosurgical pencil
Cheshire-Poole-Yankauer suction instrument
chessboard implant
chest
> c. tube
> c. tube stripper

Chester sponge forceps
Chevalier
> C. Jackson bougie
> C. Jackson bronchoesophagoscopy forceps
> C. Jackson bronchoscope
> C. Jackson dilator
> C. Jackson esophagoscope

> C. Jackson gastroscope
> C. Jackson laryngeal speculum
> C. Jackson laryngoscope
> C. Jackson scissors
> C. Jackson tracheal tube

Cheyne
> C. dissector
> C. periosteal elevator
> C. retractor

Chiba
> C. biopsy needle
> C. eye needle
> C. transhepatic cholangiography needle

Chicco breast pump
Chick
> C. CLT operating frame
> C. CLT operating table
> C. patient transfer device
> C. surgical light
> C. surgical table

chicken-bill rongeur forceps
Chick-Foster orthopaedic bed
Chick-Langren table
Chid breast pump
Chiesi powder inhaler
Chilcott venoclysis cannula
child
> C. clip-applying forceps
> c. esophagoscope
> C. intestinal forceps
> c. rectal dilator
> c. restraint device

Child-Phillips
> C.-P. forceps
> C.-P. intestinal plication needle

Children's
> C. Hospital brain spatula
> C. Hospital clip
> C. Hospital dressing forceps
> C. Hospital hand drill
> C. Hospital intestinal forceps
> C. Hospital mallet
> C. Hospital pediatric retractor
> C. Hospital screwdriver

child-resistant container
Childs Cardio-Cuff
chiller
> Geggel PRK c.

Chilli cooled ablation catheter
Chimani pharyngeal forceps

NOTES

chin
    c. implant
    c. prosthesis
    c. support
Chinese
    C. finger straps traction device
    C. fingertrap suture
    C. twisted silk suture
Chiroflex C11UB lens
ChiroFlow
    C. adjustable back support
    C. back rest
Chiron
    C. ACS microkeratome
    C. automated corneal shaper
    C. Hansatome
chiropractic adjusting instrument
Chiroslide leg discrepancy analyzer
Chirotech x-ray system
chisel
    Adson laminectomy c.
    Alexander bone c.
    Alexander mastoid c.
    Amico c.
    Andrews c.
    antral c.
    Army c.
    Artmann disarticulation c.
    Austin Moore mortising c.
    Bakelite dental c.
    Ballenger c.
    Ballenger-Hajek c.
    Basek c.
    beveled c.
    Biomet cement removal hand c.
    Bishop mastoid c.
    c. blade
    Blair nasal c.
    bone c.
    Bowen gooseneck c.
    Braithwaite nasal c.
    Brauer c.
    Brown c.
    Bruening c.
    Brunetti c.
    Brun guarded c.
    Brunner c.
    Brunswick-Mack c.
    Buckley c.
    Burns c.
    Caltagirone c.
    canal c.
    cartilage c.
    C-beveled c.
    Chermel bone c.
    Cinelli c.
    Cinelli-McIndoe c.
    Clawicz c.
    Clevedent-Gardner c.

    Cloward-Harman c.
    Cloward-Puka c.
    Cloward spinal fusion c.
    Cobb c.
    Compere bone c.
    Converse c.
    Cooley c.
    corneal c.
    costotome c.
    Cottle crossbar fishtail c.
    Cottle fishtail c.
    Cottle nasal c.
    Councilman c.
    Crane bone c.
    crossbar fishtail c.
    crurotomy c.
    Dautrey c.
    Derlacki c.
    D'Errico laminectomy c.
    disarticulation c.
    dissecting c.
    double-guarded c.
    Eicher tri-fin c.
    c. elevator
    endaural surgery c.
    ethmoid c.
    Faulkner antral c.
    fishtail c.
    Fomon nasal c.
    footplate c.
    fracture c.
    Freer bone c.
    Freer lacrimal c.
    Freer submucous c.
    French c.
    frontal sinus c.
    Gardner bone c.
    Goldman guarded c.
    gooseneck c.
    guarded c.
    Hajek septal c.
    Halle c.
    Harmon c.
    Hatch c.
    Heermann c.
    Henderson bone c.
    Hibbs bone c.
    hollow c.
    Holmes c.
    Hough c.
    House c.
    House-Derlacki c.
    Jenkins c.
    Jordan-Hermann c.
    Joseph c.
    Katsch c.
    Keyes bone-splitting c.
    Kezerian c.
    Killian-Claus c.

Killian frontal sinus c.
Killian-Reinhard c.
Kilner c.
Kos c.
Kreischer bone c.
lacrimal sac c.
Lambert-Lowman c.
Lambotte bone c.
laminectomy c.
Lebsche sternal c.
Lexer c.
Lorenz c.
Lowman c.
Lowman-Hoglund c.
Lucas c.
MacAusland c.
Magielski stapes c.
Magnum c.
Mannerfelt c.
Martin cartilage c.
mastoid c.
McIndoe nasal c.
Metzenbaum c.
Meyerding c.
Miles bone c.
Moberg c.
Moore hollow c.
Moore prosthesis-mortising c.
mortising c.
Murphy c.
nasal c.
Neivert c.
Nordent bone c.
Nordent-Ochsenbein periodontic c.
Obwegeser splitting c.
Oratek c.
Partsch bone c.
Passow c.
peapod c.
Pearson c.
Peck c.
pterygoid c.
Puka c.
Read c.
Rica mastoid c.
Richards c.
Richards-Hibbs c.
Rish c.
Roberts hip dissecting c.
Rollet c.
Rubin nasal c.

Schuknecht c.
Schwartze c.
septal c.
Sewall ethmoidal c.
Shambaugh-Derlacki c.
Sheehan nasal c.
Sheehy-House c.
Silver c.
Simmons c.
sinus c.
Skoog nasal c.
SMIC bone c.
SMIC mastoid c.
SMIC sternal c.
Smillie cartilage c.
Smillie meniscectomy c.
Smith-Petersen c.
spinal fusion c.
splitting c.
stapes c.
Stille bone c.
submucous c.
Swedish-pattern c.
Swiderski nasal c.
Troutman mastoid c.
twin-pattern c.
unibevel c.
U.S. Army bone c.
Virchow c.
vulcanite c.
Walsh footplate c.
Ward nasal c.
West lacrimal c.
West nasal c.
White bone c.
Wilmer c.
Worth c.
ChiselTip suction cautery device
Chitten-Hill retractor
chloramine catgut suture
chloride
polyvinyl c. (PVC)
Chlumsky button
choanal bur
Chocstruct chondral repair system
Cho/Dyonics two-portal endoscope
Choice PT guidewire
Cholangiocath
C. catheter
C. introducer
cholangiographic catheter

NOTES

167

cholangiography
  c. catheter
  c. clamp
cholangiograsper
  Storz c.
CholangioLAPcath catheter
cholangiopancreatography
  endoscopic retrograde c. (ERCP)
cholangioscope
  "adoptable" baby c.
  Olympus CHF-Q10 c.
  prototype c.
cholecystotomy catheter
choledochocystonephrofiberscope
  Pentax c.
choledochofiberscope
  Olympus URF-P2
    translaparoscopic c.
choledochoscope
  fiberoptic c.
  Olympus CHF-P-series c.
  Olympus CHF-series c.
choledochoscope-nephroscope
  Berci-Shore c.-n.
Cholestech LDX office lab system
Choles Trak AccuMeter
chondroplasty Beaver blade
chondrotome
  Stryker c.
Chopart
  C. brace
  C. partial foot prosthesis
Cho-Pat
  C.-P. Achilles tendon strap
  C.-P. ankle support
  C.-P. dual-action knee strap
  C.-P. elbow strap
  C.-P. knee strap
Cho 2-portal Dyonics endoscope
chopper
  Agarwal irrigating phaco c.
  Davidoff ambidextrous nucleus c.
  Fine sideport actuating quick c.
  He Hook c.
  Inamura Race c.
  Koch c.
  Koch-Minami ophthalmic c.
  McIlwain tissue c.
  Miyoshi ophthalmic c.
  Nagahara karate c.
  Nagahara ophthalmic quick c.
  Nagahara phaco c.
  Nichamin quick c.
  Nichamin triple c.
  Nichamin vertical c.
  Olson nucleus quick c.
  Olson phaco c.
  Seibel nucleus c.
  Seibel vertical safety quick c.

Shepherd Tomahawk c.
Steinert double-ended claw c.
Steinert II irrigating claw c.
Sung reverse nucleus c.
Vergs phaco c.
chorda tympani pusher
chorionic
  c. villus sampler
  c. villus sampling (CVS)
  c. villus sampling catheter
chorionscope
Chorus
  C. DDD pacemaker
  C. RM rate-responsive dual-
    chamber pacemaker
Choyce
  C. intraocular lens forceps
  C. lens inserting forceps
  C. Mark intraocular lens
  C. Mark VIII eye implant
  C. MK II keratoprosthesis
    prosthesis
Choyce-Tennant lens
Christensen
  C. articulator
  C. ophthalmic punch
  C. TMJ implant
Christie gallbladder retractor
Christmas
  C. tree adapter
  C. tree cannula
Christopher-Stille forceps
Christoudias
  C. approximator
  C. fascial closure device
Chromaser dermatology laser
chromated catgut suture
chromatograph
  Carle analytic gas c.
  column c.
  gas c.
  high-performance liquid c.
  high-pressure liquid c.
  ion c.
  Quintron Microlyzer 12 c.
  solid-phase extraction c.
  thin-layer c.
  Varian model 3600 gas c.
chromatoptometer
chromatoskiameter
ChromaVision digital analyzer
chrome-cobalt cable
Chromel-Alumel thermocouple
chromic
  c. blue dyed gut suture
  c. catgut suture
  c. collagen suture
  c. gut suture
chromicized catgut suture

chromium-cobalt alloy implant
chromoendoscope
Chromos imager system
ChromoVision video system
chronaximeter
ChroniCare TENS electrode
Chronicle implantable hemodynamic
  monitor
Chronicure wound dressing
Chronocor IV external pacemaker
ChronoFlex catheter
Chronos pacemaker
Chrys surgical CO_2 laser
CHS supracondylar bone plate
Chubb tonsillar forceps
Chubby balloon catheter
chuck
    c. adapter
    c. drill
    Gam-Mer c.
    independent jaw c.
    Jacobs snap-lock c.
    Jacobs T-handle c.
    pin c.
    press-button c.
    Steinmann pin c.
    T-handle Jacob c.
    T-handle Zimmer c.
    Trinkle c.
    Wozniak Sur-Lok c.
Chu foldable lens cutter
Chukka boot
Churchill
    C. cardiac suction cannula
    C. sucker
Church pediatric scissors
Chuter endovascular device
Chux incontinence pad
Ciaglia
    C. Blue Rhino percutaneous
    tracheostomy introducer set
    C. percutaneous tracheostomy
    introducer
Ciba
    C. Soft lens
    C. Thin lens
Ciba-Corning 2500 CO-oximeter
Cibis
    C. electrode
    C. ski needle
Cibis-Vaiser muscle retractor

CIC
    completely in canal
    completely-in-the-canal
    CIC hearing aid
    CIC listening device
Cica-Care silicone gel sheet dressing
Cicherelli
    C. bone rongeur
    C. forceps
Cida-Gel absorbent beads
CIDtech camera
CIF-4 needle
CIF needle
cigarette drain
cigar handle basket punch
Cikloid dressing
Cilacalcin double-chambered syringe
Cilco
    C. argon laser
    C. Frigitronics
    C. Frigitronics laser
    C. Hoffer Laseridge laser
    C. intraocular lens
    C. krypton laser
    C. Lasertek argon laser
    C. lens forceps
    C. MonoFlex PMMA lens
    C. ophthalmic endoscope
    C. Optiflex intraocular lens
    C. perimeter
    C. posterior chamber intraocular
    lens
    C. Slant lens
    C. ultrasound unit
    C. viscoelastic
    C. vitrector
    C. YAG laser
Cilco-Kelman Multiflex all-PMMA
    intraocular lens
Cilco-Simcoe II lens
Cilco-Sonometrics lens
cilium pacemaker
Cimino
    C. dialysis shunt
    C. fistula
    C. shunt
Cimino-Brescia arteriovenous shunt
Cimochowski cardiac cannula
cinch
    alar c.
    Daw c.

NOTES

cinch *(continued)*
    Endo c.
    joint c.
Cincinnati ACL brace
cine
    c. camera
    c. CT scanner
    c. gastrocamera
    c. magnetic resonance imaging
    c. microscope
    c. MRI
Cinelli
    C. chisel
    C. osteotome
    C. periosteal elevator
Cinelli-Fomon scissors
Cinelli-McIndoe chisel
Cineloop image review ultrasound
    system
Cinemagic diagnostic catheter
CineView Plus Freeland system
Cintor knee prosthesis
Circadia dual-chamber rate-adaptive
    pacemaker
circadian event recorder
CircAid
    C. compression bandage
    C. compression system
    C. elastic stocking
circle
    c. knife
    pediatric c.
    Randot c.
Circline magnifier lamp
CircOlectric bed
Circon
    C. ACMI cannula
    C. ACMI cutting loop electrode
    C. ACMI diagnostic laparoscope
    C. ACMI electrohydraulic
        lithotriptor probe
    C. ACMI endoscope
    C. ACMI hysteroscope
    C. ACMI lithotripter
    C. ACMI MicroDigital-I camera
    C. ACMI MR-series ureteroscope
    C. ACMI trocar
    C. arthroscope
    C. leg holder
    C. Tripolar forceps
    C. video camera
CircPlus
    C. bandage/wrap system
    C. compression dressing
    C. wrap
circuit
    AirLife heated wire c.
    Bentley Duraflo II extracorporeal
        perfusion c.

    Intertech anesthesia breathing c.
    Intertech Mapleson D
        nonrebreathing c.
    Intertech nonrebreathing modified
        Jackson-Rees c.
    Jackson-Rees c.
    low-flow c.
    Magill c.
    multipurpose breathing c.
    NMR probe c.
    phototube output c.
    Tygon tubing c.
Circulaire aerosolized drug delivery
    system
Circul'Air shoe system
circular
    c. bandage
    c. blade
    c. coil
    c. external fixator
    c. intraluminal stapler
    c. mapping catheter
    c. stapler
    c. stapling device
    c. suture
circulating water blanket
circulator
    C. boot
    c. boot therapy
    sequential c.
Circulon
    C. dressing
    C. System Step 1, 2 venous ulcer
        kit
    C. wrap
circumaortic
    c. venous collar
    c. venous ring
circumcision clamp
circumdential wire
circumductor table
circumferential dressing
circumflex artery scissors
Circumpress
    C. chin strap
    C. compression bra
    C. facelift dressing
    C. gynecomastia vest
Circumstraint
    C. circumcision restraint device
    C. infant immobilizer
    C. pediatric circumcision restraint
Circuvent aerosolized medication
    delivery device
CirKuit-Guard vascular surgery device
Cirrus
    C. composite prosthetic foot
    C. foot prosthesis
CIS-2 system

Cisco covered needle catheter
cisterna magna catheter
Citelli
C. bone punch
C. laminectomy punch
C. punch forceps
C. sphenoid rongeur
Citelli-Bruening ear forceps
Citelli-Meltzer atticus punch
CitScope arthroscope
Civiale forceps
CKS knee system
Claes scleral depressor
Clagett
C. needle
C. S-cannula
Clairborne clamp
clamp
Abadie intestinal c.
Ablaza patent ductus c.
Abramson-Allis breast c.
Acland microvascular c.
Adair breast c.
Adson c.
Adson-Brown c.
agraffe c.
Ahlquist-Durham embolism c.
air inflatable vessel occluder c.
Alfred M. Large vena caval c.
Allen intestinal anastomosis c.
Allen-Kocher c.
Allis c.
Allis tissue c.
Alyea vas c.
anastomosis c.
Anderson c.
Ando aortic c.
aneurysm c.
Ann Arbor towel c.
anterior resection c.
aortic c.
aortic aneurysm c.
aortic occlusion c.
appendage c.
arterial c.
arthrodesis c.
Asch c.
ASSI METE-series Microspike
approximator c.
ASSI METS-series Microspike
approximator c.

ASSI MKCV-series Microspike
approximator c.
ASSI MSPK-series Microspike
approximator c.
ASSI no-scalpel vasectomy fixator
ring c.
Atlee bronchus c.
A-Trac c.
AtrauGrip c.
atraumatic c.
atraumatic intestinal c.
Atraumax peripheral vascular c.
atrial c.
Ault intestinal c.
auricular appendage c.
Auto Suture Mini-CABG
occlusion c.
Auvard c.
Babcock c.
Babcock tissue c.
baby Bishop c.
baby Kocher c.
baby Payr pylorus c.
baby Satinsky c.
Backhaus-Jones towel c.
Backhaus-Kocher towel c.
Backhaus towel c.
Bahnson aortic aneurysm c.
Bahnson appendage c.
Bailey aortic c.
Bailey-Cowley c.
Bailey duckbill c.
Bailey-Morse c.
Bainbridge anastomosis c.
Bainbridge intestinal c.
Bainbridge vessel c.
Balfour c.
Ballantine c.
Bard Cunningham urinary
incontinence c.
Barraquer needle holder c.
Bartley anastomosis c.
Bartley partial-occlusion c.
bar-to-bar c.
Bauer kidney pedicle c.
Baumrucker post-TUR irrigation c.
Baumrucker urinary incontinence c.
Beall bulldog c.
Beall-Morris ascending aortic c.
Beardsley intestinal c.
Beck aortic c.
Beck-Potts aortic c.

NOTES

171

clamp *(continued)*
Beck-Potts pulmonic c.
Beck-Satinsky c.
Beck vascular c.
Beck vessel c.
Belcher c.
Benson pyloric c.
Berens muscle c.
Berke c.
Berkeley c.
Berkeley-Bonney vaginal c.
Berke ptosis c.
Berman aortic c.
Berman vascular c.
Bernhard c.
Berry pile c.
Best intestinal c.
Best right-angle colon c.
Bethune c.
Bielawski heart c.
Bigelow calvaria c.
Bihrle dorsal c.
Bircher bone-holding c.
Bircher cartilage c.
Bishop bone c.
Black meatal c.
3-bladed c.
Blair cleft palate c.
Blalock-Niedner pulmonic
  stenosis c.
Blalock pulmonary stenosis c.
Blanchard pile c.
Blasucci c.
blepharostat c.
bloodless circumcision c.
Boettcher pulmonary artery c.
Böhler os calcis c.
bone c.
bone extension c.
bone-holding c.
Bonney c.
Borge bile duct c.
Bortz c.
Boyes muscle c.
Bozeman c.
Bradshaw-O'Neill aortic c.
Bridge c.
Brock auricular c.
Brockington pile c.
Brodney urethrographic c.
bronchial c.
Bronner c.
Brown lip c.
Brunner colon c.
Brunner intestinal c.
Buie-Hirschman pile c.
Buie pile c.
bulldog c.
Bunke c.

Bunnell-Howard arthrodesis c.
Burford c.
burlisher c.
Bushey compression c.
Buxton c.
Buxton uterine c.
Cairns c.
Calandruccio c.
Calman carotid c.
Calman ring c.
calvarial c.
cannula c.
Capes c.
Cardio-Grip anastomosis c.
Cardio-Grip aortic c.
Cardio-Grip bronchus c.
Cardio-Grip pediatric c.
Cardio-Grip renal artery c.
Cardio-Grip tangential occlusion c.
Cardio-Grip vascular c.
cardiovascular anastomotic c.
Carmalt c.
Carmel c.
carotid artery c.
Carrel c.
Carter c.
Carter-Glassman resection c.
cartilage c.
caruncle c.
Casey pelvic c.
Castaneda anastomosis c.
Castaneda IMM vascular c.
Castaneda-Mixter thoracic c.
Castaneda partial-occlusion c.
Castroviejo lens c.
Castroviejo mosquito lid c.
Castroviejo needle holder c.
cautery c.
caval occlusion c.
cervical c.
chalazion c.
Charnley arthrodesis c.
Charnley bone c.
Charnley external fixation c.
Charnley pin c.
cholangiography c.
circumcision c.
Clairborne c.
Clevis c.
cloth-shod c.
coarctation c.
Codman cardiovascular c.
Codman cartilage c.
Codman towel c.
Collier thoracic c.
Collin umbilical c.
colon c.
colostomy c.
columellar c.

Conger perineal urethrostomy c.
Cooley c.
Cooley acutely-curved c.
Cooley angled pediatric c.
Cooley aortic aneurysm c.
Cooley aortic cannula c.
Cooley-Baumgarten aortic c.
Cooley-Beck vessel c.
Cooley bronchial c.
Cooley bulldog c.
Cooley carotid c.
Cooley carotid artery c.
Cooley caval occlusion c.
Cooley coarctation c.
Cooley curved cardiovascular c.
Cooley-Derra pediatric
    anastomosis c.
Cooley double-angled c.
Cooley graft c.
Cooley iliac c.
Cooley neonatal vascular c.
Cooley neonate c.
Cooley partial-occlusion c.
Cooley patent ductus c.
Cooley pediatric anastomosis c.
Cooley pediatric vascular c.
Cooley peripheral vascular c.
Cooley profunda c.
Cooley renal artery c.
Cooley-Satinsky c.
Cooley subclavian c.
Cooley tangential pediatric c.
Cooley vena caval c.
Cope crushing c.
Cope-DeMartel c.
cordotomy c.
Cottle columellar c.
cotton-roll rubber-dam c.
Crafoord auricular c.
Crafoord coarctation c.
Crafoord-Sellors auricular c.
Crenshaw caruncle c.
Crile c.
Crile crushing c.
Crile-Crutchfield c.
cross-action bulldog c.
cross-action towel c.
Cruickshank entropion c.
crushing c.
Crutchfield c.
Cunningham penile incontinence c.
Cunningham urinary incontinence c.

curved Mayo c.
curved mosquito c.
curved peripheral vascular c.
Cushing c.
Dacron graft c.
Daems bronchial c.
Dale femoral-popliteal c.
D'Allesandro c.
Dandy c.
Daniel colostomy c.
Dardik c.
David-Baker lid c.
Davidson muscle c.
Davidson pulmonary vessel c.
Davis aortic aneurysm c.
Dean MacDonald gastric
    resection c.
Deaver c.
DeBakey aortic c.
DeBakey aortic aneurysm c.
DeBakey aortic exclusion c.
DeBakey-Bahnson vascular c.
DeBakey-Bainbridge peripheral c.
DeBakey-Beck c.
DeBakey bulldog c.
DeBakey coarctation c.
DeBakey curved peripheral
    vascular c.
DeBakey-Derra anastomosis c.
DeBakey-Harken auricular c.
DeBakey patent ductus c.
DeBakey pediatric c.
DeBakey peripheral vascular c.
DeBakey ring-handled bulldog c.
DeBakey-Satinsky vena cava c.
DeBakey-Semb c.
DeBakey S-shaped peripheral
    vascular c.
DeBakey tangential occlusion c.
DeBakey vascular c.
DeCourcy goiter c.
DeMartel anastomosis c.
DeMartel vascular c.
DeMartel-Wolfson colon c.
DeMartel-Wolfson intestinal c.
Demel wire c.
Dennis anastomotic c.
Dennis intestinal c.
Derra anastomosis c.
Derra vena caval c.
Derra vestibular c.
Desmarres lid c.

NOTES

clamp *(continued)*
Devonshire-Mack c.
DeWeese vena caval c.
Dick bronchus c.
Dick pressure c.
Dieffenbach bulldog c.
Diethrich aortic c.
Diethrich graft c.
Diethrich micro bulldog c.
Diethrich micro coronary
 bulldog c.
Diethrich shunt c.
Dingman cartilage c.
Dingman sagittal bone c.
Dingman small bone c.
disposable drape c.
disposable muscle biopsy c.
dissecting c.
distraction c.
Doctor Collins fracture c.
Doctor Long c.
Dolphin cord c.
Donald c.
double-angled c.
Downes lid c.
Downing c.
Doyen intestinal c.
Doyen towel c.
duckbill c.
duodenal c.
Duval-Collin lung c.
Earle hemorrhoidal c.
C. Ease device
Eastman intestinal c.
Edwards double Softjaw c.
Edwards single Softjaw c.
Edwards spring c.
Eisenstein c.
endoaortic c.
English c.
enterostomy c.
entropion c.
Erhardt lid c.
ether screen c.
Ewald-Hudson c.
Ewing lid c.
exclusion c.
extracutaneous vas fixation c.
Falk c.
Farabeuf bone c.
Farabeuf-Lambotte bone-holding c.
Favaloro proximal anastomosis c.
feather c.
Fehland intestinal c.
femoral c.
Ferguson bone c.
Ferrier 212 gingival c.
ferrule c.
fine-tooth c.

Finochietto arterial c.
Finochietto bronchial c.
Fitzgerald aortic aneurysm c.
flexible aortic c.
flexible retractor pressure c.
flexible retractor sliding c.
flexible vascular c.
flow-regulator c.
Fogarty-Chin c.
Fogarty Hydragrip c.
Ford c.
Forrester c.
Foss anterior resection c.
Foss cardiovascular c.
Foss intestinal c.
Frahur cartilage c.
Freeman c.
Friedrich c.
Friedrich-Petz c.
Fukushima C-clamp c.
full-curved c.
Furness anastomosis c.
Furness-Clute anastomosis c.
Furness-Clute duodenal c.
gallbladder ring c.
Gam-Mer aneurysm c.
Gam-Mer occlusion c.
Gant c.
Garcia aortic c.
Gardner skull c.
Garland hysterectomy c.
Gaskell c.
gastric c.
gastroenterostomy c.
gastrointestinal c.
Gavin-Miller c.
Gemini c.
Gerald c.
Gerbode patent ductus c.
Gerster bone c.
GI c.
gingival c.
Glass liver-holding c.
Glassman-Allis c.
Glassman bowel atraumatic c.
Glassman intestinal c.
Glassman liver-holding c.
Glassman noncrushing
 gastroenterostomy c.
Glassman noncrushing
 gastrointestinal c.
Glover auricular c.
Glover auricular-appendage c.
Glover bulldog c.
Glover coarctation c.
Glover curved c.
Glover-DeBakey c.
Glover patent ductus c.
Glover spoon-shaped anastomosis c.

Glover vascular c.
goiter c.
Goldblatt c.
Goldstein Microspike
 approximator c.
Gomco bell c.
Gomco bloodless circumcision c.
Gomco umbilical cord c.
Grafco incontinence c.
Grafco umbilical cord c.
graft c.
Grant aortic aneurysm c.
grasping c.
Gray c.
Greenberg c.
green bulldog c.
Green lid c.
Green suction tube-holding c.
Gregory baby profunda c.
Gregory carotid bulldog c.
Gregory external c.
Gregory stay suture c.
Gregory vascular miniature c.
Gross coarctation c.
Grover Atra-grip c.
Grover auricular appendage c.
Gusberg hysterectomy c.
Gussenbauer c.
gut c.
Gutgemann auricular appendage c.
Guyon kidney c.
Guyon-Péan vessel c.
Guyon vessel c.
half-curved c.
Halifax interlaminar c.
Halsted curved mosquito c.
Halsted straight mosquito c.
handleless c.
Harken auricle c.
Harrah lung c.
Harrington-Carmalt c.
Harrington hook c.
Harrington-Mixter thoracic c.
Hartmann c.
Harvey Stone c.
Hatch c.
Hausmann vascular c.
Haverhill c.
Haverhill-Mack c.
Hayes anterior resection c.
Hayes colon c.
Hayes intestinal c.

Heaney c.
Heaney-Ballantine c.
Heartport endoaortic c.
Heifitz cerebral aneurysm c.
Heitz-Boyer c.
Hemoclip c.
hemorrhoidal c.
hemostatic c.
Hendren cardiovascular c.
Hendren ductus c.
Hendren megaureter c.
Hendren ureteral c.
Henley subclavian artery c.
Henley vascular c.
Herbert Adams coarctation c.
Herff c.
Herrick kidney c.
Herrick pedicle c.
Hesseltine umbilical cord c.
Hex-Fix Universal swivel c.
Heyer-Schulte Rayport muscle
 biopsy c.
Hibbs c.
hilar c.
Hirschman pile c.
Hirsch mucosal c.
Hoffmann ligament c.
Hoff towel c.
Hohmann c.
c. holder
Hollister c.
Hopener c.
Hopkins aortic occlusion c.
Hopkins hysterectomy c.
Howard-DeBakey aortic
 aneurysm c.
Hudson c.
Hufnagel aortic c.
Hume aortic c.
Humphries aortic aneurysm c.
Humphries reverse-curve aortic c.
Hunt colostomy c.
Hunter-Satinsky c.
Hurson flexible pressure c.
Hurson flexible sliding c.
Hurwitz esophageal c.
Hurwitz intestinal c.
Hymes meatal c.
hysterectomy c.
iliac c.
Iliff c.
IMP Steri-Clamp c.

NOTES

C

175

clamp *(continued)*
  incontinence c.
  Innovative Medical Products Steri-
    Clamp c.
  interlaminar c.
  intestinal c.
  intestinal anastomosis c.
  intestinal occlusion c.
  intestinal resection c.
  intestinal ring c.
  isoelastic rip c.
  Ivory rubber dam c.
  Jackson bone c.
  Jackson bone-extension c.
  Jackson bone-holding c.
  Jacobs c.
  Jacobson bulldog c.
  Jacobson-Potts vessel c.
  Jacobson vessel c.
  Jahnke anastomosis c.
  Jahnke-Cook-Seeley c.
  Jako c.
  Jameson muscle c.
  Jansen c.
  Jarit anterior resection c.
  Jarit cartilage c.
  Jarit intestinal c.
  Jarit meniscal c.
  Jarvis pile c.
  Javid bypass c.
  Javid carotid c.
  Javid shunt c.
  Jesberg laryngectomy c.
  Johns Hopkins bulldog c.
  Johns Hopkins coarctation c.
  Johns Hopkins modified Potts c.
  Johnston c.
  Jones thoracic c.
  Jones towel c.
  Joseph septal c.
  Judd c.
  Judd-Allis c.
  Juevenelle c.
  Julian-Fildes c.
  Kalt needle holder c.
  Kane obstetrical c.
  Kane umbilical cord c.
  Kantor circumcision c.
  Kantrowitz hemostatic c.
  Kantrowitz thoracic c.
  Kapp-Beck bronchial c.
  Kapp-Beck coarctation c.
  Kapp-Beck colon c.
  Kapp-Beck-Thomson c.
  Kapp microarterial c.
  Karamar-Mailatt tarsorrhaphy c.
  Kartchner carotid artery c.
  Kaufman kidney c.
  Kay aortic anastomosis c.

  Kay-Lambert c.
  Kelly c.
  Kelsey pile c.
  Kern bone-holding c.
  Kersting colostomy c.
  K-Gar umbilical c.
  Khan-Jaeger c.
  Khodadad c.
  kidney pedicle c.
  Kiefer c.
  Kindt arterial c.
  Kindt carotid c.
  King c.
  Kinsella-Buie lung c.
  Kitner c.
  Kleinert-Kutz c.
  Kleinschmidt appendectomy c.
  Klevas c.
  Klinikum-Berlin tubing c.
  Klintmalm c.
  Klute c.
  Knutsson penile c.
  Knutsson urethrography c.
  Koala c.
  Kocher intestinal c.
  Kolodny c.
  Krosnick vesicourethral
    suspension c.
  Kutzmann c.
  Ladd lid c.
  Lahey c.
  Lahey bronchial c.
  Lahey thoracic c.
  Lalonde bone c.
  Lalonde dynamic compression
    bone c.
  Lambert aortic c.
  Lambert-Kay aortic c.
  Lambert-Kay vascular c.
  Lambert-Lowman bone c.
  Lambotte bone-holding c.
  Lamis patellar c.
  Lane bone-holding c.
  Lane gastroenterostomy c.
  Lane intestinal c.
  Lane towel c.
  laparoscopic Allis c.
  laryngectomy c.
  Leahey c.
  Lee bronchus c.
  Lee microvascular c.
  Lees bronchus c.
  Lees vascular c.
  Lees wedge resection c.
  Leland-Jones vascular c.
  Lem-Blay circumcision c.
  Lewin bone-holding c.
  lid c.
  Liddle aortic c.

Life-Lok c.
ligament c.
Lillie rectus tendon c.
Lin c.
Lindner anastomosis c.
Linnartz intestinal c.
Linnartz stomach c.
lion-head c.
lion-jaw c.
lip c.
Litwak c.
Lloyd-Davies c.
Locke c.
Locke bone c.
locking c.
Lockwood c.
Longmire-Storm c.
Lorna-Edna towel c.
Lorna non-perforating towel c.
Lowman bone-holding c.
Lowman-Gerster bone c.
Lowman-Hoglund c.
Lulu c.
lung exclusion c.
MacDonald gastric c.
Madden intestinal c.
Maingot c.
Malgaigne c.
Malik cystic duct catheter c.
Malis hinge c.
Marcuse tube c.
marginal c.
Martel intestinal c.
Martin cartilage c.
Martin muscle c.
Mason vascular c.
Masters intestinal c.
Masterson pelvic c.
Masters-Schwartz intestinal c.
Masters-Schwartz liver c.
Mastin muscle c.
Matthew cross-leg c.
Mattox aortic c.
Mayfield aneurysm c.
Mayfield head c.
Mayfield three-pin skull c.
May kidney c.
Mayo c.
Mayo-Guyon kidney c.
Mayo-Guyon vessel c.
Mayo kidney c.
Mayo-Lovelace spur crushing c.

Mayo-Robson intestinal c.
Mayo vessel c.
McCleery-Miller intestinal anastomosis c.
McCullough hysterectomy c.
McDonald gastric c.
McDougal prostatectomy c.
McGuire c.
McKenzie c.
McLean c.
McNealey-Glassman c.
McNealey-Glassman-Mixter c.
McQuigg c.
meatal c.
Meeker gallstone c.
Meeker right-angle c.
meniscal c.
Michel aortic c.
Microspike approximator c.
microvascular c.
Mikulicz peritoneal c.
Mikulicz-Radecki c.
Miles rectal c.
Millard c.
Millin c.
miniature bulldog c.
mini vessel c.
Mitchel-Adam c.
Mitchel aortotomy c.
Mixter thoracic c.
Mogen circumcision c.
Mohr pinchcock c.
Moorehead lid c.
Moreno gastroenterostomy c.
Moria-France dacryocystorhinostomy c.
Morris aortic c.
mosquito c.
mosquito hemostatic c.
mosquito lid c.
mouse-tooth c.
Moynihan towel c.
Mueller aortic c.
Mueller bronchial c.
Mueller pediatric c.
Mueller vena caval c.
Muir rectal cautery c.
Mulligan anastomosis c.
muscle c.
muscle biopsy c.
Myles hemorrhoidal c.
myocardial c.

NOTES

clamp *(continued)*

Nakayama c.
Naraghi-DeCoster reduction c.
needle holder c.
neonatal vascular c.
Nichols aortic c.
Nicola tendon c.
Niedner anastomosis c.
Niedner pulmonic c.
noncrushing anterior resection c.
noncrushing bowel c.
noncrushing gastroenterostomy c.
noncrushing gastrointestinal c.
noncrushing intestinal c.
noncrushing liver-holding c.
noncrushing vascular c.
nonperforating towel c.
Noon AV fistula c.
Nunez aortic c.
Nunez auricular c.
Nussbaum intestinal c.
occluding c.
Ochsner aortic c.
Ochsner arterial c.
Ochsner artery c.
Ochsner thoracic c.
Ockerblad kidney c.
Ockerblad vessel c.
O'Connor lid c.
O'Hanlon intestinal c.
Olivecrona aneurysm c.
Olsen cholangiogram c.
Omed bulldog vascular c.
O'Neill cardiac c.
O'Shaughnessy c.
ossicle-holding c.
osteoplastic flap c.
padded c.
Pampéan vessel c.
parametrium c.
Parham-Martin bone-holding c.
Parker c.
Parker-Kerr intestinal c.
Parsonnet aortic c.
partial-occlusion c.
Partipilo c.
patellar cement c.
patent ductus c.
Payr gastrointestinal c.
Payr pylorus c.
Payr resection c.
Payr stomach c.
Péan hemostatic c.
Péan hysterectomy c.
Péan intestinal c.
pediatric bulldog c.
pediatric vascular c.
pedicle c.
Peers towel c.

pelvic c.
Pemberton sigmoid c.
Pemberton spur-crushing c.
penile c.
Pennington c.
Percy c.
pericortical c.
peripheral vascular c.
peritoneal c.
phalangeal c.
Phaneuf c.
phantom c.
Phillips rectal c.
pile c.
Pilling microanastomosis c.
Pilling pediatric c.
pinchcock c.
pin-to-bar c.
placental c.
Plastibell circumcision c.
point-of-reduction c.
Pomeranz aortic c.
Poppen aortic c.
Poppen-Blalock carotid artery c.
Poppen-Blalock-Salibi carotid c.
Posi-Grip umbilical cord c.
post-TUR irrigation c.
Potts aortic c.
Potts cardiovascular c.
Potts coarctation c.
Potts-DeBakey c.
Potts divisional c.
Potts-Niedner aortic c.
Potts patent ductus c.
Potts pulmonic c.
Potts-Satinsky c.
Potts-Smith aortic c.
Potts-Smith pulmonic c.
Poutasse renal artery c.
Presbyterian Hospital occluding c.
Preshaw c.
Price muscle c.
Price-Thomas bronchial c.
Prince muscle c.
Pringle c.
Providence Hospital c.
ptosis c.
Pudenz-Heyer c.
pulmonary arterial c.
pulmonary embolism c.
pulmonary nodulectomy c.
pulmonary vessel c.
pulmonic stenosis c.
Putterman levator resection c.
Putterman ptosis c.
pylorus c.
Quick Bend flex c.
Ralks thoracic c.
Ramstedt c.

Ranieri c.
Rankin anastomosis c.
Rankin intestinal c.
Rankin stomach c.
Ranzewski intestinal c.
ratchet c.
Ravich c.
Rayport muscle c.
reamer c.
rectal c.
Redo intestinal c.
Reich-Nechtow arterial c.
Reinhoff swan neck c.
renal artery c.
renal pedicle c.
resection c.
Reul aortic c.
reverse-curve c.
Reynolds dissecting c.
Reynolds resection c.
Reynolds vascular c.
Rhinelander c.
Rica arterial c.
Rica microarterial c.
Rica stem c.
Rica vessel c.
Richards bone c.
ring c.
ring-handled bulldog c.
ring-jawed holding c.
Robin chalazion c.
Rochester hook c.
Rochester-Kocher c.
Rochester-Péan c.
Rochester sigmoid c.
Rockey vascular c.
Roe aortic tourniquet c.
Roeder towel c.
Roosen c.
Roosevelt gastroenterostomy c.
Roosevelt gastrointestinal c.
root rubber dam c.
rubber dam c.
rubber-shod c.
Rubin bronchial c.
Rubio wire-holding c.
Rubovits c.
Rumel myocardial c.
Rumel rubber c.
Rumel thoracic c.
Rush bone c.
Salibi carotid artery c.

Santulli c.
Sarnoff aortic c.
Sarot arterial c.
Sarot bronchus c.
Satinsky anastomosis c.
Satinsky aortic c.
Satinsky pediatric c.
Satinsky vascular c.
Satinsky vena cava c.
Schaedel cross-action towel c.
Schlein c.
Schlesinger c.
Schnidt c.
Schoemaker intestinal c.
Schumacher aortic c.
Schutz c.
Schwartz arterial aneurysm c.
Schwartz bulldog c.
Schwartz intracranial c.
Schwartz vascular c.
Scoville-Lewis c.
screw occlusive c.
Scudder intestinal c.
Scudder stomach c.
Sehrt c.
Seidel bone-holding c.
Sellor c.
Selman c.
Selverstone carotid artery c.
Semb bone-holding c.
Semb bronchus c.
Senning featherweight bulldog c.
Senning-Stille c.
septal c.
serrefine c.
Sheehy ossicle-holding c.
Sheldon c.
shunt c.
shutoff c.
side-biting c.
sidewinder aortic c.
Siegler-Hellman c.
sigmoid anastomosis c.
Silber microvascular c.
Silber vasovasostomy c.
Sims-Maier c.
Singley intestinal c.
Siniscal eyelid c.
skull c.
Slim Fit flex c.
Slocum meniscal c.
slotted nerve c.

NOTES

clamp *(continued)*

SMIC intestinal c.
Smith bone c.
Smith cordotomy c.
Smith marginal c.
Smithwick anastomotic c.
Softjaw c.
soft tissue graft c.
Somers uterine c.
Somjee-Crabtree temporal bone
  support c.
Southwick c.
sponge c.
spoon anastomosis c.
spur-crushing c.
SS White c.
stainless steel c.
Stallard head c.
Stanton cautery c.
Stayce adjustable c.
Stay-Rite c.
Steinhauser bone c.
Stemp c.
stenosis c.
Stepita meatal c.
Stetten intestinal c.
Stevenson c.
Stille-Crawford coarctation c.
Stille kidney c.
Stille vessel c.
Stimson pedicle c.
Stiwer towel c.
St. Mark c.
Stockman meatal c.
Stockman penile c.
stomach c.
Stone-Holcombe anastomosis c.
Stone-Holcombe intestinal c.
Stone intestinal c.
Stone stomach c.
Stony splenorenal shunt c.
Storey c.
Storz meatal c.
straight mosquito c.
Stratte kidney c.
Strauss meatal c.
Strauss penile c.
Strauss-Valentine penile c.
Strelinger colon c.
St. Vincent tube c.
Subramanian sidewinder aortic c.
Sugarbaker retrocolic c.
Sugita head c.
Sumner c.
suprahepatic caval c.
SurgiMed c.
Swan aortic c.
swan-neck c.
Swenson ring-jawed holding c.

Swiss bulldog c.
Sztehlo umbilical c.
T c.
tangential occlusion c.
tangential pediatric c.
Tatum meatal c.
Taufic cholangiography c.
Tehl c.
tension c.
Textor vasectomy c.
Thoma c.
Thompson carotid artery c.
Thomson lung c.
thoracic c.
Thorlakson lower/upper occlusive c.
Thumb-Saver introducer c.
tissue occlusion c.
titanium vascular c.
tonsil c.
tonsillar c.
towel c.
Trendelenburg-Crafoord
  coarctation c.
Treves intestinal c.
trochanter-holding c.
truncus c.
Trusler infant vascular c.
tube-occluding c.
tubing c.
Tucker appendix c.
turkey-claw c.
Tydings tonsillar c.
Tyrrell c.
Ullrich tubing c.
umbilical cord c.
Umbilicutter umbilical cord cutter
  and c.
Universal wire c.
upper occlusive c.
ureteral c.
urethrographic cannula c.
urinary incontinence c.
uterine c.
vaginal cuff c.
Valdoni c.
Van Beek nerve approximator c.
Vanderbilt vessel c.
Varco dissecting c.
Varco gallbladder c.
vas c.
Vasconcelos-Barretto c.
VascuClamp vascular c.
vascular c.
vascular graft c.
vasovasostomy c.
Veidenheimer resection c.
vena caval c.
Verbrugge bone c.
Veridian umbilical c.

VersaClamp flex c.
Verse-Webster c.
vessel c.
vessel-occluding c.
vestibular c.
Virtus splinter c.
V. Mueller aortic c.
V. Mueller auricular appendage c.
V. Mueller bulldog c.
V. Mueller cross-action bulldog c.
V. Mueller vena caval c.
von Petz intestinal c.
Vorse tube-occluding c.
Vorse-Webster tube-occluding c.
vulsellum c.
Wadsworth lid c.
Walther-Crenshaw meatal c.
Walther kidney pedicle c.
Walther pedicle c.
Walton meniscal c.
Wangensteen anastomosis c.
Wangensteen gastric-crushing
 anastomotic c.
Wangensteen patent ductus c.
Warthen spur-crushing c.
Watts locking c.
Weaver chalazion c.
Weber aortic c.
Weck c.
Weck-Edna nonperforating towel c.
wedge resection c.
Weldon miniature bulldog c.
Wells pedicle c.
Wertheim-Cullen kidney pedicle c.
Wertheim kidney pedicle c.
Wertheim-Reverdin pedicle c.
Wester meniscal c.
West Shur cartilage c.
White c.
Whitver penile c.
Wikström gallbladder c.
Wikström-Stilgust c.
Willett c.
Williams c.
Wilman c.
Wilson c.
Winkelmann circumcision c.
Winston cervical c.
wire-tightening c.
Wirthlin splenorenal shunt c.
Wister vascular c.

Wolfson intestinal c.
Wolfson spur-crushing c.
Wood bulldog c.
Wylie hypogastric c.
Wylie J vascular c.
Wylie lumbar bulldog c.
Yasargil carotid c.
Yellen circumcision c.
Young renal pedicle c.
Zachary-Cope c.
Zachary-Cope-DeMartel colon c.
Zeppelin c.
Ziegler-Furness c.
Zimmer bone-holding c.
Zimmer cartilage c.
Zinnanti Z-clamp c.
Zipser meatal c.
Zutt c.
Zweifel appendectomy c.
Zweifel pressure c.

clamshell
  c. brace
  c. double umbrella occluder
  c. prosthesis
  c. septal occluder
  c. septal umbrella
Clar head light
ClariFlex foldable intraocular lens
Clarion
  C. CII Bionic Ear system
  C. CII BTE sound processor
  C. cochlear implant
  C. HiFocus electrode
  C. Multi-Strategy cochlear implant
  C. Platinum BTE sound processor
Claris
  C. spinal clip system
  C. titanium spinal instrumentation
Clarity newborn hearing system
clariVit
  c. Central Mag vitrectomy lens
  c. Wide Angle vitrectomy lens
Clark capsular fragment forceps
Clarke
  C. common duct dilator
  C. expanding mesh catheter
  C. eye speculum
  C. helical catheter
  C. ligator scissor forceps
  C. stereotactic instrument

NOTES

Clarke-Reich
    C.-R. laparoscopic knot pusher
    C.-R. ligator
Clark-Guyton forceps
Clark-Verhoeff capsular forceps
Clarus
    C. model 5169 peristaltic pump
    C. SpineScope spinal endoscope
clasp
    Acland c.
    Adams c.
    c. bar
    bone c.
    Charnley bone c.
    Crozat c.
    Damon c.
    Duyzings c.
    EPI-Sport epicondylitis c.
    Hahnenkratt dental c.
    c. knife
    preformed c.
    Roach c.
Classic II stethoscope
Classix pacemaker
Classon scissors
Clas von Eichen needle
Claussen fragment stabilizer
Clave needleless IV system
claw
    c. forceps
    c. retractor
Clawicz chisel
Clay Adams PE-series catheter
Clayman
    C. corneal forceps
    C. intraocular guide
    C. intraocular lens
    C. intraocular lens forceps
    C. iris hook
    C. lensholding forceps
    C. lens implant
    C. lens-inserting forceps
    C. lid retractor
    C. nucleus retractor
    C. spatula
    C. suturing forceps
Clayman-Kelman intraocular lens forceps
Clayman-Knolle irrigating lens loop
Clayman-McPherson tying forceps
Clayman-Troutman corneal scissors
Clayman-Vannas scissors
Clayman-Westcott scissors
Clayton
    C. laminectomy shears
    C. osteotome
CLC orthotic
CleanCut rotation aortic punch
Cleanlet lancet

CleanWheel disposable neurological pinwheel
Clear
    C. Advantage latex-free male external catheter
    C. Advantage pulmonary function filter
ClearCut
    C. dual-bevel line knife
    C. 2 electrosurgical handpiece
    C. ophthalmic dual bevel knife
    C. SatinSlit knife
ClearESS irrigation and suction system
Clearfix
    C. meniscal dart
    C. meniscal screw
Clearglide endoscopic vessel harvesting system
Clearpath corneal diamond knife
Clear-Plan Easy fertility monitor
ClearSite
    C. bandage
    C. bandage roll dressing
    C. borderless dressing
    C. HydroGauze dressing
    C. hydrogel absorptive borderline wound dressing
C.L.E.A.R.Sound ultrasound therapy device
ClearView
    C. CO_2 laser
    C. intracoronary shunt
    C. uterine manipulator
Cleasby
    C. iris spatula
    C. spatulated needle
cleaver
    fiber c.
    Haefliger c.
    Orton enamel c.
cleft
    c. palate elevator
    c. palate forceps
    c. palate needle
    c. palate prosthesis
    c. palate raspatory
    c. palate sharp hook
C-Leg lower limb prosthesis
Clemetson uterine forceps
Clensicair
    C. incontinence management system
    C. low-air-loss hydrotherapy bed
C-Letz conization electrode
Clevedan positive pressure respirator
Clevedent
    C. forceps
    C. retractor
Clevedent-Gardner chisel
Clevedent-Lucas curette

Cleveland
C. bone-cutting forceps
C. bone rongeur
C. IMA retractor
Clevis
C. clamp
C. dressing
CLICKline surgical instrument
climber
Fitstep II stair c.
Sprint C.
Clinac 600SR stereotactic radiation treatment system
C-line bipolar coagulator
Clini-Care low-air-loss bed
CliniCath peripherally inserted catheter
Clini-Dyne low-air-loss bed
Clini-Float flotation therapy bed system
CliniFLO breathing exerciser
Cliniguard protective dressing
Clinisert mattress
Cliniset infusion set
Clinitek 50 urine chemistry analyzer
Clinitemp fever detector
Clinitex Charles endophotocoagulator probe
Clinitron air-fluidized bed
clinometer
clip
Absolok ligating c.
Ackerman c.
Acland c.
Adams-DeWeese vena caval serrated c.
Adams orthodontic c.
Adson brain c.
Adson scalp c.
Aesculap alpha vessel c.
alligator c.
aneurysm c.
c. applier
Astro-Trace Universal adapter c.
Atrauclip ligating c.
Atraumax SofTrac bulldog spring c.
Austin c.
Autostat hemostatic c.
Autostat ligating c.
Auto Suture c.
Backhaus towel c.
bayonet aneurysm c.
Beimer-Clip aneurysm c.

Benjamin-Havas fiberoptic light c.
Biemer vessel c.
Bleier c.
blepharoplasty c.
Bonney c.
Booster c.
Boyle-Rosin c.
brain c.
Braun-Yasargil right-angle c.
butterfly c.
Callender c.
Castroviejo scleral shortening c.
Children's Hospital c.
Codman c.
Colotzmark c.
cranial aneurysm c.
crankshaft c.
cross-legged c.
Cushing c.
Cushing-McKenzie c.
Dandy c.
Delrin plastic scalp c.
Drake fenestrated aneurysm c.
Drake-Kees c.
Edslab jaw spring c.
Edwards parallel-jaw spring c.
Elgiloy c.
Elgiloy-Heifitz aneurysm c.
encircling c.
Endo GIA surgical c.
fenestrated aneurysm c.
fenestrated Drake c.
ferromagnetic intracerebral aneurysm c.
Filshie female sterilization c.
Flexi-Seal fecal collector & tail c.
c. forceps
Friedman tantalum c.
gate c.
Guilford-Wright c.
Hader bar c.
Halberg c.
Heath c.
Hegenbarth c.
Hegenbarth-Adams c.
Heifitz aneurysm c.
Heifitz-Weck c.
Hem-o-lok polymer ligating c.
hemostasis scalp c.
hemostasis silver c.
hemostatic c.
Hesseltine Umbili C.

C

NOTES

183

clip *(continued)*

Horizon surgical ligating and marking c.
House neurovascular c.
Housepian aneurysm c.
Hoxworth c.
Hulka c.
Hulka-Clemens c.
Hylinks c.
inferior vena caval c.
Ingraham-Fowler c.
Ingraham-Fowler tantalum c.
Iwabuchi c.
Janelli c.
Kapp c.
Keer aneurysm c.
Khodadad c.
Kifa c.
Koln c.
Lapra-Ty absorbable suture c.
Lapro-Clip ligating c.
LDS c.
LeRoy infant scalp c.
LeRoy-Raney scalp c.
Ligaclip endoscopic c.
Ligaclip surgical c.
L-shaped aneurysm c.
Mayfield CIS-RE aneurysm c.
Mayfield-Kees c.
McDermott c.
McFadden cross-legged c.
McFadden-Kees c.
McFadden Vari-Angle aneurysm c.
McKenzie hemostasis c.
McKenzie silver brain c.
metallic c.
Michel scalp c.
Michel skin c.
Michel suture c.
Michel-Wachtenfeldt c.
microvascular c.
Miles skin c.
Miles Teflon c.
Moren-Moretz vena caval c.
Morse towel c.
Mortson V-shaped c.
Moynihan c.
nonferromagnetic c.
Olivecrona silver c.
palmar c.
partial-occlusion inferior vena caval c.
Paterson long-shank brain c.
Penfield silver c.
Perneczky aneurysm c.
Phynox cobalt alloy c.
pivot aneurysm c.
plastic scalp c.
Poly Surgiclip absorbable c.
Pool-Pfeiffer self-locking c.
primary c.
Raney scalp c.
Raney spring steel c.
c. remover
Rica cross-action towel c.
Rica silver c.
Rica suture c.
ring c.
Samuels-Weck Hemoclip c.
scalp hemostasis c.
Scanlan aneurysm c.
Schaedel c.
Schepens tantalum c.
Schulec silver c.
Schutz c.
Schwartz c.
Schwasser brain c.
Schwasser microclip c.
scleral shortening c.
Scoville c.
Scoville-Lewis aneurysm c.
Secu c.
security c.
Selman c.
Seraphim c.
Serature spur c.
silver c.
skin c.
Smith aneurysm c.
Smithwick silver c.
Sofield retractor c.
Spetzler titanium aneurysm c.
spring c.
Stealth surgical c.
Stichs wound c.
Sugar aneurysm c.
Sugita aneurysm c.
Sugita cross-legged c.
Sugita-Ikakogyo c.
Sugita side-curved bayonet c.
Sugita temporary straight c.
Sundt booster c.
Sundt cross-legged c.
Sundt encircling c.
Sundt-Kees aneurysm c.
Sundt-Kees booster c.
Sundt-Kees encircling patch c.
Sundt-Kees Slimline c.
Sundt straddling c.
surgical c.
Surgidev iris c.
Takaro c.
tantalum hemostasis c.
Taut Safety Klip c.
Teflon c.
temporary vascular c.
temporary vessel c.
titanium aneurysm c.

Totco c.
towel c.
Tru-clip c.
Umbili C.
umbilical c.
Uni-Shunt abdominal slip c.
Uni-Shunt cranial anchoring c.
Vari-Angle c.
vascular c.
vena caval c.
vessel c.
Vitallium c.
von Petz c.
Wachtenfeldt butterfly c.
Wachtenfeldt wound c.
Weck Hemoclip ligating c.
window c.
wing c.
wound c.
Yasargil-Aesculap aneurysm c.
Yasargil cross-legged c.
Zimmer c.
Zmurkiewicz brain c.
clip-applying aneurysm forceps
clip-bending forceps
clip-cutting forceps
clip-introducing forceps
Clip-Lite clip-on headlight
clip-on occluder
clipper
Baxter surgical c.
clip-reinforced cotton sling
clip-removing
c.-r. forceps
c.-r. scissors
ClipTip reusable sensor
Clirans T-series dialyzer
CLM McCoy articulating laryngoscope blade
clock
Sonic Boom alarm c.
clogs
Hollander c.
Markell Mobility Health c.
CloneSaver card
C-loop posterior chamber lens
Cloquet needle
closed
c. iris forceps
c. Küntscher nail
c. loop tourniquet
c. suction drain

closed-circuit spirometer
closed-loop intraocular lens
Close Encounter nut
The Closer suture-mediated arterial closure device
CloseSure procedure kit
closing forceps
closure
Beta-Cap II catheter c.
Brandy scalp stretcher I, II, front c.
Brandy scalp stretcher I, II, rear c.
c. device
DuoLock curved tail pouch c.
eXit disposable puncture c.
facial compression skull cap c.
hand-sutured c.
Lowsley retractor with hand-sutured c.
Proxi-Strip skin c.
retainer c.
Steri-Strip skin c.
Steritapes c.
Sure-Closure c.
Sur-Fit/Active Life tail c.
Sur-Fit irrigation sleeve tail c.
Vacuum Assisted C. (V.A.C.)
C. vein reflux system
Clo-Sure P.A.D. hemostatic device
clot
C. Buster Amplatz thrombectomy device
c. forceps
C. Stop coating
clothesline drain
cloth-shod clamp
Cloutier unconstrained knee prosthesis
cloverleaf
c. nail
c. radiofrequency ablation catheter
Cloward
C. blade retractor
C. bone graft impactor
C. bone punch
C. cautery hook
C. cervical drill
C. cervical retractor
C. dowel ejector
C. dowel handle
C. dowel impactor
C. drill guide

NOTES

Cloward *(continued)*
C. drill shaft
C. dural hook
C. dural retractor
C. hammer
C. intervertebral disc rongeur
C. intervertebral punch
C. laminectomy retractor
C. laminectomy rongeur
C. lumbar retractor body
C. L-W gauge
C. nerve root retractor
C. osteophyte elevator
C. periosteal elevator
C. posterior lumbar interbody fusion kit
C. single-tooth retractor blade
C. spanner gauge
C. spanner wrench
C. spinal curette
C. spinal fusion chisel
C. spinal fusion osteotome
C. spreader
C. square punch
C. surgical saddle
C. tissue retractor
C. vertebral spreader
Cloward-Cone ring curette
Cloward-Cushing vein retractor
Cloward-Dowel punch
Cloward-English
C.-E. punch
C.-E. rongeur
Cloward-Harman chisel
Cloward-Harper
C.-H. cervical punch
C.-H. laminectomy rongeur
Cloward-Hoen laminectomy retractor
Cloward-Puka chisel
clubfoot splint
Clyburn Colles fracture fixator
Clyman endometrial curette
clysis cannula
CM-Band 505N rubber brace
CMI/O'Neil cup
CMI vacuum delivery system
CMS AccuProbe 450 cryosurgical system
CMSI warming system
CO
CO Sleuth carbon monoxide monitor
CO Sleuth handheld carbon monoxide analyzer
CO₂
CO_2 cylinder
CO_2 generator
CO_2 laser

CO_2 laser probe
CO_2 Sharplan laser
Coach incentive spirometer
coaching whistle
Coag-A-Mate
C.-A-M. automated coagulometer
C.-A-M. prothrombin device
CoaguChek
C. portable prothrombin time device
C. Pro DM coagulation monitor
C. system
coagulating
c. electrode
c. forceps
c. suction cannula obturator
coagulation
c. probe
c. suction tube
coagulator
American Optical c.
AO c.
argon beam c.
argon plasma c.
ball c.
Ballantine-Drew c.
Bantam Bovie c.
bipolar c.
Birtcher Hyfrecator c.
Birtcher laparoscopic c.
Bovie CSV c.
C-line bipolar c.
Codman-Shurtleff neo-coagulator c.
cold c.
Concept bipolar c.
Cut-Blot c.
electricator c.
Elmed BC digital bipolar c.
Erbe argon plasma c.
Evergreen Lasertek c.
Fukushima malleable c.
Gam-Mer bipolar c.
Grieshaber microbipolar c.
Hildreth c.
Hyfrecator c.
infrared c.
Jarit bipolar c.
Karl Storz c.
Kirwan bipolar c.
Magielski c.
Makar c.
Malis bipolar c.
Malis CMC-II PC bipolar c.
Malis solid state c.
Mentor Wet-Field cordless c.
Meyer-Schwickerath c.
Microtaze microwave c.
Mira c.
National c.

Polar-Mate bipolar c.
Poppen electrosurgical c.
Ramirez EndoForehead suction c.
Redfield IRC 2100 infrared c.
Resnick button bipolar c.
Riddle c.
Ritter c.
Ritter-Bantam Bovie c.
Scanlan bipolar c.
Tekno c.
Ultroid c.
Walker c.
wet-field c.
xenon arc c.
Zeiss c.
coagulometer
Coag-A-Mate automated c.
Coaguloop resection electrode
Coakley
C. antral curette
C. antrum trocar
C. curette
C. ethmoid curette
C. frontal sinus cannula
C. nasal curette
C. nasal probe
C. nasal speculum
C. tenaculum
C. tonsillar forceps
C. wash tube
Coakley-Allis tonsillar forceps
coaptation
c. bipolar forceps
c. plate
c. splint
coarctation
c. clamp
c. forceps
c. hook
coarse carbide cone bur
coarse-olive bur
coated
c. biopsy forceps
c. polyester suture
c. Vicryl Rapide suture
coater
Hummer V Sputter c.
Polaron sputter c.
coating
Clot Stop c.
Hydrocoat hydrophilic c.

Mardis firm stent with
HydroPlus c.
Porocoat porous c.
porous c.
Pro/Pel c.
Teflon c.
Co-Axa light
coaxial
c. cable
c. cannula
c. catheter
c. I&A nylon connector
c. microcatheter
c. sheath cut biopsy needle
c. snare
Coballoy twist drill
cobalt
c. alloy stent
c. blue light
c. chrome modular head component
c. megavoltage machine
cobalt-chromium
c.-c. alloy prosthesis
c.-c. coated implant
c.-c. femoral component
c.-c. head
cobalt-chromium-molybdenum
c.-c.-m. alloy
c.-c.-m. alloy metal implant
cobalt-chromium-tungsten-nickel alloy implant
Coban
C. bandage
C. elastic dressing
C. self-adherent wrap
Cobas
C. Fara H centrifugal analyzer
C. Helios differential analyzer
Cobaugh eye forceps
Cobb
C. bone curette
C. chisel
C. osteotome
C. periosteal elevator
C. retractor
C. spinal curette
C. spinal elevator
C. spinal gouge
C. spinal instrument
Cobbett skin graft knife
Cobb-Ragde needle

C

NOTES

Cobe

 C. cardiotomy reservoir
 C. 2991 cell processor
 C. CML oxygenator
 C. gun stapler
 C. Optima hollow-fiber membrane
  oxygenator
 C. Revolution centrifugal blood
  pump
 C. small vessel cannula
 C. Spectra apheresis system
 C. staple gun
 C. Trima automated blood
  component collection system

Cobe-Stockert heart-lung machine
Cobe-Tenckhoff peritoneal dialysis
 catheter
cobra

 c. head plate
 C. K+ cannula
 C. LASIK irrigating cannula
 c. retractor

Coburg-Connell airway
Coburn

 C. camera
 C. equiconvex lens
 C. haptic
 C. I&A system
 C. intraocular lens
 C. lensometer
 C. Mark IX eye implant
 C. Optical Industries-Feaster
  intraocular lens
 C. refractor
 C. tonometer

Coburn-Rodenstock slit lamp
Coburn-Storz intraocular lens
coccyx

 c. cushion
 c. seat cushion

Cochlea Dynamics sound processing
 technology
cochlear implant
cock

 stop c.

Cocke large flap retractor
cock-up

 c.-u. ankle splint
 c.-u. splint
 c.-u. wrist splint
 c.-u. wrist support

cocoon

 c. dressing
 c. thread suture

Co-Cr-Mo

 Co-Cr-Mo alloy
 Co-Cr-Mo alloy prosthesis material
 Co-Cr-Mo pin

Co-Cr-W-Ni

 Co-Cr-W-Ni alloy
 Co-Cr-W-Ni alloy implant metal
 Co-Cr-W-Ni alloy prosthesis

Coda titanium alloy device
Codemaster defibrillator
coder

 Chen-Smith image c.

Codere-Durette orbital floor implant
Codere orbital floor implant
Codivilla graft
cod liver oil-soaked strips dressing
Codman

 C. Accu-Flow shunt
 C. arthroscope
 C. Bicol sponge
 C. bone gouge
 C. cannula
 C. cardiovascular clamp
 C. cartilage clamp
 C. cervical rongeur
 C. clip
 C. cranioblade
 C. cranioclast
 C. cranioplastic material
 C. disposable perforator
 C. external drainage system
 C. fallopian tube forceps
 C. frame
 C. guide
 C. Hakim programmable valve
 C. ICP monitor
 C. IMA kit
 C. internal mammary artery kit
 C. laminectomy rongeur
 C. lumbar external drain
 C. magnifying loupe
 C. marker
 C. microimpactor
 C. neurological headrest
 C. osteotome
 C. ovarian forceps
 C. Rhoton dissector
 C. scissors
 C. skull perforator guard
 C. spanner
 C. sternal saw
 C. surgical patty
 C. surgical strip
 C. Ti-Frame posterior fixation
  system
 C. towel clamp
 C. vein stripper
 C. ventricular silicone catheter
 C. wire cutter
 C. wire-passing drill

Codman-Holter catheter
Codman-Kerrison laminectomy rongeur
Codman-Leksell laminectomy rongeur

Codman-Medos programmable valve
Codman-Mentor Wet-Field cautery
**Codman-Schlesinger cervical
laminectomy rongeur**
Codman-Shurtleff
    C.-S. cranial drill
    C.-S. neo-coagulator coagulator
Cody
    C. magnetic probe
    C. sacculotomy tack
Coe
    C. impression material
    C. orthodontic resin
Coe-Pak
    C.-P. paste adhesive
    C.-P. periodontal dressing
COER-24 delivery system
Coe-Rect denture reliner
Coe-Soft
    C.-S. denture reliner
    C.-S. dressing
coffer band
Coffin
    C. plate
    C. transpalatal wire
Cofield 2 total shoulder system
Coflex
    C. bandage
    C. wrap
**CoFoam hydrophilic polyurethane
composite**
Cogan-Boberg-Ans lens
Cogent
    C. light
    C. LightWear headlight
    C. XL illuminator
COGNIShunt CNS fluid shunt system
Cogswell tip aspirator
Cohan-Barraquer microscope
Cohan needle holder
Cohan-Vannas iris scissors
Cohan-Westcott scissors
Cohen
    C. corneal forceps
    C. intrauterine cannula
    C. maxillary fixation hook
    C. nasal-dressing forceps
    C. periosteal elevator
    C. retractor
    C. rongeur
    C. sinus rasp
    C. suture applicator

    C. tubal insufflation cannula
    C. uterine cannula
Cohen-Eder uterine cannula
Coherent
    C. argon laser photocoagulator
    C. carbon dioxide laser
    C. CO_2 surgical laser
    C. EPIC laser
    C. LaserLink slit lamp
    C. Medical YAG laser
    C. Novus Omni multiwavelength
    laser
    C. photocoagulator
    C. Selecta 7000 laser
    C. UltraPulse 5000C laser
    C. Versapulse device
cohesive
    c. bandage
    c. dressing
Cohn Cardiac stabilizer
Cohney scissors
Cohort
    C. anterior plate system
    C. bone brush
    C. bone screw
    C. spinal impactor
    C. Ti-Spacer
coil
    3-axis gradient c.
    bilateral breast c.
    birdcage c.
    birdcage head c.
    body c.
    circular c.
    collagen-filled interlocking
    detachable c.
    conventional head c.
    Cook detachable PDA c.
    Cook retrievable embolization c.
    crossed c.
    Dacron fiber-coated c.
    dedicated local c.
    3-dimensional Guglielmi
    detachable c.
    distal shocking c.
    DuctOcclud c.
    c. electrode
    4-element phased-array c.
    elliptical end-capped quadrature
    radiofrequency c.
    embolization c.
    endoanal c.

NOTES

coil *(continued)*

endoesophageal magnetic resonance imaging c.
endoesophageal MRI c.
endorectal-pelvic phased-array c.
endoscopic quadrature radiofrequency c.
endovaginal c.
endovascular c.
extremity c.
fat-suppressed body c.
fibered platinum c. (FPC)
flexible radiofrequency c.
flexible surface c.
Flipper detachable embolization c.
GDC-series soft c.
Gianturco occlusion c.
Gianturco steel c.
Gianturco-Wallace c.
Gianturco wool-tufted wire c.
Golay gradient c.
gradient c.
gradient sheet c.
Guglielmi detachable c. (GDC)
head c.
helical c.
Helmholtz double-surface c.
high-speed gradient c.
Hilal c.
Intercept urethral internal MR c.
interlocking detachable c. (IDC)
intraurethral c.
Ivalon wire c.
liver c.
local gradient c.
Margulies c.
Maxwell c.
MRI extremity c.
occlusion c.
opposed loop-pair quadrature NMR c.
pelvic phased-array c.
phased-array c.
phased-array extremity c.
phased-array receiver c.
phased-array torso c.
planar circular c.
platinum embolization c.
posterior neck surface c.
Prolapse c.
quadrature birdcage c.
quadrature body c.
Quadrature cervical spine c.
quadrature head c.
quadrature surface c.
radiofrequency c.
receive-only circular surface c.
RF c.
right ventricular c.

saddle c.
sensing c.
shielded gradient c.
shim c.
shoulder surface c.
solenoid surface c.
steel embolization c.
c. stent
straight-fibered Guglielmi detachable c.
Stylet internal esophageal MRI c.
surface c.
Surgi-Vision Intercept urethral c.
Surgi-Vision internal MR c.
tantalum balloon-expandable stent with helical c.
Tornado c.
torso phased-array c.
transmit-receive c.
transvenous c.
transverse gradient c.
triaxial Helmholtz c.
Vortx c.

coiled

c. catheter
c. pressure algesimeter
c. spiral pusher wire
c. spring

coil-tipped catheter
CO$_2$ject system
Colapinto

C. sheath
C. transjugular cholangiography/liver biopsy set
C. transjugular needle

CO$_3$ laser
Colclough laminectomy rongeur
Colclough-Love-Kerrison laminectomy rongeur
cold

c. beam laser
c. biopsy forceps
c. cautery
c. coagulator
c. compress mask
c. coning knife
c. conization instrument
c. cup biopsy forceps
c. knife
c. knife hook
c. pad
c. rolled rod
c. scissors

ColdHot pack
Coldite transilluminator
cold-mist humidifier
cold-weld femoral ball
Cole

C. duodenal retractor

C. endotracheal tube
C. hyperextension fracture frame
C. orotracheal tube
C. pediatric tube
C. polyethylene vein stripper
C. uncuffed endotracheal tube
Coleman
C. aspiration cannula
C. infiltration cannula
C. microinfiltration system
C. retractor
C. V-dissector
C. V-dissector infiltration cannula
Coleman-Taylor IOL forceps
Colibri
C. corneal forceps
C. eye forceps
C. mules
Colibri-Pierse forceps
Colibri-Storz corneal forceps
Colin
C. ambulatory BP monitor
C. Electronics BP-508 tonometry system
C. STBP-780 stress test blood pressure monitor
CollaCote collagen wound dressing
collagen
Bio-Oss c.
bovine biodegradable c.
Contigen glutaraldehyde cross-linked c.
c. dressing
glutaraldehyde cross-linked c.
c. hemostatic material
c. implant
InterGard knitted c.
c. membrane
microfibrillar c.
c. plug
c. scaffold
c. shield
c. sponge
c. suture
collagen-filled interlocking detachable coil
collagen-impregnated knitted Dacron velour graft
CollagENT wand
Collagraft bone graft matrix material
Collamer intraocular lens
CollaPlug wound dressing

collapsible
c. holding chamber (CHC)
c. tissue retractor
collar
Belmont c.
c. button
c. button iris retractor
cervical c.
circumaortic venous c.
Colpacs c.
cone c.
Cowboy C.
c. dressing
Exo-Static c.
Exo-Static cervical c.
foam c.
Headmaster c.
high-humidity tracheostomy c.
implant c.
MAC cervical c.
Marlin cervical c.
Miami Acute Care cervical c.
Miami J cervical c.
Minerva c.
Nec Loc cervical c.
Newport c.
Peterson cervical c.
Philadelphia cervical c.
Plastazote cervical c.
plastic c.
Plastizote c.
Pneu-trac cervical c.
c. prosthesis
Schanz c.
Thomas cervical c.
collar-button tube
collared Press-Fit femoral stem implant
collarless
c. polished taper
c. stem
Collastat
C. collagen hemostat
C. collagen hemostatic material
C. hemostat
C. OBP microfibrillar collagen hemostat
Collatamp G hemostatic sponge
CollaTape
C. tape
C. wound dressing
Colleague pump
CollectFirst system

NOTES

collecting tube
collection trap
collector
    Alden-Senturia specimen c.
    bone c.
    Carabelli cancer cell c.
    Cervex-Brush cervical cell c.
    Conveen drip c.
    Cuputi sputum c.
    Cytobrush Plus endocervical cell c.
    Cytopick cervical cell c.
    Davidson c.
    Endocell endometrial cell c.
    fetal incontinence c.
    Flexi-Seal fecal c.
    Grass force displacement fluid c.
    Herchenson esophageal cytology c.
    Hollister drainable fecal c.
    Little Ones pediatric urine c.
    Lukens c.
    Medscand Cytobrush Plus cell c.
    Misstique female external
      urinary c.
    Moffat-Robinson bone pate c.
    Papette cervical cell c.
    Pilling c.
    Sheehy Pate c.
    stool c.
    Uterobrush endometrial sample c.
    Wallach-Papette disposable cervical
      cell c.
    Ware cancer cell c.
    wound drainage c.
    Xomed sinus secretion c.
College
    C. forceps
    C. Park TruStep foot prosthesis
    C. pliers
Collen-Pozzi tenaculum
Coller
    C. arterial forceps
    C. hemostatic forceps
Colles
    C. external fixation frame
    C. needle holder
    C. sling
    C. snare
    C. splint
collet
    c. screwdriver adapter
    tibial c.
    Triton pin c.
Colley
    C. tissue forceps
    C. traction forceps
Collier
    C. hemostatic forceps
    C. needle holder
    C. thoracic clamp

Collier-DeBakey
    C.-D. hemostat
    C.-D. hemostatic forceps
Collier-Martin hook
collimated beam handpiece
collimator
    APC-3, -4 c.
    automatic c.
    CASS TrueTaper c.
    c. cone
    converging c.
    diverging c.
    Eureka c.
    external c.
    fan-beam c.
    focusing c.
    c. helmet
    high-resolution fan-beam c.
    high-resolution multileaf c.
    high-sensitivity c.
    511-keV c.
    LEAP c.
    LEUHR fan-beam c.
    Leur-par c.
    long-bore c.
    low-energy ultra high-resolution
      fan-beam c.
    Machlett c.
    micromultileaf c.
    multihole c.
    multileaf c.
    multirod c.
    parallel-hole c.
    parallel-hole medium sensitivity c.
    Picker Dyna Mo c.
    pinhole c.
    single-hole c.
    slant-hole c.
    StereoGuide c.
Collin
    C. abdominal retractor
    C. amputation knife
    C. dressing forceps
    C. intestinal forceps
    C. lung forceps
    C. mesher
    C. mucous forceps
    C. osteoclast
    C. ovarian forceps
    C. pelvimeter
    C. pleural dissector
    C. radiopaque sternal blade
    C. raspatory
    C. rib shears
    C. sternal self-retaining retractor
    C. tissue forceps
    C. tongue forceps
    C. tongue-seizing forceps
    C. umbilical clamp

C. uterine curette
C. uterine-elevating forceps
C. uterine forceps
C. vaginal speculum
Collin-Duval
C.-D. intestinal forceps
C.-D. lung grasping forceps
Collin-Duval-Crile intestinal forceps
Collings
C. electrosurgery knife
C. fulguration electrode
C. knife electrode
Collin-Hartmann retractor
Collin-Pozzi uterine forceps
Collins
C. bicycle ergometer
C. Dry spirometer
C. dynamometer
C. Eagle I spirometry unit
C. leg holder
C. respirometer
C. survey spirometer
C. SurveyTach pneumotachometer
Collins-Mayo mastoid retractor
Collis
C. anterior cervical retractor
C. microforceps
C. microscissors
C. mouthgag
C. posterior lumbar retractor
C. spirometer
C. TDR instrument
C. Universal laminectomy set
Collis-Maumenee corneal forceps
Collison
C. body drill
C. cannulated hand drill
C. screw
C. screwdriver
C. tap drill
Collis-Taylor retractor
collodion dressing
collodion-treated self-adhesive bandage
Collostat sponge
Collyer pelvimeter
colmascope
colon clamp
Colonial retractor
colonic
c. insufflator
C. Z-stent

colonofiberscope
Olympus CF-series c.
Olympus CG-P-series c.
colonoscope
ACMI fiberoptic c.
ACMI operating c.
CF-200Z Olympus c.
Eve Fujinon video c.
EVIS CF-100L video c.
Fujinon EC-series video c.
Innoflex variable stiffness c.
magnifying c.
Olympus CF-HM-series
  magnifying c.
Olympus CF-MB-series c.
Olympus CF-PL-series c.
Olympus CF-P-series c.
Olympus CF-series c.
Olympus CF-T-series c.
Olympus CF-UM3 c.
Olympus CF-VL-series c.
Olympus CV-series c.
Olympus PCF-series pediatric c.
Pentax FC-series c.
Pentax VSB-P-series pediatric c.
Toshiba TCE-M-series c.
Welch Allyn video c.
ZM-1 c.
Coloplast
C. colostomy bag
C. Conseal 1-piece, 2-piece plug
C. contoured urine leg bag
C. disposable irrigation sleeve
C. dressing
C. economy irrigation set
C. ostomy belt
C. 1-piece, 2-piece drainable pouch
C. transparent irrigation sleeve
C. urostomy pouch
C. wafer
color
c. adaptometer
C. Bar Schirmer strip
c. flow Doppler ultrasound
C. Power Angio imaging
c. spectrum CW Doppler
Colorado
C. Cycle
C. electrocautery tip
C. microdissection needle
C. microneedle

NOTES

193

ColorCards
- Basic Sequences C.
- Everyday Objects C.
- Preposition C.

ColorChecker
- Macbeth C.

color-coded therapy putty
color-flow Doppler real-time 2-D blood flow imaging
ColorFrost microslide
ColorMark microslide
ColorpHast pH indicator strip
ColorZone tape
Coloscreen VPI test kit
colostomy
- c. bag
- c. clamp
- c. irrigation set
- c. rod
- Ultra Duet c.

Colotzmark clip
Coloviras-Rumel thoracic forceps
Colpacs
- C. collar
- C. ice pack

Colpolase laser
colpomicrohysteroscope
- Hamou c.

colposcope
- Accu-Scope c.
- CooperSurgical overhead zoom c.
- Cryomedics KryMed c.
- Frigitronics c.
- Jena c.
- Leisegang c.
- MM-6000 c.
- OPMI c.
- Wallach ZoomScope c.
- Wallach ZoomStar c.
- Zeiss c.
- ZoomScope c.

colpostat
- afterload c.
- c. applicator
- dome c.
- Hejnosz radium c.
- Henschke c.
- Homiak radium c.
- Landon c.
- Regaud radium c.

Colt cannula
Coltene
- C. alloy
- C. direct inlay system
- C. impression material
- C. Magicap
- C. oven

Coltex impression material
Colton empyema tube

Colts cutting needle
Columbia
- C. scaler
- University of British C. (UBC)

Columbus
- C. McKinnon Hugger device

columellar
- c. clamp
- c. implant

column
- c. chromatograph
- disposable PD-10 c.
- Hemosorba hemoperfusion c.
- immunoadsorption c.
- NHS-activated HiTrap affinity c.
- Plasorba BR plasma perfusion c.
- Prosorba c.

Colvard pupillometer
Colver
- C. examining hook
- C. retractor hook
- C. tonsillar dissector
- C. tonsillar knife
- C. tonsillar needle
- C. tonsillar pillar-grasping forceps
- C. tonsillar retractor
- C. tonsil-seizing forceps

Colver-Coakley tonsillar forceps
Colver-Dawson tongue depressor
Colvin-Galloway Future annuloplasty band
comb
- Cottle periosteal c.
- toe c.

Combi-40 cochlear implant
Combicath telescope catheter
CombiDerm
- C. ACD
- C. nonadhesive absorbent dressing

CombiLock plate
Combi Multi-Traction system
combination gel/inflatable mammary prosthesis
CombiSit surgeon chair
Combitip Plus pipette tip
Combitrans monitoring set pressure transducer
Combitube
- C. airway
- C. endotracheal tube

Combo Cath wire-guided cytology brush
Comed
- C. footgear
- C. postoperative shoe

comedo extractor
Come-Orthotic sports replacement insole
Comet VP coronary dilation catheter

Comfeel
- C. hydrocolloid dressing
- C. Plus pressure relief dressing
- C. Purilon gel dressing

Comfit endotracheal tube

Comfort
- C. Ag prosthetic sock
- C. Care bed
- C. Cast
- C. Cast stirrup
- C. Cath catheter
- C. Classic nasal mask
- C. Cool D-ring wrist splint
- C. Cool neoprene support
- C. nylon mattress
- C. Plus cushion
- C. Quilt underpad
- C. Rite footwear
- C. Socks
- C. Take-Along wheelchair cushion
- C. wrist immobilizer

ComfortCuff blood pressure cuff

Comf-Orthotic
- C.-O. 3/4 length insole
- C.-O. sports insole

ComfortSeat
- Flofit C.

ComfortWalk$_2$ prosthetic foot

ComfortWear pouch cover

Comfy
- C. elbow orthosis
- C. knee orthosis
- C. splint
- C. walker

Command
- C. hip instrumentation system
- C. PS pacemaker

Commander
- C. Algometer
- C. angioplasty guidewire
- C. PTCA guidewire
- C. PTCA wire

commissure laryngoscope

commissurotomy knife

committed-mode pacemaker

common
- c. bile duct dilator
- c. duct probe
- c. duct stone forceps
- c. duct stone scoop
- c. McPherson forceps

Commucor A+V Patient monitor

Compacement dental cement

Compac microcentrifuge

Compact
- C. II spirometer
- C. S lithotripter
- C. spirometer

compactor
- McSpadden c.

CompaFill MH dental restorative material

CompaLay dental restorative material

CompaMolar dental restorative material

Companion
- C. 2 blood glucose monitor
- C. feeding pump
- C. papillotome
- C. 300-series nasal CPAP system

Company
- Baylis Medical C. (BMC)
- Direct Optical Research C. (DORC)

comparison eyepiece

compass
- C. CT stereotaxic adaptation system
- C. Cygnus portable frameless stereotactic system
- Mastel diamond c.
- C. stereotactic frame
- C. stereotactic phantom
- C. Universal hinge

Compat
- C. enteral feeding pump
- C. surgical feeding tube
- C. surgical gastrojejunostomy tube

Compeed Skinprotector dressing

compensating eyepiece

compensator
- multivane intensity modulation c.
- scattering foil c.
- time-gain c.

Compere
- C. bone chisel
- C. fixation wire
- C. threaded pin

Comperm tubular elastic bandage

competitive ankle board (CAB)

completely in canal (CIC)

completely-in-the-canal (CIC)
- c.-i.-t.-c. hearing aid
- c.-i.-t.-c. listening device

compliance matching stent

C

NOTES

compliant
  c. balloon
  C. pre-stress bone implant
  C. pre-stress system
Compli soft-tip catheter
ComPly panty shield
compomer
  MagicFil dual-curing c.
component
  acetabular c.
  AGC unicondylar knee c.
  Amstutz femoral c.
  Anatomical Graduated C.'s (AGC)
  Axiom knee c.
  Biodynamic acetabular c.
  Biomet AGC knee c.
  Biomet shoulder joint
    resurfacing c.
  Bio-Modular shoulder c.
  Bio-Plug c.
  Black Max mid size knee c.
  CFV wrist c.
  Charnley flat-back femoral c.
  Charnley narrow stem c.
  cobalt chrome modular head c.
  cobalt-chromium femoral c.
  Definition PM femoral implant c.
  Deyerle c.
  Duramer polyethylene c.
  Freeman femoral c.
  Harris-Galante I porous-coated
    acetabular c.
  Healey revision acetabular c.
  HGP II acetabular c.
  Hoffmann II compact external
    fixation c.
  hybrid fixation of hip
    replacement c.
  Interlok femoral c.
  Judet impactor for acetabular c.
  Kirschner Universal self-centering
    captive-head bipolar c.
  Lubinus acetabular c.
  Mallory-Head Interlok primary
    femoral c.
  MARS revision acetabular c.
  Meridian ST femoral implant c.
  Meridian TMZF femoral c.
  Metasul hip joint c.
  monoblock femoral c.
  OEC Dual-Op barrel/plate c.
  Omnifit HA femoral c.
  Opti-Fix femoral c.
  Osteolock HA femoral c.
  Osteolock NP acetabular c.
  Oxford unicompartmental knee
    femoral c.
  PCA hip c.
  PFC c.
  Press-Fit femoral c.
  Profix porous femoral c.
  Pugh barrel c.
  Reliance CM femoral c.
  Rothman Institute porous
    femoral c.
  Smith & Nephew Reflection
    Interfit acetabular cup implant c.
  Springlite G foot c.
  Springlite II foot c.
  Taperloc femoral c.
  Tharies femoral resurfacing c.
  Tharies hip c.
  Ti-Bac acetabular c.
  trial c.
  Tri-Con c.
  Tri-Lock femoral c.
  Ultima femoral c.
  Universal radial c.
  Vitallium mesh c.
  Vitalock cluster acetabular c.
  Vitalock solid-back acetabular c.
  Vitalock talon acetabular c.
composite
  CoFoam hydrophilic polyurethane c.
  c. cultured skin
  c. dental cement
  dentin-bonded resin c.
  c. dressing
  Phaseafill dental c.
  Sepramesh biosurgical c.
Composix
  C. E/X hernia mesh
  C. Kugel hernia patch
compound
  Dermatex c.
  c. dressing
  Finite dental glazing c.
  Microfil silicone-rubber injection c.
  Pediplast moldable footcare c.
  c. spectacles
  c. suture
  Tissue-Tek OCT c.
compress
  Cool Tops c.
  Cryo-Therapy eye/full face c.
  Discover cryotherapy c.
  Hydrovisage full-face hot/cold c.
**ComPreSs compliant pre-stress bone
  implant system**
compressed Ivalon patch graft
compressible acrylic intraocular lens
compression
  c. bandage
  c. belt
  c. binder
  c. boot
  c. dressing
  c. earring

c. forceps
c. garment
c. girdle
c. glove
c. hearing aid
c. hip screw
c. hook
c. instrumentation posterior
   construct
c. paddle
c. panty
c. plate
c. pump
c. rod
c. spring
c. stocking
c. U-rod instrumentation
compression-decompression
active c.-d. (ACD)
compression-molded PMMA intraocular lens
compressive internal fixation device
compressor
Adair screw c.
air c.
Anthony enucleation c.
Anthony orbital c.
Barnes c.
Beneys tonsillar c.
Berens enucleation c.
Berens orbital c.
Castroviejo c.
Charnley c.
Conn aortic c.
Deschamps c.
Easy Air 15 c.
Easy/Neb c.
external inflatable c.
Freeway Lite portable aerosol c.
medical air c.
orbital c.
Pulmo-Mist c.
Riahl coronary c.
screw c.
Sehrt c.
shot c.
tubing c.
Comprifix
C. ankle splint
C. ankle support
Compriform support stocking
Comprilan bandage

Comprol dressing
Compton
C. suppression spectrometer
C. suppression system
CompuCam digital intraoral camera
CompuMed computer-controlled local anesthetic delivery system
Compu-Neb ultrasonic nebulizer
Compuscan Hittman computerized electrocardioscanner
Compuscan-P pachymeter
computed
C. Anatomy corneal modeling system
c. tomographic scanner
c. tomography (CT)
c. tomography scan
computer
Aspect c.
CardioData Mark IV c.
Digitrace home c.
Digitron DVI/DSA c.
electromechanical slope c.
Inspiron Instromedix c.
leukocyte automatic recognition c.
on-demand analgesia c.
Scintron IV c.
Sequential Multiple Analyzer C. (SMAC)
Silicon Graphics Indigo 2 c.
C. Technology and Imaging (CTI)
thermodilution cardiac output c.
Computer-Aided
C.-A. Fluency Establishment Training (CAFET)
C.-A. Patient Information System (CAPIS)
computer-assisted
c.-a. neurosurgical navigational system
c.-a. stereotactic surgery (CASS)
c.-a. videokeratoscope
computer-controlled
c.-c. infusion pump
c.-c. infusion pump system
c.-c. neurological stimulation system
computerized
c. axial tomography scanner
c. bedside transfusion identification system
c. cycloergometer
c. isokinetic dynamometer

C

NOTES

computerized *(continued)*
 c. morphometric system
 c. pattern generator
 c. planimetry
 c. radiographic image analysis
  system
 c. rotary chair
Computon microtonometer
Comtesse medical support stocking
Comyns-Berkeley retractor
Cona-Tone office-use hearing amplifier
concave
 c. gouge
 c. rat-tooth forceps
 c. skull disc
concentration
 minimal inhibitory c. (MIC)
concentrator
 Aeris 590 c.
 Caire Breeze oxygen c.
 Keystone Plus oxygenator c.
 Millennium oxygen c.
 NewLife Elite oxygen c.
 Puritan Bennett Aeris 590 c.
 SolAiris III oxygen c.
 stem cell c.
concentric
 C. balloon guide catheter
 C. foreign body retriever
 c. needle
 c. needle electrode
Concentrix
 C. dual-aspiration pump system
 C. Fluidics technology
Concept
 C. ablator
 C. ACL/PCL graft passer
 C. arthroscopic knife
 C. arthroscopy rasp
 C. beachchair shoulder positioning
  system
 C. bipolar coagulator
 C. bone tunnel plug
 C. cannula
 C. C-reamer
 C. CTS Relief kit
 C. curette
 C. digit trap
 C. disposable cautery
 C. GraFix graft
 C. handheld cautery
 C. II rowing ergometer
 C. Intravision arthroscope
 C. mesh grafter dermatome
 C. Multi-Liner lining needle
 C. nerve stimulator
 C. Ophtho-bur
 C. 2-pin passer
 C. Precise ACL guide system

 C. PuddleVac floor suction device
 C. rotator cuff repair system
 C. self-compressing cannulated
  screw system
 C. shaver
 C. Sterling arthroscopy blade
  system
 C. suturing needle
 C. tibial guide
 C. traction tower
 C. video imaging system
 C. zone-specific cannula system
Conceptus
 C. fallopian tube catheterization
  system
 C. guidewire
 C. Robus guidewire
 C. Robust guide wire
 C. Soft Seal cervical catheter
 C. Soft Torque uterine catheter
 C. VS catheter
Concert
 C. bone cement
 C. Cranioplast
conchotome
 Hartmann nasal c.
 Henke-Stille c.
 Olivecrona c.
 Stille c.
 Struyken c.
 Watson-Williams c.
 Weil-Blakesley c.
Concise
 C. cementing sculps
 C. compression hip screw
 C. resin
 C. side plate
Conclude dental cement
Conco
 C. abdominal belt
 C. elastic bandage
Concorde
 ACS C.
 C. catheter
 C. disposable cannula
 C. disposable skin stapler
Concord line draw syringe
Concord/Portex suction catheter
condenser
 Abbe c.
 amalgam c.
 Nordent amalgam c.
condensing lens
condom
 c. catheter
 c. catheter collecting system
 female/male c.
 Reality female c.
 c. urinal

conductance catheter
conductive V-Lok cuff
conductor
    Adson c.
    Bailey saw c.
    Davis c.
    DeMartel c.
    Kanavel c.
    Martel c.
    Souttar esophageal c.
    Xomed Audiant bone c.
conduit
    Rastelli c.
    Shelhigh pulmonic valve c.
condylar
    c. implant
    c. lag screw plate
    c. neck retractor
    c. rod
cone
    c. biopsy needle
    C. bone punch
    c. bur
    c. bur bit
    C. cerebral cannula
    c. collar
    collimator c.
    c. finger separator
    C. guide
    hand c.
    C. ice-tong calipers
    C. laminectomy retractor
    MammoSpot spot c.
    McIntyre truncated c.
    C. nasal curette
    nose c.
    Placido 25-ring c.
    Posey Palm c.
    c. ring curette
    C. scalp retractor
    C. self-retaining retractor
    shielded open-end c.
    c. skull punch
    c. splint
    stacking c.
    stoma c.
    C. suction biopsy curette
    C. suction tube
    c. ventricular needle
    Visi-Flow stoma c.
    C. wire-twisting forceps

Cone-Bucy
    C.-B. cannula
    C.-B. suction cannula set
    C.-B. suction tube
Confide HIV test kit
Confidence ring
confocal
    c. laser scanning ophthalmoscope
    c. microscope
    c. optics
    c. scanning laser ophthalmoscope
    c. scanning laser polarimeter
Conform
    C. Binder submalar facial implant
    C. II w/heel-ease Nature Sleep
      pressure pad
    C. stretch bandage
Conformant
    C. 2 wound dressing
    C. 2 wound veil
Conforma 3000 proton beam treatment system
conformer
    C. diabetic boot
    Fox c.
    McGuire c.
    Moore-Wilson hyperopic c.
    silicone c.
    Trokel hyperopia c.
    Universal c.
Conger perineal urethrostomy clamp
conical
    c. bur
    c. catheter
    c. centrifuge tube
    c. eye implant
    c. probe
    c. tip
    c. tip electrode
conic bougie
conization
    c. electrode
    c. instrument
    c. instrument blade
Conjugate export pump
conjunctival
    c. fixation forceps
    c. scissors
    c. spreader
Conley
    C. mandibular prosthesis

C

NOTES

Conley *(continued)*
　　C. pin
　　C. tracheal stent
ConMed
　　C. electrosurgical pencil
　　C. Excalibur-Plus electrosurgical
　　　unit
Conn
　　C. aortic compressor
　　C. pneumatic tourniquet
　　C. Universal tourniquet
connecting
　　c. plate
　　c. tubing
connection
　　c. cord
　　internal hex-thread c.
　　Luer c.
connector
　　Accu-Flo c.
　　ACS angioplasty Y c.
　　adjustable pedicle c.
　　Beurrier c.
　　bypass c.
　　coaxial I&A nylon c.
　　Denver c.
　　Holter c.
　　Humid-Vent Port 1 elbow c.
　　Infant PRAFO 450 heel c.
　　intrinsic transverse c.
　　Luer c.
　　Luer-Lok jet ventilator c.
　　Machida light source c.
　　McIntyre nylon cannula c.
　　Olympus light source c.
　　Passy-Muir ventilator c.
　　pedicle c.
　　plastic c.
　　PMV aqua, clear, purple, white
　　　ventilator c.
　　quick c.
　　Saf-T-Flo T-tube c.
　　SpeedLink transverse c.
　　straight c.
　　suction c.
　　tandem c.
　　transverse c.
　　Tuohy-Borst c.
　　Uni-Gard piggyback c.
　　Universal c.
　　venous Y c.
　　Y c.
　　Y-port c.
Connell
　　C. airway
　　C. breathing tube
　　C. ether vapor tube
　　C. suture
Con-Nex reamer

Connor
　　C. silicone oil removal cannula
　　C. straight nonirrigating wand
**ConQuest female/male continence system
　　pressure pad with preattached flange**
**Conquest PTA balloon dilatation
　　catheter**
**Conrad-Crosby bone marrow biopsy
　　needle**
conserver
　　O$_2$ Advantage oxygen c.
　　OxiClip PC20 demand oxygen c.
　　Oxymatic electronic oxygen c.
　　PulseDose oxygen c.
　　Walkabout oxygen c.
console
　　Arrow TransAct intraaortic balloon
　　　pump c.
　　Bruker c.
　　Hitachi EUB-515C ultrasound c.
　　Siemens Satellite CT evaluation c.
constant
　　c. current stimulator
　　c. passive-motion device
　　c. passive-motion machine
Constantine flexible metal catheter
ConstaVac
　　C. autoreinfusion system
　　C. catheter
　　C. drain
Constellation mapping catheter
**constrained rotating hinged knee
　　prosthesis**
constriction ring
construct
　　AO dynamic compression plate c.
　　compression instrumentation
　　　posterior c.
　　double-rod c.
　　Edwards modular system
　　　kyphoreduction c.
　　Edwards modular system
　　　neutralization c.
　　Edwards modular system
　　　scoliosis c.
　　Guiot-Talairach c.
　　iliosacral and iliac fixation c.
　　pedicle screw c.
　　rod-hook c.
　　screw-to-screw compression c.
　　segmental compression c.
　　single-rod c.
　　tissue-engineered c.
　　titanium c.
　　triplane c.
　　TSRH double-rod c.
　　TSRH pedicle screw-laminar
　　　claw c.

upper cervical spine
anterior/posterior c.
Wiltse system H c.
Wiltse system single-rod c.
Constructa
C. foam
C. foam block
consultant
Arthroplasty Products C.'s (APC)
ConTack labral anchor
contact
C. A-scan
C. A-scan biometer
C. B-scan
c. hysteroscope
C. Laser bullet probe
C. Laser chisel probe
C. Laser conical probe
C. Laser flat probe
C. Laser interstitial probe
C. Laser round probe
C. Laser scalpel
c. lens training mirror
C. lightweight telemedicine system
c. shell implant
contact-tip laser system
container
child-resistant c.
cryogenic storage c.
Fenwal cryocyte freezing c.
instrument retrieval c.
Mini-Bag Plus c.
non-child-resistant c.
Perative enteral feeding c.
Pleatman sac specimen c.
Promoe enteral feeding c.
quartz-glass c.
Quickbox c.
contemporary
c. near-point chart
C. Products, Inc. (CPI)
Contigen
C. Bard collagen hemostatic
material
C. Bard collagen implant
C. glutaraldehyde cross-linked
collagen
C. implant collagen hemostatic
material
C. tube
contiguous spinal fluid reservoir

Contimed
C. II biofeedback device
C. II pelvic floor muscle monitor
Continental
C. cannula
C. needle
continuous
c. ambulatory drug delivery
(CADD)
c. ambulatory peritoneal dialysis
(CAPD)
c. bar retainer
c. flow resectoscope
c. insulin delivery system
c. irrigation catheter
c. microinfusion device
c. passive motion (CPM)
c. passive motion device
c. positive airway pressure (CPAP)
c. subcutaneous insulin infusion
pump
c. suction tube
C. Wave II arthroscopy pump
continuously-perfused probe
continuous-wave
c.-w. argon laser
c.-w. diode laser
c.-w. Doppler ultrasound
c.-w. high-frequency Doppler
ultrasound system
c.-w. laser spectrometer
Continuum
C. Biomedical (CB)
C. knee system
C. MR-compatible infusion system
contour
c. back cushion
C. balloon dilatation catheter
C. closed-end stent
c. deluxe nasal mask
C. Emboli artificial embolization
device
C. ERCP cannula
C. Genesis ultrasonic-assisted
liposuction system
C. II ICD system
C. implantable cardioverter-
defibrillator
C. LTV135D implantable
cardioverter-defibrillator
C. mammography system

NOTES

contour *(continued)*
    C. MD implantable single-lead cardioverter-defibrillator
    C. Profile defibrillator
    C. Profile natural saline breast implant
    C. Profile silicone breast implant prosthetic buttock c.
    C. VL Percuflex stent
contoured anterior spinal plate
contour-facilitating instrument
contractor
    Adams rib c.
    baby rib c.
    Bailey-Gibbon rib c.
    Bailey rib c.
    Cooley rib c.
    Crafoord c.
    Effenberger c.
    Finochietto-Burford rib c.
    Graham rib c.
    Lemmon rib c.
    Medicon c.
    Reinhoff-Finochietto rib c.
    rib c.
    Scanlan-Crafoord c.
    Sellor rib c.
    Stille-Bailey-Senning rib c.
    Waterman rib c.
contraflexion brace
Contrajet ERCP contrast delivery system
contrast-enhanced CT
contrast-filled catheter
Contraves stand
control
    c. bridle
    Cadogan-Hough footpedal suction c.
    CD-Chex Plus flow cytometry c.
    Cell-Chex body fluid c.
    DryTime for bladder c.
    FlexDial stimulus c.
    Generation II all-in-one-hand c.
    HepCheck whole blood c.
    Hunstad Handle flow c.
    intravascular accurate c. (IVAC)
    MegaDyne all-in-1 hand c.
    pronation spring c. (PSC)
    C. Release pop-off needle
    Sickle-Chex c.
    Sugar-Chex II glucose c.
    c. wire
controlled ankle motion (CAM)
controller
    Actis venous flow c.
    Asahi pressure c.
    Bronkhorst Hi-Tec c.
    Infant 450 EV foot/ankle c.
    IVAC 831 drip c.

    pressure c.
    shoulder c.
    vacuum c.
    venous flow c. (VFC)
    voice intensity c.
    volume c.
ControlWire guidewire
Contura medicated dressing
ConvaTec
    C. ostomy pouch
    C. Unna-Flex elastic Unna boot
    C. urostomy pouch
Conve back support
Conveen
    C. bag hanger
    C. bedside drainage bag
    C. disposable stretch brief
    C. drip collector
    C. leg bag strap
    C. net pant
    C. Security+ Conveen self-sealing Urisheath
    C. Security+ deluxe contoured leg bag
    C. Security+ self-sealing male external catheter
    C. self-sealing Urisheath
    C. tapered intermittent catheter
conventional
    c. head coil
    c. reform eye implant
    c. shell-type eye implant
    c. silicone elastomer
    c. transmission electron microscope
convergent color Doppler
converging collimator
convergiometer
Converse
    C. alar elevator
    C. alar retractor
    C. blade retractor
    C. button-end bistoury
    C. chisel
    C. double-ended alar retractor
    C. fracture-wiring button
    C. nasal knife
    C. nasal retractor
    C. nasal root rongeur
    C. nasal saw
    C. nasal tip scissors
    C. needle holder
    C. nested retractor
    C. osteotome
    C. periosteal elevator
    C. rasp
    C. raspatory
    C. retractor blade
    C. scissors
    C. skin hook

C. splint
C. sweeper curette
Converse-Lange rongeur
Converse-MacKenty periosteal elevator
Converse-Wilmer conjunctival scissors
conversion
Tilt-In-Space wheelchair c.
Converta-Litter carrier
converter
digital-to-analog c.
motion-compensating format c.
real-time format c.
sequential video c.
SRR-5 digital-analogue c.
time-to-pulse height c.
Convertible
C. trocar system
WonderBrace C.
Convertors surgical drape
convex
c. array ultrasound probe
c. obturator
c. probe
c. rasp
c. sheath
convexoconcave heart valve
Convo-Gel cushion
convoluted
c. foam mattress
c. mattress pad
c. wheelchair cushion
convolution mask
Conway
C. lid retractor
C. lid speculum
Conzett goniometer
Cooely left ventricular sump tube
Cook
C. Amplatz dilator
C. Amplatz ureteral stent
C. arterial catheter
C. balloon
C. balloon cervical cannula
C. biopsy gun
C. continence cuff
C. continence ring
C. County Hospital aspirator
C. County Hospital tracheal suction
tube
C. deflector
C. detachable PDA coil
C. drainage pouch set

C. endomyocardial needle
C. endoscopic curved needle driver
C. Enforcer balloon dilatation
catheter
C. eye speculum
C. filter
C. flexible myocardial biopsy
forceps
C. Flexi-Tip ureteral catheter
C. FlexStent stent
C. helical stone dislodger
C. helical stone extractor
C. infusion catheter
C. intracoronary stent
C. liver balloon tamponade
C. liver balloon tamponade device
C. locking stylet
C. Longdwel needle
C. micropuncture introducer
C. osteotome
C. pacemaker
C. Peel-Away introducer
C. percutaneous entry needle
C. plastic Luer-Lok adapter
C. pressure monitoring catheter
C. rectal retractor
C. rectal speculum
C. retrievable embolization coil
C. Spectrum catheter
C. stent positioner
C. stereotactic guide
C. stereotactic system
C. straight guidewire
C. tissue morcellator
C. TPN catheter
C. trocar
C. trocar needle
C. Urosoft stent
C. walking brace
C. yellow pigtail catheter
Cook-Cope loop nephrostomy catheter
cookie
c. cutter device
Gelfoam c.
metatarsal c.
Cook-Swartz Doppler flow probe
Cook-Z stent
cool
C. Comfort cold pack
c. laser
c. mist vaporizer

NOTES

cool *(continued)*
    c. pack
    C. Tops compress
Cool-Aid continuous controlled cold therapy
cooler
    Cryo/Cuff compression c.
    DermaChiller 4 dermal c.
    DermaCooler 4 dermal c.
    EMI FACT 50 MK III c.
    Hot/Ice cold therapy c.
    Thermapad cryotherapy c.
Cooley
    C. acutely-curved clamp
    C. anastomosis forceps
    C. angled pediatric clamp
    C. aortic aneurysm clamp
    C. aortic cannula clamp
    C. aortic forceps
    C. aortic retractor
    C. aortic sump tube
    C. aortic vent needle
    C. arterial occlusion forceps
    C. arteriotomy scissors
    C. atrial retractor
    C. auricular appendage forceps
    C. bronchial clamp
    C. bulldog clamp
    C. cardiac tucker
    C. cardiac tunneler
    C. cardiovascular forceps
    C. cardiovascular scissors
    C. cardiovascular suction tube
    C. carotid artery clamp
    C. carotid clamp
    C. carotid retractor
    C. caval occlusion clamp
    C. chisel
    C. clamp
    C. coarctation clamp
    C. coarctation forceps
    C. coronary dilator
    C. curved cardiovascular clamp
    C. curved forceps
    C. Dacron prosthesis
    C. double-angled clamp
    C. double-angled jaw forceps
    C. femoral retractor
    C. first-rib shears
    C. graft clamp
    C. graft forceps
    C. graft suction tube
    C. iliac clamp
    C. iliac forceps
    C. intracardiac suction tube
    C. ligature carrier
    C. mitral valve retractor
    C. MPC cardiovascular retractor

    C. neonatal instrument
    C. neonatal scissors
    C. neonatal sternal retractor
    C. neonatal vascular clamp
    C. neonatal vascular forceps
    C. neonate clamp
    C. partial-occlusion clamp
    C. patent ductus clamp
    C. patent ductus forceps
    C. pediatric anastomosis clamp
    C. pediatric aortic forceps
    C. pediatric dilator
    C. pediatric rib retractor
    C. pediatric vascular clamp
    C. peripheral vascular clamp
    C. peripheral vascular forceps
    C. pick
    C. probe-point scissors
    C. profunda clamp
    C. renal artery clamp
    C. retractor
    C. reverse-cut scissors
    C. rib contractor
    C. rib retractor
    C. rib shears
    C. sternotomy retractor
    C. sternum retractor
    C. subclavian clamp
    C. sump suction tube
    C. tangential pediatric clamp
    C. tangential pediatric forceps
    C. tissue forceps
    C. U-sutures
    C. valve dilator
    C. vascular dilator
    C. vascular suction tube
    C. vascular tissue forceps
    C. vena caval catheter
    C. vena caval clamp
    C. ventricular needle
    C. ventricular sump
    C. Vital microvascular needle holder
    C. wax carver
    C. woven Dacron graft
Cooley-Anthony suction tube
Cooley-Baumgarten
    C.-B. aortic clamp
    C.-B. aortic forceps
    C.-B. wire twister
Cooley-Beck vessel clamp
Cooley-Bloodwell-Cutter valve
Cooley-Bloodwell mitral valve prosthesis
Cooley-Cutter disc prosthetic valve
Cooley-Derra
    C.-D. anastomosis forceps
    C.-D. pediatric anastomosis clamp
Cooley-Merz sternal retractor

Cooley-Pontius
    C.-P. sternal blade
    C.-P. sternal shears
Cooley-Satinsky clamp
Cool-Flex A/K suspension belt
CoolGlide
    C. aesthetic laser system
    C. laser
Coolidge
    C. transformer
    C. x-ray tube
cooling
    c. blanket
    c. helmet
    c. machine
CoolPac hands-free unit
CoolSorb absorbent cold transfer dressing
CoolSpot light
cool-tip
    c.-t. catheter
    c.-t. laser
CoolTouch
    C. II facial laser system
    C. Nd:YAG laser
Cool-vapor vaporizer
Coombs bone biopsy system
Coonrad-Morrey total elbow prosthesis
Coons
    C. interventional wire guide
    C. Super Stiff long-tip guidewire
Cooper
    C. argon laser
    C. aspirator
    C. basal ganglia guide
    C. chemopallidectomy cannula
    C. chemopallidectomy needle
    C. cryoprobe
    C. disc cryostat
    C. double-lumen cannula
    C. endotracheal stylet
    C. herniotome
    C. implant
    C. laser adapter
    C. LaserSonics laser
    C. ligature needle
    C. pallidectomy needle
    C. spinal fusion elevator
    C. spinal fusion gouge
Cooper-Rand intraoral artificial larynx

CooperSurgical
    C. LEEP system
    C. overhead zoom colposcope
CooperVision
    C. camera
    C. Diagnostic Imaging refractor
    C. Fragmatome
    C. I&A handpiece
    C. I&A unit
    C. imaging perimeter
    C. irrigating needle
    C. microscope
    C. PMMA-ACL Flex lens
    C. refractive surgery photokeratoscope
    C. series 10,000 ocutome
    C. spatulated needle
    C. Surgeon-Plus Ultrathin blade
    C. ultrasound
    C. viscoelastic
    C. vitrector
    C. YAG laser
CooperVision-Cilco Novaflex anterior chamber intraocular lens
Coordinate complete revision knee system
CO-oximeter
    Ciba-Corning 2500 C.-o.
    IL-282 C.-o.
Copal bone cement
Copalite cavity liner
Cope
    C. crushing clamp
    C. double-ended retractor
    C. gastrointestinal suture anchor set
    C. loop nephrostomy
    C. loop nephrostomy catheter
    C. lung forceps
    C. mandril guidewire
    C. needle introducer cannula
    C. pleural biopsy needle
    C. thoracentesis needle
    C. wire
Cope-DeMartel clamp
Copeland
    C. anterior chamber intraocular lens
    C. fetal scalp electrode
    C. humeral resurfacing head
    C. radial loop intraocular lens
    C. radial panchamber UV lens
    C. 360 streak retinoscope

NOTES

Cope-Saddekni
    C.-S. catheter tip
    C.-S. introducer
copolymer
    c. ankle-foot orthosis
    c. stapler
copper
    c. band
    c. band-acrylic splint
    c. blade
    c. bromide laser
    c. mallet
    c. phosphate cement
    c. vapor pulsed laser
Copper-7 intrauterine device
copper-clad steel needle
Coppridge
    C. grasping forceps
    C. urethral forceps
coquille plano lens
Corail
    C. Corail HA-coated femoral
      implant
    C. HA-coated stem hip implant
    C. total hip replacement system
coral
    madreporic c.
coralline
    c. hydroxyapatite Goniopora
    c. PBHA bone graft
    c. porous block hydroxyapatite
      bone graft
Coratomic
    C. implantable pulse generator
    C. pacemaker
    C. prosthetic valve
    C. R-wave inhibited pacemaker
Corazonix Predictor electrocardiograph
Corbett
    C. bone-cutting forceps
    C. bone rongeur
    C. foreign body spud
Corboy
    C. hemostat
    C. needle holder
CorCap cardiac support device
cord
    Biopac gingival retraction c.
    c. blood collection device
    c. blood collection system (CBCS)
    connection c.
    Frazier monopolar cautery c.
    Poppen monopolar cautery c.
    ProSport C.
    Racestyptine c.
    Sport C.
Cordelle II sound processor
Cordes
    C. circular punch
    C. esophagoscopy forceps
    C. ethmoidal punch
    C. punch forceps tip
    C. semicircular punch
    C. sphenoidal punch
    C. square punch
Cordes-New
    C.-N. laryngeal punch elevator
    C.-N. laryngeal punch forceps
Cordguard
    C. II cord blood collection system
    C. umbilical cord sampler
Cordis
    C. Atricor pacemaker
    C. bioptome
    C. Bioptone sheath
    C. Brite Tip guiding catheter
    C. Checkmate system
    C. Chronocor IV pacemaker
    C. coronary stent
    C. Crossflex stent
    C. dilator
    C. Ducor I, II, III coronary pigtail
      catheter
    C. Ectocor pacemaker
    C. embolization device
    C. endovascular system
    C. fixed-rate pacemaker
    C. Gemini cardiac pacemaker
    C. Hakim pump
    C. implantable drug delivery pump
    C. injector
    C. lead conversion kit
    C. Lumelec catheter
    C. Multicor pacemaker
    C. multipurpose access port
    C. Omni Stanicor Theta
      transvenous pacemaker
    C. pacing lead
    C. Powerflex balloon catheter
    C. Powerflex PTA balloon
    C. Predator balloon catheter
    C. radiopaque tantalum stent
    C. Secor implantable pump
    C. Sentron transducer
    C. Sequicor cardiac pacemaker
    C. sheath
    C. SMART stent
    C. Son-II catheter
    C. Stabilizer marker wire
    C. Stanicor unipolar ventricular
      pacemaker
    C. Synchrocor pacemaker
    C. Theta Sequicor DDD pulse
      generator
    C. Trakstar PTCA balloon catheter
    C. TransTaper tip catheter
    C. Ventricor pacemaker
Cordis-Dow shunt adapter

Cordis-Hakim
  C.-H. shunt
  C.-H. valve
Cordis-Webster
  C.-W. diagnostic/ablation deflectable
  tip catheter
  C.-W. mapping catheter
Cordon Colles fracture splint
Cordostat
  Foley C.
cordotomy
  c. clamp
  c. knife
core
  C. aspiration/injection needle
  C. CO_2 insufflation needle
  C. Dynamics audible trocar
  C. Dynamics cannula system
  C. Dynamics disposable cannula
  C. Dynamics disposable trocar
  C. envelope arm sling
  C. Hibak Rest
  C. Lobak Rest
  C. Max-Relax face cushion
  c. reamer
  C. Sitback rest pillow
  C. Slimrest cushion
  C. Slimrest lumbar pillow
  c. wire
Core-Assure
  C.-A. bone biopsy kit
  C.-A. kit
Core-Check tympanic thermometer
corenal suture ring
Coretemp deep tissue thermometer
Core-Vent dental implant
Corex digital probe permeameter
Corey
  C. ovum forceps
  C. placental forceps
  C. tenaculum
**Corfit System 7000 Series lumbosacral
  support**
Cor-Flex guidewire
Corgill bone punch
Corgill-Hartmann forceps
Corgill-Shapleigh ear curette
Corin
  C. Hi-Nek total hip stem
  C. taper-fit total hip system
coring biopsy gun
Corinthian transhepatic biliary stent

Corival 400 ergometer
cork, leather, and elastic orthotic
corkscrew
  Austin Moore c.
  c. dural hook
  Filtzer c.
  C. suture anchor
Corlon
  C. angiocatheter
  C. catheter
CorIS interference screw
Cormed ambulatory infusion pump
cornea
  AlphaCor synthetic c.
cornea-holding forceps
corneal
  c. abrader
  c. block
  c. chisel
  c. curette
  c. debrider
  c. dissector
  c. erysiphake
  c. fascia lata spatula
  c. fixation forceps
  c. foreign body bur
  c. graft spatula
  c. hook
  c. implant
  c. knife
  c. light shield
  c. marker
  c. microscope
  c. monocular loupe
  c. pachymeter
  c. punch
  c. ring
  c. scissors
  c. section-enlarging scissors
  c. section spatulated scissors
  c. spatulated scissors
  c. spud
  c. suture needle
  c. suture ring
  c. suturing forceps
  c. topography system
  c. transplant centering ring
  c. transplant forceps
  c. transplant scissors
  c. trephine
  c. tube
Corneascope photokeratoscope

NOTES

CorneaSparing LTK system
cornea-splitting knife
cornea-suturing forceps
Corneo-Gage PachKnife
corneoscleral
  c. punch
  c. scissors
  c. suturing forceps
corneoscope
  IDI c.
Corner cushion
Cornet forceps
Corning 170 pH/blood gas analyzer
Cornish wool dressing
Cornman dissecting knife
Corometrics
  C. Aloka ultrasound machine
  C. Doppler scanner
  C. fetal apnea monitor
  C. maternal monitor
  C. Medical Systems Inc. fetal
    monitoring system
  C. Model 900SC in-office
    mammography machine
  C. spiral electrode tip
coronal suture
coronary
  c. anastomotic shunt
  c. angiographic catheter
  c. angiography analysis system
  c. artery button
  c. artery bypass graft (CABG)
  c. artery cannula
  c. artery forceps
  c. artery probe
  c. artery scissors
  c. atherectomy device
  c. dilatation catheter
  c. dilator
  c. endarterectomy spatula
  c. guiding catheter
  C. Imagecath angioscope
  c. perfusion cannula
  c. perfusion catheter
  c. seeking catheter
  c. sinus cannula
  c. sinus catheter
  c. sinus guiding (CSG)
  c. stent
  c. wire
Coronet
  C. alloy
  C. magnet
Coroscop C cardiac imaging system
Corpak
  C. enteral Y extension set
  C. feeding tube
  C. weighted-tip, self-lubricating
    tube

Corrigan cautery
corrugated forehead retractor
corset
  c. balloon catheter
  Boston soft c.
  Daw Industries orthopaedic c.
  Hoke lumbar c.
  lumbar c.
  lumbosacral c.
Corson
  C. myoma forceps
  C. needle electrode
  C. needle electrosurgical probe
Cortac monitoring electrode
cortex
  c. extractor
  c. retractor
  c. screw
cortex-aspirating cannula
Cortexplorer cerebral blood flow
  monitor
cortical
  c. cleaving hydrodissector
  c. cleaving hydrodissector cannula
  c. electrode
  c. pin
  c. pin screw
  c. plate
  c. screw
  c. step drill
Cortoss bone void filler
corundum ceramic implant material
Corvita
  C. endoluminal graft
  C. endoprosthesis stent graft
  C. endovascular graft
  C. graft system
  C. stent
Corwin
  C. auto wire twister
  C. knife handle
  C. tonsillar forceps
  C. tonsillar hemostat
Corwin-Hegar wire twisting forceps
Corydon HydroExpression cannula
Coryllos
  C. periosteal elevator
  C. retractor
  C. rib raspatory
  C. rib shears
  C. thoracoscope
Coryllos-Bethune rib shears
Coryllos-Doyen periosteal elevator
Coryllos-Moure rib shears
CoSeal
  C. dressing
  C. liquid plastic dressing
  C. resorbable synthetic sealant
  C. surgical sealant

Cosgrove
  C. mitral valve replacement
  C. mitral valve retractor
Cosgrove-Edwards
  C.-E. annuloplasty band
  C.-E. annuloplasty system
Cosman ICP Tele-Sensor system
Cosman-Nashold spinal stereotaxic guide
Cosman-Roberts-Wells (CRW)
cosmetic contact shell implant
CO$_2$SMO
  CO$_2$SMO Plus! capnograph/pulse
  oximeter
  CO$_2$SMO Plus continuous
  noninvasive respiratory profile
  monitor
Cosmolon hook and loop tape
Cosmos
  C. II DDD pacemaker
  C. II multiprogrammable dual-
  chamber cardiac pulse generator
  C. pulse-generator pacemaker
Cosmo-TENS wireless patch
Co-Span alloy
costal
  c. arch retractor
  c. periosteal elevator
  c. periosteotome
CoStasis
  C. dressing
  C. surgical hemostat
Costa wire suture scissors
Costen
  C. iris needle
  C. suction tube
Costenbader
  C. incision spreader
  C. retractor
Costen-Kerrison rongeur
Coston-Trent
  C.-T. cryoretractor
  C.-T. iris retractor
costotome
  c. chisel
  Tudor-Edwards c.
  Vehmehren c.
cot
  finger c.
  Kenwood finger c.
  O'Connor rectal finger c.
  Profex finger c.
  rubber finger c.

Cotrel
  C. pedicle screw
  C. traction
Cotrel-Dubousset
  C.-D. distraction system
  C.-D. dynamic transverse traction
  device
  C.-D. hook
  C.-D. hook-rod
  C.-D. orthopaedic brace
  C.-D. pediatric rod
  C.-D. pedicle screw instrumentation
  C.-D. pedicular instrumentation
  C.-D. screw-rod system
  C.-D. spinal instrumentation
Cottingham punch
Cottle
  C. alar elevator
  C. alar retractor
  C. angled skin hook
  C. bone crusher
  C. bone guide
  C. bone lever
  C. bulldog scissors
  C. calipers
  C. cartilage crusher
  C. cartilage guide
  C. columellar clamp
  C. crossbar fishtail chisel
  C. dorsal scissors
  C. double hook
  C. dressing scissors
  C. fishtail chisel
  C. forceps
  C. heavy septal scissors
  C. hook retractor
  C. insertion forceps
  C. knife guide
  C. lower lateral forceps
  C. mallet
  C. nasal chisel
  C. nasal elevator
  C. nasal hook
  C. nasal knife
  C. nasal rasp
  C. nasal retractor
  C. nasal speculum
  C. needle holder
  C. osteotome
  C. periosteal comb
  C. periosteal elevator
  C. pillar retractor

NOTES

Cottle *(continued)*
  C. profilometer
  C. pronged retractor
  C. 4-prong retractor
  C. protected knife handle
  C. scissors
  C. septum elevator
  C. septum speculum
  C. sharp prong retractor
  C. single-blade retractor
  C. skin elevator
  C. skin hook
  C. soft palate retractor
  C. speculum
  C. spicule sweeper
  C. spring scissors
  C. suction tube
  C. tenaculum
  C. tenaculum hook
  C. tissue forceps
  C. Universal nasal saw
  C. upper lateral exposing retractor
  C. weighted retractor
Cottle-Arruga cartilage forceps
Cottle-Jansen
  C.-J. forceps
  C.-J. rongeur
Cottle-Joseph
  C.-J. double hook
  C.-J. retractor
  C.-J. saw
Cottle-Kazanjian
  C.-K. bone-cutting forceps
  C.-K. nasal forceps
  C.-K. rongeur
Cottle-MacKenty
  C.-M. elevator
  C.-M. rasp
Cottle-Neivert nasal retractor
Cottle-Walsham
  C.-W. septal straightener
  C.-W. septum forceps
  C.-W. septum-straightening forceps
cotton
  c. applicator
  c. ball
  c. ball sponge
  c. batting
 . c. bolster dressing
  C. cannulatome
  c. carrier
  C. cartilage graft
  c. crepe bandage
  c. Deknatel suture
  c. elastic bandage
  c. elastic dressing
  C. graduated dilation catheter
  c. nonabsorbable suture
  c. pledget

  c. pledget dressing
  C. sphincterotome
cotton-ball dressing
cotton-covered tourniquet
Cotton-Huibregtse double-biliary pigtail stent
Cotton-Leung
  C.-L. biliary stent
  C.-L. biliary stent set
Cotton-Loader position cast
cottonoid
  c. dissector
  neurosurgical c.
  c. patty
  c. pledget
cotton-roll rubber-dam clamp
cotton-tipped applicator
cotton-wadding dressing
cotton-wool bandage
cottony Dacron tape suture
couch
  Boston neurosurgical c.
couching needle
couch-mounted head frame
coudé
  c. bag
  c. catheter
  c. fulgurating electrode
coudé-tip demeure catheter
CoughAssist In-Exsufflator
Coulter
  C. Channelyser cell analyzer
  C. counter
  C. Epics C-flow flow cytometer
  C. Epics Elite flow cytometer
  C. HmX hematology flow cytometer
  C. MD 16 hemocytometer
  C. S-Plus 5 automated red cell counter
  C. STKS hematology analyzer
Coumatrak prothrombin time device
Councill retention catheter
Councilman chisel
Counsellor
  C. plug
  C. vaginal mold
counter
  automated gamma c.
  beta scintillation c.
  boron c.
  Capintec gamma c.
  Coulter c.
  Coulter S-Plus 5 automated red cell c.
  gamma ray c.
  gamma well c.
  Geiger c.
  Geiger-Müller c.

Gill pressor c.
ionization c.
joule c.
Linson electronic cell c.
LKB/Wallach 1277 automatic
  gamma c.
pacing c.
pill c.
RackBeta scintillation c.
scintillation c.
Sysmex R-1000 reticulocyte c.
time-based c.
whole-body c.
Wizard gamma c.
countercurrent heat exchanger
CounterForce osteoarthritis knee brace
counteroccluder
Counterpoint electromyograph
counterpressor
Acland-Bunke c.
Bruni c.
Gill c.
counterpulsation
c. balloon
c. catheter
Counter Rotational System (CRS)
counterrotation splint
countersink bur
Count'R-Force arch brace
coupeur
capsule c.
Coupland
C. elevator
C. suction tube
coupler
Acutome 2000 Reich-Hasson
  laparoscopic CO_2 laser c.
Ferrier c.
Precise anastomotic c.
coupling head
Cournand
C. arteriography needle
C. cardiac device
C. quadpolar electrode catheter
Cournand-Grino needle
Cournand-Potts needle
CoVac
C. 50, 70 ArthroWands
C. Wand
Covaderm
C. Plus adhesive barrier dressing
C. Plus tube site dressing

C. Plus VAD dressing
C. Plus vascular access dressing
Coventry stapler
cover
AquaShield reusable orthopaedic
  cast c.
Bili mask phototherapy eye c.
bur hole c.
ComfortWear pouch c.
Expo Bubble eye c.
E-Z Flap burr hole c.
Hollister replacement filters
  pouch c.
I.V. House wound c.
Medipore dressing c.
MIP reusable c.
OxiLink oximetry probe c.
protective mattress c.
c. screw
Sheathes ultrasound probe c.
ShowerSafe waterproof cast and
  bandage c.
Show'rbag cast and dressing c.
SofStep wheelchair footplate c.
TiMesh burrhole c.
Ultra Cover transducer c.
covering
Permalume c.
Coverlet
C. OR adhesive surgical dressing
C. Strips adhesive dressing
Cover-Pad dressing
Cover-Roll
C.-R. adhesive gauze
C.-R. dressing
C.-R. gauze adhesive
C.-R. stretch bandage
Coverslipper
Jung CV 5000 Robotic C.
Cover-Strip wound closure strip
Covertell composite secondary dressing
CovRSite dressing
Cowboy Collar
cowhorn tooth-extracting forceps
Co-Wrap dressing
Cox
C. cytology brush
C. III LaserSecure shield
C. II ocular laser shield
C. metatarsal spreader
C. polypectomy snare

NOTES

Cox *(continued)*
    C. sterilizer
    C. Uphoff International (CUI)
Coxeter urologic catheter
Cox-Uphoff implant
Coyne spoon
Coyote OTW balloon catheter
Cozean
    C. angled lens forceps
    C. bipolar forceps
    C. implantation forceps
Cozean-McPherson
    C.-M. angled lens forceps
    C.-M. tying forceps
CP2
    CP2 Inflat-A-Mask inflatable sinus mask
    CP2 Inflat-A-Wrap cold pad
CPAP
    continuous positive airway pressure
    Aladdin II nasal CPAP
    DeVilbiss CPAP
    Down's continuous flow CPAP
    Polaris CPAP
    Sullivan III CPAP
    Tranquility Quest CPAP
    CPAP ventilator
CPCA2000 counterpulsation device
C-PET scanner
CPHV OptiForm mitral valve
CPI
    Contemporary Products, Inc.
    CPI 6260 aspirator
    CPI Astra pacemaker
    CPI automatic implantable defibrillator
    CPI DDD pacemaker
    CPI endocardial defibrillation rate-sensing pacing lead
    CPI Endotak electrode
    CPI Endotak SQ electrode lead
    CPI #9100 insulin pump
    CPI Maxilith pacemaker
    CPI Microthin DI, DII lithium-powered programmable pacemaker
    CPI Minilith pacemaker
    CPI porous tined-tip bipolar pacing lead
    CPI PRx pulse generator
    CPI Sentra endocardial lead
    CPI Sweet Tip lead
    CPI tunneler
    CPI Ultra II pacemaker
    CPI Ventak AICD
    CPI Ventak PRx cardioverter-defibrillator
    CPI Vigor pacemaker
    CPI Vista-T pacemaker

CPM
    continuous passive motion
    CPM device
    CPM machine
CPR
    cardiopulmonary resuscitation
Cr6-45NMf retinal camera
Crabtree
    C. attic dissector
    C. dissector pick
cracker
    Dodick nucleus c.
    Ernest nucleus c.
    LeVeen plaque c.
    Newsom side port nucleus c.
    nucleus c.
cradle
    alpha c.
    c. arm sling
    c. boot
    CT scan c.
    foot c.
    Posey bed c.
Crafoord
    C. auricular clamp
    C. bronchial forceps
    C. coarctation clamp
    C. coarctation forceps
    C. contractor
    C. hemostat
    C. lobectomy scissors
    C. lung scissors
    C. pulmonary forceps
    C. retractor
    C. thoracic scissors
    C. tunneler
Crafoord-Cooley tucker
Crafoord-Sellors
    C.-S. auricular clamp
    C.-S. forceps
Crafoord-Senning heart-lung machine
Cragg
    C. Convertible wire
    C. endoluminal graft
    C. EndoPro nitinol stent
    C. Endopro System I stent
    C. FX wire
    C. infusion wire
    C. thrombolytic brush
Craig
    C. abduction splint
    C. biopsy needle
    C. headrest
    C. nasal-cutting forceps
    C. pin
    C. scissors
    C. septum forceps
    C. tonsil-seizing forceps

C. vertebral body biopsy
instrument set
**Craig-Domnick septum bone-cutting
forceps**
Craig-Scott orthosis
Craig-Sheehan retractor
Cramer wire splint
**Crampton-Tsang percutaneous
endoscopic biliary stent set**
Crane
C. bone chisel
C. dental pick
C. gouge
C. mallet
C. osteotome
C. pick elevator
cranial
c. aneurysm clip
c. bone rongeur
c. bur
c. clip-applying forceps
c. drill
c. forceps
c. Jacobs hook
c. osteosynthesis system
c. perforator
c. plating system
c. retractor
c. rongeur
c. suture
cranioblade
Codman c.
Kirwan c.
CranioCap
C. craniofacial orthosis
C. helmet
craniocervical plate
cranioclast
Auvard c.
Braun c.
Codman c.
Rica c.
Tarnier c.
Zweifel-DeLee c.
craniofacial
c. fracture appliance
c. instrumentation
CranioFIX device
craniomaxillofacial
c. mesh
c. plate
c. plating system

c. screw
c. sheet
Cranioplast
Concert C.
cranioplastic acrylic material
cranioplasty
dynamic orthotic c. (DOC)
craniotome
Anspach c.
DeMartel c.
Midas Rex c.
Verbrugge-Souttar c.
Williams c.
craniotomy scissors
Craniovac drain
crank
c. frame retractor
c. table
crankshaft clip
Cranwall laryngoscope blade
Crapeau nasal snare
cravat bandage
Crawford
C. aortic retractor
C. canaliculus probe
C. dural elevator
C. epidural needle
C. fascial forceps
C. fascial needle
C. fascial stripper
C. head frame
C. hook
C. lacrimal set
C. suture ring
C. tube
Crawford-Adams acetabular cup
Crawford-Beaver retractor
Crawford-Cooley tunneler
Crawford-Knighton forceps
C-reamer
Concept C-r.
Creative diabetic socks
Creech aortoiliac graft
Creed dissector
Creevy
C. biopsy forceps
C. bladder evacuator
C. calyx stone dislodger
C. urethral dilator
Crego
C. periosteal elevator
C. periosteal retractor

NOTES

C

Crego-Gigli saw
Crego-McCarroll traction bow
Cremer-Ikeda
    C.-I. papillotome
    C.-I. sphincterotome
Crenshaw
    C. caruncle clamp
    C. caruncle forceps
crenulated tantalum wire
crepe
    c. bandage
    c. bandage dressing
crescent
    c. blade
    c. broach
    C. graft
    C. memory pillow
    C. plaster knife
    c. snare
crescentic blade
crib
    c. splint
    TiMesh mandibular c.
Cribier-Letac
    C.-L. aortic valvuloplasty balloon
    C.-L. catheter
Crib-O-Gram neonatal screening
  audiometer
Cricket
    C. disposable skin stapler
    C. pulse oximetry monitor
    C. recording pulse oximeter
    C. stapling device
cricothyrotomy
    c. cannula
    c. trocar tube
Crigler evacuator
Crile
    C. arterial forceps
    C. blade
    C. clamp
    C. cleft palate knife
    C. crushing clamp
    C. gall duct forceps
    C. gasserian ganglion dissector
    C. gasserian ganglion knife
    C. hemostatic forceps
    C. Micro-Line arterial forceps
    C. needle holder
    C. nerve hook
    C. retractor
    C. spatula
    C. thyroid double-ended retractor
    C. vagotomy stripper
    C. wire passer
Crile-Barnes hemostatic forceps
Crile-Crutchfield clamp
Crile-Duval lung-grasping forceps
Crile-Murray needle holder

Crile-Rankin forceps
Crile-Wood
    C.-W. needle holder
    C.-W. Vital needle holder
crimped
    c. Dacron prosthesis
    c. toric lens
crimped-wire prosthesis
crimper
    Caparosa wire c.
    ENT wire c.
    Farrior wire c.
    Gruppe wire c.
    Juers wire c.
    McGee-Caparosa wire c.
    McGee-Priest wire c.
    McGee wire c.
    pin c.
    Schuknecht wire c.
    Sheer wire c.
    washer c.
    wire c.
crimping forceps
Crinotene dressing
Cripps obturator
Cristobalite investment material
Critchett eye speculum
Crites laryngeal cotton screw
Critical
    C. Care mattress
    C. Care ventilator
Criticare
    C. ETCO$_2$/SpO$_2$ monitor
    C. HN-Isocal tube feeding set
    C. 506N2 vital signs monitor
    C. pulse oximeter
    C. sensor probe
    C. 507-series noninvasive blood
      pressure monitor
    C. 8100 vital signs monitor
CritiCath
    C. flow-directed thermodilution
      catheter
    C. pulmonary artery catheter
CritiCore monitoring system
Critikon
    C. balloon thermodilution catheter
    C. balloon wedge pressure catheter
    C. blood pressure cuff
    C. Optiva IV catheter
    C. oximeter
    C. pressure infuser
Critikon-Berman angiographic balloon
  catheter
Crit-Line whole blood diagnostic
  instrument
CritSpin
    C. centrifuge
    C. hematocrit system

crochet hook
Crockard
    C. ligament grasping forceps
    C. microdissector
    C. midfacial osteotomy retractor
    plate
    C. odontoid peg-grasping forceps
    C. pharyngeal retractor
    C. retractor
    C. retractor system
    C. small-tongue retractor blade
    C. sublaminar wire guide
    C. suction tube holder
    C. transoral retractor body
crocodile biopsy forceps
CROM
    cervical range-of-motion
    CROM device
Cronin
    C. cleft palate elevator
    C. cleft palate knife
    C. mammary implant
    C. palate elevator
    C. palate knife
    C. Silastic mammary prosthesis
Crookes
    C. glasses
    C. lens
Crookes-Hittorf tube
Crosby
    C. biopsy needle
    C. knife
Crosby-Kugler biopsy capsule
cross
    c. bar
    c. bar handle
    C. corneal bur
    C. needle trocar
    C. osteotome
    C. Top replacement oxygen sensor
cross-action
    c.-a. bulldog clamp
    c.-a. capsular forceps
    c.-a. towel clamp
crossbar fishtail chisel
cross-bracing
    spinal rod c.-b.
cross-clamp
    aortic c.-c.
crossed coil
crossed-loop resonator
Crossen puncturing tenaculum forceps

Crossfire polyethylene bearing material
CrossFlex LC coronary stent
Cross-Jones
    C.-J. aortic valve
    C.-J. caged mitral valve
    C.-J. disc valve prosthesis
    C.-J. mitral valve prosthesis
cross-legged clip
crosslinked glaucoma filtration device
CrossPoint TransAccess catheter
cross-Polaroid projection chart
CrossSail coronary dilatation catheter
cross-sectional anal sphincter probe
cross-slot screwdriver
cross-table leg immobilizer
cross-talk pacemaker
crosstrainer
    Sprint c.
Crosswire
    C. nitinol hydrophilic-coated
    guidewire
    C. PTCA guidewire
crotchless compression garment
Crotti
    C. goiter retractor
    C. thyroid retractor
Crouch corneal protector
croupette tent
croup tent
Crowe-Davis
    C.-D. mouthgag
    C.-D. mouth retractor
Crowe pilot point
Crowe-tip pin
Crowley shank
crown
    Alfred Becht temporary c.
    c. amalgamator
    Bosworth temporary c.
    c. drill
    c. drill screw
    freestanding single c.
    Getz c.
    Hahnenkratt temporary c.
    C. high-profile cushion
    Kontack temporary c.
    C. mattress system
    C. needle
    PD preformed c.
    C. quadtro cushion
    C. recliner system
    Royal c.

NOTES

crown *(continued)*
    Safco polycarbonate c.
    c. saw
    c. scissors
    stainless steel c.
    C. stent
    temporary c.
Crown-A-Matic crown and bridge remover
crown-crimping pliers
Crozat
    C. clasp
    C. orthodontic wire
    C. removable orthodontic appliance
C-R resin syringe
CRS
    Counter Rotational System
    CRS brace
    CRS tibial torsion system
CrTmEr:YAG laser
cruciate
    c. head bone screw
    c. ligament guide
    c. punch
cruciate-retaining prosthesis
cruciate-sacrificing prosthesis
cruciform
    c. anterior spinal hyperextension (CASH)
    c. anterior spinal hyperextension orthosis
    c. head bone screw
    c. screwdriver
Cruickshank entropion clamp
Cruiser hip abduction brace
crumpled aluminum foil
crural
    c. hook
    c. nipper forceps
Cruricast dressing
crurotomy
    c. chisel
    c. saw
crus guide fork
crusher
    baby spur c.
    Berger spur c.
    bone c.
    cartilage c.
    Cottle bone c.
    Cottle cartilage c.
    Gross spur c.
    Lieberman phaco c.
    Lowsley stone c.
    Mayo-Lovelace spur c.
    Mikulicz c.
    Ochsner-DeBakey spur c.
    Proud fascia c.
    Stetten spur c.
    ultrasonic stone c.
    Warthen spur c.
    Wolfson spur c.
    Wurth spur c.
crushing clamp
crutch
    c. and belt femoral closed nail
    EuroCuff forearm c.
    Everett c.
    Hardy aluminum c.
    iWALKfree c.
    Kenny c.
    Lofstrand c.
    Warm Springs c.
crutched stick-type polyurethane endoprosthesis
Crutchfield
    C. bone drill
    C. cervical traction
    C. clamp
    C. hand drill
    C. skeletal traction
    C. skeletal traction tongs
    C. skull-tip pin
    C. tongs
    C. tongs prosthesis
    C. traction bow
Crutchfield-Raney skull traction tongs
CRW
    Cosman-Roberts-Wells
    CRW MRI stereotactic ring
    CRW stereotactic frame
    CRW stereotactic system
CRx valve
Cryer
    C. dental root elevator
    C. Universal forceps
cryoablation catheter
Cryo-Barrages vitreous implant
Cry-O-Cadet
    Kelman C.-O.-C.
CRYOcare cryoablation system
CryoCath catheter
cryocatheter
    Freezor c.
CryoCor
    C. cardiac cryoablation catheter
    C. cardiac cryoablation system
    C. system
Cryo/Cuff
    Aircast C./C.
    C./C. compression cooler
    C./C. knee compression dressing
    C./C. pressure boot
Cryocup ice massager
Cryo-Cut microtome
cryoenucleator
    Gallie c.

cryoextractor
> Alcon c.
> Amoils c.
> Beaver cataract c.
> Bellows c.
> Frigitronics Mark II c.
> Keeler c.
> Kelman c.
> Rubinstein c.
> Thomas c.

cryoflex envelope
CryoGenetics CryoPrism
cryogenic
> c. probe
> c. storage container

CryoGuide ultrasound guidance system
CryoHit
> C. cryotherapy system
> C. probe

Cryojet
> Torre C.

CryoLife
> C. homograft
> C. homograft graft
> C. vascular graft

CryoLife-O'Brien stentless heart valve
cryomagnet
CryoMed freezer
Cryomedics
> C. disposable LLETZ electrode
> C. electrosurgery system
> C. KryMed colposcope

CryoNeedles needle
cryopencil
> Amoils c.
> Mira endovitreal c.

CryoPen cryosurgical system
cryopexy probe
cryophake
> Alcon c.
> Amoils c.
> Bellows c.
> Keeler c.
> Kelman c.
> Rubinstein c.

cryopreserved homograft valve
CryoPrism
> CryoGenetics C.

cryoprobe
> Amoils c.
> Cooper c.
> cryoptor c.

> Erbe c.
> Frigitronics c.
> intravitreal c.
> Lee c.
> Linde c.
> MST c.
> Rubinstein c.
> Spembly c.
> Sudarsky c.
> Thomas c.

cryoptor
> c. cryoprobe
> Thomas c.

cryoretractor
> Coston-Trent c.
> Hartstein iris c.
> Thomas c.

cryostat
> Cooper disc c.
> c. frozen sectioning aid
> Tissue Tek-II c.

cryosurgical
> c. apparatus
> c. instrument
> c. unit

cryosystem
> Keeler-Amoils ophthalmic c.

cryotherapy
> c. probe
> c. system

Cryo-Therapy eye/full face compress
cryotome
cryotube
> Nunc c.

Cryo-Vac-Away cryostat vacuum system
CryoValve SG allograft heart valve
CryoVein saphenous vein allograft
Cryovial system
crypt hook
cryptoscope
> Satvioni c.

cryptotome
> Blanchard c.
> Pierce c.

crystal
> C. adjusting exam lift table
> C. cannula
> Cardiometrics FloWire Doppler
> echo c.
> c. gamma camera
> piezoelectric c.
> C. Tone hearing aid

NOTES

217

Crystalase Erbium2 laser
CrystalEyes endoscopic video system
crystalline lens
Crystar porcelain kit
CSC3 cervical support cushion
CSF
    cerebrospinal fluid
      CSF prosthesis
      CSF reservoir
      CSF shunt-introducing forceps
      CSF T-tube shunt
      CSF valve
CSG
    coronary sinus guiding
C-shaped
      C-s. microplate
      C-s. plate
      C-s. resistive magnet
CSI lens
C-sponge sponge
CSV Bovie electrosurgical unit
CSZ Electri-Cool cold therapy system
CT
    computed tomography
      CT body scanner
      contrast-enhanced CT
      CT densitometer
      HeartView CT
      HearTwave CT
      helical CT
      CT Max 640 scanner
      multidetector CT
      CT scan
      CT scan cradle
      CT scan gantry
      spiral CT
      spiral multidetector CT
      triphasic spiral CT
      twin-beam CT
CT-1000 cardiotachometer
CT-10 computerized tonometer
CT1 needle
CTDx electrostimulation system
C-Tek anterior cervical plate system
CTEV brace
CTE:YAG laser
CTI
    Computer Technology and Imaging
      CTI Cyclotron system
      CTI 933/04 ECAT PET scanner
      CTI infusion pump
      CTI positron emission tomography
      scanner
C.Ti.2 brace
CTI-Siemens 933/08-12 PET camera
CTM
    cardiac transplant monitoring
CT/MRI-compatible stereotactic
  headframe

CT-MRI-compatible stereotactic head
  frame system
C-Trak
    C-T. analyzer
    C-T. handheld gamma detector
    C-T. handheld gamma probe
    C-T. surgical guidance system
CTS
    carpal tunnel syndrome
    CTS gauge
    CTS Gripfit splint
    CTS relief kit
C-type acupuncture needle
Cu-7 intrauterine device
CU-8 needle
Cubbins
    C. screw
    C. screwdriver
cube
    Gelfoam c.
    c. pessary
    Temper Foam c.
    tumbling E c.
Cuchica syringe
Cuda
    C. endoscope
    C. laparoscope
    C. laparoscope
    C. retractor
    C. shaver
Cueva
    C. cranial nerve electrode
    C. cranial nerve electrode
      monitoring device
cuff
    antimicrobial catheter c.
    Astropulse c.
    blood pressure c.
    blood warmer c.
    calibrated V-Lok c.
    ComfortCuff blood pressure c.
    conductive V-Lok c.
    Cook continence c.
    Critikon blood pressure c.
    Dacron c.
    Dinamap blood pressure c.
    Ducker-Hayes nerve c.
    c. electrode
    endotracheal tube c.
    endovascular aortic graft c.
    Ethox blood pressure c.
    Falk vaginal c.
    Finapres finger c.
    finger c.
    hand c.
    Honan c.
    inflatable tourniquet c.
    inflatable tracheal tube c.
    joint distraction c.

Kendall endotracheal tube c.
C. Link orthopaedic device
nerve c.
oscillometric blood pressure c.
Papercuff disposable blood
  pressure c.
pneumatic c.
Polmedco endotracheal tube c.
Portex SS endotracheal tube c.
Portex XL endotracheal tube c.
pressure c.
push c.
Push-Ease Quad c.
PyMaH pre-gaged c.
Safe-Cuff blood pressure c.
Sheridan endotracheal tube c.
shoulder c.
c. sphygmomanometer
sphygmomanometer c.
Steri-Cuff disposable tourniquet c.
SureCuff tissue ingrowth c.
C. Tack anchor
Temp-Kuff blood pressure c.
tourniquet c.
tracheal tube c.
VitaCuff antimicrobial c.
V-Lok disposable blood pressure c.
Watzke c.

cuffed
c. endotracheal tube
c. esophageal endoprosthesis
Rusch endotracheal tube c.
c. tracheostomy tube

Cufflator
Posey C.

CUI
Cox Uphoff International
CUI artificial breast prosthesis
CUI catheter
CUI chin prosthesis
CUI columellar implant
CUI dorsal implant
CUI eye sphere prosthesis
CUI gel-filled breast prosthesis
CUI joint
CUI malar implant
CUI myringotomy tube
CUI nasal prosthesis
CUI rhinoplasty implant
CUI saline mammary prosthesis
CUI shunt
CUI tendon prosthesis

CUI testicular prosthesis
CUI tissue expander
CUI urological drain

Cuidant system

cuirass
c. jacket
c. respirator
c. ventilator

Cukier nasal forceps

Culbertson canal knife

cul-de-sac
c.-d.-s. irrigating vectis
c.-d.-s. irrigation T-tube

culdoscope
Decker fiberoptic c.

Culler
C. eye forceps
C. fixation forceps
C. iris spatula
C. iris speculum
C. lens spoon
C. rectus muscle hook

Culley ulna splint

Cullom-Mueller adenotome

Cullom septal forceps

Culp biopsy needle

CultiSpher-G microcarrier

CultiSpher macroporous gel
  microcarrier

culturette
Mini-tip c.

Cummings
C. folding forceps
C. four-wing Malecot retention
  catheter
C. nephrostomy catheter

Cummings-Pezzer catheter

CunMeter accupuncture aid

Cunningham
C. brace
C. penile incontinence clamp
C. urinary incontinence clamp

Cunningham-Cotton
C.-C. sleeve
C.-C. sleeve coaxial dilator

cup
AccuPressure heel c.
acetabular c.
acetabular trial c.
Alivium prosthesis c.
APR acetabular c.
Arthopor acetabular c.

NOTES

cup *(continued)*
    Aufranc c.
    Bard alligator c.
    Bard oval c.
    Berkeley suction c.
    Bicon-Plus c.
    c. biopsy forceps
    Bird OP c.
    Breinin suction c.
    Buchholz acetabular c.
    c. catheter
    Centaur trial c.
    Chambers intrauterine c.
    Charnley acetabular c.
    Charnley offset-bore c.
    CMI/O'Neil c.
    Crawford-Adams acetabular c.
    c. curette
    Dual Geometry HA c.
    Duraloc acetabular c.
    ear c.
    Flo-Trol drinking c.
    c. forceps
    Galin silicone bleb c.
    Gap c.
    Harris-Galante c.
    heel c.
    HGP II acetabular c.
    Instead feminine protection c.
    Integrity acetabular c.
    Interseal acetabular c.
    iodine c.
    Judet impactor for acetabular c.
    Kennedy spillproof c.
    Laing concentric hip c.
    Lord c.
    magnetic c.
    Mahnstrom c.
    Malström c.
    McBride c.
    McGoey-Evans acetabular c.
    McKee-Farrar acetabular c.
    Mityvac cup vacuum extractor c.
    Mityvac obstetric vacuum
      extractor c.
    Mityvac Super M c.
    Mityvac vacuum extractor c.
    MMS low-profile acetabular c.
    Mueller-type acetabular c.
    multipolar bipolar c.
    Natural-Lok acetabular c.
    New England Baptist acetabular c.
    Newhart-Smith c.
    O'Connor finger c.
    ocular c.
    Ogee acetabular c.
    O'Harris-Petruso c.
    Omnifit acetabular c.
    ophthalmic c.

    Opti-Fix acetabular c.
    c. palm manual percussor
    PCA acetabular c.
    c. pessary
    Pierce nasal c.
    Polysorb heel c.
    c. positioner
    PQ premium heel c.
    prosthetic c.
    c. pusher shaft
    Reflection acetabular c.
    Restoration GAP acetabular c.
    Rickham c.
    Rotalok acetabular c.
    Silastic obstetrical vacuum c.
    Silipos silicone wonder c.
    slit-lamp c.
    Smith-Petersen c.
    Soft Touch c.
    Sorbuthane II heel c.
    S-ROM acetabular c.
    stainless steel c.
    suction c.
    Super M vacuum extractor c.
    Tender Touch Ultra vacuum c.
    Ti-Bac I, II acetabular c.
    Trilogy acetabular c.
    TuliGel heel c.
    Tuli heel c.
    University of California
      Biomechanics Laboratory heel c.
    Veenema-Gusberg prostatic
      biopsy c.
    Vitallium c.
    wet c.
    ZTT acetabular c.

cupped
    c. curette
    c. forceps

cup-shaped
    c.-s. electrode
    c.-s. forceps
    c.-s. inner ear forceps
    c.-s. middle ear forceps

Cuputi sputum collector

Curad
    C. bandage
    C. surgical adhesive dressing

Curaderm hydrocolloid dressing

Curafil
    C. hydrogel impregnated gauze
    C. hydrogel wound dressing

Curafoam Plus island dressing

Curagel
    C. hydrogel island dressing
    C. wafer

Curasol gel sterile wound dressing

Curasorb calcium alginate dressing

Curdy
   C. blade
   C. sclerotome
   C. sclerotome knife
Curdy-Hebra blade
curettage
   Guyon c.
   Gynaspir vacuum c.
curette, curet
   Abraham rectal c.
   Accurette endometrial suction c.
   Acu-Dispo-Curette disposable
     dermal c.
   adenoid c.
   Alvis foreign body eye c.
   Anderson c.
   Angell c.
   AngleLoop c.
   antral c.
   apicitis c.
   aspirating c.
   Austin oval c.
   Auto Suture c.
   Ballantine uterine c.
   Ballenger ethmoidal c.
   banjo c.
   Bardic c.
   Barnhill adenoid c.
   Barnhill-Jones c.
   bayonet c.
   Beaver c.
   Beckmann adenoid c.
   Bellucci c.
   Berlin c.
   Billeau ear wax c.
   Billroth c.
   biopsy suction c.
   Blake uterine c.
   blunt-ring c.
   bone c.
   bowl c.
   box c.
   Bozeman c.
   Bromley uterine c.
   Bronson-Ray pituitary c.
   Brun ear c.
   Brun mastoid bone c.
   Buck bone c.
   Buck ear c.
   Buck-House c.
   Buck mastoid c.
   Buck wax c.

   Bumm placental c.
   Bumm uterine c.
   Bunge c.
   Bush intervertebral c.
   Carlens c.
   Carmack ear c.
   Carroll hook c.
   Carter submucous elevator c.
   CeraSpoon c.
   cervical biopsy c.
   chalazion c.
   Charnley double-ended bone c.
   Clevedent-Lucas c.
   Cloward-Cone ring c.
   Cloward spinal c.
   Clyman endometrial c.
   Coakley c.
   Coakley antral c.
   Coakley ethmoid c.
   Coakley nasal c.
   Cobb bone c.
   Cobb spinal c.
   Collin uterine c.
   Concept c.
   Cone nasal c.
   cone ring c.
   Cone suction biopsy c.
   Converse sweeper c.
   Corgill-Shapleigh ear c.
   corneal c.
   cup c.
   cupped c.
   cylindrical uterine c.
   Daubenspeck bone c.
   Daviel chalazion c.
   Dawson-Yuhl c.
   DeLee c.
   Dench ear c.
   Dench uterine c.
   dental c.
   DePuy bone c.
   Derlacki ear c.
   dermal c.
   disc c.
   double-ended bone c.
   double-ended dental c.
   double-ended stapes c.
   double-lumen c.
   down-biting Epstein c.
   Duncan endometrial biopsy c.
   Dunning c.
   ear c.

NOTES

curette *(continued)*

embolectomy c.
endaural c.
endocervical biopsy c.
endodontic c.
endometrial c.
endometrial biopsy c.
endotracheal c.
Epstein down-biting c.
Epstein spinal fusion c.
ethmoid c.
Farrior angulated c.
Farrior ear c.
Faulkner antral c.
Faulkner double-end ring c.
Faulkner ethmoidal c.
Faulkner nasal c.
fenestration c.
Ferguson bone c.
fine-angled c.
Fink chalazion c.
FlexLoop c.
foreign body c.
Fowler double-end c.
Fox dermal c.
Franklin-Silverman c.
Freimuth ear c.
Frenckner-Stille c.
frontal sinus c.
Fukushima-Giannotta c.
Gam-Mer spinal fusion c.
Gifford corneal c.
Gillquist suction c.
Gill-Welsh c.
Goldman c.
Goldstein c.
Goodhill double-end c.
Gracey c.
Green corneal c.
Greene endocervical c.
Greene placental c.
Greene uterine c.
Gross ear c.
Guilford-Wright c.
Gusberg cervical cone biopsy c.
Gusberg endocervical biopsy c.
GynoSampler endometrial c.
Halle bone c.
Halle ethmoid c.
Halle sinus c.
Hannon endometrial c.
Hardy bayonet c.
Hardy hypophysial c.
Hardy modification of Bronson-
   Ray c.
Harrison-Shea c.
Hartmann adenoidal c.
Hatfield bone c.
Hayden tonsillar c.

Heaney endometrial biopsy c.
Heaney uterine c.
Heath chalazion c.
Hebra chalazion c.
Hebra corneal c.
Helix endocervical c.
Helix uterine biopsy c.
Heyner c.
Hibbs bone c.
Hibbs spinal c.
Hibbs-Spratt spinal fusion c.
Hofmeister endometrial biopsy c.
Holden uterine c.
Holtz endometrial c.
hook-type dermal c.
horizontal ring c.
Hough c.
House-Buck c.
House ear c.
House-Paparella stapes c.
House-Saunders middle ear c.
House-Sheehy knife c.
House stapes c.
House tympanoplasty c.
Houtz endometrial c.
Howard spinal c.
Hunter uterine c.
hypophysial c.
Ingersoll adenoid c.
Innomed bone c.
intervertebral c.
irrigating uterine c.
Jacobson c.
Jansen bone c.
Jarit reverse adenoid c.
Jones adenoid c.
Jordan-Rosen c.
Juers ear c.
Kelly c.
Kelly-Gray uterine c.
Kerpel bone c.
Kevorkian endocervical c.
Kevorkian endometrial c.
Kevorkian-Younge endocervical
   biopsy c.
Kevorkian-Younge uterine c.
Kezerian c.
Kirkland c.
Kos c.
Kraff capsule polisher c.
Kuhn-Bolger angled c.
Kushner-Tandatnick endometrial
   biopsy c.
labyrinth c.
Laufe aspirating c.
Laufe-Novak gynecologic c.
Laufe-Randall gynecologic c.
Lempert bone c.
Lempert endaural c.

Lempert fine c.
Lounsbury placental c.
Lucas alveolar c.
Luer bone c.
Luongo c.
Lynch c.
Magnum c.
Majewski nasal c.
Malis c.
Marino transsphenoidal c.
Maroon lip c.
Martin dermal c.
Martini bone c.
mastoid c.
Mayfield spinal c.
McCain TMJ c.
McCaskey antral c.
McElroy c.
Meigs endometrial c.
Meigs uterine c.
meniscal c.
Meyerding saw-toothed c.
Meyhöffer bone c.
Meyhöffer chalazion c.
Microsect c.
Middleton adenoid c.
Milan uterine c.
Miles antral c.
Miller c.
Misdome-Frank c.
Moe bone c.
Molt c.
Moorfields c.
Mosher ethmoid c.
Moult c.
Mueller c.
Munchen endometrial biopsy c.
Myles antral c.
nasal c.
Noland-Budd cervical c.
Nordent bone c.
Novak-Schoeckaert endometrial c.
Novak uterine biopsy c.
O'Connor double-edged c.
optical aspirating c.
Orban c.
oval window c.
ovum c.
Paparella angled-ring c.
Paparella-House c.
Paparella mastoid c.
Paparella stapes c.

periapical c.
Piffard dermal c.
Piffard placental c.
Pipelle-deCornier endometrial c.
Pipelle endometrial c.
pituitary c.
placental c.
Pratt antral c.
Pratt ethmoid c.
Pratt nasal c.
Randall endometrial biopsy c.
Randall uterine c.
Rand bayonet ring c.
Raney spinal fusion c.
Raney stirrup-loop c.
Ray pituitary c.
Read facial c.
Read oral c.
Récamier uterine c.
Reich c.
Reich-Nechtow cervical biopsy c.
Reiner c.
resectoscope c.
retrograde c.
reverse-angle skid c.
reverse-curve adenoid c.
Rheinstaedter flushing c.
Rheinstaedter uterine c.
Rhoton blunt-ring c.
Rhoton horizontal-ring c.
Rhoton loop c.
Rhoton pituitary c.
Rhoton spoon c.
Rhoton vertical ring c.
Rica ear c.
Rica lipoma c.
Rica mastoid c.
Rica uterine c.
Richards bone c.
Richards ethmoid c.
Richards mastoid c.
Ridpath ethmoid c.
Rock endometrial suction c.
Rosen knife c.
Rosenmüller c.
ruptured disc c.
salpingeal c.
saw-toothed c.
scarifying c.
Schaefer ethmoid c.
Schaefer mastoid c.
Schede bone c.

C

NOTES

curette *(continued)*
Schroeder uterine c.
Schuletz antral c.
Schuletz-Simmons ethmoidal c.
Schwartz endocervical c.
Scoville ruptured disc c.
Semmes c.
serrated c.
Shambaugh adenoidal c.
Shapleigh c.
Shapleigh ear wax c.
Sharman c.
sharp dermal c.
sharp loop c.
Shea c.
Sheehy-House c.
Simon bone c.
Simon cup uterine c.
Simon spinal c.
Simpson antral c.
Sims irrigating uterine c.
sinus c.
Skeele chalazion c.
Skeele corneal c.
Skeele eye c.
skid c.
SMIC ear c.
SMIC mastoid c.
SMIC pituitary c.
Smith-Petersen c.
soft rubber c.
spinal fusion c.
sponge ear c.
spoon c.
Sprague ear c.
Spratt ear c.
Spratt mastoid c.
stapes c.
St. Clair-Thompson adenoidal c.
stirrup-loop c.
Stiwer c.
Storz resectoscope c.
stout-neck c.
straight ring c.
Strully ruptured-disc c.
Stubbs adenoidal c.
submucous c.
suction biopsy c.
suction tip c.
Sweaper c.
Synthes facial c.
Tabb ear c.
Tamsco c.
Taylor c.
Temens c.
T-handle cup c.
Thomas uterine c.
Thompson adenoid c.
Thomson adenoid c.

Thorpe c.
tonsillar c.
Townsend endocervical biopsy c.
toxemia c.
Toynbee c.
transsphenoidal c.
Uffenorde bone c.
Ulbrich wart c.
Ultra-Cut Cobb c.
Unimar Pipelle c.
uterine c.
uterine biopsy c.
uterine irrigating c.
uterine suction c.
uterine vacuum aspirating c.
Vabra suction c.
Vacurette suction c.
vacuum c.
Vakutage c.
VersaLoop c.
vertical ring c.
Visitec capsule polisher c.
V. Mueller mastoid c.
Vogel infant adenoid c.
Volkmann bone c.
Voller c.
Walker ring c.
Walker ruptured-disc c.
Wallich bone c.
Walsh dermal c.
Walsh hook-type dermal c.
Walton c.
wax c.
Weaver chalazion c.
Weisman ear c.
West-Beck spoon c.
Whiting mastoid c.
Whitney single-use plastic c.
Williger bone c.
Williger ear c.
Wolf dermal c.
Wright-Guilford c.
Wullstein ring c.
Yankauer ear c.
Yankauer salpingeal c.
Yasargil c.
Younge endocervical c.
Younge endometrial c.
Zielke c.
Z-Sampler endometrial suction c.
Curity
C. ABD pad
C. cover sponge
C. disposable laparotomy sponge
C. dressing
C. gauze sponge
C. ureteral drainage bag
C. urine leg bag
curl-back shell eye implant

Curl Cath peritoneal catheter
Curlin 2000 Plus pump
Curon dressing
Curran knife needle
current
    high-voltage pulsed c. (HVPC)
Curry
    C. cerebral needle
    C. hip nail
    C. intravascular retriever
    C. walking splint
currycomb instrument
Curschmann trocar
Curtis tissue forceps
curved
    c. array transducer
    c. dissecting forceps
    c. intraluminal stapler
    c. iris forceps
    c. iris scissors
    c. Kelly hemostat
    c. knot-tying forceps
    c. laryngeal mirror
    c. Mayo clamp
    c. mosquito clamp
    c. mosquito hemostat
    c. nasal prongs
    c. needle spud
    c. operating scissors
    c. peripheral vascular clamp
    c. retinal probe
    c. spring-handled microscissors
    c. tenotomy scissors
curved-on-flat scissors
curved-tip bipolar forceps
curvilinear chin implant
CurvTek
    C. bone tunneling system
    C. TSR bone drill
CUSA
    Cavitron Ultrasonic Surgical Aspirator
    CUSA CEM system
    CUSA electrosurgical module
    (CEM)
    CUSA Excel ultrasonic surgical
    aspirator
    CUSA laparoscopic tip
    CUSA system 200 straight
    autoclavable handpiece
CUSALap
    C. device
    C. ultrasonic accessory needle

Cusco vaginal speculum
Cushing
    C. aluminum retractor
    C. artery forceps
    C. bayonet forceps
    C. bipolar forceps
    C. bivalve retractor
    C. bone rongeur
    C. brain depressor
    C. brain forceps
    C. brain retractor
    C. brain spatula
    C. clamp
    C. clip
    C. cranial bur
    C. cranial drill
    C. cranial perforator
    C. cranial rongeur forceps
    C. decompression forceps
    C. decompression retractor
    C. Diamond-Points thumb forceps
    C. disc rongeur
    C. dissecting forceps
    C. dressing forceps
    C. dural hook
    C. dural hook knife
    C. flat drill
    C. forceps
    C. gasserian ganglion hook
    C. Gigli-saw guide
    C. laminectomy rongeur
    C. little joker periosteal elevator
    C. loop retractor
    C. monopolar forceps
    C. nerve hook
    C. nerve retractor
    C. nerve root retractor
    C. perforator drill
    C. periosteal elevator
    C. pituitary elevator
    C. pituitary rongeur
    C. pituitary spoon
    C. raspatory
    C. self-retaining retractor
    C. spatula spoon
    C. S-shaped brain spatula
    C. S-shaped retractor
    C. staphylorrhaphy elevator
    C. straight retractor
    C. subtemporal retractor
    C. thumb forceps
    C. tissue forceps

C

NOTES

Cushing *(continued)*
  C. vein retractor
  C. ventricular needle
Cushing-Brown tissue forceps
Cushing-Gutsch
  C.-G. dressing forceps
  C.-G. tissue forceps
Cushing-Hopkins periosteal elevator
Cushing-Kocher retractor
Cushing-Landolt transsphenoidal speculum
Cushing-McKenzie clip
Cushing-Taylor carbide-jaw forceps
Cushing-Vital tissue forceps
cushion
  AirKair seat c.
  Air-1517 vacuum-formed static air wheelchair c.
  Akros DFD wheelchair wedge c.
  Back Bull lumbar support c.
  Back-Huggar lumbar support c.
  Backjoy spine repositioning c.
  Bauerfeind ViscoSpot heel c.
  birth c.
  breakaway lap c.
  Butterfly c.
  Carter immobilization c.
  Checkerboard wheelchair c.
  coccyx c.
  coccyx seat c.
  Comfort Plus c.
  Comfort Take-Along wheelchair c.
  contour back c.
  Convo-Gel c.
  convoluted wheelchair c.
  Core Max-Relax face c.
  Core Slimrest c.
  Corner c.
  Crown high-profile c.
  Crown quadtro c.
  CSC3 cervical support c.
  Disc-O-Sit Jr. c.
  dry flotation wheelchair c.
  Easy Up c.
  Elasto-Gel c.
  enhancer c.
  EZ-Dish pressure relief c.
  Ezo denture c.
  Flexseat c.
  Flofit c.
  foam c.
  foam wedge wheelchair c.
  Foot Waffle c.
  gel c.
  Gel-Foam Ultra-Wedge c.
  Geo-Matt gel contour c.
  Geo-Matt PRT c.
  Geo-Matt wheelchair c.
  Healthier gel seating c.

  heel c.
  HeelCare c.
  Hudson Hydro-Float c.
  hydrofloat c.
  Invacare Comfort-Mate extra c.
  invalid c.
  Isch-Dish c.
  Isch-Dish Plus c.
  Jay Rave c.
  Jay Triad c.
  Jay Xtreme c.
  LapTop c.
  latex wheelchair c.
  MagneZorb magnetic heel c.
  MaxiFloat wheelchair c.
  Medline gel/foam wheelchair c.
  Medline Lap-pal safety c.
  Memory II c.
  Movin' Step Gait c.
  Novex wedged wheelchair c.
  Passavant c.
  Pedi-Cushions c.
  Pediplast c.
  Peri-Comfort seating c.
  pommel c.
  Position Plus c.
  Posture Curve lumbar c.
  Posture Wedge seat c.
  Premier pincore latex c.
  pressure-relief c.
  Prop'r Toes hammer toe c.
  Pro Relief gel/foam wheelchair c.
  Quadtro c.
  Response c.
  ring c.
  Roho enhancer c.
  Roho high-profile c.
  Roho Pack-It c.
  Roho quadtro c.
  sacral Dish pressure relief back c.
  Samadhi c.
  Sat-A-Lite contoured wedge seat c.
  scintimammography prone breast c.
  ShockMaster heel c.
  Side Rester c.
  Sit Straight coccyx relief wheelchair c.
  SkareKare silicon gel-filled c.
  Skil-Care Alarm c.
  Snug denture c.
  Sof-Care chair c.
  Sof-Care Plus c.
  Span-American wheelchair c.
  Stop-Leak gel flotation c.
  Sullivan bubble c.
  suture c.
  Temper Foam c.
  Tempur-Med wheelchair c.
  T-Foam c.

T-Gel c.
trilaminate c.
UltraFoam seating c.
Vac-Lok immobilization c.
ViscoSpot heel c.
Waffle seating c.
wheelchair c.
Wool'n Gel seating c.
Xact c.
Y B Sore c.
Cushman drain
Cusick goniotomy knife
Cusp-Lok
    C.-L. bracket
    C.-L. cuspid traction system
Custodis implant
custom-contoured implant
CustomCornea wavefront measurement
system
Custom Ultrasonic automatic endoscope
reprocessor
cut
    c. biopsy needle
    c. taper needle
cutaneous punch
Cut-Blot coagulator
cutdown catheter
cuticle
    c. nipper
    c. scissors
Cutifilm Plus waterproof wound
dressing
Cutinova
    C. alginate dressing
    C. cavity foam dressing
    C. cavity wound filler
    C. hydroactive dressing
Cutiplast sterile wound dressing
Cutler
    C. eye implant
    C. forceps
    C. forceps thoracoscope
    C. lens spoon
cutout
    c. patellar brace
    c. table
cutter
    adenoid c.
    AMO vitreous aspiration c.
    Anspach diamond dissecting c.
    arch bar c.
    Bantam wire c.

Beaver ring c.
Bi-Pol endoscopic c.
bone c.
Breck pin c.
Buettner-Parel vitreous c.
cannulated pin c.
Chu foldable lens c.
Codman wire c.
diamond pin c.
diamond wire c.
double-action plate c.
Douvas vitreous c.
dowel c.
Dual Geometry c.
Endopath ELC35 endoscopic
  linear c.
Endopath endoscopic linear c.
Endopath ETS-Flex endoscopic
  articulating linear c.
Endopath EZ-series endoscopic
  linear c.
endoscopic linear c.
Ethicon endoscopic linear c.
fascial c.
finger ring c.
Gator meniscal c.
Guilford-Wright wire c.
guillotine-type c.
Heath wire c.
Hefty Bite pin c.
Horsley bone c.
Horsley spine c.
Hough Teflon c.
C. implant
infusion suction vitreous c.
Jarit pin c.
Kirschner wire c.
Kleinert-Kutz bone c.
Kloti vitreous c.
Koo foldable intraocular lens c.
Leibinger Micro System plate c.
Lempert malleus c.
lens glide c.
Lindemann bone c.
Luhr microfixation system plate c.
Machemer vitreous c.
Maguire-Harvey vitreous c.
malleus c.
Martin diamond wire c.
membrane peeler c. (MPC)
meniscal c.
Microvit vitrectomy c.

NOTES

cutter *(continued)*
Millenium Lightning vitrectomy c.
M-Pact cast c.
Nu-Hope hole c.
O'Malley-Heintz vitreous c.
Parel-Crock vitreous c.
Pendula cast c.
Polaris reusable c.
Porter-O-Surgical c.
Premiere vitreous c.
Pro-Vit c.
Proximate linear c.
Reflex articulating endoscopic c.
rib c.
Rochester harvest bone c.
Rochester recipient bone c.
Rogers wire c.
Schuknecht c.
Sheets lens c.
Sklar pin c.
Spartan jaw wire c.
Stille cast c.
Stryker cast c.
Szulc bone c.
TC pin c.
Tolentino vitreoretinal c.
Utrata foldable lens c.
Vanadium arch bar c.
Verner-Joel c.
Vernon wire c.
Vit Commander vitreous c.
vitreoretinal infusion c.
vitreous infusion suction c.
wire c.
Wright-Guilford wire c.
Cutter-Smeloff
C.-S. aortic valve prosthesis
C.-S. cardiac valve prosthesis
C.-S. mitral valve
cutting
c. balloon
c. balloon catheter
c. board
c. bur
c. cautery
c. forceps
c. jig
c. loop
c. loop electrode
c. needle
4-in-1 cutting block
CVA sling
C-Vest radiation detection system
CVIS
Cardiovascular Imaging Systems
CVIS imaging catheter instrument
CVIS information system
CVIS intravascular US imaging
catheter

CVIS/InterTherapy intravascular ultrasound system
CVP
central venous pressure
CVP catheter
CVS
chorionic villus sampling
CVS catheter
CVX-300 excimer laser
C-wire Serter
cyanoacrylate
c. fixed orbital silicone sleds
implant material
c. glue
c. tissue adhesive
CyberKnife
C. SRS hypofractionated stereotactic
radiosurgery
C. stereotactic radiosurgery system
Cyberlith
C. demand pacemaker
C. multiprogrammable pulse
generator
Cyberscanner 3-D digitizer
Cybertach antiarrhythmic pacemaker
Cyberware Cyberscanner 3-D digitizer
Cybex
C. cycle ergometer
C. finger-clip pulse meter
C. isokinetic dynamometer
C. isokinetic exerciser
C. Norm testing and rehabilitation
system
C. trunk extension/flexion unit
cycle
Colorado C.
Ergociser exercise c.
Exer-Pedic c.
Power Trainer c.
recumbent c.
Saratoga c.
Upper Body C. (UBC)
cyclodialysis
c. cannula
c. spatula
cyclodiathermy
Castroviejo-Scheie c.
c. electrode
c. needle
cycloergometer
computerized c.
isokinetic c.
Mijnhard electrical c.
upright foot pedal c.
cyclohexane scintillator
cyclophorometer
Cyclotech medication dosing device
cyclotron
Eclipse ST c.

medical c.
multiparticle c.
Cygnet Laboratories fetal monitoring system
Cygnus PFS image-guided system
cylinder
    abdominal compression c.
    AMS CX penile prosthesis c.
    Arthrotek calibrated c.
    Bodenham dermabrasion c.
    Burnett c.
    CO_2 c.
    Delclos c.
    drill stop c.
    Feldenkrais c.
    Fletcher-Delclos dome c.
    Mitroflow PeriPatch c.
    c. penile distensible prosthesis
    c. penile nondistensible prosthesis
    suction c.
    TPS-coated c.
    Ultrex c.
    vaginal c.
cylinder-type implant
cylindrical
    c. balloon
    c. bougie
    c. bur
    c. diffuser
    c. diffusing balloon catheter
    c. lens
    c. sponge
    c. uterine curette
cymba conchal cartilage graft
Cymetra
    C. tissue
    C. tissue replacement graft
Cynosar catheter
Cynosure laser
Cypher sirolimus-eluting coronary stent
cystic
    c. duct forceps
    c. duct scoop
    c. hook
cystitome (*var. of* cystotome)
Cystocath catheter
cystofiberscope
    Olympus CYF-series OES c.
cystogastrotome
cystometer
    Lewis recording c.
    Uroflo c.

cystonephroscope
    ACMI ACN-2 flexible c.
cystopanendoscope
cystoresectoscope
    anterior-posterior c.
    Damon-Julian c.
    Julian c.
cystoscope
    Albarran laser c.
    Braasch direct catheterization c.
    Braasch-Kaplan direct vision c.
    Brown-Buerger c.
    Broyles retrograde c.
    Butterfield c.
    French c.
    Hamou c.
    InjecTx c.
    Judd c.
    Kelly c.
    Kidd c.
    Laidley double-catheterizing c.
    Lowsley-Peterson c.
    McCarthy-Campbell miniature c.
    McCarthy foroblique panendoscope c.
    McCrea c.
    Miller c.
    Morganstern continuous-flow operating c.
    National general purpose c.
    Nesbit c.
    Olympus neonatal c.
    Storz c.
    Surgitek graduated c.
    Young c.
cystoscopic
    c. forceps
    c. fulgurating electrode
cystotome, cystitome
    air c.
    Alcon c.
    Atkinson G-series short curved c.
    Azar c.
    Beard c.
    Beaver Ocu-1 curved c.
    Blumenthal irrigating c.
    Capsitome c.
    Drews c.
    formed c.
    Graefe flexible c.
    guarded irrigating c.
    Holth c.

C

NOTES

cystotome *(continued)*
 irrigating c.
 Kelman c.
 Kelman air c.
 Kelman double-bladed c.
 Kelman knife c.
 Knapp c.
 knife c.
 knife cannula c.
 Knolle-Kelman cannulated c.
 Knolle-Kelman sharp c.
 Kratz c.
 Lewicky formed c.
 Lieppman sharp c.
 Look c.
 McIntyre guarded c.
 McIntyre reverse c.
 Mendez c.
 Mendez ultrasonic c.
 Moorfields c.
 Neuhann c.
 Nevyas double sharp c.
 reverse c.
 Sharp point-tip c.
 side-cutting irrigating c.
 Visitec double-cutting c.
 von Graefe c.
 Wheeler c.
 Wilder c.
 Worth c.
 Zawadzki c.
cystourethropexy
 In-Fast c.
cystourethroscope
 ACMI c.
 Microlens c.
 O'Donoghue c.
 Wappler microlens c.
cyst puncture device
Cytobrush
 C. Plus brush
 C. Plus endocervical cell collector
 C. Plus endocervical cell sampler
 C. spatula
 Zelsmyr C.

cytocentrifuge
 Cytopro c.
 Cyto-Tek c.
CytoFlex membrane
CytoFluor II fluorometer
CytoGuard aerosol containment device
cytokeratin filament
cytological brush
cytology brush
Cytomax brush cytology system
cytometer
 Bayer/Technicon H1 automated
  flow c.
 CAS-200 image c.
 CD-Chex CD4 LOW flow c.
 Coulter Epics C-flow flow c.
 Coulter Epics Elite flow c.
 Coulter HmX hematology flow c.
 Dickinson FACS 400-series flow c.
 Epics C-flow flow c.
 Epics Elite flow c.
 Epics Profile II flow c.
 FACScan flow c.
 flow c.
 HmX hematology flow c.
 Ortho Cytofluorograf 50-H flow c.
Cytopick cervical cell collector
Cytopro cytocentrifuge
CytoRich
 C. cervical cytology monolayer
  preparation system
 C. cervical cytology slide
Cyto-Tek cytocentrifuge
Czaja-McCaffrey rigid stent introducer
Czapski microscope
Czermak keratome
Czerny
 C. rectal speculum
 C. retractor
 C. suture
 C. tenaculum forceps
Czerny-Lembert suture

3D
   3D Accuscan facial implant
   3D Accuscan facial prosthesis
   3D surface digitizer scanner
da
   d. Vinci robot
   d. Vinci surgical system
Dacomed snap gauge
Dacron
   D. arterial prosthesis
   D. bifurcation prosthesis
   D. bolstered suture
   D. catheter
   D. cuff
   D. fiber-coated coil
   D. graft
   D. graft clamp
   D. implant
   knitted D.
   D. knitted graft
   D. mesh
   D. mesh sling
   D. mesh synthetic ligament
   D. onlay patch graft
   D. patch
   D. pledget
   D. preclotted knitted graft
   D. prosthesis
   D. Sauvage graft
   D. shield
   D. tape
   D. tightly-woven graft
   D. traction suture
   D. tube graft
   D. tubular graft
   D. velour graft
   D. Weave Knit graft
Dacron-backed implant
dacryocystorhinostomy
   d. cannula
   d. needle
   d. retractor
dacryolith
   Desmarres d.
D.A.D. mattress
Daems bronchial clamp
Dafilon suture
Dagger dilator
Dagrofil suture
Dahlberg hearing aid
Dahlgren
   D. iris scissors
   D. rongeur
   D. skill-cutting forceps
Dahlgren-Hudson cranial forceps

Daicoff
   D. needle-pulling forceps
   D. vascular forceps
Daig screw-in lead pacemaker
Daily
   D. cataract needle
   D. cooling jacket
   D. fixation hook
   D. keratome
Daimas Blue
Dainer-Kaupp needle holder
Daisy I&A instrument
Daiwa dental needle
Dakin
   D. Biograft
   D. catheter
   D. dressing
   D. tube
Dale
   D. abdominal binder
   D. drainage bulb and G-tube
      holder
   D. femoral-popliteal clamp
   D. first rib rongeur
   D. Foley catheter legband holder
   D. gastrostomy tube holder
   D. nasal dressing holder
   D. oxygen cannula support
   D. surgical binder
   D. tapeless wound dressing holder
   D. thoracic rongeur
   D. tracheostomy tube holder
   D. ventilator tubing support
Dalkon
   D. shield
   D. shield intrauterine device
Dalla Bona ball and socket abutment
Dallas
   D. lens-inserting forceps
   D. retractor
D'Allesandro
   D. clamp
   D. serial suture-holding forceps
Dall-Miles
   D.-M. cable
   D.-M. cable system
   D.-M. cerclage wire
   D.-M. plate
Dallop-type fascial prosthesis
dam
   d. drain
   nonlatex dental d.
Damato
   D. campimeter
   D. curved catheter

D

Damian
>D. inverter
>D. lumen finder

Damon clasp

Damon-Julian
>D.-J. cystoresectoscope
>D.-J. ring remover

Damshek
>D. needle
>D. sternal trephine

Dana shoulder prosthesis

Danberg iris forceps

dancer pad

Dan chalazion forceps

Dandy
>D. arterial forceps
>D. artery forceps
>D. clamp
>D. clip
>D. nerve hook
>D. probe
>D. scalp forceps
>D. scalp hemostat
>D. suction tube
>D. trigeminal scissors
>D. ventricular needle

Dandy-Cairns
>D.-C. brain needle
>D.-C. ventricular needle

Dandy-Kolodny hemostatic forceps

Danek
>D. cervical fusion plate
>D. rod
>D. self-retaining retractor

Dan-Gradle ciliary forceps

Daniel
>D. colostomy clamp
>D. double-punch laser laparoscope
>D. EndoForehead instrument

Daniels
>D. adenotome
>D. hemostatic tonsillectome

Danis retractor

Dankner Panariello cortex cannula

Dannheim eye implant

Danniflex
>D. CPM exerciser
>D. CPM machine
>D. CPM system

Dann-Jennings mouthgag

Dann respirator

Dansac
>D. Colo F mini cap
>D. colostomy irrigation set
>D. Combi Colo F pouch
>D. Combi micro cap
>D. Contour I mini cap
>D. Contour 1 pouch
>D. irrigation system

Dantec
>D. 12-channel Urocolor video system
>D. Etude system
>D. Menuet urodynamic analyzer
>D. rotating disc flowmeter
>D. Urodyn 1000 flowmeter
>D. Urodyn uroflowmeter

DAR breathing system

Darby surgical shoe

d'Arcet metal alloy

Darco
>D. Body Armor walker
>D. MedSurg shoe
>D. moldable insole
>D. OrthoWedge healing shoe
>D. toe alignment splint

DarcoGel ankle brace

Dardik
>D. Biograft
>D. clamp
>D. umbilical vein graft

Darin lens

Darkos boot

Darling
>D. capsulotome
>D. popliteal retractor

Darox cutaneous patch electrode

Darrach retractor

d'Arsonval galvanometer

dart
>Arthrex meniscal d.
>Clearfix meniscal d.
>D. coronary stent
>D. pacemaker

Dartigues
>D. kidney-elevating forceps
>D. uterine-elevating forceps

Das Angel Wings atrial septal defect closure device

Dasco Pro angle finder

Dasher guidewire

Dash single-chamber rate-adaptic pacemaker

DAS single-pass dialyzer

DataHand system

Datascope
>D. Accusat pulse oximeter
>D. Accutor bedside monitor
>D. balloon
>D. DL-II percutaneous translucent balloon catheter
>D. intraaortic balloon pump catheter
>D. System 90 intraaortic balloon pump

Datel endoscopy travel cart

Datex
  D. relaxograph
  D. Ultima spirometer
Datex-Ohmeda
  D.-O. infrared sensor
  D.-O. 3800 pulse oximeter
  D.-O. S/5 oxygen saturation
    module
Daubenspeck bone curette
Dautrey
  D. chisel
  D. retractor
Dautrey-Munro osteotome
David-Baker
  D.-B. lid clamp
  D.-B. lid retractor
Davidoff
  D. ambidextrous nucleus chopper
  D. blade
  D. cordotomy knife
  D. trigeminal retractor
David pharyngolaryngectomy tube
Davidson
  D. bur
  D. collector
  D. erector spinae retractor
  D. muscle clamp
  D. periosteal elevator
  D. pneumothorax apparatus
  D. pulmonary vessel clamp
  D. pulmonary vessel forceps
  D. scapular retractor
  D. syringe
  D. trocar
Davidson-Alexander rib raspatory
Daviel
  D. cataract spoon
  D. chalazion curette
  D. chalazion knife
  D. lens loupe
  D. lens scoop
  D. lens spoon
Davis
  D. aortic aneurysm clamp
  D. bayonet forceps
  D. blade
  D. bone skid
  D. brain retractor
  D. brain spatula
  D. bronchoscope
  D. capsular forceps
  D. catheter

  D. coagulating forceps
  D. coagulation electrode
  D. conductor
  D. diathermy forceps
  D. dissector
  D. double-ended retractor
  D. foreign body spud
  D. graft
  D. guide
  D. hemostat
  D. hook
  D. interlocking sound
  D. knife needle
  D. lamp
  D. loop stone dislodger
  D. loop stone extractor
  D. metacarpal splint
  D. modified Finochietto rib
    spreader
  D. monopolar bayonet forceps
  D. nerve separator
  D. pin
  D. rhytidectomy scissors
  D. rib spreader
  D. root tip pick
  D. saw guide
  D. scalp retractor
  D. sterilizer forceps
  D. tissue forceps
  D. tonsillar needle
  D. trephine
Davis-Crowe
  D.-C. mouthgag
  D.-C. tongue blade
Davis-Geck suture
Davol
  D. bag
  D. canal wall punch
  D. dermatome
  D. irrigation system
  D. pacemaker introducer
  D. rongeur forceps
  D. sterile intermittent red rubber
    catheter
  D. suction drain
  D. sump drain
  D. tube
  D. tunneler
Davol-Simon dermatome
Daw
  D. cinch

D

NOTES

Daw (*continued*)
    D. Industries orthopaedic corset
    D. Strap-Pad
DawSkin flexible protective skin system
Dawson-Mueller drainage catheter
Dawson-Yuhl
    D.-Y. curette
    D.-Y. gouge
    D.-Y. impactor
    D.-Y. osteotome
    D.-Y. periosteal elevator
    D.-Y. rongeur forceps
    D.-Y. suction tube
Dawson-Yuhl-Kerrison
    D.-Y.-K. rongeur
    D.-Y.-K. rongeur forceps
Dawson-Yuhl-Leksell
    D.-Y.-L. rongeur
    D.-Y.-L. rongeur forceps
Day
    D. attic cannula
    D. ear hook
    D. stapler
    D. tonsillar knife
Daya double-ended lamellar dissector
DayTimer carpal tunnel support
Daytona cervical orthosis
DBM
    demineralized bone matrix
DCI-S automated coronary analysis system
DCS
    dynamic condylar screw
    DCS condylar screw system
    DCS dynamic hip system
DC Squid sensor
DDD pacemaker
DDI mode pacemaker
de
    d. la Caffiniére trapeziometacarpal prosthesis
    d. la Cruz stapes implant
    d. la Plaza transconjunctival retractor
    d. la Vega lens pusher
    d. la Vega vitreous-aspirating cannula
    d. Pezzer mushroom-tipped catheter
    d. Pezzer self-retaining catheter
    d. Signeux dilator
Dean
    D. antral needle
    D. antral trocar
    D. applicator
    D. blade
    D. bone rongeur
    D. dissecting scissors
    D. iris knife
    D. iris needle

    D. iris scissors
    D. knife holder
    D. knife needle
    D. MacDonald gastric resection clamp
    D. periosteal elevator
    D. periosteotome
    D. rasp
    D. tonsillar forceps
    D. tonsillar hemostat
    D. tonsillar knife
    D. tonsillar scissors
    D. wash tube
Deane
    D. tube
    D. unconstrained knee prosthesis
Deaver
    D. blade
    D. clamp
    D. hemostat
    D. operating scissors
    D. retractor
    D. T-tube
    D. tube
DeBakey
    D. aortic aneurysm clamp
    D. aortic clamp
    D. aortic exclusion clamp
    D. aortic forceps
    D. Autraugrip forceps
    D. ball-valve prosthesis
    D. blade
    D. bulldog clamp
    D. chest retractor
    D. coarctation clamp
    D. curved peripheral vascular clamp
    D. Dacron graft
    D. dissecting forceps
    D. endarterectomy scissors
    D. heart pump oxygenator
    D. implant
    D. infant rib spreader
    D. intraluminal stripper
    D. ligature carrier
    D. needle holder
    D. patent ductus clamp
    D. pediatric clamp
    D. peripheral vascular clamp
    D. prosthetic heart valve
    D. ring-handled bulldog clamp
    D. S-shaped brain spatula
    D. S-shaped peripheral vascular clamp
    D. stitch scissors
    D. suction tube
    D. tangential occlusion clamp
    D. tangential occlusion forceps
    D. thoracic tissue forceps

D. tissue forceps
D. tunneler
D. VAD
D. VAD continuous-axial-flow pump
D. valve hook
D. valve prosthesis
D. valve scissors
D. vascular clamp
D. vascular dilator
D. vascular scissors
D. vascular tissue forceps
D. vascular tunneler
D. ventricular assist device
D. Vital needle holder
DeBakey-Adson suction tube
DeBakey-Bahnson vascular clamp
DeBakey-Bainbridge
D.-B. intenstinal forceps
D.-B. peripheral clamp
D.-B. vascular forceps
DeBakey-Beaver blade
DeBakey-Beck
D.-B. clamp
D.-B. multipurpose forceps
DeBakey-Cooley
D.-C. cardiovascular forceps
D.-C. Deaver-type retractor
D.-C. dissecting forceps
D.-C. valve dilator
DeBakey-Derra
D.-D. anastomosis clamp
D.-D. anastomosis forceps
DeBakey-Diethrich
D.-D. coronary artery forceps
D.-D. vascular forceps
DeBakey-Harken auricular clamp
DeBakey-Metzenbaum scissors
DeBakey-Mixter thoracic forceps
DeBakey-NASA
D.-NASA axial flow ventricular assist device
D.-NASA miniature heart assist device
DeBakey-Péan cardiovascular forceps
DeBakey-Potts scissors
DeBakey-Satinsky vena cava clamp
DeBakey-Semb
D.-S. clamp
D.-S. forceps
D.-S. ligature carrier
DeBakey-Surgitool prosthetic valve

DeBastiani
D. distractor
D. external fixator
DebioClip single-dose delivery system
Deblasio LASIK marker
debonding pliers
debridement needle
debrider
corneal d.
Sauer corneal d.
Debrisan dressing
decalcified freeze-dried bone allograft
decapolar
d. electrode catheter
d. pacing catheter
decelerator
graduated electronic d.
decentered spectacles
Decker
D. fiberoptic culdoscope
D. microsurgical forceps
D. microsurgical rongeur
D. microsurgical scissors
D. photoculdoscope
D. retractor
deck plate
decoder
TeleCaption d.
decompression
d. catheter
d. retractor
decompressive enteroclysis catheter
decompressor
Savage d.
Sims vaginal d.
decortication bur
DeCourcy goiter clamp
DeCube
D. therapeutic mattress
D. therapeutic surface
Decubi-Care pad dressing
decubitus
d. bed pad
d. boot shoe
dedicated
d. head scanner
d. local coil
d. PET scanner
d. push enteroscope
Dedo
D. laryngoscope
D. laser retractor

D

NOTES

235

Dedo-Jako
    D.-J. laryngoscope
    D.-J. microlaryngoscope
Dedo-Pilling laryngoscope
Dee
    D. elbow hinge
    D. elbow prosthesis
deep
    d. abdominal retractor
    d. blunt rake retractor
    d. brain extension
    d. Deaver retractor
    d. dermal suture
    d. ligature carrier
    d. spreader blade
    d. surgery forceps
    d. vein thrombosis (DVT)
    d. vessel forceps
Dees
    D. holder
    D. renal needle
    D. suture needle
defibrillation paddle
defibrillator
    AED automatic external d.
    Alert Companion II d.
    atrioverter implantable d.
    automatic external d. (AED)
    automatic implantable d.
    Birtcher d.
    Cadence d.
    Cadet d.
    Cambridge d.
    CardioServ d.
    Codemaster d.
    Contour Profile d.
    CPI automatic implantable d.
    Endotak d.
    FirstSave automated external d.
    ForeRunner semiautomatic
      external d.
    Guidant d.
    Heartstream ForeRunner d.
    Heartstream XL, XLT d.
    Hewlett-Packard d.
    Hewlett-Packard Codemaster d.
    d. implant
    implantable atrial d.
    implantable cardioverter d.
    Ipco-Partridge d.
    Jewel AF implantable d.
    Lifepak d.
    LifeVest wearable d.
    Marquette Responder 1500
      multifunctional d.
    Medtronic Gem automatic
      implantable d.
    Medtronic Jewel Plus Active
      Can d.

    d. paddle
    d. patch
    Porta Pulse 3 portable d.
    Prizm d.
    transvenous implantable d.
    Ventak Mini II, III d.
    Zoll PD1200 external d.
**Definition PM femoral implant
  component**
deflectable quadripolar catheter
deflector
    Albarran d.
    Cook d.
Deflux system implant
Defourmental
    D. bone rongeur
    D. forceps
    D. nasal rongeur
degradable polyglycolide rod
0-degree laparoscope
4-degree-of freedom manipulator
6-degrees-of-freedom electrogoniometer
45-degree spinal wedge
Degucast alloy
Degudent alloy
dehumidifier
    Grand Sahara d.
    Sonoran d.
Dejerine percussion hammer
Deklene II polypropylene suture
Deknatel
    D. autotransfusion system
    D. K-needle needle
    D. silk suture
    D. wound closure tape
**Dekompressor percutaneous diskectomy
  probe**
Del
    D. Mar Avionics 3-channel
      recorder
    D. Mar Avionics scanner
Delcath double-balloon catheter
Delclos
    D. cylinder
    D. dilator
    D. ovoid
Deldent
    D. Delsonic 2000 scaler
    D. Jetsonic 2000 polisher
    D. Miniblaster
DeLee
    D. cervix-holding forceps
    D. corner retractor
    D. curette
    D. dressing forceps
    D. infant catheter
    D. laparotrachelotomy knife
    D. meconium aspirator
    D. obstetrical forceps

D. ovum forceps
D. pelvimeter
D. shuttle forceps
D. speculum
D. spoon tissue forceps
D. stethoscope
D. suction catheter
D. trap
D. Universal retractor
D. uterine forceps
D. uterine-packing forceps
D. vaginal retractor
D. vesical retractor
DeLee-Hillis fetal stethoscope
DeLee-Simpson forceps
Delgado electrode
delicate
  d. grasping forceps
  d. intervertebral disc rongeur
  d. thumb-dressing forceps
Delitala T-nail nail
delivery
  d. assistance sleeve
  d. balloon
  continuous ambulatory drug d. (CADD)
  d. guidewire
  d. wire
Dell
  D. astigmatism marker
  D. ophthalmic fixation ring
Della Badia laparoscopic suturing device
DeLorme boot
Delphia II massage and microdermabrasion system
Delrin
  D. applicator
  D. biomaterial joint replacement prosthesis
  D. cutting block
  D. disc heart valve
  D. joint
  D. joint replacement biomaterial
  D. locking-handle forceps
  D. plastic scalp clip
  D. push rod
Delrin-handle bone saw
Delta
  D. dermatoscope
  D. 32 digital stereotactic system
  D. external fixation frame

D. Recon nail
D. reconstruction nail
D. reconstruction proximal drill guide
D. rod
D. 32 TACT 3-dimensional breast imaging system
D. TRS pacemaker
D. valve
D. walker
Deltafit keel
Delta-Lite
  D.-L. casting tape
  D.-L. FlashCast
Deltaloc anterior cervical plate system
DELTAmanager MedImage system
Delta-Rol cast padding
DeltaTrac II metabolic monitor
Deltec-Pharmacia CADD pump
Deltec portable external infusion device
Deltoid-Aid arm counterbalance system
Deltran disposable transducer
deluxe
  d. FIN extractor
  d. FIN pin
  d. FIN pin inserter
  d. head halter
  d. leg bag strap
demand
  d. cardiac pacemaker
  d. flow machine
demarcator
  flap d.
DeMartel
  D. anastomosis clamp
  D. appendix forceps
  D. conductor
  D. conductor saw
  D. craniotome
  D. neurosurgical scissors
  D. scalp flap forceps
  D. self-retaining brain retractor
  D. trephine
  D. T-wire saw
  D. vascular clamp
  D. vascular scissors
DeMartel-Wolfson
  D.-W. closing forceps
  D.-W. colon clamp
  D.-W. holder
  D.-W. intestinal clamp
  D.-W. intestinal-holding forceps

D

NOTES

237

Dembone
- D. demineralized cortical dental block
- D. demineralized cortical powder Pastegraft
- D. demineralized cortical powder Pulvograft
- D. demineralized freeze-dried cortical bone

Demel
- D. twisting forceps
- D. wire clamp
- D. wire guide
- D. wire-tightening forceps

demigauntlet
- d. bandage
- d. dressing

demineralized
- d. bone
- d. bone matrix (DBM)
- d. flexible laminar bone strip

demodulator
demonstration eyepiece
Denar articulator
denatured homograft
Dench
- D. ear curette
- D. ear forceps
- D. ear knife
- D. insufflator
- D. nebulizer
- D. rongeur
- D. uterine curette
- D. vaporizer

Denham
- D. external fixation device
- D. pin

Denhardt mouthgag
Denis
- D. bipolar cautery
- D. Browne abdominal retractor
- D. Browne abdominal retractor blade
- D. Browne bar
- D. Browne bucket
- D. Browne cleft palate needle
- D. Browne clubfoot splint
- D. Browne-Hendren pediatric retractor blade
- D. Browne hip splint
- D. Browne malleable copper retractor blade
- D. Browne mastoid pediatric retractor blade
- D. Browne needleholder
- D. Browne pouch
- D. Browne retractor oval sprocket frame
- D. Browne ring retractor
- D. Browne talipes hobble splint
- D. Browne tonsillar forceps
- D. Browne tray

Denker
- D. trocar
- D. tube

DenLite illuminated handheld mirror
Dennen forceps
Dennis
- D. anastomotic clamp
- D. blade
- D. intestinal clamp
- D. intestinal forceps
- D. tube

Denniston dilator
Densco
- D. bur
- D. dental handpiece
- D. ultrasonic scaler

Densilay alloy
densitometer
- accuDEXA bone d.
- Achilles d.
- bone d.
- Cavitat ultrasonograph bone d.
- CT d.
- DEXA bone d.
- digital OsteoView d.
- Discovery QDR bone d.
- dual-energy x-ray absorptiometry bone d.
- dual-photon d.
- Expert-XL bone d.
- Hoefer GS 300 laser d.
- Hologic QDR-series d.
- Lunar DPX d.
- Lunar Expert d.
- Norland XR26 bone d.
- OsteoAnalyzer bone d.
- OsteoView 2000 digital bone d.
- pDEXA x-ray peripheral bone d.
- Pixi bone d.
- Prodigy bone d.
- QDR-series bone d.
- Sahara portable bone d.
- single-photon d.

Dent
- D. manometry system
- D. sleeve catheter

Dentaflex wire
Dentaform band
dental
- d. amalgam packer
- d. apparatus
- d. arch bar
- d. arch bar facial fracture appliance
- d. bur
- d. capsule

d. cement
d. curette
d. dressing forceps
d. drill
d. excavator
d. explorer
d. implant
d. implant cover screw
d. pick
d. pliers
D. Pro II camera
d. retractor
d. rongeur
d. scaler
d. shield
d. wax
d. wax carver
DentaScan
D. imager
D. scan
dentate bur
Dentatus
D. articulator
D. reamer
D. screw
DentCAM dental camera
Dentemp filling material
Dentex acrylic
DentiCAD system
Dentifix denture repair kit
dentin-bonded resin composite
DentiPatch lidocaine transoral delivery system
Dentloid impression material
Dento-Infuser infuser
Dentomat amalgamator
Dentsply
D. alloy
D. FlexoFiles file
D. implant
D. implant system
D. MVS evacuator
D. resin
denture
Astron d.
full lower d.
full upper d.
implant-retained d.
maxillary removable implant-retained d.
Nesbit removable partial d.
partial lower d.

partial upper d.
removable partial d.
soft-lined d.
unilateral removable partial d.
d. vulcanite bur
Dentus x-ray film
Dent-X
D.-X dental imaging system
D.-X digital imaging
Denver
D. ascites shunt
D. connector
D. hydrocephalus shunt
D. nasal splint
D. peritoneovenous shunt
D. pleural effusion shunt
D. pleuroperitoneal shunt
D. reservoir
D. shunt
D. splint
D. valve
D. valve shunt
Denver-Wells
D.-W. atrial retractor
D.-W. sternal retractor
Deon
D. hip prosthesis
D. stem
Depage-Janeway gastrostomy
DePalma
D. hip prosthesis
D. knife
D. staple
DePaul tube
Depilase laser
depilatory forceps
depolarizing electrode
depressor
Andrews-Pynchon tongue d.
Andrews tongue d.
Balmer tongue d.
Beatty tongue d.
Blakesley tongue d.
Boebinger tongue d.
Bosworth tongue d.
brain d.
Braun uterine d.
Bruening tongue d.
Buchwald tongue d.
Chamberlain tongue d.
Claes scleral d.
Colver-Dawson tongue d.

NOTES

D

depressor *(continued)*
    Cushing brain d.
    Dorsey tongue d.
    Dunn d.
    Farlow tongue d.
    Flynn scleral d.
    Fraser d.
    Granberry tongue d.
    Hamilton tongue d.
    humeral head d.
    Israel tongue d.
    Jobson-Pynchon tongue d.
    Kellogg tongue d.
    Kocher d.
    Layman tongue d.
    Lewis tongue d.
    metal tongue d.
    Mullins tongue d.
    O'Connor scleral d.
    orbital d.
    Pirquet tongue d.
    Proetz tongue d.
    Pynchon-Lillie tongue d.
    Pynchon tongue d.
    Schepens scleral d.
    Schocket scleral d.
    scleral d.
    Sims uterine d.
    Titus tongue d.
    Tobold tongue d.
    tongue d.
    Urrets-Zavalia d.
    Urrets-Zavalia scleral d.
    Weider tongue d.
    Wilder scleral d.
    wood tongue d.

depth
    d. check drill
    d. electrode
    d. gauge
    d. plate

Depthalon depth electrode

DePuy
    D. acetabular liner
    D. aeroplane splint
    D. any-angle splint
    D. awl
    D. bolt
    D. 1 bone cement
    D. bone curette
    D. Bremer AirFlo halo vest system
    D. cannulated reamer
    D. drill
    D. extractor
    D. Global Advantage shoulder eccentric humeral head
    D. head halter
    D. hip prosthesis

    D. interference screw
    D. Isola hook
    D. Kaneda system
    D. Keystone graft instrument
    D. Lumbar I/V cage
    D. M-2 Anterior Plate system
    D. Moss Miami hook
    D. open-thimble splint
    D. orthopaedic implant
    D. Peak anterior compression plate
    D. pituitary rongeur
    D. Profile system
    D. rainbow fracture frame
    D. retractor
    D. rocking leg splint
    D. rolled Colles splint
    D. screwdriver
    D. small-joint arthroscopy instrument set
    D. Songer cable system
    D. Summit rod
    D. support
    D. TiMX comprehensive low back system
    D. total hip system
    D. University Plate system
    D. VertiGraft bone wedge
    D. VSP plate and screw system

Derek-Harwood-Nash catheter

Derf
    D. forceps
    D. needle holder
    D. scissors
    D. Vital needle holder

Derlacki
    D. capsular knife
    D. chisel
    D. duckbill elevator
    D. ear curette
    D. ear mobilizer
    D. gouge
    D. ossicle holder

Derma
    D. Cool hydrocolloid wound dressing
    D. 20 Er:YAG laser
    D. Peel

Dermablate
    D. hair transplantation system
    D. skin rejuvenation laser

Dermabond topical skin adhesive

dermabrader
    diamond d.
    high-speed d.
    HydroBrader irrigating-aspirating d.
    sandpaper d.
    Schumann-Schreus d.

dermabrasion bur

DermaCare
    D. dressing
    D. electrosurgical forceps
dermacarrier
    Tanner mesh graft d.
Dermacea alginate dressing
DermaChiller 4 dermal cooler
DermaCooler 4 dermal cooler
DermaFilm dressing
Dermafit massage mat
DermaGard
    D. II seating surface
    D. prism
    D. spectrum
    D. Triad seating surface
Derma-Gel hydrogel sheet
DermaGlide cosmetic surgery suture
Dermagraft
    D. graft
    D. skin substitute
Dermagraft-TC temporary skin substitute
Dermagran-B hydrophilic wound dressing
Dermagran zinc-saline hydrogel wound dressing
Derma-K
    D.-K CO_2 laser
    D.-K Er:YAG laser
    D.-K laser system
dermal
    d. curette
    d. regeneration template
    d. suture
DermaLase
    D. laser
    D. laser system
Dermalogen material
Dermalon cuticular suture
DermaMend
    D. barrier
    D. foam
    D. foam wound dressing
    D. hydrogel dressing
DermaNet wound contact layer dressing
Dermaplant dermal allograft
Dermapor glove
Dermapulse wound management system
DermaScan
    D. laser scanner
    D. machine
Derma-Sil impression material

DermaSite transparent film dressing
Dermasoft mattress
DermaSorb hydrocolloid/alginate wound dressing
DermAssist
    D. glycerin hydrogel dressing
    D. hydrocolloid dressing
    D. hydrogel packing strip
    D. wound filling material
DermaStat
    D. calcium alginate wound dressing
    D. handpiece
    Variable Spot D.
Dermatell hydrocolloid dressing material
DermaTemp infrared thermographic sensor
Dermatex compound
dermatologic ultraviolet light
dermatome
    air d.
    Bard-Parker d.
    Barker Vacu-tome d.
    d. blade
    Brown air d.
    Brown-Blair d.
    Castroviejo d.
    d. cement
    Concept mesh grafter d.
    Davol d.
    Davol-Simon d.
    Down hand d.
    drum d.
    Duval disposable d.
    electric d.
    Goulian d.
    Hall d.
    hand d.
    Hood manual d.
    Jordan-Day d.
    manual d.
    Meek-Wall d.
    mesh graft d.
    Padgett-Hood d.
    Padgett manual d.
    Pitkin d.
    Reese d.
    Reese-Drum d.
    Reuse Expanda-graft d.
    Rica d.
    Rolodermatome d.
    Schink d.
    Simon d.

NOTES

D

dermatome *(continued)*
    single-use d.
    SMIC d.
    Strempel d.
    Tanner-Vandeput mesh d.
    Weck d.
    Zimmer d.
dermatoscope
    Delta d.
    Heine d.
Derma-Wand device
Dermicare hypoallergenic paper tape
Dermicel
    D. cloth tape dressing
    D. hypoallergenic cloth tape
    D. Montgomery strap
Dermiclear tape
Dermiform hypoallergenic knitted tape
dermis-fat passer
Dermiview hypoallergenic transparent tape
DermMaster macrodermabrasion system
Dermo-Jet high-pressure injector
dermoplasty cast
Dermostat
    D. eye implant material
    D. orbital implant
DermX cosmetic surgery needle
Dero hole-in-one prosthetic sock
derotation
    d. boot
    d. brace
    d. knee cage
    d. orthosis
DeRoyal
    D. cannula
    D. catheter tube holder
    D. Grab Bag specimen retrieval pouch
    D. laparotomy sponge
    D. mattress overlay
DeRoyal/LMB finger splint
Derra
    D. anastomosis clamp
    D. cardiac valve dilator
    D. cardiovascular forceps
    D. commissurotomy knife
    D. guillotine knife
    D. urethral forceps
    D. valvulotome
    D. vena caval clamp
    D. vestibular clamp
D'Errico
    D. bayonet pituitary forceps
    D. brain spatula
    D. dressing forceps
    D. hypophyseal forceps
    D. laminar knife
    D. laminectomy chisel

    D. nerve root retractor
    D. perforating bur
    D. perforating drill
    D. perforator
    D. periosteal elevator
    D. skull trephine
    D. tissue forceps
    D. ventricular needle
Desai VectorCath mapping catheter
Desault
    D. apparatus
    D. dressing
    D. ligature
    D. wrist bandage
Descemet membrane punch
Deschamps
    D. compressor
    D. ligature carrier
    D. ligature needle
Deseret
    D. angiocatheter
    D. flow-directed thermodilution catheter
    D. sump drain
desiccation needle
DesignLine orthotic
Desilets
    D. catheter
    D. introducer
Desilets-Hoffman
    D.-H. catheter
    D.-H. pacemaker introducer
    D.-H. sheath
Desjardins
    D. dilator
    D. gall duct forceps
    D. gall duct scoop
    D. gallstone forceps
    D. gallstone probe
    D. gallstone scoop
    D. kidney pedicle forceps
Desk-Rest arm support
Desmarres
    D. cardiovascular retractor
    D. chalazion forceps
    D. corneal dissector
    D. dacryolith
    D. eye dissector
    D. eye speculum
    D. fixation pick
    D. iris knife
    D. lid clamp
    D. lid elevator
    D. lid forceps
    D. lid retractor
    D. marker
    D. paracentesis knife
    D. paracentesis needle
    D. paracentesis needle dilator

D. scarifier
D. valve retractor
D. vein retractor
desmin filament
destructive obstetrical hook
detector
AddOn-Bucky direct x-ray d.
anular d.
Ausculscope carotid bruit d.
cadmium iodide d.
cesium fluoride scintillation d.
Clinitemp fever d.
C-Trak handheld gamma d.
digital amorphous silicon flat-panel d.
digital x-ray d.
diode d.
Dionex 450 Data System amperometric d.
direct digital x-ray d.
Doptone fetal pulse d.
electrical resistance d.
electrochemical d.
electron capture d.
element-specific d.
emission spectrometric d.
flame ionization d.
flame photometric d.
flat-panel d.
flat-plate d.
fluorescence d.
gamma probe radiation d.
Geiger-Müller d.
glass tract d.
high-purity germanium d.
Isometer bone graft placement site d.
kinestatic charge d.
NeoProbe radioactivity d.
nitrogen-phosphorus d.
passive track d.
Pendoppler ultrasonic fetal heart d.
phase-sensitive d.
photoionization d.
Pocket-Dop blood-flow d.
pulsed ultrasonic velocity d.
quadrature d.
quadrature phase d.
radiation d.
scintillation d.
Si(Li) d.
slot-scanning d.

sodium iodide d.
solid-state nuclear track d.
thermal conductivity d.
TubeChek esophageal intubation d.
ultraviolet d.
Wang-Binford edge d.
Waters M-440 fixed wavelength d.
deuterium-tritium generator
Deutschman cataract knife
device
abdominal aortic counterpulsation d.
Abdominal Left Ventricular Assist D. (ALVAD)
Abiomed BVAD 5000 left ventricular assist d.
ablative d.
Ablatr temperature control d.
Acapella chest physical therapy d.
Accutorr oscillometric d.
Ace Trippi-Wells tongs cervical traction d.
Ace Universal tongs cervical traction d.
ACMI ulcer-measuring d.
A1cNow glucose monitoring d.
Acorn CorCap cardiac support d.
AcroMed Isola d.
ACS Anchor exchange d.
Actis venous flow d.
Acucise cutting balloon d.
Acufex Suretac fixation d.
AcuSnare polypectomy d.
AcuTrainer bladder retraining d.
AeroChamber spacing d.
Agee 4-pin fixation d.
AIS CELLector d.
alternative communication d. (ACD)
Altona finger extension d.
Amplatzer VSD occluder d.
Amplatz thrombectomy d.
Amplatz ventricular septal defect d.
Anchor soft tissue biopsy d.
AngelWings d.
Ange-Med Sentinel ICD d.
Angioguard guidewire filter d.
AngioJet thrombectomy d.
AngioLink vascular closure d.
Angio-Seal hemostatic puncture closure d.
Angio-Seal puncture closure d.
Antense antitension d.
anterior internal fixation d.

D

NOTES

device *(continued)*

AOR check traction d.
Aprema II d.
Aqua-Flow collagen glaucoma
  drainage d.
AquaMED hydrotherapy d.
Aqua-Purator suction d.
AquaTrek d.
Arnoff external fixation d.
AromaScan aroma analysis d.
arrhythmia control d.
Arrow emergency infusion d.
Arrow-Trerotola percutaneous
  thrombectomy d.
ArtAssist arterial assist d.
ArtAssist pneumatic compression d.
ArthroCare Rubo-Vac d.
Arthroscrew arthroscopic suturing d.
ArthroSew arthroscopic suturing d.
Arthrotek tibial fixation d.
Asta-Cath catheter d.
Atad cervical ripening d.
Atad ripener d.
augmentative communication d.
AutoAdjust CPAP d.
Autoclix fingerstick lancet d.
Autolet fingerstick d.
automatic stapling d.
automatic suction d.
Automator computerized
  distraction d.
AutoPap automated screening d.
autostapling d.
Auto Suture d.
Auto Suture endoscopic suction-
  irrigation d.
Auto Suture One-Shot
  anastomotic d.
Auto Suture SurgiStitch d.
autotitration d.
AVA 3Xi triple-lumen venous
  access d.
Babyhaler spacer d.
BackCycler continuous passive
  motion d.
BackMaster d.
back range-of-motion d.
Baim-Turi cardiac d.
balloon catheter sealing d.
balloon-on-a-wire d.
band ligator d.
Bard ambulatory PCA d.
Bard FCD fecal containment d.
Bard Federal containment d.
Barton traction d.
Bassett electrical stimulation d.
BAS-300 transurethral
  thermotherapy d.
battery-assisted heart assist d.

Baxter ambulatory PCA d.
BeasyTrans transfer d.
Becker orthotic d.
behind-the-ear listening d.
BetaSorb hemodialysis d.
bilateral ventricular assist d.
  (BIVAD)
bilevel positive pressure d.
bioabsorbable closure d.
bioartificial liver support d.
Biocare portable handheld
  irrigation d.
BioDerm external continence d.
biofeedback galvanic skin
  response d.
Bioglass middle ear d.
BioScrew XtraLok tibial fixation d.
BioStinger fixation d.
BioStinger-V bioabsorbable meniscal
  repair d.
biventricular assist d.
Bivona-Colorado sizing d.
Bivona cuff maintenance d.
blade plate fixation d.
Blanchard traction d.
Block cardiac d.
Boing exercise d.
BoneCollector d.
bone fixation d.
Bovie electrocautery d.
Bovie suction d.
Boyden chamber assay d.
braided occlusion d.
Brannock foot measuring d.
Breas PV10 CPAP d.
BreastAlert DTS breast cancer
  screening d.
Brockenbrough cardiac d.
BTE listening d.
Bucky digital x-ray d.
Burnett bidirectional TMJ d.
Burnett mouth positioning d.
buttoned d.
button gastrostomy d.
Button One-Step gastrostomy d.
BVM d.
Calandruccio II compression d.
Calandruccio triangular compression
  fixation d.
Cameco syringe pistol aspiration d.
Cameron fracture d.
Camino intraparenchymal
  fiberoptic d.
Candela dynamic cooling d.
Capio CL suture-capturing d.
Capio transvaginal suture-
  capturing d.
CarboMedics valve d.
Carden jetting d.

CardioGrip exercise d.
Cardiomemo d.
CardioSeal septal occlusion d.
CathLink implantable vascular
access d.
Cath-Lok catheter locking d.
CaverMap surgical d.
Cavi-Jet dental prophylaxis d.
C-D instrumentation d.
Cell Sweep cervical cytology d.
Cellugel ophthalmologic
viscosurgical d.
Centermark vascular access d.
Ceprate SC Instrument II cell-
separation d.
CerviSoft cytology collection d.
Cervitrak d.
Champ cardiac d.
Charnley deepening d.
Chick patient transfer d.
child restraint d.
Chinese finger straps traction d.
ChiselTip suction cautery d.
Christoudias fascial closure d.
Chuter endovascular d.
CIC listening d.
circular stapling d.
Circumstraint circumcision
restraint d.
Circuvent aerosolized medication
delivery d.
CirKuit-Guard vascular surgery d.
Clamp Ease d.
C.L.E.A.R.Sound ultrasound
therapy d.
closure d.
Clo-Sure P.A.D. hemostatic d.
Clot Buster Amplatz
thrombectomy d.
Coag-A-Mate prothrombin d.
CoaguChek portable prothrombin
time d.
Coda titanium alloy d.
Coherent Versapulse d.
Columbus McKinnon Hugger d.
completely-in-the-canal listening d.
compressive internal fixation d.
Concept PuddleVac floor suction d.
constant passive-motion d.
Contimed II biofeedback d.
continuous microinfusion d.
continuous passive motion d.

Contour Emboli artificial
embolization d.
cookie cutter d.
Cook liver balloon tamponade d.
Copper-7 intrauterine d.
CorCap cardiac support d.
cord blood collection d.
Cordis embolization d.
coronary atherectomy d.
Cotrel-Dubousset dynamic transverse
traction d.
Coumatrak prothrombin time d.
Cournand cardiac d.
CPCA2000 counterpulsation d.
CPM d.
CranioFIX d.
Cricket stapling d.
CROM d.
crosslinked glaucoma filtration d.
Cueva cranial nerve electrode
monitoring d.
Cuff Link orthopaedic d.
Cu-7 intrauterine d.
CUSALap d.
Cyclotech medication dosing d.
cyst puncture d.
CytoGuard aerosol containment d.
Dalkon shield intrauterine d.
Das Angel Wings atrial septal
defect closure d.
DeBakey-NASA axial flow
ventricular assist d.
DeBakey-NASA miniature heart
assist d.
DeBakey ventricular assist d.
Della Badia laparoscopic
suturing d.
Deltec portable external infusion d.
Denham external fixation d.
Derma-Wand d.
Deyerle fixation d.
Dialock port d.
DiaPhine corneal trephination d.
Diasys Novacor cardiac d.
Digiflator digital inflation d.
Digital Add-On Bucky x-ray d.
Digit-grip d.
Dinamap automated blood
pressure d.
directional coronary atherectomy d.
DirectRay direct-to-digital x-ray
capture d.

D

NOTES

245

device (continued)

Disk-Criminator nerve stimulation measuring d.
Dispenstir d.
displacement sensing d.
Dispo-sand d.
distal targeting d.
distraction d.
DIV laparoscopic morcellator d.
Dolphin d.
Donnez endometrial ablation d.
Doppler d.
double-headed P190 stapling d.
Drionic electrical iontophoresis d.
Duett arterial closure d.
Duett closure d.
Duett sealing d.
Duett vascular sealing d.
Dunn fracture d.
DuraGen neurosurgical d.
Dwyer d.
dynamic cooling d.
DynaVox 2 communication d.
DynaWell medical compression d.
Echocheck hearing screening d.
echo-tracking d.
Econo-Cerv traction d.
Econolith d.
Eder cord blood collection d.
Edwards modular system sacral fixation d.
EEA surgical stapling d.
Elecath circulatory support d.
electroacupuncture d.
electronic portal imaging d.
electronic summation d.
Elscint Planar d.
eNclose proximal anastomosis d.
Endermologie noninvasive body contouring d.
Endo Babcock surgical grasping d.
Endo-Bender bending d.
endocut cautery d.
Endoflip d.
Endograsp d.
EndoLift d.
EndoPaddle d.
Endopath EZ-RF linear cutter and coagulation d.
EndoPearl bioabsorbable fixation d.
endoscopically deliverable tissue-transfixing d.
endoscopic Hemoclip d.
Endostitch laparoscopic suturing d.
EpiE-Z Pen injection d.
EpiPen injection d.
EpiPen-Jr injection d.
Epi-Stay d.
ErecAid vacuum erection d.

Ergolift d.
Erlangen magnetic colostomy d.
Eros-CTD clitoral therapy d.
esophageal detection d.
esophageal variceal ligation d.
E-Trap surgical filter d.
EVS hemostasis d.
EX-FI-RE external fixation d.
eXit disposable puncture closure d.
external counterpressure d.
external tachyarrhythmia control d.
external vascular compression d.
extracorporeal liver assist d. (ELAD)
extraction atherectomy d.
ExtreSafe phlebotomy d.
EZ Flex jaw exercising d.
Facial-Flex Ultra d.
FemAssist continence d.
Femcept d.
FemoStop inflatable pneumatic compression d.
ferromagnetic monitoring d.
FilterWire EX embolic d.
finger photoplethysmograph d.
flexible delivery d.
flexible Olympus GF-eUM3 d.
Flexi-Trak skin anchoring d.
Flexor Ansel introducer d.
Flexor Balkin Up & Over introducer d.
Flexor Shuttle introducer d.
Flo-Restors backbleeding control d.
FloTem IIe fluid-warming d.
Flutter mucus clearance d.
fog reduction/elimination d.
foot orthotic d.
ForeRunner automatic external defibrillator d.
Fox internal fixation d.
fracture fixation d.
galvanic skin response d.
GelPort laparoscopic hand access d.
GenJect injection d.
Georgiade fixation d.
Gerster traction d.
GIA stapling d.
glaucoma drainage d.
Glucolet lancet d.
GlucoWatch glucose monitoring d.
Goetz cardiac d.
Golgi d.
Goodale-Lubin cardiac d.
Gore thyroplasty d.
Gould polygraph gastric motility measuring d.
Graftmaster d.
Grass pressure-recording d.

green sleeve compression d.
Grip-Ease d.
G-suit d.
Gyno Sampler endometrial sampling d.
Hakim shunt reprogramming d.
Hall intrauterine d.
halo gravity traction d.
halo hoop d.
Handisizer exercise d.
Handisol phototherapy d.
HandPort d.
Hare splint d.
Hare traction d.
Harrington-Kostuik distraction d.
head fixation d.
HeartMate implantable ventricular assist d.
HeatProbe d.
hemostatic puncture closure d.
Hemovac suction d.
Hershey left ventricular assist d.
Heyer-Schulte antisiphon d.
HiSonic ultrasonic bone conduction hearing d.
Hoffmann external fixation d.
Hoffmann traction d.
Hoffmann-Vidal external fixation d.
Hollister circumcision d.
Hollister collecting d.
horizontal drain attachment d.
horizontal tube attachment d.
Hotline fluid-warming d.
HumatroPen injection d.
Hunstad Quik-Clik d.
Ideal cardiac d.
Ikuta fixation d.
Ilizarov fixation d.
Illi intracranial fixation d.
Illi intracranial pressure monitoring d.
implantable vascular access d.
implantable venous access d. (IVAD)
implantable ventricular assist d. (IVAD)
ImPulse Elite electronic oxygen conserving d.
ImPulse Select oxygen conserving d.
indwelling transcutaneous vascular access d.

Infiltrator local drug delivery d.
Infrasonic QIGong 5.5 pain management d.
Infuse bone graft d.
infusion d.
InjecTx transurethral injection d.
InnerVasc vascular access d.
InnovaTome microkeratome d.
Inspiron inspiratory training d.
Insta-Mold ear protection d.
Insta-Nerve d.
insufflation d.
Insuflon insulin delivery d.
InSurg LapTie needle driver suturing d.
Inter Fix RP threaded spinal fusion cage d.
internal fixation d.
interrogation d.
in-the-ear listening d.
intraaortic balloon assist d.
Intracell mechanical muscle d.
Intracell myofascial trigger-point d.
intramedullary fixation d.
intraoral titanium mandibular distraction d.
IntraSonix Tulip laser d.
intrauterine d. (IUD)
intravenous accurate control d.
inverted buttoned d.
Isobar barostat distension d.
ITE listening d.
IVAC d.
Jace W550 continuous passive motion wrist d.
JAS elbow d.
Jewel atrial fibrillation dual chamber d.
Kaneda anterior spine stabilizing d.
Kaneda distraction d.
Kaufman incontinence d.
Keller cephalometric d.
Kendall sequential compression d.
Kennedy ligament augmentation d.
Keratolux fixation d.
Kerboull acetabular reinforcement d.
keyed filling d.
Kin-Con d.
kinetic continuous passive motion d.
kinetic rehabilitation d.
King interlocking d.

D

NOTES

device *(continued)*

Kronner external fixation d.
Kuhlman cervical traction d.
Küntscher traction d.
Lancet laser d.
language acquisition d.
Laparofan pneumoperitoneum d.
Laparomed suture-applier d.
Lapro-Loop d.
LaserPen d.
LaTeX d.
lead locking d.
left ventricular assist d. (LVAD)
Legasus Sport CPM d.
leg-holding d.
Leksell stereotactic d.
Leslie Parachute stone retrieval d.
Lewis intramedullary d.
Lewis suspension d.
Lewy suspension d.
Libbe lower bowel evacuation d.
LiftALERT electronic d.
LiftMate patient transfer d.
ligament augmentation d. (LAD)
ligation d.
linear stapling d.
Linx-EZ cardiac d.
Lippes loop intrauterine d.
Liss CES d.
Lite-Gait partial weight-bearing gait therapy d.
LithoCatch stone retrieval d.
LithoCath immobilization d.
Lixiscope inspection d.
Lock Clamshell d.
locking d.
Loewi suspension d.
Look micropuncture d.
Lorenz Blue multi-vector external distraction d.
LT-cage lumbar tapered fusion d.
Luque fixation d.
Macroplastique implantable d.
Magna-Finder locating d.
magnetic induction d.
magnetic jaw tracking d.
Makler insemination d.
Makler sperm counting d.
malleable microsurgical suction d.
Mammotome core biopsy d.
mandibular advancement d.
mandibular positioning d.
Margulies intrauterine d.
Mazlin intrauterine d.
McAtee olecranon compression screw d.
McCleery-Miller locking d.
McLaughlin osteosynthesis d.
M-cup vacuum extraction d.

mechanical d.
Medelec five-channel neurophysiological d.
Medi-Breather IPPB d.
Medical Intelligence BodyFix d.
Medicamat ultrasound d.
Medicon ultrasonic liposuction d.
Mediflex-Bookler d.
MediPort infusion vascular access d.
MediRule measuring d.
Medtronic external tachyarrhythmia control d.
Medtronic Jewel ICD d.
Medtronic tremor control therapy d.
MedX physical therapy d.
Mic-Key button gastrostomy d.
MicroAire power-assisted lipoplasty d.
MicroDigitrapper-S apnea screening d.
MicroEnhancer UL micropigmentation d.
MicroFet2 muscle testing d.
Microgyn II urinary incontinence d.
Microjet-based cutting and debriding d.
MicroMed DeBakey ventricular assist d.
MicroStim 100 TENS d.
Microvolt T-wave alternans d.
Miniguard stress incontinence d.
Minnesota thermal disc temperature testing d.
Mitek QuickAnchor d.
3M microvascular anastomotic coupling d.
Mobilimb CPM d.
Modulock posterior spinal fixation d.
Molteno implant glaucoma drainage d.
Monojector fingerstick d.
Montgomery Stomeasure d.
Mosher Life Saver antichoke suction d.
motorized transducer pullback d.
Mueller fixation d.
Multiclip disposable ligating clip d.
Multifire Endo GIA stapling d.
Multiload Cu-375 intrauterine d.
Multiple Parameter telemetry d.
Multispatula cervical sampling d.
MurphyScope neurologic d.
Myoexorciser II, III portable EMG d.
MyoTRac biofeedback incontinence training d.

Nachlas-Linton esophagogastric balloon tamponade d.
Nauth traction d.
Navarre interventional radiology d.
NBIH cardiac d.
Necktrac traction d.
Needle-Ease d.
Needle-Pro needle protection d.
needlescope d.
Nemdi tweezer epilation d.
NeoNaze nasal function restoration d.
Neuro-Aide testing d.
Neuromed Octrode implantable pain management d.
neurometer d.
Neuropath biofeedback d.
Neurotone biofeedback d.
Neuro Vasx interventional d.
Nicolet Pathfinder I recording d.
Nimbus Hemopump cardiac assist d.
Niplette d.
NMR LipoProfile d.
noise reduction d.
nonferromagnetic positioning d.
noninvasive immobilization d.
nonthoracotomy system antitachycardia d.
notcher d.
Novacor Diasys left ventricular assist d.
Nozovent anti-snoring d.
NuPulse d.
Nu-Thor thoracostomy d.
Nu-Trake cricothyrotomy d.
Ogden Anchor soft tissue d.
Olympus clip-fixing d.
Olympus UES-series snare cautery d.
Ommaya reservoir d.
Omniport hand-assisted laparoscopic d.
One-Shot ablation d.
On2 lateral transfer d.
OraSure HIV-1 oral specimen collection d.
Oratek d.
Orthofix external fixation d.
Orthofix lengthening d.
Ortholav irrigation and suction d.
OrthoNail intramedullary fixation d.

orthopaedic fixation d.
OtoScan d.
Oxylator EM-100 emergency resuscitation d.
Oxymizer d.
Pain Care 3000 pain management d.
Palpagraph breast density mapping d.
Panoramic 200 Ultra-Widefield ophthalmic imaging d.
Panos G. Koutrouvelis, M.D. stereotactic d.
Parachute stone retrieval d.
ParaGard intrauterine d.
Parascan scanning d.
passive motion d.
patient self-administration d.
Pavenik monodisk d.
Pennig minifixator d.
Penn State ventricular assist d.
Perc-D SpineWand d.
Perclose closure d.
Perclose percutaneous vascular surgery d.
Perclose PVS d.
Perclose suture d.
Perclose vascular closure d.
percutaneous arterial closure d.
percutaneous thrombolytic d. (PTD)
PercuTx percutaneous injection d.
PerDUCER pericardial access d.
peripheral indwelling intermediate infusion d.
PET balloon Simpson atherectomy d.
PGK stereotactic d.
phased-array ultrasonographic d.
phonologic acquisition d.
PhotoDerm PL, VL pulsed light d.
Pierce-Donachy Thoratec ventricular assist d.
Pigg-O-Stat immobilization d.
Pillo-Boot lower leg positioning d.
Pisces spinal cord stimulation d.
Plastazote orthotic d.
Plastibell circumcision d.
PlegiaGuard safety d.
Pleura-Stay chest tube securement d.
Pleur-evac d.

D

NOTES

device *(continued)*

PlexiPulse pneumatic sequential compression d.
PMT InVac in-line suction control d.
PMT MicroVac suction d.
Pocket Starter d.
Polar Bair forced-air active cooling d.
Polar Care 500 cryotherapy d.
PolyGIA stapling d.
portable monitoring d.
Port-A-Cath d.
Portex Neo-Vac meconium suction d.
Portnoy DPV d.
PortSaver PercLoop d.
posterior reduction d.
Pos-T-Vac vacuum erection d.
precise lesion measuring d.
Premium CEEA circular stapling d.
PressureEasy cuff inflation d.
Pressurefuse automatic constant pressure d.
Presto cardiac d.
Progestasert intrauterine d.
Pronex pneumatic d.
Pronex traction d.
Pron-Pillo head positioning d.
Prostar-Plus percutaneous closure d.
Prostar XL percutaneous closure d.
Prostatron transurethral thermotherapy d.
Protector suturing d.
ProTrac cruciate reconstruction measurement d.
Provider 5500 patient-controlled analgesia d.
PuddleVac floor suction d.
Putterman-Chaflin ocular asymmetry d.
Q-Maxx side-firing laser d.
Quantum biliary inflation d.
Quartzo d.
QuickSeal arterial closure d.
Quickswitch irrigation-aspiration ophthalmic d.
Quikcoff d.
RaAct NMES d.
radiative hyperthermia d.
Radstat hemostasis d.
RapidFlap d.
Rapid Loc d.
Rashkind double-umbrella d.
Ray TFC d.
ReAct NMES d.
Reliance d.
ReliefBand RB-EL Explorer d.
Resistex PEP therapy d.

ResMed CPAP Sullivan III d.
Resnick Tone Emitter I intraoral electrolarynx d.
Res-Q arrhythmia control d.
Rezaian interbody external fixation d.
Richards lag screw compression d.
right ventricular assist d.
rigid internal fixation d.
Rigiflator handheld inflation/deflation d.
RigiScan d.
ring-type rigidity measuring d.
Rinn XCP radiographic paralleling d.
Roboprep G d.
robotic-automated assist d.
Rochester bone trephine d.
Roentgen knife stereotaxic radiosurgical d.
Roger Anderson external skeletal fixation d.
Roll-A-Bout mobility d.
RollerBack self-massage d.
Rosen incontinence d.
Rotablator atherectomy d.
Rotacs rotational atherectomy d.
RotaLink Plus rotational atherectomy d.
rotational atherectomy d.
Roth Net retrieval d.
Rotosnare d.
Rudolf-Buck suturing d.
Russell traction d.
sacral fixation d.
Saf-T-Coil intrauterine d.
Sarns ventricular assist d.
scaling d.
ScopeTrac support d.
Scram emergency escape breathing d.
Seirin LaserPen d.
Sensation vacuum assist d.
Senso listening d.
SensorHand d.
sequential compression d. (SCD)
Servox d.
ShotBlocker pain reduction d.
Shug male contraceptive d.
Sideris adjustable buttoned d.
Silent Nite snore prevention d.
Simpson directional coronary atherectomy d.
Simpson PET balloon atherectomy d.
single-needle d.
SkinTech medical tattooing d.
Sleep Right d.
Slot distraction d.

SmartFlow Multiple Lesion d.
SmartNeedle vascular access d.
smoke Controller d.
Snap EEG d.
Snap-Gauge impotence screening d.
SnorNoMor d.
Snyder suction d.
Soehendra stent retrieval d.
SofPulse electrotherapy d.
Softepil tweezer epilation d.
SofTouch vacuum erection d.
Soft Touch lancet d.
SomaSensor d.
SomnoStar apnea testing d.
SOMNOvent S sleep apnea
 therapy d.
Sonablate ablation d.
SonoSite imaging d.
Sono-Stat Plus sound d.
Sonotron electronic therapeutic d.
Sorbothane orthotic d.
Spenco orthotic d.
Spitz-Holter flushing d.
SplintsRite stabilization d.
SporTX stimulation d.
StairClimber assist d.
Statak soft tissue attachment d.
Stat-Temp II temperature d.
Stellbrink fixation d.
1-step button gastrostomy d.
Stepty P hemostasis d.
Steri-Oss dental implant d.
St. Jude cardiac d.
stoma-measuring d.
Stone clamp-locking d.
Stone Cone nitinol retrieval d.
Stonetome stone removal d.
Stress-Ray varus-valgus d.
Stretch cardiac d.
STx Saunders lumbar disc d.
Sub-Q-Set subcutaneous continuous
 infusion d.
Sukhtian-Hughes fixation d.
superconducting quantum
 interference d.
Super Pinky pressure d.
SuperQuad assistive d.
SuperStitch vascular closure d.
Suretac fixation d.
Surgicutt incision d.
SurgiScope navigational d.
Surgitron 3000 ultrasound d.

Surgiwand suction/irrigation d.
Sutter-CPM knee d.
Sutura Superstitch vascular
 closure d.
Suture Lok d.
SutureMate suture assist d.
Swedish Helparm d.
Swiss Kiss intrastent balloon
 inflation d.
Symbion biventricular assist d.
SynchroMed drug administration d.
Synergist vacuum erection d.
Tacticon peripheral neuropathy
 screening d.
TandemHeart ventricular assist d.
TaperSeal hemostatic d.
targeted cryoablation d.
Tatum Tee intrauterine d.
Taylor halter d.
TEC atherectomy d.
Techstar percutaneous closure d.
Tekscan in-shoe monitoring d.
Telos stress d.
Tenderfoot incision-making d.
Tenderlett d.
The Closer suture-mediated arterial
 closure d.
Thermedics HeartMate 10001P left
 anterior assist d.
Thermex-II transurethral prostate
 heating d.
Thermo Cardiosystems left
 ventricular assist d.
The Rope stretch/traction d.
Thoratec biventricular assist d.
Thoratec right ventricular assist d.
thread-locking d.
Threshold IMT d.
Threshold PEP d.
Throat-E-Vac suction d.
Tibbs semi-automatic suturing d.
tiered-therapy antiarrhythmic d.
Tissomat d.
Tis-U-Trap tissue retrieval d.
titanium fixation d.
tongue-retaining d.
tooth-borne distraction d.
Trach-Talk d.
traction d.
Trak Back II digital pullback d.
Tranquility Quest CPAP d.
Trapper exchange d.

D

NOTES

device *(continued)*
TraumaSeal topical wound
closure d.
TriggerWheel d.
Trimedyne Optilase 1000 d.
T-Scan 2000 breast imaging d.
TULIP aspiration d.
U-Clip anastomotic d.
U-Control training d.
Umbilicup umbilical cord blood
collection d.
Unilink anastomotic d.
Universal joint d.
Uri-Drain male incontinence d.
Urosheath incontinence d.
Uterine Explora Curette endometrial
sampling d.
UV-Flash ultraviolet germicidal
exchange d.
Vacuconstrictor erection d.
vacuum constriction d.
vacuum entrapment d.
vacuum erection d.
vacuum extraction d.
Vapotherm 2000i respiratory
therapy d.
Vapr coagulation and cautery d.
Vasceze vascular access/flush d.
vascular access d. (VAD)
vascular hemostatic d.
vascular sealing d.
VasoSeal ES arterial sealing d.
VasoSeal VHD extravascular
sealing d.
Vasotrax handheld monitoring d.
Venodyne pneumatic
compression d.
venous access d. (VAD)
ventricular assist d. (VAD)
Ventritex Cadence d.
Venture demand oxygen delivery d.
Versa-Fx femoral d.
Versalok low-back fixation d.
VersaTack stapling d.
Viking IV nerve monitoring d.
VitaCuff infection control d.
Vitallium d.
Vita-Stat automatic d.
Voyager Aortic IntraClusion d.
V-Vac suction d.
Wagner distraction d.
Wagner leg-lengthening
distraction d.
Wallstent delivery d.
WasherLoc tibial graft fixation d.
wearable cardioverter-defibrillator d.
Wedge electrosurgical resection d.
Williams cardiac d.
wire-guided metal spiral retrieval d.

Wizard cardiac d.
Wolf Piezolith 2300 lithotripsy d.
Wolvek fixation d.
Wright Care-TENS d.
Xercise Tube resistive d.
XT cardiac d.
Y-Knot d.
Zipper antidisconnect d.
Z Strong blood pressure d.
Zucker-Myler cardiac d.
DeVilbiss
D. aerosol syringe
D. atomizer
D. CPAP
D. cranial forceps
D. cranial rongeur
D. eye irrigator
D. I&A unit
D. Mini-Dop fetal monitor
D. OB-Dop fetal monitor
D. plastic powder blower
D. Pulmo-Aide nebulizer
D. skull trephine
D. suction pump
D. suction tube
D. Vacu-Aide aspirator
D. vaginal speculum
Devon-Pura stent
Devonshire
D. catheter
D. knife
D. needle
D. roller
Devonshire-Mack
D.-M. cannula
D.-M. catheter
D.-M. clamp
D.-M. stop
Dewald halo hoop apparatus
Dewar
D. elevator
D. flask
DeWecker
D. eye implant
D. forceps
D. iridectomy scissors
D. iris spatula
D. syringe cannula
DeWeese
D. axis traction obstetrical forceps
D. caval catheter
D. vena caval clamp
Dewey obstetrical forceps
DEXA
dual-energy x-ray absorptiometry
DEXA bone densitometer
DEXA scan
Dexide
D. disposable cannula

D. laparoscopic trocar
D. locking trocar
Dexon
D. absorbable suture
D. II suture
D. mesh
D. Plus suture
D. surgically knitted mesh
DexTBrush
D. brush
D. toothbrush
Dexterity
D. protractor
D. Surgical Pneumo Sleeve
dextrose stick
Deyerle
D. apparatus
D. bone graft plate
D. component
D. drill
D. fixation device
D. pin
D. punch
D. screw
D/Flex filter
DFP+/DXP+
DFS 2 mattress replacement system
DGH-KOI diamond knife
DG Softgut suture
DH pressure relief walker
Diab-A-Foot
D.-A.-F. protection system
D.-A.-F. rocker insole
Diab-A-Pad insole
Diab-A-Sheet ThermoThotic sheet
Diab-A-Sole insole
Diab-A-Thotics orthotic
diabetic
D. Diagnostic Insole
D. D-Sole foot orthosis
d. orthosis kit
d. pressure relief shoe
d. sock
DiaB Gel hydrogel dressing
diacrylate resin
Diaflex
D. cytology brush
D. dilator
D. grasping forceps
D. retrieval loop
D. ureteral dilatation catheter

DIAGNOdent
D. caries detection system
D. dental laser
diagnostic
d. duodenoscope
d. hysteroscope
d. tube
d. tympanometer
d. ultrasound catheter
Diaket root canal cement
dial
Mendez astigmatism d.
Regan-Lancaster d.
dialer
intraocular lens d.
IOL d.
irrigating d.
Visitec intraocular lens d.
Dialix dialyzer
dial-lock orthosis
Dialock
D. access port
D. port device
Dialog pacemaker
Dialy-Nate catheter
Dialys-Aids system
dialysate
d. bag
d. preparation module
d. tubing
dialysis
d. catheter
continuous ambulatory peritoneal d.
(CAPD)
d. shunt
d. tube
d. tubing
dialyzer
AM-UP-75WET d.
AN69 membrane d.
Asahi Biomembrane hollow-fiber d.
Asahi hollow fiber d.
Baxter d.
Baxter PSN d.
CA membrane hollow-fiber d.
capillary flow d.
CA-series d.
C-Dak d.
Clirans T-series d.
DAS single-pass d.
Dialix d.
Digi-Dyne d.

D

NOTES

dialyzer *(continued)*
    Filtryzer d.
    Fresenius AG d.
    F-series d.
    Gambro d.
    Gambro-Lundia coil d.
    Hemoclear d.
    HF d.
    high flux d.
    hollow fiber d.
    Idecap d.
    low-flux cuprammonium d.
    Nephross d.
    parallel flow d.
    parallel plate d.
    Polyflux S d.
    polysulfone d.
    Renaflo hollow fiber d.
    Renalin d.
    Renal systems d.
    Renatron II d.
    Sorbiclear d.
    TAF175 d.
    Terumo d.
    Terumo-Clirans d.
    twin-coil d.
Diamatrix trapezoidal diamond knife
Diamed leg bag
diamond
    D. biomechanical table
    d. blade knife
    d. bur
    d. dermabrader
    d. electrode
    d. finishing bur
    d. fraise
    d. high-speed air drill
    D. II DDDR pacemaker
    D. II DDR pacemaker
    d. inlay bone graft
    d. micrometer knife
    d. nail
    d. nail file
    d. phaco knife
    d. pin cutter
    D. pocket maker
    d. pyramid indenter
    d. rasp
    d. saw blade
    D. SharpPoint needle
    D. valve
    D. Valve flow-regulating shunt
    d. wafering saw
    d. wire cutter
diamond-coated bur
diamond-dust bur
diamond-dusted knife
diamond-edge scissors

Diamond-Flex
    D.-F. forceps
    D.-F. trocar
Diamond-Jaw
    D.-J. Babcock grasper
    D.-J. needle holder
DiamondLite restorative material
Diamond-Lite titanium thumb forceps
diamond-point suture needle
Diamontek knife
Diapact CRRT system
diaper
    BiliBottoms light-permeable
      phototherapy d.
    Nature Boy & Girl d.
diaphanoscope
    Binner d.
DiaPhine
    D. corneal trephination device
    D. trephine
diaphragm
    Bucky d.
    d. inserter
    Ortho All-Flex d.
    d. pessary
    Potter-Bucky d.
    Ramses d.
    wide-seal d.
Diapulse
    D. electromagnetic therapy machine
    D. machine
    D. wound treatment system
Dia pump aspirator
DiaryCard
    Micro D.
diascope
Diasensor 1000 sensor
Diasonics
    D. Cardiovue SectOR scanner
    D. catheter
    D. DRF ultrasound unit
    D. Sonotron Vingmed CFM 800
      imaging system
    D. Therasonic lithotripter
    D. transducer
    D. ultrasound
Diastat vascular access graft
diastolic fluttering aortic valve
Diasys Novacor cardiac device
DiaTap vascular access button
Diatek 9000 Insta-Temp thermometer
diathermic snare
diathermocoagulator
diathermy
    d. electrode
    d. forceps
    d. knife
    Mira d.
    d. needle

d. scissors
d. snare
underwater d.
d. wire
Diatube-H Vacutainer tube
DIC
disposable inner cannula
DIC tracheostomy tube
dichroic filter system
dichromate dosimeter
Dick
D. bronchus clamp
D. cardiac valve dilator
D. pressure clamp
Dickinson
Becton D.
D. FACS 400-series flow
cytometer
Dickson paraffin bath
Dicon ocular blood flow analyzer
die
pin-deburring d.
Schuknecht-Paparella wire-
bending d.
Dieckmann intraosseous needle
Dieffenbach
D. bulldog clamp
D. forceps
D. scalpel
D. serrefine
D. tenotome
Diener forceps
Dieter
D. malleus forceps
D. nipper
Dieter-House nipper
Diethrich
D. aortic clamp
D. circumflex artery scissors
D. coronary artery bypass kit
D. coronary artery scissors
D. graft clamp
D. micro bulldog clamp
D. micro coronary bulldog clamp
D. right-angled hemostatic forceps
D. shunt clamp
D. valve scissors
Diethrich-Hegemann scissors
Diethrich-Potts scissors
Dieulafoy aspirator
Difco ESP testing system

differential
d. scanning calorimeter
d. temperature sensor
DiffSpin slide spinner
diffuser
cylindrical d.
diffusion-weighted MR imaging
Digi-Dyne
D.-D. cardiopulmonary bypass
oxygenator
D.-D. dialyzer
Digiflator digital inflation device
Digi-Flex
D.-F. exercise system
D.-F. finger exerciser
D.-F. hand exerciser
Digiflex
D. cannula
D. high-flow catheter
Digi-Grip hand exerciser
Digikit finger tourniquet
Digilab
D. FTS 40A spectrometer
D. perimeter
D. tonometer
Digirad
D. gamma camera
D. 2020tc imager
DigiScope
D. camera
Direx D.
D. handheld USB microscope
Digi-Sleeve pressure garment
digit
D. Aid splint
D. finger oximeter
d. splint
d. wrap
d. wrap adhesive flap
digital
d. acuity card
D. Add-On Bucky x-ray device
d. amorphous silicon flat-panel
detector
d. autofluoroscope
D. B system
d. calipers
d. cardiotachometer
d. constant-current pacing box
d. goniometer
d. holography system
d. imaging spectrophotometer

D

NOTES

digital *(continued)*
d. inflection rigidometer
d. OsteoView densitometer
D. Response HbA1c patient monitor
d. selenium-based chest imaging system
d. slide scanner
d. slit-lamp imager
d. stadiometer
D. Traumex system
d. voltmeter
d. x-ray detector
digital-to-analog converter
Digit-grip device
Digitimer pattern reversal stimulator
digitizer
BitPad d.
Cyberscanner 3-D d.
Cyberware Cyberscanner 3-D d.
3-dimensional sonic d.
Hough-Powell d.
laser d.
Metrecom d.
optical d.
Pixsys FlashPoint d.
Polhemus Liberty 3D d.
Scanmaster D, DX x-ray film d.
Digitrace home computer
DigiTrace sleep/EEG monitoring syringe
Digitrapper
D. III EGG recorder
D. Mark III sleep monitor
D. Mark II pH recorder
Synthetics dual-channel, solid-state D.
Digitron
D. dialysis chair scale
D. digital subtraction imaging system
D. DVI/DSA computer
Dignity
D. Plus briefmates guard
D. Plus briefmates pad
D. Plus liner
D. Plus regular pant
D. Plus underpad
Dilamezinsert
D. dilator
D. inserter
D. penile prosthesis
D. surgical instrument
Dilapan laminaria
Dilapan-S hygroscopic cervical dilator
Dilaprobe dilator
dilatation catheter
dilating
d. bougie
d. bulb

d. forceps
d. pressure balloon catheter
d. probe
dilator
achalasia d.
Achiever balloon d.
Ackrad Cervicet d.
Alm d.
Ambler d.
American Endoscopy d.
American Hanks uterine d.
Amplatz fascial d.
anal d.
Anthony quadrisected d.
argon vessel d.
Arnott d.
Atlee uterine d.
Avenida d.
Avenida-Torres d.
Backhaus d.
Bailey d.
Bakes bile duct d.
Bakes common duct d.
Bakes-Pearce d.
balloon d.
Bard urethral d.
Barnes cervical d.
Barnes common duct d.
Beardsley aortic d.
Béniqué d.
Bennett common duct d.
Berens punctum d.
biliary duct balloon d.
bisected minigraft d.
Black-Wylie obstetric d.
bladder d.
2-bladed d.
Bonney cervical d.
Bossi cervical d.
bougie d.
Bowman lacrimal d.
Bozeman d.
Braasch ureteral d.
Bransford-Lewis ureteral d.
Brock cardiac d.
bronchial d.
Brown-Buerger d.
Brown-McHardy pneumatic d.
Broyles esophageal d.
canaliculus d.
cardioesophageal junction d.
cardiospasm d.
Castroviejo-Galezowski d.
Castroviejo lacrimal d.
Catalano d.
d. catheter
Celestin graduated d.
cervical d.
Chevalier Jackson d.

child rectal d.
Clarke common duct d.
common bile duct d.
Cook Amplatz d.
Cooley coronary d.
Cooley pediatric d.
Cooley valve d.
Cooley vascular d.
Cordis d.
coronary d.
Creevy urethral d.
Cunningham-Cotton sleeve
  coaxial d.
Dagger d.
DeBakey-Cooley valve d.
DeBakey vascular d.
Delclos d.
Denniston d.
Derra cardiac valve d.
de Signeux d.
Desjardins d.
Desmarres paracentesis needle d.
Diaflex d.
Dick cardiac valve d.
Dilamezinsert d.
Dilapan-S hygroscopic cervical d.
Dilaprobe d.
disposable cervical d.
Dittel uterine d.
Dotter d.
double-ended d.
Dourmashkin d.
duct d.
Eder-Puestow esophageal d.
Einhorn esophageal d.
Eliminator PET biliary balloon d.
Encapsulon vessel d.
ERCP d.
esophageal balloon d.
expandable cervical d.
expansile d.
Falope-ring d.
fascial d.
Feldbausch nasal d.
Fenton uterine d.
Ferris biliary duct d.
Ferris filiform d.
fixed cervical d.
fluoroscopy-guided balloon d.
French lacrimal d.
frontal sinus d.
Galezowski lacrimal d.

gall duct d.
gallstone d.
Garrett d.
Gerbode mitral valvulotomy d.
Gillquist-Oretorp-Stille d.
Glover modification of Brock
  aortic d.
Gohrbrand cardiac d.
Goodell uterine d.
Gouley d.
Grüntzig balloon d.
Guyon d.
Hanks-Bradley uterine d.
Hanks uterine d.
Hayman d.
Hearst d.
Heath punctum d.
Hegar double-ended d.
Hegar-Goodell d.
Hegar rectal d.
Hegar uterine d.
Henley d.
Henning cardiac d.
Heyner d.
Hiebert vascular d.
Hohn vessel d.
Hopkins d.
Hosford double-ended lacrimal d.
House lacrimal d.
Hurst bullet-tip esophageal d.
Hurst-Maloney d.
Hurst mercury-filled d.
Hurst-Tucker pneumatic d.
Hurtig d.
hydrophilic d.
hydrostatic d.
Iglesias d.
implant site d.
incision d.
infant d.
Ivinsco cervical d.
Jackson bronchial d.
Jackson esophageal d.
Jackson-Mosher cardiospasm d.
Jackson-Plummer d.
Jackson tracheal d.
Jackson triangular brass d.
Jackson-Trousseau d.
Jewett uterine d.
Johnston infant d.
Jolly uterine d.
Jones lacrimal canaliculus d.

D

NOTES

dilator *(continued)*
Jones punctum d.
Jordan wire loop d.
Kahn uterine d.
Kearns bladder d.
Kelly orifice d.
Kelly sphincter d.
Kelly uterine d.
Keuch pupil d.
KeyMed d.
Kleegman d.
Kohlman urethral d.
K-Pratt d.
Krol esophageal d.
Krol-Koski tracheal d.
Kron bile duct d.
Laborde tracheal d.
lacrimal canaliculus d.
laminaria seaweed obstetrical
  cervical d.
Landau d.
laryngeal d.
Laufe cervical d.
Leader-Kohlman d.
LeFort d.
LeMaitre-Bookwalter d.
Lucchese mitral valve d.
Mahoney d.
Mahorner d.
Maloney-Hurst d.
Maloney mercury-filled
  esophageal d.
Maloney tapered-tip d.
mandrin d.
Mantz rectal d.
Marax d.
Marritt d.
McCrea d.
meatal d.
Medi-Tech fascial d.
mercury-filled d.
mercury-weighted d.
Microvasive controlled radial
  expansion esophageal d.
Microvasive Rigiflex balloon d.
Miller d.
mitral valve d.
Moersch cardiospasm d.
Mosher d.
Murphy common duct d.
myocardial d.
nasal d.
Nettleship canaliculus d.
Nettleship-Wilder lacrimal d.
Nottingham One-Step tapered d.
Nottingham ureteral d.
Olbert balloon d.
olive-tipped d.
Optilume prostate balloon d.

Otis bougie à boule d.
Ottenheimer common duct d.
Outerbridge uterine d.
over-the-endoscope Witzel d.
over-the-guidewire esophageal d.
Palmer uterine d.
Parsonnet d.
Patton esophageal d.
pediatric rectal d.
Percor d.
Pharmaseal disposable cervical d.
Phillips d.
Pilling d.
Plummer-Vinson esophageal d.
Plummer water-filled pneumatic
  esophageal d.
pneumatic balloon d.
pneumostatic d.
polyvinyl d.
Porges Neoflex d.
Potts expansile d.
Potts-Riker d.
Pratt rectal d.
Pratt uterine d.
d. probe
probe d.
progressive d.'s
Puestow d.
punctal d.
punctum d.
pupil d.
pyloric stenosis d.
quadrisected minigraft d.
Quantum TTC biliary balloon d.
Ramstedt pyloric stenosis d.
Ravich ureteral d.
rectal d.
Reich-Nechtow d.
Richards-Moeller pneumatic air-
  filled d.
Rider-Moeller d.
Rigiflex achalasia balloon d.
Ritter meatal d.
Rockert d.
Roland d.
Rolf punctum d.
Royal Hospital d.
Rubbs aortic d.
Ruedemann lacrimal d.
Russell hydrostatic d.
Russell peel-away sheath d.
Saint Mark d.
Savary esophageal d.
Savary-Gilliard esophageal d.
Savary-Gilliard metal olive-tipped d.
Savary-Gilliard over-the-wire d.
Savary tapered thermoplastic d.
Scanlan vessel d.
Simpson lacrimal d.

Simpson uterine d.
Sims uterine d.
Sinexon d.
sinus d.
Sippy esophageal d.
Sisler punctum d.
Smedberg d.
Soehendra rotary d.
sphincter d.
Spielberg d.
stapes d.
Starck d.
Starlinger uterine d.
Steele bronchial d.
Stille uterine d.
synthetic hygroscopic cervical d.
Szulc vascular d.
Taylor pulmonary d.
Theobald lacrimal d.
through-the-scope balloon d.
tracheal d.
tracheoesophageal puncture d.
transventricular d.
Trousseau-Jackson esophageal d.
Trousseau-Jackson tracheal d.
Trousseau tracheal d.
Tubbs aortic d.
Tubbs mitral valve d.
Tubbs two-bladed d.
Tucker cardiospasm d.
urethral female d.
urethral male d.
urethral meatal d.
uterine d.
vaginal d.
valve d.
Van Buren d.
Vantec d.
vascular d.
vein d.
vessel d.
Wales rectal d.
Walther urethral d.
Weiss gold d.
Whylie uterine d.
Wilder lacrimal d.
Williams lacrimal d.
wire-guided oval intracostal d.
wire loop stapes d.
Wise d.
Wylie uterine d.
Young pediatric rectal d.

Young vaginal d.
Ziegler lacrimal d.
Zipser meatal d.
dilator-sheath system
Dimaq integrated ultrasound system
Dimension
    D. hip prosthesis
    D. hip system
2-dimensional
    2-d. MRA slab
    2-d. ultrasound machine
3-dimensional
    3-d. biocompatible scaffold
    3-d. fast spin-echo magnetic
      resonance imaging
    3-d. fast spin-echo magnetic
      resonance imaging
    3-d. GDC
    3-d. Guglielmi detachable coil
    3-d. laparoscope
    3-d. magnetic sensor
    3-d. MRA slab
    3-d. sonic digitizer
    3-d. SPECT phantom
    3-d. Viewnix software system
Dimension-C femoral stem prosthesis
Dimisil gel sheeting
Dimitry
    D. chalazion trephine
    D. dacryocystorhinostomy trephine
    D. erysiphake
Dinamap
    D. automated blood pressure device
    D. blood pressure cuff
    D. Plus vital signs monitor
    D. Pro 100 vital signs monitor
    D. ultrasound blood pressure
      manometer
Dine
    D. digital scanner
    D. SLR digital camera
Dingman
    D. abrader
    D. bone-holding forceps
    D. breast dissector
    D. cartilage clamp
    D. cheek blade
    D. flexible retractor
    D. Flexsteel retractor
    D. malleable passing needle
    D. mouthgag
    D. oral retraction system

D

NOTES

Dingman *(continued)*
> D. osteotome
> D. otoabrader
> D. periosteal elevator
> D. sagittal bone clamp
> D. small bone clamp
> D. wire passer
> D. zygoma elevator
> D. zygomatic hook

Dingman-Denhardt mouthgag
diode
> Apogee 100 long pulse d.
> d. detector
> d. endolaser
> infrared light-emitting d.
> laser d.
> light-emitting d. (LED)
> Microlase transpupillary d.
> Pin d.
> positive-intrinsic-negative d.
> d. pumped Nd:YAG laser
> Zener d.

DioLite 532 laser
Diomed surgical diode laser
Dionex 450 Data System amperometric detector
DioPexy probe
diopsimeter
diopter
> d. lens
> d. prism

Dioptimum system
diploscope
dipstick
> Fyodorov d.
> Kelman d.
> Knolle d.
> Rapid One Ecstasy d.
> Rapid One OXY d.

direct
> d. current generator
> d. digital x-ray detector
> d. electrical nerve stimulator
> d. forward-vision telescope
> d. gonioscopic lens
> d. laryngoscope
> D. Optical Research Company (DORC)
> d. retainer
> d. vision spectroscope

direct-current bone growth stimulator
DirectFlow arterial cannula
directional
> d. atherectomy catheter
> d. coronary atherectomy device

director
> Brodie d.
> Brodie fistula d.
> Doyen d.

> Dr. Quickert d.
> grooved d.
> D. Guidewire system
> Kocher goiter d.
> Kocher grooved d.
> Koenig grooved d.
> Larry rectal d.
> laser fiber d.
> Leksell grooved d.
> ligature d.
> Ormco ligature d.
> Payr grooved d.
> plain-end grooved d.
> Pratt rectal d.
> probe-ended grooved d.
> Putti-Platt d.
> Stiwer grooved d.
> Toennis d.
> ultrasonic flow d.

DirectRay direct-to-digital x-ray capture device
DirectView CR 900 imaging system
direct-vision
> d.-v. adenotome
> d.-v. prism
> d.-v. telescope

Direx
> D. digiscope
> D. Tripter lithotripter
> D. Tripter X-1 lithotripter

disarticulation chisel
DISA S-Flex coronary stent
DISC
> dynamic integrated stabilization chair

disc, disk
> AcroFlex artificial d.
> concave skull d.
> d. curette
> Double-hesive adhesive d.
> Eigon d.
> d. electrode
> d. endoscope
> d. forceps
> Horico d.
> Krupin eye d.
> d. lens intraocular lens
> Molnar d.
> Moore d.
> Moran-Karaya d.
> d. oxygenator
> Placido da Costa d.
> planoconvex d.
> Prodisc prosthetic lumbar d.
> d. rongeur
> Tracho-Foam adhesive d.

Disc-Criminator
> Mackinnon-Dellon D.-C.

discectomy forceps
DisCide disinfecting towel

discission
    d. blade
    d. knife
    d. needle
Discofix stopcock
discographic needle
disconnect wedge
discoscope
    percutaneous d.
Disc-O-Sit Jr. cushion
Discover
    D. cryotherapy compress
    D. Cryo-Therapy unit
Discovery
    D. DDDR pacemaker
    D. elbow prosthesis
    D. handheld spirometer
    D. LS fusion imaging
    D. PET/CT imaging system
    D. QDR bone densitometer
Discrene breast form
discriminator
    EMI Aped amplifier d.
    2-point d.
    Sweet two-point d.
disease
    thromboembolic d. (TED)
Disetronic infuser syringe pump
dish
    insemination d.
    Lux culture d.
    panning d.
    Petri d.
    scoop d.
    Side-Fire reflecting d.
    Uri-Two petri d.
disimpaction forceps
DisIntek reagent strip
disk (*var. of* disc)
Diskard head halter
Disk-Criminator
    D.-C. discrimination instrument
    D.-C. nerve stimulation measuring
      device
Diskhaler inhaler
diskoscope
dislocator
    Kirby lens d.
dislodger
    Cook helical stone d.
    Creevy calyx stone d.
    Davis loop stone d.

    Dormia ureteral stone d.
    Ellik loop stone d.
    Evans loop stone d.
    filiform stone d.
    Gibson stone d.
    Howard-Flaherty spiral stone d.
    Howard spiral stone d.
    Jimmy d.
    Johnson stone d.
    Levant stone d.
    Mitchell ureteral stone d.
    Morton stone d.
    Ortved stone d.
    Pfister-Schwartz stone d.
    Porges stone d.
    Robinson stone d.
    spiral stone d.
    stone d.
    Storz stone d.
    Tessier d.
    ureteral basket stone d.
    Wullen stone d.
Dispatch
    D. balloon
    D. balloon catheter
    D. infusion catheter
dispenser
    Baxa oral d.
    DropTainer d.
    Exacta-Med oral d.
    Jet Vac cement d.
    Metron Plus d.
    PressPak d.
Dispenstir device
Dispersalloy dental amalgam
dispersing
    d. electrode
    d. lens
displacement sensing device
display
    virtual reality head-mounted d.
    virtual retinal d.
disposable
    d. acupuncture needle
    d. airway kit
    d. aortic rotating punch
    d. aspiration needle
    d. biopsy forceps
    d. biopsy needle
    d. cannula
    d. cautery
    d. cervical dilator

D

NOTES

disposable *(continued)*
- d. coaxial Endostat
- d. concentric needle
- d. cystotome cannula
- d. cytology brush
- d. Doppler-constant thermocouple sensor
- d. drape
- d. drape clamp
- d. electrode pad
- d. forceps
- d. head halter
- d. injection needle
- d. inner cannula (DIC)
- d. iris retractor
- d. measuring guide
- d. microclamp
- d. muscle biopsy clamp
- d. nasal speculum
- d. ocutome
- d. one-piece osteotome
- d. PD-10 column
- d. perforator
- d. probe
- d. scalpel
- d. scissors
- d. sculptured Endostat
- d. sheathed flexible sigmoidoscope
- d. skin stapler
- d. Styrofoam block
- d. surface EMG electrode
- d. surgical electrode
- d. suturing needle
- d. trephine
- d. trocar
- d. TUR drape
- d. Yankauer aspirating tube
- d. Yankauer suction tube

disposable-sheath flexible gastroscope
Disposa-Hood disposable infant oxygen hood
Dispos-a-ject microinjection system
Dispo-sand device
Disposashielf sheath
Dispos-a-trode disposable electrode
Dispos-A-Ture single-use surgical needle
dissecting
- d. chisel
- d. clamp
- d. diathermy forceps
- d. forceps
- d. hook
- d. probe
- d. scissors

dissection
- d. forceps
- d. knife
- d. probe
- d. scissors

dissector
- Adson d.
- Agris-Dingman submammary d.
- Allerdyce d.
- Allis dry d.
- aneurysm neck d.
- Angell-James d.
- Aspiradeps d.
- aspirating d.
- ASSI breast d.
- attic d.
- Aufranc d.
- Austin attic d.
- ball d.
- balloon d.
- Barraquer corneal d.
- bat-wing d.
- Beaver d.
- Berens corneal d.
- Brunner goiter d.
- Butte d.
- Carpenter d.
- Castroviejo corneal d.
- Cavitron d.
- channel d.
- Cherry Secto d.
- Cheyne d.
- Codman Rhoton d.
- Collin pleural d.
- Colver tonsillar d.
- corneal d.
- cottonoid d.
- Crabtree attic d.
- Creed d.
- Crile gasserian ganglion d.
- Davis d.
- Daya double-ended lamellar d.
- Desmarres corneal d.
- Desmarres eye d.
- Dingman breast d.
- dolphin-nose monopolar electrosurgical d.
- double-ended d.
- double-ended lamellar d.
- Doyen rib d.
- ear d.
- Effler double-ended d.
- Effler-Groves d.
- endarterectomy d.
- Endo-Assist cutting d.
- Endo Dissect d.
- Endo-Right Angle d.
- endoscopic d.
- facial nerve d.
- Falcao suction d.
- Feild suction d.
- Fisher tonsillar d.
- flap knife d.
- Freer d.

Freer dural d.
Fukushima d.
Fukushima-Giannotta d.
goiter d.
Gorney d.
Green corneal d.
Haines arachnoid d.
Hajek-Ballenger septal d.
Hamrick suction d.
Hardy pituitary d.
Harris d.
Hartmann tonsillar d.
Heath trephine flap d.
Henke tonsillar d.
Herczel d.
Hitselberger-McElveen neural d.
Holinger laryngeal d.
Hood d.
hook d.
House d.
House-Crabtree d.
House-Urban vacuum rotary d.
Hunt arachnoid d.
Hurd-Morrison d.
Hurd tonsillar d.
Hurd-Weder tonsillar d.
hydrostatic d.
Inaba and Ezaki d.
Israel tonsillar d.
Jackson-Pratt d.
Jannetta aneurysm neck d.
Jazbi tonsillar d.
Jimmy d.
joker d.
Judet d.
Kennerdell-Maroon d.
Killian d.
King-Hurd tonsillar d.
Kittner d.
Kleinert-Kutz d.
knife d.
d. knife
Kocher goiter d.
Kocher periosteal d.
Kurze d.
Kuttner d.
laminar d.
Lane d.
Lang d.
laryngeal d.
Lemmon intimal d.
Lewin bunion d.

Lewin sesamoidectomy d.
Logan d.
Lopez-Reinke tonsillar d.
Lothrop d.
Luetje stimulating d.
Lynch blunt d.
Lynch laryngeal d.
Lynch tonsillar d.
MacAusland d.
MacDonald d.
Madden d.
Malis d.
Manhattan Eye & Ear corneal d.
Maroon-Jannetta d.
Martinez double-ended corneal d.
Maryland monopolar
  electrosurgical d.
Mason tonsil suction d.
McCabe facial nerve d.
McCabe flap knife d.
McDonald d.
McElveen-Hitselberger neural d.
McWhinnie tonsillar d.
Meeker monopolar electrosurgical d.
Milette-Tyding d.
Miller tonsillar d.
Milligan double-ended d.
Mixter d.
Molt d.
Moorehead d.
Morrison-Hurd tonsillar d.
Mulligan d.
needle d.
Neivert d.
nerve root laminectomy d.
neural d.
neurosurgical d.
Niblitt d.
Oldberg d.
Olivecrona d.
Olivecrona-Stille d.
olive-tipped monopolar
  electrosurgical d.
Paton corneal d.
Peanut Secto d.
Penfield d.
Pennington septal d.
Pierce submucous d.
pleural d.
Polaris reusable d.
Potts d.
prostatic d.

D

NOTES

dissector *(continued)*
    Ramirez EndoFaceLift d.
    Raney d.
    Reinhoff d.
    Resposable Spacemaker surgical
      balloon d.
    Rhode Island Secto d.
    Rhoton ball d.
    Rhoton round d.
    Rhoton spatula d.
    Rochester laminar d.
    Roger submucous d.
    Rosebud d.
    Rosen d.
    rotary d.
    round d.
    Ruddy d.
    Sachs-Freer d.
    SaphFinder surgical balloon d.
    SAPHtrak balloon d.
    Schmieden-Taylor d.
    Secto d.
    Sens d.
    septal d.
    sesamoidectomy d.
    Sheldon-Pudenz d.
    Silverstein arachnoid d.
    Silverstein auditory canal d.
    Sloan goiter flap d.
    Smith tonsillar d.
    Smithwick nerve d.
    Spacemaker breast balloon d.
    Spacemaker hernia balloon d.
    spatula d.
    Spetzler d.
    sponge d.
    spud d.
    square-tipped arterial d.
    Stallard blunt d.
    Stiwer tendon d.
    Stolte tonsillar d.
    straight monopolar electrosurgical d.
    submammary d.
    submucous d.
    suction d.
    synovial d.
    teardrop d.
    Toennis d.
    Toennis-Adson d.
    Toledo d.
    tonsil d.
    Touma d.
    transsphenoidal d.
    Troutman corneal d.
    Troutman nonincisional lamellar d.
    Troutman wave-edge corneal d.
    Truszkowski dural d.
    ultrasonic d.
    vascular d.

    walker suction tonsillar d.
    Wangensteen d.
    Watson-Cheyne dry d.
    Weder d.
    West blunt d.
    West hand d.
    West plastic d.
    Wieder tonsillar d.
    Woodson double-ended d.
    Wynne-Evans tonsillar d.
    Yasargil d.
    Yoshida tonsillar d.
    Young urological d.
Dissectron ultrasonic aspirator
Distaflex
    D. balloon
    D. dental attachment
Distaflo bypass graft
distal
    d. femoral cutting guide
    d. locking screw
    d. over-shoulder strap
    d. perfusion system10000
    d. radioulnar joint (DRUJ)
    d. radioulnar joint prosthesis
    d. shocking coil
    d. stimulation generator
    d. targeting device
distending obturator
Disten-U-Flo fluid system
distometer
    Haag-Streit d.
distraction
    d. bar
    d. clamp
    d. device
    d. hook
    d. instrumentation
    d. pin
    rigid external d. (RED)
    d. rod
    d. screw
distractor
    Ace/Normed bidirectional d.
    Ace OsteoGenic d.
    Anderson d.
    AO femoral d.
    ArthroDistractor d.
    Beckman d.
    bidirectional telescopic d.
    Bliskunov implantable femoral d.
    Caspar d.
    DeBastiani d.
    femoral d.
    hip d.
    hook d.
    Ilizarov d.
    intramedullary skeletal kinetic d.
      (ISKD)

Kaneda d.
Kessler metacarpal d.
Mark II distal femur d.
Molina mandibular d.
Monticelli-Spinelli d.
multidirectional d.
MultiGuide mandibular d.
multiplanar mandibular d.
Orthofix M-100 d.
d. pin
Pinto d.
telescopic d.
turnbuckle d.
Zurich pediatric maxillary d.
Dittel
D. dilating urethral bougie
D. urethral sound
D. uterine dilator
D. uterine sound
Dittrich plug
DIVA laparoscopic morcellator
divergent outlet forceps
diverging collimator
diversion stent
diverticuloscope
Holinger-Benjamin laser d.
DIV laparoscopic morcellator device
Dix
D. double-ended instrument
D. eye spud
D. foreign body spud
D. gouge
D. needle
D. spud probe
Dixey spatula
Dixon
D. blade
D. center-blade retractor
D. collar scissors
D. flamingo forceps
DK 201 cryotherapy wrap
DLP
DLP aortic root cannula
DLP cardiac sling
DLP cardioplegic catheter
DLP cardioplegic needle
DLP infant ventricular catheter
DLP left atrial pressure monitoring catheter
DLP pericardial sump
DM-400 tape Holter recorder
DMetrix digital slide scanner

DMR2 disposable manual resuscitator
DMV contact lens remover
DN acupuncture needle
Dobbhoff
D. biliary stent
D. bipolar coagulation probe
D. gastrectomy feeding tube
D. gastric decompression tube
D. G/J system
D. nasogastric feeding tube
D. PEG tube
DOBI
Dynamic Optical Breast Imaging
DOBI breast cancer diagnostic system
DOC
dynamic orthotic cranioplasty
DOC band
DOC guidewire extension
Dockhorn retractor
docking needle
Docktor
D. needle
D. suture
D. tissue forceps
Doc's Proplug earplug
Doctor
D. Collins fracture clamp
D. Long clamp
D. Plymale lift fracture frame
Docustar fundus camera
Dodd perforator
Dodick
D. laser Photolysis system
D. lens-holding forceps
D. nucleus cracker
D. Nucleus Cracker forceps
Doesel-Huzly
D.-H. bronchoscope
D.-H. bronchoscopic tube
Dogbone ACFS
Doherty
D. sphere
D. spherical eye implant
Dohlman
D. endoscope
D. esophagoscope
D. incus hook
D. plug
DoLi S lithotripter
dolorimeter
Chatillon d.

D

NOTES

Dolphin
> D. cord clamp
> D. device
> D. II fluid management system

dolphin-nose
> d.-n. dissecting forceps
> d.-n. grasping forceps
> d.-n. monopolar electrosurgical
> dissector

Dolwick-Reich diamond rasp

dome
> d. colpostat
> d. hole plug
> d. hole plug grommet
> d. plunger
> D. wand

Donald
> D. clamp
> D. vulsellum

Donaldson
> D. drain tube
> D. eustachian tube
> D. eye patch
> D. fundus camera
> D. myringotomy tube
> D. ventilation tube

Donate-A-Gel impregnated gauze hydrogel dressing

DonJoy
> D. ALP ankle brace
> D. Defiance CI brace
> D. Goldpoint hinged knee brace
> D. knee splint
> D. Legend ACL knee brace
> D. 4-point ACL Super Sport knee brace

Donnez endometrial ablation device

Donnheim
> D. implant
> D. lens

Dontrix
> D. gouge
> D. intraoral gauge

Dopcord recorder

Doppler
> Acuson color D.
> Aloka 2000 color D.
> D. 4-beam laser probe
> D. blood flow monitor
> CardioBeat vascular D.
> Carolina color spectrum CW D.
> D. Cavin monitor
> color spectrum CW D.
> convergent color D.
> D. coronary catheter
> 2D D.
> D. device
> Dopplette D.
> Dopplex fetal D.

> Elite vascular D.
> FetalPulse Plus fetal D.
> D. fetal stethoscope
> D. flow echocardiographic probe
> D. FloWire guidewire
> FreeDop cordless D.
> Hadeco ES100VX mini D.
> Hadeco intraoperative D.
> Hadeco MiniDop D.
> Haemoson ultrasound D.
> Imex Pocket-Dop OB D.
> IntraDop intraoperative D.
> D. laser velocimeter
> Medasonics transcranial D.
> Minidop ES-100VX Pocket D.
> Mizuho surgical D.
> Multi Dopplex II D.
> Neuroguard transcranial D.
> Nicolet Elite obstetrical D.
> penile D.
> pulsed D.
> pulsed-range gated D.
> pulse wave D.
> D. Quantum color flow system
> Siemens Quantum 2000 Color D.
> Smartdop D.
> spectral D.
> D. transesophageal color flow
> imaging
> Ultrascope obstetrical D.
> D. ultrasonic fetal heart monitor
> D. ultrasonic flowmeter
> D. ultrasonic probe
> D. ultrasound
> D. ultrasound stethoscope

Doppler-tipped angioplasty guidewire

Dopplette Doppler

Dopplex fetal Doppler

Doptone
> D. fetal monitor
> D. fetal pulse detector
> D. fetal stethoscope
> D. ultrasound

DORC
> Direct Optical Research Company
> DORC diathermy system
> DORC fast freeze cryosurgical
> system
> DORC microforceps
> DORC microscissors
> DORC surgical instrument
> DORC vitreous shaver

Doriot handpiece

Dormed cranial electrotherapy stimulator

Dormia
> D. biliary stone basket
> D. extracorporeal shockwave
> lithotripsy system

D. gallstone basket
D. gallstone lithotripter
D. stone basket catheter
D. ureteral stone basket
D. ureteral stone dislodger
D. waterbath lithotripter

Dornier
D. compact lithotripter
D. Compact S lithotripter
D. Epos Ultra lithotripter
D. extracorporeal shock wave lithotripter
D. HM-series lithotripter
D. Medilas H holmium:YAG laser
D. MPL 9000 gallstone lithotripter
D. scanner
D. Urotract cysto table

Dorros
D. brachial internal mammary guiding catheter
D. infusion/probing catheter

dorsal
d. columellar implant
d. column stimulator
d. scissors
d. wrist splint

Dorsey
D. cervical foraminal punch
D. dural separator
D. forceps
D. irrigation tubing
D. needle
D. nerve root retractor
D. screwdriver
D. spatula
D. tongue depressor
D. transorbital leukotome
D. ventricular cannula

Dorsiwedge night splint
dose
targeted d. (TD)

Dosick
D. bellows assembly
D. tunneler

dosimeter
dichromate d.
Gardray d.
LiF thermoluminescence d.
Rosenthal-French nebulization d.
silicone diode d.
single-channel in vivo light d.

thermoluminescent d.
Victoreen d.

dosimetrist radiation beam monitor
Dos Santos lumbar aortography needle
dot-plotted probe
Dott
D. mouthgag
D. retractor

Dott-Dingman self-retaining cleft palate gag
Dotter
D. catheter
D. coaxial catheter
D. dilator
D. intravascular retriever set

Dott-Kilner mouthgag
Doubilet sphincterotome
double-action
d.-a. bone-cutting forceps
d.-a. forceps
d.-a. plate cutter
d.-a. rongeur

double-angled
d.-a. blade
d.-a. blade plate
d.-a. clamp

double-armed suture
double-articulated
d.-a. bronchoscopic forceps
d.-a. forceps tip

double-balloon perfusion catheter
double-barreled
d.-b. irrigating-aspirating cannula
d.-b. needle

double-bent Hohmann acetabular retractor
double-cannula tracheostomy tube
double-catheterizing
d.-c. sheath and obturator
d.-c. telescope

double-channel
d.-c. endoscope
d.-c. irrigating bronchoscope
d.-c. operating sheath
d.-c. sphincterotome
d.-c. videoendoscope

double-cuff urinary sphincter
double-cupped forceps
double-current catheter
double-dome reservoir
double-edged sickle knife

D

NOTES

267

double-ended
- d.-e. bone curette
- d.-e. chrome probe
- d.-e. dental curette
- d.-e. dilator
- d.-e. dissector
- d.-e. flap knife
- d.-e. forceps
- d.-e. lamellar dissector
- d.-e. nail
- d.-e. needle forceps
- d.-e. nickelene probe
- d.-e. retractor
- d.-e. root tip dental pick
- d.-e. silver probe
- d.-e. stapes curette
- d.-e. suture forceps
- d.-e. tissue forceps

double-fixation forceps
double-focus tube
double-guarded chisel
double-headed
- d.-h. P190 stapling device
- d.-h. stereotactic carrier

Double-hesive adhesive disc
double-hinge cervical retractor handle
double-hub emulsifying needle
double-J
- d.-J dangle stent
- d.-J indwelling catheter
- d.-J indwelling catheter stent
- d.-J silicone internal ureteral catheter stent
- d.-J stent
- d.-J ureteral catheter
- d.-J ureteral stent

double-L spinal rod
double-lumen
- d.-l. balloon stone extractor catheter
- d.-l. breast implant
- d.-l. cannula
- d.-l. catheter
- d.-l. central venous catheter
- d.-l. curette
- d.-l. endobronchial tube
- d.-l. endoprosthesis
- d.-l. endotracheal tube
- d.-l. gastric laryngeal mask airway
- d.-l. injection catheter
- d.-l. irrigation cannula
- d.-l. needle
- d.-l. Silastic catheter
- d.-l. subclavian catheter
- d.-l. Swan-Ganz catheter
- d.-l. tapered-tip papillotome
- d.-l. wire-guided papillotome

double-pigtail
- d.-p. endoprosthesis
- d.-p. prosthesis
- d.-p. ureteral stent

double-plate Molteno implant
double-pronged
- d.-p. Cottle hook
- d.-p. Fomon hook
- d.-p. forceps
- d.-p. fork
- d.-p. ligature carrier
- d.-p. pick

double-ring frame
double-rod construct
double-running penetrating keratoplasty suture
double-spoon
- d.-s. biopsy forceps
- d.-s. forceps

double-stem implant
DoubleStent biliary endoprosthesis
doublet
- Wollaston d.

double-tenaculum hook
double-tooth tenaculum
double-vector
- d.-v. blade
- d.-v. brain spatula

double-velour knitted graft
double-walled incubator
Dougherty anterior chamber cannula
doughnut
- d. headrest
- d. magnet
- d. pessary
- d. tip suction tube
- d. transformer

doughnut-shaped balloon
Douglas
- D. antrum trocar
- D. bag
- D. bag spirometer
- D. cannula
- D. ciliary forceps
- D. eye dressing
- D. eye forceps
- D. graft
- D. measuring plate pelvimeter
- D. mucosal speculum
- D. nasal scissors
- D. nasal snare
- D. nasal trocar
- D. suture needle
- D. tonsillar knife
- D. tonsillar snare

Dourmashkin
- D. dilator
- D. tunneled bougie

Douvas
- D. rotoextractor

D. Roto-extractor extractor
D. vitreous cutter
Dover
D. abdominal belt
D. midstream urine collection kit
D. Premium teflon-coated latex
Foley catheter
D. Texas disposable male catheter
dovetail stress broken abutment
Dow
D. Corning antifoam agent dressing
D. Corning cannula
D. Corning external breast form
D. Corning hollow-fiber analyzer
D. Corning ileal pouch catheter
D. Corning implant
dowel
d. cutter
d. grip
Thompson d.
threaded cortical d.
Down
D. epiphyseal knife
D. flow generator
D. hand dermatome
down-biting Epstein curette
Downes
D. cautery
D. lid clamp
D. nasal speculum
Downing
D. cartilage knife
D. cartilage scalpel
D. clamp
D. II laminectomy retractor
D. stapler
Down's continuous flow CPAP
Doyen
D. abdominal retractor
D. abdominal scissors
D. bone mallet
D. costal elevator
D. costal periosteotome
D. cylindrical bur
D. cylindrical drill
D. director
D. electrode
D. gallbladder forceps
D. intestinal clamp
D. intestinal clamp forceps
D. mouthgag
D. myoma screw

D. needle
D. needle holder
D. periosteal elevator
D. rib dissector
D. rib elevator
D. rib hook
D. rib rasp
D. rib raspatory
D. rib spreader
D. rib stripper
D. spatula
D. spherical bur
D. towel clamp
D. towel forceps
D. uterine forceps
D. uterine scissors
D. vaginal retractor
D. vaginal speculum
D. vulsellum forceps
Doyen-Collin mouthgag
Doyle
D. bi-valved airway splint
D. Combo nasal airway splint
D. ear dressing
D. II silicone stent
D. intranasal airway splint
D. Shark nasal splint
D. spacer splint
D. vein stripper
Dozier radiolucent Bennett retractor
Dr.
Dr. Bruecke aspirating tube
Dr. Gibaud thermal health support
Dr. Hays bite guard
Dr. Joseph's original footbrush
Dr. Kho's CMC Support
Dr. Quickert director
Dr. Scholl exercise sandal
Dr. Twiss duodenal tube
Dr. White trocar
Draeger
D. forceps
D. high-vacuum erysiphake
D. modified keratome
D. tonometer
Dräger
D. MTC transducer
D. respirometer
D. thermal gel mattress
D. ventilator
D. volumeter

D

NOTES

269

Dragstedt
    D. graft
    D. implant
drain
    Abramson sump d.
    accordion d.
    ACMI Pezzer d.
    Angle-Pezzer d.
    Axiom d.
    Baker continuous flow capillary d.
    Bardex d.
    Bardex-Bellini d.
    Bartkiewicz two-sided d.
    Blair silicone d.
    Blake silicone d.
    butterfly d.
    Chaffin-Pratt d.
    Charnley suction d.
    cigarette d.
    closed suction d.
    clothesline d.
    Codman lumbar external d.
    ConstaVac d.
    Craniovac d.
    CUI urological d.
    Cushman d.
    dam d.
    Davol suction d.
    Davol sump d.
    Deseret sump d.
    dual-sump silicone d.
    DuoDERM d.
    ERCP nasobiliary d.
    filtered dual-sump d.
    filtered mediastinal sump d.
    fluted d.
    fluted J-Vac d.
    Foley straight d.
    glove d.
    Gomco d.
    Guardian stoma irrigator d.
    Guibor lacrimal d.
    Hemaduct wound d.
    Hemovac Hydrocoat d.
    Hendrickson suprapubic d.
    Heyer-Robertson suprapubic d.
    Heyer-Schulte wound d.
    high-capacity silicone d.
    Hollister irrigator d.
    Hysto-vac d.
    intercostal d.
    Jackson-Pratt flat d.
    Jackson-Pratt Gold wound d.
    Jackson-Pratt Hemaduct d.
    Jackson-Pratt round PVC d.
    Jackson-Pratt silicone flat d.
    Jackson-Pratt silicone round d.
    Jackson-Pratt suction d.
    Jackson-Pratt T-tube d.

    J-Vac d.
    Keith d.
    Lahey d.
    large-volume round silicone d.
    latex d.
    Leydig d.
    Liguory endoscopic nasal biliary d.
    Malecot 2-wing d.
    Malecot 4-wing d.
    Mantisol d.
    Marion d.
    mediastinal d.
    Medpor coated tear d.
    Mikulicz d.
    Mikulicz-Radecki d.
    Monaldi d.
    Morris Silastic thoracic d.
    Mosher d.
    Nagaraja endoscopic nasal
      biliary d.
    nasobiliary d.
    nasocystic d.
    Nélaton rubber tube d.
    papilla d.
    pencil d.
    Penrose d.
    Penrose sump d.
    Pezzer d.
    Pharmaseal closed d.
    pigtail nephrostomy d.
    polyethylene d.
    polyvinyl d.
    PVC d.
    quarantine d.
    Ragnell d.
    Redivac suction d.
    Redon d.
    Relia-Vac d.
    Ritter suprapubic suction d.
    Robertson suprapubic d.
    rubber dam d.
    Sacks biliary d.
    Salem sump d.
    seton d.
    Shirley wound d.
    Silastic thoracic d.
    Silastic thyroid d.
    silicone hubless flat d.
    silicone round d.
    silicone sump d.
    silicone thoracic d.
    Snyder Hemovac silicone sump d.
    Sof-Wick d.
    Sovally suprapubic suction cup d.
    spaghetti d.
    stab-wound d.
    Steri-Vac d.
    stoma irrigator d.
    Stryker d.

subgaleal d.
suction d.
sump d.
Surgivac d.
Taut capillary d.
Teflon nasobiliary d.
thoracic d.
TLS suction d.
transnasal pancreaticobiliary d.
transpapillary d.
triple-lumen sump d.
T-tube d.
T-tube round suction d.
U-tube d.
Vacutainer d.
van Sonnenberg sump d.
Varidyne d.
Wangensteen d.
Waterman sump d.
water-seal d.
water-trap d.
whistle-tip d.
2-wing Malecot d.
4-wing Malecot d.
Wolf d.
wolffian d.
wound d.
Wylie d.
Y d.
Yeates d.
Younken double-lumen d.
drainage
    d. bag
    d. catheter
    percutaneous transhepatic biliary d.
    (PTBD)
    Snyder Surgivac d.
drain-to-wall suction tube
Drake
    D. fenestrated aneurysm clip
    D. tourniquet
    D. uroflowmeter
Drake-Kees clip
Drake-Willock
    D.-W. automatic delivery system
    D.-W. dialysis machine
drape
    adhesive plastic d.
    Alcon disposable d.
    AliMed surgical d.
    Auto-Band Steri-Drape d.
    Bard absorption d.

Barrier laparoscopy d.
Bioclusive d.
Blair head d.
Convertors surgical d.
disposable d.
disposable TUR d.
Eye-Pak d.
fenestrated sterile d.
Gator d.
Hough d.
Incise d.
Ioban antimicrobial incise d.
Johnson & Johnson Band-Aid
  sterile d.
Lingeman 3-in-1 procedure d.
Lingeman TUR d.
3M d.
3M small aperture Steri-Drape d.
NeuroDrape surgical d.
O'Connor d.
OPMI microscopic d.
Opraflex incise d.
OpSite d.
paper d.
plastic d.
Pro-Ophtha d.
Qualtex surgical d.
Richards d.
Rusch perineal d.
Secureline operating room
  camera d.
sewn-in waterproof d.
small aperture Steri-Drape d.
split d.
Steri-Drape 2 incise d.
sterile d.
surgical d.
Surgikos disposable d.
Surgi-Site Incise d.
Thompson d.
towel d.
Transelast surgical d.
transparent d.
Vi-Drape incise d.
Visidrape Mini Aperture d.
Visidrape Mini Incise d.
Visidrape ophthalmic d.
Visiflex d.
V. Mueller TUR d.
Zeiss OPMI d.
draw-over vaporizer
drawsheet

NOTES

Dream
  D. pillow
  D. Ride car seat
DreamSeal mask
Dremel Moto-tool
DressFlex orthotic
Dressinet tubular bandage
dressing
  absorbent cover d. (ACD)
  Ace-Hesive d.
  Ace longitudinal strips d.
  Acquacel Hydrofiber d.
  AcryDerm border island d.
  AcryDerm sheet wound d.
  AcryDerm Strands absorbent
    wound d.
  Acry Island border d.
  acrylic resin d.
  Acticoat composite d.
  Acticoat foam d.
  Acticoat silver-based burn d.
  Acu-Derm IV/TPN d.
  Acu-Derm wound d.
  Adaptic gauze d.
  Adaptic nonadhering d.
  Adaptic petroleum gauze d.
  Adaptic PG gauze d.
  Adaptic X Xeroform gauze
    nonadhering d.
  Ad-Hese-Away d.
  adhesive absorbent d.
  Aeroplast d.
  Airstrip composite d.
  AlgiDerm wound d.
  alginate wound d.
  AlgiSite alginate wound d.
  Algisorb wound d.
  Algosteril alginate d.
  Alldress multilayer wound d.
  Allevyn adhesive hydrocellular d.
  Allevyn cavity wound d.
  Allevyn hydrophilic polyurethane d.
  Allevyn island d.
  Allevyn polyurethane foam d.
  Allevyn tracheostomy d.
  antiseptic d.
  Aquacel Ag Hydrofiber wound d.
  Aquacel Hydrofiber wound d.
  Aquaflo hydrogel wound d.
  Aquaphor gauze d.
  Aquaplast tie-down d.
  Aquasorb Border hydrogel d.
  Aquasorb hydrogel d.
  Aquasorb transparent hydrogel d.
  Arglaes wound d.
  ArtAssist compression d.
  Aureomycin gauze d.
  Bactigras d.

Band-Aid sterile adhesive
  surgical d.
Bard absorption d.
Bard AlgiDerm d.
Barnes-Hind ophthalmic d.
barrel d.
Barton d.
Baynton d.
BD butterfly swab d.
BGC Matrix d.
bias-cut stockinette d.
Biatain foam d.
binocular eye d.
Biobrane biosynthetic d.
Biobrane/HF wound d.
Bioclusive MVP Select
  transparent d.
Biocol d.
BioCore collagen d.
Biodrape d.
Biolex wound cleanser d.
Biopatch antimicrobial d.
Bishop-Harman d.
Blenderm surgical tape d.
BlisterFilm transparent wound d.
blue sponge d.
bolus d.
Borsch d.
brassiere-type d.
BreakAway wound d.
Breast Vest Exu-Dry one-piece
  wound d.
bulky compressive d.
bulky hand d.
bulky pressure d.
Bunnell d.
Bunnell-Littler d.
Burn Jel d.
butterfly d.
calcium sodium alginate wound d.
Calgitrol d.
Carasyn hydrogel wound d.
CarboFlex odor-control d.
CarraFilm transparent film d.
CarraGauze d.
CarraSorb H wound d.
Carrasyn V viscous hydrogel
  wound d.
Castex rigid d.
Catrix wound d.
Cecil d.
cellophane d.
Chronicure wound d.
Cica-Care silicone gel sheet d.
Cikloid d.
CircPlus compression d.
Circulon d.
circumferential d.
Circumpress facelift d.

ClearSite bandage roll d.
ClearSite borderless d.
ClearSite HydroGauze d.
ClearSite hydrogel absorptive
  borderline wound d.
Clevis d.
Cliniguard protective d.
Coban elastic d.
cocoon d.
cod liver oil-soaked strips d.
Coe-Pak periodontal d.
Coe-Soft d.
cohesive d.
CollaCote collagen wound d.
collagen d.
CollaPlug wound d.
collar d.
CollaTape wound d.
collodion d.
Coloplast d.
CombiDerm nonadhesive
  absorbent d.
Comfeel hydrocolloid d.
Comfeel Plus pressure relief d.
Comfeel Purilon gel d.
Compeed Skinprotector d.
composite d.
compound d.
compression d.
Comprol d.
Conformant 2 wound d.
Contura medicated d.
CoolSorb absorbent cold transfer d.
Cornish wool d.
CoSeal d.
CoSeal liquid plastic d.
CoStasis d.
cotton-ball d.
cotton bolster d.
cotton elastic d.
cotton pledget d.
cotton-wadding d.
Covaderm Plus adhesive barrier d.
Covaderm Plus tube site d.
Covaderm Plus VAD d.
Covaderm Plus vascular access d.
Coverlet OR adhesive surgical d.
Coverlet Strips adhesive d.
Cover-Pad d.
Cover-Roll d.
Covertell composite secondary d.
CovRSite d.

Co-Wrap d.
crepe bandage d.
Crinotene d.
Cruricast d.
Cryo/Cuff knee compression d.
Curaderm hydrocolloid d.
Curad surgical adhesive d.
Curafil hydrogel wound d.
Curafoam Plus island d.
Curagel hydrogel island d.
Curasol gel sterile wound d.
Curasorb calcium alginate d.
Curity d.
Curon d.
Cutifilm Plus waterproof wound d.
Cutinova alginate d.
Cutinova cavity foam d.
Cutinova hydroactive d.
Cutiplast sterile wound d.
Dakin d.
Debrisan d.
Decubi-Care pad d.
demigauntlet d.
DermaCare d.
Dermacea alginate d.
Derma Cool hydrocolloid wound d.
DermaFilm d.
Dermagran-B hydrophilic wound d.
Dermagran zinc-saline hydrogel
  wound d.
DermaMend foam wound d.
DermaMend hydrogel d.
DermaNet wound contact layer d.
DermaSite transparent film d.
DermaSorb hydrocolloid/alginate
  wound d.
DermAssist glycerin hydrogel d.
DermAssist hydrocolloid d.
DermaStat calcium alginate
  wound d.
Dermicel cloth tape d.
Desault d.
DiaB Gel hydrogel d.
Donate-A-Gel impregnated gauze
  hydrogel d.
Douglas eye d.
Dow Corning antifoam agent d.
Doyle ear d.
Drilac surgical d.
dry-and-occlusive d.
dry pressure d.
dry sterile d.

D

NOTES

dressing *(continued)*
    dry textile d.
    Dual-Dress wound d.
    DuoDERM CGF gel d.
    DuoDERM hydrocolloid d.
    Dynaflex compression d.
    Eakin cohesive seal d.
    Elastikon wristlet d.
    Elasto d.
    Elasto-Gel hydrogel occlusive d.
    Elasto-Gel island d.
    Elastomull gauze support d.
    Elastoplast d.
    Elta dermal hydrogel d.
    Epigard synthetic skin d.
    Episeal wound d.
    Esmarch roll d.
    ethylene oxide d.
    Expo Bubble d.
    ExuDerm RCD hydrocolloid d.
    Exu-Dry absorptive d.
    Exu-Dry oncology d.
    eye pad d.
    EZ Derm porcine biosynthetic
      wound d.
    Fabco gauze d.
    felt d.
    Ferris polyostomy wound d.
    Fibracol collagen alginate wound d.
    figure-of-8 d.
    filiform d.
    film wound d.
    fine-mesh d.
    finger cot d.
    Flexderm wound d.
    Flexfilm wound d.
    Flex Foam d.
    FlexiGel gel sheet d.
    Flexigrid d.
    Flexinet d.
    Flexzan Extra topical wound d.
    fluff d.
    fluffed gauze d.
    foam wound d.
    d. forceps
    Fowler d.
    Fricke scrotal d.
    Fuller rectal d.
    Furacin gauze d.
    FyBron calcium alginate d.
    Galen d.
    Gamgee d.
    Garretson d.
    gauze stent d.
    Gauztex d.
    Gelfilm d.
    Geliperm gel d.
    Gelocast d.
    GelPad d.

    Gel-Syte wound d.
    gel wound d.
    Gentell foam wound d.
    Gentell hydrogel d.
    Gentell isotonic saline wet d.
    Gibney d.
    Gibson d.
    Glasscock ear d.
    GraftCyte moist wound d.
    GRX-Wound gel d.
    Gypsona plaster d.
    hammock d.
    Harman eye d.
    Hexcel cast d.
    hip spica d.
    hourglass d.
    Hueter perineal d.
    hyCure collagen hemostatic
      wound d.
    hyCure G hydrogel d.
    Hydragran absorption d.
    Hydrasorb foam wound d.
    Hydrasorb Plus d.
    hydroactive d.
    hydrocolloid occlusive d.
    Hydrocol sacral wound d.
    HydroDerm transparent d.
    Hydrofera Blue PVA d.
    hydrogel wound d.
    hydrophilic polyurethane foam d.
    HyFil hydrogel d.
    Hypergel hydrogel wound d.
    Hyperion wound gel d.
    Hysorb wound d.
    impermeable d.
    impregnated d.
    Inerpan flexible burn d.
    InteguDerm d.
    Intelligent d.
    IntraSite gel wound d.
    Iodoflex absorptive d.
    Iodosorb absorptive d.
    IPOP cast d.
    Ivalon d.
    Jelonet d.
    Jobst facelift d.
    Jobst mammary support d.
    Jobst UlcerCare d.
    Johnson & Johnson d.
    Jones d.
    Kalginate calcium alginate
      wound d.
    Kaltostat calcium sodium alginate
      wound d.
    Kaltostat Fortex d.
    Karaya d.
    Kelikian foot d.
    Kerlix d.
    Kirkland cement d.

Kling adhesive d.
Kling gauze d.
Koagamin d.
Koch-Mason d.
Komform coated gauze d.
Koylon foam rubber d.
Larrey d.
Lipisorb d.
Lister d.
Lubafax d.
Lukens bone wax d.
LYOfoam A, C, T water resistant d.
Macropro Beta-Glucan gel d.
mammary support d.
Manchu cotton d.
many-tailed d.
Martin rubber d.
mastoid d.
Maxorb alginate wound d.
mechanic's waste d.
Medical Resources hydrophilic wound d.
Medici aerosol adhesive tape remover d.
Medifil collagen hemostatic wound d.
Mediplex with Safetac d.
Medipore Dress-it d.
Medi-Rip d.
Mediskin porcine biological wound d.
Medline Derma-Gel d.
Mefilm d.
Mepiform self-adherent silicone d.
Mepilex foam d.
Mepitel contact-layer wound d.
Mepitel nonadherent silicone d.
Mepore absorptive d.
MeroGel d.
Merthiolate d.
Mesalt sodium chloride-impregnated d.
Metaline d.
Microdon d.
Microfoam d.
Micropore surgical tape d.
Mills d.
Mitraflex sterile spyrosorbent multilayer wound d.
Mitraflex wound d.
Mitrathane wound d.

3M Microdon d.
modified Robert Jones d.
moistened fine-mesh gauze d.
moist interactive d.
moisture-retentive d.
moleskin traction hitch d.
monocular eye d.
Montgomery strap d.
Mother Jones d.
moustache d.
MPM conductive hydrogel wound d.
MPM GelPad d.
MPM hydrogel d.
MPM multilayer d.
MPM Regenecare wound care gel d.
3M SoftCloth adhesive wound d.
3M Tegaderm HP high MVTR transparent d.
3M Tegasorb hydrocolloid d.
Multidex maltodextrin wound d.
MultiPad absorptive d.
muslin d.
mustache d.
nasal-tip d.
NDM adhesive wound d.
NeoDerm d.
neoprene d.
nonadhesive d.
nonocclusive d.
Normlgel protective wound d.
N-Terface contact-layer wound d.
Nu-Derm foam island d.
Nu Gauze d.
Nu-Gel wound d.
NutraCol hydrocolloid wound d.
NutraDress zinc-saline d.
NutraFil hydrophilic B d.
NutraGauze hydrophilic wound d.
NutraStat calcium alginate wound d.
NutraVue hydrogel d.
Nu-wrap roll d.
Oasis wound d.
occlusive collodion d.
occlusive moisture-retentive d.
occlusive semipermeable d.
O'Donoghue d.
odor-absorbent d.
oiled silk d.

D

NOTES

dressing *(continued)*

Omiderm transparent adhesive film d.
Opraflex d.
OpSite Flexifix transparent film d.
OpSite Flexigrid d.
OpSite occlusive d.
OpSite Plus wound d.
OriGHel hydrogel d.
Orthoflex d.
Orthoplast d.
OsmoCyte island wound care d.
OsmoCyte PCA pillow wound d.
Ostic plaster d.
Owen cloth d.
Owen gauze d.
Owen nonadherent surgical d.
Oxycel d.
oxyquinoline d.
Pak-Its hydrogel gauze d.
Panogauze d.
Panoplex hydrogel wound d.
Paracine d.
paraffin d.
peacock d.
PEG self-adhesive elastic d.
Peries medicated hygienic wipe d.
petrolatum gauze d.
Photo Derma wound gel d.
Piedmont all-cotton elastic d.
Pillo Pro d.
plaster-of-Paris d.
plastic d.
pledget d.
Polyderm foam wound d.
PolyFlex traction d.
PolyMem adhesive surgical wound d.
Polyskin II d.
PolyTrach d.
PolyWic d.
Pope halo d.
postauricular ear d.
postnasal d.
Preptic d.
Presso-Elastic d.
Pressoplast compression d.
Presso-Superior d.
pressure applied d. (PAD)
pressure patch d.
Priessnitz d.
Primaderm foam d.
Primapore absorptive wound d.
Primer compression d.
Pro-Clude transparent wound d.
Procol hydrocolloid wound d.
ProCyte transparent film d.
proflavine wool d.
Profore four-layer wound d.

Promogran matrix wound d.
Pro-Ophtha d.
propylene d.
protective d.
pulped muscle d.
PuraPly wound d.
Purilon gel d.
Quadro d.
Queen Anne d.
Quinaband d.
Qwik-Clean d.
Ray-Tec d.
Red Cross adhesive d.
Release nonadhering d.
RepliCare Thin hydrocolloid d.
Repliderm d.
Reston hydrocolloid d.
Restore CalciCare d.
Restore calcium alginate wound d.
Restore Cx wound care d.
Restore hydrocolloid d.
Restore Plus wound care d.
Rezifilm d.
Reziplast spray-on d.
Rhino Rocket d.
Ribble d.
ribbon gauze d.
Richet d.
Robert Jones bulky soft compressive d.
Rochester d.
roller d.
Rondic sponge d.
Rose bed d.
Royl-Derm wound hydrogel nonadherent d.
rubber Scan spray d.
Saf-Gel hydrating dermal wound d.
SaliCept d.
saline d.
saline-saturated wool d.
Sayre d.
scan spray d.
scarlet red gauze d.
d. scissors
scrotal d.
SeaSorb alginate wound d.
Sellotape d.
Sellotape tie-over d.
Selofix d.
Selopor d.
semicompressive d.
semiocclusive moisture-retentive d.
semipermeable membrane d.
semipressure d.
Septisol soap d.
Septopack periodontal d.
Setopress d.
Shah aural d.

Shantz d.
sheepskin d.
sheet-wadding d.
SignaDress hydrocolloid d.
Silastic foam d.
Silastic gel d.
silicone d.
Silon Dual-Dress wound d.
Silon wound d.
Siloskin d.
Silverstein d.
SiteGuard MVP transparent d.
Skin-Prep protective d.
SkinTegrity hydrogel d.
SkinTemp biosynthetic skin d.
sling d.
Snugs d.
Sof-Foam d.
Sof-Rol d.
SofSorb absorptive d.
SoftCloth absorptive d.
Sof-Wick d.
SoloSite hydrogel d.
SorbaView composite wound d.
SorbaView window d.
Sorbex hydrocolloid wound d.
Sorb-It II d.
Sorbsan calcium alginate d.
Sorbsan gel block topical
  wound d.
Spand-Gel primary hydrogel d.
spica d.
sponge d.
Spray Band d.
Spyrogel hydrogel wound d.
starch-based copolymer d.
Sta-Tite gauze d.
stent d.
Stericare copolymer absorbent d.
Stericare hydrogel gauze d.
Steri-Pad d.
d. stick
Stimson d.
stockinette d.
StrataSorb composite d.
Stretch Net wound d.
Styrofoam d.
super-absorptive polymer d.
Superflex elastic d.
SuperSkin thin film d.
Super-Trac adhesive traction d.
SurePress compression d.

SureSite transparent adhesive
  film d.
Surfasoft d.
surgical d.
Surgicel gauze d.
Surgicel Nu-Knit d.
Surgifix d.
Surgiflex d.
Surgilast tubular elastic d.
Surgi-Pad combined d.
Surgitube d.
suspensory d.
Sween-A-Peel wound d.
Synthaderm occlusive wound d.
4-tailed d.
tap water wet d.
T-bandage d.
T-binder pressure d.
Tegaderm semipermeable
  occlusive d.
Tegagel hydrogel d.
Tegagen HG, HI alginate
  wound d.
Tegapore contact-layer wound d.
Tegasorb occlusive d.
Telfa Clear nonadherent wound d.
Telfa island d.
Telfamax ultra absorbent d.
Telfa Plus barrier island d.
Telfa Xtra absorbent island d.
TenderCups postoperative breast d.
Tenoplast elastic adhesive d.
Tensor elastic d.
Tes Tape d.
TheraSkin wound d.
Thillaye d.
ThinSite border hydrogel d.
ThinSite topical wound d.
Tielle absorptive d.
Tielle hydropolymer d.
Tielle Plus d.
Tomac foam rubber traction d.
Tomac knitted rubber elastic d.
Transeal d.
Transeal transparent adhesive
  film d.
TransiGel woven gauze d.
Transorbent hydrogel topical
  wound d.
Transorb wound d.
transparent adhesive film d.
Transpore surgical tape d.

D

NOTES

dressing *(continued)*
  Triad hydrophilic wound d.
  triangular d.
  Tube-Lok tracheotomy d.
  tube site d.
  Tubex gauze d.
  Tubigrip d.
  tubular d.
  tulle gras d.
  twill d.
  Ultec Pro alginate hydrocolloid d.
  Ultex thin extra thin
    hydrocolloid d.
  Ultrafera wound d.
  Uniflex polyurethane adhesive
    surgical d.
  Unna-Flex Plus compression d.
  Usher Marlex mesh d.
  V.A.C. d.
  vapor-permeable d.
  Varick elastic d.
  Vari/Moist wound d.
  Vaseline gauze d.
  Vaseline wick d.
  Veingard d.
  Velpeau sling d.
  Veni-Gard stabilization d.
  Ventex d.
  Ventifoam traction d.
  VersaDerm d.
  Viasorb absorbent d.
  Victorian collar d.
  VigiFOAM d.
  Vigilon primary wound d.
  Vioform gauze d.
  Viscopaste PB7 gauze d.
  VitaCuff d.
  Wangensteen d.
  water d.
  Webril d.
  Weck-Cel d.
  wet d.
  wet-to-dry d.
  whisk-packets d.
  wick d.
  wood roll d.
  wound d.
  Woun'Dres collagen hydrogel
    wound d.
  WoundSpan Bridge II d.
  wraparound d.
  Xeroflo d.
  Xeroform d.
  Y-bandage d.
  Yield nonadherent gauze d.
  Zephyr rubber elastic d.
  Zim-Flux d.
  Zimocel d.
  Zipzoc stocking compression d.
  Zobec sponge d.
  Zonas porous adhesive tape d.
  Zoroc resin plaster d.

DressSkin skin replacement

Drews
  D. cataract needle
  D. cystotome
  D. inclined prism
  D. intraocular forceps
  D. iris retractor
  D. irrigating cannula
  D. irrigating vectis
  D. lavage needle
  D. lens
  D. needle holder
  D. posterior capsule polisher

Drews-Knolle reverse irrigating vectis

Drew-Smythe catheter

Drews-Rosenbaum iris retractor

Drews-Sato
  D.-S. capsular fragment spatula
  D.-S. suture-pickup hook
  D.-S. suture-pickup spatula
  D.-S. tying forceps

DRG Sherlock threaded suture anchor

Dri-flo underpad

Drilac surgical dressing

drill
  ACL d.
  Acufex d.
  Adson-Rogers perforating d.
  Adson spiral d.
  Adson twist d.
  Aesculap d.
  air d.
  air-powered d.
  Albee d.
  Amico d.
  Amsco Orthairtome d.
  Anspach 65K d.
  anticavitation d.
  Archimedean d.
  Arthrex biointerference d.
  autotome d.
  Bailey d.
  bar d.
  Björk rib d.
  bone hand d.
  Bosworth crown d.
  Bowen suture d.
  Brunswick-Mack rotating d.
  Buckingham d.
  Bucky hand d.
  Bunnell bone d.
  Bunnell hand d.
  bur d.
  Calcitek d.
  Canal Master d.
  Carmody perforator d.

Carroll-Bunnell d.
Caspar d.
Cebotome d.
cement eater d.
centering d.
d. chamber
Championnière bone d.
Charnley centering d.
Charnley femoral condyle d.
Charnley pilot d.
Charnley starting d.
Cherry d.
Cherry-Austin d.
Children's Hospital hand d.
chuck d.
Cloward cervical d.
Coballoy twist d.
Codman-Shurtleff cranial d.
Codman wire-passing d.
Collison body d.
Collison cannulated hand d.
Collison tap d.
cortical step d.
cranial d.
crown d.
Crutchfield bone d.
Crutchfield hand d.
CurvTek TSR bone d.
Cushing cranial d.
Cushing flat d.
Cushing perforator d.
dental d.
depth check d.
DePuy d.
D'Errico perforating d.
Deyerle d.
diamond high-speed air d.
Doyen cylindrical d.
driver nail d.
Elan d.
Elan-E power d.
electric d.
fingernail d.
Fisch d.
flat d.
Galt hand d.
Gates-Glidden d.
glenoid d.
Gray bone d.
Grosse-Kempf bone d.
d. guard
d. guide

d. guide forceps
Hall air d.
Hall-Dundar d.
Hall Micro-Aire d.
Hall Neurairtome d.
Hall Orthairtome d.
Hall power d.
Hall step-down d.
Hall Surgairtome II d.
Hall surgical d.
Hall Versipower d.
Hamby twist d.
hand d.
Harold Crowe d.
Harris-Smith anterior interbody d.
Hewson d.
high-speed d.
high-speed air d.
Hudson bone d.
Hudson cranial d.
intramedullary d.
Jacobs chuck d.
Jordan-Day d.
Kerr electro-torque d.
Kerr hand d.
Kirschner bone d.
Kirschner wire d.
Kodex d.
Küntscher d.
Lentulo spiral d.
Light-Veley cranial d.
Loth-Kirschner d.
Luck bone d.
Lusskin bone d.
Macewen d.
Magnuson twist d.
Mathews hand d.
Mathews load d.
McKenzie cranial d.
McKenzie perforating twist d.
Michelson-Sequoia air d.
Micro-Aire d.
MicroMax speed d.
Midas Rex d.
Minos air d.
Mira d.
Modny d.
Moore bone d.
nail d.
Neil-Moore perforator d.
Neurairtome d.
Orthairtome II d.

D

NOTES

drill *(continued)*
orthopaedic Universal d.
OsseoCare d.
Osseodent surgical d.
Osteon d.
ototome otological d.
Patrick d.
Pease bone d.
pencil-tip d.
penetrating d.
Penn finger d.
perforating d.
perforating twist d.
perforator d.
pilot d.
pistol-grip hand d.
pneumatic d.
Portmann d.
Posi-Stop d.
power d.
Powerforma surgical d.
pronator d.
Rainbow d.
Ralks bone d.
Ralks fingernail d.
Raney bone d.
Raney cranial d.
Raney-Crutchfield d.
Raney perforator d.
retention d.
Rica bone d.
Richards-Lovejoy bone d.
Richards pistol-grip d.
Richmond subarachnoid twist d.
Richter bone d.
Romano curved surgical d.
root canal d.
Shea ear d.
Sherman-Stille d.
Skeeter otologic d.
Sklar bone d.
skull traction d.
SMIC sternal d.
Smith d.
spiral d.
Spirec d.
step d.
step-down d.
Stille bone d.
Stille cranial d.
Stille hand d.
Stille-Sherman bone d.
Stiwer hand d.
d. stop cylinder
Stryker d.
Surgairtome air d.
surgical orthopaedic d.
suture hole d.
Synthes d.

tap d.
Thornwald antral d.
Toti trephine d.
Treace stapes d.
trephine d.
Trinkle bone d.
Trinkle Super-Cut twist d.
Trowbridge-Campau bone d.
Trowbridge triple-speed d.
twist d.
Uniflex calibrated step d.
Universal two-speed hand d.
Vitallium d.
Warren-Mack rotating d.
wire d.
Wolferman d.
Wullstein d.
Xcalibur otologic d.
Xoman d.
Zimalate twist d.
Zimmer hand d.
Zimmer-Kirschner hand d.
Zimmer Universal d.
drill-tipped guidewire
D-ring strap
Drinker tank respirator
Drionic electrical iontophoresis device
drip chamber
driver
Apex Universal d.
Cook endoscopic curved needle d.
D. coronary stent
Eby band d.
endoscopic curved needle d.
femoral head d.
Flatt d.
graft d.
Hall d.
Haney needle d.
Harrington hook d.
Jewett d.
Ken d.
Küntscher nail d.
K wire d.
laparoscopic needle d.
Laurus needle d.
Linvatec d.
Lloyd nail d.
Massie d.
Maxi-Driver d.
McNutt d.
McReynolds d.
Micro series wire d.
Milewski d.
Moore d.
Moore-Blount d.
d. nail drill
needle d.
Neufeld d.

Nystroem nail d.
Nystroem-Stille d.
orthodontic band d.
ParaMax angled d.
Pereyra needle d.
polyethylene-faced d.
Pugh d.
Put-In d.
Rush d.
Schneider nail d.
Sharbaro d.
Sven Johansson d.
Szabo-Berci needle d.
Talon curved needle d.
tibial d.
TLC-II portable VAD d.
Torx d.
universal fixation d.
wire d.

driver-extractor
Sage d.-e.
Schneider d.-e.

Dromos pacemaker

drop
d. foot brace
d. foot splint

DropTainer dispenser

drug
d. infusion pump
d. infusion sleeve

drug-coated stent

DRUJ
distal radioulnar joint
DRUJ prosthesis

drum
d. dermatome
d. elevator knife
d. probe
d. scraper

Drummond
D. button
D. hook
D. hook holder
D. wire

dry
d. flotation wheelchair cushion
d. heat sterilizer
d. pressure dressing
d. spirometer
d. sterile dressing
d. sterile gauze

d. textile dressing
d. textile gauze

dry-and-occlusive dressing
dry-powder inhaler
Drysdale nucleus manipulator
Drystar dry imager
DryTime for bladder control
DryView laser imaging system
D-shaped implant
DSIS orthotic
D-Soles
D-S. foot sole
D-S. insole
D-S. orthotic

DSP Micro Diamond-Point microsurgery set
DSX
DSX ELISA system
DSX Sopha camera

D-Tach removable needle
DTR-one UltraSure imaging ultrasound system
D-Tron insulin pump
DTU-series cardiac digital stimulator
Dua
D. antireflux valve
D. stent

dual
d. coil transvenous lead
D. Geometry cutter
D. Geometry HA cup
d. leg immobilizer
d. nerve root suction retractor
d. octapolar lead
d. quadrapolar lead
D. Quattrode spinal cord stimulation system
D. Range Limiter system
d. square-ended Harrington rod

dual-chamber
d.-c. flushing valve
d.-c. ICD
d.-c. Medtronic Kappa pacemaker
d.-c. pacemaker
d.-c. rate-responsive pacemaker

Dual-Dress wound dressing
dual-energy
d.-e. digital linear accelerator
d.-e. x-ray absorptiometry (DEXA)
d.-e. x-ray absorptiometry bone densitometer

Dualer Plus system

NOTES

D

dual-head
   d.-h. coincidence camera
   d.-h. gamma camera
Dualine digital hearing instrument
Duall 88 cement
dual-lead electrode
dual-lock total hip prosthesis
dual-lumen
   d.-l. catheter
   d.-l. hemodialysis catheter
   d.-l. nasogastric tube
   d.-l. papillotome
DualMesh
   D. biomaterial
   D. hernia mesh
   D. material
   D. Plus biomaterial
dual-mode, ventricular inhibited (DVI)
dual-photon
   d.-p. densitometer
   d.-p. electrospinal orthosis
dual-sensing, dual-pacing, dual-mode pacemaker
DualStim TENS unit
dual-sump silicone drain
Dualtherm dual-thermistor thermodilution catheter
Duane
   D. retractor
   D. U-clip
Dubecq-Princeteau angulating needle holder
Dubois decapitation scissors
Duchenne trocar
duckbill
   d. clamp
   d. elevator
   d. forceps
   d. rongeur
   d. speculum
   d. voice prosthesis
Ducker-Hayes nerve cuff
Ducor
   D. angiographic catheter
   D. balloon catheter
   D. cardiac catheter
   D. HF catheter
   D. tip
Ducournau fine gripping forceps
duct
   d. dilator
   main pancreatic d. (MPD)
   d. scoop
DuctOcclud coil
Dudley
   D. rectal hook
   D. tenaculum hook

Duet
   D. coronary stent
   D. glucose control monitor
Duett
   D. arterial closure device
   D. catheter
   D. closure device
   D. sealing device
   D. vascular sealing device
Duette
   D. basket
   D. double lumen ERCP instrument
Duffield cardiovascular scissors
Duke
   D. boot
   D. cannula
   D. trocar
   D. tube
Duke-Elder lamp
Dulaney
   D. antral cannula
   D. intraocular implant lens
   D. LASIK marker
Dumbach
   D. mandibular reconstruction system
   D. mini mesh
   D. regular mesh
   D. titanium mesh
dummy
   d. source
   d. spacer
Dumon
   D. rigid bronchoscope
   D. silicone stent
   D. tracheobronchial stent
Dumon-Gilliard
   D.-G. endoprosthesis system
   D.-G. prosthesis introducer
Dumon-Harrell bronchoscope
Dumont
   D. dissecting forceps
   D. jeweler's forceps
   D. retractor
   D. thoracic scissors
   D. tweezers
Dumontpallier pessary
Duncan
   D. dural film
   D. endometrial biopsy curette
   D. loop
   D. shoulder brace
Dundas-Grant tube
Dunhill forceps
Dunlap cold compression wrap system
Dunlop
   D. sleeve
   D. thrombus stripper
   D. traction
   D. tractor

Dunn
D. depressor
D. fracture device
Dunn-Dautrey osteotome
Dunning
D. curette
D. elevator
DuoCeph cephalostat
Duo-Cline contoured bed wedge
Duocondylar knee prosthesis
duodecapolar catheter
duodenal
d. clamp
d. pin
d. retractor
duodenofiberscope
Olympus d.
Pentax FD-series d.
duodenoscope
ACMI d.
d. cannula
diagnostic d.
Fujinon ED-series d.
Fujinon FD-series d.
GF-UM3 d.
large-channel therapeutic d.
Olympus EW-series fiberoptic d.
Olympus JF-series video d.
Olympus JF-V-series video d.
Olympus JT-series video d.
Olympus PJF-series pediatric d.
Olympus video d.
Pentax d.
side-viewing d.
standard d.
therapeutic side-viewing d.
video d.
DuoDERM
D. CGF gel dressing
D. drain
D. hydrocolloid dressing
D. SCB sustained compression
bandage
Duo-Flow catheter
DuoLock curved tail pouch closure
Duoloid impression system
Duo-Patellar knee prosthesis
Duostat rotating hemostatic valve
Duotrak blade
Duovisc viscoelastic system
Dupel iontophoretic drug delivery system

Du Pen long-term epidural catheter
Duplay
D. nasal speculum
D. uterine tenaculum
D. uterine tenaculum forceps
duplex
d. scan
d. ultrasound
duplicator
cardiac pulse d.
DuPont
D. Cronex x-ray film
D. rare earth imaging system
D. scanner
Dupuytren
D. knife
D. splint
D. suture
D. tourniquet
Dura
D. II concealable penile implant
D. II positionable penile prosthesis
Durabase soft rebase acrylic
durable medical equipment
DuraBoot boot
Duracell Activair hearing aid battery
Duracon
D. knee implant
D. prosthesis
D. PS total knee system
Durafill dental restorative material
Duraflow heart valve
Duragel lens
DuraGen
D. absorbable dural graft matrix
D. dural graft
D. neurosurgical device
DuraGlide3 catheter
DURAglide³ stone removal balloon
Dura-Guard patch
Durahesive
D. moldable convex skin barrier
D. Wafer pouch
Dura-Kold reusable compression ice wrap
dural
d. elevator
d. forceps
d. hook
d. implant
d. needle
d. protector

D

NOTES

dural *(continued)*
    d. retractor
    d. scissors
    d. separator
    d. substitute
Duralay acrylic
Dura-Liner acrylic
Duralite tube
Duraloc
    D. acetabular cup
    D. acetabular cup system
Duralon-UV nylon membrane
DuraMatrix collagen dura substitute membrane
Duramer polyethylene component
Duran annuloplasty ring
DuraNeb
    D. portable nebulizer
    D. portable nebulizer pump
durapatite
    d. bone replacement material
    D. graft
    d. implant
DuraPhase
    D. inflatable penile prosthesis
    D. semirigid penile prosthesis
Durapore tape
Durashield dural substitute
Dur-A-Sil
    D.-A.-S. ear impression material
    D.-A.-S. silicone impression system
Durasoft
    D. 2 contact lens
    D. toric lens
Dura-Soft soft-compression reusable ice or heat wrap
Dura-Stick adhesive electrode
Durasul
    D. acetabular insert
    D. large diameter head system
DuraTilt wheeled shower/commode chair
DuraView OL-1 flexible nasopharyngeoscope
Duray-Read gouge
Durelon dental cement
Durette
    D. dental shield
    D. external ocular laser shield
Durham
    D. needle
    D. tracheostomy tube
    D. tracheotomy trocar
    D. tube
Durkan CTS gauge
Duromedics
    D. bileaflet mitral valve
    D. valve prosthesis
Duros leuprolide implant
Durotip scissors

Durrani dorsal vein complex ligation needle
Dutchman's roll
Dutch pessary
duToit
    d. shoulder staple
    d. stapler
Duval
    D. bag
    D. disposable dermatome
    D. intestinal forceps
    D. lung forceps
    D. tissue forceps
Duval-Allis forceps
Duval-Collin
    D.-C. intestinal forceps
    D.-C. lung clamp
Duval-Crile
    D.-C. intestinal forceps
    D.-C. lung forceps
    D.-C. lung-grasping forceps
    D.-C. tissue forceps
Duyzings clasp
DVI
    dual-mode, ventricular inhibited
    DVI pacemaker
    DVI Simpson coronary AtheroCath catheter
DVT
    deep vein thrombosis
Dwellcath cannula
Dwyer
    D. device
    D. instrument
    D. instrumentation
    D. spinal mechanical stapler
    D. spinal screw
DX-PC spirometry system
Dycem roll matting
Dycor prosthetic foot
dye
    ABI fluorescence d.
    fluorescence d.
Dymedix
    D. airflow/snore sensory
    D. pediatric airflow sensor
    D. precision chin patch
    D. sleep sensor
Dymer
    D. excimer delivery probe
    D. excimer excimer laser delivery system
Dynabond resin
Dyna-Care pressure pad system
Dynacor
    D. ear syringe
    D. enema cleansing kit
    D. Foley catheter
    D. leg bag

D. suction catheter
D. ulcer syringe
D. vaginal irrigator set
D. vaginal speculum

DynaDisc exercise equipment
Dynafill graft biomedium mineralized bone matrix
DynaFix external fixation system
Dynaflex
D. compression dressing
D. elastic bandage
D. multilayer compression system
D. penile implant

DynaGraft
D. bioimplant
D. putty

Dynagrip blade handle
DynaGuard
D. APM alternating pressure mattress
D. LAL low-air-loss pressure management system

DynaHeat hot pack
DynaLator ultrasound unit
Dynalink
D. 0.035 biliary self-expanding stent
D. biliary self-expanding stent system

Dyna-Lok plating system
Dynalyzer equipment
Dyna Med anti-shock trousers
dynamic
d. angioplasty catheter
d. axial fixator
d. bed
d. bridging plate
d. compression plate
d. compression plating
d. condylar screw (DCS)
d. contrast-enhanced magnetic resonance imaging
d. contrast-enhanced MRI
d. cooling device
d. digit extensor tube
d. elbow orthosis
d. flotation mattress
d. foot stabilizer
d. hip screw
d. integrated stabilization chair (DISC)
d. knee orthosis

D. Optical Breast Imaging (DOBI)
d. optical breast imaging system
d. orthotic cranioplasty (DOC)
d. orthotic cranioplasty band
d. penile prosthesis
d. spatial reconstructor scanner
d. splint
d. wrist orthosis
d. Y stent

Dynamite mattress system
dynamometer
back-leg-chest d.
Baseline d.
bicycle d.
Biodex isokinetic d.
bulb d.
Collins d.
computerized isokinetic d.
Cybex isokinetic d.
electromechanical d.
handheld d.
Harpenden handgrip d.
hydraulic hand d.
Isobex d.
Jamar hydraulic hand d.
Lido Multi Joint II isokinetic d.
MicroFET isometric force d.
orthopaedic d.
Padgett hydraulic hand d.
Smedley d.
Spark handheld d.

DynaPak electrode kit
Dynaphor iontophoresis
DynaPulse 5000A 24-hour ambulatory blood pressure monitor
DynaRad portable x-ray system
dynascope
Fukuda DS-5800NX d.

Dynaslipper night shoe
Dynasplint
D. knee extension unit
D. shoulder system

Dynastat surgical hemostat
Dynasty delivery system
DynaSurg electric handpiece
DynaTorq wrench
Dynatron
D. electrotherapy
D. TX 900 electrotherapy
D. 150 ultrasound

Dynatronics Model 1620 laser
DynaVox 2 communication device

D

NOTES

DynaWell medical compression device
DynaWraps strap
DyoBrite illuminator
DyoCam 550 arthroscopic video camera
Dyonics
- D. arthroplasty bur
- D. arthroscope
- D. arthroscopic blade
- D. arthroscopic instrument
- D. basket forceps
- D. DyoBrite light source
- D. Dyosite office arthroscopy system

- D. full-radius resector
- D. IntelliJet fluid management system
- D. meniscotome
- D. needle
- D. rod lens arthroscope
- D. rod lens laparoscope
- D. suction punch
- D. syringe injector

DyoPneumatic insufflator
DyoVac suction punch

E

E Clips computer eyewear
E Wildcat orthodontic wire

Eagle

E. II survey spirometer
E. straight-ahead arthroscope

EaglePlug tapered-shaft punctum plug
EagleVision Freeman punctum plug
Eakin cohesive seal dressing
E-A-R

E-A-R Hi-Fi earplug
E-A-R Link eartips

ear

e. applicator
e. bougie
e. cannula
e. cup
e. curette
e. dissector
e. dressing forceps
e. forceps with suction
e. furuncle knife
e. hook
e. knife handle
e. loop
e. magnet
e.'s, nose, throat (ENT)
e. oximeter
e. pinna prosthesis
e. piston prosthesis
e. polyp forceps
e. polyp snare
e. probe
e. prosthesis
e. punch forceps
e. putty ear plug
e. rasp
e. scissors
e. snare wire
e. snare wire carrier
e. speculum
e. spoon
e. syringe

EarCheck

E. monitor
E. Pro instrument

Earle

E. hemorrhoidal clamp
E. rectal probe

EarPlanes silicone earplug
earplug

Doc's Proplug e.
E-A-R Hi-Fi e.
EarPlanes silicone e.

Insta-Putty silicone e.
Mack's e.

earring

Brent pressure e.
compression e.
Glori pressure e.
pressure e.
pressure-producing e.

Earscope otoscope
eartips

E-A-R Link e.

Ear-Tronics hearing aid
Easi-Breathe inhaler
Easi-Lav gastric lavage
East-Grinstead

E.-G. needle
E.-G. scissors

Eastman

E. cystic duct forceps
E. dental cement
E. intestinal clamp
E. Kodak scanner
E. suction tube
E. vaginal retractor
E. vaginal speculum

Easy

E. Access foot splint
E. Air 15 compressor
E. Analysis system
E. Introduction system
E. Lok ankle brace
E. Rider catheter
E. sleeve
E. Up cushion
E. Wallstent stent

EasyChair massage chair
**EasyGuide Neuro image-guided surgery
system**
Easy/Neb compressor
Easy-On elbow brace
EasyPivot patient lift
EasyStand 6000 glider
EasyStep walker
Easytrak coronary venous lead
eater

cement e.

Eaton

E. nasal speculum
E. trapezium finger joint
replacement prosthesis

EBCT

electron beam computed tomography

E. Benson Hood Laboratories

E. B. H. L. esophageal tube
E. B. H. L. salivary bypass tube

Eber
E. holder
E. needle-holder forceps
EBI
EBI bone healing system
EBI external fixator
EBI gravity cold therapy system
EBI Omega21 expandable screw
EBI SPF-2 implantable bone stimulator
EBI SpineLink anterior cervical spinal system
EBI Temptek blanket
EBI XFix DynaFix system
EBT
electron beam tomography
EBT scanner
Eby
E. band driver
E. band setter
EC-5000 excimer laser
EC50 Toxco breath carbon monoxide monitor
E.CAM
E.CAM dual-head emission imaging system
E.CAM photon emission camera
E-cath catheter
ECAT Reveal PET/CT scanner
eccentric
e. drill guide
e. dynamic compression plate
E. Isotac tibial guide
E. locked rib shears
e. monocuspid tilting-disc prosthetic valve
E. Y finger retractor
Eccocee CX ultrasound system
EccoVision
E. acoustic pharyngometer
E. acoustic rhinometry system
ECG
electrocardiogram (*See also* EKG)
AT-2 ECG
KoKo Rhythm PC-Based ECG
ECG trigger unit
Echlin
E. bone rongeur
E. duckbill rongeur
E. laminectomy rongeur
E. rongeur forceps
echo
e. catheter
e. probe
e. transponder electrode catheter
echocardiograph
Acuson e.
Biosound Surgiscan e.
Siemens Sonoline SL-2 e.

echocardiographic probe
Echocheck hearing screening device
Echo-Coat ultrasound biopsy needle
echocolonoscope
CF-UM3 e.
echoendoscope
FG-36UX scanning e.
GF-UM30P linear-oriented radial scanning e.
linear array e.
mechanical longitudinal e.
oblique-viewing e.
Olympus CF-UM-series e.
Olympus GF-UM30P e.
Olympus GF-UM-series e.
Olympus GIF-EUM-series e.
Olympus JF-UM-series e.
Olympus VU-M-series e.
Olympus XIF-UM-series e.
Pentax FG-36UX scanning e.
radial sector scanning e.
scanning e.
sector scanning e.
EchoEye
E. imaging system
E. ultrasound
EchoFlow blood velocity meter system
echogastroscope
echogenic needle
EchoMark
E. salpingography catheter
E. SSG catheter
echoplanar magnetic resonance imaging
echoprobe
Olympus XMP-U2 catheter e.
EchoScan
Nidek E.
Echosight
E. Jansen-Anderson intrauterine catheter set
E. Patton coaxial catheter set
Echotip
E. Baker amniocentesis needle set
E. Dominion needle set
E. Kato-Asch coaxial needle set
echo-tracking
e.-t. device
e.-t. probe
Echovar Doppler system
Eckardt
E. backflush instrument
E. Heme-Stopper instrument
E. temporary keratoprosthesis
Eclipse
E. Axcis PTMR system
E. blood collection needle
E. gel ankle brace
E. gel elbow strap
E. gel wrist splint

E. Highfield MRI system
E. holmium laser
E. infusion system
E. magnetic resonance system
E. ST cyclotron
E. TENS unit
E. TMR holmium laser

ECMO
extracorporeal membrane oxygenation
ECMO cannula
ECMO pump
EcoCheck oxygen monitor
Econo-Cerv traction device
Econo-Float water flotation mattress
Econolith device
Econo Vienna nasal speculum
E-cotton bandage
EC Proline cephalostat
ECT
electroconvulsive therapy
ECT internal fracture fixation
ECT pacemaker
ectopic atrial pacemaker
ECTRA
Endoscopic Carpal Tunnel Release
Assembly
ECTRA system
Edap LT.2 lithotripter
edema sock
EdenTec 2000W in-home
cardiorespiratory monitor
Edentrace sleep system
Eder
E. cord blood collection device
E. esophagoscope
E. forceps
E. gastroscope
E. insufflator
E. laparoscope
E. sigmoidoscope
Eder-Bernstein gastroscope
Eder-Hufford
E.-H. esophagoscope
E.-H. gastroscope
Eder-Palmer
E.-P. gastroscope
E.-P. semiflexible fiberoptic
endoscope
Eder-Puestow
E.-P. esophageal dilator
E.-P. guidewire
E.-P. metal olive

Edge
E. blade
E. dilatation catheter
E. III hydrogel contact lens
E. knee brace
E. needle electrode
The E. coated blade
EdgeAhead
E. IOL knife
E. MVR knife
EDG system
Edinburgh
E. brain retractor
E. suture
Edison fluoroscope
EDM infusion catheter
Edmonton extension tongs
Edslab
E. cholangiography catheter
E. jaw spring clip
E. pressure gauge
EDTA Vacutainer blood collection tube
Eductor fluid management system
Edwards
E. diagnostic catheter
E. D-L modular fixator
E. double Softjaw clamp
E. instrumentation
E. modular spinal system
E. modular system kyphoreduction
construct
E. modular system neutralization
construct
E. modular system sacral fixation
device
E. modular system scoliosis
construct
E. parallel-jaw spring clip
E. Prima Plus valve
E. raspatory
E. rectal hook
E. sacral screw
E. seamless heart valve
E. seamless prosthesis
E. single Softjaw clamp
E. spring clamp
E. Teflon intracardiac patch
implant material
E. Teflon intracardiac patch
prosthesis
E. Universal rod

E

NOTES

Edwards *(continued)*
  E. woven Teflon aortic bifurcation
    graft
**Edwards-Duromedics bileaflet heart
valve**
Edwards-Levine
  E.-L. hook
  E.-L. rod
  E.-L. sleeve
EDXRF
  Energy Dispersive X-ray Fluorescence
  EDXRF spectrometer
EEA
  EEA Auto Suture
  EEA disposable loading unit
  EEA stapler
  EEA surgical stapling device
EEG
  electroencephalogram
  electroencephalograph
  Equinox digital EEG
  EEG and PSG instrumentation
  Xltek EEG
eel
  e. cobra tip
  e. wire
Efer-Dumon bronchoscope
Effapoxy resin
Effenberger
  E. contractor
  E. retractor
Efficere embryo transfer catheter
Effler
  E. double-ended dissector
  E. tack
Effler-Groves
  E.-G. cardiovascular forceps
  E.-G. dissector
  E.-G. hook
Efica CC dynamic air therapy unit
EfosLite curing light
eggcrate
  e. foam
  e. mattress
  e. mattress pad
  e. positioner
  e. protector
Eggers
  E. bone plate
  E. contact splint
  E. screw
Eggsercizer resistive hand exerciser
Egnell
  E. breast pump
  E. uterine aspirator
  E. vacuum extractor
egress
  e. cannula
  e. needle

EG-series clear corneal knife
Ehmke
  E. ear prosthesis
  E. platinum Teflon implant
Eichelter-Schenk vena cava catheter
Eicher
  E. hip prosthesis
  E. rasp
  E. tri-fin chisel
**EID percutaneous central venous large-
bore catheter**
EIE
  EIE 150F operating microscope
  EIE MiniEndo piezoelectric
    ultrasonic unit
Eigon
  E. CardioLoop recorder
  E. disc
Einhorn
  E. esophageal dilator
  E. tube
Einthoven string galvanometer
Eiselsberg ligature scissors
Eiselsberg-Mathieu needle holder
Eisenhammer speculum
Eisenstein
  E. clamp
  E. hysterectomy forceps
ejector
  Cloward dowel e.
  Johnson & Johnson saliva e.
EKG
  electrocardiogram *(See also* ECG)
  EKG calipers
Eklund breast positioning system
Ela
  E. Chorus DDD pacemaker
  E. Medical Elatec V 3.03A
    arrhythmia analyzer
  E. ventricular pacing lead
ELAD
  extracorporeal liver assist device
  ELAD cartridge
Elan
  E. drill
  E. electrosurgical unit
Elan-E
  E.-E electronic motor system
  E.-E power drill
Elastafit tubing kit
Elastalloy
  E. esophageal endoprosthesis
  E. esophageal stent
ElastaTrac
  E. home lumbar traction system
  E. home lumbar traction unit
elastic
  e. bougie
  e. bowel forceps

e. foam-backed bandage
e. O-ring
Spandage e.
e. stable intramedullary nail
e. stocking
e. suspensor
e. suture
elastic-hinge knee brace
Elastikon
E. bandage
E. elastic tape
E. wristlet dressing
Elasto dressing
Elasto-Gel
E.-G. cushion
E.-G. heel/ankle boot
E.-G. hot and cold therapy
cervical neck wrap
E.-G. hydrogel occlusive dressing
E.-G. hydrogel sheet
E.-G. island dressing
E.-G. pressure pad
E.-G. shoulder therapy wrap
elastomer
American Heyer-Schulte e.
conventional silicone e.
e. shell
silicone e.
thermoplastic e. (TPE)
elastomeric pump
Elastomull
E. bandage
E. gauze support dressing
Elastoplast
E. bandage
E. dressing
E. eye occlusor
Elastylon glove
elbow
e. extension splint
e. flexion splint
e. hinge
e. magnet
e. sleeve
elbowed
e. bougie
e. catheter
elbow-wrist-hand orthosis
Eldridge-Green lamp
Elecath
E. circulatory support device

E. ECMO cannula
E. pacemaker
E. switch box
E. thermodilution catheter
Electra 1000C coagulation analyzer
electric
e. bed
e. dermatome
e. drill
General E. (GE)
e. generator
e. probe
e. syringe
e. tissue morcellator
electrical
e. brain stimulator
e. implant
e. muscle stimulation (EMS)
e. nerve stimulator
e. resistance detector
e. sector scanner
electricator
e. coagulator
National e.
Electri-Cool
E.-C. cold therapy system
E.-C. continuous controlled cold
therapy
electroacupuncture device
Electro-Acuscope
E.-A. myopulse therapy system
E.-A. scope
Electro-Blend epilator
electrocardioanalyzer
electrocardiogram (ECG, EKG)
electrocardiograph
Arrhythmia Research 1200 EPX e.
Cambridge e.
CardioMatic e.
Cardiotest portable e.
Corazonix Predictor e.
MAC-Vu e.
Marquette e.
Megacart e.
Mingograf 62 6-channel e.
PocketView e.
signal-averaged e.
Welch Allyn Schiller AT-1, AT-
2 e.
electrocardiographic transtelephonic
monitor

E

NOTES

electrocardioscanner
    Compuscan Hittman
      computerized e.
electrocautery
    AmpErase e.
    Aspen e.
    bipolar e.
    Bovie e.
    Bugbee e.
    EndoClip monopolar e.
    Fine micropoint e.
    Geiger e.
    Hildreth e.
    Mira e.
    monopolar e.
    Mueller e.
    needlepoint e.
    Neomed e.
    ophthalmic e.
    Op-Temp disposable e.
    Parker-Heath e.
    Rommel e.
    Rommel-Hildreth e.
    Schanz e.
    Scheie e.
    Valleylab e.
    von Graefe e.
    Wadsworth-Todd e.
    wet-field e.
    Ziegler e.
electrochemical detector
electrocoagulating biopsy forceps
electrocoagulator
electroconvulsive therapy (ECT)
electrode
    abdominal patch e.
    ACMI biopsy loop e.
    ACMI cutting loop e.
    ACMI monopolar e.
    ACMI retrograde e.
    acromioplasty e.
    AE-series implantable pronged
      unipolar e.
    Ag/AgCl e.
    air-spaced e.
    Alfa II e.
    all-in-one laparoscopic e.
    AMS Coaguloop resection e.
    antimony pH e.
    Arrowsmith e.
    Arruga surface e.
    Arzbaecher pill e.
    Arzco Tapsul pill e.
    Aspen laparoscopic e.
    atrial e.
    atrial endocardial e.
    Ballenger follicle e.
    e. balloon
    Bard e.

Bard-Hamm fulgurating e.
Bard nonsteerable bipolar e.
Baumrucker e.
Beaver tail-tip e.
Beckman stomach e.
Berens bident e.
Berkovits-Castellanos hexapolar e.
BICAP monopolar e.
BioKnit garment e.
Bioplus dispersive e.
biopotential skin e.
biopsy loop e.
BioTac ECG e.
Biotronik pacemaker e.
bipolar e.
bipolar clip e.
bipolar glass e.
bipolar needle e.
bipolar pacemaker e.
Birtcher e.
Bisping e.
BIS Sensor e.
biterminal e.
blade e.
Bovie conization e.
Bugbee fulgurating e.
Buie fulgurating e.
Burian-Allen contact lens e.
button e.
calomel e.
Cambridge jelly e.
Cameron-Miller e.
CAPSure e.
CAPSure steroid-eluting e.
Care e.
Castroviejo surface e.
e. catheter
cautery e.
cautery knife e.
Cecar e.
central terminal e.
cervical conization e.
ChroniCare TENS e.
Cibis e.
Circon ACMI cutting loop e.
Clarion HiFocus e.
C-Letz conization e.
coagulating e.
Coaguloop resection e.
coil e.
Collings fulguration e.
Collings knife e.
concentric needle e.
conical tip e.
conization e.
Copeland fetal scalp e.
Corson needle e.
Cortac monitoring e.
cortical e.

coudé fulgurating e.
CPI Endotak e.
Cryomedics disposable LLETZ e.
Cueva cranial nerve e.
cuff e.
cup-shaped e.
cutting loop e.
cyclodiathermy e.
cystoscopic fulgurating e.
Darox cutaneous patch e.
Davis coagulation e.
Delgado e.
depolarizing e.
depth e.
Depthalon depth e.
diamond e.
diathermy e.
disc e.
dispersing e.
disposable surface EMG e.
disposable surgical e.
Dispos-a-trode disposable e.
Doyen e.
dual-lead e.
Dura-Stick adhesive e.
Edge needle e.
Electro-Mesh e.
El-Naggar-Nashold right-angled
  nucleus caudalis DREZ e.
EMG e.
endocardial e.
Endotak transvenous e.
EnGuard PFX lead e.
ENT e.
epicardial sock e.
epidural peg e.
epilation e.
Eppendorf needle e.
equipotential e.
ESA acromioplasty e.
ESA electrosurgical arthroscopy e.
ESA hook e.
ESA jet stream ball e.
ESA Smillie e.
esophageal pill e.
Excel Plus e.
exploring e.
external e.
eye diathermy e.
EZ Clean laparoscopic e.
fetal scalp e.
fine-needle e.

fine-wire e.
flat spatula e.
flat-tip e.
flat-wire eye e.
flexible fulgurating e.
flexible radiothermal e.
flexible wire e.
follicle e.
fulgurating e.
Geuder corneal e.
glass pH e.
e. glove
Goetz bipolar e.
Gradle needle e.
Grantham lobotomy e.
Greenwald Control Tip
  cystoscopic e.
Greenwald flexible endoscopic e.
Guyton e.
Haiman tonsillar e.
Hamm fulgurating e.
Hamm resectoscope e.
Hildreth e.
hook e.
Hubbard e.
Hughes fulguration e.
Hurd bipolar diathermy e.
Hurd turbinate e.
Hymes-Timberlake e.
Iglesias e.
impedance e.
implantable e.
impregnated e.
inactive e.
indifferent e.
Innsbruck e.
intracerebral depth e.
intraluminal reference e.
intrameatal e.
intravascular catheter e.
Iomed Phoresor e.
ion-selective e.
iontophoresis e.
Jewett e.
J-loop e.
J orthogonal e.
Josephson quadpolar mapping e.
J-shaped pacemaker e.
Kalk e.
Karaya e.
knife e.
Kontron e.

E

NOTES

electrode *(continued)*

Kronfeld surface e.
LaCarrere e.
lancet-shaped e.
Lane ureteral meatotomy e.
large-loop e.
large-tip e.
Laserdish e.
LEEP active loop e.
LeVeen needle e.
Levin thermocouple cordotomy e.
Lifeline e.
Littmann ECG e.
LLETZ loop e.
lobotomy e.
localizing e.
loop e.
loop ball e.
LSI Gold self-adhesive e.
LSI Silver self-adhesive e.
Lynch e.
Mansfield Polaris e.
McCarthy coagulation e.
McCarthy diathermic knife e.
McCarthy fulgurating e.
McCarthy loop operating e.
McCarthy miniature loop e.
McWhinnie e.
meatotomy e.
Medelec DMG 50 Teflon-coated
   monopolar e.
Medi-Trace e.
Meditrode iontophoresis
   Transvene e.
MegaDyne arthroscopic hook e.
MegaDyne/Fann E-Z clean
   laparoscopic e.
meniscectomy e.
Microglass pH e.
midgastric e.
midoccipital e.
Moersch e.
monopolar loop e.
monopolar temporary e.
multilead e.
multiple-point e.
Multi-Ply reusable e.
multipurpose ball e.
Myerson e.
myocardial e.
Myowire II cardiac e.
Nashold TC e.
National cautery e.
needle e.
Neil-Moore meatotomy e.
Neotrode II neonatal e.
Nesbit e.
neutral e.
New York Hospital e.

Numby Stuff e.
Nyboer esophageal e.
ophthalmic cautery e.
optically transparent e.
Osypka Cereblate e.
pacemaker e.
pacing wire e.
e. pad
pad e.
panendoscope e.
parallel-loop e.
e. paste
patch e.
pencil-tip e.
percutaneous epidural e.
periaqueductal gray e.
PE-series implantable pronged
   unipolar e.
pH e.
Pisces e.
Pischel e.
platinum blade meatotomy e.
platinum-iridium e.
platinum oxygen e.
PMT Cortac cortical e.
PMT Depthalon depth e.
pointed-tip e.
Polaris e.
polarographic needle e.
Polystim e.
Prizm Electro-Mesh Sock e.
proctological ball e.
proctoscopic fulguration e.
prostatic aluminum e.
Prosurg RollerLoop e.
pyramidal e.
Quadpolar e.
Quinton Quik-Prep e.
Ray rhizotomy e.
Ray RRE-TM thermistor e.
recording e.
reference e.
Reflex e.
reimplanted e.
REM PolyHesive II patient
   return e.
renal sympathetic nerve activity
   recording e.
Re-Ply TENS e.
Resume e.
retinal diathermy e.
retrograde e.
Riba electrourethrotome e.
ring e.
Ringenberg e.
rod e.
roller e.
rollerball e.
roller-bar e.

roller-barrel e.
RollerLoop e.
rotating disc e.
Rychener-Weve e.
saturated calomel e.
scalp e.
scalpel e.
Schepens surface e.
screw-in epicardial e.
screw-in sutureless myocardial e.
semiflat tip e.
Severinghaus e.
sew-on e.
Shank e.
Shealy facet rhizotomy e.
silver bead e.
silver-silver chloride e.
single-fiber EMG e.
single-use e.
single-wire e.
Skylark surface e.
Sluder cautery e.
Sluder-Mehta e.
small-loop e.
Smith endoscopic e.
e. sock
Soderstrom-Corson e.
Soft-EZ reusable e.
Softrace gel e.
Somatics monitoring e.
Spencer probe depth e.
spiral e.
SportStim muscle stimulation e.
stab e.
stab-in epicardial e.
Stat-Trace e.
Stern-McCarthy e.
steroid-eluting e.
stick-on e.
Stimitrode e.
stimulating e.
St. Mark pudendal e.
Stockert cardiac pacing e.
Storz cystoscopic e.
straight-blade e.
straight-needle e.
straight-tip e.
straight-wire e.
subcutaneous patch e.
subdural grid e.
subdural strip e.
surface e.

surgical e.
Surgicraft-Copeland fetal scalp e.
Surgicraft pacemaker e.
sutured plaque e.
sutureless pacemaker e.
Tapcath esophageal e.
Tapsul pill e.
temporal e.
temporary percutaneous SCS e.
Teq-Trode e.
terminal e.
Thymapad stimulus e.
Timberlake e.
tined ventricular e.
e. tip
tip e.
tissue desiccation needle e.
TransQFlex iontophoresis e.
Transvene tripolar e.
transvenous e.
trigeminal e.
tripolar coil defibrillation e.
turbinate e.
ultrasonic e.
UltraStim e.
underwater e.
unipolar e.
unipolar glass e.
ureteral meatotomy e.
Uroloop vaporizing cutting e.
USCI Goetz bipolar e.
USCI NBIH bipolar e.
USCI pacing e.
vaginal aluminum e.
Valleylab ball e.
Valleylab loop e.
VaporTome resection e.
VaporTrode roller e.
Vitatron catheter e.
Walker coagulating e.
Walker ureteral meatotomy e.
Wappler e.
Weve e.
Williams tonsillar e.
Wilson-Cook coagulation e.
Wilson-Cook needle e.
Wolfe loop e.
Wolfram needle e.
wraparound inactive e.
Wyler subdural strip e.
Ziegler cautery e.

E

NOTES

electrode *(continued)*
    Zuker bipolar pacing e.
    Zywiec e.
electrodermatome
    Brown e.
    Hood e.
    Padgett e.
    e. sterile blade
electrodiaphake
    LaCarrere e.
Electrodyne pacemaker
electroejaculator
    G&S e.
electroencephalogram (EEG)
    Xltek e.
electroencephalograph (EEG)
    biofeedback e.
    BMSI 5000 e.
    Galileo evoked potential e.
    Grass e.
    Neurofax e.
    Nihon-Kohden e.
electrogoniometer
    6-degrees-of-freedom e.
electrogustometer
    Nagashima e.
electrohemostasis catheter
electrohydraulic
    e. lithotripsy probe
    e. lithotripter
electrokeratotome
    Castroviejo e.
Electro-Link joint wrap
electromagnet
    spring-mounted e.
    structured coil e.
electromagnetic
    e. blood flowmeter
    e. field probe
    e. flow probe
    e. flow transducer
    e. lithotripter
electromechanical
    e. artificial heart
    e. dynamometer
    e. impactor
    e. morcellator
    e. slope computer
Electro-Mesh
    E.-M. electrode
    E.-M. electrode sock
    E.-M. glove
    E.-M. sleeve
electrometer
    vibrating-reed e.
electromucotome
    Castroviejo e.
    Steinhauser e.
    Steinhauser-Castroviejo e.

electromyogram
    kinesiological e.
    e. sensor
electromyograph
    Counterpoint e.
electromyography (EMG)
    integrated e.
electromyometer
    biofeedback e.
electron
    e. beam computed tomography (EBCT)
    e. beam tomography (EBT)
    e. beam tomography scanner
    e. beam x-ray CT scanner
    e. capture detector
    e. diffraction camera
    e. gun
    e. linear accelerator
    e. microscope
    e. multiplier tube
    e. probe x-ray microanalyzer
electronic
    e. aggregometer
    American Medical E.'s (AME)
    e. artificial larynx
    e. calipers
    e. endoscope
    e. goniometer
    e. inclinometer
    e. microanalyzer
    e. muscle stimulator
    e. portal imaging device
    e. summation device
    e. voltmeter
electronic-amplified stethoscope
electronystagmogram
    Nystar Plus e.
electro-oculogram apparatus
electroretinograph
    Ganzfeld e.
electroscope
    Bruening e.
Electroscope disposable scissors
Electroshield
    E. cylindrical conductive shield
    E. monitoring system
    E. reusable sheath
electrospinal orthosis
electrostatic generator
electrosurgery
    e. forceps
    e. snare
electrosurgical
    E. Arthroscopy (ESA)
    e. blade
    e. filter
    e. forceps
    e. generator

e. monopolar spatula probe
e. needle
e. pencil
e. probe needle
e. scalpel
e. scissors
e. spatula
e. spatula blade
e. unit

Electro Surgical Instruments (ESI)
electrotherapy
Dynatron e.
Dynatron TX 900 e.
Mettler e.
electrothermal catheter
electrotome
McCarthy infant e.
McCarthy miniature e.
McCarthy punctate e.
Nesbit e.
Stern-McCarthy e.
Timberlake obturator e.
Elekta
E. stereotactic body frame
E. stereotactic head frame
E. viewing wand
Elema pacemaker
element
beam-splitter optimal e.
4-e. phased-array coil
Mira encircling e.
element-specific detector
elevated rim acetabular liner
elevating forceps
elevator
Abbott e.
Abraham e.
Adson-Love periosteal e.
Adson periosteal e.
Alexander e.
Alexander-Farabeuf e.
Allerdyce e.
Allis periosteal e.
amalgam plugger e.
Amerson bone e.
Anderson e.
angular e.
Anthony e.
Apexo e.
Arenberg dural palpator e.
Artmann e.
Ashley cleft palate e.

Aufranc periosteal e.
Aufricht nasal e.
Austin duckbill e.
Austin footplate e.
Austin right-angle e.
ball-end e.
Ballenger-Hajek e.
Ballenger septal e.
Barsky e.
Batson-Carmody e.
Behrend periosteal e.
Bellucci e.
Bennett bone e.
Berry-Lambert periosteal e.
Bethune periosteal e.
Blair cleft palate e.
blunt e.
Boise nasal fracture e.
bone e.
Bowen periosteal e.
Boyle uterine e.
Bristow periosteal e.
Brophy periosteal e.
Brophy tooth e.
Brown tooth e.
Buck periosteal e.
Cameron e.
Cameron-Haight periosteal e.
Cameron periosteal e.
Campbell periosteal e.
Cannon-Rochester lamina e.
Carmody-Batson e.
Carroll-Legg periosteal e.
Carroll periosteal e.
Carter submucous e.
Chandler bone e.
Cheyne periosteal e.
chisel e.
Cinelli periosteal e.
cleft palate e.
Cloward osteophyte e.
Cloward periosteal e.
Cobb periosteal e.
Cobb spinal e.
Cohen periosteal e.
Converse alar e.
Converse-MacKenty periosteal e.
Converse periosteal e.
Cooper spinal fusion e.
Cordes-New laryngeal punch e.
Coryllos-Doyen periosteal e.
Coryllos periosteal e.

E

NOTES

elevator *(continued)*

costal periosteal e.
Cottle alar e.
Cottle-MacKenty e.
Cottle nasal e.
Cottle periosteal e.
Cottle septum e.
Cottle skin e.
Coupland e.
Crane pick e.
Crawford dural e.
Crego periosteal e.
Cronin cleft palate e.
Cronin palate e.
Cryer dental root e.
Cushing-Hopkins periosteal e.
Cushing little joker periosteal e.
Cushing periosteal e.
Cushing pituitary e.
Cushing staphylorrhaphy e.
Davidson periosteal e.
Dawson-Yuhl periosteal e.
Dean periosteal e.
Derlacki duckbill e.
D'Errico periosteal e.
Desmarres lid e.
Dewar e.
Dingman periosteal e.
Dingman zygoma e.
Doyen costal e.
Doyen periosteal e.
Doyen rib e.
duckbill e.
Dunning e.
dural e.
Ellik e.
endaural e.
Endotrac e.
ESI lighted suction e.
Farabeuf periosteal e.
Fay suction e.
Federspiel periosteal e.
Fomon nostril e.
Fomon periosteal e.
footplate e.
fracture reducing e.
Frazier dural e.
Frazier suction e.
Freer double-end e.
Freer periosteal e.
Freer septal e.
Friedman e.
Friedrich rib e.
Gam-Mer periosteal e.
Gillies malar e.
Gillies zygoma e.
Goldman septal e.
Gorney septal suction e.
Graham scalene e.

Guilford-Wright drum e.
Guilford-Wright duckbill e.
Haberman suction e.
Hajek e.
Hajek-Ballenger septal e.
Halle septal e.
Hamrick suction e.
Hargis periosteal e.
Harper periosteal e.
Harrington spinal e.
Hatt golf-stick e.
Hayden palate e.
Hedblom costal e.
Heel Minder foot e.
Henahan e.
Henner endaural e.
Herczel periosteal e.
Herczel raspatory e.
Herczel rib e.
Hibbs chisel e.
Hibbs costal e.
Hibbs periosteal e.
Hoen periosteal e.
Hopkins-Cushing periosteal e.
Horsley e.
Hough spatula e.
House ear e.
House endaural e.
House stapes e.
House Teflon-coated e.
Howorth e.
Hu-Friedy e.
Hulka-Kenwick uterine e.
Hurd septal e.
Iowa University periosteal e.
Jackson perichondrial e.
Jacobson counter-pressure e.
Jannetta angular e.
Jannetta duckbill e.
Jarit periosteal e.
joker e.
Jordan canal e.
Jordan-Rosen e.
Joseph-Killian septal e.
Joseph nasal e.
Joseph periosteal e.
J-periosteal e.
Kahre-Williger periosteal e.
Kartush stimulus dissection e.
Kennerdell-Maroon duckbill e.
Key periosteal e.
Killian septal e.
Kilner e.
Kinsella periosteal e.
Kirmisson periosteal e.
Kleesattel e.
Kleinert-Kutz e.
Kocher periosteal e.
Koenig e.

Kos e.
Krego e.
Kritzinger-Updegraff e.
Ladd e.
Lambotte e.
laminar e.
Lamont e.
Lane periosteal e.
Lange bone e.
Langenbeck periosteal e.
Lee-Cohen septal e.
Lemmon sternal e.
lemon-squeezer obstetrical e.
Lempert heavy e.
Lempert narrow e.
Lempert periosteal e.
Lewin e.
Lewis periosteal e.
Lindholm-Stille e.
Lindo-Levian dental e.
Logan periosteal e.
Louisville e.
Love-Adson periosteal e.
Lowis periosteal e.
L-shaped e.
lumbosacral fusion e.
Luongo septal e.
MacDonald periosteal e.
MacKenty-Converse periosteal e.
MacKenty periosteal e.
MacKenty septal e.
Magielski e.
Malis e.
Matson-Alexander rib e.
Matson rib e.
McClamary e.
McCollough e.
McGee canal e.
McGlamry e.
McIndoe e.
Mead periosteal e.
Melt e.
MGH periosteal e.
Miller-Apexo e.
Miller dental e.
Miltex Cottle skin e.
Molt No. 4 e.
Molt periosteal e.
Monks malar e.
Moore bone e.
Moorehead e.
mucosal e.

Murphy-Lane bone e.
Netterville double-ended e.
Neurological Institute periosteal e.
Norcross periosteal e.
Nordent oral surgery e.
Norrbacka bone e.
Ohl periosteal e.
Oldberg e.
orthopaedic e.
OSI extremity e.
osteophyte e.
Overholt periosteal e.
Pace periosteal e.
palatorrhaphy e.
Paparella duckbill e.
Pennington septum e.
periosteal e.
Perkins e.
Phemister raspatory e.
Pierce e.
Polcyn e.
Pollock-Dingman e.
Pollock sweetheart periosteal e.
Pollock zygoma e.
Poppen periosteal e.
Potts dental e.
Presbyterian Hospital
  staphylorrhaphy e.
Pritchard e.
Proctor mucosal e.
Quervain e.
Ramirez periosteal e.
Raney periosteal e.
Ray-Parsons-Sunday
  staphylorrhaphy e.
Read periosteal e.
Rhoton e.
rib e.
Richards-Cobb spinal e.
Richardson periosteal e.
Rissler periosteal e.
Roberts-Gill periosteal e.
Rochester lamina e.
Rochester spinal e.
Roger septal e.
Rolyan arm e.
Rosen angular e.
Rowe bone e.
Rowe zygomatic e.
Rubin-Lewis periosteal e.
Rudderman Frelevator fragment e.
Sabbatsberg septum e.

E

NOTES

elevator *(continued)*
    Sauerbruch-Frey rib e.
    Sauerbruch rib e.
    Sayre double-end periosteal e.
    Scheer knife e.
    Schuknecht e.
    Scott-McCracken periosteal e.
    Sebileau periosteal e.
    Sédillot periosteal e.
    Seldin e.
    Seldin periosteal e.
    septal e.
    Sewall ethmoidal e.
    Sewall mucoperiosteal e.
    Shambaugh-Derlacki duckbill e.
    Shambaugh narrow e.
    Shea e.
    Silverstein dural e.
    Sisson fracture-reducing e.
    skin e.
    skull e.
    SMIC periosteal e.
    Smith-Petersen e.
    Sokolec e.
    Soonawalla uterine e.
    Spurling periosteal e.
    stapes e.
    staphylorrhaphy e.
    Steele periosteal e.
    Stille-Langenbeck e.
    Stille periosteal e.
    Stolte-Stille e.
    Story orbital e.
    straight inclined plane e.
    straight periosteal e.
    suction e.
    Sunday staphylorrhaphy e.
    Suraci zygoma hook e.
    Swanson e.
    Tabb ear e.
    Tarlov nerve e.
    Tenzel double-end periosteal e.
    Tessier e.
    T-handle e.
    Tobolsky e.
    Toriumi sharp and dull suction e.'s
    Traquair periosteal e.
    Tronzo e.
    Turner cord e.
    Turner periosteal e.
    upper lid e.
    Urquhart periosteal e.
    uterine e.
    von Langenbeck periosteal e.
    Wadia e.
    walker submucous e.
    Ward periosteal e.
    Warwick-James dental e.
    Watson-Jones e.
    West blunt e.
    Willauer-Gibbon periosteal e.
    Williger e.
    Winter e.
    Woodson dental periosteal e.
    Wright-Guilford drum e.
    Wurzelheber dental e.
    zygoma e.

El Gamal coronary bypass catheter
Elgiloy
    E. clip
    E. clip material
    E. frame
    E. lead-tip pacemaker
Elgiloy-Heifitz aneurysm clip
Eliminator
    E. ArthroWands
    E. biliary stent
    E. dilatation balloon
    E. nasal biliary catheter
    E. PET biliary balloon dilator
    E. stone extraction basket
Elite
    E. Farley retractor
    E. Farley retractor for spinal surgery
    E. guide catheter
    E. hip system
    E. knee brace
    E. pacemaker
    E. System rotating resectoscope
    E. vascular Doppler
Ellik
    E. bladder evacuator
    E. elevator
    E. kidney stone basket
    E. loop stone dislodger
    E. meatotome
    E. resectoscope
    E. sound
Elliot
    E. corneal trephine
    E. femoral condyle holder
    E. knee plate
    E. trephine blade
    E. trephine handle
Elliott
    E. blade plate
    E. gallbladder forceps
    E. hemostatic forceps
    E. obstetrical forceps
Ellipse compact spacer
ellipsometer
    retinal laser e.
elliptical end-capped quadrature radiofrequency coil
Elliptosphere cardiac catheter set

Ellis
  E. buttress plate
  E. foreign body spud
  E. foreign body spud probe
  E. needle holder
Ellison
  E. fixation staple
  E. glenoid rim punch
Ellman
  E. press-form system
  E. rotary scaler
Ellsner gastroscope
Elmed
  E. BC digital bipolar coagulator
  E. diagnostic/operating laparoscope
  E. hysteroscope
  E. peristaltic irrigation pump
Elmiskop 101 electron microscope
Elmo camera
El-Naggar-Nashold right-angled nucleus caudalis DREZ electrode
Elsberg ventricular cannula
Elschnig
  E. capsular forceps
  E. cataract knife
  E. cataract spoon
  E. corneal knife
  E. cyclodialysis forceps
  E. cyclodialysis spatula
  E. extrusion needle
  E. eye spoon
  E. fixation forceps
  E. lens scoop
  E. lens spoon
  E. lid retractor
  E. pterygium knife
  E. refractor
  E. secondary membrane forceps
  E. tissue-grasping forceps
  E. trephine
Elschnig-O'Brien
  E.-O. fixation forceps
  E.-O. tissue-grasping forceps
Elschnig-O'Connor fixation forceps
Elschnig-Weber
  E.-W. loop
  E.-W. loupe
Elscint
  E. dual-detector cardiac camera
  E. ESI-3000 ultrasound
  E. Excel 905 CT scanner
  E. MR scanner

  E. Planar device
  E. tomography system
  E. Twin CT scanner
Elta
  E. dermal hydrogel dressing
  E. dermal sterile impregnated hydrogel gauze pad
eluting stent
Elvarex garment
E-Mac laryngoscope blade
Embarc bone repair material
Embletta portable diagnostic system
embolectomy
  e. catheter
  e. curette
embolization coil
Embol-X
  E.-X arterial cannula
  E.-X arterial cannula and filter system
Embosphere microsphere
Embryon
  E. GIFT introducer
  E. GIFT transfer catheter
  E. HSG catheter
embryotome
  obstetrical decapitating e.
Emcee lens
Emed
  E. insole
  E. scanner
  E. SF pedobarograph
Emerald implantation system
Emergence Profile implant system
emergency
  e. oxygen mask assembly
Emerson
  E. bronchoscope
  E. postoperative ventilator
  E. respirator
  E. vein stripper
Emery lens
Emesay suture button
Emesco handpiece
EMG
  electromyography
  EMG electrode
  FlexComp/DSP EMG
  MyoDac 2 EMG
  Nicolet Viking Iie EMG
  Nordotrack motion EMG
  ProComp EMG

E

NOTES

EMG *(continued)*
    Regain personal trainer EMG
    EMG stimulator
EMHI galvanic electrode stimulator
EMI
    EMI Aped amplifier discriminator
    EMI 9813B photomultiplier
    EMI brain scanner
    EMI CT scanner
    EMI FACT 50 MK III cooler
    EMI 7070 scanner
Emiks heart valve
Emir
    E. razor
    E. razor blade
emission
    e. computerized axial tomography
    e. spectrometric detector
emitter
    alpha-particle e.
    Auger-electron e.
    gamma e.
Emmet
    E. cervical tenaculum
    E. hemostatic bag
    E. hook
    E. needle
    E. obstetrical forceps
    E. obstetrical retractor
    E. ovarian trocar
    E. uterine probe
    E. uterine scissors
Emory EndoPlastic retractor
Empire needle
EMS
    electrical muscle stimulation
    EMS 2000 neuromuscular
        stimulator
EnAbl thermal ablation system
Enac ultrasonic endodontic system
enamel rod
Encapsulon
    E. epidural catheter
    E. sheath introducer
    E. TFX-Medical bacterial filter
    E. vessel dilator
encased screw
encircling
    e. band
    e. clip
eNclose proximal anastomosis device
enclosure
    air-flow e.
Encore
    E. ceramic hip joint replacement
        system
    E. ceramic knee joint replacement
        system
    E. inflator

    E. microptic powder-free latex
        surgical glove
    E. PASS
    E. Poly-Axial Spine System
Encor pacemaker
endarterectomy
    e. dissector
    e. spatula
endaural
    e. curette
    e. elevator
    e. retractor
    e. speculum
    e. surgery chisel
Endeavor nondetachable silicone balloon catheter
end-end stapler
Ender
    E. fixation
    E. nail
    E. pin
    E. rod
Endermologie
    E. adipose destruction system
    E. noninvasive body contouring
        device
Endex apex sensor
end-fire
    e.-f. transducer
    e.-f. transrectal probe
Endius
    E. Atavi spine surgery system
    E. EndoFusion system
    E. endoscopic access system
    E. MiCOR precision bone allograft
    E. spinal camera
    E. spinal endoscope
    E. TiTLE implant and instrument
        system
    E. WAVE polyaxial plate system
Endless Pool physical therapy pool
Endo
    E. Babcock grasper
    E. Babcock stapler
    E. Babcock surgical grasping
        device
    E. cinch
    E. Clip applier
    E. Dissect dissector
    E. GIA surgical clip
    E. GIA 30 suture stapler
    E. Grasp instrument
    E. hinged knee prosthesis
    E. Multi-Mode stimulator
    E. Optics MicroProbe
    E. rotating knee joint prosthesis
    E. sled prosthesis
    E. Stitch
    E. Stitch instrument

E. stop
E. Tip port system
E. Tip Storz trocar
E. zoom lens camera
Endo-AID suction irrigation
endoanal
  e. coil
  e. ultrasound
EndoAnchor anchor
endoaortic clamp
Endo-Assist
  E.-A. cutting dissector
  E.-A. endoscopic knot pusher
  E.-A. endoscopic ligature carrier
  E.-A. endoscopic needle holder
  E.-A. retractable blade
  E.-A. retractable scalpel
  E.-A. sponge aspirator
EndoAvitene
  E. collagen hemostatic material
  E. disposable applicator
  E. microfibrillar collagen hemostat
Endobag
  E. laparoscopic specimen retrieval system
  E. specimen bag
Endo-Bender bending device
endobiliary stent
EndoBlade
  LaserSonics E.
endobronchial tube
endobrow push screw
Endobutton 6 button
Endocam
  E. digital camera
  E. endoscope
  E. video camera system
endocamera
  Olympus e.
  Polaroid instant e.
endocapsular
  e. artificial lens
  e. balloon
endocardial
  e. balloon lead
  e. bipolar pacemaker lead
  e. cardiac lead
  e. electrode
  e. screw-in lead
  e. wire
Endocare Horizon prostatic stent
Endocatch II bag

endocavitary
  e. applicator
  e. applicator system
  e. probe
Endocavity V33W probe
Endocell
  E. disposable endometrial cell sampler
  E. endometrial cell collector
endocervical
  e. aspirator
  e. biopsy curette
  e. probe
EndoCinch suturing system
EndoClamp ST aortic catheter
EndoClip
  E. ML/Surgiport System pack
  E. monopolar electrocautery
Endoclose suture carrier
endocoagulator laser system
  ophthalmic e.
  Semm e.
EndoCoil-T biliary stent
EndoCPB catheter
EndoCurette
  Fowler E.
endocut cautery device
Endocutter
  Long45 E.
Endodermologie LPG system
endodiathermy
EndoDissect instrument
endodontic
  e. broach
  e. bur
  e. curette
  e. endosteal implant
  e. file
  e. pin
  e. plugger
  e. reamer
EndoDynamics
  E. AdzorbStar
  E. glutameter
  E. suction polyp trap
endoesophageal
  e. magnetic resonance imaging coil
  e. MRI coil
  e. tube
Endofit vessel occluder
EndoFix absorbable interference screw

E

NOTES

Endoflex
 E. below-knee prosthesis
 E. endoscopic instrument system
 E. endoscopic retractor
 E. endoscopy instrument
Endoflip device
Endo-Flo irrigator
EndoGauge gauge
endograft
 AneuRx stent e.
 Endologix aortic e.
 Prograft Exluder bifurcated e.
 Talent bifurcated e.
 Vanguard e.
Endograsp device
endograsper
Endo-Gripper endodontic handpiece
endohernia stapler
endo-illuminator
 Grieshaber e.-i.
endo-irrigator
Endoknot suture
EndoLase laser
endolaser
 diode e.
 e. probe
EndoLift device
EndoLive 3-D stereo video endoscope
Endologix aortic endograft
Endoloop suture
EndoLumina bougie
endoluminal
 e. stent
 e. stent graft
endolymphatic shunt tube introducer
endolymphatic-subarachnoid shunt
EndoMax
 E. advanced laparoscopic instrument
 E. endoscope
 E. endoscopic instrumentation
EndoMed LSS laparoscopy system
endometrial
 e. ablator
 e. aspirator
 e. biopsy curette
 e. cannula
 e. curette
 e. polyp forceps
Endo-Model
 E.-M. total hinge knee
EndoNet
 Pentax E.
EndoOctopus stabilizer
endo-osseous dental implant
EndoPaddle device
Endopap endometrial sampler
Endopath
 E. bladeless trocar
 E. disposable surgical trocar

E. ELC35 endoscopic linear cutter
E. EMS hernia stapler
E. endoscopic articulating stapler
E. endoscopic linear cutter
E. ES endoscopic stapler
E. ETS-Flex endoscopic articulating
 linear cutter
E. EZ45 No knife
E. EZ-RF linear cutter and
 coagulation device
E. EZ-series endoscopic linear
 cutter
E. laparoscopic trocar
E. needle tip electrosurgery probe
E. Optiview laparoscopic obturator
E. Optiview system
E. Stealth stapler
E. surgical trocar
E. surgical trocar reducer
E. TriStar trocar
E. Ultra Veress needle
EndoPearl
 E. bioabsorbable ACL implant
 E. bioabsorbable fixation device
Endo-Pool suction cannula
Endopore
 E. dental implant system
 E. implant
Endopost
 Kerr E.
Endopouch Pro specimen retrieval bag
Endo-P-Probe endorectal probe
endoprobe
 rotating e.
endoprosthesis
 Atkinson e.
 Austin Moore e.
 Austin Moore curved e.
 Austin Moore straight-stem e.
 Averett total hip e.
 Bateman e.
 Bateman UPF II bipolar e.
 biliary e.
 Celestin e.
 Centrax bipolar e.
 crutched stick-type polyurethane e.
 cuffed esophageal e.
 double-lumen e.
 double-pigtail e.
 DoubleStent biliary e.
 Elastalloy esophageal e.
 Excluder bifurcated e.
 expandable biliary e.
 expandable metal mesh e.
 femoral e.
 Gore Viatorr e.
 hip e.
 IntraCoil e.
 IntraStent DoubleStent biliary e.

IntraStent DoubleStrut biliary e.
large-bore bile duct e.
Leinbach head and neck e.
Matchett-Brown hip e.
metallic biliary e.
metatarsophalangeal e.
Moore hip e.
nonporous-coated e.
pancreatic e.
Passager e.
pigtail e.
plastic e.
Proctor-Livingston e.
Ring-Derlan TM biliary e.
Schneider Wallstent biliary e.
self-expandable stainless steel
  braided e.
self-expanding metallic e.
self-expanding Wallstent e.
Thompson XL e.
tibial e.
Titan e.
transpapillary e.
tumor-replacement e.
Unitrax modular e.
Viabahn e.
Viatorr e.
Wallgraft e.
Wallstent biliary e.
Wallstent iliac e.
Wilson-Cook e.
endoprosthetic flange
endorectal
  e. coil magnetic resonance imaging
  e. coil MRI
  e. surface coil MR imaging
endorectal-pelvic phased-array coil
EndoRetract retractor
Endo-Right Angle dissector
Endo-Ring surgical retraction system
Endosac specimen bag
EndoSaph vein harvest system
endoscope
  e. ACMI e.
  ACMI e.
  Agee e.
  battery-powered e.
  cap-fitted e.
  Cho/Dyonics two-portal e.
  Cho 2-portal Dyonics e.
  Cilco ophthalmic e.
  Clarus SpineScope spinal e.

Cuda e.
disc e.
Dohlman e.
double-channel e.
Eder-Palmer semiflexible
  fiberoptic e.
electronic e.
Endius spinal e.
Endocam e.
EndoLive 3-D stereo video e.
EndoMax e.
end-viewing e.
ETB e.
EUM-series e.
EVIS Exera 160 e.
EVIS Q-series e.
FG-series 2-channel e.
fiberoptic e.
flexible fallopian tube e.
foroblique e.
forward-viewing e.
Fujinon EG-FP-series e.
Fujinon EG-series e.
Fujinon EVE-series e.
Fujinon EVG-CT-series e.
Fujinon EVG-FP-series e.
Fujinon EVG-F-series e.
Fujinon EVG-series e.
Fujinon FP-series e.
Fujinon UGI-FP-series video e.
Gaab e.
Hamou e.
Haslinger e.
Insight 40000 e.
Jarit Rotator e.
J-shaped e.
Karl Storz Calcutript e.
Karl Storz flexible e.
Kelly e.
large-channel e.
Lowsley-Peterson e.
lung imaging fluorescence e.
Machida flexible e.
magnetic resonance e.
McCarthy e.
Messerklinger e.
MicroLap e.
MicroProbe ophthalmic laser e.
mother-baby e.
mother-daughter e.
Navigator flexible e.
near-infrared electronic e.

E

NOTES

endoscope *(continued)*
Needlescoper e.
Neuro Navigational flexible e.
nonrigid e.
oblique-viewing e.
Olympus CF-UM20 ultrasonic e.
Olympus CHF-BP30 e.
Olympus EU-series e.
Olympus EUS-series e.
Olympus EVIS Q-series e.
Olympus forward-viewing e.
Olympus GF-UM-series e.
Olympus GIF-HM-series e.
Olympus GIF-J-series e.
Olympus GIFK-XQ-series e.
Olympus GIF-Q-series e.
Olympus GIF-XP-series e.
Olympus GIF-XV-series e.
Olympus JF-T-series e.
Olympus JF-TV-series e.
Olympus P-series e.
Olympus Q-series e.
Olympus side-viewing e.
Olympus S20-20R e.
Olympus TJF-series e.
Olympus XCF-XK-series e.
Olympus XP-series e.
ophthalmic e.
oral e.
Padgett e.
pediatric e.
Pentax EC-series video e.
Pentax EG-series video e.
Pentax EndoNet digital e.
Pentax FG-series ultrasound e.
Pentax flexible e.
Pentax side-viewing e.
percutaneous spinal e.
rigid intranasal e.
Rockey e.
Satellite ear e.
semiflexible e.
semirigid e.
Sensatec e.
side-viewing e.
Simpson e.
Sine-U-View nasal e.
Storz e.
Storz Sine-U-View e.
Surgenomic e.
Toshiba video e.
transpapillary e.
UGI e.
variable stiffness e.
velolaryngeal e.
Visicath e.
Weerda e.
Welch Allyn video e.
Wolf e.
Zeiss Endolive e.
endoscopic
e. access port
e. Babcock grasper
e. band ligator
e. BICAP probe
e. biopsy forceps
E. Carpal Tunnel Release
  Assembly (ECTRA)
e. carpal tunnel release system
e. color Doppler ultrasonography
e. curved needle driver
e. dissector
e. electrode handle
e. flowprobe
e. grasping forceps
e. heat probe
e. Hemoclip device
e. irrigator
e. laser
e. linear cutter
e. quadrature radiofrequency coil
e. retrograde
  cholangiopancreatography (ERCP)
e. retrograde
  cholangiopancreatography catheter
e. scissors
e. sewing machine
e. suture-cutting forceps
e. telescope
e. threaded imaging port
e. ultrasonogram
e. washing pipe
endoscopically deliverable tissue-transfixing device
endoscopy
laserlight-induced fluorescence e.
  (LIFE)
Polavision Land camera for e.
Endo-Set
Haag-Streit E.-S.
EndoShears instrument
EndoSheath
E. endoscopy system
Slide-On E.
EndoShield
E. mask
E. mask and goggles
endoskeleton
stationary ankle flexible e.
Endo-Sock specimen retrieval bag
Endo-Sof double pigtail stent
EndoSonics
E. IVUS/balloon dilatation catheter
E. ultrasound-guided catheter
endosonography
e. instrument
e. probe

endosonoprobe
EndoSound
 E. endoscopic ultrasound
 E. endoscopic ultrasound catheter
 E. ultrasound probe
endospeculum
 e. forceps
 Gynex e.
 Kogan e.
endosseous HA implant
endostapler stapler
EndoStasis probe
Endostat
 E. calibration pod insert
 disposable coaxial E.
 disposable sculptured E.
 E. disposable sterile fiber
 E. fiber stripper
 E. II bipolar/monopolar
 electrosurgical generator
endosteal implant
Endostitch laparoscopic suturing device
Endo-Suction sinus microstat
Endotak
 E. C transvenous lead
 E. C tripolar
 pacing/sensing/defibrillation lead
 E. defibrillator
 E. DSP lead
 E. Endurance EZ lead
 E. Endurance RX lead
 E. lead system
 E. nonthoracotomy implantable
 cardioverter-defibrillator
 E. Picotip
 E. Reliance defibrillator lead
 E. transvenous electrode
Endotec spreader
Endotek
 E. machine
 E. OM-3 Urodata monitor
 E. UDS-1000 monitor
 E. urodynamics system
endothelial specular microscope
endothelin-1 microcoil
Endo-therapy disposable biopsy forceps
EndoTIP
 E. access cannula
 E. imaging port
Endotrac
 E. blade system
 E. cannula

 E. elevator
 E. endoscopic carpal tunnel release
 system
 E. endoscopy instrument
 E. ligament probe
 E. ligament rasp
 E. obturator
 E. retractor
endotracheal (ET)
 e. cardiac output monitor
 e. catheter
 e. curette
 e. forceps
 e. stylet
 e. tube
 e. tube brush
 e. tube cuff
 e. tube forceps
Endotrol endotracheal tube
Endotron-Lipectron ultrasonic scalpel
Endo-Tube nasal jejunal feeding tube
endovaginal
 e. coil
 e. transducer
endovascular
 e. aortic graft
 e. aortic graft cuff
 e. coil
 e. photoacoustic recanalization
 (EPAR)
 e. stent-graft
Endovasix
 E. endovascular photoacoustic
 recanalization system
 E. EPAR system
Endovations disposable cytology brush
EndoVideo-Five endoscopic camera
EndoView camera
Endowel
 E. dental post
 E. post
EndoWrist instrument
EndoZime sponge
Endur
 E. bonding material
 E. resin
Endura
 E. coronary dilation catheter
 E. dressing forceps
EnduraFix tape
Endurance bone cement
EnduraSplint splint

NOTES

E

EnduraSports tape
EnduraTape tape
Enduron acetabular liner
end-viewing
    e.-v. endoscope
    e.-v. gastroscope
Enemette enema cleansing kit
energometer
Energy Dispersive X-ray Fluorescence (EDXRF)
Engel plaster saw
Engen
    E. palmar finger orthosis
    E. palmar wrist splint
engine
    Acrotorque hand e.
    Robbins Acrotorque hand e.
engineering
    Arterial Vascular E. (AVE)
English
    E. anvil nail nipper
    E. brace
    E. clamp
    E. hospital reflex percussor
    E. lock
    E. MacIntosh fiberoptic laryngoscope blade
    E. profile laryngoscope blade
    E. tissue forceps
Engstrom
    E. multigas monitor
    E. respirator
EnGuard
    E. double-lead ICD system
    E. pacing and defibrillation lead system
    E. PFX lead electrode
enhanced
    e. external counterpulsation unit
    e. MRI
Enhanced Torque guiding catheter
enhancer
    Aerosol Cloud E. (ACE)
    e. cushion
enlarging bur
Ensi syringe
EnSite
    E. cardiac catheter
    E. 3000 cardiac mapping system
    E. 3000 electrophysiology workstation
ENT
    ears, nose, throat
    ENT bite block
    ENT electrode
    ENT scope
    ENT speculum
    ENT wire crimper
ENTaxis packing

ENTec
    E. Coblator Plasma Surgery system
    E. Plasma Wands
Entegra prosthesis
Entera-Flo enteral feeding pump
enteroclysis tube
Enteroport feeding pump
enteroscope
    dedicated push e.
    Goldberg MPC operative e.
    Olympus SIF-M-series video e.
    Olympus SIF-series video e.
    Olympus SIF-SW-series video e.
    Olympus SSIF-series video e.
    Olympus XSIF-series video e.
    Sonde e.
    video push e.
enterostomy clamp
Entero-Test
    E.-T. capsule
    E.-T. Hp capsule
enterotomy scissors
Enterra
    E. pacemaker
    E. therapy
Entity pacemaker
entor injector gun
Entos vascular and abdominal intraoperative scanhead
Entre II trocar and cannula system
Entract
    E. dilation and occlusion catheter
    E. stent
    E. stone retriever
ENTrak electromagnetic surgical navigation system
entrapment sack
Entree
    E. disposable CO_2 insufflation needle
    E. II cannula
    E. II laparoscopic trocar system
    E. II trocar and cannula system
    E. Plus cannula
    E. Plus trocar
    E. Plus trocar and cannula system
Entrex small-joint arthroscopy instrument set
EntriStar
    E. percutaneous endoscopic gastrostomy tube
    E. skin level gastrostomy system
entropion
    e. clamp
    e. forceps
EntSol nasal wash system
enucleation
    e. scissors

e. scoop
e. wire snare
enucleator
Botvin-Bradford e.
Bradford snare e.
Castroviejo snare e.
Foster snare e.
Hardy bayonet e.
Hardy microsurgical e.
Marino rotatable transsphenoidal e.
Rhoton e.
snare e.
Young prostatic e.
enuresis alarm
envelope
e. arm sling
cryoflex e.
Envision
E. lens
E. targeted dose drug delivery system
E. TD implantable drug delivery system
Envoy middle ear implantable system
EOC goniometer
EPAR
endovascular photoacoustic recanalization
EPAR laser system
Epic
E. laser
E. ophthalmic 3-in-1 laser system
E. wheelchair
epicardial
e. Doppler flow sector transducer
e. lead
e. pacemaker
e. patch
e. retractor
e. sock electrode
Epicel skin graft material
Epics
E. C-flow flow cytometer
E. Elite flow cytometer
E. Profile II flow cytometer
Epi-Derm silicone gel sheeting
epidural peg electrode
EpiE-Z
E.-Z Pen epinephrine injector
E.-Z Pen injection device
E.-Z Pen-Jr. pen
EpiFilm
E. film

E. graft
E. otologic lamina
EpiFlex heel and elbow protector
EPIfoam adhesive foam pad
EPI foam pad
Epigard synthetic skin dressing
epiglottis retractor
Epigrip material
epi-illuminated microscope
EpiLaser
E. hair removal laser
E. laser-based hair removal system
epilation
e. electrode
e. forceps
e. needle
epilator
Electro-Blend e.
Epilot high-frequency needle-type e.
Epitron Super high-frequency e.
high-frequency tweezer-type e.
Removatron e.
Thermaderm e.
Trichodemolus e.
Epilatron hair-removal machine
epilepsy implant
EpiLight hair removal system
EpiLock
E. tennis elbow strap
E. tennis elbow support
Epilot high-frequency needle-type epilator
EpiPen injection device
EpiPen-Jr injection device
Epiquick syringe
epiretinal delamination diamond knife
episcleral forceps
Episeal wound dressing
episiotomy scissors
EPI-Sport epicondylitis clasp
Epistar
E. diode laser
E. magnetic resonance imaging
E. subtraction angiogram
Epistat double balloon
epistaxis balloon
Epi-Stay device
epithelial
e. rete peg
e. scraper
Epitome scalpel

NOTES

EpiTouch ruby SilkLaser hair removal system
Epitrain active elastic elbow support
Epitron Super high-frequency epilator
Epoca custom offset shoulder prosthesis
Epos Ultra orthopaedic shock wave therapy
Epoxylite CBA dental resin cement
Eppendorf
  E. angiocatheter
  E. cardiac catheter
  E. catheter
  E. centrifuge
  E. cervical biopsy forceps
  E. microelectrode
  E. needle electrode
  E. Repeater Pro pipette
  E. tube
Eppendorfer
  E. biopsy punch
  E. uterine biopsy forceps
Epstein
  E. bone rasp
  E. collar stud acrylic lens
  E. down-biting curette
  E. hemilaminectomy blade
  E. needle
  E. neurological hammer
  E. osteotome
  E. posterior chamber intraocular lens
  E. spinal fusion curette
EPT-1000 XP cardiac ablation system
EPT Dx steerable diagnostic catheter
ePTFE
  expanded polytetrafluoroethylene
  ePTFE augmentation membrane
  ePTFE graft prosthesis
  ePTFE implant
  ePTFE vascular suture
  ePTFE ventricular shunt catheter
Epworth Sleepiness scale
Equalizer air walker
Equen stomach magnet
Equiflex bandage
Equinox
  E. balloon occlusion balloon catheter
  E. digital EEG
  E. EEG neuromonitoring system
equipment
  Bodyblade exercise e.
  Body Solid exercise e.
  bubble chamber e.
  durable medical e.
  DynaDisc exercise e.
  Dynalyzer e.
  Galileo training circuit e.
  Invertrac e.

Luxar Silhouette noninvasive body appearance e.
OsseoCare drilling e.
OsteoStat single-use power surgical e.
StereoGuide breast biopsy e.
equipotential electrode
ERA resectoscope sheath
eraser
  e. cautery
  hemostatic e.
  Mentor Wet-Field e.
  Tano ·e.
Eraser-tip cautery
Erbe
  E. argon plasma coagulator
  E. bipolar laparoscopic forceps
  E. cryoprobe
  E. ICC generator
erbium
  e. CrystaLase laser
  e. Renaissance laser
  e. SilkLaser
erbium:YAG infrared laser
ERCP
  endoscopic retrograde cholangiopancreatography
  ERCP balloon extractor
  ERCP cannula
  ERCP catheter
  ERCP dilator
  ERCP guidewire
  ERCP nasobiliary drain
  ERCP sphincterotome
ERCPeel Away catheter
ErCr:YAG laser
ErecAid
  E. Esteem external vacuum therapy system
  E. vacuum erection device
erector spinae retractor
ERG-Jet disposable contact lens
Er:glass dermatologic laser
Ergo
  E. bipolar forceps
  E. Cush back support
  E. irrigation system
  E. microaspirator
  E. style flexion table
Ergociser
  Cateye E.
  E. exercise cycle
ErgoForm contoured cold pack
Ergolift device
Ergoline bicycle ergometer
ErgoLogic keyboard
ergometer
  bicycle e.
  Bosch ERG 501 e.

Collins bicycle e.
Concept II rowing e.
Corival 400 e.
Cybex cycle e.
Ergoline bicycle e.
Excalibur sport cycle e.
Gauthier bicycle e.
Monark bicycle e.
pedal-mode e.
Siemens-Albis bicycle e.
Siemens-Elema AG bicycle e.
Tunturi EL400 bicycle e.

ergonomic vascular access needle (EVAN)

Ergos
E. O_2 dual-chamber rate-responsive pacemaker
E. work simulator

ErgoTec vitreoretinal instrument system

Erhardt
E. ear speculum
E. eyelid forceps
E. lid clamp

Eric
E. Lloyd extractor
E. Lloyd introducer

Erich
E. facial fracture frame
E. laryngeal biopsy forceps
E. malleable dental arch bar
E. maxillary splint
E. nasal splint
E. swivel

Eriksson
E. guide
E. knee prosthesis
E. muscle biopsy cannula

Erlangen
E. magnetic colostomy device
E. papillotome

Erlanger sphygmomanometer
Ermold needle holder
Ernest-McDonald
E.-M. II folding forceps
E.-M. soft intraocular lens-folding forceps
E.-M. soft intraocular lens inserter

Ernest nucleus cracker
eroder
facet e.

Erosa
E. amnioscope
E. disposable hypodermic needle

Ero-Scan otoacoustic emissions test system
Eros-CTD clitoral therapy device
Er:YAG laser
erysiphake
Barraquer e.
Bell e.
Castroviejo e.
corneal e.
Dimitry e.
Draeger high-vacuum e.
Falcao e.
Harken e.
Harrington e.
Johnson e.
Johnson-Bell e.
Kara e.
L'Esperance e.
Maumenee e.
Maumenee-Park e.
New York e.
nucleus e.
Nugent e.
Nugent-Green-Dimitry e.
Post-Harrington e.
Sakler e.
Searcy oval cup e.
Simcoe nucleus e.
Storz-Bell e.
Viers e.
Welsh rubber bulb e.
Welsh Silastic e.

ESA
Electrosurgical Arthroscopy
ESA acromioplasty electrode
ESA electrosurgical arthroscopy electrode
ESA hook electrode
ESA jet stream ball electrode
ESA Smillie electrode

escape pacemaker
Eschenbach
E. low-vision rehabilitation guide
E. monocular telescope

Eschenback Optik lens
Eschmann
E. blade
E. endotracheal tube introducer

E-Scope electronic stethoscope

E

NOTES

Escort
- E. 300A defibrillator/pacer monitor
- E. balloon stone extractor

E-series
- E-s. bipolar forceps
- E-s. hip system
- E-s. needle holder
- E-s. scissors

ESI
- Electro Surgical Instruments
- ESI bite block
- ESI fiberoptic light source
- ESI laryngoscope
- ESI Lav gastric lavage system
- ESI lighted suction elevator
- ESI Lite-Pipe fiberoptic cable
- ESI Lite-Pipe fiberoptic instrument
- ESI long, narrow mammoplasty retractor
- ESI sigmoidoscope

ESKA-Jonas silicone-silver penile prosthesis

Esmarch
- E. bandage
- E. bandage scissors
- E. plaster knife
- E. plaster shears
- E. roll dressing
- E. tin bullet probe
- E. tourniquet

EsophaCoil
- E. prosthesis
- E. self-expanding esophageal stent

esophageal
- e. balloon
- e. balloon catheter
- e. balloon dilator
- e. balloon tamponade
- e. detection device
- e. manometry catheter
- e. motility catheter
- e. obturator airway
- e. pH probe
- e. pill electrode
- e. prosthesis
- e. retractor
- e. scissors
- e. stent
- e. stethoscope
- e. Strecker stent
- e. temperature probe
- e. variceal ligation device
- e. Z-stent
- E. Z-Stent stent

esophagofiberscope
- Olympus e.

esophagoprobe
- Olympus ultrasonic e.

esophagoscope
- ACMI fiberoptic e.
- ballooning e.
- Blom-Singer e.
- Boros e.
- Broyles e.
- Bruening e.
- Chevalier Jackson e.
- child e.
- Dohlman e.
- Eder e.
- Eder-Hufford e.
- fiberoptic e.
- Foregger rigid e.
- foroblique fiberoptic e.
- Haslinger e.
- Holinger infant e.
- Hufford e.
- infant e.
- Jackson e.
- Jasbee e.
- Jesberg oval e.
- Jesberg upper e.
- J-scope e.
- Kalk e.
- Lell e.
- LoPresti fiberoptic e.
- Mosher e.
- Moure e.
- Olympus e.
- optical e.
- oval-open e.
- pediatric e.
- Roberts folding e.
- Roberts-Jesberg e.
- Roberts oval e.
- Sam Roberts e.
- Schindler optical e.
- standard full-lumen e.
- Storz operating e.
- Storz optical e.
- Storz pediatric e.
- Tesberg e.
- Tucker e.
- Universal e.
- Yankauer e.

esophagoscopic
- e. cannula
- e. catheter
- e. forceps

E-Spart analyzer

Espe
- E. Ketac-Bond Aplicap
- E. Photac-Bond Aplicap

E-speed intraoral film
Espocan combined spinal/epidural needle
ESP radiation reduction examination glove

ESPrit
    E. ear level speech processor
Esprit
    E. critical care ventilator
    E. microdermabrasion system
Esquire dental sterilizer
ESRA-10 erythrocyte sedimentation rate analyzer
ESR-Auto Plus erythrocyte sedimentation rate analyzer
ESSential shaver system
Esser
    E. graft
    E. implant
    E. prosthesis
Essrig
    E. dissecting scissors
    E. tissue forceps
Essure sterilization system
EST40 electronic stethoscope
EsteLux dermatological laser
Esterman scale
esthesiometer
    manual e.
esthetic
    e. CO_2 laser
    e. Taylor mandibular angle implant
Estilux
    E. dental restorative material
    E. ultraviolet system
Estring
    E. estradiol vaginal ring
    E. silicone vaginal ring
ESU dispersive pad
ET
    endotracheal
    ET tube
etafilcon A disposable contact lens
ETB endoscope
Etch-Master
    E.-M. electronic stencil
    E.-M. felt pad
    E.-M. kit
ETE
    external tissue expander
ether
    e. guard
    e. screen
    e. screen clamp
Ethezyme papain-urea debriding ointment

Ethibond
    E. polybutilate-coated polyester suture
    E. polyester suture
Ethicon
    E. BV-75-3 needle
    E. clip applier
    E. disposable cannula
    E. disposable trocar
    E. endoscopic linear cutter
    E. Endo-Surgery circular stapler
    E. mesh
    E. Micropoint suture
    E. Polytef paste prosthesis
    E. Sabreloc suture
    E. silk suture
    E. ST-4 straight taper-point needle
    E. TG Plus needle
    E. TGW needle
Ethiguard needle
Ethilon nylon suture
Ethi-pack suture
ethmoid
    e. chisel
    e. curette
    e. forceps
    e. punch
ethmoid-Blakesley forceps
Ethox
    E. bite block
    E. blood pressure cuff
    E. rectal tube
    E. Surgi-Press pressure infuser
Ethrone
    E. implant
    E. prosthesis
ethyl cyanoacrylate glue
ethylene
    e. oxide (ETO)
    e. oxide dressing
ETO
    ethylene oxide
ETO Sleuth
E-Trap surgical filter device
Etude cystometer uroflowmeter
E-type dental implant
EUB-series portable ultrasound
EUE tonsillar snare
EUM-series endoscope
Eureka collimator
EuroCuff forearm crutch
Euro-Med FNA-21 aspiration needle

E

NOTES

European
    E. bipolar cable
    E. in-the-bag lens
EuroPeel system
Eurotech
    E. Diamond table
    E. Emerald table
    E. Platinum table
    E. Sapphire table
EUSN-1 EchoTip needle
eustachian
    e. bougie
    e. bur
    e. catheter
    e. probe
    e. tube
euthyscope
    AC-powered e.
EVac Plasma wand
evacuator
    Bard e.
    Bigelow e.
    bladder e.
    Creevy bladder e.
    Crigler e.
    Dentsply MVS e.
    Ellik bladder e.
    high-volume e.
    Hutch e.
    ice clot e.
    Iglesias e.
    Kennedy-Cornwell bladder e.
    Laparofan smoke e.
    Laufe portable uterine e.
    Lavacuator gastric e.
    McCarthy bladder e.
    McKenna Tide-Ur-Ator e.
    Ortho-evac e.
    oval-window piston e.
    Plume-Away e.
    Sklar e.
    smoke e.
    SmokEvac smoke e.
    Snyder Hemovac e.
    Solcovac suction e.
    Thompson e.
    Timberlake e.
    Toomey bladder e.
    Urovac bladder e.
    uterine e.
evaluator
    Touch-Test sensory e.
EVAN
    ergonomic vascular access needle
Evans
    E. loop stone dislodger
    E. tissue forceps

Evazote
    E. cushioning material
    E. foam
Eve Fujinon video colonoscope
event recorder
Everett
    E. crutch
    E. eustachian catheter
    E. fallopian cannula
    E. fallopian catheter
    E. forceps
Ever-Flex insole
Evergreen
    E. Lasertek coagulator
    E. Lasertek laser
Evermed catheter
Evershears
    E. bipolar forceps
    E. bipolar laparoscopic scissors
    E. LP bipolar scissors
everter
    Berens lid e.
    Berke double-end lid e.
    lid e.
    Luther-Peter lid e.
    Pess lid e.
    Roveda lid e.
    Schachne-Desmarres lid e.
    Siniscal-Smith lid e.
    Strubel lid e.
    Vail lid e.
    walker lid e.
Evert-O-Cath drug delivery catheter
Everyday
    E. Objects ColorCards
    E. self-adhering urinary external
    catheter
Eves tonsillar snare
EVIS
    EVIS CF-100L video colonoscope
    EVIS Exera 160 endoscope
    EVIS Q-series endoscope
evisceration spoon
Evolution
    E. EBCT scanner
    E. hip prosthesis
    E. scanner
    E. XP scanner
Evolve orthopaedic implant
EVS hemostasis device
Ewald
    E. elbow prosthesis
    E. gastroscope
    E. tissue forceps
    E. tube
Ewald-Hudson
    E.-H. brain forceps
    E.-H. clamp

E.-H. dressing forceps
E.-H. tissue forceps
Ewing
  E. capsular forceps
  E. eye implant
  E. lid clamp
ExAblate 2000 MR scanner/ultrasound delivery system
Exacta-Med oral dispenser
ExacTech blood glucose meter
Exact-Fit ATH hip replacement system
Exakt
  E. cutting/grinding system
  E. cutting/grinding unit
Exami-Gown gown
examination retractor
eXamine cholangiography catheter
examining
  e. arthroscope
  e. gastroscope
  e. hysteroscope
  e. lamp
  e. telescope
Excalibur
  Bard Safety E.
  E. sport cycle ergometer
excavating bur
excavator
  Austin e.
  dental e.
  Farrior oval-window e.
  fenestration e.
  Henry Schein e.
  Hough oval-window e.
  Hough-Saunders e.
  Hough whirlybird e.
  House e.
  House-Hough e.
  Lempert e.
  Merlis obstetrical e.
  Nordent e.
  oval-window e.
  Paparella-Hough e.
  PD e.
  Schuknecht whirlybird e.
  sinus tympani e.
  SMIC e.
  stapes e.
  whirlybird stapes e.
Excel
  E. disposable biopsy forceps
  E. electric hospital bed

E. GE blood glucose monitoring test strip
E. Plus electrode
E. Plus underpad
E. quilted underpad
Excel-14 microcatheter
Excelart short-bore MRI
eXcel-DR
  e.-DR disposable/reusable Glasser laparoscopic needle
  e.-DR pneumothorax needle
Excell
  E. polishing point
  E. polishing wheel
Excelsior 1018 microcatheter
Exceltech imaging
exchange guidewire
exchanger
  countercurrent heat e.
  heat and moisture e.
  heat/moisture e.
  HumidFilter heat and moisture e.
  hygroscopic heat and moisture e.
  moisture e.
  Portex Thermovent heat and moisture e.
  Provox FreeHands heat/moisture e.
  ThermoVent heat/moisture e.
Excilon dressing sponge
ExciMed UV200 excimer laser
excimer
  e. laser
  e. sheath
Excluder
  E. bifurcated endoprosthesis
  E. endovascular stent-graft
exclusion clamp
Excursiometer
  Mandibular E.
executive bifocal
Exel Zero Dead Space syringe
exenteration
  e. forceps
  e. spoon
Exerball kit
ExerBand therapy band
exercise
  Back atYa rebounder for plyometric e.
  e. band
  Cardiac Assessment System for E. (CASE)

E

NOTES

exercise *(continued)*
   e. sandal
   e. treadmill
exerciser
   AnkleCiser e.
   Böhler e.
   Builder Grip hand e.
   carpal care e.
   Cat's Paw e.
   ChairCiser e.
   Chattanooga e.
   CliniFLO breathing e.
   Cybex isokinetic e.
   Danniflex CPM e.
   Digi-Flex finger e.
   Digi-Flex hand e.
   Digi-Grip hand e.
   Eggsercizer resistive hand e.
   Exer-Cor e.
   ExtendaFLEX e.
   Finger Helper hand e.
   Finger Platter hand e.
   Flextender Plus hand e.
   Grahamizer II e.
   Gripp squeeze ball hand e.
   Hand Helper hand e.
   isokinetic Unex III e.
   Iso-Quadron e.
   Jace shoulder e.
   jaw e.
   Jux-A-Cisor e.
   Kegel e.
   Kinetec clubfoot CPM e.
   Knead-A-Ball hand e.
   KneeThing e.
   Lordoticiser e.
   microcomputer upper limb e.
    (MULE)
   MiniMedBall hand e.
   Morpho e.
   Motivator FTR2000 e.
   MULE upper limb e.
   NordiCare Enabler e.
   NordiCare Strider e.
   NordicTrack ski e.
   NuStep e.
   Omni-Flexor wrist e.
   Oppociser hand e.
   Orthotron e.
   Physio-Roll-R-Cise e.
   PlyoSled e.
   Posture Pump Lordoticiser e.
   Powerflex CMP e.
   Power Pogo stationary e.
   Power Web hand e.
   Preston Traveler CPM e.
   ProStretch e.
   Pul-Ez e.
   Relax-a-Cizor e.

   Resistex expiratory resistance e.
   resistive e.
   Rickshaw Rehab e.
   Rotaflex e.
   Roylan ergonomic hand e.
   Soft Touch hand e.
   Stronghands hand e.
   Stryker CPM e.
   Stryker leg e.
   Swanson Grip-X isometric e.
   Therabite jaw e.
   Thera Cane shoulder e.
   Thera-Fit e.
   Theraflex wrist e.
   Ther-A-Hoop e.
   Thera-Loop e.
   Toronto Medical CPM e.
   Tuf Nex neck e.
   Tunturi hand e.
   Universal Fitstep e.
   Walk-'n-tone e.
Exer-Cor exerciser
Exer-Pedic cycle
Exerstrider machine
Exertools gym ball
Exeter
   E. intramedullary bone plug
   E. ophthalmoscope
EX-FI-RE external fixation device
eXit
   e. disposable puncture closure
   e. disposable puncture closure
    device
Exmoor plastics aural grommet
Exo-Bed traction
exocervical probe
Exogen 2000+ ultrasound fracture
  healing system
Exonix Ultrasonic Surgical system
Exo-Overhead traction unit
exophthalmometer
   Hertel e.
   Krahn e.
   Luedde e.
   Marco prism e.
   Naugle orbitometer e.
exoplant
   scleral e.
   silicone e.
Exo-Static
   E.-S. cervical collar
   E.-S. collar
   E.-S. overhead traction
   E.-S. overhead tractor
Exotec brace
expandable
   e. access catheter
   e. biliary endoprosthesis
   e. blade

e. breast implant
e. cervical dilator
e. esophageal stent
e. intrahepatic portacaval shunt
  stent
e. LeMaitre valvulotome
e. metallic stent
e. metal mesh endoprosthesis
e. prosthesis
Expandacell
E. nasal pack
E. sponge
expanded
e. polytetrafluoroethylene (ePTFE)
e. polytetrafluoroethylene-covered
  stent
e. polytetrafluoroethylene implant
e. polytetrafluoroethylene suture
e. polytetrafluoroethylene vascular
  graft
expander
AccuSpan tissue e.
Becker tissue e.
Beehler irrigating pupil e.
Biospan anatomical tissue e.
Biospan breast tissue e.
CUI tissue e.
external tissue e. (ETE)
field e.
Graether pupil e.
Hextend plasma volume e.
Heyer-Schulte tissue e.
Integra tissue e.
irrigating pupil e.
Man facelift e.
McGhan tissue e.
Mentor Spectrum contour e.
Mentor tissue e.
Meshgraft skin e.
Osmed hydrogel tissue e.
PMT AccuSpan tissue e.
PMT Integra breast e.
Radovan tissue e.
Ruiz-Cohen round e.
saline-filled e.
self-inflating tissue e.
skin graft e.
slow palatal e.
subperiosteal tissue e.
tissue e.
T-Span tissue e.

expanding
e. reamer
e. valvotome
expansile
e. dilator
e. forceps
expansion screw
Expert-XL bone densitometer
expiratory valve
expirograph
Godart e.
explorer
E. common bile duct exploration
  system
E. coronary dilatation catheter
E. 360-degree rotational diagnostic
  catheter
dental e.
Nordent e.
E. precurved diagnostic EP catheter
SMIC e.
Steri-Probe e.
E. ST fixed-curve diagnostic
  catheter
E. X 70 intraoral radiography
  system
exploring
e. cannula
e. electrode
e. needle
Expo
E. Bubble dressing
E. Bubble eye cover
E. Bubble eye shield
E. diagnostic catheter
Export aspiration catheter
eXpose retractor
exposure meter
Express
E. 2 balloon catheter
E. 2 coronary stent system
E. over-the-wire balloon catheter
E. Plus PTCA catheter
expressor
Arroyo e.
Arruga eye e.
Arruga lens e.
Bagley-Wilmer lens e.
Berens lens e.
follicle e.
Fyodorov lens e.
Goldmann e.

E

NOTES

expressor *(continued)*
Heath follicle e.
Hess tonsil e.
Heyner e.
hook e.
e. hook
Hosford meibomian gland e.
intracapsular lens e.
iris e.
Kirby hook e.
Kirby intracapsular lens e.
lens e.
lid e.
McDonald e.
Medallion lens e.
meibomian gland e.
nucleus e.
Osher nucleus stab e.
ring lens e.
Rizzuti iris e.
Rizzuti lens e.
Smith lens e.
Smith lid e.
Stahl nucleus e.
Wilmer-Bagley iris e.
Wilmer-Bagley lens e.

EXS femoropopliteal bypass graft

Extend
E. stem
E. total hip system

ExtendaFLEX exerciser

extended
e. anatomical high-profile malar
implant
e. needle
e. sector ultrasonic probe
E. Wear self-adhering urinary
external catheter starter kit

extended-wear soft contact lens

extender
Ahmed glaucoma valve tube e.
Blomqvist external tissue e.
rear-tip e.
Rousek e.
Superstabilizer cemented stem e.
Superstabilizer press-fit stem e.
Sven Johansson e.
Taq e.

Extend-It finger splint

extension
e. apparatus
bifurcated drain e.
e. bow
Buck e.
deep brain e.
DOC guidewire e.
Hudson cerebellar e.
Jackson-Pratt bifurcated drain e.
Linx guidewire e.

Loc guidewire e.
NexGen offset stem e.
Orascoptic loupe e.
radiolucent operating room table e.
e. tube

extensometer
laser e.

external
e. asynchronous pacemaker
e. auditory larynx
e. biliary drainage catheter
e. cardioverter-defibrillator
e. collimator
e. counterpressure device
e. demand pacemaker
e. drug infusion pump
e. electrode
e. fixator
e. functional neuromuscular
stimulator
e. inflatable compressor
e. monitor
e. orthosis
e. pacemaker
e. pacemaker battery
e. retractor
e. ring fixator
e. sequential pneumatic compression
boot
e. spinal skeletal fixator
e. tachyarrhythmia control device
e. tissue expander (ETE)
e. transthoracic pacemaker
e. ureteral catheter
e. urethral barrier
e. vascular compression device
e. vein stripper

extra
e. large (XL)
E. Sport coronary guidewire
e. stiff Amplatz wire

extracapsular forceps

extracardiac right-to-left shunt

extracoronal retainer

extracorporeal
e. liver assist device (ELAD)
e. membrane oxygenation (ECMO)
e. membrane oxygenation system
e. membrane oxygenator
e. piezoelectric lithotripter
e. pump
e. pump oxygenator
e. shockwave lithotripsy system
e. shock wave lithotripter

extraction
e. atherectomy device
e. balloon
e. forceps
e. generator

e. hook
e. pliers
e. trap
Extract-N-Amp blood PCR kit
extractor
 Andrews comedo e.
 Applied Biosystems 340A nucleic
  acid e.
 Austin Moore e.
 ball e.
 balloon stone e.
 Bellows cryoextractor e.
 Bilos pin e.
 Bird vacuum e.
 broach e.
 cataract rotoextractor e.
 Cherry screw e.
 comedo e.
 Cook helical stone e.
 cortex e.
 Davis loop stone e.
 deluxe FIN e.
 DePuy e.
 Douvas Roto-extractor e.
 Egnell vacuum e.
 ERCP balloon e.
 Eric Lloyd e.
 Escort balloon stone e.
 femoral trial e.
 fetal head e.
 fetal vacuum e.
 food e.
 Gill-Welsh cortex e.
 Glassman stone e.
 Hallach comedo e.
 head e.
 infant mucus e.
 Intraflex intramedullary pin e.
 Jarit comedo e.
 Jewett bone e.
 Kalish Duredge wire e.
 Kobayashi vacuum e.
 Krwawicz cataract e.
 Küntscher e.
 Lewicky cortex e.
 Lloyd nail e.
 Look cortex e.
 Luxator e.
 magnetic e.
 Malström vacuum e.
 Mark II femoral component e.
 Mark II tibial component e.

Massie e.
McDermott e.
McNutt e.
McReynolds e.
Mignon cataract e.
Mityvac e.
Moore-Blount e.
Moore hooked e.
Moore nail e.
Moore prosthesis e.
Murless fetal head e.
Rush e.
Rutner balloon dilation stone e.
Saalfeld comedo e.
Schamberg comedo e.
Schneider e.
Silastic cup e.
Silc e.
Simcoe cortex e.
Smirmaul nucleus e.
Smith-Petersen e.
Soehendra stent e.
Southwick screw e.
stem e.
Take-Out e.
Tender Touch e.
Torpin vectis e.
Trizol RNA e.
Troutman cataract e.
Unna comedo e.
ureteral stone e.
vacuum e.
Vantos vacuum e.
Visitec cortex e.
Walton comedone e.
Welsh cortex e.
Wilson-Cook eight-wire basket
 stone e.
E. XL triple-lumen retrieval
 balloon
Zimmer e.
extracutaneous vas fixation clamp
extra-depth shoe
extra-flexible wire
extrahepatic shunt
extramedullary
 e. alignment guide
 e. tibial alignment jig
extraoral
 e. bone-anchored implant
 e. fracture appliance
 e. sigmoid notch retractor

E

NOTES

ExtraSafe butterfly infusion needle
extra-stiff guidewire
extra-support guidewire
extrathoracic ventilator
ExtraView balloon
Extreme
    E. laser catheter
    E. orthotic
    E. peripheral catheter
    E. Select ligament brace
extremity
    e. coil
    e. mobilization strap
    e. pump
ExtreSafe phlebotomy device
extruded bar polyethylene
extrusion
    e. balloon catheter
    e. needle
exudate disposal bag
ExuDerm RCD hydrocolloid dressing
Exu-Dry
    E.-D. absorptive dressing
    E.-D. oncology dressing
Exxcel ePTFE soft vascular graft
eye
    artificial e.
    e. bandage
    e. blade
    e. calipers
    e. diathermy electrode
    e. dressing forceps
    e. fixation forceps
    e. irrigator
    e. knife
    e. knife guard
    e. magnet
    e. movement measuring apparatus
    e. needle holder
    e. pad
    e. pad dressing
    e. patch
    e. probe
    e. protector
    e. scissors
    e. shield
    e. spear
    e. speculum
    e. spherical implant
    e. stitch scissors
    e. suture scissors
6-eye catheter
EyeClose
    E. adhesive strip
    E. external eyelid weight
Eyecor camera
eyed suture needle
eyeFix speculum system
eyeglass hearing aid

eyeless
    e. atraumatic suture needle
    e. needle
eyelid
    e. forceps
    e. retractor
    e. spacer
    e. speculum
EyeMap EH-290 corneal tomography system
Eye-Pak drape
eyepiece
    comparison e.
    compensating e.
    demonstration e.
    huygenian e.
    Huygens e.
    negative e.
    positive e.
    Ramsden e.
    wide-field e.
EyeSys
    E. 2000 corneal topographic mapping system
    E. videokeratoscope
eyetracker
    Visx STAR S3 ActiveTrak e.
eyewear
    E Clips computer e.
E-Z
    E-Z Flap burr hole cover
    E-Z 'Jector injector
EZ
    EZ arm abduction orthosis
    EZ band hemostasis band
    EZ Cath catheter
    EZ Clean cautery tip
    EZ Clean laparoscopic electrode
    EZ Derm porcine biosynthetic wound dressing
    EZ Flap titanium miniplate system
    EZ Flex bed
    EZ Flex jaw exercising device
    EZ hand pump
    EZ hold adhesive catheter tube holder pad
    EZ Lift table
    EZ reacher
    EZ Rider support chair
    EZ Splint mouthpiece
    EZ Splint PM mouthpiece
    EZ syringe
    EZ Tac system
    EZ Temp thermometer
EZ.1 multifocal contact lens
EZ45 No Knife
EZ-Dish pressure relief cushion
EZE-Fit IOL system
Ezeform splint

E-Z-EM
    E-Z-EM BioGun automated biopsy
    system
    E-Z-EM cut biopsy needle
    E-Z-EM PercuSet amniocentesis
    tray
E-Z-Guard mouthpiece
EZ-Guide SL light bar
EZ-Ject injector

Ezo denture cushion
EZ-On
    EZ-On traction belt system
    EZ-On vest
EZ-Splint PM TMJ splint
EZVue violet haptic intraocular lens
Ezy
    E. Wrap lumbosacral support
    E. Wrap shoulder immobilizer

NOTES

E

F2L Multineck femoral stem
Fabco
    F. gauze bandage
    F. gauze dressing
face
    f. mask
    f. rest
    f. shield
facebow
    Asher high-pull f.
    Hanau f.
    Kinematic f.
    Kloehn f.
    Ortho-Yomy f.
    Rickett f.
Face-It protective shield
facelift
    f. flap marker
    f. retractor
    f. scissors
faceplate
    Sur-Fit irrigation adapter f.
facet
    f. eroder
    f. rasp
    f. screw system
facial
    f. compression skull cap closure
    f. fracture appliance dental arch
    bar
    f. nerve dissector
    f. nerve knife
    f. nerve stimulator
    f. plastic surgery scissors
Facial-Flex
    F.-F. therapy
    F.-F. Ultra device
FACScan flow cytometer
FACSVantage cell sorter
FACT-22 coronary balloon angioplasty
   catheter
Fahrenheit flat bath thermometer
Fairdale orthodontic appliance
Falcao
    F. erysiphake
    F. fixation forceps
    F. suction dissector
Falcon
    F. coronary catheter
    F. filter
    F. lens
    F. plastic flask
    F. single-operator exchange balloon
    catheter

Falk
    F. appendectomy spoon
    F. clamp
    F. lion-jaw forceps
    F. needle
    F. vaginal cuff
    F. vaginal retractor
fallopian
    f. cannula
    f. tube forceps
falloposcope
    f. endoscopic instrument
Falope
    F. ring
    F. tubal sterilization ring
Falope-ring
    F.-r. applicator
    F.-r. dilator
    F.-r. tubal occlusion band
fan
    f. elevator retractor
    f. liver retractor
    Schmitt f.
fan-beam collimator
Fanelli laparoscopic endobiliary stent
fan-shaped liver retractor
Fansler
    F. anoscope
    F. proctoscope
    F. rectal speculum
Fansler-Ives rectal speculum
Farabeuf
    F. bone clamp
    F. bone-holding forceps
    F. bone rasp
    F. double-ended retractor
    F. periosteal elevator
    F. raspatory
    F. rugine
    F. saw
Farabeuf-Collin rasp
Farabeuf-Lambotte
    F.-L. bone-holding clamp
    F.-L. bone-holding forceps
    F.-L. raspatory
Faraday
    F. cage
    F. shield
    F. shielded resonator
Farlow
    F. tongue depressor
    F. tonsillar snare
Farr
    F. self-retaining retractor

F

Farr *(continued)*
  F. spring retractor
  F. wire retractor
Farrington
  F. nasal polyp forceps
  F. septal forceps
Farrior
  F. angulated curette
  F. anterior footplate pick
  F. blunt palpator
  F. bur
  F. ear curette
  F. ear speculum
  F. mushroom raspatory
  F. otoplasty knife
  F. oval speculum
  F. oval-window excavator
  F. oval-window pick
  F. posterior footplate pick
  F. rasp
  F. septal cartilage stripper knife
  F. sickle knife
  F. suction applicator
  F. triangular knife
  F. wire crimper
  F. wire-crimping forceps
Fasanella
  F. double-ended iris retractor
  F. lacrimal cannula
fascia
  f. lata implant
  f. lata prosthesis
  f. lata stripper
fascial
  f. cutter
  f. dilator
  f. needle
  f. press
  f. snare
  f. stripper
Fascian human fascia lata
fasciatome
  Lane f.
  Luck f.
  Masson f.
  Moseley f.
Fasplint splint
FAST
  flow-assisted short-term
  FAST balloon flotation catheter
  FAST right heart cardiovascular
    catheter
**F.A.S.T.1 adult intraosseous infusion
  system**
FASTak suture anchor
fast-breeder reactor
Fast-Cath
  F.-C. catheter

F.-C. Duo hemostasis introducer
F.-C. Trio hemostasis introducer
fastener
  ball f.
  Brown-Mueller T-bar f.
  Cath-Strip recloseable catheter f.
  Intrafix tibial f.
  NG strip nasal tube f.
  Percu-Stay catheter f.
  Roc suture f.
  Roc XS suture f.
  SmartPins f.
  UC strip catheter tubing f.
  Velcro f.
Fast-Fit compression stocking
**Fast Fourier Transform spectrum
  analyzer**
**fast-imaging steady precession sequence
  3-dimensional magnetic resonance
  imaging**
FastIn threaded anchor
FastPack system
Fast-Pass endocardial lead
FasTrac
  F. hydrophilic-coated guidewire
  F. introducer
FasTracker-18 infusion catheter
FastRNA, Green kit
fast-setting acrylic
fastSTART
  f. EMS neuromuscular stimulator
  f. HVPC pulsed stimulator
**FastTake blood glucose monitoring
  system**
fat
  f. pad retractor
  f. towel
Fat-O-Meter skinfold calipers
fat-suppressed body coil
faucet aspirator
Faught sphygmomanometer
Faulkner
  F. antral chisel
  F. antral curette
  F. double-end ring curette
  F. ethmoidal curette
  F. folder
  F. nasal curette
  F. trocar
Faure
  F. peritoneal forceps
  F. uterine biopsy forceps
Favaloro
  F. atrial retractor
  F. coronary scissors
  F. ligature carrier
  F. proximal anastomosis clamp
  F. saphenous vein bypass graft
  F. self-retaining sternal retractor

Faxitron x-ray machine
Fay
    F. suction elevator
    F. suction tube
FCP2 laser
Feaster
    F. Accura diamond knife
    F. Dualens intraocular lens
    F. dual-placement intraocular lens
    F. K7-5460 hydrodissecting cannula
    F. lens holding forceps
    F. lens hook
    F. lens manipulator
    F. radial keratotomy knife
    F. RK diamond knife
feather
    F. carbon breakable blade
    f. clamp
    F. clear cornea knife
    f. scalpel
feathered extended malar implant
FeatherTouch
    F. automated rasp
    F. CO_2 laser
    F. SilkLaser
    F. SilkLaser system
Fechtner
    F. conjunctival forceps
    F. intraocular lens
    F. ring forceps
    F. trabeculectomy marker
Federspiel
    F. cheek retractor
    F. needle
    F. periosteal elevator
    F. scissors
feeder
    Brecht f.
    Haberman f.
    offset suspension f.
    Rancho Los Amigos f.
    Tumble Forms f.
feeding
    f. gastrostomy
    f. tube
feeler
    O'Donoghue cartilage f.
Fehland
    F. intestinal clamp
    F. intestinal forceps
Feilchenfeld splinter forceps

Feild
    F. retractable blade assembly
    F. suction dissector
Feild-Lee biopsy needle
Fein
    F. antral trocar
    F. cannula
    F. needle
Feldbausch nasal dilator
Feldenkrais cylinder
Feldman
    F. adaptometer
    F. aortic stenosis catheter
    F. bur
    F. lid retractor
    F. lip retractor
    F. radial keratotomy marker
Felig insulin pump
Fell-O'Dwyer apparatus
felt
    f. dressing
    f. pledget
    f. shears
    Teflon f.
female
    f. sound
    f. urinary pouch
    f. washer
female/male condom
FemAssist continence device
Femcept device
Feminal female urinal
Femina vaginal weight
femoral
    f. aligner
    f. artery cannula
    f. broach
    f. canal restrictor
    f. cerebral catheter
    f. clamp
    f. distractor
    f. endoprosthesis
    f. guide pin
    f. guiding catheter
    f. head bone removal reamer
    f. head driver
    f. hemodialysis catheter
    f. impactor
    f. intramedullary guide
    f. introducer sheath
    f. neck retractor
    f. notch guide

NOTES

F

femoral *(continued)*
  f. perfusion cannula
  f. plug
  f. rasp
  f. retractor
  f. shaft reamer
  f. stem
  f. trial extractor
femorofemoral crossover prosthesis
FemoStop
  F. femoral artery compression arch
  F. inflatable pneumatic compression
    device
FemRx laparoscopic morcellator
FemSoft
  F. continence insert
  F. urethral insert
FemTone vaginal weight
femtosecond laser system
fence
  Kirklin f.
  f. splint
Fenelli guide
fenestrated
  f. aneurysm clip
  f. blade forceps
  f. bowel grasper
  f. catheter
  f. compression plate
  f. cup biopsy forceps
  f. Drake clip
  f. ellipsoid spiked biopsy forceps
  f. Moore-type femoral stem
  f. sterile drape
  f. tracheostomy tube
  f. tube
fenestration
  f. bur
  f. curette
  f. excavator
  f. hook
fenestrator
  Montgomery tracheal f.
  Rosen f.
fenestrometer
  Guilford-Wright f.
  Paparella f.
  Rosen f.
  Wright-Guilford f.
Fenger
  F. gall duct probe
  F. spiral gallstone probe
Fenlin total shoulder system
Fenton
  F. bulldog vulsellum
  F. tibial bolt
  F. uterine dilator
Fenwal
  F. blood warmer

  F. cryocyte freezing container
  F. CS3000 Plus cell separator
  F. hemapheresis pump
FEP-ringed Gore-Tex vascular graft
Ferciot
  F. tip-toe splint
  F. wire guide
Ferguson
  F. abdominal scissors
  F. angiotribe
  F. angiotribe forceps
  F. bone clamp
  F. bone curette
  F. bone holder
  F. bone-holding forceps
  F. esophageal probe
  F. gallstone scoop
  F. implant
  F. mouthgag
  F. retractor
  F. round-body needle
  F. stone basket
  F. suction
  F. suture needle
Ferguson-Ackland mouthgag
Ferguson-Frazier suction tube
Ferguson-Metzenbaum scissors
Ferguson-Moon rectal retractor
Fergusson tubular vaginal speculum
Ferno
  F. AquaCiser II underwater
    treadmill system
  F. Recline-a-Bath bathing system
Ferran awl
Ferree-Rand perimeter
Ferrier
  F. coupler
  F. 212 gingival clamp
  F. separator
Ferris
  F. biliary duct dilator
  F. chart
  F. colporrhaphy forceps
  F. common duct scoop
  F. disposable bone marrow
    aspiration needle
  F. filiform dilator
  F. polyostomy wound dressing
Ferris-Robb tonsillar knife
Ferris-Smith
  F.-S. bone-biting forceps
  F.-S. cup rongeur forceps
  F.-S. fragment forceps
  F.-S. intervertebral disc rongeur
  F.-S. needle holder
  F.-S. orbital retractor
  F.-S. pituitary cup jaw rongeur
  F.-S. rongeur forceps
  F.-S. tissue forceps

Ferris-Smith-Gruenwald rongeur
Ferris-Smith-Halle sinus bur
Ferris-Smith-Kerrison
    F.-S.-K. bone punch
    Ferris-Smith-Lyman periosteotome
    F.-S.-K. forceps
    F.-S.-K. laminectomy rongeur
Ferris-Smith-Sewall orbital retractor
Ferris-Smith-Spurling
    F.-S.-S. disc rongeur
    F.-S.-S. intervertebral disc forceps
Ferris-Smith-Takahashi forceps
Ferris-Smith-Takahashi rongeur
Ferrolite crown remover
ferromagnetic
    f. intracerebral aneurysm clip
    f. monitoring device
ferrule clamp
Ferszt
    F. dissecting hook
    F. ligature passer
fetal
    F. Dopplex II FD2+ monitor
    f. head extractor
    f. heart rate monitor
    f. incontinence collector
    f. scalp electrode
    f. stethoscope
    f. vacuum extractor
FetalPulse
    F. Plus fetal Doppler
    F. Plus monitor
Fetasonde fetal monitor
fetoscope
    Pinard horn f.
Feuerstein
    F. drainage tube
    F. split ventilation tube
F&F machine
FG-36UX scanning echoendoscope
FG diamond bur
FHT
    Fox Hollow Technologies
    FHT Reform coronary catheter
fiber
    Bard Urolase f.
    Bare-Tip f.
    braided polyester f.
    carbon f.
    f. cleaver
    C. R. Bard Urolase f.
    Endostat disposable sterile f.

    FiberLase flexible f.
    hollow f. (HF)
    Indigo diffuser f.
    laser f.
    Laserscope disposable Endostat f.
    f. mallet
    Micro Link endoscope f.
    Pinnacle contact Nd:YAG f.
    Prolase f.
    SLT FiberTact/Contact laser f.
    UltraLine Nd:YAG laser f.
    Urolase neodymium:YAG laser f.
fibercolonoscope
    Olympus CF-20 f.
fibered platinum coil (FPC)
fiberendoscope
    flexible f.
    laser f.
    Olympus transnasal f.
    ultrasonic f.
fibergastroscope
    fluorescence f.
fiberglass
    f. bandage
    f. graft
FiberLase
    F. beam delivery system
    F. flexible fiber
    F. laser
Fiberlite microscope
fiberoptic
    f. anoscope
    f. arthroscope
    f. bronchoscope
    f. catheter delivery system
    f. choledochoscope
    f. endoscope
    f. esophagoscope
    f. gastroscope
    f. hysteroscope
    f. lens
    f. light cable
    f. light carrier
    f. lighted mirror
    f. light pipe
    f. light projector
    f. light source
    f. loupe
    f. microscope
    f. otoscope
    f. oximeter catheter
    f. PCO_2 sensor

F

NOTES

fiberoptic *(continued)*
  f. pick
  f. pressure catheter
  f. probe
  f. proctosigmoidoscope
  f. retractor
  f. right-angle telescope
  f. sheath
  f. sigmoidoscope
  f. slide laryngoscope
  f. suction tube
  f. surgical field illuminator
  f. vaginal speculum
  f. videoendoscope
  f. video glasses
fiberscope
  Hirschowitz gastroduodenal f.
  nasopharyngeal f.
  Olympus OES f.
  Olympus XK-series oblique-viewing
    flexible f.
  Pentax sigmoid f.
  side-viewing f.
  superfine f.
fiberTome system
FiberWire suture
**Fibracol collagen alginate wound
  dressing**
Fibra Sonics phaco aspirator
Fibrel gelatin matrix implant
fibrin
  f. glue
  f. glue adhesive
  f. sealant adhesive
fibrin-film stent
fibrin-soaked Gelfoam
fibroid hook
fibrotome
  Pelosi f.
Fichman surgical ophthalmic guide
Ficoll-Hypaque gradient centrifuge
Fidelity intraaortic balloon catheter
fiducial marker
field
  F. blade
  f. emission tube
  f. expander
  f. tourniquet
field-effect transistor
field-of-view camera
figure-of-8
  f.-o.-8 bandage
  f.-o.-8 brace
  f.-o.-8 clavicle strap
  f.-o.-8 dressing
  f.-o.-8 suture
filament
  Charcot-Bottcher f.
  cytokeratin f.

  desmin f.
  Semmes-Weinstein pressure
    aesthesiometer f.
  f. suture
  f. transformer
  vimentin f.
filamentary keratome
**Filcard temporary removable vena
  caval filter**
file
  bone f.
  Charnley trochanter f.
  Dentsply FlexoFiles f.
  diamond nail f.
  endodontic f.
  Flex-R-File f.
  Hedstrom f.
  Kerr K-Flex f.
  K-Flexofile f.
  Kleinert-Kutz bone f.
  K root canal f.
  Miller bone f.
  Mity Gates Glidden f.
  Mity Hedström f.
  Mity Turbo File f.
  nickel-titanium f.
  Nordent bone f.
  Onyx-R NiTi f.
  orthopaedic bone f.
  ProFile f.
  pulp canal f.
  Putti bone f.
  root canal f.
  Schwed Flexicut f.
  scrub f.
  SMIC bone f.
  SMIC periodontal f.
  S root canal f.
  SureFlex nickel-titanium f.
  surgical f.
  taper hand f.
filiform
  f. bougie
  f. bougie probe
  f. catheter
  f. dressing
  f. and follower
  f. guide
  LeFort f.
  Rusch f.
  f. steel needle
  f. stone dislodger
filiform-tipped catheter
Fillauer
  F. bar
  F. dorsiflexion assist ankle joint
  F. endoskeletal alignment system
  F. night splint
  F. PDC ankle joint

F. prosthesis liner
F. Scottish Rite orthosis kit
F. silicone suspension liner
F. Tiny Titans pediatric knee
  brace

filler

Bio-Oss maxillofacial bone f.
BonePlast bone void f.
Cortoss bone void f.
Cutinova cavity wound f.
Orthoss resorbable bone void f.
OsteoSet bone f.
ProOsteon implant 500 coralline
  hydroxyapatite bone void f.
spiral f.

film

absorbable gelatin f.
AccuFilm articulating f.
Accu-Flo dural f.
f. alternator
autoradiographic f.
Bard protective barrier f.
Biobrane transparent f.
f. changer
Dentus x-ray f.
Duncan dural f.
DuPont Cronex x-ray f.
EpiFilm f.
E-speed intraoral f.
Ioban 2 incise f.
Knuttsen bending f.
Kodak XAR-5 x-ray f.
Kodak XRP-1 x-ray f.
MDS Truspot articulating f.
3M No Sting barrier f.
No Sting barrier f.
Nuvo barrier f.
orthogonal f.
Repel-CV bioresorbable adhesion
  barrier f.
Softopac intraoral f.
soft x-ray f.
vaginal contraceptive f.
f. wound dressing

Filshie

F. clip minilaparotomy applicator
F. female sterilization clip

filter

Ace autografter bone f.
Adams kidney stone f.
Affinity arterial f.
Amicon D-20 f.

arterial f.
bacterial f.
bandpass f.
Baxter CA-series f.
Berkefeld f.
bidirectional Butterworth digital f.
Biospal f.
bird's nest IVC f.
Butterworth bidirectional four-pole
  high-pass digital f.
Centricon-10 f.
charcoal f.
Clear Advantage pulmonary
  function f.
Cook f.
D/Flex f.
electrosurgical f.
Encapsulon TFX-Medical
  bacterial f.
Falcon f.
Filcard temporary removable vena
  caval f.
flattening f.
fluorescence excitation f.
Fresenius F-40 f.
Gambro FH88H f.
GeneScreen nylon membrane f.
Gianturco-Roehm bird's nest vena
  caval f.
Greenfield titanium IVC f.
Greenfield vena caval f.
Günther Tulip vena caval
  MReye f.
Günther Tulip vena caval MRI f.
Haag-Streit 900 cobalt blue f.
Hamming-Hahn f.
Hann f.
HEPA f.
high-pass f.
Holter in-line shunt f.
Hybond-N f.
inferior vena caval umbrella f.
inherent f.
Interface arterial blood f.
interference barrier f.
Jostra arterial blood f.
Kalman f.
K-edge f.
Kim-Ray Greenfield antiembolus f.
Kim-Ray Greenfield vena caval f.
KoKo Moe f.
leukocyte reduction f.

F

NOTES

329

filter *(continued)*
 LeukoNet f.
 LGM f.
 Liposorber cholesterol f.
 low-pass f.
 f. maintainer
 mediastinal sump f.
 Medi-Tech IVC f.
 Millex GS-series f.
 Millex GV-series f.
 Millipore ultrafree-CL centrifugal f.
 Mobin-Uddin umbrella vena caval f.
 monomer f.
 MReye f.
 MultiSPIRO Clear Advantage pulmonary function f.
 Nalgene capsule f.
 neutral density f.
 Pall Biomedical heat- and moisture-exchanging f.
 Pall leukocyte removal f.
 Pall PL-series leukocyte removal f.
 Pall RC-series leukocyte removal f.
 Pall transfusion f.
 Percoll f.
 Portex bacterial f.
 power peak f.
 PreVENT Anti-Reflux f.
 red-free f.
 Re/Flex f.
 Renal Systems HF250 f.
 rhodium f.
 Rubicon embolic f.
 shunt f.
 Simon nitinol inferior vena caval f.
 Steriflex-Braun bacterial f.
 suprarenal Greenfield f.
 Swank high-flow arterial blood f.
 Thoreau f.
 TrapEase permanent vena caval f.
 TULIP vena caval MReye f.
 tunable notch f.
 umbrella f.
 UV-blocking f.
 vena caval f.
 Vena Tech dual vena caval f.
 Vena Tech LGM vena caval f.
 Vena Tech LP vena caval f.
 Vitalograph bacterial/viral f.
 wedge f.
 Wiener MRI f.
 William Harvey arterial blood f.
 Wratten 6B f.
 Zeta probe nylon f.
filtered
 f. dual-sump drain

 f. mediastinal sump drain
 f. specimen trap
FilterWatch sensor
FilterWire EX embolic device
Filtresse surgical smoke filtration system
Filtryzer dialyzer
Filtzer
 F. corkscrew
 F. interbody rasp
Finapres
 F. blood pressure monitor
 F. Dinamap blood pressure machine
 F. finger cuff
finder
 Acupoint f.
 Carabelli lumen f.
 Damian lumen f.
 Dasco Pro angle f.
 gravity-driven angle f.
 hamate f.
 Hedwig lumen f.
 IMP Femur f.
 lumen f.
 Moore direction f.
 pedicle f.
Findley folding pessary
fine
 f. arterial forceps
 F. bimanual ophthalmic handpiece set
 f. chromic suture
 F. corneal carrying case
 F. crescent fixation ring
 F. dissecting forceps
 F. folding block
 F. gripping forceps
 F. head-tilt capsulorrhexis forceps
 f. intestinal needle
 F. magnetic implant
 F. micropoint cautery
 F. micropoint electrocautery
 f. olive bur
 F. sideport actuating quick chopper
 F. sideport capsulorrhexis forceps
 f. silk suture
 F. suture scissors
 F. suture-tying forceps
 F. toric/limbal relaxing incision marker
fine-angled curette
fine-line tissue marker
fine-mesh dressing
fine-needle electrode
Finesse
 F. dilating trocar system
 F. large-lumen guiding catheter
Fine-Thornton scleral fixation ring

fine-tipped mosquito hemostat
fine-tooth
    f.-t. clamp
    f.-t. forceps
fine-wire
    f.-w. electrode
    f.-w. speculum
Fin & Flipper exercise log
finger
    f. circumference gauge
    f. clip sensor
    f. cot
    f. cot dressing
    f. cot splint
    f. cuff
    f. extension clockspring splint
    6th F. knot pusher
    F. Fitness spring ball
    f. flexion glove
    f. flexion splint
    f. gauze
    f. goniometer
    F. Helper hand exerciser
    f. hook
    f. indicator
    f. joint implant
    f. ladder
    f. loop
    mechanical f.
    f. orthosis
    F. Phantom pulse oximeter testing system
    f. photoplethysmograph device
    f. plate
    F. Platter hand exerciser
    f. rake retractor
    f. ring cutter
    f. ring saw
    f. separator
    f. sling
    f. splint
Finger-Hugger splint
fingernail drill
FingerPrint handheld pulse oximeter
fingertrap
    Japanese f.
    MicroDigitrapper-HR f.
    MicroDigitrapper-S f.
    MicroDigitrapper-V f.
    f. suture
finisher
    Küntscher f.

finishing bur
Finite dental glazing compound
Fink
    F. biprong marker
    F. cataract aspirator
    F. chalazion curette
    F. cul-de-sac cannula
    F. cul-de-sac irrigator
    F. fixation forceps
    F. lacrimal retractor
    F. laryngoscope
    F. muscle marker
    F. oblique muscle hook
    F. refractor
    F. tendon tucker
    F. tendon-tucker forceps
    F. valve
Finn
    F. chamber
    F. hinged knee replacement prosthesis
finned pacemaker lead
finned-stem punch
Finney
    F. mask
    F. penile implant
Finnoff
    F. laryngoscope
    F. sinus transilluminator
Finochietto
    F. arterial clamp
    F. bronchial clamp
    F. clamp carrier
    F. hand retractor
    F. infant rib retractor
    F. infant rib spreader
    F. laminectomy retractor
    F. lobectomy forceps
    F. lobectomy scissors
    F. needle
    F. needle holder
    F. stirrup
    F. thoracic forceps
    F. thoracic scissors
Finochietto-Burford
    F.-B. rib contractor
    F.-B. rib spreader
Fino vascular catheter
Finsen
    F. bath
    F. lamp
    F. retractor

F

NOTES

Finsen *(continued)*
  F. tracheal hook
  F. wound hook
Finsterer
  F. myringotomy split tube
  F. suction tube
Firlit-Sugar intermittent catheter I-Cath
Firm D-Ring wrist support
FirmFlex Plus custom orthotic
first
  F. Beat ultrasound stethoscope
  F. knee prosthesis
  F. Option uterine cryoblation
    therapy
  F. Quality belted undergarment
  F. Response manual resuscitator
  f. rib shears
  F. Step Select low-air overlay
  F. Temp Genius 3000A tympanic
    thermometer
FirstChoice
  F. postoperative drainable pouch
  F. urostomy pouch
FirstSave
  F. AED
  F. automated external defibrillator
FirstStep
  F. mattress
  F. tibial osteotomy instrument
FirstTemp Genius tympanic
  thermometer
Fisch
  F. bone drill irrigator
  F. cutting bur
  F. drill
  F. dural hook
  F. dural retractor
  F. microcrurotomy scissors
Fischer
  F. modular stereotaxic system
  F. nasal rasp
  F. pneumothorax needle
  F. tendon stripper
Fish
  F. antral probe
  F. grasping forceps
  F. infusion cannula
  F. inlet
  F. nasal-dressing forceps
  F. sinus probe
  The F. Glassman viscera retainer
Fisher
  F. Accumet pH meter
  F. advancement forceps
  F. bed
  F. brace
  F. capsular forceps
  F. double-ended retractor
  F. eye needle

  F. eye spoon
  F. fenestrated lid retractor
  F. half pin
  F. iris forceps
  F. lid retractor
  F. microcapillary tube reader
  F. & Paykel HC-series heated
    humidifier
  F. spud
  F. tape board
  F. tonsillar dissector
  F. tonsillar knife
  F. tonsil retractor
Fisher-Paykel
  F.-P. MR290 water-feed chamber
  F.-P. RD1000 resuscitator
Fisher-plus slide
Fisher-Smith spatula
fishhook
  f. lead
  f. needle
fishtail
  f. burnisher
  f. chisel
  f. spatula
  f. spatula raspatory
Fiskars scissors
Fisons
  F. indirect binocular
    ophthalmoscope
  F. nebulizer
fissure
  f. bur
  f. burnisher
fistula
  Brescia-Cimino AV f.
  Cimino f.
  Gore-Tex AF f.
  f. hook
  f. needle
  f. probe
  f. scissors
fistulotome
  needle-knife f.
Fit-Lastic therapy band
Fitnet joint testing system
Fits-All sling
Fitstep II stair climber
fitting
  Luer lock f.
  Shrader f.
Fitz-all fabric leg strap
Fitzgerald
  F. aortic aneurysm clamp
  F. aortic aneurysm forceps
Fitzwater
  F. ligature carrier
  F. peanut sponge-holding forceps

Fixateur
F. Interne fixation system
F. Interne rod
F. Interne screw
fixation
AO spinal internal f.
f. apparatus
Arthrex Bio-Transfix cross pin f.
Arthrex Transfix II cross pin f.
Association for the Study of
Internal F. (ASIF)
f. bandage
f. binocular forceps
f. button
ECT internal fracture f.
Ender f.
f. forceps
f. jig
Kempf internal screw f.
Kirschner pin f.
Kirschner wire f.
LactoSorb resorbable
craniomaxillofacial f.
microplate f.
Obwegeser-Dalpont internal screw f.
OrthoFrame external f.
OrthoSorb pin f.
Pariefix mesh f.
f. pick
f. pin
ReUnite hand f.
ReUnite VersaTile f.
f. ring
f. screw
Seidel intramedullary f.
Spiessel internal screw f.
Steinhauser internal screw f.
Turvy internal screw f.
f. twist hook
Wolvek sternal approximation f.
fixator
Ace-Fischer external f.
AO internal f.
articulated external f.
Bay external f.
BioSymMetRic PIP f.
biplanar f.
circular external f.
Clyburn Colles fracture f.
DeBastiani external f.
dynamic axial f.
EBI external f.

Edwards D-L modular f.
external f.
external ring f.
external spinal skeletal f.
Herbert screw f.
Hex-Fix monolateral external f.
hinged articulated f.
Hoffmann external f.
HTO f.
Ilizarov circular external f.
Ilizarov external ring f.
Ilizarov hybrid f.
Kessler external f.
K-Fix f.
Monofixateur external f.
Olerud internal f.
Orthofix monolateral femoral
external f.
Oxford f.
Pennig dynamic wrist f.
spanning external f.
Stableloc Colles fracture external f.
Stuhler-Heise f.
thin-wire Ilizarov f.
Thomas f.
True/Lok external f.
Vermont spinal f.
fixed
f. arch bar
f. cervical dilator
f. expansion prosthesis
f. femoral head prosthesis
f. mandibular implant
f. ring retractor
fixed-beam portal
fixed-bearing knee implant
fixed-focus scope
fixed-offset guide
fixed-rate
f.-r. asynchronous atrial pacemaker
f.-r. asynchronous ventricular
pacemaker
f.-r. pacemaker
fixed-wire
f.-w. balloon
f.-w. catheter
Fixion
F. IL nailing system
F. IM nail
F. interlocking medullary proximal
femoral nail

F

NOTES

333

Fixion *(continued)*
    F. PF hip peg
    F. PF nailing system
fixture
    VersaLap lapping f.
Fizeau-Tolansky interferometer
Flagg laryngoscope
FlairCair mattress
flame
    f. bur
    f. ionization detector
    f. photometric detector
Flamingo stent
flange
    adhesive f.
    Callahan f.
    ConQuest female/male continence
      system pressure pad with
      preattached f.
    endoprosthetic f.
    Scuderi-Callahan f.
4-flanged nail
flanged Teflon tube
flap
    f. demarcator
    digit wrap adhesive f.
    f. knife
    f. knife dissector
    Leibinger E-Z f.
    peg f.
FLAPmaker
    F. disposable microkeratome
flared
    f. ABS tip
    f. patch mesh
    f. spinal rod
FlashCast
    Delta-Lite F.
flashlamp pulsed Nd:YAG laser
FlashPoint optical localizer
Flash portable spirometer
flask
    Dewar f.
    Falcon plastic f.
    tissue culture f.
flat
    f. bottom reservoir
    f. brain spatula support
    f. burnisher
    f. drill
    f. eye bandage
    f. needle spud
    f. probe
    f. spatula
    f. spatula electrode
    f. spatula needle
    f. tenotomy hook
    f. wire coil stent
flat-bladed nasal speculum

FlatFoot insole
Flatow-Bigliani shoulder prosthesis
flat-panel
    f.-p. detector
    f.-p. megavoltage imager
flat-plate detector
Flatt
    F. driver
    F. finger prosthesis
    F. implant
flattened irrigating cannula
flattening filter
flat-tip electrode
flat-wire eye electrode
Flaxedil suture
Fleischer-Kayser fixation ring
Fleisch pneumotachograph
Fleming
    F. afterloading tandem
    F. conization instrument
    F. ovoid
Flents breast comfort pack
Fletcher
    F. afterloader
    F. dressing forceps
    F. sponge forceps
    F. tonsillar knife
Fletcher-Delclos dome cylinder
Fletcher-Suit
    F.-S. afterloading tandem
    F.-S. applicator
    F.-S. polyp forceps
    F.-S. tandem and ovoid
Fletcher-Suit-Delclos
    F.-S.-D. brachytherapy applicator
    F.-S.-D. system
    F.-S.-D. tandem
Fletcher-Van
    F.-V. Doren sponge-holding forceps
    F.-V. Doren uterine polyp forceps
Fleurant bladder trocar
Flex
    F. Foam brace
    F. Foam dressing
    F. Foam orthosis
    F. H/A total ossicular prosthesis
    F. Tip guidewire
Flexacryl hard rebase acrylic
Flexblock cranial implant
Flex-Cath double-lumen intraaortic
    balloon catheter
FlexComp/DSP EMG
Flexcon lens
Flexderm
    F. hydrogel sheet
    F. wound dressing
FlexDial stimulus control
flexer
    X-Tend-O knee f.

Flex-E-Z wax
Flexfilm wound dressing
FlexFinder guidewire
Flex-Foot prosthesis
Flexiblade laryngoscope
flexible
  f. angioscope
  f. aortic clamp
  f. arm micro retractor
  f. aspiration needle
  f. bandage
  f. biopsy needle
  f. blade osteotome
  f. bronchoscopy simulator
  f. cardiac valve
  f. coil stent
  f. delivery device
  f. digital implant
  f. Dualens implant
  f. endoscopic overtube
  f. endosonography probe
  f. fallopian tube endoscope
  f. fiberendoscope
  f. fiberoptic bronchoscope
  f. fluoropolymer
  f. fluoropolymer contact lens
  f. foreign body forceps
  f. forward-viewing panendoscope
  f. fulgurating electrode
  f. gastroscope
  f. guidewire
  f. hysteroscope
  f. injection needle
  f. intramedullary nail
  f. laminar bone strip
  f. loop anterior chamber intraocular lens
  f. loop posterior chamber intraocular lens
  f. nasopharyngolaryngoscope
  f. neck rake retractor
  f. neck retractor
  f. Olympus GF-eUM3 device
  f. optical biopsy forceps
  f. pump
  f. radiofrequency coil
  f. radiothermal electrode
  f. reamer
  f. retractor pressure clamp
  f. retractor sliding clamp
  f. rod penile implant

  f. sigmoidoscope
  f. socket
  f. sound
  f. stent
  f. surface coil
  f. surface-coil-type resonator
  f. translimbal iris retractor
  f. ureteroscope
  f. vascular clamp
  f. video laparoscope
  f. wand
  f. wire electrode
Flexicair
  F. eclipse low air loss therapy unit
  F. II low-air-loss therapy unit bed
  F. MC3 low-air-loss therapy unit bed
Flexi-Cath
  F.-C. double-lumen intraaortic balloon catheter
  F.-C. silicone subclavian cannula
  F.-C. straight dual-lumen catheter
Flexicon gauze bandage
FlexiCut coronary catheter
Flexi-Flate
  F.-F. I, II penile prosthesis
  F.-F. penile implant
Flexiflo
  F. Companion enteral nutrition pump
  F. enteral feeding tube
  F. feeding pump
  F. gastrostomy tube enteral delivery system
  F. Inverta-PEG gastrostomy kit
  F. Inverta-PEG tube
  F. Lap G laparoscopic gastrostomy kit
  F. Lap J laparoscopic jejunostomy kit
  F. over-the-guidewire gastrostomy kit
  F. Sacks-Vine tube
  F. Stomate low-profile gastrostomy tube
  F. suction feeding tube
  F. tap-fill enteral tube
  F. Taptainer tube
  F. tungsten-weighted feeding tube
  F. Versa-PEG tube

F

NOTES

FlexiGel
>F. gel sheet dressing
>F. strands

Flexigrid dressing
Flexi-Guard splint
Flexilite conforming elastic bandage
Flexima
>F. biliary drainage catheter
>F. biliary stent
>F. nephrostomy catheter
>F. ureteral catheter

Flexinet dressing
flexion glove
Flexipost dental post
Flexi-Rod
>F.-R. II penile implant
>F.-R. II penile prosthesis

Flexi-Seal
>F.-S. fecal collector
>F.-S. fecal collector & tail clip

Flexisplint arm board
Flexistone impression material
Flexi-Therm
>F.-T. diabetic diagnostic insole
>F.-T. liquid crystal system

Flexi-Tip ureteral catheter
Flexi-Trak skin anchoring device
Flexlase 600 laser
Flexlens lens
FlexLite hinged knee support
FlexLoop curette
flexometer
>Moeltgen f.

Flexon steel suture
flexor
>F. Ansel introducer device
>F. Balkin Up & Over introducer
> device
>f. hinge hand splint brace
>F. Shuttle introducer device

Flexoreamer Batt tip
Flexo wax
FlexPosure endoscopic retractor
Flex-R-File file
Flexseat cushion
Flexsteel ribbon retractor
FlexStent
>F. flexible esophageal stent
>F. flexible esophageal stent system
>F. memory stent

FlexStrand cable
Flextender Plus hand exerciser
Flextend glove
FlexTip intervertebral rongeur
Flex-Walk foot prosthesis
Flex-Wrap self-adherent wrap
Flexxicon
>F. Blue dialysis catheter
>F. II PC internal jugular catheter

Flexzan Extra topical wound dressing
Flieringa
>F. fixation ring
>F. scleral ring

Flimm Fighter percussor
Flint glass speculum
flip-flap
>Mathieu-Horton-Devine f.-f.

Flip-Flop pillow
flipper
>F. detachable embolization coil
>MacRae flap f.

Floam ankle stirrup brace
floating
>f. disc heart valve
>f. lead
>f. table

Flocare 500 feeding pump
Flofit
>F. ComfortFluid seat
>F. ComfortSeat
>F. cushion

Flo-Gard pump
FloMap
>F. guidewire
>F. velocimeter

floor-standing surgical light
floppy guidewire
floppy-tipped guidewire
Flo-Restors backbleeding control device
Florex medical compression stocking
Florida
>F. back brace
>F. cervical brace
>F. contraflexion brace
>F. extension brace
>F. hyperextension brace
>F. J-series brace
>F. postfusion brace
>F. spinal brace
>F. urinary pouch

FloSeal matrix hemostatic sealant
Flo-Stat
>F.-S. fluid management system
>F.-S. fluid monitor

flotation
>f. catheter
>f. gel pad

Flo-Tech prosthetic socket
FloTem IIe fluid-warming device
Flo-Thru intraluminal shunt
Flo-Trol drinking cup
**FloVAC Hi-Flo laparoscopic suction-
  irrigation system**
flow
>f. cytometer
>f. probe
>F. Rider neurovascular catheter
>f. wire

Flow-20-push method gastrostomy
flow-assisted
    f.-a. short-term (FAST)
    f.-a. short-term balloon catheter
flow-directed
    f.-d. balloon cardiovascular catheter
    f.-d. balloon-tipped catheter
    f.-d. thermodilution catheter
Flowers
    F. dorsal nasal implant
    F. Extended Tear Trough implant
    F. Mandibular Glove implant
    F. Tear Trough implant
FlowGel barrier material
FlowGun suction-irrigator
FloWire
    F. Doppler catheter
    F. Doppler guidewire
    F. Doppler wire
    F. guidewire
flowmeter
    AirZone f.
    Asmalert Lo-Range peak f.
    Assess peak f.
    Astech peak f.
    AsthmaMentor peak f.
    blood f.
    Dantec rotating disc f.
    Dantec Urodyn 1000 f.
    Doppler ultrasonic f.
    electromagnetic blood f.
    Gould electromagnetic f.
    Heidelberg retinal f.
    infrared laser-Doppler f.
    laser Doppler f.
    Life-Tech f.
    MBF3 infrared laser-Doppler f.
    Mini-Wright peak f.
    Narcomatic f.
    Parks bidirectional Doppler f.
    Periflux laser Doppler f.
    Personal Best peak f.
    Pocketpeak peak f.
    preVent Pneumotach f.
    pulsed Doppler ultrasonic f.
    Respalert peak f.
    Spir-O-Flow peak f.
    Statham electromagnetic f.
    transit-time f.
    Transonic f.
    TruZone peak f.
    Wright peak f.

flow-over vaporizer
flow-oximetry catheter
FlowPlus therapeutic pneumatic
  compression system
flowprobe
    endoscopic f.
flow-regulated suction tube
flow-regulating shunt
flow-regulator clamp
flow-sensing spirometer
Flowtron
    F. DVT prophylactic deep venous
    thrombosis unit
    F. Excel DVT prophylaxis system
Floxite mirror light
Floyd
    F. loop cannula
    F. pneumothorax needle
Floyd-Barraquer wire speculum
fluff dressing
fluffed gauze dressing
Fluftex gauze roll
Fluhrer bullet rectal probe
fluid
    cerebrospinal f. (CSF)
    f. control trauma pad
    f. warmer
Fluid-Air Plus bed
fluid-filled
    f.-f. balloon-tipped flow-directed
    catheter
    f.-f. pigtail catheter
    f.-f. pressure monitoring guidewire
fluorescence
    f. detector
    f. dye
    Energy Dispersive X-ray F.
    (EDXRF)
    f. excitation filter
    f. fibergastroscope
fluorescence-activated cell sorter
fluorescence-guided "smart" laser
fluorescent
    f. lamp
    f. optode
    f. probe
    f. pulsed light (FPL)
    f. in situ hybridization
Fluorescite syringe
fluoride
    argon f. (ArF)
Fluor-i-Strip ophthalmic strip

F

NOTES

fluorodopa positron emission
tomographic scan
Fluorognost HIV-1 IFA assay kit
fluorometer
    CytoFluor II f.
    scanning f.
    96-well scanning f.
FluoroNav virtual fluoroscopy system
fluoronephelometer
Fluoropassiv thin-wall carotid patch
graft
fluorophotometer
    Fluorotron Master f.
    slit-lamp f.
FluoroPlus
    F. angiogram
    F. Roadmapper digital fluoroscopy
fluoropolymer
    flexible f.
Fluoroptic
    F. thermometry probe
    F. thermometry system
FluoroScan C-arm fluoroscope
fluoroscope
    C-arm f.
    Edison f.
    FluoroScan C-arm f.
    Xi-scan f.
fluoroscopic
    f. foreign body forceps
    f. imaging chair
fluoroscopy (FX)
    FluoroPlus Roadmapper digital f.
fluoroscopy-guided balloon dilator
Fluoro Tip ERCP cannula
FluoroTrak 3500 navigation system
Fluorotron Master fluorophotometer
Fluotec vaporizer
flush chamber
flushing
    f. reservoir
    f. valve
flute
    f. cannula
    f. needle
fluted
    f. drain
    f. finishing bur
    f. J-Vac drain
    f. reamer
    f. Sampson nail
    f. titanium nail
fluted-stem punch
Flutter mucus clearance device
Fluvog
    F. aspirator
    F. irrigator
flying spot excimer laser system

Flynn
    F. lens loop
    F. scleral depressor
F-Mat screening system
F/M base curve contact lens
FMS Intracell stick
FNA-21 syringe
foam
    CarraSmart f.
    f. collar
    Constructa f.
    f. cube mattress
    f. cushion
    DermaMend f.
    eggcrate f.
    Evazote f.
    hi-density f.
    Ivalon f.
    Neoplush f.
    nonadherent f.
    Pedilen polyurethane f.
    polyethylene f.
    polyvinyl alcohol f.
    prosthetic f.
    Reston polyurethane f.
    Reston self-adhering f.
    f. ring
    f. rubber vaginal stent
    Sandia Decon f.
    Super Constructa f.
    f. tape
    tube f.
    f. tubing
    f. wedge wheelchair cushion
    f. wound dressing
Foamart foot impression system
FoaMTrac traction bandage
FocalSeal-L
    F.-L. lung sealant
FocalSeal liquid sealant
FocalSeal-R neurosurgical stent
FocalSeal-S surgical sealant
focused, segmented, ultrasound machine
focusing collimator
Focus Night & Day contact lens
Focustent coronary stent
Foerster
    F. abdominal retractor
    F. capsulotomy knife
    F. enucleation snare
    F. forceps
    F. gallbladder forceps
    F. iris forceps
    F. sponge forceps
    F. sponge-holding forceps
    F. surgical support brassiere
    F. tissue forceps
    F. uterine forceps
Foerster-Bauer sponge-holding forceps

Fogarty
F. adherent clot catheter
F. arterial embolectomy catheter
F. arterial irrigation catheter
F. balloon
F. balloon biliary catheter
F. balloon embolectomy catheter
F. biliary balloon probe
F. bulldog clamp-applying forceps
F. calibrator
F. dilation catheter
F. embolectomy catheter
F. gallstone catheter
F. graft thrombectomy catheter
F. Hydragrip clamp
F. insert
F. occlusion catheter
F. Thru-Lumen catheter
F. venous irrigation catheter
F. venous thrombectomy catheter
Fogarty-Chin
F.-C. clamp
F.-C. extrusion balloon catheter
F.-C. peripheral dilatation catheter
Fogarty-Hydragrip insert
fog reduction/elimination device
foil
f. carrier
crumpled aluminum f.
scattering f.
f. sheet
Shimstock occlusion f.
titanium f.
Folatex catheter
foldable intraocular lens
folder
Faulkner f.
intraocular lens f.
folding
f. blade
f. forceps
f. lens
fold-over finger splint
Foley
F. acorn-bulb catheter
F. balloon
F. balloon catheter
F. catheter
F. catheter holder
F. cone-tip catheter
F. Cordostat
F. hemostatic bag

F. plate
F. straight drain
F. vas isolation forceps
F. 3-way catheter
Foley-Alcock
F.-A. bag
F.-A. catheter
follicle
f. electrode
f. expressor
follower
filiform and f.
Le Fort f.
Rusch f.
Foltz
F. catheter
F. flushing reservoir
F. needle
Fome-Cuf
F.-C. endotracheal tube
F.-C. laser kit
F.-C. pediatric tracheostomy tube
Fomon
F. angular scissors
F. double-edge knife
F. double-hook retractor
F. facelift scissors
F. hook retractor
F. lower lateral scissors
F. nasal chisel
F. nasal hook
F. nasal rasp
F. nasal retractor
F. nostril elevator
F. osteotome
F. periosteal elevator
F. periosteotome
F. saber-back scissors
F. upper lateral scissors
Fonar
F. 360-degree MRI
F. Quad MRI scanner
F. Standing Ovation MRI system
F. Stand-Up MRI scanner
Fonix
F. 6500-CX hearing aid test system
F. hearing aid
food extractor
foot
Beachcomber prosthetic f.
Cirrus composite prosthetic f.

F

NOTES

foot *(continued)*
ComfortWalk$_2$ prosthetic f.
f. cradle
f. drop night splint
f. drop stop
Dycor prosthetic f.
Freedom prosthetic f.
f. holder
F. Hugger foot support
Kingsley Steplite f.
F. Levelers custom orthotic
F. Levelers orthosis
Lo Rider prosthetic f.
f. magnet
multiaxis f.
f. orthotic device
Otto Bock 1D25 Dynamic Plus f.
f. pillow
f. rest
SACH f.
single-axis Syme DYCOR f.
f. splint
Springlite Lo Rider prosthetic f.
f. stabilizer
Sure-Flex III prosthetic f.
Syme Dycor prosthetic f.
Trowbridge TerraRound f.
Vari-Flex prosthetic f.
f. volumeter
F. Waffle cushion
F. Waffle positioner
foot-ankle brace
footbed
Orthofeet-Gel f.
footbrush
Dr. Joseph's original f.
footdrop brace
3-footed lens intraocular lens
Footfax-SL portable foot scanner
footgear
Comed f.
FootHugger
footplate
f. chisel
f. elevator
f. hook
f. pick
FootPrinter box
Foot-Station 3-D foot imaging system
footwear
Ambulator biomechanical f.
Comfort Rite f.
Mobils Professionals pedorthic f.
Forbes
F. esophageal speculum
F. uterine-dressing forceps
force
F. balloon
F. 2 CEM generator

f. fulcrum retractor
F. FX generator
F. GSU argon-enhanced electrosurgery system
F. wire
forceps
Abbott-Mayfield f.
Abernaz strut f.
abscess f.
Absolok f.
ACMI Martin endoscopic f.
Acufex curved basket f.
Acufex rotary basket f.
Acufex straight basket f.
AcuTouch tissue f.
Adair-Allis tissue f.
Adair breast tenaculum f.
Adair tissue f.
Adair tissue-holding f.
Adair uterine f.
adenoid f.
Adler bone f.
Adlerkreutz f.
Adler punch f.
adnexal f.
Adson f.
Adson arterial f.
Adson bayonet dressing f.
Adson-Biemer f.
Adson bipolar f.
Adson brain f.
Adson-Brown tissue f.
Adson-Callison tissue f.
Adson clip-applying f.
Adson dressing f.
Adson hemostatic f.
Adson hypophyseal f.
Adson microbipolar f.
Adson microdressing f.
Adson microtissue f.
Adson-Mixter neurosurgical f.
Adson monopolar f.
Adson scalp clip-applying f.
Adson thumb f.
Adson tissue f.
Adson tooth f.
Adson-Vital tissue f.
advancement f.
Aesculap f.
Akahoshi phaco prechopper f.
Akins valve re-do f.
Alabama University f.
Alderkreutz tissue f.
Alexander dressing f.
Alexander-Farabeuf f.
Alio MICS capsulorrhexis f.
Allen-Barkan f.
Allen-Braley f.
Allen intestinal f.

Allen tenaculum f.
Allen uterine f.
alligator f.
alligator crimper f.
alligator cup f.
alligator ear f.
alligator jaw f.
alligator nasal f.
Allis f.
Allis-Abramson breast biopsy f.
Allis-Adair intestinal f.
Allis-Adair tissue f.
Allis-Coakley tonsillar f.
Allis-Coakley tonsil-seizing f.
Allis-Duval f.
Allis intestinal f.
Allis Micro-Line pediatric f.
Allis-Ochsner tissue f.
Allis-Ochsner tonsillar f.
Allis thoracic f.
Allis tissue f.
Allis-Willauer thoracic f.
Allis-Willauer tissue f.
Almeida f.
Alvis fixation f.
Ambrose eye f.
Ambrose suture f.
Amdur lid f.
Amenabar capsular f.
AMO phacoemulsification lens-folder f.
anastomosis f.
Andrews-Hartmann f.
Andrews tonsillar f.
Andrews tonsil-seizing f.
aneurysm f.
Angell-James hypophysectomy f.
Angell-James punch f.
angiotribe f.
Anis capsulotomy f.
Anis corneal f.
Anis corneoscleral f.
Anis intraocular lens f.
Anis microsurgical tying f.
Anis straight corneal f.
Anis tying f.
anterior capsule f.
anterior segment f.
Anthony-Fisher f.
antral f.
AO reduction f.
aortic aneurysm f.

aortic occlusion f.
Apfelbaum bipolar f.
Apple Medical bipolar f.
applicator f.
approximation f.
Archer splinter f.
Arrow articulation paper f.
Arrowsmith fixation f.
Arroyo f.
Arruga curved capsular f.
Arruga-Gill f.
Arruga-McCool capsular f.
arterial f.
ArthroForce basket cutting f.
Arthur splinter f.
articulating paper f.
Artilk f.
Asch septal f.
Asch septum-straightening f.
Ashby fluoroscopic foreign body f.
Ash dental f.
Ash septum-straightening f.
ASICO capsulorrhexis f.
ASSI f.
ASSI bipolar coagulating f.
ASSI no-scalpel vasectomy f.
Athens f.
AtrauGrip dissecting f.
atraumatic f.
atraumatic tissue f.
atraumatic visceral f.
aural f.
auricular appendage f.
Austin f.
Auto Suture f.
Autraugrip tissue f.
Auvard-Zweifel f.
axis-traction f.
Ayers chalazion f.
Azar intraocular f.
Azar lens f.
Azar tying f.
Babcock-Beasley f.
Babcock intestinal f.
Babcock lung-grasping f.
Babcock thoracic tissue-holding f.
Babcock tissue f.
Babcock-Vital atraumatic tissue f.
Babcock-Vital intestinal f.
baby Adson f.
baby Allis f.
baby Babcock f.

F

NOTES

341

forceps *(continued)*
baby Crile f.
baby dressing f.
baby hemostatic f.
baby intestinal tissue f.
baby Lane bone-holding f.
baby Mikulicz f.
baby Mixter f.
baby mosquito f.
baby Overholt f.
BackBiter f.
backbiting f.
Backhaus f.
Backhaus-Roeder f.
Bacon cranial f.
Baer bone-cutting f.
Bahnson-Brown f.
Bailey aortic valve-cutting f.
Bailey chalazion f.
Bailey-Williamson obstetrical f.
Bainbridge hemostatic f.
Bainbridge intestinal f.
Bainbridge resection f.
Bainbridge thyroid f.
Baird chalazion f.
Baker tissue f.
Ball f.
Ballantine hysterectomy f.
Ballantine-Peterson hysterectomy f.
Ballen-Alexander f.
Ballenger-Foerster f.
Ballenger hysterectomy f.
Ballenger sponge f.
Ballenger tonsillar f.
Bane rongeur f.
Bangerter muscle f.
Bansal LASIK f.
Bard f.
Bardeleben bone-holding f.
Bard-Parker transfer f.
Barkan iris f.
Barlow f.
Barnes-Crile hemostatic f.
Barnes-Hill f.
Barnes-Simpson obstetrical f.
Baron f.
Barraquer ciliary f.
Barraquer-Colibri f.
Barraquer conjunctival f.
Barraquer corneal f.
Barraquer fixation f.
Barraquer hemostatic mosquito f.
Barraquer-Katzin f.
Barraquer-Troutman corneal f.
Barraquer-von Mandach capsular f.
Barraquer-von Mandach clot f.
Barraya tissue f.
Barrett-Allen placental f.
Barrett-Allen uterine f.

Barrett intestinal f.
Barrett lens f.
Barrett-Murphy intestinal f.
Barrett placental f.
Barrett tenacular f.
Barrett uterine tenaculum f.
Barrie-Jones angled crocodile f.
Barsky f.
Barton obstetrical f.
basket f.
basket-cutting f.
basket-punch f.
basket-type crushing f.
Bauer dissecting f.
Bauer sponge f.
Baumberger f.
Baumgartner f.
Baum-Hecht tarsorrhaphy f.
Bausch articulation paper f.
bayonet f.
bayonet bipolar f.
bayonet monopolar f.
bayonet root tip f.
BB shot f.
Bead ethmoidal f.
beaked cowhorn f.
bean f.
Beardsley f.
bearing-seating f.
Beasley-Babcock tissue f.
Beaupre ciliary f.
Beaupre epilation f.
Bechert lens-holding f.
Bechert-McPherson tying f.
Beck f.
Beebe hemostatic f.
Beebe wire-cutting f.
Beer ciliary f.
Behen ear f.
Behrend cystic duct f.
Bellucci ear f.
Benaron scalp-rotating f.
Bengolea arterial f.
Bennell f.
Bennett ciliary f.
Bennett epilation f.
Berens capsular f.
Berens corneal transplant f.
Berens muscle recession f.
Berens ptosis f.
Berens recession f.
Berens suturing f.
Berger biopsy f.
Bergeron pillar f.
Bergh ciliary f.
Berghmann-Foerster sponge f.
Bergman tissue f.
Berke chalazion f.
Berke ciliary f.

Berkeley Bioengineering ptosis f.
Berkeley-Bonney hysterectomy f.
Berke ptosis f.
Bernard uterine f.
Berne nasal f.
Bernhard towel f.
Berry uterine-elevating f.
Best common duct stone f.
Best gallstone f.
Bettman-Noyes fixation f.
Bevan gallbladder f.
Bevan hemostatic f.
Beyer f.
BiCoag bipolar laparoscopic f.
Bierer ovum f.
Bigelow f.
Billroth tumor f.
Bill traction handle f.
Binkhorst capsular f.
Binkhorst lens f.
binocular fixation f.
biopsy f.
biopsy punch f.
biopsy specimen f.
bipolar f.
bipolar bayonet f.
bipolar coagulating f.
bipolar coaptation f.
bipolar cutting f.
bipolar diathermy f.
bipolar electrocautery f.
bipolar eye f.
bipolar laparoscopic f.
bipolar transsphenoidal f.
Bircher-Ganske cartilage f.
Birkett hemostatic f.
Birks Mark II grooved f.
Birks Mark II needle-holder f.
Birks Mark II suture-tying f.
Birks Mark II toothed f.
Birks suture-tying f.
Birtcher endoscopic f.
Bishop-Harman dressing f.
Bishop-Harman foreign body f.
Bishop-Harman iris f.
Bishop-Harman tissue f.
Bi-tec f.
biting f.
Björk-Stille diathermy f.
bladder specimen f.
Blade-Wilde ear f.
Blake ear f.

Blake embolus f.
Blake gallstone f.
Blakesley ethmoid f.
Blakesley nasal f.
Blakesley septal bone f.
Blakesley septal compression f.
Blakesley-Weil upturned
  ethmoidal f.
Blakesley-Wilde ear f.
Blakesley-Wilde ethmoidal f.
Blakesley-Wilde nasal f.
Blalock f.
Blalock-Kleinert f.
Blanchard hemorrhoidal f.
Bland cervical traction f.
Bland vulsellum f.
Blaydes angled lens f.
Blaydes corneal f.
Blaydes lens-holding f.
blepharochalasis f.
Block-Potts intestinal f.
Blohmka tonsillar f.
Bloodwell-Brown f.
Bloodwell tissue f.
Bloodwell vascular f.
Bloomberg lens f.
Blum f.
Blumenthal uterine dressing f.
blunt f.
Boer craniotomy f.
Boerma obstetrical f.
Boettcher arterial f.
Boettcher pulmonary artery f.
Boettcher-Schnidt f.
Boettcher tonsillar artery f.
Boise cutting f.
Bolton f.
Bonaccolto cup-jaw f.
Bonaccolto fragment f.
Bonaccolto jeweler's f.
Bonaccolto magnet tip f.
Bonaccolto splinter f.
Bonaccolto strabismus f.
Bonaccolto utility f.
Bond placental f.
bone-biting f.
bone-cutting double-action f.
bone-holding f.
bone punch f.
bone-reduction f.
bone rongeur f.
bone-splitting f.

F

NOTES

forceps (*continued*)

Bonn European suturing f.
Bonney tissue f.
Bonn iris f.
Bonn peripheral iridectomy f.
Bonn suturing f.
Bores corneal fixation f.
Bores U-shaped fixation f.
Boruchoff f.
Boston Lying-In cervical f.
Botvin iris f.
Botvin vulsellum f.
Bouchayer grasping f.
Bovie coagulating f.
Bovino scleral-spreading f.
bowel f.
Bowen suction loose body f.
box joint f.
Boys-Allis tissue f.
Bozeman f.
Bozeman-Douglas f.
Bozeman Lorenz-Barmesh
   holding f.
Bozeman LR packing f.
Bozeman LR uterine-dressing f.
Bozeman uterine dressing f.
Bozeman uterine packing f.
B-P transfer f.
Braasch bladder specimen f.
Bracken fixation f.
Bracken-Forkas corneal f.
Bracken iris f.
Bracken scleral fixation f.
Bradford thyroid f.
brain clip f.
brain dressing f.
brain spatula f.
brain tissue f.
brain tumor f.
Braithwaite f.
Brand passing f.
Brand shunt-introducing f.
Brand tendon-holding f.
Brand tendon-passing f.
Brannon extracapsular cleaving f.
Brannon extracapsular removal f.
Braun f.
Brenner f.
Bridge deep surgery f.
Bridge hemostatic f.
Bridge intestinal f.
Brigham brain tumor f.
Brigham dressing f.
Brigham tissue f.
Brigham 1x2 teeth f.
Brock biopsy f.
Brock cardiovascular f.
bronchial biopsy f.
bronchial grasping f.

bronchoscopic f.
bronchoscopic biopsy f.
Bronson-Magnion f.
Brophy dressing f.
Brophy tissue f.
Brown-Adson side-grasping f.
Brown-Adson tissue f.
Brown-Bahnson bayonet f.
Brown-Buerger f.
Brown-Cushing f.
Brown-Grabow capsulorrhexis f.
Brown ophthalmic insertion f.
Brown side-grasping f.
Brown-Swan f.
Brown thoracic f.
Brown tissue f.
Broyles optical f.
Bruening-Citelli f.
Bruening cutting-tip f.
Bruening ethmoid exenteration f.
Bruening nasal-cutting septal f.
Bruening septal f.
Brunner intestinal f.
Brunner sigmoid anastomosis f.
Brunner tissue f.
Brunschwig arterial f.
Brunschwig visceral f.
Bryant nasal f.
Buck foreign body f.
Buerger-McCarthy bladder f.
Buie biopsy f.
Buie rectal f.
Buie specimen f.
bulldog clamp-applying f.
bullet f.
Bumpus specimen f.
Bunim urethral f.
Bunker modification of Jackson
   laryngeal f.
Buratto flap f.
Buratto LASIK f.
Buratto ophthalmic f.
Burch biopsy f.
Burford coarctation f.
Burnham biopsy f.
Burns bone f.
Butler bayonet f.
Cairns-Dandy hemostasis f.
Cairns dissection f.
Cairns hemostatic f.
Calibri f.
Callahan scleral fixation f.
Callison-Adson tissue f.
Cameron-Miller monopolar f.
Campbell ligature-carrier f.
Campbell ureteral f.
Cane bone-holding f.
capsular f.
capsular fragment f.

capsule-grasping f.
capsulorrhexis f.
capsulotomy f.
caput f.
Carb-Bite tissue f.
carbide-jaw f.
Cardio-Grip iliac f.
Cardio-Grip tissue f.
cardiovascular tissue f.
Cardona corneal prosthesis f.
Cardona threading lens f.
Carlens f.
Carmalt arterial f.
Carmalt hemostatic f.
Carmalt hysterectomy f.
Carmalt splinter f.
Carmalt thoracic f.
Carmody thumb tissue f.
carotid artery f.
Carrel hemostatic f.
Carrel mosquito f.
Carroll-Adson dural f.
Carroll bone holding f.
Carroll dressing f.
Carroll tendon-passing f.
Carroll tendon-pulling f.
Carroll tissue f.
cartilage f.
cartilage-holding f.
Cartman lens insertion f.
caruncle f.
Casebeer capsulorrhexis f.
Caspar alligator f.
Cassidy-Brophy dressing f.
Castaneda-Mixter f.
Castaneda vascular f.
Castroviejo-Arruga capsular f.
Castroviejo capsular f.
Castroviejo clip-applying f.
Castroviejo-Colibri corneal f.
Castroviejo cornea-holding f.
Castroviejo corneoscleral f.
Castroviejo cross-action capsular f.
Castroviejo fixation f.
Castroviejo-Furness cornea-
  holding f.
Castroviejo lid f.
Castroviejo scleral fold f.
Castroviejo-Simpson f.
Castroviejo straight tying f.
Castroviejo suture f.
Castroviejo transplant f.

Castroviejo wide-grip handle f.
Catalano capsular f.
Catalano corneoscleral f.
Catalano tying f.
catheter introducing f.
Cavanaugh-Wells tonsillar f.
center-action f.
cephalic blade f.
cervical biopsy f.
cervical grasping f.
cervical hemostatic f.
cervical punch f.
cervical traction f.
cesarean f.
chalazion f.
Chamberlen obstetrical f.
Championnière f.
Chandler iris f.
Chandler spinal-perforating f.
Chang bone-cutting f.
Chaput tissue f.
Charnley-Riches arterial f.
Charnley suture f.
Charnley wire-holding f.
Cheatle sterilizing f.
Cheron uterine dressing f.
Cherry f.
Cherry-Adson f.
Cherry-Kerrison f.
Chester sponge f.
Chevalier Jackson
  bronchoesophagoscopy f.
chicken-bill rongeur f.
Child clip-applying f.
Child intestinal f.
Child-Phillips f.
Children's Hospital dressing f.
Children's Hospital intestinal f.
Chimani pharyngeal f.
Choyce intraocular lens f.
Choyce lens inserting f.
Christopher-Stille f.
Chubb tonsillar f.
Cicherelli f.
Cilco lens f.
Circon Tripolar f.
Citelli-Bruening ear f.
Citelli punch f.
Civiale f.
Clark capsular fragment f.
Clarke ligator scissor f.
Clark-Guyton f.

F

NOTES

forceps *(continued)*
  Clark-Verhoeff capsular f.
  claw f.
  Clayman corneal f.
  Clayman intraocular lens f.
  Clayman-Kelman intraocular lens f.
  Clayman lensholding f.
  Clayman lens-inserting f.
  Clayman-McPherson tying f.
  Clayman suturing f.
  cleft palate f.
  Clemetson uterine f.
  Clevedent f.
  Cleveland bone-cutting f.
  clip f.
  clip-applying aneurysm f.
  clip-bending f.
  clip-cutting f.
  clip-introducing f.
  clip-removing f.
  C. L. Jackson head-holding f.
  C. L. Jackson pin-bending
    costophrenic f.
  closed iris f.
  closing f.
  clot f.
  coagulating f.
  Coakley-Allis tonsillar f.
  Coakley tonsillar f.
  coaptation bipolar f.
  coarctation f.
  coated biopsy f.
  Cobaugh eye f.
  Codman fallopian tube f.
  Codman ovarian f.
  Cohen corneal f.
  Cohen nasal-dressing f.
  cold biopsy f.
  cold cup biopsy f.
  Coleman-Taylor IOL f.
  Colibri corneal f.
  Colibri eye f.
  Colibri-Pierse f.
  Colibri-Storz corneal f.
  College f.
  Coller arterial f.
  Coller hemostatic f.
  Colley tissue f.
  Colley traction f.
  Collier-DeBakey hemostatic f.
  Collier hemostatic f.
  Collin dressing f.
  Collin-Duval-Crile intestinal f.
  Collin-Duval intestinal f.
  Collin-Duval lung grasping f.
  Collin intestinal f.
  Collin lung f.
  Collin mucous f.
  Collin ovarian f.
  Collin-Pozzi uterine f.
  Collin tissue f.
  Collin tongue f.
  Collin tongue-seizing f.
  Collin uterine f.
  Collin uterine-elevating f.
  Collis-Maumenee corneal f.
  Coloviras-Rumel thoracic f.
  Colver-Coakley tonsillar f.
  Colver tonsillar pillar-grasping f.
  Colver tonsil-seizing f.
  common duct stone f.
  common McPherson f.
  compression f.
  concave rat-tooth f.
  Cone wire-twisting f.
  conjunctival fixation f.
  Cook flexible myocardial biopsy f.
  Cooley anastomosis f.
  Cooley aortic f.
  Cooley arterial occlusion f.
  Cooley auricular appendage f.
  Cooley-Baumgarten aortic f.
  Cooley cardiovascular f.
  Cooley coarctation f.
  Cooley curved f.
  Cooley-Derra anastomosis f.
  Cooley double-angled jaw f.
  Cooley graft f.
  Cooley iliac f.
  Cooley neonatal vascular f.
  Cooley patent ductus f.
  Cooley pediatric aortic f.
  Cooley peripheral vascular f.
  Cooley tangential pediatric f.
  Cooley tissue f.
  Cooley vascular tissue f.
  Cope lung f.
  Coppridge grasping f.
  Coppridge urethral f.
  Corbett bone-cutting f.
  Cordes esophagoscopy f.
  Cordes-New laryngeal punch f.
  Corey ovum f.
  Corey placental f.
  Corgill-Hartmann f.
  cornea-holding f.
  corneal fixation f.
  corneal suturing f.
  corneal transplant f.
  cornea-suturing f.
  corneoscleral suturing f.
  Cornet f.
  coronary artery f.
  Corson myoma f.
  Corwin-Hegar wire twisting f.
  Corwin tonsillar f.
  Cottle f.
  Cottle-Arruga cartilage f.

Cottle insertion f.
Cottle-Jansen f.
Cottle-Kazanjian bone-cutting f.
Cottle-Kazanjian nasal f.
Cottle lower lateral f.
Cottle tissue f.
Cottle-Walsham septum f.
Cottle-Walsham septum-
  straightening f.
cowhorn tooth-extracting f.
Cozean angled lens f.
Cozean bipolar f.
Cozean implantation f.
Cozean-McPherson angled lens f.
Cozean-McPherson tying f.
Crafoord bronchial f.
Crafoord coarctation f.
Crafoord pulmonary f.
Crafoord-Sellors f.
Craig-Domnick septum bone-
  cutting f.
Craig nasal-cutting f.
Craig septum f.
Craig tonsil-seizing f.
cranial f.
cranial clip-applying f.
Crawford fascial f.
Crawford-Knighton f.
Creevy biopsy f.
Crenshaw caruncle f.
Crile arterial f.
Crile-Barnes hemostatic f.
Crile-Duval lung-grasping f.
Crile gall duct f.
Crile hemostatic f.
Crile Micro-Line arterial f.
Crile-Rankin f.
crimping f.
Crockard ligament grasping f.
Crockard odontoid peg-grasping f.
crocodile biopsy f.
cross-action capsular f.
Crossen puncturing tenaculum f.
crural nipper f.
Cryer Universal f.
CSF shunt-introducing f.
Cukier nasal f.
Culler eye f.
Culler fixation f.
Cullom septal f.
Cummings folding f.
cup f.

cup biopsy f.
cupped f.
cup-shaped f.
cup-shaped inner ear f.
cup-shaped middle ear f.
Curtis tissue f.
curved dissecting f.
curved iris f.
curved knot-tying f.
curved-tip bipolar f.
Cushing f.
Cushing artery f.
Cushing bayonet f.
Cushing bipolar f.
Cushing brain f.
Cushing-Brown tissue f.
Cushing cranial rongeur f.
Cushing decompression f.
Cushing Diamond-Points thumb f.
Cushing dissecting f.
Cushing dressing f.
Cushing-Gutsch dressing f.
Cushing-Gutsch tissue f.
Cushing monopolar f.
Cushing-Taylor carbide-jaw f.
Cushing thumb f.
Cushing tissue f.
Cushing-Vital tissue f.
Cutler f.
cutting f.
cystic duct f.
cystoscopic f.
Czerny tenaculum f.
Dahlgren-Hudson cranial f.
Dahlgren skill-cutting f.
Daicoff needle-pulling f.
Daicoff vascular f.
Dallas lens-inserting f.
D'Allesandro serial suture-holding f.
Danberg iris f.
Dan chalazion f.
Dandy arterial f.
Dandy artery f.
Dandy-Kolodny hemostatic f.
Dandy scalp f.
Dan-Gradle ciliary f.
Dartigues kidney-elevating f.
Dartigues uterine-elevating f.
Davidson pulmonary vessel f.
Davis bayonet f.
Davis capsular f.
Davis coagulating f.

F

NOTES

forceps *(continued)*

Davis diathermy f.
Davis monopolar bayonet f.
Davis sterilizer f.
Davis tissue f.
Davol rongeur f.
Dawson-Yuhl-Kerrison rongeur f.
Dawson-Yuhl-Leksell rongeur f.
Dawson-Yuhl rongeur f.
Dean tonsillar f.
DeBakey aortic f.
DeBakey Autraugrip f.
DeBakey-Bainbridge intenstinal f.
DeBakey-Bainbridge vascular f.
DeBakey-Beck multipurpose f.
DeBakey-Cooley cardiovascular f.
DeBakey-Cooley dissecting f.
DeBakey-Derra anastomosis f.
DeBakey-Diethrich coronary
  artery f.
DeBakey-Diethrich vascular f.
DeBakey dissecting f.
DeBakey-Mixter thoracic f.
DeBakey-Péan cardiovascular f.
DeBakey-Semb f.
DeBakey tangential occlusion f.
DeBakey thoracic tissue f.
DeBakey tissue f.
DeBakey vascular tissue f.
Decker microsurgical f.
deep surgery f.
deep vessel f.
Defourmental f.
DeLee cervix-holding f.
DeLee dressing f.
DeLee obstetrical f.
DeLee ovum f.
DeLee shuttle f.
DeLee-Simpson f.
DeLee spoon tissue f.
DeLee uterine f.
DeLee uterine-packing f.
delicate grasping f.
delicate thumb-dressing f.
Delrin locking-handle f.
DeMartel appendix f.
DeMartel scalp flap f.
DeMartel-Wolfson closing f.
DeMartel-Wolfson intestinal-
  holding f.
Demel twisting f.
Demel wire-tightening f.
Dench ear f.
Denis Browne tonsillar f.
Dennen f.
Dennis intestinal f.
dental dressing f.
depilatory f.
Derf f.

DermaCare electrosurgical f.
Derra cardiovascular f.
Derra urethral f.
D'Errico bayonet pituitary f.
D'Errico dressing f.
D'Errico hypophyseal f.
D'Errico tissue f.
Desjardins gall duct f.
Desjardins gallstone f.
Desjardins kidney pedicle f.
Desmarres chalazion f.
Desmarres lid f.
DeVilbiss cranial f.
DeWecker f.
DeWeese axis traction obstetrical f.
Dewey obstetrical f.
Diaflex grasping f.
Diamond-Flex f.
Diamond-Lite titanium thumb f.
diathermy f.
Dieffenbach f.
Diener f.
Dieter malleus f.
Diethrich right-angled hemostatic f.
dilating f.
Dingman bone-holding f.
disc f.
discectomy f.
disimpaction f.
disposable f.
disposable biopsy f.
dissecting f.
dissecting diathermy f.
dissection f.
divergent outlet f.
Dixon flamingo f.
Docktor tissue f.
Dodick lens-holding f.
Dodick Nucleus Cracker f.
dolphin-nose dissecting f.
dolphin-nose grasping f.
Dorsey f.
double-action f.
double-action bone-cutting f.
double-articulated bronchoscopic f.
double-cupped f.
double-ended f.
double-ended needle f.
double-ended suture f.
double-ended tissue f.
double-fixation f.
double-pronged f.
double-spoon f.
double-spoon biopsy f.
Douglas ciliary f.
Douglas eye f.
Doyen gallbladder f.
Doyen intestinal clamp f.
Doyen towel f.

Doyen uterine f.
Doyen vulsellum f.
Draeger f.
dressing f.
Drews intraocular f.
Drews-Sato tying f.
drill guide f.
duckbill f.
Ducournau fine gripping f.
Dumont dissecting f.
Dumont jeweler's f.
Dunhill f.
Duplay uterine tenaculum f.
dural f.
Duval-Allis f.
Duval-Collin intestinal f.
Duval-Crile intestinal f.
Duval-Crile lung f.
Duval-Crile lung-grasping f.
Duval-Crile tissue f.
Duval intestinal f.
Duval lung f.
Duval tissue f.
Dyonics basket f.
ear dressing f.
ear polyp f.
ear punch f.
Eastman cystic duct f.
Eber needle-holder f.
Echlin rongeur f.
Eder f.
Effler-Groves cardiovascular f.
Eisenstein hysterectomy f.
elastic bowel f.
electrocoagulating biopsy f.
electrosurgery f.
electrosurgical f.
elevating f.
Elliott gallbladder f.
Elliott hemostatic f.
Elliott obstetrical f.
Elschnig capsular f.
Elschnig cyclodialysis f.
Elschnig fixation f.
Elschnig-O'Brien fixation f.
Elschnig-O'Brien tissue-grasping f.
Elschnig-O'Connor fixation f.
Elschnig secondary membrane f.
Elschnig tissue-grasping f.
Emmet obstetrical f.
endometrial polyp f.
endoscopic biopsy f.

endoscopic grasping f.
endoscopic suture-cutting f.
endospeculum f.
Endo-therapy disposable biopsy f.
endotracheal f.
endotracheal tube f.
Endura dressing f.
English tissue f.
entropion f.
epilation f.
episcleral f.
Eppendorf cervical biopsy f.
Eppendorfer uterine biopsy f.
Erbe bipolar laparoscopic f.
Ergo bipolar f.
Erhardt eyelid f.
Erich laryngeal biopsy f.
Ernest-McDonald II folding f.
Ernest-McDonald soft intraocular
  lens-folding f.
E-series bipolar f.
esophagoscopic f.
Essrig tissue f.
ethmoid f.
ethmoid-Blakesley f.
Evans tissue f.
Everett f.
Evershears bipolar f.
Ewald-Hudson brain f.
Ewald-Hudson dressing f.
Ewald-Hudson tissue f.
Ewald tissue f.
Ewing capsular f.
Excel disposable biopsy f.
exenteration f.
expansile f.
extracapsular f.
extraction f.
eye dressing f.
eye fixation f.
eyelid f.
Falcao fixation f.
Falk lion-jaw f.
fallopian tube f.
Farabeuf bone-holding f.
Farabeuf-Lambotte bone-holding f.
Farrington nasal polyp f.
Farrington septal f.
Farrior wire-crimping f.
Faure peritoneal f.
Faure uterine biopsy f.
Feaster lens holding f.

F

NOTES

forceps *(continued)*

Fechtner conjunctival f.
Fechtner ring f.
Fehland intestinal f.
Feilchenfeld splinter f.
fenestrated blade f.
fenestrated cup biopsy f.
fenestrated ellipsoid spiked
  biopsy f.
Ferguson angiotribe f.
Ferguson bone-holding f.
Ferris colporrhaphy f.
Ferris-Smith bone-biting f.
Ferris-Smith cup rongeur f.
Ferris-Smith fragment f.
Ferris-Smith-Kerrison f.
Ferris-Smith rongeur f.
Ferris-Smith-Spurling intervertebral
  disc f.
Ferris-Smith-Takahashi f.
Ferris-Smith tissue f.
fine arterial f.
Fine dissecting f.
Fine gripping f.
Fine head-tilt capsulorrhexis f.
Fine sideport capsulorrhexis f.
Fine suture-tying f.
fine-tooth f.
Fink fixation f.
Fink tendon-tucker f.
Finochietto lobectomy f.
Finochietto thoracic f.
Fisher advancement f.
Fisher capsular f.
Fisher iris f.
Fish grasping f.
Fish nasal-dressing f.
Fitzgerald aortic aneurysm f.
Fitzwater peanut sponge-holding f.
fixation f.
fixation binocular f.
Fletcher dressing f.
Fletcher sponge f.
Fletcher-Suit polyp f.
Fletcher-Van Doren sponge-
  holding f.
Fletcher-Van Doren uterine
  polyp f.
flexible foreign body f.
flexible optical biopsy f.
fluoroscopic foreign body f.
Foerster f.
Foerster-Bauer sponge-holding f.
Foerster gallbladder f.
Foerster iris f.
Foerster sponge f.
Foerster sponge-holding f.
Foerster tissue f.
Foerster uterine f.

Fogarty bulldog clamp-applying f.
folding f.
Foley vas isolation f.
Forbes uterine-dressing f.
foreign body cystoscopy f.
foreign body eye f.
foreign body-retrieving f.
Förster iris f.
forward-grasping f.
Foss cardiovascular f.
Foss clamp f.
Foster-Ballenger bone f.
Fox bipolar electrocautery f.
fragment f.
Francis spud chalazion f.
Frangenheim biopsy punch f.
Frangenheim hook f.
Fränkel cutting-tip f.
Fränkel esophagoscopy f.
Fränkel laryngeal f.
Fränkel tampon f.
Frankfeldt grasping f.
Fraser f.
Freer septal f.
French-pattern f.
Fricke arterial f.
Friedman rongeur f.
Fuchs capsular f.
Fuchs capsulotomy f.
Fuchs extracapsular f.
Fuchs iris f.
Fujinon biopsy f.
Furness cornea-holding f.
Furness polyp f.
Gabriel Tucker f.
gallbladder f.
gall duct f.
gallstone f.
Gam-Mer bone-cutting f.
Gardner bone f.
Gardner hysterectomy f.
Garland hysterectomy f.
Garrigue uterine-dressing f.
Garrison f.
Gaskin fragment f.
gastrointestinal f.
Gavin-Miller colon f.
Gavin-Miller intestinal f.
Gavin-Miller tissue f.
Gaylor uterine biopsy f.
Geissendorfer uterine f.
Gelfilm f.
Gelfoam pressure f.
Gelhorn biopsy f.
Gellhorn uterine biopsy f.
Gelpi hysterectomy f.
Gelpi-Lowrie hysterectomy f.
Gemini gall duct f.
Gemini hemostatic f.

Gemini-Mixter f.
Gemini thoracic f.
general tissue f.
general wire f.
Gerald bayonet microbipolar
  neurosurgical f.
Gerald brain f.
Gerald dressing f.
Gerald monopolar f.
Gerald straight microbipolar
  neurosurgical f.
Gerald tissue f.
Gerbode cardiovascular tissue f.
GI f.
Gifford fixation f.
Gifford iris f.
Gilbert cystic duct f.
Gildenberg biopsy f.
Gill-Arruga capsular f.
Gill-Chandler iris f.
Gill curved iris f.
Gill-Fuchs capsular f.
Gill-Hess iris f.
Gillies dissecting f.
Gillies tissue f.
Gill incision-spreading f.
Gill iris f.
Gillquist-Oretorp-Stille f.
Gill-Welsh capsular f.
Ginsberg tissue f.
giraffe biopsy f.
Girard corneoscleral f.
Glassman f.
Glassman-Allis intestinal f.
Glassman-Allis noncrushing common
  duct f.
Glassman-Allis noncrushing
  intestinal f.
Glenn diverticular f.
Glenner vaginal hysterectomy f.
Glover anastomosis f.
Glover coarctation f.
Glover curved f.
Glover infundibular rongeur f.
Glover patent ductus f.
Glover spoon-shaped f.
goiter vulsellum f.
Gold deep-surgery f.
gold hemostatic f.
Goldman-Kazanjian nasal f.
Goldmann capsulorrhexis f.
Gomco f.

Goodhill tonsillar f.
Good obstetrical f.
Gordon bead f.
Gordon ciliary f.
Gordon uterine f.
Gordon vulsellum f.
Grabow capsulorrhexis f.
Gradle ciliary f.
Graefe curved iris f.
Graefe dressing f.
Graefe eye-fixation f.
Graefe straight iris f.
Graefe tissue f.
Graefe tissue-grasping f.
grasping f.
grasping biopsy f.
grasping tripod f.
Graspit stone retrieval f.
Gray arterial f.
Gray cystic duct f.
Green-Armytage hemostatic f.
Green capsular f.
Green chalazion f.
Green fixation f.
Green suction tube f.
Green tissue-grasping f.
Green tube-holding f.
Greenwood bipolar coagulation-
  suction f.
Gregory f.
Greven alligator f.
Grey Turner f.
Grieshaber diamond-coated f.
Grieshaber internal limiting
  membrane f.
Grieshaber iris f.
Grieshaber manipulator f.
grooved tying f.
Gross dressing f.
Gross hyoid-cutting f.
Gross sponge f.
Gruenwald bayonet dressing f.
Gruenwald-Bryant nasal-cutting f.
Gruenwald dissecting f.
Gruenwald dressing f.
Gruenwald Durogrip f.
Gruenwald ear f.
Gruenwald-Jansen f.
Gruenwald-Love neurosurgical f.
Gruenwald nasal-cutting f.
Gruenwald nasal-dressing f.
Gruenwald tissue f.

F

NOTES

forceps *(continued)*
Gruppe wire-crimping f.
Guggenheim adenoidal f.
Guilford-Wright f.
Guist fixation f.
Gunderson bone f.
Gunderson muscle recession f.
Gunnar-Hey roller f.
Guppe f.
Gusberg uterine f.
Gutgemann auricular appendage f.
Gutglass hemostatic cervical f.
Gutierrez-Najar grasping f.
Guyton-Clark fragment f.
Guyton-Noyes fixation f.
Guyton suturing f.
Haberer gastrointestinal f.
Haberer-Gili f.
Hagenbarth clip-applying f.
Haig-Ferguson obstetrical f.
Haig obstetrical f.
Hajek antral punch f.
Hajek-Koffler bone punch f.
Hajek-Koffler sphenoidal f.
Hakler f.
Halberg contact lens f.
Hale obstetrical f.
Halifax placement f.
Hallberg f.
hallux f.
Halsey mosquito f.
Halsted arterial f.
Halsted curved mosquito f.
Halsted hemostatic mosquito f.
Halsted Micro-Line arterial f.
Halsted-Swanson tendon-passing f.
Hamby clip-applying f.
Hamilton deep-surgery f.
hammer f.
Hank-Dennen obstetrical f.
Hannahan f.
Hardy bayonet dressing f.
Hardy bayonet neurosurgical
  bipolar f.
Hardy microbipolar f.
harelip f.
Harken auricle f.
Harken cardiovascular f.
Harken-Cooley f.
Harman fixation f.
Harms corneal f.
Harms microtying f.
Harms-Tubingen tying f.
Harms tying f.
Harms utility f.
Harms vessel f.
Harrington clamp f.
Harrington lung-grasping f.
Harrington-Mayo tissue f.

Harrington-Mixter thoracic f.
Harrington thoracic f.
Harrington vulsellum f.
Harrison bone-holding f.
Harris suture-carrying f.
Hartmann alligator f.
Hartmann-Citelli alligator f.
Hartmann-Citelli ear punch f.
Hartmann-Corgill ear f.
Hartmann ear-dressing f.
Hartmann ear polyp f.
Hartmann-Gruenwald nasal-cutting f.
Hartmann hemostatic mosquito f.
Hartmann-Herzfeld ear f.
Hartmann mosquito hemostatic f.
Hartmann nasal-cutting f.
Hartmann nasal-dressing f.
Hartmann nasal polyp f.
Hartmann-Noyes nasal-dressing f.
Hartmann-Proctor ear f.
Hartmann tonsillar punch f.
Hartmann uterine biopsy f.
Hartmann-Weingärtner ear f.
Hartmann-Wullstein ear f.
Haslinger tip f.
Hasner lid f.
Hasson bullet-tip f.
Hasson grasping f.
Hasson needle-nose f.
Hasson ring f.
Hasson spike-tooth f.
Haugh ear f.
Hawkins cervical biopsy f.
Hawks-Dennen obstetrical f.
Hayes anterior resection f.
Hayes Martin f.
Hayes-Olivecrona f.
Hayton-Williams disimpaction f.
Hayton-Williams maxillary f.
Healy gastrointestinal f.
Healy intestinal f.
Healy suture-removing f.
Healy uterine biopsy f.
Heaney-Ballantine hysterectomy f.
Heaney hysterectomy f.
Heaney-Kantor hysterectomy f.
Heaney-Rezek f.
Heaney-Simon hysterectomy f.
Heaney-Stumf f.
Heaney tissue f.
Heath chalazion f.
Heath clip-removing f.
Heath nasal f.
Hecht fascia lata f.
Heermann alligator f.
Heermann ear f.
Hegenbarth clip-applying f.
Hegenbarth-Michel clip-applying f.
Heidelberg fixation f.

Heifitz cup serrated ring f.
Heiming kidney stone f.
Heiss artery f.
Heiss hemostatic f.
Heiss vulsellum f.
Heller biopsy f.
Hemoclip-applying f.
hemorrhoidal f.
hemostatic f.
hemostatic cervical f.
hemostatic clip-applying f.
hemostatic neurosurgical f.
hemostatic tissue f.
hemostatic tonsillar f.
hemostatic tracheal f.
Hendren cardiovascular f.
Hendren pediatric f.
Henke punch f.
Henrotin vulsellum f.
Henry ciliary f.
Herff membrane-puncturing f.
Herget biopsy f.
Hermann bone-holding f.
Herrick kidney f.
Hersh LASIK retreatment f.
Hertel kidney stone f.
Hertel rigid dilator stone f.
Hertel rigid kidney stone f.
Herzfeld ear f.
Herz meniscal tendon f.
Hess-Barraquer iris f.
Hessburg lens-inserting f.
Hess capsular f.
Hess-Gill iris f.
Hess-Horwitz iris f.
Hess iris f.
Hevesy polyp f.
Heyman-Knight nasal dressing f.
Heyman nasal f.
Heyman nasal-cutting f.
Heyner f.
Heywood-Smith dressing f.
Heywood-Smith gallbladder f.
Heywood-Smith sponge-holding f.
Hibbs biting f.
Hibbs bone-cutting f.
Hibbs bone-holding f.
Hildebrandt uterine hemostatic f.
Hildyard nasal f.
Himalaya dressing f.
Hinderer cartilage f.
Hirsch hypophysis punch f.

Hirschman hemorrhoidal f.
Hirschman jeweler's f.
Hirschman lens f.
Hirst-Emmet obstetrical f.
Hirst-Emmet placental f.
Hirst obstetrical f.
Hirst placental f.
Hodge obstetrical f.
Hoen alligator f.
Hoen bayonet f.
Hoen dressing f.
Hoen grasping f.
Hoen hemostatic f.
Hoen scalp f.
Hoen tissue f.
Hoffmann ear punch f.
Hoffmann-Pollock f.
holding f.
Holinger specimen f.
Holmes fixation f.
Holth punch f.
Holzbach hysterectomy f.
hook f.
Hopkins aortic f.
Horsley bone-cutting f.
Horsley-Stille bone-cutting f.
Horsley-Stille rib shears f.
Hosemann choledochus f.
Hosford-Hicks transfer f.
Hoskins beaked Colibri f.
Hoskins-Colibri f.
Hoskins-Dallas intraocular lens-inserting f.
Hoskins fine straight f.
Hoskins fixation f.
Hoskins-Luntz f.
Hoskins microstraight f.
Hoskins-Skeleton fine f.
Hoskins-Skeleton grooved broad-tipped f.
Hoskins suture f.
hot biopsy f.
hot flexible f.
Hot Sampler disposable hot biopsy f.
House alligator crimper f.
House alligator grasping f.
House alligator strut f.
House cup f.
House-Dieter eye f.
House ear f.
House Gelfoam pressure f.

F

NOTES

forceps *(continued)*

House grasping f.
House miniature f.
House oval-cup f.
Housepian clip-applying f.
House pressure f.
House strut f.
House-Wullstein alligator f.
House-Wullstein cup ear f.
Houspian clip-applying f.
Howard closing f.
Howard tonsillar f.
Howard tonsil-ligating f.
Howmedica Microfixation System f.
Hoxworth f.
Hoyt deep-surgery f.
Hoytenberger tissue f.
Hoyt hemostatic f.
Hubbard corneoscleral f.
Hudson brain f.
Hudson cranial f.
Hudson dressing f.
Hudson-Ewald tissue f.
Hudson rongeur f.
Hudson tissue f.
Hufnagel mitral valve f.
Hulka clip f.
Hulka-Kenwick uterine-elevating f.
Hulka tenaculum f.
hump f.
Hunt angled serrated ring f.
Hunt bipolar f.
Hunt chalazion f.
Hunter splinter f.
Hunt grasping f.
Hunt tumor f.
Hunt vessel f.
Hunt-Yasargil pituitary f.
Hurd bone f.
Hurd bone-cutting f.
Hurdner tissue f.
Hurd septal bone-cutting f.
Hurd septum-cutting f.
Hurteau f.
Hyde double-curved corneal f.
hypophysectomy f.
hysterectomy f.
Ikeda capsulorrhexis f.
Ilg capsular f.
Ilg insertion f.
iliac f.
Iliff blepharochalasis f.
IM Jaws alligator f.
Imperatori laryngeal f.
implantation f.
Inamura small incision
  capsulorrhexis f.
infant biopsy f.
infundibular f.

Ingraham-Fowler clip-applying f.
inlet f.
insertion f.
insulated bayonet f.
insulated monopolar f.
insulated tissue f.
intervertebral disc f.
intestinal anastomosis f.
intestinal closing f.
intestinal holding f.
intestinal tissue f.
intracapsular lens f.
intraocular irrigating f.
intraocular lens f.
intrathoracic f.
introducing f.
Iowa membrane f.
Iowa-Mengert membrane f.
Iowa State fixation f.
iris f.
iris bipolar f.
iris tissue f.
Iselin f.
isolation f.
I-tech intraocular foreign body f.
I-tech splinter f.
I-tech tying f.
Jackson alligator grasping f.
Jackson approximation f.
Jackson biopsy f.
Jackson broad staple f.
Jackson button f.
Jackson conventional foreign
  body f.
Jackson cross-action f.
Jackson cylindrical-object f.
Jackson double-concave rat-tooth f.
Jackson double-prong f.
Jackson down-jaw f.
Jackson dressing f.
Jackson dull-pointed f.
Jackson endoscopic f.
Jackson fenestrated f.
Jackson fenestrated peanut-
  grasping f.
Jackson flexible upper lobe
  bronchus f.
Jackson forward-grasping f.
Jackson globular object f.
Jackson head-holding f.
Jackson hemostatic f.
Jackson hollow-object f.
Jackson infant biopsy f.
Jackson laryngeal applicator f.
Jackson laryngeal basket f.
Jackson laryngeal-dressing f.
Jackson laryngeal-grasping f.
Jackson laryngeal punch f.
Jackson laryngeal ring-rotation f.

Jackson laryngofissure f.
Jackson papilloma f.
Jackson pin-bending costophrenic f.
Jackson punch f.
Jackson ring-jaw f.
Jackson ring-rotation f.
Jackson sharp-pointed rotation f.
Jackson side-curved f.
Jackson sister-hook f.
Jackson tendon-seizing f.
Jackson tracheal hemostatic f.
Jackson triangular-punch f.
Jacob capsular fragment f.
Jacobs biopsy f.
Jacobs capsular fragment f.
Jacobson bipolar f.
Jacobson dressing f.
Jacobson hemostatic f.
Jacobson mosquito f.
Jacobs vulsellum f.
Jaffe capsulorrhexis f.
Jaffe suturing f.
Jaffe tying f.
Jager meniscal f.
Jako laryngeal f.
Jako microlaryngeal cup f.
Jako microlaryngeal grasping f.
Jameson muscle recession f.
Jameson strabismus f.
Jameson tracheal muscle f.
James wound-approximation f.
Jannetta alligator grasping f.
Jannetta bayonet f.
Jannetta microbayonet f.
Jansen bayonet dressing f.
Jansen bayonet ear f.
Jansen bayonet nasal f.
Jansen dissecting f.
Jansen dressing f.
Jansen-Gruenwald f.
Jansen-Middleton nasal-cutting f.
Jansen-Middleton punch f.
Jansen-Middleton septal f.
Jansen-Middleton septotomy f.
Jansen-Middleton septum-cutting f.
Jansen monopolar f.
Jansen-Mueller f.
Jansen nasal-dressing f.
Jansen-Struyken septal f.
Jansen thumb f.
Jarcho tenaculum f.
Jarell f.

Jarit-Allis tissue f.
Jarit brain f.
Jarit-Crafoord f.
Jarit-Dandy f.
Jarit-Liston bone-cutting f.
Jarit microsuture tying f.
Jarit mosquito f.
Jarit sterilizer f.
Jarit tendon-pulling f.
Jarit tube-occluding f.
Jarit wire-pulling f.
Jarvis hemorrhoidal f.
Javerts placental f.
Javerts polyp f.
jaw f.
Jawz disposable biopsy f.
Jayles f.
Jensen intraocular lens f.
Jensen lens-inserting f.
Jerald f.
Jervey capsular fragment f.
Jervey iris f.
Jesberg grasping f.
jeweler's bipolar f.
jeweler's pickup f.
Johns Hopkins f.
Johns Hopkins gallbladder f.
Johns Hopkins gall duct f.
Johns Hopkins hemostatic f.
Johns Hopkins occluding f.
Johns Hopkins serrefine f.
Johnson brain tumor f.
Johnson ptosis f.
Johnson thoracic f.
John Weiss f.
Jones hemostatic f.
Jones IMA f.
Jones towel f.
Joplin bone-holding f.
Jordan strut f.
Judd-Allis intestinal f.
Judd-Allis tissue f.
Judd-DeMartel gallbladder f.
Judd strabismus f.
Judd suture f.
Juers crimper f.
Juers-Lempert rongeur f.
Juers lingual f.
Julian-Damian thoracic f.
Julian splenorenal f.
Julian thoracic artery f.
Jurasz laryngeal f.

F

NOTES

forceps *(continued)*

Kadesky f.
Kahler bronchial biopsy f.
Kahler bronchoscopic f.
Kahler bronchus-grasping f.
Kahler laryngeal biopsy f.
Kahler polyp f.
Kahn tenaculum f.
Kalman occluding f.
Kalman tube-occluding f.
Kalt capsular f.
Kansas University corneal f.
Kantor f.
Kantrowitz dressing f.
Kantrowitz thoracic f.
Kantrowitz tissue f.
Kapp f.
Kapp-Beck f.
Karp aortic punch f.
Katena f.
Katzin-Barraquer Colibri f.
Katzin-Barraquer corneal f.
Kaufman ENT f.
Kazanjian bone-cutting f.
Kazanjian-Cottle f.
Kazanjian cutting f.
Kazanjian nasal f.
Kazanjian nasal hump f.
Keeler extended round tip f.
Keeler intraocular foreign body grasping f.
Keen Edge disposable biopsy f.
Kelly arterial f.
Kelly dressing f.
Kelly-Gray uterine f.
Kelly hemostatic f.
Kelly-Murphy f.
Kelly ovum f.
Kelly placental f.
Kelly polypus f.
Kelly-Rankin f.
Kelly tissue f.
Kelly urethral f.
Kelman implantation f.
Kelman intraocular f.
Kelman irrigator f.
Kelman-McPherson corneal f.
Kelman-McPherson suture f.
Kelman-McPherson tissue f.
Kelman-McPherson tying f.
Kennedy vulsellum f.
Kennerdell bayonet f.
Kent f.
keratotomy f.
Kern bone-holding f.
Kern-Lane bone-holding f.
Kerrison f.
Kershner LASIK flap f.

Kershner one-step micro capsulorrhexis f.
Kevorkian uterine biopsy f.
Kevorkian-Younge cervical biopsy f.
Kevorkian-Younge uterine biopsy f.
Khodadad microclip f.
kidney elevating f.
kidney pedicle f.
kidney stone f.
Killian-Jameson f.
Killian septal compression f.
Kinder Design pedodontic f.
King-Prince muscle f.
King-Prince recession f.
Kingsley grasping f.
King tissue f.
King wound f.
Kirby-Arthus fixation f.
Kirby-Bracken iris f.
Kirby capsular f.
Kirby corneoscleral f.
Kirby eye tissue f.
Kirby fixation f.
Kirby intracapsular lens f.
Kirby iris f.
Kirby lens f.
Kirkpatrick tonsillar f.
Kirschner-Ullrich f.
Kirwan-Adson ophthalmic bipolar f.
Kirwan bipolar electrosurgical f.
Kirwan coaptation ophthalmic bipolar f.
Kirwan jeweler's ophthalmic bipolar f.
Kirwan-Nadler coaptation ophthalmic bipolar f.
Kirwan-Tenzel ophthalmic bipolar f.
Kitner goiter f.
Kitner thyroid-packing f.
Kjelland-Barton f.
Kjelland-Luikart obstetrical f.
Kjelland obstetrical f.
KleenSpec f.
Kleinert-Kutz bone-cutting f.
Kleinert-Kutz rongeur f.
Kleinert-Kutz tendon f.
Kleinert-Kutz tendon-passing f.
Kleinert-Kutz tendon-retrieving f.
Kleppinger bipolar f.
KLI bipolar f.
KLI monopolar f.
Knapp-Luer trachoma f.
Knapp trachoma f.
Knight nasal-cutting f.
Knight nasal septum-cutting f.
Knighton-Crawford f.
Knight polyp f.
Knight septal f.

Knight septum-cutting f.
Knight-Sluder nasal f.
Knight turbinate f.
Knolle lens implantation f.
Knolle-Shepard lens-holding f.
Knolle-Volker lens-holding f.
knotting f.
knot-tying f.
Koby cataract f.
Kocher arterial f.
Kocher artery f.
Kocher hemostatic f.
Kocher kidney-elevating f.
Kocher Micro-Line intestinal f.
Kocher-Ochsner hemostatic f.
Koeberlé f.
Koenig vascular f.
Koerte gallstone f.
Koffler-Lillie septal f.
Koffler septal f.
Kogan endospeculum f.
Kolb bronchial f.
Kolodny f.
Korte gallstone f.
Kos crimper f.
Kraff intraocular utility f.
Kraff lens-inserting f.
Kraff-Osher lens f.
Kraff suturing f.
Kraff tying f.
Kraff-Utrata capsulorrhexis f.
Kraff-Utrata intraocular utility f.
Kraff-Utrata tear capsulotomy f.
Kramer f.
Kratz lens-inserting f.
Krause biopsy f.
Krause esophagoscopy f.
Krause punch f.
Krause Universal f.
Kremer fixation f.
Kremer 2-point fixation f.
Kronfeld micropin f.
Kronfeld suturing f.
Krönlein hemostatic f.
Krukenberg pigment spindle f.
K/S-Allis f.
Kuhnt capsular f.
Kuhnt fixation f.
Kulvin-Kalt iris f.
Kurze microbiopsy f.
Kurze micrograsping f.
Kurze pickup f.

Küstner uterine tenaculum f.
Kwapis interdental f.
Laborde f.
Lahey arterial f.
Lahey-Babcock f.
Lahey dissecting f.
Lahey gall duct f.
Lahey goiter-seizing f.
Lahey goiter vulsellum f.
Lahey hemostatic f.
Lahey lock arterial f.
Lahey-Sweet dissecting f.
Lahey thoracic f.
Lahey thyroid tenaculum f.
Lahey thyroid traction vulsellum f.
Lajeune hemostatic f.
Lalonde delicate hook f.
Lambert chalazion f.
Lambert-Kay anastomosis f.
Lambotte bone-holding f.
Lambotte fibular f.
Lancaster-O'Connor f.
lancet-shaped biopsy f.
Landers vitrectomy lens f.
Landolt spreading f.
Landon f.
Lane bone-holding f.
Lane gastrointestinal f.
Lane intestinal f.
Lane screw-holding f.
Lane tissue f.
Lange approximation f.
Langenbeck bone-holding f.
Lang iris f.
laparoscopic f.
Laplace f.
LaRoe undermining f.
Larsen tendon f.
Larsen tendon-holding f.
laryngeal applicator f.
laryngeal basket f.
laryngeal biopsy f.
laryngeal bronchial grasping f.
laryngeal curette f.
laryngeal grasping f.
laryngeal punch f.
laryngeal rotation f.
laryngeal sponging f.
laryngofissure f.
laser microlaryngeal cup f.
laser microlaryngeal grasping f.
laser ovary f.

F

NOTES

forceps *(continued)*

Laufe-Barton-Kjelland obstetrical f.
Laufe-Barton-Kjelland-Piper
  obstetrical f.
Laufe-Barton obstetrical f.
Laufe divergent outlet f.
Laufe obstetrical f.
Laufe-Piper obstetrical f.
Laufe-Piper uterine polyp f.
Laufe uterine polyp f.
Laufman f.
Laurer f.
Laval advancement f.
Lawrence deep f.
Lawrence hemostatic f.
Lawton f.
Lawton-Schubert biopsy f.
Lawton-Wittner cervical biopsy f.
Lazar microsuction f.
Leader vas isolation f.
Leahey chalazion f.
Leahey marginal chalazion f.
Leahey suture f.
Leasure nasal f.
Leaver sclerotomy f.
Lebsche f.
Lees arterial f.
Lees nontraumatic f.
Lefferts bone-cutting f.
Leibinger Micro System plate-
  holding f.
Leigh capsular f.
Lejeune thoracic f.
Leksell rongeur f.
Leland-Jones f.
Lemmon-Russian f.
Lemoine f.
Lempert rongeur f.
lens implantation f.
lens loop f.
lens-threading f.
Leonard f.
Leo Schwartz sponge-holding f.
Leriche hemostatic f.
Leriche tissue f.
LeRoy clip-applying f.
Lester fixation f.
Lester muscle f.
Levenson tissue f.
Levora fixation f.
Levret f.
Lewin bone-holding f.
Lewin spinal-perforating f.
Lewis septal f.
Lewis tonsillar hemostatic f.
Lewis ureteral stone isolation f.
Lewkowitz lithotomy f.
Lewkowitz ovum f.
Lewkowitz placental f.

Lexer tissue f.
Leyro-Diaz thoracic f.
lid f.
Lieberman-Pollock double corneal f.
Lieberman suturing f.
Lieberman tying f.
Lieb-Guerry f.
ligament-grasping f.
ligamentum flavum f.
ligature f.
ligature-carrying f.
Lillehei valve-grasping f.
Lillie intestinal f.
Lillie-Killian septal f.
Lillie tissue-holding f.
Lindsay-Rea f.
Lindstrom lens-insertion f.
lingual f.
Linnartz f.
Linn-Graefe iris f.
lion f.
lion-jaw bone-holding f.
Lister conjunctival f.
Liston bone-cutting f.
Liston-Key bone-cutting f.
Liston-Key-Horsley f.
Liston-Littauer bone-cutting f.
Liston-Stille bone-cutting f.
lithotomy f.
Littauer bone-cutting f.
Littauer ciliary f.
Littauer ear-dressing f.
Littauer ear polyp f.
Littauer-Liston bone-cutting f.
Littauer nasal-dressing f.
Littauer-West cutting f.
Littlewood tissue f.
Livernois lens-holding f.
Livernois-McDonald f.
Livernois pickup and folding f.
Livingston f.
Llobera fixation f.
Llorente dissecting f.
Lloyd-Davies occlusion f.
lobectomy f.
lobe-grasping f.
lobe-holding f.
Lobenstein-Tarnier f.
Lockwood-Allis intestinal f.
Lockwood-Allis tissue f.
Lockwood intestinal f.
Lockwood tissue f.
Lombard-Beyer f.
London tissue f.
Long Island College Hospital
  placental f.
long tissue f.
loose body suction f.
Lordan chalazion f.

Lore subglottic f.
Lorna-Edna towel f.
Lothrop ligature f.
Love-Gruenwald alligator f.
Love-Gruenwald pituitary f.
Love-Kerrison rongeur f.
Lovelace bladder f.
Lovelace gallbladder traction f.
Lovelace hemostatic f.
Lovelace lung-grasping f.
Lovelace thyroid-traction
  vulsellum f.
Lovelace tissue f.
Lovelace traction lung f.
Lovelace traction tissue f.
Löw-Beer f.
Löwenberg f.
lower gall duct f.
lower lateral f.
Lowis intervertebral disc f.
Lowman bone-holding f.
Lowsley grasping f.
Lowsley-Luc f.
Lowsley prostatic f.
Lucae bayonet dressing f.
Lucae bayonet ear f.
Lucae bayonet tissue f.
Lucae dissecting f.
Luc ethmoidal f.
Luc nasal-cutting f.
Luc septal f.
Luc septum-cutting f.
Luer curette f.
Luer hemorrhoidal f.
Luer rongeur f.
Luer-Whiting f.
Luer-Whiting rongeur f.
Luhr microfixation system plate-
  holding f.
Luikart f.
Luikart-Bill f.
Luikart-Kjelland obstetrical f.
Luikart-McLane obstetrical f.
Luikart-Simpson obstetrical f.
lung f.
lung-grasping f.
lung tissue f.
Lutz septal f.
Lynch cup-shaped curette f.
Lynch laryngeal f.
Lyon f.
MacCarty f.

MacGregor conjunctival f.
Machemer diamond-dust-coated
  foreign body f.
Machemer diamond-dusted f.
MacKenty tissue f.
MacQuigg-Mixter f.
Madden f.
Madden-Potts intestinal f.
Madden-Potts tissue f.
Magielski coagulating f.
Magielski-Heermann strut f.
Magielski tonsillar f.
Magielski tonsil-seizing f.
Magill catheter f.
Magill endotracheal f.
Maier dressing f.
Maier polyp f.
Maier sponge f.
Maier uterine f.
Mailler colon f.
Mailler cut-off f.
Mailler intestinal f.
Mailler rectal f.
Maingot hysterectomy f.
Malis angled bayonet f.
Malis bipolar coagulation f.
Malis bipolar cutting f.
Malis bipolar irrigating f.
Malis cup f.
Malis-Jensen bipolar f.
Malis-Jensen microbipolar f.
Malis jeweler's bipolar f.
Malis titanium microsurgical f.
malleus f.
Manche LASIK f.
Manhattan Eye & Ear suturing f.
Mann f.
Manning f.
Mansfield f.
Mantis retrograde f.
March-Barton f.
Marcuse f.
marginal chalazion f.
Markwalder rib f.
Marshik tonsillar f.
Marshik tonsil-seizing f.
Martin bipolar coagulation f.
Martin cartilage f.
Martin meniscal f.
Martin nasopharyngeal biopsy f.
Martin thumb f.
Martin tissue f.

F

NOTES

forceps *(continued)*

Martin uterine tenaculum f.
Maryan biopsy punch f.
Maryland f.
Masket f.
Masterson hysterectomy f.
Mastin goiter f.
Mastin muscle f.
Mathieu foreign body f.
Mathieu tongue f.
Mathieu urethral f.
matte black f.
Matthew f.
Maumenee capsular f.
Maumenee-Colibri corneal f.
Maumenee corneal f.
Maumenee cross-action capsular f.
Maumenee straight-action
  capsular f.
Maumenee Suregrip f.
Maumenee tissue f.
Max Fine tying f.
maxillary disimpaction f.
maxillary fracture f.
Maxum Carr-Locke angled f.
Maxum reusable endoscopic f.
Mayer f.
Mayfield aneurysm f.
Mayo bone-cutting f.
Mayo-Harrington f.
Mayo kidney pedicle f.
Mayo-Ochsner f.
Mayo-Robson gastrointestinal f.
Mayo-Russian gastrointestinal f.
Mayo tissue f.
Mayo ureter isolation f.
Mazzariello-Caprini stone f.
Mazzocco flexible lens f.
McCain TMJ f.
McCarthy-Alcock f.
McCarthy visual hemostatic f.
McClintock placental f.
McClintock uterine f.
McCollough tying f.
McCoy septal f.
McCoy septum-cutting f.
McCullough strabismus f.
McCullough suture-tying f.
McCullough suturing f.
McDonald lens-folding f.
McGannon lens f.
McGee-Paparella wire-crimping f.
McGee-Priest-Paparella f.
McGee-Priest wire-closure f.
McGee wire-closure f.
McGee wire-crimping f.
McGill f.
McGivney hemorrhoidal f.
McGravey tissue f.

McGregor conjunctival f.
McGuire marginal chalazion f.
McHenry tonsillar f.
McIndoe bone-cutting f.
McIndoe diathermy f.
McIndoe dissecting f.
McIndoe dressing f.
McIndoe rongeur f.
McIntosh suture-holding f.
McKay ear f.
McKenzie clip-applying f.
McKerman-Adson f.
McKerman-Potts f.
McKernan f.
McKernan-Adson f.
McKernan-Potts f.
McLane-Luikart obstetrical f.
McLane obstetrical f.
McLane pile f.
McLane-Tucker-Kjelland f.
McLane-Tucker-Luikart f.
McLane-Tucker obstetrical f.
McLean capsular f.
McLean muscle-recession f.
McLean ophthalmic f.
McLearie bone f.
McNealey-Glassman-Mixter f.
McNealy-Glassman-Babcock f.
McPherson angled f.
McPherson bent f.
McPherson-Castroviejo f.
McPherson corneal f.
McPherson irrigating f.
McPherson lens f.
McPherson microbipolar f.
McPherson microcorneal f.
McPherson microiris f.
McPherson microsuture f.
McPherson-Pierse microcorneal f.
McPherson-Pierse microsuturing f.
McPherson straight bipolar f.
McPherson suture-tying f.
McPherson tying iris f.
McQueen vitreous f.
McQuigg f.
McQuigg-Mixter bronchial f.
McWhorter tonsillar f.
Meacham-Scoville f.
meat f.
mechanical finger f.
Medicon-Jackson rectal f.
Medicon-Packer mosquito f.
Medicon wire-twister f.
Meeker deep-surgery f.
Meeker gallbladder f.
Meeker hemostatic f.
Meeker intestinal f.
meibomian expressor f.
membrane f.

membrane-puncturing f.
Mendel ligature f.
Mendez multi-purpose LASIK f.
Mengert membrane-puncturing f.
meniscal basket f.
Mentor-Maumenee Suregrip f.
Merlin stone f.
Mermoud nonpenetrating
  glaucoma f.
Merriam f.
Merz hysterectomy f.
Metico f.
Metzel-Wittmoser f.
Metzenbaum tonsillar f.
Metzenbaum-Tydings f.
MGH uterine vulsellum f.
Michel clip-applying f.
Michel clip-removing f.
Michel tissue f.
Michigan University intestinal f.
Micrins f.
microbipolar f.
microclip applying f.
microdissecting f.
micro-jewelers monopolar f.
microlaryngeal grasping f.
Micro-Line arterial f.
Micro-One dissecting f.
Microsnap hemostatic f.
microsurgical grasping f.
microsurgical tying f.
Microtek cupped f.
micro tissue f.
Micro-Two f.
microtying f.
microvascular clamp-applying f.
microvascular tying f.
Microvasive disposable alligator-
  shaped f.
Microvasive radial jaw biopsy f.
MIC Thermal Option biopsy f.
midcavity f.
middle ear f.
Mighty Bite Zimmon lateral biopsy
  cup f.
Mikulicz peritoneal f.
Mikulicz tonsillar f.
Miles punch biopsy f.
Milex f.
Miller articulating paper f.
Miller bayonet f.
Miller rectal f.

Millin capsular f.
Millin ligature-guiding f.
Millin prostatectomy f.
Millin T-shaped f.
Mill-Rose RiteBite biopsy f.
Mill-Rose SureBite biopsy f.
Mills tissue f.
Miltex Cushing bayonet f.
Mitchell-Diamond biopsy f.
Mixter arterial f.
Mixter artery f.
Mixter baby hemostatic f.
Mixter gallbladder f.
Mixter gallstone f.
Mixter-McQuigg f.
Mixter mosquito f.
Mixter-O'Shaughnessy dissecting f.
Mixter-O'Shaughnessy hemostatic f.
Mixter-Paul arterial f.
Mixter-Paul hemostatic f.
Mixter pediatric hemostatic f.
Mixter thoracic f.
Moberg f.
Moberg-Stille f.
modified Younge f.
Moehle corneal f.
Moersch bronchoscopic f.
Molt pedicle f.
Monod punch f.
monopolar f.
monopolar coagulating f.
monopolar diathermy f.
monopolar insulated f.
monopolar tissue f.
Montenovesi cranial f.
Moody fixation f.
Moolgaoker f.
Moore lens-inserting f.
Morgenstein blunt f.
Moritz-Schmidt laryngeal f.
Morris f.
Morson f.
Mosher ethmoid punch f.
mosquito hemostatic f.
Mount intervertebral disc f.
Mount-Mayfield aneurysmal f.
Mount-Olivecrona f.
mouse-tooth f.
Moynihan intestinal f.
Moynihan kidney pedicle f.
Moynihan-Navratil f.
Moynihan towel f.

F

NOTES

forceps *(continued)*
    MPC coagulation f.
    Muck tonsillar f.
    Mueller f.
    Mueller-Markham patent ductus f.
    Muir hemorrhoidal f.
    Muldoon meibomian f.
    Multibite multiple sample biopsy f.
    Mundie placental f.
    Murless head extractor f.
    Murphy-Péan hemostatic f.
    Murphy tonsillar f.
    Murray f.
    muscle f.
    Museholdt nasal-dressing f.
    Museux-Collins uterine vulsellum f.
    Museux tenaculum f.
    Museux uterine f.
    Museux vulsellum f.
    Musial tissue f.
    Mustarde f.
    Myerson bronchial f.
    Myerson laryngeal f.
    Myles hemorrhoidal f.
    Myles nasal f.
    Nadler bipolar coaptation f.
    Naegele obstetrical f.
    nail-cutting f.
    nail-extracting f.
    nail-pulling f.
    Nakao Ejector biopsy f.
    nasal alligator f.
    nasal cutting f.
    nasal dressing f.
    nasal hump-cutting f.
    nasal packing f.
    nasal polyp f.
    nasal septal f.
    nasopharyngeal biopsy f.
    Natvig wire-twister f.
    needle-holder f.
    Negus-Green f.
    Negus tonsillar f.
    Nelson lung f.
    Nelson-Martin f.
    Nelson tissue f.
    nephrolithotomy f.
    Neubauer foreign body f.
    Neubauer vitreous micro-extractor f.
    Neubuser tube-seizing f.
    neurosurgical dressing f.
    neurosurgical ligature f.
    neurosurgical suction f.
    neurosurgical tissue f.
    neurovascular f.
    Neuwirth-Palmer f.
    Neville-Barnes f.
    Nevins dressing f.
    Nevins tissue f.

    Nevyas lens f.
    New biopsy f.
    Newman uterine tenaculum f.
    New Orleans Eye & Ear fixation f.
    New tissue f.
    New York Eye and Ear Hospital fixation f.
    Nicola f.
    Niedner dissecting f.
    NIH mitral valve f.
    Niro bone-cutting f.
    Niro wire-twister f.
    Niro wire-twisting f.
    Nisbet eye f.
    Nisbet fixation f.
    Nissen cystic f.
    Nissen gall duct f.
    Nissen hassux f.
    Noble iris f.
    noncrushing common duct f.
    noncrushing intestinal f.
    noncrushing pickup f.
    noncrushing tissue-holding f.
    nonfenestrated f.
    nonmagnetic dressing f.
    nonmagnetic tissue f.
    nonperforating towel f.
    nonslipping f.
    nontoothed f.
    nontraumatizing visceral f.
    Nordan-Colibri f.
    Nordan tying f.
    Norris sponge f.
    Norwood f.
    Noto dressing f.
    Noto ovum f.
    Noto polypus f.
    Noto sponge f.
    Novak fixation f.
    Noyes ear f.
    Noyes nasal f.
    Noyes nasal-dressing f.
    Nugent fixation f.
    Nugent rectus f.
    Nugent superior rectus f.
    Nugent utility f.
    Nugowski f.
    Nussbaum intestinal f.
    Nyhus-Potts intestinal f.
    Nystroem tumor f.
    Oberhill obstetrical f.
    O'Brien-Elschnig f.
    O'Brien fixation f.
    O'Brien tissue f.
    obstetrical f.
    occluding f.
    Ochsner cartilage f.
    Ochsner-Dixon arterial f.

Ochsner hemostatic f.
Ochsner tissue f.
Ockerblad f.
O'Connor biopsy f.
O'Connor-Elschnig fixation f.
O'Connor eye f.
O'Connor grasping f.
O'Connor iris f.
O'Connor lid f.
O'Connor sponge f.
O'Dell spicule f.
odontoid peg-grasping f.
O'Gawa-Castroviejo tying f.
O'Gawa suture f.
O'Gawa suture-fixation f.
O'Gawa tying f.
Ogura cartilage f.
Ogura tissue f.
O'Hanlon f.
O'Hara f.
Oldberg intervertebral disc f.
Oldberg pituitary rongeur f.
Olivecrona aneurysm f.
Olivecrona clip-applying/removing f.
Olivecrona rongeur f.
Olivecrona-Toennis clip-applying f.
Olsen bayonet monopolar f.
Olympus alligator-jaw endoscopic f.
Olympus basket-type endoscopic f.
Olympus Endo-Therapy disposable
  biopsy f.
Olympus FBK-series f.
Olympus FB-series biopsy f.
Olympus FG-series f.
Olympus FS-K-series endoscopic
  suture-cutting f.
Olympus FS-series endoscopic
  suture-cutting f.
Olympus grasping rat-tooth f.
Olympus hot biopsy f.
Olympus magnetic extractor f.
Olympus pelican-type endoscopic f.
Olympus rat-tooth endoscopic f.
Olympus reusable oval cup f.
Olympus shark-tooth endoscopic f.
Olympus W-shaped endoscopic f.
Ombrédanne f.
optical biopsy f.
oral f.
Orr gall duct f.
orthopaedic f.
O'Shaughnessy artery f.

Osher bipolar coaptation f.
Osher capsular f.
Osher conjunctival f.
Osher foreign body f.
Osher haptic f.
Osher superior rectus f.
ossicle-holding f.
Ossoff-Karlan laser f.
ostrum punch f.
otologic cup f.
Otto tissue f.
Oughterson f.
outlet f.
oval cup f.
ovary f.
Overholt clip-applying f.
Overholt dissecting f.
Overholt-Geissendörfer arterial f.
Overholt-Mixter dissecting f.
Overstreet polyp f.
ovum f.
Pace-Potts f.
Packer mosquito f.
packing f.
Page tonsillar f.
Palmer biopsy f.
Palmer cutting f.
Palmer-Drapier f.
Palmer grasping f.
Palmer ovarian biopsy f.
Pang biopsy f.
Pang nasopharyngeal f.
Panje-Shagets tracheoesophageal
  fistula f.
papilloma f.
parametrium f.
Parker fixation f.
Parker-Kerr f.
Park lens implantation f.
partial-occlusion f.
Passarelli one-pass capsulorrhexis f.
passing f.
patent ductus f.
Paterson brain clip f.
Paterson laryngeal f.
Paton anterior chamber lens
  implant f.
Paton capsular f.
Paton corneal f.
Paton corneal transplant f.
Paton extra-delicate f.
Paton suturing f.

F

NOTES

forceps *(continued)*

Paton tying/stitch removal f.
Patterson bronchoscopic f.
Patterson specimen f.
Paufique suturing f.
Paulson infertility microtissue f.
Paulson infertility microtying f.
Pauwels fracture f.
Pavlo-Colibri corneal f.
Payne-Ochsner arterial f.
Payne-Péan arterial f.
Payne-Rankin arterial f.
Payr pylorus f.
Péan arterial f.
Péan hemostatic f.
Péan hyserectomy f.
Péan intestinal f.
Péan sponge f.
peanut-fenestrated f.
peanut grasping f.
peanut sponge-holding f.
peapod intervertebral disc f.
pediatric f.
pedicle f.
Peet mosquito f.
Peet splinter f.
pelican biopsy f.
Pelkmann foreign body f.
Pelkmann gallstone f.
Pelkmann sponge f.
Pelkmann uterine f.
pelvic reduction f.
pelvic tissue f.
Pemberton f.
Penfield watchmaker suture f.
Penn-Anderson scleral fixation f.
Pennington hemorrhoidal f.
Pennington hemostatic f.
Pennington tissue f.
Pennington tissue-grasping f.
Percy intestinal f.
Percy tissue f.
Percy-Wolfson gallbladder f.
Perdue tonsillar hemostat f.
Perez-Castro f.
peripheral blood vessel f.
peripheral iridectomy f.
peripheral vascular f.
peritoneal f.
Perman cartilage f.
Perone LASIK flap f.
Perritt fixation f.
Perritt lens f.
Perry f.
Peter-Bishop f.
Peters tissue f.
Peyman-Green vitreous f.
Peyman intraocular f.
Peyman vitreous-grasping f.

Pfau polyp f.
Pfister-Schwartz basket f.
phalangeal f.
Phaneuf arterial f.
Phaneuf hysterectomy f.
Phaneuf peritoneal f.
Phaneuf uterine artery f.
Phaneuf vaginal f.
Phillips fixation f.
Phillips swan neck f.
phimosis f.
Phipps f.
phrenicectomy f.
Pierse-Colibri corneal f.
Pierse corneal f.
Pierse fixation f.
Pierse-Hoskins f.
Pierse tip f.
Pigott f.
Pike jawed f.
pillar f.
pillar-grasping f.
Pilling f.
Pilling-Liston bone utility f.
Pilling Weck Y-stent f.
pin-bending f.
pinch f.
pin-seating f.
Piper obstetrical f.
Piranha uteroscopic biopsy f.
Pischel micropin f.
Pistofidis cervical biopsy f.
Pitanguy f.
Pitha foreign body f.
Pitha urethral f.
pituitary f.
placement f.
placenta previa f.
plain f.
plastic f.
plate-holding f.
platform f.
pleurectomy f.
Pley extracapsular f.
Plondke uterine f.
point f.
Polack corneal fixation f.
Polaris reusable f.
Polk placental f.
Polk sponge f.
Pollock double corneal f.
polyp f.
polypus f.
Poppen intervertebral disc f.
Porter duodenal f.
posterior f.
posterior segment f.
postmortem f.
postnasal sponge f.

Potta coarctation f.
Potter sponge f.
Potter tonsillar f.
Potts bronchial f.
Potts bulldog f.
Potts coarctation f.
Potts fixation f.
Potts intestinal f.
Potts-Nevins dressing f.
Potts patent ductus f.
Potts-Smith bipolar f.
Potts-Smith dressing f.
Potts-Smith monopolar f.
Potts-Smith thumb f.
Potts-Smith tissue f.
Poutasse renal artery f.
Pozzi tenaculum f.
Pratt hemostatic f.
Pratt-Smith hemostatic f.
Pratt tissue f.
Pratt T-shaped hemostatic f.
Pratt vulsellum f.
Precisor Direct Bite biopsy f.
Prentiss f.
prepuce f.
Presbyterian Hospital f.
pressure f.
Preston ligamentum flavum f.
Price-Thomas bronchial f.
Primbs suturing f.
Prince advancement f.
Prince muscle f.
Prince trachoma f.
proctological grasping f.
proctological polyp f.
Proctor phrenectomy f.
Proctor phrenicectomy f.
3-prong grasping f.
prostatectomy f.
prostatic lobe f.
protological biopsy f.
Proud adenoidectomy f.
Providence Hospital artery f.
ptosis f.
pulmonary arterial f.
pulmonary vessel f.
punch f.
Puntenney f.
Puntenney tying f.
Puntowicz arterial f.
pupil spreader f.
QSA dressing f.

quadripolar cutting f.
Quervain cranial f.
Quevedo conjunctival f.
Quevedo suturing f.
Quinones-Neubüser uterine-grasping f.
Quinones uterine-grasping f.
Quire foreign body f.
Quire mechanical finger f.
Raaf f.
Raaf-Oldberg intervertebral disc f.
Radial Jaw bladder biopsy f.
Radial Jaw hot biopsy f.
Raimondi scalp hemostatic f.
Ralks ear f.
Ralks splinter f.
Ralks wire-cutting f.
Rampley sponge f.
Rand f.
Randall kidney stone f.
Randall stone f.
Raney rongeur f.
Raney scalp clip-applying f.
Raney straight coagulating f.
Rankin arterial f.
Rankin-Crile f.
Rankin hemostatic f.
Rankow f.
Rapp f.
Rappazzo intraocular foreign body f.
Ratliff-Blake gallstone f.
Ratliff-Mayo gallstone f.
rat-tooth f.
Ray kidney stone f.
reach-and-pin f.
Read f.
recession f.
rectal f.
Reese advancement f.
Reese muscle f.
Reich-Nechtow f.
Reich-Nechtow hypogastric artery f.
Reill f.
Reiner-Knight ethmoid-cutting f.
Reinhoff arterial f.
Reisinger lens-extracting f.
renal artery f.
Resano sigmoid f.
resection intestinal f.
retrieval f.
Reul coronary f.

F

NOTES

forceps *(continued)*
reverse-action hypophysectomy f.
Rezek f.
Rhein capsulorrhexis cystotome f.
Rhoton-Adson dressing f.
Rhoton-Adson tissue f.
Rhoton bipolar f.
Rhoton cup f.
Rhoton-Cushing tissue f.
Rhoton dural f.
Rhoton grasping f.
Rhoton microcup f.
Rhoton microdissecting f.
Rhoton microtying f.
Rhoton microvascular f.
Rhoton ring tumor f.
Rhoton-Tew bipolar f.
Rhoton tissue f.
Rhoton transsphenoidal bipolar f.
Rhoton tying f.
Riba-Valeira f.
Rica-Adson f.
Rica clip-applying f.
Rica hemostatic f.
Rich f.
Richards f.
Richards-Andrews f.
Richards tonsillar f.
Riches diathermy f.
Riches diathermy artery f.
Richmond f.
Richter f.
Richter-Heath clip-removing f.
ridge f.
Ridley f.
rigid biopsy f.
ring f.
ringed formed f.
Ringenberg stapedectomy f.
ring rotation f.
ring-tip f.
Ripstein arterial f.
Ripstein tissue f.
Ritch-Krupin-Denver eye valve
  insertion f.
RiteBite biopsy f.
Ritter f.
Rizzuti double-prong f.
Rizzuti fixation f.
Rizzuti-Furness cornea-holding f.
Rizzuti scleral f.
Rizzuti superior rectus f.
Rizzuti-Verhoeff f.
Robb tonsillar f.
Roberts artery f.
Roberts bronchial f.
Roberts hemostatic f.
Robertson tonsillar f.
Roberts-Singley dressing f.

Roberts-Singley thumb f.
Robson intestinal f.
Rochester-Carmalt hemostatic
  arterial f.
Rochester-Carmalt hysterectomy f.
Rochester-Davis f.
Rochester-Ewald tissue f.
Rochester gallstone f.
Rochester-Harrington f.
Rochester-Mixter arterial f.
Rochester-Mixter gall duct f.
Rochester-Mueller f.
Rochester-Ochsner f.
Rochester oral tissue f.
Rochester-Péan f.
Rochester-Péan hysterectomy f.
Rochester-Rankin arterial f.
Rochester Russian tissue f.
Rochester tissue f.
Rockey f.
Roeder towel f.
Roeltsch f.
Roger vascular-toothed
  hysterectomy f.
Rolf jeweler's f.
Rolf utility f.
roller f.
rongeur f.
Ronis cutting f.
Rose disimpaction f.
rotating f.
Roubaix f.
round punch f.
Rovenstine catheter-introducing f.
Rowe bone-drilling f.
Rowe disimpaction f.
Rowe-Harrison bone-holding f.
Rowe-Killey f.
Rowe maxillary disimpaction f.
Rowe modified-Harrison f.
Rowland double-action f.
Rowland hump f.
Royce f.
rubber-shod f.
Rudd Clinic hemorrhoidal f.
Rugby deep-surgery f.
Rugelski arterial f.
Rumel dissecting f.
Rumel lobectomy f.
Rumel thoracic f.
Ruskin bone-cutting f.
Ruskin-Liston bone-cutting f.
Ruskin rongeur f.
Ruskin-Rowland bone-cutting f.
Russell f.
Russell-Davis f.
Russell hysterectomy f.
Russian Péan f.
Russian thumb f.

Russian tissue f.
Russ tumor f.
Russ vascular f.
Rycroft tying f.
Sachs tissue f.
Saenger ovum f.
Saenger placental f.
Sajou laryngeal f.
Sam Roberts bronchial biopsy f.
Samuels Hemoclip-applying f.
Sanders-Castroviejo suturing f.
Sanders vasectomy f.
Sandt suture f.
Sandt utility f.
Saqalain dressing f.
Sarot arterial f.
Sarot intrathoracic f.
Sarot pleurectomy f.
Satellight needle holder f.
Satinsky f.
Satterlee advancement f.
Satterlee muscle f.
Sauerbruch pickup f.
Sauerbruch rib f.
Sauer outer ring f.
Sauer suture f.
Sawtell arterial f.
Sawtell-Davis f.
Sawtell gallbladder f.
Sawtell tonsillar f.
scalp f.
scalp clip-applying f.
scalp flap f.
Scanlan laparoscopic f.
Scanzoni f.
Schaaf foreign body f.
Schaefer fixation f.
Schanzioni craniotomy f.
Scharff bipolar f.
Schatz utility f.
Scheer crimper f.
Scheie-Graefe fixation f.
Scheinmann esophagoscopy f.
Scheinmann laryngeal f.
Schepens f.
Schick f.
Schindler peritoneal f.
Schlesinger cervical punch f.
Schlesinger intervertebral disc f.
Schlesinger meniscus-grasping f.
Schlesinger rongeur f.
Schnidt gall duct f.

Schnidt-Rumpler f.
Schnidt thoracic f.
Schnidt tonsillar f.
Schoenberg intestinal f.
Schoenberg uterine f.
Scholten endomyocardial biopsy f.
Schroeder-Braun uterine f.
Schroeder tissue f.
Schroeder uterine vulsellum f.
Schroeder-Van Doren tenaculum f.
Schroeder vulsellum f.
Schubert cervical biopsy f.
Schubert uterine biopsy f.
Schumacher biopsy f.
Schutz f.
Schwartz clip-applying f.
Schwartz multipurpose f.
Schwartz obstetrical f.
Schwartz temporary vessel clamp-applying f.
Schweigger capsular f.
Schweigger extracapsular f.
Schweizer cervix-holding f.
Schweizer uterine f.
scissors f.
scleral twist-grip f.
sclerectomy punch f.
Scobee-Allis f.
Scott lens-insertion f.
Scoville brain f.
Scoville clip-applying f.
Scoville-Greenwood bipolar f.
Scoville-Hurteau f.
screw-holding f.
Scudder intestinal f.
Scuderi bipolar coagulating f.
Searcy capsular f.
Segond hysterectomy f.
Segond-Landau hysterectomy f.
Segond tumor f.
Seiffert esophagoscopy f.
Seiffert laryngeal f.
Seitzinger tripolar cutting f.
seizing f.
Seletz foramen-plugging f.
self-opening f.
self-retaining bone holding f.
Selman lung tissue f.
Selman nonslip tissue f.
Selman peripheral blood vessel f.
Selman vessel f.
Selverstone embolus f.

F

NOTES

forceps (*continued*)

Selverstone intervertebral disc f.
Selverstone rongeur f.
Semb bone-cutting f.
Semb bone-holding f.
Semb dissecting f.
Semb-Ghazi dissecting f.
Semb ligature f.
Semb ligature-carrying f.
Semb rib-holding f.
Semb rongeur f.
Semken bipolar f.
Semken dressing f.
Semken infant f.
Semken microbipolar
  neurosurgical f.
Semken thumb f.
Semken tissue f.
Semmes dural f.
Senning cardiovascular f.
Senturia f.
septal bone f.
septal compression f.
septal ridge f.
septum-cutting f.
septum-straightening f.
sequestrum f.
serrated conjunctival f.
serrefine f.
Sewall brain clip-applying f.
Seyfert f.
Shaaf eye f.
Shaaf foreign body f.
Shallcross cystic duct f.
Shallcross-Dean gall duct f.
Shallcross gallbladder f.
Shallcross nasal f.
Shapshay-Healy laryngeal
  alligator f.
Shark disposable biopsy f.
shark-tooth f.
sharp-pointed f.
Shea f.
Shearer chicken-bill f.
Sheehy ossicle-holding f.
Sheets lens f.
Sheets-McPherson angled f.
Sheets-McPherson tying f.
Sheinmann laryngeal f.
Shepard bipolar f.
Shepard curved intraocular lens f.
Shepard lens f.
Shepard-Reinstein intraocular lens f.
Shepard tying f.
Shields f.
Shimano stainless steel cutting f.
Shoemaker intraocular lens f.
short tooth f.
Shuppe biting f.

Shuster suture f.
Shuster tonsillar f.
Shutt Aggressor f.
Shutt alligator f.
Shutt basket f.
Shutt B-scoop f.
Shutt grasping f.
Shutt Mantis retrograde f.
Shutt Mini-Aggressor f.
Shutt retrograde f.
Shutt shovel-nosed f.
Shutt suction f.
side-biting Stammberger punch f.
side-curved f.
side-cutting basket f.
side-grasping f.
side-lip f.
Siegler biopsy f.
Silcock dissection f.
silicone rod and sleeve f.
silicone sponge f.
Silver endaural f.
Simcoe implantation f.
Simcoe lens-inserting f.
Simcoe nucleus f.
Simcoe posterior chamber f.
Simcoe superior rectus f.
Simons stone-removing f.
Simpson f.
Simpson-Braun obstetrical f.
Simpson-Luikart obstetrical f.
Simpson obstetrical f.
Sims-Maier dressing f.
single-tooth f.
Singley intestinal f.
Singley tissue f.
Singley-Tuttle dressing f.
Singley-Tuttle intestinal f.
Singley-Tuttle tissue f.
Sinskey intraocular lens f.
Sinskey-McPherson f.
Sinskey microtying f.
Sinskey tying f.
Sinskey-Wilson foreign body f.
Sisson f.
sister-hook f.
Skeleton fine f.
Skene tenaculum f.
Skene uterine f.
Skene vulsellum f.
Skillern phimosis f.
Skillman arterial f.
Skillman mosquito f.
Skillman prepuce f.
sleeve-spreading f.
sliding capsular f.
Sluder-Ballenger tonsillar punch f.
Smellie obstetrical f.
Smith grasping f.

Smith-Leiske cross-action intraocular
  lens f.
Smith lion-jaw f.
Smith & Nephew Richards
  bipolar f.
Smith obstetrical f.
Smith-Petersen f.
Smithwick clip-applying f.
Smithwick-Hartmann f.
smooth-tipped jeweler's f.
smooth-tooth f.
Snellen entropion f.
Snyder corneal spring f.
Somers uterine f.
Songer tonsillar f.
Soonawalla vasectomy f.
Sopher ovum f.
Sourdille f.
Spaleck f.
spatula f.
specimen f.
speculum f.
Spence-Adson f.
Spencer biopsy f.
Spencer chalazion f.
Spence rongeur f.
Spencer-Wells arterial f.
Spencer-Wells chalazion f.
Spero meibomian f.
Spetzler f.
sphenoidal punch f.
spicule f.
spinal-perforating f.
spiral f.
splinter f.
splitting f.
sponge f.
sponge-holding f.
spoon f.
spoon-shaped f.
spreading f.
spring-handled f.
Spurling intervertebral disc f.
Spurling-Kerrison rongeur f.
Spurling tissue f.
square specimen f.
squeeze-handle f.
stainless steel jaw f.
Stammberger side-biting punch f.
Stamm bone-cutting f.
standard arterial f.
stapedectomy f.

stapes f.
staple f.
Stark vulsellum f.
Starr fixation f.
Staude-Moore uterine tenaculum f.
Staude tenaculum f.
Stavis fixation f.
St. Clair f.
St. Clair-Thompson adenoidal f.
St. Clair-Thompson peritonsillar
  abscess f.
Steinmann intestinal f.
Steinmann tendon f.
Stephens soft IOL-inserting f.
sterilizer f.
sterilizing f.
sternal punch f.
Stern-Castroviejo locking f.
Stern-Castroviejo suturing f.
Stevens fixation f.
Stevens iris f.
Stevenson alligator f.
Stevenson cupped-jaw f.
Stevenson grasping f.
Stevenson microsurgical f.
Stieglitz splinter f.
Stille-Adson f.
Stille-Babcock f.
Stille-Barraya intestinal f.
Stille-Barraya vascular f.
Stille-Björk f.
Stille-Crafoord f.
Stille-Crile f.
Stille gallstone f.
Stille-Halsted f.
Stille-Horsley bone-cutting f.
Stille-Horsley rib f.
Stille kidney f.
Stille-Liston bone f.
Stille-Liston rib-cutting f.
Stille-Luer rongeur f.
Stille rongeur f.
Stille-Russian f.
Stille tissue f.
Stille-Waugh f.
Stiwer biopsy f.
Stiwer bone-holding f.
Stiwer dressing f.
Stiwer sponge f.
Stiwer tissue f.
S&T Lalonde hook f.
St. Martin eye f.

F

NOTES

forceps *(continued)*
    St. Martin suturing f.
    Stolte capsulorrhexis f.
    stone f.
    Stone clamp-applying f.
    stone-crushing f.
    stone-extraction f.
    stone-grasping f.
    Stone intestinal f.
    Stoneman f.
    Stone tissue f.
    Storey gall duct f.
    Storey-Hillar dissecting f.
    Storey thoracic f.
    Storz biopsy f.
    Storz-Bonn suturing f.
    Storz bronchoscopic f.
    Storz capsular f.
    Storz ciliary f.
    Storz corneal f.
    Storz curved f.
    Storz cystoscopic f.
    Storz esophagoscopic f.
    Storz grasping biopsy f.
    Storz kidney stone f.
    Storz miniature f.
    Storz nasopharyngeal biopsy f.
    Storz optical biopsy f.
    Storz sinus biopsy f.
    Storz stone-crushing f.
    Storz stone-extraction f.
    Storz-Utrata f.
    strabismus f.
    straight coagulating f.
    straight-end cup f.
    straight knot-tying f.
    straight line bayonet f.
    straight Maryland f.
    straight microbipolar f.
    straight micromonopolar f.
    straight single tenaculum f.
    straight-tip bipolar f.
    straight tying f.
    Strassburger tissue f.
    Strassmann uterine f.
    Stratte f.
    2-stream irrigating f.
    Streli f.
    Strelinger catheter-introducing f.
    Stringer catheter-introducing f.
    Stringer newborn throat f.
    Strow corneal f.
    Struempel ear alligator f.
    Struempel ear punch f.
    Struempel-Voss ethmoidal f.
    Struempel-Voss nasal f.
    Strully dressing f.
    Strully tissue f.
    strut f.

    Struyken ear f.
    Struyken nasal f.
    Struyken nasal-cutting f.
    Struyken turbinate f.
    St. Vincent tube-occluding f.
    Styles f.
    subglottic f.
    suction f.
    Suker iris f.
    superior rectus f.
    SureBite biopsy f.
    Sutherland-Grieshaber f.
    Sutherland rotatable intraocular f.
    Sutherland vitreous f.
    suture clip f.
    suture tag f.
    suture-tying platform f.
    suturing f.
    Swan-Brown arterial f.
    Sweet clip-applying f.
    Sweet dissecting f.
    Sweet ligature f.
    Syark vulsellum f.
    synovium biopsy f.
    Szuler vascular f.
    Szultz corneal f.
    tack-and-pin f.
    Takahashi cutting f.
    Takahashi ethmoidal f.
    Takahashi iris retractor f.
    Takahashi nasal f.
    Takahashi neurosurgical f.
    Take-apart grasping f.
    tampon f.
    Tamsco f.
    tangential f.
    tangential occlusion f.
    Tarnier axis-traction f.
    Tarnier obstetrical f.
    Taylor-Cushing dressing f.
    Taylor dissecting f.
    Taylor tissue f.
    Teale tenaculum f.
    Teale vulsellum uterine f.
    Tekno f.
    tenaculum f.
    tenaculum-reducing f.
    tendon f.
    tendon-holding f.
    tendon-passing f.
    tendon-pulling f.
    tendon-retrieving f.
    tendon-seizing f.
    Tennant-Colibri corneal f.
    Tennant intraocular lens f.
    Tennant lens f.
    Tennant-Maumenee f.
    Tennant titanium suturing f.
    Tennant-Troutman superior rectus f.

Tennant tying f.
Tenzel bipolar f.
Terson capsular f.
Terson extracapsular f.
Thackray dental f.
Therma Jaw hot urologic f.
The Shark disposable biopsy f.
Theurig sterilizer f.
Thomas fixation f.
Thomas shot compression f.
Thompson hip prosthesis f.
Thoms-Allis intestinal f.
Thoms-Allis tissue f.
Thoms-Allis vulsellum f.
Thoms-Gaylor uterine biopsy f.
thoracic f.
thoracic artery f.
thoracic tissue f.
Thorek gallbladder f.
Thorek-Mixter gallbladder f.
Thornton episcleral f.
Thornton fixation f.
Thornton intraocular f.
Thorpe-Castroviejo corneal f.
Thorpe-Castroviejo fixation f.
Thorpe conjunctival f.
Thorpe corneal f.
Thorpe corneoscleral f.
Thorpe foreign body f.
Thrasher intraocular f.
Thrasher lens implant f.
throat f.
thumb-dressing f.
thumb tissue f.
Thurston-Holland fragment f.
thyroid f.
Tickner tissue f.
Tiemann bullet f.
Tiger Shark f.
Tilley dressing f.
Tilley-Henckel f.
Tischler cervical biopsy punch f.
Tischler-Morgan uterine biopsy f.
tissue f.
tissue-grasping f.
tissue-holding f.
tissue-spreading f.
titanium microsurgical bipolar f.
Tivnen tonsillar f.
Tobey f.
Tobold-Fauvel grasping f.
Tobold laryngeal f.

Toennis-Adson f.
Toennis tumor-grasping f.
Tomac f.
tongue f.
tonsillar f.
tonsillar abscess f.
tonsillar artery f.
tonsillar grasping f.
tonsillar punch f.
tonsil-seizing f.
Tooke corneal f.
Toomey f.
2-toothed f.
toothed thumb f.
toothed tissue f.
tooth-extracting f.
toothless f.
Torchia capsular f.
Torchia-Colibri f.
Torchia lens implantation f.
Torchia microbipolar f.
Torchia tissue f.
Torchia tying f.
Torres cross-action f.
torsion f.
towel f.
Tower muscle f.
Townley tissue f.
tracheal dilating f.
trachoma f.
traction f.
transfer f.
transsphenoidal bipolar f.
traumatic grasping f.
triangular f.
triangular jaw f.
Tricep hooked-prong grasping f.
tripod grasping f.
Troeltsch dressing f.
Troeltsch ear f.
Trotter f.
Trousseau dilating f.
Troutman-Barraquer-Colibri f.
Troutman-Barraquer corneal
 fixation f.
Troutman-Barraquer iris f.
Troutman corneal f.
Troutman-Llobera fixation f.
Troutman-Llobera-Flieringa f.
Troutman microsurgery f.
Troutman superior rectus f.
Troutman tying f.

F

NOTES

forceps *(continued)*
TruLine f.
Trush grasping f.
Trylon hemostatic f.
tube-occluding f.
Tubinger gall stone f.
tubing introducer f.
tubular f.
Tucker bead f.
Tucker hallux f.
Tucker-McLane axis-traction f.
Tucker-McLane obstetrical f.
Tucker reach-and-pin f.
Tucker staple f.
Tudor-Edwards bone-cutting f.
Tuffier arterial f.
tumor f.
tumor-grasping f.
turbinate f.
Turnbull adhesion f.
Turner-Babcock tissue f.
Turner-Warwick-Adson f.
Turner-Warwick stone f.
Turrell biopsy f.
Turrell specimen f.
Turrell-Wittner rectal biopsy f.
Tuttle dressing f.
Tuttle obstetrical f.
Tuttle-Singley thoracic f.
Tuttle thoracic thumb f.
Tuttle tissue f.
Twisk f.
Tydings-Lakeside tonsillar f.
Tydings tonsil-seizing f.
tying f.
tympanoplasty f.
Tyrrell foreign body f.
Ullrich-Aesculap f.
Ullrich bone-holding f.
Ullrich dressing f.
Ullrich-St. Gallen f.
Ulrich bone-holding f.
Ultrata capsulorrhexis f.
Universal f.
University of Kansas corneal f.
University of Michigan Mixter
  thoracic f.
upbiting f.
upbiting bean f.
upbiting cup f.
upcupped f.
upcurved basket f.
Uppsala gall duct f.
upturned f.
upward-bent f.
Urbantschitsch nasal f.
ureteral stone f.
urethral f.
U-shaped f.

uterine artery f.
uterine biopsy punch f.
uterine-dressing f.
uterine-elevating f.
uterine-grasping f.
uterine-holding f.
uterine-manipulating f.
uterine-packing f.
uterine polyp f.
uterine specimen f.
uterine tenaculum f.
uterine vulsellum f.
utility f.
Utrata capsulorrhexis f.
vaginal hysterectomy f.
Valin f.
Van Buren bone-holding f.
Van Buren sequestrum f.
Vanderbilt arterial f.
Vanderbilt deep-vessel f.
Vanderbilt University hemostatic f.
Vanderbilt University vessel f.
Vander Pool sterilizer f.
Van Doren uterine biopsy punch f.
Vannas fixation f.
Van Ruben f.
Van Struyken nasal f.
Vantage tube-occluding f.
Vantec grasping f.
Varco f.
Varco gallbladder f.
vascular tissue f.
vasectomy f.
vas isolation f.
Vaughn sterilizer f.
vectis cesarean f.
vena caval f.
Verbrugge bone-holding f.
Verhoeff capsular f.
Verhoeff cataract f.
vertical f.
vessel f.
Vick-Blanchard hemorrhoidal f.
Vickerall round ringed f.
Vickers ring-tip f.
Victor-Bonney f.
Vigger-5 eye f.
Virtus splinter f.
viscera-holding f.
visceral f.
vise f.
Vital-Adson tissue f.
Vital-Babcock tissue f.
Vital-Cushing tissue f.
Vital-Duval intestinal f.
Vital-Evans pelvic tissue f.
Vital general tissue f.
Vital intestinal f.
Vital lung-grasping f.

Vital needle holder f.
Vital-Potts-Smith f.
Vital-Wangensteen tissue f.
vitreous-grasping f.
V. Mueller biopsy f.
V. Mueller bone-cutting f.
V. Mueller laser Allis f.
V. Mueller laser Backhaus towel f.
V. Mueller laser Crile micro-
arterial f.
V. Mueller laser Rhoton
microtying f.
V. Mueller laser Singley tissue f.
V. Mueller nonperforating towel f.
V. Mueller tying f.
V. Mueller-Vital laser Babcock f.
V. Mueller-Vital laser Potts-
Smith f.
Vogler hysterectomy f.
Vogt toothed capsular f.
vomer septal f.
von Graefe fixation f.
von Graefe iris f.
von Graefe tissue f.
Von Mandach capsule fragment f.
Von Mandach clot f.
von Petz f.
Voris-Oldberg intervertebral disc f.
Vorse tube-occluding f.
Vorse-Webster f.
VPI-Ambrose resectoscope f.
vulsellum f.
Wachenfeldt clip-applying f.
Wachenfeldt suture clip f.
Wadsworth lid f.
Wainstock eye suturing f.
Waldeau fixation f.
Waldenstrom laryngeal f.
Waldeyer f.
walker f.
Wallace cesarean f.
Walsham nasal septal f.
Walsham septum-straightening f.
Walsh tissue f.
Walter splinter f.
Walther tissue f.
Walton-Allis tissue f.
Walton-Liston f.
Walton meniscal f.
Walton-Schubert uterine biopsy f.
Walzl hysterectomy f.
Wangensteen intestinal f.

Wangensteen tissue f.
Warthen f.
watchmaker f.
Watson duckbill f.
Watson tonsil-seizing f.
Watson-Williams ethmoid-biting f.
Watson-Williams nasal polyp f.
Watzke f.
Waugh-Brophy f.
Waugh dissecting diathermy f.
Waugh dressing f.
Waugh tissue f.
wave-tooth f.
Weaver chalazion f.
Weck-Harms f.
Weck hysterectomy f.
Weck rectal biopsy f.
Weck towel f.
Weck uterine biopsy f.
Weeks eye f.
Weiger-Zollner f.
Weil-Blakesley ear f.
Weil-Blakesley ethmoidal f.
Weil ethmoidal f.
Weiner uterine biopsy f.
Weingartner ear f.
Weis chalazion f.
Weisman f.
Weiss f.
Welch Allyn anal biopsy f.
Weller cartilage f.
Weller meniscal f.
Wells f.
Welsh ophthalmic f.
Welsh pupil-spreader f.
Wertheim-Cullen compression f.
Wertheim-Cullen hysterectomy f.
Wertheim-Cullen kidney pedicle f.
Wertheim hysterectomy f.
Wertheim-Navratil f.
Wertheim uterine f.
Wertheim vaginal f.
Westermark-Stille f.
Westermark uterine dressing f.
Westmacott dressing f.
West nasal dressing f.
Westphal gall duct f.
Westphal hemostatic f.
Wheeler plaque f.
Wheeler vessel f.
White-Lillie tonsillar f.
White-Oslay prostatic f.

F

NOTES

forceps *(continued)*

White-Smith f.
White tonsillar f.
Whitney superior rectus f.
Wickman uterine f.
Wiener hysterectomy f.
Wies chalazion f.
Wiet otologic cup f.
Wikström arterial f.
Wilde-Blakesley ethmoidal f.
Wilde ear f.
Wilde ethmoidal f.
Wilde laminectomy f.
Wilde nasal-cutting f.
Wilde nasal-dressing f.
Wilder dilating f.
Wilde septal f.
Wilde-Troeltsch f.
Wilkerson intraocular lens-insertion f.
Willauer intrathoracic f.
Willett placental f.
Willett placenta previa f.
Willett scalp flap f.
Williamsburg f.
Williams discectomy f.
Williams gastrointestinal f.
Williams intestinal f.
Williams splinter f.
Williams tissue f.
Williams uterine f.
Williams vessel-holding f.
Wills Eye Hospital ophthalmic f.
Wilmer iris f.
Wilson-Cook bronchoscope biopsy f.
Wilson-Cook colonoscopy biopsy f.
Wilson-Cook gastroscopy biopsy f.
Wilson-Cook grasping f.
Wilson-Cook hot biopsy f.
Wilson-Cook retrieval f.
Wilson-Cook tripod grasping f.
Wilson foreign body f.
Winter-Nassauer placental f.
Winter ovum f.
Winter placental f.
wire-closure f.
wire-crimping f.
wire-holding f.
wire-pulling f.
wire-twisting f.
Wittner uterine biopsy f.
Wolf biopsy f.
Wolf biting-basket f.
Wolf cataract delivery f.
Wolf curved-basket f.
Wolf eye f.
Wolfson f.
Wolf uterine cuff f.
Woodward f.
Woodward-Potts intestinal f.
Woodward thoracic artery f.
Worth advancement f.
Worth muscle f.
Worth strabismus f.
wound-clip f.
wound closure f.
Wright-Rubin f.
Wrigley f.
W-shaped f.
Wullstein ear f.
Wullstein-House f.
Wullstein-Paparella f.
Wullstein tympanoplasty f.
Wylie tenaculum f.
Wylie uterine f.
X-long cement f.
Yankauer ethmoidal f.
Yankauer-Little f.
Yasargil applying f.
Yasargil arterial f.
Yasargil bipolar f.
Yasargil clip-applying f.
Yasargil flat serrated ring f.
Yasargil microvessel clip-applying f.
Yasargil neurosurgical bipolar f.
Yeoman uterine f.
Yeoman uterine biopsy f.
Yeoman-Wittner rectal f.
Younge-Kevorkian f.
Younge uterine f.
Young intestinal f.
Young lobe f.
Young prostatectomy f.
Young prostatic f.
Young tongue f.
Young uterine f.
Zaldivar iridectomy f.
Zaldivar reverse capsulorrhexis f.
Z-Clamp hysterectomy f.
Zeeifel angiotribe f.
Zenker f.
Zeppelin obstetrical f.
Ziegler ciliary f.
Zimmer-Hoen f.
Zimmer-Schlesinger f.
Zollinger multipurpose tissue f.

Ford

F. clamp
F. Hospital ventricular cannula

Ford-Deaver retractor

forearm

f. flexion control strap
f. tourniquet

forefoot compression sleeve

Foregger

F. bronchoscope

F. laryngoscope
F. rigid esophagoscope
foreign
  f. body bur
  f. body curette
  f. body cystoscopy forceps
  f. body eye forceps
  f. body locator
  f. body loop
  f. body magnet
  f. body needle
  f. body needle spud
  f. body probe
  f. body remover
  f. body retriever
  f. body-retrieving forceps
  f. body screw
  f. body spud
ForeRunner
  F. automatic external defibrillator device
  F. coronary sinus guiding catheter
  F. semiautomatic external defibrillator
fork
  broadbill hemostat with push f.
  Burch fixation f.
  crus guide f.
  double-pronged f.
  Gardiner-Brown neurological tuning f.
  f. hammer
  Hardy implant f.
  Hardy 3-prong f.
  Hartmann tuning f.
  Jacobson f.
  Jannetta double-pronged f.
  Jarit tuning f.
  knife and f.
  Leasure tuning f.
  magnesium tuning f.
  McCabe crus guide f.
  neurological tuning f.
  Okonek-Yasargil tumor f.
  Penn tuning f.
  3-prong f.
  Ralks tuning f.
  Rhoton 3-prong f.
  Rica tuning f.
  Rydel-Seiffert tuning f.
  SMIC tuning f.
  tuning f.

form
  Amoena breast f.
  breast f.
  Discrene breast f.
  Dow Corning external breast f.
  mastopexy f.
  Nearly Me breast f.
  Roth arch f.
  SoLight breast f.
  Spenco external breast f.
  Trulife silicone breast f.
  Yours Truly asymmetrical external breast f.
Forma water-jacketed incubator
formboard
  Seguin f.
formed cystotome
FormFlex
  F. formocresal lens
  F. intraocular lens
  F. lens loop
formocresol lens
foroblique
  f. bronchoscope
  f. bronchoscopic telescope
  f. endoscope
  f. fiberoptic esophagoscope
  f. lens
  f. microlens resectoscope
  f. panendoscope
Forrester
  F. cervical collar brace
  F. clamp
  F. head halter
  F. head splint
Förster
  F. enucleation snare
  F. iris forceps
  F. photometer
  F. photoptometer
FortaFlex bioengineered collagen matrix
FortaGen mesh
FortaPerm surgical sling
Fortuna syringe
forward-grasping forceps
forward-viewing endoscope
forward-vision telescope
Foss
  F. anterior resection clamp
  F. bifid gallbladder retractor
  F. biliary retractor
  F. cardiovascular clamp

F

NOTES

Foss *(continued)*
F. cardiovascular forceps
F. clamp forceps
F. intestinal clamp
Fossa ureteral stone sweeper
FossFill Health pillow
Foster
F. bed
F. fracture frame
F. scissors
F. snare enucleator
F. suture
Foster-Ballenger
F.-B. bone forceps
F.-B. nasal speculum
Fotofil
F. dental restorative material
F. light
Fotona
F. Novalis Er:YAG laser
F. Novalis R ruby laser
Foundation
F. 4-part fracture system
F. total hip system
F. total knee system
F. total shoulder system
fountain
F. design prosthesis
F. infusion catheter
xenon cold light f.
Fourier
F. harmonic analysis
F. transformation spectrum analyzer
F. transform infrared microspectroscopy
F. transform infrared spectroscopy
Fournier tip
Fowler
F. double-end curette
F. dressing
F. EndoCurette
F. self-retaining retractor
F. urethral sound
Fox
F. aluminum eye shield
F. bipolar electrocautery forceps
F. clavicular splint
F. conformer
F. dermal curette
F. eyelid implant
F. eye speculum
F. Hollow Technologies (FHT)
F. hydrostatic irrigator
F. I&A unit
F. impactor-extractor
F. internal fixation device
F. LASIK spatula
F. postnasal balloon

F. prosthesis
F. spherical eye implant
FPC
fibered platinum coil
FPL
fluorescent pulsed light
FRACAS
fracture computer-aided surgery
Frackelton
F. fascial needle
F. wire threader
FracSure
F. apparatus
F. splint
F. total hip system
F. unit
Fractomed splint
Fractura
F. Flex bandage
F. Flex cast
fracture
f. band
f. bar
f. bed
f. boot
f. brace
f. chisel
f. computer-aided surgery (FRACAS)
f. fixation device
f. frame
f. reducing elevator
f. splint
f. table
Fragen
F. anterior commissure microlaryngoscope
F. carrier
F. laryngoscope
F. laryngoscope fiberoptic light
Fragmatome
CooperVision F.
F. flute syringe
Gill-Hess F.
Girard F.
F. tip
fragmentation probe
fragment forceps
fragmentor
Lieberman f.
Frahm carver
Frahur
F. cartilage clamp
F. scissors
fraise
diamond f.
frame
Ace-Fischer f.

Alexian Brothers overhead
  fracture f.
Andrews spinal f.
anterior quadrilateral triplane f.
Balkan fracture f.
Boehler-Braun fracture f.
Böhler-Braun fracture f.
Böhler reducing fracture f.
Boston Children's f.
Bradford fracture f.
Braun f.
Brown-Roberts-Wells head f.
Brown-Roberts-Wells stereotactic f.
Buck extension f.
Budde-Greenberg-Sugita stereotactic
  head f.
Charest head f.
Chick CLT operating f.
Codman f.
Cole hyperextension fracture f.
Colles external fixation f.
Compass stereotactic f.
couch-mounted head f.
Crawford head f.
CRW stereotactic f.
Delta external fixation f.
Denis Browne retractor oval
  sprocket f.
DePuy rainbow fracture f.
Doctor Plymale lift fracture f.
double-ring f.
Elekta stereotactic body f.
Elekta stereotactic head f.
Elgiloy f.
Erich facial fracture f.
Foster fracture f.
fracture f.
fusion f.
Gardner-Wells fixation f.
Goldthwait fracture f.
Granberry hyperextension fracture f.
Greenberg retractor f.
Hall-Relton f.
halo fracture f.
halo head f.
Hastings f.
head f.
Heffington lumbar seat spinal
  surgery f.
Herzmark fracture f.
Hibbs fracture f.

Hitchcock stereotactic
  immobilization f.
Horsley-Clarke stereotactic f.
hyperextension fracture f.
Ilizarov f.
Irby head f.
Janes fracture f.
Jewett f.
Jones abduction f.
Joseph septal f.
Kessler traction f.
Laitinen stereotactic head f.
laminectomy f.
Leksell D-shaped stereotactic f.
Leksell-Elekta stereotactic f.
Leksell Model G stereotactic f.
Lex-Ton lumbar laminectomy f.
Malcolm-Lynn C-RXF cervical
  retractor f.
Malcolm-Rand cranial x-ray f.
Mayfield fixation f.
Monticelli-Spinelli f.
mouth gag f.
MTL trial f.
Mussen f.
nitinol mesh-covered f.
nonferromagnetic MR-compatible f.
OBT f.
occluding fracture f.
Oculus trial f.
Olivier-Bertrand-Tipal f.
Ostby dam f.
overhead fracture f.
Pearson attachment to Thomas f.
Pelorus stereotactic f.
phantom f.
Pittsburgh triangular f.
4-poster f.
Putti f.
quadraplegic standing f.
radiolucent spine f.
Radionics CRW stereotactic head f.
Rainbow fracture f.
Rand-Malcolm cranial x-ray f.
reducing fracture f.
Reichert-Mundinger-Fischer
  stereotactic f.
Reichert-Mundinger stereotactic
  head f.
Relton-Hall spinal f.
retractor oval sprocket f.
Richards Colles fracture f.

F

NOTES

frame *(continued)*
    Risser f.
    robotics-controlled stereotactic f.
    Russell f.
    self-retaining brain retractor f.
    Slatis f.
    sling f.
    spinal f.
    spinal turning f.
    Stealth f.
    stereotactic coordinate f.
    stereotactic head f.
    stereotactic localization f.
    Stryker CircOlectric fracture f.
    Stryker turning fracture f.
    Sugita multipurpose head f.
    Talairach stereotactic f.
    Taylor spinal f.
    Thompson hyperextension
      fracture f.
    Todd-Wells stereotaxis f.
    triangular ankle fusion f.
    vasocillator fracture f.
    Vidal-Hoffman fixator f.
    Watson-Jones f.
    Whitman fracture f.
    Wilson spinal f.
    Wingfield fracture f.
    Young rubber dam fracture f.
    Zimcode traction f.
    Zimmer fracture f.
frameless
    f. air support therapy
    f. stereotaxy system
Framer
    F. finger extension bow
    F. splint
    F. tendon passer
    F. tendon-passing needle
Franceschetti corneal trephine
Franceschetti-type blade
Francis
    F. knife spud
    F. spud
    F. spud chalazion forceps
Francke needle
Franco triflange ventilation tube
Frangenheim
    F. biopsy punch forceps
    F. hook forceps
    F. hook punch
    F. laparoscope
Frank
    F. EKG lead placement system
    F. XYZ orthogonal lead
Fränkel
    F. appliance
    F. cutting-tip forceps
    F. esophagoscopy forceps

    F. head band
    F. laryngeal forceps
    F. sinus probe
    F. speculum
    F. tampon forceps
Frankfeldt
    F. diathermy snare
    F. grasping forceps
    F. hemorrhoidal needle
    F. rectal snare
    F. sigmoidoscope
Franklin
    F. glasses
    F. liver puncture needle
    F. malleable retractor
    F. spectacles
Franklin-Silverman
    F.-S. biopsy cannula
    F.-S. curette
    F.-S. prostatic biopsy needle
Franseen
    F. liver biopsy needle
    F. needle
Franz
    F. abdominal retractor
    F. monophasic action potential
      catheter
Franzen needle guide
Fraser
    F. depressor
    F. forceps
Fraser-Harlake respirometer
Frater
    F. intracardiac retractor
    F. suture
Frazier
    F. aspirating tube
    F. brain-exploring cannula
    F. brain-exploring trocar
    F. brain suction tube
    F. Britetrac nasal suction tube
    F. cerebral retractor
    F. cordotomy hook
    F. cordotomy knife
    F. dural elevator
    F. dural guide
    F. dural hook
    F. dural scissors
    F. dural separator
    F. fiberoptic suction tube
    F. laminectomy retractor
    F. lighted retractor
    F. mastoid suction tube
    F. modified suction tube
    F. monopolar cautery cord
    F. nasal suction tube
    F. nerve hook
    F. osteotome
    F. pituitary capsulectomy knife

F. skin hook
F. stylet
F. suction
F. suction cannula
F. suction elevator
F. suction tip
F. suction tip aspirator
F. suction tube
F. suction tube obturator
F. ventricular cannula
F. ventricular needle
Frazier-Ferguson
F.-F. aspirating tube
F.-F. ear suction tube
Frederick
F. pneumothorax needle
F. sleeve spreader
Frederick-Miller tube
free
F. & Active incontinence pad
F. & Active incontinence panty
f. implant
Freedom
F. arthritis support
F. arthritis support for hand
F. back support
F. Cath
F. Clear external catheter
F. coronary stent
F. dental unit
F. Elastic Long Wrist Support
F. external catheter
F. knife
F. leg bag collection system
F. memory thumb spica cast
F. Micro Pro stimulator
F. Neutral Position splint
F. Omni progressive splint
F. Pak seven catheter
F. Palm guard
F. Progressive resting splint
F. prosthetic foot
F. Sportsfit splint
F. Thumbkeeper
F. Thumb spica cast
F. Thumb stabilizer
F. T-tap leg bag
F. T-tap leg bag kit
F. Ultimate Grip splint
F. USA Wristlet
FreeDop
F. cordless Doppler

F. Doppler monitor
F. portable Doppler unit
FreeFlo stent-graft
Free-Flow system prosthesis
Freegenol cement
freehand
F. neuroprosthetic system
f. probe
Freeman
F. Blue-Max cannula
F. clamp
F. cookie cutter areola marker
F. facelift retractor
F. femoral component
F. frontal sinus stent
F. modular total hip prosthesis
F. positioning cannula
F. posterior capsule polisher
F. pudendal needle
F. punctum plug
F. rhytidectomy scissors
F. transorbital leukotome
Freeman-Samuelson knee prosthesis
Freeman-Swanson knee prosthesis
Freer
F. bone chisel
F. dissector
F. double-end elevator
F. dural dissector
F. dural retractor
F. lacrimal chisel
F. nasal gouge
F. nasal spatula
F. nasal submucous knife
F. periosteal elevator
F. periosteotome
F. septal elevator
F. septal forceps
F. septal knife
F. skin hook
F. skin retractor
F. submucous chisel
F. submucous retractor
freestanding
f. implant
f. single crown
f. stent
Freestyle
F. aortic root bioprosthesis
F. CAPD catheter adapter
F. stentless bioprosthesis
F. stentless valve

F

NOTES

FreeStyle Tracker diabetes management system
Freeway
    F. Lite portable aerosol compressor
    F. PTCA
    F. PTCA balloon catheter
freezer
    CryoMed f.
    Gentle Jane Snap f.
freezing point osmometer
Freezor cryocatheter
Freiberg
    F. cartilage knife
    F. hip retractor
    F. meniscectomy knife
    F. nerve root retractor
    F. traction
    F. tractor
Freiburg
    F. biopsy set
    F. mediastinoscope
Freimuth ear curette
Freitag stent
Frejka
    F. cast
    F. hip pillow
    F. jacket
    F. orthosis
    F. pillow splint
    F. traction
French
    F. angiographic catheter
    F. catheter gauge
    F. chisel
    F. Cope loop nephrostomy catheter
    F. curve out-of-plane catheter
    F. cystoscope
    F. double-lumen catheter
    F. Foley catheter
    F. Gesco catheter
    F. hook spatula
    F. in-plane guiding catheter
    F. JR4 Schneider catheter
    F. lacrimal dilator
    F. lacrimal probe
    F. lacrimal spatula
    F. lock
    F. MBIH catheter
    F. mushroom-tip catheter
    F. needle holder
    F. Pharmacovigilance system
    F. pigtail nephrostomy catheter
    F. red rubber Robinson catheter
    F. Robinson catheter
    F. rod bender
    F. SAL catheter
    F. scoop
    F. shaft catheter
    F. sheath

    F. Silastic Foley catheter
    F. sizing of catheter
    F. spring-eye needle
    F. S-shaped brain retractor
    F. steel sound
    F. stent
    F. Swan-Ganz balloon
    F. Teflon catheter
    F. Teflon pyeloureteral catheter
    F. T-tube
French-eye
    F.-e. needle
    F.-e. Vital needle holder
French-pattern
    F.-p. forceps
    F.-p. osteotome
    F.-p. raspatory
    F.-p. spatula
Frenckner-Stille
    F.-S. curette
    F.-S. punch
Frenta
    F. enteral feeding bag
    F. Mat feeding pump
    F. System II feeding pump
frequency
    f. doubled neodymium:yttrium-aluminum-garnet laser
    f. shifter
Fresenius
    F. AG dialyzer
    F. dialysis machine
    F. Euro-Collins kit
    F. F-40 filter
    F. volumetric dialysate balancing system
fresh frozen allograft
FreshStart mammary support garment
Fresnel
    F. goggles
    F. lens
    F. lens pusher
    F. manipulating hook
    F. nystagmus glasses
    F. nystagmus spectacles
    F. prism
    F. zone plate
Frey-Sauerbruch rib shears
Frialit-2 system dental implant system
Frialoc transgingival threaded dental implant
Friatec
    F. implant
    F. manual arthroscopy instrument
Fricke
    F. arterial forceps
    F. bandage
    F. scrotal dressing

friction-fit
  f.-f. adapter
  F.-f. adapter from Stiegmann-Goff
    endoscopic ligator
friction grip diamond bur
friction-reduced segmented table
Friedenwald
  F. funduscope
  F. ophthalmoscope
Friedlander marker
Friedman
  F. bone rongeur
  F. elevator
  F. handheld Hruby lens
  F. knife guide
  F. lens manipulator
  F. olive-tip vein stripper
  F. perineal retractor
  F. rasp
  F. rongeur forceps
  F. splint
  F. splint brace
  F. tantalum clip
  F. vaginal retractor
  F. visual field analyzer
Friedman-Otis bougie à boule
Friedrich
  F. clamp
  F. raspatory
  F. rib elevator
Friedrich-Petz
  F.-P. clamp
  F.-P. machine resector
Friesner ear knife
Frigitronics
  Cilco F.
  F. colposcope
  F. cryoprobe
  F. cryosurgical unit
  F. disposable cryosurgical stylet
  F. freeze-thaw cryopexy probe
  F. Mark II cryoextractor
  F. nitrous oxide cryosurgery
    apparatus
  F. vitrector
Frimberger-Karpiel
  F.-K. 12 o'clock papillotome
  F.-K. 12 o'clock sphincterotome
Fritsch
  F. abdominal retractor
  F. catheter

Fritz
  F. aspirator
  F. vitreous transplant needle
frog
  f. cortex remover
  f. splint
front
  f. build-up implant
  f. support strap
  f. wall needle
frontal
  f. sinus cannula
  f. sinus chisel
  f. sinus curette
  f. sinus dilator
  f. sinus probe
  f. sinus rasp
  f. sinus wash cannula
Frontrunner coronary catheter
front-wheeled walker
Frost
  F. scissors
  F. stitch
  F. suture
Frosted Flex earmold material
Frostline linear cryoablation system
Frydman catheter
Frykholm
  F. bone rongeur
  F. goniometer
**F-Scan foot force and gait analysis
  system**
F-series
  F-s. dialyzer
  F-s. fluorescence spectrophotometer
Fuchs
  F. capsular forceps
  F. capsulotomy forceps
  F. extracapsular forceps
  F. iris forceps
  F. lancet-type keratome
  F. retinal detachment syringe
  F. surgical stool
  F. 2-way eye syringe
Fugo blade
Fuji
  F. AC2 storage phosphor computed
    radiology system
  F. dental cement
  F. FCR9000 computed radiology
    system
Fujica camera

NOTES

F

Fujinon
- F. biopsy forceps
- F. CEG-FP-series videoelectroscope
- F. diagnostic laparoscope
- F. EC-series video colonoscope
- F. ED-series duodenoscope
- F. ED7-XU2 videoduodenoscope
- F. EG-FP-series endoscope
- F. EG-series endoscope
- F. EG-series gastroscope
- F. EG7-series videoelectroscope
- F. ES-series sigmoidoscope
- F. EVE-series endoscope
- F. EVG-CT-series endoscope
- F. EVG-FP-series endoscope
- F. EVG-F-series endoscope
- F. EVG-series endoscope
- F. FD-series duodenoscope
- F. flexible bronchoscope
- F. flexible fiberoptic laparoscope
- F. flexible hysteroscope
- F. flexible sigmoidoscope
- F. FP-series endoscope
- F. FS-series sigmoidoscope
- F. GF-series gastroscope
- F. operating laparoscope
- F. 400-series super image video gastroscope
- F. Sonoprobe
- F. SP-501 sonoprobe system
- F. UGI-FP-series video endoscope
- F. variceal injector
- F. 310XU videoduodenoscope

Fujita
- F. snake retractor
- F. suction cannula

Fukasaku pupil snapper hook

Fukuda
- F. DS-5800NX dynascope
- F. humeral head retractor

Fukushima
- F. C-clamp clamp
- F. dissector
- F. malleable brain spatula
- F. malleable coagulator
- F. microdissector
- F. retractor
- F. ring-curette
- F. rongeur

Fukushima-Giannotta
- F.-G. curette
- F.-G. dissector
- F.-G. needle holder
- F.-G. scissors

Fukuyama limbal relaxing incision marker

fulgurating electrode

full
- f. lower denture
- f. spine board
- f. upper denture

full-circle goniometer

full-curved clamp

Fuller
- F. bivalve trach tube
- F. perianal shield
- F. rectal dressing
- F. Shield perineal binder
- F. silicone sponge

Fullerview flexible iris retractor

full-field digital mammography system

FullFlow perfusion dilation catheter

full-occlusal splint

full-radius resector

full-ring scanner

full-wave rectifier

fully
- f. automatic erythrocyte aggregometer
- f. constrained tricompartmental knee prosthesis

Fulton
- F. laminectomy rongeur
- F. pediatric scissors
- F. retractor

Ful-Vue
- F.-V. ophthalmoscope
- F.-V. spot retinoscope
- F.-V. streak retinoscope

functional
- f. electronic peroneal brace
- f. fracture brace
- f. MRI
- f. orthotic
- f. resting position splint

fundal
- f. contact lens
- f. laser lens

fundamental frequency indicator

fundus
- f. camera
- f. contact lens
- f. focalizing lens
- f. laser lens

funduscope
- Friedenwald f.

funnelform taper

Furacin
- F. gauze dressing
- F. gauze holder

Furness
- F. anastomosis clamp
- F. catheter
- F. cornea-holding forceps
- F. polyp forceps

Furness-Clute
- F.-C. anastomosis clamp

F.-C. duodenal clamp
F.-C. pin
fused bifocal lens
fused-tip catheter
fusiform bougie
fusion
f. cage
f. frame
f. plate
Futrex analyzer
Futura resectoscope sheath
Futuro
F. splint

F. wrist brace
F. wrist support
FX
fluoroscopy
FyBron calcium alginate dressing
Fyodorov
F. dipstick
F. lens expressor
F. 4-loop iris clip intraocular lens
F. type I, II intraocular lens
F. type I, II lens implant

NOTES

F

G5

G5 Fleximatic massage/percussion unit
G5 Flimm-Fighter percussor
G5 massage and percussion machine
G5 Mist-Ease nebulizer
G5 Neocussor percussor
G5 Porta-Plus muscle stimulator
G5 Vari-Tilt Adjustable Tilt-Board
G5 Vibracare massager

Gaab endoscope

GaAs laser

Gabarro

G. board
G. retractor

Gabbay-Frater suture guide

Gabor probe

Gabriel

G. proctoscope
G. syringe
G. Tucker bougie
G. Tucker forceps
G. Tucker tube

gadolinium scan

Gaeltec catheter-tip pressure transducer

Gaffney

G. ankle prosthesis
G. joint

gag

Brophy g.
Dott-Dingman self-retaining cleft palate g.

Gaillard-Arlt suture

gain

body oscillation integrates neuromuscular g.

gait

g. belt
g. lock splint
g. lock splint brace
g. plate

Galand

G. disc lens
G. in-the-bag lens
G. lens manipulating hook

Galante

G. hip guide
G. hip prosthesis

Galaxy

G. 900HS adjusting table
G. IVUS system
G. McManis hylo table
G. pacemaker

Galen

G. bandage
G. dressing
G. Scan scanner
G. teleradiology system

Galetti articulator

Galezowski lacrimal dilator

Galilean

G. loupe
G. microscope

Galileo

G. computerized measurement unit
G. evoked potential electroencephalograph
G. III intravascular radiotherapy system
G. rigid hysteroscope
G. training circuit equipment
G. ventilator

Galin

G. intraocular implant lens
G. intraocular lens implant
G. lens spatula
G. silicone bleb cup

gall

g. duct dilator
g. duct forceps
g. duct probe
g. duct scoop

Gallagher

G. antral rasp
G. bipolar mapping probe
G. trocar

gallbladder

g. aspirator
g. cannula
g. forceps
g. retractor
g. ring clamp
g. scissors
g. scoop
g. spoon

Gallie

G. cryoenucleator
G. fusion-using cable
G. tendon passer

Gallini bone marrow aspiration needle

gallium-aluminum-arsenide laser

gallium-arsenide laser

gallows

Killian suspension g.
G. splint

gallstone

g. basket
g. dilator

G

gallstone *(continued)*
   g. forceps
   g. lithotripter
   g. probe
   g. scoop
Galt
   G. aspirating cannula
   G. hand drill
   G. skull trephine
Galton
   G. ear whistle
   G. galvanometer
galvanic
   g. electrode stimulator
   g. probe
   g. skin response device
   g. skin response meter
galvanometer
   d'Arsonval g.
   Einthoven string g.
   Galton g.
Galveston
   G. metacarpal brace
   G. plate
   G. splint
Gambale-Degeorge (GD)
Gambee suture
Gamboscope scope
Gambro
   G. AK10 machine
   G. catheter
   G. dialyzer
   G. dialyzer holder
   G. FH88H filter
   G. freezing bag
   G. hemodialyzer
   G. hemofiltration system
   G. Liendia plate
   G. Lundia plate
   G. oxygenator
Gambro-Lundia
   G.-L. coil dialyzer
   G.-L. Minor hemodialyzer
Gamgee dressing
gamma
   g. camera
   g. detection probe
   g. emitter
   g. knife
   G. locking nail system
   g. probe
   g. probe radiation detector
   g. ray counter
   g. ray scanner
   g. ray spectrometer
   g. scintillation camera
   G. trochanteric locking nail
   g. well counter

Gam-Mer
   G.-M. aneurysm clamp
   G.-M. bipolar coagulator
   G.-M. bone-cutting forceps
   G.-M. bur
   G.-M. chuck
   G.-M. clip applier
   G.-M. gouge
   G.-M. groover
   G.-M. medial esophageal retractor
   G.-M. minimallet
   G.-M. miniosteotome
   G.-M. nerve hook
   G.-M. oblique raspatory
   G.-M. occipital retractor
   G.-M. occlusion clamp
   G.-M. periosteal elevator
   G.-M. rasp
   G.-M. rongeur
   G.-M. spinal fusion curette
   G.-M. vise
Gammex
   G. RMI DAP meter
   G. RMI scanner
ganglion
   g. injection needle
   g. scissors
Ganley splint
Gans cyclodialysis cannula
Gant
   G. clamp
   G. gallbladder retractor
   G. rectal probe
gantry
   CT scan g.
   LINAC g.
gantry-free gamma camera
Ganzfeld
   G. electroretinograph
   G. stimulator
Gap cup
Garceau
   G. bougie
   G. ureteral catheter
Garcia
   G. aortic clamp
   G. endometrial biopsy set
Gardiner-Brown neurological tuning fork
Gardner
   G. bone chisel
   G. bone forceps
   G. chair
   G. headholder
   G. headrest
   G. hysterectomy forceps
   G. needle
   G. needle holder
   G. skull clamp

Gardner-Wells
   G.-W. fixation frame
   G.-W. headrest
   G.-W. traction tongs
Gardray dosimeter
Gariel pessary
Garland
   G. hysterectomy clamp
   G. hysterectomy forceps
garment
   Canfield facial plastics g.
   Caromed surgical g.
   compression g.
   crotchless compression g.
   Digi-Sleeve pressure g.
   Elvarex g.
   FreshStart mammary support g.
   HK Breast/Torso g.
   Jobskin pressure g.
   Jobst pressure g.
   Marena Comfortwear
      compression g.
   Medical Z post surgery g.
   pneumatic g.
   PresSsion pneumatic g.
   surgical compression g.
Garren-Edwards gastric balloon
Garretson
   G. bandage
   G. dressing
Garrett
   G. dilator
   G. peripheral vascular retractor
   G. vein passer
Garrigue
   G. uterine-dressing forceps
   G. vaginal retractor
   G. weighted vaginal speculum
Garrison forceps
garter
   Goffman blue eye shield g.
   G. shield
Gärtner tonometer
Garty diamond trephine
gas
   G. Check blood analyzer
   g. chromatograph
   g. chromatography/mass
      spectroscopy
   g. discharge lamp
   g. insufflator

   g. isotope ratio mass spectrometer
   g. laser
GaSampler multilaminate bag
Gaskell clamp
gasket
   Seal-Tite adhesive g.
Gaskin fragment forceps
Gas-Lyte
   G.-L. ABG syringe
   G.-L. arterial blood gas syringe
GasPak jar
Gass
   G. cataract-aspirating cannula
   G. cervical punch
   G. corneoscleral punch
   G. dye applicator
   G. I&A unit
   G. muscle hook
   G. neurosurgical light
   G. retinal detachment cannula
   G. retinal detachment hook
   G. scleral marker
   G. scleral punch
   G. sclerotomy punch
   G. vitreous-aspirating cannula
gastric
   g. balloon
   g. clamp
   g. resection retractor
   g. shield
   g. tube
gastrocamera
   Bolex g.
   cine g.
   Olympus g.
gastroenterostomy
   g. catheter
   g. clamp
gastrofiberscope
   Pentax FG-series ultrasound g.
GastrograpH
   G. ambulatory pH monitoring
      system
   G. Mark III pH analyzer
gastrointestinal (GI)
   g. anastomosis (GIA)
   g. clamp
   g. forceps
   g. needle
   g. surgical gut suture
   g. surgical linen suture
   g. surgical silk suture

G

NOTES

gastrointestinal *(continued)*
    g. suture
    upper g. (UGI)
gastrojejunostomy
    g. catheter
    g. tube
Gastrolyzer breath hydrogen monitor
gastroplasty stapler
Gastro-Port II feeding tube
Gastroscan motility system
gastroscope
    ACMI g.
    Benedict operating g.
    Bernstein g.
    Cameron omni-angle g.
    Chevalier Jackson g.
    disposable-sheath flexible g.
    Eder g.
    Eder-Bernstein g.
    Eder-Hufford g.
    Eder-Palmer g.
    Ellsner g.
    end-viewing g.
    Ewald g.
    examining g.
    fiberoptic g.
    flexible g.
    Fujinon EG-series g.
    Fujinon GF-series g.
    Fujinon 400-series super image
      video g.
    Herman-Taylor g.
    Hirschowitz g.
    Housset-Debray g.
    Janeway g.
    Jenning-Streifeneder g.
    Kelling g.
    Krentz g.
    Mancke flex-rigid g.
    Olympus GF-series g.
    Olympus GIF-K-series g.
    Olympus GIF-series g.
    Olympus GIF-XQ-series flexible g.
    Olympus GTF-series g.
    Olympus OES-series g.
    Olympus 2T-2000 twin-channel
      therapeutic g.
    Olympus XQ-series g.
    pediatric g.
    Pentax EG-2900 video g.
    peroral g.
    Schindler g.
    Sielaff g.
    Taylor g.
    Tomenius g.
    Universal g.
    Wolf-Henning g.
    Wolf-Knittlingen g.
    Wolf-Schindler g.

gastrostomy
    Beck g.
    g. button
    g. catheter
    g. catheter kit
    Depage-Janeway g.
    feeding g.
    g. feeding tube
    Flow-20-push method g.
    Glassman g.
    Kader g.
    Olympus g.
    percutaneous endoscopic g. (PEG)
    g. plug
    Russell percutaneous endoscopic g.
    Surgitek One Step percutaneous
      endoscopic g.
    g. tube
    Witzel g.
Gastro-Test capsule
Gatch bed
gate clip
Gates-Glidden
    G.-G. bur
    G.-G. drill
Gator
    G. drape
    G. meniscal cutter
    G. plastic orthosis
    G. resector
    G. shaver
Gauderer-Ponsky PEG
gauge
    American wire g.
    Austin measuring g.
    Boley g.
    bone screw depth g.
    Bourdon tube pressure g.
    Broggi-Kelman dipstick g.
    calibrated depth g.
    carpal tunnel syndrome g.
    Charnley femoral condyle radius g.
    Charnley socket g.
    Cloward L-W g.
    Cloward spanner g.
    CTS g.
    Dacomed snap g.
    depth g.
    Dontrix intraoral g.
    Durkan CTS g.
    Edslab pressure g.
    EndoGauge g.
    finger circumference g.
    French catheter g.
    Harris femoral head g.
    isometric strain g.
    Jamar hydraulic pinch g.
    Knolle lens g.
    Kundin wound measurement g.

leaf g.
LeVeen inflator with pressure g.
manual dermatome thickness g.
Marco radius g.
measuring g.
Mendez degree g.
mercury-in-Silastic strain g.
Neumann depth g.
orthopaedic depth g.
Padgett baseline pinch g.
pain threshold g.
Philips toe force g.
Pilling Excalibur g.
pinch g.
pressure g.
Preston pinch g.
Reichert radius g.
Rocabado posture g.
screw depth g.
Shepard incision depth g.
Silastic strain g.
spanner g.
Stahl lens g.
standard wire g.
Steinert-Deacon incision g.
Synthes mini-depth g.
Tinnant g.
Tycos g.
uniaxial strain g.
Universal g.
water g.
Zaldivar degree g.
gauntlet bandage
Gauthier
  G. bicycle ergometer
  G. retractor
gauze
  Adaptic g.
  Aquaphor g.
  Avant nonwoven g.
  g. bandage
  BIPP ribbon g.
  Cover-Roll adhesive g.
  Curafil hydrogel impregnated g.
  g. dissector sponge
  dry sterile g.
  dry textile g.
  finger g.
  GraftCyte g.
  Intersorb fine mesh g.
  Intersorb 6-ply absorbent roll stretch g.

Intersorb wide mesh g.
iodoform g.
KBM absorbent g.
Kling g.
g. neck tie
Oxycel g.
g. pack
g. packer
g. pad carrier
Panogauze hydrogel-impregnated g.
paraffin g.
petrolatum g.
petroleum g.
plain g.
g. rosebud sponge
Safe-Wrap g.
g. scissors
sodium chloride-impregnated g.
Sof-Form conforming g.
g. sponge
Sta-Tite 2ply elastic roll g.
g. stent dressing
Surgicel g.
Surgitube tubular g.
tantalum g.
Teletrast g.
Telfa g.
g. tissue bag
Topper nonadherent g.
TransiGel hydrogel-impregnated g.
White Plume absorbent g.
g. wick
woven cotton g.
Xeroform g.
Gauztape bandage
Gauztex
  G. bandage
  G. dressing
Gavin-Miller
  G.-M. clamp
  G.-M. colon forceps
  G.-M. intestinal forceps
  G.-M. tissue forceps
Gavriliu gastric tube
Gaylor uterine biopsy forceps
Gaymar
  G. Thermacare warming unit
  G. water-circulating blanket
Gazayerli
  G. endoscopic retractor
  G. knot pusher
Gazelle balloon dilatation catheter

NOTES

G-C

G-C diamond point
G-C polishing strip
G-C syringe
G-C Vest investment material
G-C wax carver

GD

Gambale-Degeorge
GD Regainer system

GDC

Guglielmi detachable coil
3-dimensional GDC

GDC-series soft coil
GDLH posterior spinal system
GDx nerve fiber analyzer
GE

General Electric
GE Advance PET scanner
GE CT Advantage scanner
GE CT Hi-Speed Advantage
system
GE CT Max scanner
GE CT Pace scanner
GE CT/T scanner
GE Genesis CT scanner
GE 9800 high-resolution CT
scanner
GE HiSpeed Advantage helical CT
scanner
GE Maxicamera gamma camera
GE MR Max scanner
GE MR Signa scanner
GE MR Vectra scanner
GE NMR spectrometer
GE Omega 500-MHz scanner
GE pacemaker
GE RT 3200 Advantage II
ultrasound
GE Senographe 2000D
mammography system
GE Signa Genesis MR imager
GE Signa Horizon EchoSpeed MR
imager
GE Signa 1.5-T magnet
GE single-axis SR-230 echoplanar
scanner
GE single-detector SPECT-capable
camera
GE Spiral CT scanner
GE Starcam single-crystal
tomographic scintillation camera

gear shift pedicle probe
Geenan

G. biliary cytology brush
G. Endotorque guidewire
G. graduated dilation catheter
G. pancreatic stent

Geggel

G. corneal transplant marker
G. PRK chiller

Gehrung pessary
Geiger

G. cautery
G. counter
G. electrocautery

Geiger-Müller

G.-M. counter
G.-M. detector
G.-M. tube

Geissendorfer

G. rib retractor
G. uterine forceps

gel

g. cushion
g. mammary prosthesis
G. Mark Ultra biopsy site marker
g. pack
g. pad
g. sheeting
G. Sole shoe insert
g. stump sock
g. suspension sleeve
g. tubing
g. warmer
g. wound dressing

Gelastic bed
gelatin

g. compression boot
g. sponge
g. sponge pad

gelatin-resorcin-formalin

g.-r.-f. glue
g.-r.-f. tissue glue adhesive

gelatin-subbed slide
GelBand arm band
gel-filled

g.-f. bladder
g.-f. breast prosthesis
g.-f. implant

Gelfilm

G. cap
G. dressing
G. forceps
G. plate
G. retinal implant
G. stent

Gelfoam

G. cookie
G. cube
fibrin-soaked G.
G. pad
G. pledget
G. pressure forceps
G. punch
G. sponge

thrombin-soaked G.

G. torpedo

Gel-Foam Ultra-Wedge cushion

Gelhorn biopsy forceps

Geliperm gel dressing

Gellhorn

G. pessary

G. uterine biopsy forceps

G. uterine biopsy punch

GellyComb bed

Gelocast

G. dressing

G. Unna boot

GelPad dressing

Gelpi

G. hysterectomy forceps

G. perineal retractor

G. self-retaining abdominal retractor

G. vaginal retractor

Gelpi-Lowrie

G.-L. hysterectomy forceps

G.-L. retractor

GelPort laparoscopic hand access device

gel-saline Surgitek mammary prosthesis

Gel-Syte wound dressing

Gel-U-Sleep series III floatation
  mattress system

Gély suture

Gem

G. II DR/VR implantable
  cardioverter-defibrillator

G. III AT implantable cardioverter-
  defibrillator

G. PCL Plus coagulation system

G. Premier Plus whole blood
  analyzer

G. SensiCath blood gas
  mesaurement system

Gemini

G. clamp

G. combined PET/CT system

G. DDD pacemaker

G. gall duct forceps

G. helical wire basket

G. hemostatic forceps

G. hip

G. hip system prosthesis

G. PC1 IV pump

G. syringe

G. thoracic forceps

Gemini-Mixter forceps

GeneAmp RNA PCR kit

general

g. closure needle

g. closure suture

G. Electric (GE)

G. Electric Advantx system

G. Electric pacemaker

G. Electric Pass-C echocardiograph
  machine

g. probe

g. retractor

g. tissue forceps

g. utility scissors

g. wire forceps

Generation

G. 4 bone cement

G. II all-in-one-hand control

G. II KAFO

G. II Matrix knee brace

Zest Anchor Advanced G. (ZAAG)

generator

Angeion 2000 ICD g.

Aurora pulse g.

ballistic energy g.

bipolar g.

Bird neonatal CPAP g.

Birtcher electrosurgical g.

carbon dioxide g.

Chardack-Greatbatch implantable
  cardiac pulse g.

CO_2 g.

computerized pattern g.

Coratomic implantable pulse g.

Cordis Theta Sequicor DDD
  pulse g.

Cosmos II multiprogrammable dual-
  chamber cardiac pulse g.

CPI PRx pulse g.

Cyberlith multiprogrammable
  pulse g.

deuterium-tritium g.

direct current g.

distal stimulation g.

Down flow g.

electric g.

electrostatic g.

electrosurgical g.

Endostat II bipolar/monopolar
  electrosurgical g.

Erbe ICC g.

extraction g.

Force 2 CEM g.

Force FX g.

G

NOTES

generator *(continued)*
Grass visual pattern g.
high-voltage g.
implantable pulse g.
implanted NCP g.
Instant Response technology g.
Intec AID cardioverter-
defibrillator g.
Itrel II quadripolar pulse g.
LithoClast ballistic energy g.
Maxilith pacemaker pulse g.
Medstone STS shockwave g.
Medtronic Cardiorhythm Atakr g.
Medtronic pulse g.
Meniett low-pressure pulse g.
Microlith pacemaker pulse g.
Microny SR+ single-chamber, rate-
responsive pulse g.
Minilith pacemaker pulse g.
molybdenum-99 g.
molybdenum-technetium g.
multiprogrammable dual-chamber
cardiac pulse g.
multiprogrammable pulse g.
Neuro N-50 lesion g.
Optima pulse g.
Pacesetter Synchrony III pulse g.
Pacesetter Trilogy DR+ pulse g.
Parama pulse wave g.
Pegasys electrosurgical g.
3-phase g.
polyphase g.
programmable pulse g.
6-pulse g.
12-pulse g.
radio frequency g.
radiofrequency g.
Radionics radiofrequency lesion g.
Radionics stimulus g.
rate-responsive pulse g.
Regency SR+ pulse g.
resonance g.
Res-Q ICD g.
RFG-3C Plus lesion g.
RF2000 radiofrequency g.
scan pattern g.
single-chamber pulse g.
small-particle aerosol g.
spark-gap shock wave g.
Stilith implantable cardiac pulse g.
supervoltage g.
Symmetry endobipolar g.
g. system
tantalum-178 g.
Trilogy DC, DR, SR pulse g.
Triphasix g.
Valleylab Force 1C
electrosurgical g.
van de Graaf g.

ventricular demand pulse g.
Ventritex Contour pulse g.
Vivalith II pulse g.
in vivo g.
waveform g.
x-ray g.
GenESA closed-loop delivery system
Gene scissors
GeneScreen
G. nylon membrane filter
G. Plus nylon membrane
Genesis
G. 2000 carbon dioxide laser
G. diamond blade
G. II foot/ankle system
G. II total knee system
G. lens
GenesisXP neurostimulation system
**Genesys Vertex variable angle gamma
camera**
Genetra seedless brachytherapy
Genie resin
genioplate
Synthes g.
Genisis dual-chamber pacemaker
GenJect
G. injection device
G. injector
Genotropin
G. 2-chamber cartridge
G. MiniQuick
G. pen
G. system
GenProbe collection kit
Gensini
G. coronary arteriography catheter
G. Teflon catheter
gentamicin-impregnated Biodel bead
Gentell
G. foam wound dressing
G. hydrogel dressing
G. isotonic saline wet dressing
Gentex PDQ polycarbonate lens
gentian violet marking pen
Gentle
G. Jane Snap freezer
G. Jet pediatric injector
G. Threads interference screw
G. Touch colostomy appliance
G. Touch colostomy/ileostomy
postoperative kit
G. Touch colostomy/ileostomy
postoperative system
G. Touch loop ostomy system
G. Touch urostomy postoperative
kit
Gentle-Flo suction catheter
GentleLASE
G. laser

G. laser system
G. Plus laser
G. Plus laser system
GentlePeel skin exfoliation system
GentleStep shoe
Genucom
G. ACL laxity analysis system
G. arthrometer
G. knee flexion analysis system
Genutrain
G. knee brace
G. P3 active knee support
Genzyme Hind Site 20/20 system
GeoFlex knee
Geo-Matt
G.-M. 30-degree body aligner
G.-M. gel contour cushion
G.-M. mattress
G.-M. PRT cushion
G.-M. therapeutic foam overlay
G.-M. wheelchair cushion
Geometric total knee prosthesis
Georgiade
G. breast prosthesis
G. fixation device
G. rasp
G. visor cervical traction
GEO Structure spinal implant
Gerald
G. bayonet microbipolar neurosurgical forceps
G. brain forceps
G. clamp
G. dressing forceps
G. monopolar forceps
G. straight microbipolar neurosurgical forceps
G. tissue forceps
Gerbode
G. cardiovascular tissue forceps
G. mitral valvulotome
G. mitral valvulotomy dilator
G. modified Burford rib spreader
G. patent ductus clamp
G. rib spreader
G. sternal retractor
Gerdy interatrial loop
geriatric
g. chair
g. chair trunk support
GeriMend skin tear therapy

Gerster
G. bone clamp
G. fracture appliance
G. traction bar
G. traction device
Gertie ball
Gerzog
G. bone hammer
G. bone mallet
G. ear knife
G. nasal speculum
Gesco
G. aspirator
G. cannula
G. catheter
G. Umbili-Cath catheter
Gess cannula tip
Getz
G. crown
G. root canal pin
G. rubber base
Geuder
G. corneal electrode
G. corneal needle
G. implanter
G. keratoplasty needle
GFH alloy
GFS Mark II inflatable penile prosthesis
GF-UM3
GF-UM3 duodenoscope
GF-UM3 scanner
GF-UM30P linear-oriented radial scanning echoendoscope
GFX coronary stent
GFX2 coronary stent system
Ghajar guide
Gherini-Kauffman endo-otoprobe laser
GHM
GHM KLE II x-ray film holder
GHM polishing strip
GI
gastrointestinal
GI clamp
GI forceps
GI pop-off silk suture
GIA
gastrointestinal anastomosis
GIA II loading unit
GIA staple
GIA stapling device

G

NOTES

Gianturco
- G. expandable metallic biliary stent
- G. metal urethral stent
- G. occlusion coil
- G. prosthesis
- G. steel coil
- G. wool-tufted wire coil
- G. zigzag stent
- G. Z-stent

Gianturco-Roehm bird's nest vena caval filter
Gianturco-Rosch
- G.-R. metallic stent
- G.-R. self-expandable biliary Z stent

Gianturco-Roubin
- G.-R. flexible coil stent
- G.-R. FlexStent coronary stent
- G.-R. II stent

Gianturco-Wallace coil
Gibbon
- G. indwelling ureteral stent
- G. urethral catheter

Gibney
- G. boot
- G. dressing
- G. fixation bandage

Gibson
- G. anterior chamber irrigator
- G. bandage
- G. dressing
- G. I&A unit
- G. inner ear shunt
- G. splint
- G. stone dislodger

Gibson-Cooke sweat test apparatus
Giebel blade plate
Giertz
- G. rib guillotine
- G. rib shears

Giertz-Shoemaker rib shears
Giertz-Stille
- G.-S. rib shears
- G.-S. scissors

Gifford
- G. corneal applicator
- G. corneal curette
- G. fixation forceps
- G. iris forceps
- G. mastoid retractor
- G. needle holder
- G. scalp retractor

Gigli
- G. saw
- G. saw guide
- G. solid-handle saw
- G. spiral saw wire
- G. wire saw

Gigli-saw
- G.-s. blade
- G.-s. handle

Gigli-Strully saw
G II Unloader ADJ knee brace
Gilbert
- G. cystic duct forceps
- G. pediatric balloon catheter
- G. plug-sealing catheter
- G. prosthesis

Gildenberg biopsy forceps
Giliberty acetabular prosthesis
Gill
- G. biopsy brush
- G. blade
- G. corneal knife
- G. counterpressor
- G. curved iris forceps
- G. double I&A cannula
- G. double Luer-Lok cannula
- G. incision spreader
- G. incision-spreading forceps
- G. intraocular implant lens
- G. I respirator
- G. iris forceps
- G. iris knife
- G. needle
- G. pop-up arcuate diamond knife
- G. pressor counter
- G. renal tourniquet
- G. scissors
- G. sinus cannula

Gill-Arruga capsular forceps
Gill-Chandler iris forceps
Gillette
- G. Blue blade
- G. brace
- G. double-flexure ankle joint system
- G. joint orthosis
- G. joint prosthesis

Gill-Fuchs capsular forceps
Gill-Hess
- G.-H. blade
- G.-H. Fragmatome
- G.-H. iris forceps
- G.-H. knife
- G.-H. mules
- G.-H. scissors

Gillies
- G. bone hook
- G. dissecting forceps
- G. dural hook
- G. hook
- G. horizontal dermal suture
- G. implant
- G. malar elevator
- G. nasal hook
- G. needle holder

G. prosthesis
G. single-hook skin retractor
G. skin hook
G. suture scissors
G. tissue forceps
G. zygoma elevator
G. zygomatic hook
Gillies-Converse skin hook
Gillmore needle
Gillquist
G. suction curette
G. suction tube
Gillquist-Oretorp-Stille
G.-O.-S. dilator
G.-O.-S. forceps
G.-O.-S. knife
G.-O.-S. needle holder
G.-O.-S. probe
Gills-Welsh-Morrison lens loop
Gill-Thomas locator
Gillum nucleus splitter
Gill-Welsh
G.-W. capsular forceps
G.-W. capsular polisher
G.-W. cortex extractor
G.-W. curette
G.-W. double cannula
G.-W. guillotine port
G.-W. irrigation-aspiration cannula
G.-W. knife
G.-W. lens loop
G.-W. olive-tip cannula
G.-W. scissors
G.-W. spatula
Gill-Welsh-Vannas
G.-W.-V. angled microscissors
G.-W.-V. capsulotomy scissors
Gilmer
G. dental splint
G. tooth splint
G. wire
Gilmore
G. intraocular implant lens
G. probe
Gil-Vernet lumbotomy retractor
Gilvernet retractor
Gimbel
G. fountain cannula
G. glove
G. stabilization ring
G. stabilizing ring
gingival clamp

gingivectomy knife
Ginsberg
G. eye speculum
G. tissue forceps
Giotto Image mammography unit
GIP/Medi-Globe prototype needle
giraffe
g. biopsy forceps
G. incubator
G. OmniBed
Girard
G. anterior chamber needle
G. cataract-aspirating needle
G. corneoscleral forceps
G. corneoscleral scissors
G. Fragmatome
G. Fragmatome probe
G. irrigating cannula
G. irrigating tip
G. keratoprosthesis prosthesis
G. scleral ring
G. synechia spatula
G. ultrasonic unit
Girard-Swan
G.-S. knife
G.-S. needle
girdle
Ace halo pelvic g.
compression g.
Lipo-Medi g.
male compression g.
girth hitch
Gish
G. autoinfuser
G. micro YAG laser
Gissane
G. spike
G. spike nail
Given diagnostic imaging system
Gizmo catheter
glabellar rasp
Glacier
G. ceramic 4-in-1 knee cutting guide
G. Pack
Glasgold Wafer chin implant
glass
G. abdominal retractor
g. bead
g. bead sterilizer
g. ionomer cement
G. liver-holding clamp

NOTES

G

glass *(continued)*
 g. penile prosthesis
 g. pH electrode
 g. retracting rod
 g. sphere eye implant
 g. tract detector
 g. vaginal plug
Glasscock
 G. ear dressing
 G. scissors
glasses
 bifocal g.
 Crookes g.
 fiberoptic video g.
 Franklin g.
 Fresnel nystagmus g.
 Grafco magnifying g.
 Hallauer g.
 hyperbolic g.
 magnifying g.
 Masselon g.
 nystagmus g.
 presbyopia g.
 protective g.
 safety g.
 trifocal g.
 Wood g.
 Worst corneal contact g.
Glassman
 G. basket
 G. bowel atraumatic clamp
 G. brush
 G. forceps
 G. gastrostomy
 G. grasper
 G. intestinal clamp
 G. liver-holding clamp
 G. noncrushing gastroenterostomy
  clamp
 G. noncrushing gastrointestinal
  clamp
 G. stone extractor
 G. thin-point scissors
Glassman-Allis
 G.-A. clamp
 G.-A. intestinal forceps
 G.-A. noncrushing common duct
  forceps
 G.-A. noncrushing intestinal forceps
glaucoma
 g. drainage device
 g. pencil
 g. wick
Gleason
 G. headband
 G. rasp
 G. speculum
Glegg nasal polyp snare

Glenn
 G. diverticular forceps
 G. shunt
Glenner
 G. vaginal hysterectomy forceps
 G. vaginal retractor
glenoid
 g. alignment peg
 g. drill
 g. drill guide
 g. fin broach
 g. fixation screw
Gliadel wafer
**GliaSite RTS balloon brachytherapy
  applicator**
glide
 Hessburg intraocular lens g.
 intraocular lens g.
 mushroom-shaped walker g.
 Pearce intraocular g.
 Sheets intraocular g.
 Sheets lens g.
Glidecath hydrophilic coated catheter
glider
 EasyStand 6000 g.
Glidewire
 angled G.
 angle-tip G.
 G. catheter
 G. Gold surgical guide wire
 G. Gold surgical guidewire
 G. guidewire
 G. hydrophilic coated guidewire
 long taper shaft G.
 Microvasive G.
 Radiofocus G.
 stiff shaft G.
 Terumo G.
gliding hinge joint
global
 G. Advantage total shoulder system
 g. force applicator
 G. Fx shoulder fracture system
 G. Healthcare disposable vaginal
  speculum
 G. Therapeutics Freedom stent
 G. Therapeutics V-Flex stent
 G. total shoulder arthroplasty
Glori pressure earring
Glo-Tip ERCP catheter
glottic prosthesis
glottiscope
 Zeitels UM g.
 Zeitels universal modular g.
glove
 Biobrane g.
 Biogel orthopaedic surgical g.
 Biogel Reveal surgical g.
 Biogel Sensor surgical g.

Biogel Surgeons g.
compression g.
Dermapor g.
g. drain
Elastylon g.
electrode g.
Electro-Mesh g.
Encore microptic powder-free latex
  surgical g.
ESP radiation reduction
  examination g.
finger flexion g.
flexion g.
Flextend g.
Gimbel g.
Handeze therapeutic support g.
impact g.
Isotoner g.
Jobst g.
Kevlar g.
Life Liner stick-resistant and cut-
  resistant g.
Maxxus orthopaedic latex
  surgical g.
Medarmor puncture-resistant g.
Necelon surgical g.
neoprene g.
New ultra-thick powder-free latex
  surgical g.
nitrile g.
peripheral nerve g.
Polymed exam g.
pressure g.
Push-Ease wheelchair g.
radial nerve g.
Repela surgical g.
Satin Plus g.
SensiCare synthetic powder-free
  surgical g.
Skinsense g.
Smartglove orthopaedic wrist g.
Surgtech g.
Tactyl 1 g.
Tactylon synthetic surgical g.
Thermal responsive nitrile
  surgical g.
Thermoskin arthritic wrap-around g.
vinyl g.
weighted g.
Glove-n-Gel amniotome
Glover
G. anastomosis forceps

G. auricular-appendage clamp
G. auricular clamp
G. bulldog clamp
G. coarctation clamp
G. coarctation forceps
G. curved clamp
G. curved forceps
G. infundibular rongeur forceps
G. modification of Brock aortic
  dilator
G. patent ductus clamp
G. patent ductus forceps
G. rongeur
G. spoon-shaped anastomosis clamp
G. spoon-shaped forceps
G. suction tube
G. vascular clamp
Glover-DeBakey clamp
Gloves
Glow 'N Tell tape
Gluck rib shears
Glucolet lancet device
glucometer
Accu-Chek II, III g.
Accu-Chek InstantPlus g.
Advantage g.
G. DEX blood glucose monitor
GlucoWatch g.
G. II home glucose monitoring
  system
Miles Encore QA g.
Mills Glucometer II g.
One Touch basic g.
GlucoScan 2000 monitor
GlucoWatch
G. Biographer
G. bloodless glucose monitor
G. glucometer
G. glucose monitoring device
glue
Beriplast P fibrin tissue g.
Biolex wound g.
Body g.
butyl cyanoacrylate g.
cyanoacrylate g.
ethyl cyanoacrylate g.
fibrin g.
gelatin-resorcin-formalin g.
Histoacryl g.
methyl cyanoacrylate g.
g. patch
Tisseel fibrin g.

G

NOTES

glue *(continued)*
    Tisseel surgical g.
    tissue g.
glued-on hard contact lens
glue-in suture
glutameter
    EndoDynamics g.
glutaraldehyde cross-linked collagen
glutaraldehyde-tanned
    g.-t. bovine collagen tube
    g.-t. bovine graft
    g.-t. bovine heart valve
    g.-t. porcine heart valve
glycerine syringe
glycol
    polyethylene g.
glycolide trimethylene carbonate material
GlyMed Camouflage system
gnathograph
gnatholator
gnathologic instrument
gNomos stereotactic system
go-cart
    Chailey g.-c.
Godart expirograph
Godina vessel-fixation instrument
Godiva wax
Goelet double-ended retractor
Goetz
    G. bipolar electrode
    G. cardiac device
Goffman
    G. blue eye garter shield
    G. blue eye shield garter
    G. occluder
goggles
    EndoShield mask and g.
    Fresnel g.
    stenopaic g.
    swimmer's g.
Gohrbrand
    G. cardiac dilator
    G. valvulotome
goiter
    g. clamp
    g. dissector
    g. hook
    g. ligature carrier
    g. retractor
    g. scissors
    g. vulsellum forceps
Golaski
    G. graft
    G. vascular prosthesis
Golay gradient coil
Gold
    G. deep-surgery forceps

    G. pessary
    G. portable CO_2 laser
gold
    g. bur
    g. burnisher
    g. eyelid load implant
    g. hemostatic forceps
    g. needle
    g. probe
    G. probe bipolar hemostasis catheter
    g. probe hemostasis therapy
    g. ring
    g. saw
    g. weight
    g. weight and wire spring implant material
Goldbacher
    G. anoscope
    G. anoscope speculum
    G. proctoscope
    G. rectal needle
Goldberg
    G. MPC mediastinoscope
    G. MPC operative enteroscope
    G. side port splitter
Goldblatt clamp
Golden
    G. Comfort orthotic
    G. Fitness orthotic
    G. Retriever
Goldenberg
    G. footplate shoe
    G. implant system
    G. Snarecoil bone marrow biopsy needle
Golden-Drain
    MMG G.-D.
Goldman
    G. bar
    G. campimeter
    G. cartilage punch
    G. curette
    G. guarded chisel
    G. guillotine nerve knife
    G. knife guide
    G. saw
    G. septal elevator
    G. septal scissors
    G. Universal nerve hook
    G. vaporizer
Goldman-Fox
    G.-F. gum scissors
    G.-F. knife
    G.-F. probe
Goldman-Kazanjian
    G.-K. nasal forceps
    G.-K. rongeur
Goldman-McNeill blepharostat

Goldmann
- G. applanation tonometer
- G. applanator
- G. capsulorrhexis forceps
- G. contact lens prism
- G. expressor
- G. goniolens
- G. knife needle
- G. macular contact lens
- G. 3-mirror gonioscopy lens
- G. multimirror lens
- G. multimirror lens implant
- G. perimeter

GoldSeal nasal mask
Goldsmith inflatable airway splint
Goldstein
- G. anterior chamber cannula
- G. anterior chamber irrigator
- G. anterior chamber syringe
- G. curette
- G. golf club spud
- G. Grasp atraumatic cervical stabilizer
- G. irrigating cannula
- G. lacrimal cannula
- G. lacrimal sac retractor
- G. lacrimal syringe
- G. Microspike approximator clamp
- G. refractor
- G. septal speculum

Goldthwait
- G. bar
- G. brace
- G. fracture appliance
- G. fracture frame

golf
- g. exercise system
- g. tee hollow titanium cannula

golf-club spud
Golgi
- G. apparatus
- G. device

Goligher
- G. modification of the Berkeley-Bonney retractor
- G. modified Berkeley-Bonney retractor
- G. speculum
- G. sternal-lift retractor

Gomco
- G. bell clamp
- G. bloodless circumcision clamp
- G. circumcision bell
- G. drain
- G. forceps
- G. suction tube
- G. thoracic drainage pump
- G. umbilical cord clamp
- G. uterine aspirator

Gomez gastric retractor
gonad shield
Gonin
- G. cautery
- G. marker

goniolaser
- Thorpe 4-mirror g.

goniolens
- Allen-Thorpe g.
- Barkan g.
- Cardona focalizing g.
- Goldmann g.
- Koeppe g.
- g. lens
- 4-mirror g.
- PF Lee pediatric g.
- single-mirror g.
- Thorpe 4-mirror g.
- Zeiss g.

goniometer
- 2-arm g.
- Bailliart g.
- Carroll finger g.
- Conzett g.
- digital g.
- electronic g.
- EOC g.
- finger g.
- Frykholm g.
- full-circle g.
- Grafco g.
- International standard g.
- Jarit finger g.
- Mottgen g.
- orthopaedic g.
- Osborne g.
- Polk finger g.
- portable electronic g.
- Sammons biplane g.
- Sceratti g.
- Sedan g.
- Thole g.
- Tomac g.
- Universal g.
- Zimmer g.

G

NOTES

Goniopora
coralline hydroxyapatite G.
gonioprism
Allen-Thorpe g.
Jacob-Swan g.
Posner diagnostic/surgical g.
goniopuncture knife
gonioscope
Barkan g.
Heine g.
Jacob-Swan g.
Maine g.
Nevada g.
Sussman 4-mirror g.
Thorpe surgical g.
Troncoso g.
University of Michigan g.
Zeiss g.
gonioscopic
g. implant
g. lens
g. prism
goniotomy
g. knife
g. knife cannula
g. needle holder
Gooch
G. mastoid retractor
G. splint
Good
G. antral rasp
G. 'N Bed wedge
G. obstetrical forceps
G. retractor
G. tonsillar scissors
Goodale-Lubin
G.-L. cardiac catheter
G.-L. cardiac device
Goode
G. Magne-Splint magnetic nasal splint
G. Trim tube
G. T-tube ventilating tube
Goodell uterine dilator
Goodhill
G. cautery
G. double-end curette
G. hook
G. knife
G. prosthesis
G. retractor
G. strut introducer
G. tonsillar forceps
Goodhill-Pynchon tonsillar suction tube
GoodKnight
G. nasal auto-PAP system
G. nasal CPAP system

Goodyear
G. tonsillar knife
G. tonsillar retractor
gooseneck
g. chisel
g. rongeur
g. snare
Goosen vascular punch
Gordh needle
Gordon
G. bead forceps
G. ciliary forceps
G. splint
G. uterine forceps
G. vulsellum forceps
Gore
G. cast liner
G. cast liner material
G. Excluder endovascular stent-graft
G. EZE-Sit valvulotome
G. Eze-Sit valvulotome kit
G. Resolut Adapt regenerative membrane
G. Smoother crucial tool
G. subcutaneous augmentation material
G. suture passer
G. thyroplasty device
G. Viatorr endoprosthesis
Gore-Tex
G.-T. AF fistula
G.-T. alloplastic material
G.-T. baffle
G.-T. bifurcated vascular graft
G.-T. cardiovascular patch
G.-T. DualMesh Plus biomaterial
G.-T. FEP-ringed vascular graft
G.-T. jump graft
G.-T. knee prosthesis
G.-T. MycroMesh Plus biomaterial
G.-T. nasal implant
G.-T. periodontal material
G.-T. peritoneal catheter
G.-T. regenerative material
G.-T. SAM facial implant
G.-T. shunt
G.-T. soft tissue patch
G.-T. stretch vascular graft
G.-T. strip
G.-T. surgical membrane
G.-T. suture
G.-T. tapered vascular graft
G.-T. vascular graft
G.-T. vascular implant
G.-T. waterproof cast liner
gorget
Anthony g.
Teale g.
Gorlin pacing catheter

Gorney
 G. dissector
 G. facelift scissors
 G. rhytidectomy scissors
 G. septal suction elevator
Gorsch
 G. needle
 G. sigmoidoscope
Gosnell scale
Gosset
 G. abdominal retractor
 G. appendectomy retractor
 G. self-retaining retractor
Gotfried percutaneous compression plating
Gott
 G. butterfly heart valve
 G. cannula
 G. implant
 G. low-profile prosthesis
 G. malleable retractor
 G. shunt
 G. tube
Gott-Daggett heart valve prosthesis
Gottschalk
 G. middle ear aspirator
 G. transverse saw
Gouffon hip pin
gouge
 Alexander mastoid g.
 Andrews g.
 Andrews mastoid g.
 antral g.
 anular g.
 AO g.
 Army bone g.
 Aufranc arthroplasty g.
 Ballenger g.
 Bishop mastoid g.
 Boley dental g.
 bone g.
 Bowen g.
 Bowls septal g.
 Buch-Gramcko g.
 Campbell arthroplasty g.
 Capner g.
 Cave scaphoid g.
 Charnley g.
 Chermel bone g.
 Cobb spinal g.
 Codman bone g.
 concave g.

Cooper spinal fusion g.
Crane g.
Dawson-Yuhl g.
Derlacki g.
Dix g.
Dontrix g.
Duray-Read g.
Freer nasal g.
Gam-Mer g.
Guy g.
Hibbs bone g.
Hibbs spinal fusion g.
hip arthroplasty g.
Hoen laminar g.
Holmes cartilage g.
Hough g.
hump g.
Jewett g.
Kezerian g.
Killian g.
Kuhnt g.
lacrimal sac g.
Lahey Clinic spinal fusion g.
Lexer g.
Lillie g.
long-handle offset g.
Lucas g.
Mannerfelt g.
Martin hip g.
mastoid g.
Metzenbaum g.
Meyerding curved g.
Moe g.
Moore spinal fusion g.
Morgenstein g.
Murphy g.
nasal g.
Neivert rocking g.
Newport cartilage g.
Nicola g.
orthopaedic g.
Parkes hump g.
Partsch bone g.
Petanguy-McIndoe g.
Pilling g.
Putti arthroplasty g.
Read g.
Rica mastoid g.
Richards-Cobb spinal g.
Richards-Hibbs g.
Rowen spinal fusion g.
Rubin g.

G

NOTES

gouge *(continued)*
- Schuknecht g.
- semicircular g.
- Sheehan g.
- SMIC mastoid g.
- Smith-Petersen bone g.
- Smith-Petersen curved g.
- spinal fusion g.
- g. spud
- spud g.
- Stacke g.
- Stagnara g.
- Stille bone g.
- Stille-Stiwer g.
- surgical g.
- swan-neck g.
- tendon g.
- Todd foreign body g.
- Trough g.
- Tworek Universal g.
- Ultra-Cut Cobb spinal g.
- Ultra-Cut Hibbs g.
- U.S. Army g.
- U X-Acto g.
- vomerine g.
- Walton foreign body g.
- Watson-Jones bone g.
- West nasal bone g.
- Zielke scoliosis g.

Gould
- G. electromagnetic flowmeter
- G. ES 1000 recorder
- G. Godard pneumotachograph
- G. intraocular implant lens
- G. PentaCath thermodilution catheter
- G. pneumotachograph
- G. polygraph
- G. polygraph gastric motility measuring device
- G. Statham pressure transducer
- G. suture

Gould-Brush 481 8-channel recorder
Gouley
- G. dilator
- G. guide
- G. tunneled urethral sound
- G. whalebone filiform catheter

Goulian
- G. blade
- G. dermatome
- G. knife

Gowen decompression tube
gown
- barrier g.
- Exami-Gown g.

GPX rotary instrument

grab
- G. Bag specimen retrieval pouch
- g. bar

grabber
- Apple laparoscopic stone g.
- meniscal suture g.
- SunVideo frame g.

Graber appliance
Grabow capsulorrhexis forceps
Grace plate 4-hole adapter
Gracey curette
gradient
- g. amplifier
- g. coil
- G. Index (GRIN)
- g. index lens
- g. sheet coil

gradiometer
- axial g.

Gradle
- G. ciliary forceps
- G. corneal trephine
- G. eyelid retractor
- G. needle electrode
- G. refractor
- G. stitch scissors

graduated
- g. catheter
- g. compression stocking
- g. electronic decelerator

Graefe
- G. cataract knife
- G. cataract spoon
- G. curved iris forceps
- G. cystotome knife
- G. dressing forceps
- G. eye-fixation forceps
- G. eye speculum
- G. flexible cystotome
- G. instrument
- G. iris hook
- G. iris knife
- G. iris needle
- G. mules
- G. scarifier
- G. strabismus hook
- G. straight iris forceps
- G. tissue forceps
- G. tissue-grasping forceps

Graether
- G. mushroom hook
- G. pupil expander
- G. refractor
- G. retractor

Graf
- G. cervical cordotomy knife
- G. stabilization system

Grafco
- G. breast pump

G. cannula
G. colostomy bag
G. cotton tip applicator
G. eye shield
G. goniometer
G. head mirror
G. ileostomy bag
G. incontinence clamp
G. laryngeal mirror
G. magnet
G. magnifying glasses
G. Martin laryngectomy tube
G. ophthalmoscope
G. otoscope
G. pelvic traction belt
G. percussion hammer
G. perineal lamp
G. pinwheel
G. seizure stick
G. tourniquet
G. tracheal tube brush
G. umbilical cord clamp
G. x-ray apron

GraFix graft
Graflex material
graft

accordion g.
G. ACE fixed-wire balloon catheter
albumin-coated vascular g.
albuminized woven Dacron tube g.
AlloDerm dermal tissue g.
AlloDerm processed tissue g.
aortic bifurcation g.
aortic tube g.
Apligraf g.
Aria prosthetic coronary artery
  bypass g.
Artegraft bovine g.
Artegraft natural collagen
  vascular g.
Atrium hemodialysis g.
autogenic g.
autogenous g.
AV Gore-Tex g.
Banks bone g.
Bard Composix mesh g.
Bard PTFE g.
batten g.
Berens g.
bifurcated vascular g.
Biobrane g.
Biocoral g.

Bioglass synthetic bone g.
Biograft g.
BioGran resorbable synthetic
  bone g.
Bionit vascular g.
BioPolyMeric femoropopliteal
  bypass g.
BioPolyMeric vascular g.
Björk-Shiley g.
Blair-Brown g.
g. board
BonePlast g.
Bonfiglio bone g.
Boplant g.
bovine pericardium dural g.
Boyd bone g.
Braun g.
Braun-Wangensteen g.
brephoplastic g.
Brett bone g.
cable g.
Calcitite bone g.
Campbell g.
Carbo-Seal cardiovascular
  composite g.
cartilage g.
g. clamp
Codivilla g.
collagen-impregnated knitted Dacron
  velour g.
compressed Ivalon patch g.
Concept GraFix g.
Cooley woven Dacron g.
coralline PBHA bone g.
coralline porous block
  hydroxyapatite bone g.
coronary artery bypass g. (CABG)
Corvita endoluminal g.
Corvita endoprosthesis stent g.
Corvita endovascular g.
Cotton cartilage g.
Cragg endoluminal g.
Creech aortoiliac g.
Crescent g.
CryoLife homograft g.
CryoLife vascular g.
cymba conchal cartilage g.
Cymetra tissue replacement g.
Dacron g.
Dacron knitted g.
Dacron onlay patch g.
Dacron preclotted knitted g.

G

NOTES

graft *(continued)*

Dacron Sauvage g.
Dacron tightly-woven g.
Dacron tube g.
Dacron tubular g.
Dacron velour g.
Dacron Weave Knit g.
Dardik umbilical vein g.
Davis g.
DeBakey Dacron g.
Dermagraft g.
diamond inlay bone g.
Diastat vascular access g.
Distaflo bypass g.
double-velour knitted g.
Douglas g.
Dragstedt g.
g. driver
DuraGen dural g.
Durapatite g.
Edwards woven Teflon aortic
  bifurcation g.
endoluminal stent g.
endovascular aortic g.
EpiFilm g.
Esser g.
expanded polytetrafluoroethylene
  vascular g.
EXS femoropopliteal bypass g.
Exxcel ePTFE soft vascular g.
Favaloro saphenous vein bypass g.
FEP-ringed Gore-Tex vascular g.
fiberglass g.
Fluoropassiv thin-wall carotid
  patch g.
glutaraldehyde-tanned bovine g.
Golaski g.
Gore-Tex bifurcated vascular g.
Gore-Tex FEP-ringed vascular g.
Gore-Tex jump g.
Gore-Tex stretch vascular g.
Gore-Tex tapered vascular g.
Gore-Tex vascular g.
GraFix g.
Grafton DBM bone g.
Graftpatch g.
Hancock pericardial valve g.
Hancock vascular g.
Hapset hydroxyapatite bone g.
Hemashield collagen-enhanced g.
Hemashield collagen-impregnated g.
Hemashield Gold Microvel knitted
  double velour g.
Hemashield Vantage vascular g.
H. Vantage g.
hybrid g.
IMA g.
Impra bypass g.
Impra Carboflo ePTFE vascular g.

Impra Flex vascular g.
Impra microporous PTFE
  vascular g.
Inclan g.
Infuse bone g.
inlay bone g.
InterGard heparin vascular g.
Interpore g.
Ionescu-Shiley vascular g.
Ivalon compressed patch g.
Jeb g.
Kebab g.
Kiel g.
Kimura cartilage g.
knitted g.
knitted Dacron velour g.
Koenig g.
Krause-Wolfe g.
latex sponge g.
Lee g.
LifeCell AlloDerm acellular
  dermal g.
Lo-Por vascular g.
Lyodura dura mater g.
lyophilized g.
mandrel g.
Mangoldt epithelial g.
Marlex mesh g.
Marqez-Gomez conjunctival g.
Martius g.
McFarland tibial g.
McMaster bone g.
Meadox Microvel arterial g.
Meadox Microvel double-velour
  Dacron g.
Meadox vascular g.
g. measuring instrument
Mediform dural g.
Medtronic AneuRx stent g.
Mersilene g.
mesh g.
methyl methacrylate g.
Meyerding bone g.
Microknit vascular g.
Microvel double velour g.
Milliknit g.
modular stent g.
Nicoll bone g.
NovaBone bone g.
NovaBone-C/M bone g.
NuVasc stent g.
Ollier g.
Ollier-Thiersch g.
OsteoGen bone g.
Ostrup vascularized rib g.
Padgett mesh skin g.
Papineau bone g.
paraffin g.
Paritene mesh g.

g. passing guide pin
patch g.
Peri-Guard vascular g.
PerioGlas synthetic bone g.
Perma-Flow coronary bypass g.
Perma-Seal dialysis access g.
Phemister onlay bone g.
pigskin g.
plasma TFE vascular g.
Plexiglas g.
Plystan g.
polyethylene g.
Poly-Plus Dacron vascular g.
polytetrafluoroethylene stent g.
polyurethane g.
polyvinyl g.
porcine g.
portacaval H g.
Possis Perma-Seal dialysis
  access g.
Powerlink endoluminal g.
Proplast g.
prosthetic g.
PTFE Gore-Tex g.
Rapidgraft radial artery g.
Rastelli g.
Red Cross g.
Repliform g.
Reverdin g.
Ruese bone g.
Sauvage Bionit g.
Sauvage Dacron g.
Sauvage filamentous velour g.
seamless g.
Seddon nerve g.
Sheen tip g.
Shiley Tetraflex vascular g.
sieve g.
Silastic g.
Silovi saphenous vein g.
Siloxane g.
Solvang g.
Speed osteotomy g.
sponge g.
spongiosa bone g.
spreader g.
St. Jude composite valve g.
strut g.
g. suction tube
Supramid g.
SurgiSis Gold hernia repair g.
Talent stent g.

tarsoconjunctival composite g.
Teflon g.
Thiersch g.
Thomas extrapolated bar g.
triple-branched stent g.
tube g.
tunnel g.
Vantage g.
Varivas loop g.
Varivas vein g.
VascuLink vascular access g.
Vascutek Gelseal vascular g.
Vascutek knitted vascular g.
Vascutek woven vascular g.
Vectra vascular access g.
velour collar g.
VenaFlow vascular g.
VertiGraft textured allograft
  bone g.
Viabahn g.
Vitagraft vascular g.
Weaveknit vascular g.
Wesolowski bypass g.
Wesolowski Teflon g.
Wheeler g.
Wolf g.
Wölfe-Krause g.
woven Dacron fabric g.
woven Dacron tube g.
XenoDerm g.
Zenith AAA endovascular g.
Zenotech g.
Graftac absorbable skin tack
Graftac-S skin stapler
GraftCyte
  G. gauze
  G. moist wound dressing
Graftmaster device
Grafton
  G. bone grafting material
  G. DBM bone graft
  G. flexible sheet
  G. moldable putty
Graftpatch graft
Graftskin
  Apligraf G.
Graham
  G. blunt hook
  G. catheter
  G. Clark silicone sponge
  G. dural hook
  G. muscle hook

G

NOTES

405

Graham *(continued)*
    G. nerve hook
    G. pediatric scissors
    G. rib contractor
    G. scalene elevator
Grahamizer II exerciser
Grams
    G. nylon nonabsorbable suture
    G. polypropylene nonabsorbable
    suture
    G. silk nonabsorbable suture
Gramsorb suture
Granberg cervical traction system
Granberry
    G. finger traction bow
    G. hyperextension fracture frame
    G. splint
    G. tongue depressor
Grand
    G. Sahara dehumidifier
    G. stand support stand
Grandon-Barraquer eye speculum
Grandview laryngoscope blade
GraNee needle
Granger articulator
Grant
    G. aortic aneurysm clamp
    G. dural separator
    G. gallbladder retractor
    G. needle holder
Grantham
    G. lobotomy electrode
    G. lobotomy needle
graphic level recorder
Graseby
    G. anesthesia pump
Grason-Stadler Inc. (GSI)
Grasp
    Babcock Endo G.
grasper
    atraumatic g.
    atraumatic curved g.
    Babcock g.
    Blakesley g.
    bowel g.
    Diamond-Jaw Babcock g.
    Endo Babcock g.
    endoscopic Babcock g.
    fenestrated bowel g.
    Glassman g.
    Hansen g.
    Hasson g.
    laparoscopic g.
    Lion's Claw g.
    Lion's Paw g.
    loose body g.
    MetraGrasp ligament g.
    mother-in-law g.
    Polaris reusable g.

    3-pronged g.
    Raptor surgical g.
    ratcheted g.
grasping
    g. biopsy forceps
    g. clamp
    g. forceps
    g. forceps tip
    G. Stitcher system
    g. tripod forceps
Graspit stone retrieval forceps
Grass
    G. electroencephalograph
    G. force displacement fluid
    collector
    G. Model S9 stimulator
    G. Neurodata system
    G. neurostimulator
    G. pressure-recording device
    G. S88 muscle stimulator
    G. visual pattern generator
Grasshopper positioner
grater
    acetabular g.
Graves
    G. bivalve speculum
    G. Britetrac vaginal speculum
    G. Coldlite speculum
    G. open-side vaginal speculum
gravity
    g. cold therapy system
    g. infusion cannula
    G. Lumbar Traction system
gravity-driven angle finder
Gravlee jet washer
Gray
    G. arterial forceps
    G. bone drill
    G. clamp
    G. cystic duct forceps
    G. flexible intramedullary reamer
    G. surgical retractor
gray-scale ultrasonogram
great
    G. Ormond Street pediatric
    tracheostomy tube
    g. toe implant
    g. toe prosthesis
green
    G. automatic corneal trephine
    g. braided suture
    g. bulldog clamp
    G. capsular forceps
    G. cataract knife
    G. chalazion forceps
    G. corneal curette
    G. corneal dissector
    G. corneal knife
    G. corneal marker

G. double spatula
G. eye calipers
G. eye needle holder
G. eye shield
G. fixation forceps
G. goiter retractor
G. iris replacer
g. laser
G. lens scoop
G. lens spatula
G. lid clamp
g. Mersilene suture
g. monofilament polyglyconate suture
G. muscle hook
G. muscle tucker
G. optical crater marker
G. pendulum scalpel
G. refractor
G. replacer spatula
g. sleeve compression device
G. strabismus hook
G. strabismus tucker
G. suction tube forceps
G. suction tube-holding clamp
G. thyroid retractor
G. tissue-grasping forceps
G. tube-holding forceps

Green-Armytage
G.-A. hemostatic forceps
G.-A. polythene rod
G.-A. reamer
G.-A. syringe

Greenberg
G. bar
G. clamp
G. Maxi-Vise adapter
G. retracting system
G. retractor frame
G. Universal retractor

Greene
G. endocervical curette
G. needle
G. placental curette
G. uterine curette

Greenfield
G. caval catheter
G. needle
G. titanium IVC filter
G. vena caval filter

Greenwald
G. Control Tip cystoscopic electrode
G. cutting loop
G. flexible endoscopic electrode
G. needle
G. retractor
G. Roth Grip-Tip suture guide
G. sound

Greenwood
G. bipolar coagulation-suction forceps
G. spinal trephine

Greer Seroma-Cath catheter
Gregg cannula
Gregory
G. baby profunda clamp
G. carotid bulldog clamp
G. external clamp
G. forceps
G. stay suture clamp
G. vascular miniature clamp

Greissinger
G. foot prosthesis
G. multi-axis joint
G. multi-axis joint implant

grenade
bulb g.

Greven alligator forceps
Grey Turner forceps
Grice
G. laparoscopic sump
G. lift
G. retractor
G. suture needle

grid
Amsler g.
Bernell g.
g. cabinet
Hirji-Callandar g.
oscillating g.
radiographic g.
Shar-Tek foot positioning g.

Grierson
G. meniscal shaver
G. tendon stripper

Grieshaber
G. blade
G. calibrated corneal trephine
G. corneal needle
G. diamond-coated forceps
G. endo-illuminator

G

NOTES

Grieshaber *(continued)*
G. flexible iris retractor
G. internal limiting membrane
  forceps
G. iris forceps
G. iris needle
G. manipulator forceps
G. microbipolar coagulator
G. needle holder
G. power injector system
G. ruby knife
G. self-retaining retractor
G. spring wire retractor
G. three-function manipulator
G. two-function manipulator
G. Ultrasharp knife
G. vertical cutting scissors
G. vitreous scissors
GRII coronary stent
GRIN
Gradient Index
GRIN lens
grinder
Sani-Grinder g.
skin g.
Grinfeld cannula
**Gringnolo-Tagliasco-Zingirian projection
campimeter**
grip
dowel g.
polly power g.
Posey g.
screw g.
Skil-Care cushion g.
Grip-Ease device
Gripp
G. squeeze ball
G. squeeze ball hand exerciser
Gripper
G. acetabular cup prosthesis
G. needle
Steeper Powered G.
Grip-Tip suture guide
GripTrack hand instrument
Grizzard subretinal cannula
Groenholm
G. lid retractor
G. refractor
Groff electrosurgical knife
Grollman
G. pigtail catheter
G. pulmonary artery-seeking
  catheter
grommet
g. bone liner
dome hole plug g.
g. drain tube
Exmoor plastics aural g.
g. myringotomy tube

Shah g.
Shepard g.
Silastic g.
Szulc g.
Twardon g.
g. ventilating tube
Groningen
G. button
G. voice prosthesis
grooved
g. director
g. silicone implant
g. silicone sponge
g. tying forceps
groover
Alway g.
Gam-Mer g.
groove suture
Groshong double-lumen catheter
Gross
G. brain spatula
G. coarctation clamp
G. dressing forceps
G. ductus spreader
G. ear curette
G. ear hook
G. ear spoon
G. ear spud
G. hyoid-cutting forceps
G. iris retractor
G. patent ductus retractor
G. probe
G. sponge forceps
G. spur crusher
Grosse-Kempf
G.-K. bone drill
G.-K. femoral nail
G.-K. locking nail
G.-K. tibial nail
Gross-Pomeranz-Watkins atrial retractor
Grotena
G. abdominal belt
G. abdominal support
G. lumbar belt
Group
Medical Marketing G. (MMG)
Grover
G. Atra-grip clamp
G. auricular appendage clamp
G. meniscotome
G. meniscus knife
Gruber
G. bougie
G. ear speculum
Gruca
G. hip reamer
G. spring
Gruca-Weiss spring

Gruenwald
    G. bayonet dressing forceps
    G. dissecting forceps
    G. dressing forceps
    G. Durogrip forceps
    G. ear forceps
    G. nasal-cutting forceps
    G. nasal-dressing forceps
    G. nasal punch
    G. pituitary rongeur
    G. retractor
    G. tissue forceps
Gruenwald-Bryant nasal-cutting forceps
Gruenwald-Jansen forceps
Gruenwald-Love
    G.-L. intervertebral disc rongeur
    G.-L. neurosurgical forceps
Grüning magnet
Grüntzig
    G. arterial balloon catheter
    G. balloon
    G. balloon angiography catheter
    G. balloon dilator
    G. femoral stiffening cannula
    G. G, S dilating catheter
    G. steerable catheter
Gruppe
    G. wire crimper
    G. wire-crimping forceps
    G. wire prosthesis
GRX-Wound gel dressing
GS-9
    GS-9 blade
    GS-9 needle
GSB
    Gschwend, Scheier, Bahler
    GSB elbow prosthesis
    GSB knee prosthesis
Gschwend, Scheier, Bahler (GSB)
G&S electroejaculator
2G-series 3-channel endoscope
GSI
    Grason-Stadler Inc.
    GSI 16 audiometer
G-suit device
G-tube
    button-type G-t.
guard
    Albany eye g.
    BandageGuard half-leg g.
    cataract knife g.
    Codman skull perforator g.

    Dignity Plus briefmates g.
    Dr. Hays bite g.
    drill g.
    ether g.
    eye knife g.
    Freedom Palm g.
    Hansen keratome g.
    intracardiac sucker g.
    Joseph g.
    keratome g.
    Kneed-It knee g.
    LASIK eye g.
    McDavid ankle g.
    McDavid hinged knee g.
    Omed vented instrument g.
    palm g.
    Peri-Guard vascular graft g.
    pin g.
    plastic mouth g.
    Platypus AV Fistula needle g.
    Pro-Designed wrist g.
    Progressive palm g.
    Rubin-Wright forceps g.
    scalpel g.
    Somatics mouth g.
    tip g.
    tooth g.
    Twist-Lock drill g.
    UltraPower bur g.
    Wright-Rubin forceps g.
guarded
    g. bur
    g. chisel
    g. irrigating cystotome
    g. osteotome
Guardian
    G. AICD
    G. ICD
    G. limb salvage system
    G. pacemaker
    G. 2-piece ostomy system
    G. stoma irrigator drain
    G. walker
guard-ring tocodynamometer
Guardsman femoral interference screw
GuardWire Plus system
Guastella/Mantovani internal nasal
    splint
Guedel
    G. airway
    G. laryngoscope
    G. laryngoscope blade

G

NOTES

Guepar II hinged knee prosthesis
Guggenheim
    G. adenoidal forceps
    G. scissors
Guglielmi detachable coil (GDC)
Guibor
    G. bubble bandage
    G. canaliculus intubation set
    G. Expo flat eye bandage
    G. lacrimal drain
    G. Silastic tube
Guidant
    G. balloon
    G. CRM pacemaker
    G. defibrillator
    G. guidewire
    G. guiding catheter
    G. Heart Rhythm Technologies Linear Ablation system
    G. lead
    G. Multi-Link Tetra coronary stent system
    G. stent
    G. Triad 3-electrode energy defibrillation system
guide
    Accu-Cut osteotomy g.
    acetabular shell g.
    ACL drill g.
    Acufex alignment drill g.
    Adapteur multifunctional drill g.
    Adson drill g.
    Adson Gigli-saw g.
    AGC dual-pivot resection g.
    Amplatz tube g.
    anterior cruciate ligament g.
    antirotation g.
    AO stopped-drill g.
    Arrow true torque wire g.
    Arthrex drill g.
    Arthrex suture anchor g.
    Asta-Cath female catheter g.
    Augustine g.
    Bailey Gigli-saw g.
    Barraquer wire g.
    barrel g.
    Blair Gigli-saw g.
    bone g.
    Borchard Gigli-saw g.
    bougie g.
    Bow & Arrow cannulated drill g.
    Brown-Roberts-Wells stereotactic g.
    BRW CT stereotaxic g.
    Bullseye femoral g.
    Caldwell g.
    cartilage g.
    catheter g.
    g. catheter
    cervical drill g.

chamfer g.
Clayman intraocular g.
Cloward drill g.
Codman g.
Concept tibial g.
Cone g.
Cook stereotactic g.
Coons interventional wire g.
Cooper basal ganglia g.
Cosman-Nashold spinal stereotaxic g.
Cottle bone g.
Cottle cartilage g.
Cottle knife g.
Crockard sublaminar wire g.
cruciate ligament g.
Cushing Gigli-saw g.
Davis g.
Davis saw g.
Delta reconstruction proximal drill g.
Demel wire g.
disposable measuring g.
distal femoral cutting g.
drill g.
eccentric drill g.
Eccentric Isotac tibial g.
Eriksson g.
Eschenbach low-vision rehabilitation g.
extramedullary alignment g.
femoral intramedullary g.
femoral notch g.
Fenelli g.
Ferciot wire g.
Fichman surgical ophthalmic g.
filiform g.
fixed-offset g.
Franzen needle g.
Frazier dural g.
Friedman knife g.
Gabbay-Frater suture g.
Galante hip g.
Ghajar g.
Gigli saw g.
Glacier ceramic 4-in-1 knee cutting g.
glenoid drill g.
Goldman knife g.
Gouley g.
Greenwald Roth Grip-Tip suture g.
Grip-Tip suture g.
guidepin g.
gutter g.
Guyon curved catheter g.
handheld drill g.
Harrison forked-type strut g.
Harris precoat neck osteotomy g.
House strut g.

House wire g.
humeral cutting g.
IM/EM tibial resection g.
Impingement-Free tibial g.
Interson biopsy needle g.
intramedullary g.
Iowa pudendal needle g.
Iowa trumpet needle g.
Jonesco bone wire g.
Joseph saw g.
Kazanjian g.
Lebsche saw g.
LeFort filiform g.
Levin drill g.
ligature g.
Lipscomb-Anderson drill g.
long nail-mounted drill g.
Lunderquist extra-stiff wire g.
Lunderquist-Ring torque wire g.
Maggi disposable biopsy needle g.
measuring g.
Modny g.
Morrissey Gigli-saw g.
Mumford Gigli-saw g.
Navigus trajectory g.
Neivert knife g.
nut alignment g.
Oshukova collapsible bougie g.
Palmer cruciate ligament g.
patellar drill g.
patellar reamer g.
patellar resection g.
picket fence g.
Pilotip catheter g.
Pilot suturing g.
pin g.
Poppen Gigli saw g.
protector g.
ProTrac ACL tibial g.
pudendal needle g.
punch g.
Rand-Wells
 pallidothalmomectomy g.
Raney Gigli-saw g.
rear-entry ACL drill g.
Reece osteotomy g.
Rhinelander g.
Richards drill g.
Roth Grip-Tip suture g.
Savary-Gilliard wire g.
Scanlan ligature g.
scaphoid screw g.

Schlesinger Gigli-saw g.
Scott-RCE osteotomy g.
Slick stylette endotracheal tube g.
Slidewire extension g.
Stader pin g.
stationary angle g.
Stewart cruciate ligament g.
Stille Gigli-saw g.
stoma-centering g.
straight catheter g.
Strategy coronary wire g.
surgical instrument g.
suture g.
targeting drill g.
Tefcor core wire g.
TEGwire g.
telescopic view g.
telescoping g.
tibial g.
tibial cutter g.
tip-deflecting wire g.
tissue anchor g.
Todd stereotaxic g.
Todd-Wells stereotactic g.
Todt-Heyer cannula g.
TraceHybrid wire g.
Tracer hybrid wire g.
trumpet needle g.
tunnel drill g.
Tworek screw g.
Urbanski strut g.
Van Buren catheter g.
Vista Brite tip IG introducer g.
Wilson-Cook Protector wire g.
Wilson-Cook Tracer wire g.
wire g.
g. wire
Guidefather catheter
guideline
Böhler g.
Letournel g.
guidepin
AO g.
g. guide
guidewire, guide wire
ACS Amplatz g.
ACS Hi-Torque Balance
 middleweight g.
ACS Hi-Torque Iron Man g.
ACS LIMA g.
Amplatz g.
Amplatz Super Stiff g.

G

NOTES

guidewire *(continued)*
  angled g.
  angle-tip g.
  argon g.
  Athlete coronary g.
  Bard Commander PTCA g.
  beaded g.
  Beath g.
  Bentson g.
  Bentson floppy-tip g.
  Bentson Glidewire g.
  Bentson straight g.
  Bentson-type Glidewire g.
  CannuFlex g.
  Cardiometrics FloWire g.
  catheter g.
  Choice PT g.
  Commander angioplasty g.
  Commander PTCA g.
  Conceptus g.
  Conceptus Robus g.
  ControlWire g.
  Cook straight g.
  Coons Super Stiff long-tip g.
  Cope mandril g.
  Cor-Flex g.
  Crosswire nitinol hydrophilic-
    coated g.
  Crosswire PTCA g.
  Dasher g.
  delivery g.
  Doppler FloWire g.
  Doppler-tipped angioplasty g.
  drill-tipped g.
  Eder-Puestow g.
  ERCP g.
  exchange g.
  Extra Sport coronary g.
  extra-stiff g.
  extra-support g.
  FasTrac hydrophilic-coated g.
  FlexFinder g.
  flexible g.
  Flex Tip g.
  FloMap g.
  floppy g.
  floppy-tipped g.
  FloWire g.
  FloWire Doppler g.
  fluid-filled pressure monitoring g.
  Geenan Endotorque g.
  Glidewire g.
  Glidewire Gold surgical g.
  Glidewire hydrophilic coated g.
  Guidant g.
  Headliner g.
  heparin-coated g.
  Hi-Per Flex exchange g.
  Hi-Torque Balance middleweight g.

  Hi-Torque Cross-It g.
  Hi-Torque Flex-T g.
  Hi-Torque Floppy II g.
  Hi-Torque Intermediate g.
  Hi-Torque Memcore g.
  Hi-Torque Spartacore g.
  Hi-Torque Steel core g.
  Hi-Torque Supra Core g.
  Hi-Torque Wiggle g.
  HPC g.
  Hydronol hydrophilic g.
  hydrophilic polymer-coated
    steerable g.
  Hydro Plus coated g.
  Hyperflex flexible g.
  HyTek g.
  inclination g.
  Intercept Vascular g.
  J g.
  Jagwire g.
  J exchange g.
  Jometrics SmartWire pressure g.
  J Rosen g.
  J-tipped g.
  Kadir Hi-Torque g.
  Lubriglide coated g.
  Lumenator injectable g.
  Lumina g.
  Lunderquist g.
  Magic Torque g.
  Magnum g.
  MAPwire J-tip g.
  Medi-Tech g.
  Microvasive stiff piano wire g.
  Mirage g.
  movable-core g.
  Mustang steerable g.
  Newton LLT g.
  New Yorker g.
  nitinol g.
  nonconductive g.
  Pathfinder g.
  PDT g.
  Phantom cardiac g.
  Placer g.
  Platinum Plus g.
  Preceder interventional g.
  Premo g.
  Pressure Guard g.
  Prima laser g.
  Puestow g.
  QuickSilver hydrophilic-coated g.
  Radiofocus g.
  Reflex SuperSoft steerable g.
  Roadrunner PC g.
  Rosen J-guide g.
  Rotacs g.
  RotaWire floppy gold g.
  Safe-Steer g.

safety g.
Saf-T J g.
Schwarten LP g.
Seeker g.
Segway hydrophilic g.
Sensor surgical g.
silk g.
SilverSpeed hydrophilic g.
slipper-tipped g.
Sniper Elite hydrophilic g.
Sof-T g.
solid-core g.
Sones g.
spring-tipped g.
stainless steel g.
steerable angioplastic g.
stiff g.
Storq g.
straight g.
Superselector Y-K g.
super-stiff g.
Surpass g.
TAD tapered steerable g.
Taper g.
tapered torque g.
Teflon-coated g.
Terumo g.
Terumo hydrophilic g.
Terumo/Meditech g.
TherOx infusion g.
tip-deflecting g.
TomCat PTCA g.
Ultra-Select nitinol PTCA g.
USCI Hyperflex g.
variable stiffness g.
VascuLink vascular access g.
Veriflex g.
VeriSoft steerable g.
VertiGraft extured allograft bone g.
WaveWire g.
WaveWire pressure g.
Whisper g.
Wholey Hi-Torque floppy g.
Wholey Hi-Torque modified J g.
Wiggle coronary g.
Zebra exchange g.
guiding
g. cannula
g. catheter
coronary sinus g. (CSG)

Guilford
G. brace
G. scissors
Guilford-Wright
G.-W. bivalve speculum
G.-W. bur
G.-W. clip
G.-W. crurotomy knife
G.-W. curette
G.-W. cutting block
G.-W. double-edged knife
G.-W. drum elevator
G.-W. duckbill elevator
G.-W. elevator knife
G.-W. fenestrometer
G.-W. flap knife
G.-W. forceps
G.-W. incudostapedial knife
G.-W. meatal retractor
G.-W. middle ear instrument
G.-W. prosthesis
G.-W. roller knife
G.-W. scissors
G.-W. stapes pick
G.-W. suction tube
G.-W. Teflon wire piston
G.-W. wire cutter
guillotine
g. adenotome
Ballenger-Sluder g.
Charnley femoral inlay g.
g. cutting tip
Giertz rib g.
g. knife
Lilienthal rib g.
Myles g.
Poppers tonsillar g.
Sauerbruch rib g.
g. scissors
Sluder-Sauer tonsillar g.
Sluder tonsillar g.
SMIC tonsillar g.
tonsillar g.
Van Osdel g.
g. vitrectomy instrument
Zipster rib g.
guillotine-type cutter
Guimaraes
G. implantable contact lens manipulator
G. ophthalmic flap spatula
Guiot-Talairach construct

NOTES

G

413

Guisez tube
Guist
G. enucleation hemostat
G. enucleation scissors
G. fixation forceps
G. speculum
G. sphere eye implant
Guist-Black eye speculum
Guist-Bloch speculum
Gulani
G. globe stabilizer and flap restrainer
G. ophthalmic edge lifter
G. triple function laser-assisted intrastromal keratomileusis cannula
G. triple function LASIK cannula
Gulden red and green slip-ins
Guldmann Overhead Trac system
Guleke bone rongeur
Gullstrand
G. lens
G. lens loupe
G. ophthalmoscope
G. slit lamp
G. slit-lamp
G. 6-surface eye model
Gullstrand-Zeiss lens loupe
gum
g. elastic bougie introducer
G. Machine oral irrigator
gun
Arthrex meniscal dart g.
automated biopsy g.
Bard Biopty g.
BD g.
Biofix arrow g.
biopsy g.
Biopty biopsy g.
BioStinger g.
bone injection g.
caulking g.
Cobe staple g.
Cook biopsy g.
coring biopsy g.
electron g.
entor injector g.
Harris cement g.
Heaf g.
heat g.
introducer g.
Lidge cement g.
Messing root canal g.
Miltex g.
Moss T-anchor needle introducer g.
Promag 2.2 biopsy g.
Reflex g.
rivet g.
seam-sealer g.
skin g.

spring-loaded biopsy g.
surgical stapling g.
Gunderson
G. bone forceps
G. muscle recession forceps
Gundry cannula
Gunnar-Hey roller forceps
Gunning jaw splint
GunSlinger shoulder orthosis
Gunston-Hult knee prosthesis
Gunston polycentric knee prosthesis
Günther
G. catheter
G. Tulip vena caval MReye filter
G. Tulip vena caval MRI filter
Guppe forceps
gurney
SafetySURE transfer g.
Gusberg
G. cervical cone biopsy curette
G. endocervical biopsy curette
G. endocervical biopsy punch
G. hysterectomy clamp
G. uterine forceps
Gussenbauer
G. clamp
G. suture
Gustilo knee prosthesis
Gustilo-Kyle
G.-K. cementless total hip arthroplasty
G.-K. total hip
G.-K. total knee
gut
g. clamp
g. suture
Gutgemann
G. auricular appendage clamp
G. auricular appendage forceps
Gutglass
G. hemostat
G. hemostatic cervical forceps
Guthrie
G. card
G. fixation hook
G. iris hook
G. retractor
G. skin hook
Guthrie-Smith
G.-S. apparatus
G.-S. bed
Gutierrez-Najar grasping forceps
gutta-percha point
gutter
g. guide
G. speculum
Guttmann
G. obstetrical retractor

G. vaginal retractor
G. vaginal speculum
Guy
G. gouge
G. tenotomy knife
Guyon
G. curettage
G. curved catheter guide
G. dilating bougie
G. dilating sound
G. dilator
G. exploratory bougie
G. kidney clamp
G. ureteral catheter
G. urethral sound
G. vessel clamp
Guyon-Béniqué urethral sound
Guyon-Péan vessel clamp
Guyton
G. corneal transplant trephine
G. electrode
G. scissors
G. suturing forceps
Guyton-Clark fragment forceps
Guyton-Friedenwald suture
Guyton-Lundsgaard
G.-L. cataract knife
G.-L. keratome
G.-L. scalpel
G.-L. sclerotome
Guyton-Maumenee speculum
Guyton-Minkowski potential acuity meter
Guyton-Noyes fixation forceps
Guyton-Park eye speculum
Guzman-Blanco epiglottic retractor
Gwathmey
G. hook
G. suction tube
G/W Heel Lift, Inc. orthosis
Gx-99 vibratory endermatherapie system
gym
g. ball
hand g.
limb g.
Total G.
Zuni g.
Gymnastik ball

Gymnic
G. ball
G. Plus ball
Gyn-A-Lite vaginal speculum
Gynaspir vacuum curettage
Gynecare
G. tension-free vaginal tape system
G. Thermachoice uterine balloon therapy system
G. Verascope hysteroscopy system
G. X-Tract tissue morcellator
Gynefold
G. prolapse pessary
G. retrodisplacement pessary
GyneLase diode laser
GyneSys Dx diagnostic catheter
Gynex
G. angle hook
G. Emmett tenaculum
G. endospeculum
G. extended-reach needle
G. iris hook
Gynkotek pump
GynoSampler
G. endometrial aspirator
G. endometrial curette
Gyno Sampler endometrial sampling device
Gynoscann cell sampler
Gynos perineometer
Gypsona
G. cast
G. plaster dressing
G. rapid-setting cast material
Gyroscan
G. ACS NT MRI scanner
G. HP Philips 15S whole-body system
G. NT-series MR scanner
Philips ACS-NT G.
G. S-series scanner
G. superconducting MRI
G. T5-NT MR scanner
T Philips ACS-II G.
Gyrotwister laboratory shaker
Gyrus endourology system
Gysi articulator

G

NOTES

H-1 MR spectroscopy
HA
    hyaluronic acid
      HA adhesive
      HA membrane
      Proplast HA
Haab
    H. after-cataract knife
    H. eye knife
    H. eye magnet
    H. knife needle
    H. scleral resection knife
Haag-Streit
    H.-S. 900 cobalt blue filter
    H.-S. distometer
    H.-S. Endo-Set
    H.-S. keratometer
    H.-S. ophthalmometer
    H.-S. pacemeter
    H.-S. slit lamp
Haberer
    H. gastrointestinal forceps
    H. spatula
Haberer-Gili forceps
Haberman
    H. feeder
    H. suction elevator
HA-biointegrated dental implant system
Hackett sacroiliac cinch belt
HA-coated
    HA-c. hip implant
    HA-c. Micro-Vent implant
    HA-c. root-form dental implant
    HA-c. stem
Hadeco
    H. ES100VX mini Doppler
    H. intraoperative Doppler
    H. MiniDop Doppler
Hader
    H. aneroid sphygmomanometer
    H. bar clip
    H. dental attachment
    H. implant bar
Hadfield hand board
Hadlock table
Hadow balloon
Haefliger cleaver
Haeggstrom antral trocar
Haemolite autologous blood recovery system
Haemonetics Cell Saver
Haemoson ultrasound Doppler
Haenig irrigating scissors

Haering
    H. esophageal prosthesis
    H. tube
Haftelast self-adhering bandage
Hagan surface suction tube
Hagar probe
Hagedorn
    H. needle holder
    H. operation suture needle
Hagenbarth clip-applying forceps
Hagfer needle holder
Hagie
    H. pin
    H. wrench
Haglund
    H. plaster scissors
    H. plaster spreader
    H. vaginal speculum
Haglund-Stille
    H.-S. plaster spreader
    H.-S. vaginal speculum
Hagner
    H. bag catheter
    H. hemostatic bag
    H. urethral bag
Hague cataract lamp
Hahn
    H. bone nail
    H. cannula
    H. screw
Hahnenkratt
    H. aspirator
    H. dental clasp
    H. lingual bar
    H. matrix band
    H. orthodontic wire
    H. retainer
    H. root canal pin
    H. root canal post
    H. temporary crown
Haid
    H. cervical plate
    H. Universal bone plate
Haidinger brush
Haifa camera
Haig-Ferguson obstetrical forceps
Haight
    H. baby rib spreader
    H. pediatric rib spreader
    H. pulmonary retractor
    H. rib retractor
    H. rib spreader
Haight-Finochietto
    H.-F. rib retractor
    H.-F. rib spreader

H

Haig obstetrical forceps
Haik eye implant
Haiman tonsillar electrode
Haimovici arteriotomy scissors
Haines arachnoid dissector
hair transplant punch
Haitz canaliculus punch
Hajek
    H. antral punch forceps
    H. antral retractor
    H. antral rongeur
    H. cannula
    H. downbiting rongeur
    H. elevator
    H. lip retractor
    H. mallet
    H. septal chisel
    H. upbiting rongeur
Hajek-Ballenger
    H.-B. septal dissector
    H.-B. septal elevator
Hajek-Claus rongeur
Hajek-Koffler
    H.-K. bone punch forceps
    H.-K. laminectomy rongeur
    H.-K. reversible punch
    H.-K. sphenoidal forceps
    H.-K. sphenoidal punch
    H.-K. sphenoidal rongeur
Hajek-Skillern sphenoidal punch
Hakansson bone rongeur
Hakansson-Olivecrona rongeur
Hakim
    H. catheter
    H. high-pressure valve
    H. precision valve
    H. programmable valve
    H. reservoir
    H. shunt
    H. shunt reprogramming device
    H. tube
    H. valve system
Hakim-Cordis pump
Hakko Dwellcath catheter
Hakler forceps
Halberg
    H. clip
    H. contact lens forceps
    H. indirect ophthalmoscope
    H. trial clip occluder
Haldane-Priestley tube
Haldane tube
Hale obstetrical forceps
half
    h. Jimmie
    h. ring
half-and-half nail
half-circle plate
half-curved clamp

half-intensity needle
half-moon retractor
Halifax
    H. interlaminar clamp
    H. placement forceps
    H. wrench
Hall
    H. air drill
    H. arthrotome
    H. bone bur
    H. dermatome
    H. double-hole spinal stapler
    H. driver
    H. intrauterine device
    H. mandibular implant system
    H. mastoid bur
    H. Micro-Aire drill
    H. modified Moe hook
    H. modular acetabular reamer system
    H. Neurairtome drill
    H. Orthairtome drill
    H. Osteon drill system
    H. Osteon irrigation kit
    H. power drill
    H. prosthetic heart valve
    H. sacral anchor
    H. sagittal saw
    H. screwdriver
    H. spinal screw
    H. step-down drill
    H. Surgairtome II drill
    H. surgical drill
    H. valve
    H. valvulotome
    H. Versipower drill
    H. Versipower oscillating saw
    H. Versipower reamer
    H. Versipower reciprocating saw
Hallach comedo extractor
Hallauer glasses
Hallberg forceps
Hall-Chevalier stripper
Hall-Dundar drill
Halle
    H. bone curette
    H. chisel
    H. dural knife
    H. ethmoid curette
    H. infant nasal speculum
    H. septal elevator
    H. septal needle
    H. sinus curette
    H. trigeminus knife
    H. vascular spatula
Hall-effect strain transducer
Halle-Tieck nasal speculum
Hall-Fish Hyfrecator
Hallin carotid endarterectomy shunt

Hall-Kaster
    H.-K. heart valve
    H.-K. tilting-disc valve prosthesis
Hallman tunneler
Hall-Morris biphase screw
Hallpike-Blackmore ear microscope
Hall-Relton frame
hallux
    h. forceps
    h. valgus orthosis
halo
    Ace low-profile MR h.
    Ace Mark III h.
    h. brace
    Bremer h.
    Brown-Roberts-Wells head ring h.
    H. catheter
    h. cervical orthosis
    h. cervical traction system
    H. CO_2 laser system
    h. fracture frame
    h. gravity traction device
    h. head frame
    h. hoop device
    Houston h.
    Lerman noninvasive h.
    h. retractor
    h. traction
    h. vest
Halocath catheter
halogen
    h. coaxial ophthalmoscope
    h. dual light source
    h. lamp
    h. otoscope
halo-Ilizarov distraction instrumentation
halo-ring adapter
Haloscale respirometer
haloscope
    phase-difference h.
halothane analyzer
halo-vest orthosis
Halsey
    H. mosquito forceps
    H. nail scissors
    H. needle
    H. Vital needle holder
Halsey-Webster needle holder
Halsted
    H. arterial forceps
    H. curved mosquito clamp
    H. curved mosquito forceps

    H. hemostatic mosquito forceps
    H. mattress suture
    H. Micro-Line arterial forceps
    H. mosquito hemostat
    H. mules
    H. strabismus scissors
    H. straight mosquito clamp
Halsted-Swanson tendon-passing forceps
halter
    Cerva crane h.
    deluxe head h.
    DePuy head h.
    Diskard head h.
    disposable head h.
    Forrester head h.
    head h.
    Repro head h.
    standard head h.
    TMJ h.
    Upper 7 model head h.
    Zimfoam head h.
    Zyler head h.
Hamas upper limb prosthesis
hamate finder
Hamblin minimagnet
Hamburger-Brennan-Mahorner thyroid retractor
Hamby
    H. brain retractor
    H. clip-applying forceps
    H. right-angle clip applier
    H. rod
    H. twist drill
    H. wire threader
Hamby-Hibbs retractor
Hamer scalpel
Hamilton
    H. bandage
    H. deep-surgery forceps
    H. pelvic traction screw tractor
    H. tongue depressor
    H. ventilator
Hamilton-Forewater amniotomy hook
Hamilton-Steward catheter
Hamilton-Thorn motility analyzer
Hamm
    H. fulgurating electrode
    H. resectoscope electrode
hammer
    Babinski percussion h.
    Berliner neurological percussion h.
    Buck neurological percussion h.

NOTES

H

hammer *(continued)*
    Cloward h.
    Dejerine percussion h.
    Epstein neurological h.
    h. forceps
    fork h.
    Gerzog bone h.
    Grafco percussion h.
    Hibbs h.
    House tapping h.
    intranasal h.
    Kirk bone h.
    Kirk orthopaedic h.
    Küntscher h.
    Millet test h.
    Monreal reflex h.
    neurological percussion h.
    orthopaedic h.
    percussion h.
    Quisling intranasal h.
    Rabiner neurological h.
    reflex h.
    Rica bone h.
    slide h.
    sliding h.
    SMIC bone h.
    Smith-Petersen h.
    surgical h.
    tapping h.
    Taylor reflex percussion h.
    Traube neurological h.
    Tromner percussion h.
    Wartenberg neurological h.
    Williger h.
Hammer mini-tubular external fixation system
Hammersmith mitral valve prosthesis
hammer-type acupuncture needle
Hamming-Hahn filter
hammock
    h. bandage
    h. dressing
    Mersilene gauze h.
Hammond
    H. alloy
    H. orthodontic splint
    H. winged retractor blade
Hamou
    H. colpomicrohysteroscope
    H. contact microhysteroscope
    H. cystoscope
    H. endoscope
    H. hysteroflator
    H. hysteroscope
    H. microcolpohysteroflator
    H. microhysteroflator
Hampton
    H. electrosurgical unit
    H. needle holder

Hamrick
    H. suction dissector
    H. suction elevator
Hanafee catheter
Hanau
    H. 130-21 articulator
    H. facebow
Hancke/Vilmann biopsy handle
Hancock
    H. aortic valve prosthesis
    H. bioprosthetic heart valve
    H. coronary perfusion catheter
    H. embolectomy catheter
    H. fiberoptic catheter
    H. heterograft heart valve
    H. hydrogen detection catheter
    H. II aortic bioprosthesis
    H. II mitral bioprosthesis
    H. II porcine bioprosthesis
    H. II tissue valve
    H. luminal electrophysiologic recording catheter
    H. mitral valve prosthesis
    H. modified orifice valve
    H. MO II aortic bioprosthesis
    H. MO II porcine bioprosthesis
    H. pericardial valve graft
    H. porcine heterograft
    H. porcine valve
    H. temporary cardiac pacing wire
    H. thermodilution catheter
    H. vascular graft
    H. wedge-pressure catheter
hand
    h. block
    h. brace
    Brueckmann lead h.
    h. cock-up snare
    h. cock-up splint
    h. cone
    h. cuff
    h. dermatome
    h. drill
    h. exercise ball
    Freedom arthritis support for h.
    h. gym
    H. Helper hand exerciser
    lead h.
    Myobock artificial h.
    Naeser laser home treatment program for the h.
    pediatric retractor malleable wire h.
    h. retractor
    h. trephine
    Vaduz h.
    h. volumeter
    Winter Helping H.

Hand-Aid
>   H.-A. arterial wrist support
>   H.-A. strapping material

HandClens instant hand sanitizer
hand-control cautery
hand-crimped stent
Handeze therapeutic support glove
handheld
>   h. cautery
>   h. diagnostic tympanometer
>   h. Doppler probe
>   h. drill guide
>   h. dynamometer
>   h. exploring electrode probe
>   h. eye magnet
>   h. fundus camera
>   h. Hruby lens
>   h. mapping probe
>   h. nebulizer
>   h. pulse oximeter
>   h. retractor
>   h. rotary prism
>   h. trephine

HandiCare adult disposable pant and pad system
Handi-Cath catheter kit
Handisizer exercise device
Handisol phototherapy device
handle
>   autopsy h.
>   Bard-Parker h.
>   Barron scalpel h.
>   Barton traction h.
>   bayonet h.
>   Beaver h.
>   B-P surgical h.
>   Cardioblate BP surgical h.
>   Charnley brace h.
>   Cloward dowel h.
>   Corwin knife h.
>   Cottle protected knife h.
>   cross bar h.
>   double-hinge cervical retractor h.
>   Dynagrip blade h.
>   ear knife h.
>   Elliot trephine h.
>   endoscopic electrode h.
>   Gigli-saw h.
>   Hancke/Vilmann biopsy h.
>   Hardy lateral knife h.
>   hexagonal h.
>   House myringotomy knife h.

>   Huber forceps h.
>   insulated knife h.
>   Klein-Delrin Luer-Lok h.
>   knife h.
>   knurled h.
>   Luikart-Bill traction h.
>   Lynch laryngeal knife h.
>   Marlow Primus h.
>   Ortho-Grip silicone rubber h.
>   Parker-Bard h.
>   protected knife h.
>   Rusch laryngoscope h.
>   safety h.
>   saw h.
>   scalpel blade h.
>   Stiwer scalpel h.
>   Strully Gigli-saw h.
>   surgical h.
>   Thera-Band h.
>   Therap-Loop door h.
>   Tip-Trol h.
>   T-pin h.
>   traction h.
>   tympanum perforator h.
>   Universal chuck h.
>   V. Mueller Tip-Trol h.
>   V. Mueller Universal h.

handleless clamp
HandMaster system
hand-mounted stent
handpiece
>   A-Dec h.
>   Avit h.
>   Cavitron I&A h.
>   Chayes h.
>   ClearCut 2 electrosurgical h.
>   collimated beam h.
>   CooperVision I&A h.
>   CUSA system 200 straight autoclavable h.
>   Densco dental h.
>   DermaStat h.
>   Doriot h.
>   DynaSurg electric h.
>   Emesco h.
>   Endo-Gripper endodontic h.
>   Hexascan computerized dermatology h.
>   Imperator h.
>   infusion h.
>   irrigation-aspiration h.
>   Kaessman h.

NOTES

H

421

handpiece *(continued)*
    KaVo dental h.
    Kelman irrigating h.
    Kerr M4 safety h.
    Kurtin h.
    Lares dental h.
    Lightning high-speed vitrectomy h.
    Litton dental h.
    McIntyre infusion h.
    Medtronic ClearCut 2 h.
    MicroSeal phaco h.
    Microstat h.
    M4 safety h.
    Neuroguide optical h.
    Nu-Abrasion microdermabrasion h.
    oral surgery h.
    Packer Wick extrusion h.
    phacoemulsification h.
    ProFinesse II ultrasonic h.
    reciprocating power h.
    Revelation h.
    rotosteotome rotary h.
    Sabra OMS 45 h.
    Sonic Air h.
    StraightShot Magnum h.
    SureScan scanning h.
    Surgitek h.
    Titan slow-speed h.
HandPort
    H. device
    H. laparoscopic instrument
hand-roller
    Lundy tubing h.-r.
Hands Free knee retractor system
Hands-Off thermodilution cardiac
  catheter
1-hand speculum
hand-sutured closure
Handy
    H. II articulator
    H. non-mydriatic video fundus
      camera
Handy-Buck extension tractor
HandyStep electronic repeating pipette
Haney needle driver
Hanger
    H. ComfortFlex socket system
    H. prosthesis
hanger
    Adjusta-Rak h.
    Conveen bag h.
hanging cast sling
Hank-Dennen obstetrical forceps
Hankins lucite ovoid
Hanks-Bradley uterine dilator
Hanks uterine dilator
Hanley-McDermott pelvimeter

Hannahan
    H. bur
    H. forceps
Hanna trephine
Hann filter
Hannon endometrial curette
Hannover needle holder
Hans
    H. Rudolph full face mask
    H. Rudolph 3-way valve
Hansa ophthalmic speculum
Hansatome
    Chiron H.
    H. microkeratome
Hanscom transscleral cannula
Hansen
    H. grasper
    H. keratome
    H. keratome guard
    H. ophthalmic shell
Hansen-Street
    H.-S. anchor plate
    H.-S. pin
    H.-S. self-broaching nail
    H.-S. solid intramedullary nail
Hanslik patellar prosthesis
Hanson speed bracket
Hapad
    H. felt shoe insert
    H. longitudinal metatarsal arch pad
    H. metatarsal insole
Hapex bioactive material
Happy podiatric bur
Hapset
    H. bone graft plaster material
    H. hydroxyapatite bone graft
    H. hydroxyapatite bone graft
      plaster
haptic
    h. area implant
    h. area lens
    Coburn h.
    modified C-loop h.
    modified J-loop h.
    h. plate lens
    PMMA h.
    Slant h.
haptic-fixated intraocular lens
hard
    h. contact lens
    h. mallet
    h. palate retractor
    h. socket
    h. tissue replacement (HTR)
    h. tissue replacement-malleable
      facial implant (HTR-MFI)
    h. tissue replacement-patient
      matched implant (HTR-PMI)
    h. x-ray imaging spectrometer

Hardesty
- H. tendon hook
- H. tenotomy hook

Hardt-Delima osteotome

Hardy
- H. aluminum crutch
- H. bayonet curette
- H. bayonet dressing forceps
- H. bayonet enucleator
- H. bayonet neurosurgical bipolar forceps
- H. bivalve speculum
- H. hypophysial curette
- H. implant fork
- H. lateral knife handle
- H. lensometer
- H. lip retractor
- H. microbipolar forceps
- H. microdissector
- H. microsurgical enucleator
- H. modification of Bronson-Ray curette
- H. nasal bivalve speculum
- H. pituitary dissector
- H. pituitary spoon
- H. 3-prong fork
- H. rongeur
- H. sellar punch
- H. suction tube
- H. transsphenoidal mirror

Hardy-Duddy
- H.-D. speculum
- H.-D. vaginal retractor

Hardy-Rand-Rittler plate

Hardy-Sella pump

Hare
- H. compact traction splint
- H. splint device
- H. traction device

harelip
- h. forceps
- h. needle
- h. traction bow

Har-el pharyngeal tube

Hargin antral trocar

Hargis periosteal elevator

Hariri-Heifetz microsurgical system

Harken
- H. auricle clamp
- H. auricle forceps
- H. ball heart valve
- H. cardiovascular forceps
- H. erysiphake
- H. heart needle
- H. prosthesis
- H. prosthetic valve
- H. rib retractor
- H. rib spreader
- H. valvulotome

Harken-Cooley forceps

Harken-Starr valve

Harloff cart

Harlow
- H. plate
- H. Wood spinal biopsy needle

Harm
- H. cage
- H. posterior cervical plate

Harman
- H. eye dressing
- H. fixation forceps

Harmon chisel

harmonic
- h. attenuation table
- H. Scalpel II curved shears
- h. scissors

Harmonie
- H. Classic Plus brief
- H. underpad

Harms
- H. corneal forceps
- H. microtying forceps
- H. trabeculotome
- H. trabeculotomy probe
- H. tying forceps
- H. utility forceps
- H. vessel forceps

Harms-Moss anterior thoracic instrumentation

Harms-Tubingen tying forceps

harness
- Heart Hugger sternum support h.
- Kicker Pavlik h.
- Pavlik h.
- Rhino Cruiser Pavlik h.
- Rhino Kicker Pavlik h.
- SecureEasy endotracheal h.
- Wheaton Pavlik h.
- Zuni h.

Harold
- H. Crowe drill
- H. Hayes eustachian bougie

Harpenden
- H. handgrip dynamometer

NOTES

H

Harpenden *(continued)*
- H. skinfold calipers
- H. stadiometer

Harper
- H. cervical laminectomy punch
- H. periosteal elevator

Harpoon suture anchor
Harrah lung clamp
Harrell Y stent
Harrington
- H. bladder retractor
- H. Britetrac retractor
- H. clamp forceps
- H. deep surgical scissors
- H. distraction instrumentation
- H. dual square-ended rod
- H. erysiphake
- H. flat wrench
- H. hook clamp
- H. hook driver
- H. lung-grasping forceps
- H. pedicle hook
- H. protractor
- H. rod
- H. rod and hook system
- H. rod instrumentation
- H. spinal elevator
- H. spinal instrumentation
- H. splanchnic retractor
- H. spreader
- H. strut
- H. sympathectomy retractor
- H. thoracic forceps
- H. tonometer
- H. vulsellum forceps

Harrington-Carmalt clamp
Harrington-Deaver retractor
Harrington-Flocks multiple pattern
Harrington-Kostuik distraction device
Harrington-Mayo
- H.-M. scissors
- H.-M. tissue forceps

Harrington-Mixter
- H.-M. thoracic clamp
- H.-M. thoracic forceps

Harrington-Pemberton sympathectomy retractor
Harris
- H. band
- H. brace-type reamer
- H. broach
- H. catheter
- H. cemented hip prosthesis
- H. cement gun
- H. center-cutting acetabular reamer
- H. condylocephalic nail
- H. condylocephalic rod
- H. dissector
- H. femoral head gauge

- H. footprint mat
- H. Hemi Arm sling
- H. implant
- H. medullary nail
- H. Micromini prosthesis
- H. modified J-loop intraocular lens
- H. plate
- H. precoat neck osteotomy guide
- H. precoat prosthesis
- H. protrusio shell
- H. rigid quadriped intraocular lens
- H. separator
- H. snare
- H. splint sling
- H. suture-carrying forceps
- H. tonsillar knife
- H. trephine
- H. uterine injector (HUI)
- H. wire tightener

Harris-Galante (HG)
- H.-G. cup
- H.-G. I porous-coated acetabular component
- H.-G. porous (HGP)
- H.-G. porous hip prosthesis

Harris-Kronner
- H.-K. uterine manipulator
- H.-K. uterine manipulator-injector (HUMI)

Harrison
- H. bone-holding forceps
- H. capsular knife
- H. chalazion retractor
- H. forked-type strut guide
- H. implant
- H. interlocked mesh prosthesis
- H. myringoplasty knife
- H. suture-removing scissors
- H. tucker

Harrison-Nicolle polypropylene peg
Harrison-Shea
- H.-S. curette
- H.-S. knife

Harris-Sinskey microlens hook
Harris-Smith anterior interbody drill
Hart
- H. extension finger splint
- H. pediatric 3-mirror lens

Hartinger Coincidence refractionometer
Hartley
- H. implant
- H. mammary prosthesis

Hartmann
- H. adenoidal curette
- H. alligator forceps
- H. biopsy punch
- H. bone rongeur
- H. clamp
- H. dewaxer speculum

H. ear-dressing forceps
H. ear polyp forceps
H. ear punch
H. ear rongeur
H. ear speculum
H. eustachian catheter
H. hemostat
H. hemostatic mosquito forceps
H. knife
H. mastoid rongeur
H. mosquito hemostatic forceps
H. nasal conchotome
H. nasal-cutting forceps
H. nasal-dressing forceps
H. nasal polyp forceps
H. nasal punch
H. nasal speculum
H. tonsillar dissector
H. tonsillar punch
H. tonsillar punch forceps
H. tuning fork
H. uterine biopsy forceps
Hartmann-Citelli
H.-C. alligator forceps
H.-C. ear punch
H.-C. ear punch forceps
Hartmann-Corgill ear forceps
Hartmann-Gruenwald nasal-cutting
forceps
Hartmann-Herzfeld
H.-H. ear forceps
H.-H. ear rongeur
Hartmann-Noyes nasal-dressing forceps
Hartmann-Proctor ear forceps
Hartmann-Weingärtner ear forceps
Hartmann-Wullstein ear forceps
Hartshill rectangle
Hartstein
H. iris cryoretractor
H. irrigating iris retractor
H. irrigator
H. refractor
Hartzler
H. ACS coronary dilatation
catheter
H. ACX II catheter
H. dilatation catheter
H. Excel catheter
H. LPS dilatation catheter
H. Micro-600 catheter
H. Micro II angioplasty balloon
catheter

H. Micro XT catheter
H. rib retractor
H. RX-14 balloon catheter
Harvard
H. cannula
H. 2 dual-syringe pump
H. needle
harvester
Brandel cell h.
multiple automated sample h.
OsteoHarvester bone h.
TomTec cell h.
Harvey
H. Elite stethoscope
H. Stone clamp
H. vapor sterilizer
H. wire-cutting scissors
Hashizume endoscopic ligator
Hashmat shunt
Hashmat-Waterhouse shunt
Haslinger
H. bronchoscope
H. endoscope
H. esophagoscope
H. headholder
H. headrest
H. laryngoscope
H. palate retractor
H. soft palate retractor
H. tip forceps
H. tracheobronchoesophagoscope
H. tracheoscope
H. uvular retractor
Hasner
H. lid forceps
H. valve
Hasson
H. balloon uterine elevator cannula
H. blunt-end cannula
H. blunt port
H. bullet-tip forceps
H. cannula
H. grasper
H. grasping forceps
H. laparoscope
H. laparoscopic trocar
H. needle-nose forceps
H. open-laparoscopy cannula
H. retractor
H. ring forceps
H. spike-tooth forceps

NOTES

H

Hasson *(continued)*
    H. stable access cannula
    H. uterine manipulator
Hasson-Eder laparoscopy cannula
Hastings frame
Hasund appliance
hat
    measuring h.
Hatch
    H. catheter
    H. chisel
    H. clamp
Hatcher pin
hatchet
    black h.
    California h.
    Nordent h.
Hatfield bone curette
HA-threaded hexlock implant
Hatt
    H. golf-stick elevator
    H. spoon
Haugh ear forceps
Hausmann
    H. vascular clamp
    H. weight rack
    H. Work-Well work hardening
    system
Hautmann ileoneobladder
Haven skin graft hook
Haverfield
    H. brain cannula
    H. hemilaminectomy retractor
Haverfield-Scoville hemilaminectomy
   retractor
Haverhill
    H. clamp
    H. dermal abrader
    H. needle
Haverhill-Mack clamp
Havlicek
    H. spiral cannula
    H. trocar
Hawkeye suture needle
Hawkins
    H. breast localization needle
    H. cervical biopsy forceps
Hawkins-Akins needle
Hawkins-Bell retractor
Hawks-Dennen obstetrical forceps
Hawksley random zero mercury
   sphygmomanometer
Hawley
    H. bite plate
    H. chart
    H. retainer
    H. table
Hayden
    H. footplate pick

    H. palate elevator
    H. probe
    H. tonsillar curette
Hayek oscillator
Hayes
    H. anterior resection clamp
    H. anterior resection forceps
    H. colon clamp
    H. intestinal clamp
    H. Martin forceps
    H. vaginal speculum
Hayes-Olivecrona forceps
Hayman dilator
Haynes
    H. brain cannula
    H. pin
    H. retractor
    H. scissors
Haynes-Griffin mandibular splint
Haynes-Stellite implant metal prosthesis
Hays
    H. finger retractor
    H. hand retractor
    H. pharyngoscope
Hayton-Williams
    H.-W. disimpaction forceps
    H.-W. maxillary forceps
    H.-W. mouthgag
HBT Sleuth hydrogen breath test
   instrument
HCH
    hygroscopic condenser humidifier
HCMI
    Healthcare Manufacturing Inc.
    HCMI chiropractic system
HDI
    Huntleigh Diagnostics Inc.
    HDI cardiovascular ultrasound
    system
HDI-series color Doppler imaging
   ultrasound
head
    Austin Moore h.
    Biolox ball h.
    h. brace
    Bruening-Storz diagnostic h.
    Bruening-Work diagnostic h.
    cobalt-chromium h.
    h. coil
    Copeland humeral resurfacing h.
    coupling h.
    DePuy Global Advantage shoulder
    eccentric humeral h.
    h. extractor
    h. fixation device
    h. frame
    h. halter
    h. halter cervical traction
    h. holder

J-FX bipolar h.
h. lamp
Matroc femoral h.
h. mirror
modular h.
Rhoton-Merz rotatable coupling h.
h. ring
Series-II humeral h.
h. sling
h. spoon separator
Storz-Bruening diagnostic h.
Vitox femoral h.
Work-Bruening diagnostic h.
Ziramic femoral h.
zirconia orthopaedic prosthetic h.
Zyranox femoral h.
headband
Bosworth h.
Gleason h.
plagiocephaly h.
Pynchol h.
Sluder h.
Worrall h.
4-head camera
Headcam headlight
headframe
CT/MRI-compatible stereotactic h.
headgear
horizontal pull h.
Kloehn h.
Kurz pulsation orthodontic h.
ProtectaCap h.
ProtectaCap + Plus h.
headholder
Amsco h.
Bayless neurosurgical h.
Gardner h.
Haslinger h.
integrated h.
Malcolm-Rand carbon-composite h.
Mayfield-Kees h.
Mayfield radiolucent h.
Mayfield skull-pin h.
Mayfield tic h.
Parkinson h.
pin h.
pinion h.
radiolucent cranial pin h.
Shampaine h.
Headhunter visceral angiography catheter

headlamp
Keeler Magnalite fiberoptic h.
Keeler video h.
MightyLite h.
MTA h.
headlight
Clip-Lite clip-on h.
Cogent LightWear h.
Headcam h.
Heine UBL 100 h.
high beam fiberoptic h.
Keeler fiberoptic h.
Klaar h.
LightWear h.
Orascoptic fiberoptic h.
Ultra Lite II h.
Welch Allyn single fiber illumination h.
Headliner guidewire
Headmaster collar
headrest
adjustable h.
Adson h.
Brown-Roberts-Wells h.
Codman neurological h.
Craig h.
doughnut h.
Gardner h.
Gardner-Wells h.
Haslinger h.
horseshoe h.
Lempert rongeur h.
Light h.
Light-Veley h.
Mayfield-Kees h.
Mayfield pediatric horseshoe h.
Mayfield radiolucent h.
Mayfield swivel horseshoe h.
McConnell orthopaedic h.
Multipoise h.
neurosurgical h.
pin h.
pinion h.
Richards h.
Roberts h.
Shea h.
Storz adjustable h.
Veley h.
Whitmyer h.
heads-up imaging system
Heaf gun
Healey revision acetabular component

NOTES

H

healing
    h. screw
    h. shoe
Healon injection cannula
Healos bone graft substitute material
health
    National Institutes of H. (NIH)
HealthCam 2 camera
Healthcare Manufacturing Inc. (HCMI)
Healthdyne
    H. apnea monitor
    H. pulse oximeter
    H. ventilator
Healthflex orthotic
Healthier gel seating cushion
HealthShield antimicrobial mediastinal
    wound drainage catheter
Healthy Back system
HealWell night splint
Healy
    H. gastrointestinal forceps
    H. intestinal forceps
    H. suture-removing forceps
    H. uterine biopsy forceps
Healy-Jako pediatric subglottiscope
Heaney
    H. clamp
    H. endometrial biopsy curette
    H. hysterectomy forceps
    H. hysterectomy retractor
    H. suture
    H. tissue forceps
    H. uterine curette
    H. vaginal retractor
    H. Vital needle holder
Heaney-Ballantine
    H.-B. clamp
    H.-B. hysterectomy forceps
Heaney-Kantor hysterectomy forceps
Heaney-Rezek forceps
Heaney-Simon
    H.-S. hysterectomy forceps
    H.-S. hysterectomy retractor
    H.-S. vaginal retractor
Heaney-Stumf forceps
hearing
    h. aid
    h. aid amplifier
    h. aid microphone
    h. protector
Hearn needle
Hearst dilator
heart
    AbioCor replacement h.
    air-driven artificial h.
    Akutsu III total artificial h.
    ALVAD partial artificial h.
    artificial h.
    Baylor total artificial h.

    electromechanical artificial h.
    Hershey total artificial h.
    H. Hugger sternum support harness
    implantable artificial h.
    Jarvik-7, -8, 2000 artificial h.
    H. Laser 2 CO_2 laser
    Liotta total artificial h.
    H. nebulizer
    h. needle
    orthotopic biventricular artificial h.
    orthotopic univentricular artificial h.
    h. pacemaker
    Penn State total artificial h.
    Phoenix total artificial h.
    H. pillow
    H. pillow infuser
    h. prosthesis
    h. pump
    H. Rate 1-2-3 monitor
    RTV total artificial h.
    Symbion/CardioWest 100 mL total
      artificial h.
    Symbion Jarvik-7 artificial h.
    H. Technology Rotablator
    total artificial h.
    University of Akron artificial h.
    Utah total artificial h.
    h. valve
HeartCard
    H. cardiac event recorder
    H. monitor
Heartflow automated anastomosis system
heart-lung resuscitator
HeartMate
    H. implantable ventricular assist
      device
    H. portable pump
Heartport
    H. endoaortic clamp
    H. endocoronary sinus catheter
    H. endovenous drainage cannula
    H. Precision-OP system
Heartport-Endoclamp balloon cannula
HEARTrac I cardiac monitoring system
HeartSaver VAD
Heartstream
    H. ForeRunner defibrillator
    H. XL, XLT defibrillator
HeartView CT
HeartWatch cardiac event recorder
HearTwave CT
heat
    h. gun
    h. killed (HK)
    h. and moisture exchanger
    h. pad
heat-activated recoverable temporary
    stent

heater
    h. probe
    resistance wire h.
    SlidePro 15 compact slide h.
    Snowden-Pencer internal h.
heat-expandable stent
Heath
    H. chalazion curette
    H. chalazion forceps
    H. clip
    H. clip-removing forceps
    H. clip-removing scissors
    H. follicle expressor
    H. mallet
    H. mules
    H. nasal forceps
    H. punctum dilator
    H. suture-cutting scissors
    H. suture scissors
    H. trephine flap dissector
    H. wire cutter
    H. wire-cutting scissors
heat/moisture exchanger
HeatProbe
    H. catheter
    H. device
    H. unit
    H. water irrigation/lavage system
HeatWrap
    ThermaCare H.
heavy
    h. cross-slot screwdriver
    h. monofilament suture
    h. retention suture
    h. septal scissors
    h. silk retention suture
    h. wire suture
heavy-duty pliers with side-cutter
heavy-gauge suture material
HeavyMed ball
Hebra
    H. blade
    H. chalazion curette
    H. corneal curette
    H. hook
Hecht fascia lata forceps
Heck screw
Hedblom
    H. costal elevator
    H. rib retractor

Hedrocel
    H. bone substitute material
    H. trabecular metal
Hedstrom file
Hedwig
    H. introducer
    H. lumen finder
heel
    h. cup
    h. cushion
    H. Free splint
    H. Hugger therapeutic heel
      stabilizer
    h. lift
    H. Minder foot elevator
    h. pillow
    rubber walking h.
    h. sleeve
    solid ankle-cushion h. (SACH)
    H. Spur Special orthotic
    Thomas h.
    walking h.
    wedge adjustable cushioned h.
Heelbo decubitus protector
HeelCare cushion
Heeler
    H. inflatable heel protector
    The H. inflatable heel protector
Heelfit orthosis
Heelift suspension boot
HeelWedge healing shoe
Heermann
    H. alligator forceps
    H. chisel
    H. ear forceps
Heffernan nasal speculum
Heffington
    H. lumbar seat
    H. lumbar seat spinal surgery
      frame
Hefty Bite pin cutter
Hegar
    H. bougie
    H. double-ended dilator
    H. needle
    H. rectal dilator
    H. uterine dilator
Hegar-Baumgartner needle
Hegar-Goodell dilator
Hegar-Mayo-Seeley needle holder
Hegar-Olsen needle holder
Hegemann scissors

NOTES

H

Hegenbarth
    H. clip
    H. clip-applying forceps
Hegenbarth-Adams clip
Hegenbarth-Michel clip-applying forceps
Hegge pin
He Hook chopper
Heidbrink expiratory spill valve
Heidelberg
    H. angulator
    H. arm
    H. fixation forceps
    H. laser tomographic scanner
    H. retinal angiograph
    H. retinal flowmeter
Heidelberg-R table
Heifitz
    H. aneurysm clip
    H. carotid occluder
    H. cerebral aneurysm clamp
    H. clip applier
    H. cup serrated ring forceps
    H. microclip
    H. retractor
    H. skull perforator
    H. spatula
Heifitz-Weck clip
Heightronic stadiometer
Heiming kidney stone forceps
Heimlich
    H. chest drainage valve
    H. heart valve
    H. tube
    H. Vygon pneumothorax valve
Heimlich-Gavrilu gastric tube
Hein
    H. raspatory
    H. rongeur
Heine
    H. dermatoscope
    H. gonioscope
    H. HSL 100 handheld slit lamp
    H. Lambda 100 retinometer
    H. penlight
    H. UBL 100 headlight
Heinkel sigmoidoscope
Heiss
    H. artery forceps
    H. hemostatic forceps
    H. mastoid retractor
    H. soft tissue retractor
    H. vulsellum forceps
Heister
    H. jaw opener
    H. mouthgag
Heitz-Boyer clamp
Hejnosz radium colpostat
Helanca seamless tube prosthesis
Helex septal occluder

Helfrick anal retractor
helical
    h. coil
    h. coil stent
    h. computed tomographic angiogram
    h. CT
    h. PTCA dilatation catheter
    h. suture
    h. tube saw
helical-ridged ureteral stent
helical-tip Halo catheter
helicoid endosteal implant
Helio cortical lag screw
Heliodent dental x-ray unit
Heliodorus bandage
Helios diagnostic imaging system
Helioseal dental sealant
Helistat absorbable collagen hemostatic
    sponge
Helitene absorbable collagen hemostatic
    sponge
helium-cadmium diagnostic laser
helium-filled balloon catheter
helium-neon laser
helix
    h. balloon
    H. camera
    H. endocervical curette
    H. multihead nuclear imaging
        system
    H. PTCA dilatation catheter
    H. uterine biopsy curette
Helixcision cardiovascular catheter
Heller
    H. biopsy forceps
    H. probe
Hellige electrocardiographic recorder
helmet
    collimator h.
    cooling h.
    CranioCap h.
    plagiocephaly h.
Helmholtz
    H. double-surface coil
    H. keratometer
    H. ophthalmoscope
    H. speculum
Helmont speculum
Helmstein balloon
HELP
    heparin-induced extracorporeal
    lipoprotein precipitation
    HELP system
Helsper
    H. laryngectomy button
    H. tracheostomy vent tube
Helveston
    H. "Great Big Barbie" retractor
    H. scleral marking ruler

Helvestoon hook
hemacytometer
Hemaduct wound drain
hemadynamometer
Hemaflex
H. PTCA sheath with obturator
H. pure collage hemostat
H. sheath
Hemagard collection tube
Hemaquet
H. introducer
H. PTCA sheath
Hemaseel APR fibrin sealant
Hemashield
H. collagen-enhanced graft
H. collagen-impregnated graft
H. Gold Microvel knitted double velour graft
H. Vantage vascular graft
HemAssist blood substitute
HemataSTAT portable microhematocrit centrifuge
hematology rocker
Hematome system
Hemex prosthetic valve
hemiambulator walker
Hemi-Arc surgical navigator
hemi-interpositional implant
hemiknee
hemilaminectomy
h. blade
h. retractor
hemiprosthesis
single-stemmed silicone h.
Hemi sling
hemisphere eye implant
hemispherical pusher
Hemobahn endovascular prosthesis
Hemocal hemoperfusion cartridge
Hemo-Cath catheter
Hemoccult Sensa slide
Hemochron P214 glass-activated ACT tube
Hemoclear dialyzer
Hemoclip-applying forceps
Hemoclip clamp
hemoconcentrator
Biofilter cardiovascular h.
Hemocor HPH high-performance h.
Hemocor HPH high-performance hemoconcentrator

HemoCue
H. B-hemoglobin system
H. blood glucose analyzer
H. blood hemoglobin analyzer
H. Glucose 201 photometer
H. Glucose 201+ photometer
H. microcurette
hemocytometer
Coulter MD 16 h.
MD 16 h.
Neubauer h.
hemodialysis catheter
hemodialyzer
Altra Flux h.
Baxter h.
Biospal h.
2008E h.
Gambro h.
Gambro-Lundia Minor h.
Polyflux h.
Redy h.
hemofilter
Hemofreeze blood bag
hemoheater
Vickers Treonic h.
Hemoject
H. injection catheter
H. needle
Hemokart hemoperfusion cartridge
Hem-o-lok
H.-o-l. polymer ligating clip
H.-o-l. polymer ligation clip system
HemoMatic blood collection monitor
Hemo-Nate blood filtration system
Hemopad
H. collagen hemostatic material
H. sterile absorbable collagen hemostat
Hemophan membrane
hemopump
H. cardiac assist system
Johnson & Johnson h.
Hemopure oxygen-based therapeutic system
hemorrhoidal
h. clamp
h. forceps
h. ligator
h. needle
HemoSonic monitor
Hemosorba hemoperfusion column
HemoSplit dialysis catheter

NOTES

H

hemostasis
- h. band
- h. scalp clip
- h. silver clip

hemostat
- Adson h.
- Allis h.
- Avitene microfibrillar collagen h.
- Avitene Ultrafoam collagen h.
- blackened.
- Blohmka tonsillar h.
- blunt-nose h.
- Boettcher h.
- Carmalt h.
- Collastat h.
- Collastat collagen h.
- Collastat OBP microfibrillar collagen h.
- Collier-DeBakey h.
- Corboy h.
- Corwin tonsillar h.
- CoStasis surgical h.
- Crafoord h.
- curved Kelly h.
- curved mosquito h.
- Dandy scalp h.
- Davis h.
- Dean tonsillar h.
- Deaver h.
- Dynastat surgical h.
- EndoAvitene microfibrillar collagen h.
- fine-tipped mosquito h.
- Guist enucleation h.
- Gutglass h.
- Halsted mosquito h.
- Hartmann h.
- Hemaflex pure collage h.
- Hemopad sterile absorbable collagen h.
- Hemotene absorbable collagen h.
- Instat MCH microfibrillar collagen h.
- Jackson tracheal h.
- Kelly h.
- Kocher h.
- Lahey h.
- Lewis h.
- Lothrop h.
- Lowsley h.
- Mathrop h.
- Mayo h.
- McWhorter h.
- Meigs h.
- microfibrillar collagen h.
- Mixter h.
- mosquito h.
- Nu-Knit absorbable h.
- Ochsner h.

- Ormco orthodontic h.
- orthopaedic h.
- Perdue h.
- Providence Hospital h.
- Raimondi h.
- Rankin h.
- Rochester-Ochsner h.
- Rochester-Péan h.
- Sawtell h.
- Sawtell-Davis h.
- scalp h.
- Schnidt h.
- Shallcross h.
- straight mosquito h.
- Surgicel fibrillar absorbable h.
- Surgicel Nu-Knit absorbable h.
- Thrombogen absorbable h.

hemostatic
- h. bag
- h. catheter
- h. cervical forceps
- h. clamp
- h. clip
- h. clip-applying forceps
- h. eraser
- h. forceps
- h. neurosurgical forceps
- h. puncture closure device
- h. suture
- h. tissue forceps
- h. tonsillar forceps
- h. tonsillectome
- h. tracheal forceps

Hemostatix thermal scalpel system

HemoTec
- H. activated clotting time monitor
- H. ACT machine

Hemotene
- H. absorbable collagen hemostat
- H. collagen hemostatic material

Hemovac
- H. Hydrocoat drain
- H. suction device
- H. suction tube

Henahan elevator

Hendel guided osteotome

Henderson
- H. bone chisel
- H. clamp approximator
- H. self-retaining retractor

Henderson-Haggard inhaler

Hendon venoclysis cannula

Hendren
- H. cardiovascular clamp
- H. cardiovascular forceps
- H. ductus clamp
- H. megaureter clamp
- H. pediatric forceps
- H. pediatric retractor blade

H. self-retaining retractor
H. ureteral clamp
Hendrickson
H. bag
H. lithotrite
H. suprapubic drain
HeNe laser
Henke
H. punch forceps
H. tonsillar dissector
Henke-Stille conchotome
Henley
H. carotid retractor
H. dilator
H. retractor blade
H. subclavian artery clamp
H. vascular clamp
Henner
H. endaural elevator
H. T-model endaural retractor
Henning
H. cardiac dilator
H. cast spreader
H. instrument set
H. mallet
H. meniscal retractor
Henning-Keinkel stomach probe
Henny laminectomy rongeur
Henrotin
H. retractor
H. vulsellum
H. vulsellum forceps
H. weighted vaginal speculum
Henry
H. ciliary forceps
H. Schein excavator
Henschke
H. afterloader
H. colpostat
H. seed applicator
Henschke-Mauch SNS lower limb
prosthesis
Henson CFS 2000 perimeter
Henton
H. suture needle
H. tonsillar needle
H. tonsillar suture hook
HepaCoat end-point attachment
Hepacon
H. cannula
H. catheter
HEPA filter

Hepamed-coated Wiktor stent
Heparinase test cartridge
heparin-bonded Bott-type tube
heparin-coated
h.-c. catheter
h.-c. guidewire
h.-c. Palmaz-Schatz stent
heparin-flushing needle
heparin-induced extracorporeal
lipoprotein precipitation (HELP)
heparin lock
HepatAssist
H. bioartificial liver
H. bioartificial liver system
HEPAtech Air Purification system
hepatic artery infusion pump
hepatofugal porto-systemic venous shunt
HepCheck whole blood control
Heraeus
H. LaserSonics InfraGuide
H. LaserSonics laser
Herbert
H. Adams coarctation clamp
H. bone screw
H. knee prosthesis
H. scaphoid screw
H. sclerotomy knife
H. screw fixator
Herbert-Whipple bone screw
Herbst Cradle orthosis
Herchenson esophageal cytology
collector
Hercules
H. drop-adjusting table
H. 7000 mobile x-ray unit
H. plaster shears
H. power injector
H. table
Herculite XRV lab system
Herculon suture
Herczel
H. dissector
H. periosteal elevator
H. raspatory elevator
H. rib elevator
H. rib rasp
Herff
H. clamp
H. membrane-puncturing forceps
Herget biopsy forceps
Heritage hip system
Hermann bone-holding forceps

NOTES

H

Herman-Taylor gastroscope
**Hermes Evolution tricompartmental
    knee system**
Hermes-Ready pump
hermetically sealed pacemaker
**Hermetic II drainage management
    system**
Hermitex bandage
Hernandez-Ros bone staple
hernia
    h. retractor
    h. stapler
Herniamesh
    H. surgical mesh
    H. surgical plug
herniotome
    Cooper h.
Heros chiropody sponge
HerpeSelect test kit
Herrick
    H. kidney clamp
    H. kidney forceps
    H. lacrimal plug
    H. pedicle clamp
    H. silicone lacrimal implant
Herring tube
**Hersbury anterior chamber intraocular
    lens**
Hersh
    H. LASIK retreatment forceps
    H. LASIK retreatment spatula
Hershey
    H. left ventricular assist device
    H. total artificial heart
Hertel
    H. bougie urethrotome
    H. exophthalmometer
    H. kidney stone forceps
    H. nephrostomy speculum
    H. ophthalmometer
    H. rigid dilator stone forceps
    H. rigid kidney stone forceps
Hertzler
    H. baby rib retractor
    H. rib spreader
Hertzog
    H. lens spatula
    H. pliable probe
Herzenberg bolt
Herzfeld ear forceps
Herzmark fracture frame
Herz meniscal tendon forceps
Hess
    H. capsular forceps
    H. diplopia screen
    H. iris forceps
    H. lens scoop
    H. lens spoon
    H. Memory Lens inserter

    H. nerve root retractor
    H. serrefine
    H. tonsil expressor
Hess-Barraquer iris forceps
Hessburg
    H. corneal shield
    H. eye shield
    H. intraocular lens glide
    H. lacrimal needle
    H. lens-inserting forceps
    H. subpalpebral lavage system
    H. vacuum trephine
Hessburg-Barron vacuum trephine
Hessel-Nystrom pin
Hesseltine
    H. umbilical cord clamp
    H. Umbili Clip
Hess-Gill iris forceps
Hess-Horwitz iris forceps
Hessing brace
Hess-Lee screen
heterograft
    bovine h.
    Hancock porcine h.
    h. implant
    h. prosthesis
heteroscope
Hetherington circular saw
Hetter pyramid tip
Hevesy polyp forceps
Hewitt mouthgag
Hewlett-Packard (HP)
    H.-P. Codemaster defibrillator
    H.-P. color flow imager
    H.-P. defibrillator
    H.-P. ear oximeter
    H.-P. Echo-Doppler machine
    H.-P. 5 MHz phased-array TEE
      system
    H.-P. omniplane 5-MHz probe
    H.-P. Sonos 1000, 1500 ultrasound
      system
Hewson
    H. breakaway pin
    H. drill
    H. suture passer
Hewson-Richards reamer
hex
    h. bar
    H. heat applicator
    h. implant
    h. socket wrench
hexagonal
    h. handle
    h. handle osteotome
    h. wrench
hexagon snare
hexapolar catheter

Hexascan computerized dermatology handpiece
Hexcel
    H. cast dressing
    H. total condylar prosthesis
Hexcelite
    H. cast
    H. mesh
    H. sheet splint
Hex-Fix
    H.-F. Add-A-Clamp
    H.-F. monolateral external fixator
    H.-F. system
    H.-F. Universal swivel clamp
hexhead
    h. bolt
    h. pin
    h. screwdriver
Hex-Lock abutment
Hexon illumination system
Hextend plasma volume expander
Heyer-Pudenz valve
Heyer-Robertson suprapubic drain
Heyer-Schulte
    H.-S. antisiphon device
    H.-S. brain retractor
    H.-S. breast implant
    H.-S. breast prosthesis
    H.-S. catheter
    H.-S. disposal bag
    H.-S. hydrocephalus shunt
    H.-S. Jackson-Pratt wound-drainage reservoir
    H.-S. lens implant
    H.-S. microscope
    H.-S. Pour-Safe exudate bag
    H.-S. PVC kit
    H.-S. Rayport muscle biopsy clamp
    H.-S. rhinoplasty implant
    H.-S. silicone kit
    H.-S. Small-Carrion sizing set
    H.-S. tissue expander
    H.-S. valve
    H.-S. wedge-suction reservoir
    H.-S. wound drain
Heyer-Schulte-Fischer ventricular cannula
Heyer-Schulte-Ommaya CSF reservoir
Heyer-Schulte-Pudenz cardiac catheter
Heyer-Schulte-Spetzler lumbar peritoneal shunt

Hey-Groves needle
Heyman
    H. nasal-cutting forceps
    H. nasal forceps
Heyman-Knight nasal dressing forceps
Heymann nasal scissors
Heyman-Paparella angular scissors
Heyman-Simon
    H.-S. capsule
    H.-S. source
Heyner
    H. cannula
    H. curette
    H. dilator
    H. double needle
    H. expressor
    H. forceps
Heyns abdominal decompression apparatus
Hey skull saw
Heywood-Smith
    H.-S. dressing forceps
    H.-S. gallbladder forceps
    H.-S. sponge-holding forceps
HF
    hollow fiber
    HF dialyzer
    HF infrared laser
H-file
    Mity engine H-f.
HG
    Harris-Galante
HGM
    HGM argon green laser
    HGM intravitreal laser
    HGM ophthalmic laser
    HGM Spectrum K1 krypton yellow & green laser
HG Multilock hip prosthesis
HGN
    human glucose monitoring
HGP
    Harris-Galante porous
    HGP II acetabular component
    HGP II acetabular cup
H-H
    H-H neonatal shunt
    H-H open-end alimentation catheter
    H-H Rickham cerebrospinal fluid reservoir
    H-H shunt introducer

NOTES

H

Hi
- H. Speed Pulse lavage
- H. Vac tubing

Hi5 Torq Flow catheter

Hibbs
- H. biting forceps
- H. bone chisel
- H. bone curette
- H. bone-cutting forceps
- H. bone gouge
- H. bone-holding forceps
- H. chisel elevator
- H. clamp
- H. costal elevator
- H. fracture appliance
- H. fracture frame
- H. hammer
- H. mallet
- H. mouthgag
- H. osteotome
- H. periosteal elevator
- H. scoop
- H. self-retaining laminectomy retractor
- H. spinal curette
- H. spinal fusion gouge
- H. spinal retractor blade
- H. sponge

Hibbs-Spratt spinal fusion curette

Hi-Care pulmonary hygiene system

Hickman
- H. catheter
- H. line
- H. tunneled catheter

Hicks lugged plate

Hicor angiography machine

Hidalgo catheter

hi-density foam

Hiebert
- H. esophageal suture spoon
- H. vascular dilator

Hieshima coaxial catheter

Higbee vaginal speculum

Higgins
- H. bag
- H. catheter

Higginson irrigation syringe

high
- h. beam fiberoptic headlight
- h. density polyethylene
- H. Flex D 700 S bubble oxygenator
- h. flux dialyzer
- h. heat capacity x-ray tube
- H. Oxygen PRM resuscitator
- h. tibial osteotomy (HTO)

high-capacity
- h.-c. fluid warmer
- h.-c. silicone drain

high-energy
- h.-e. bent-beam linear accelerator
- h.-e. laser

high-fidelity micromanometer catheter

high-field
- h.-f. MRI system
- h.-f. open MRI scanner

high-flow
- h.-f. catheter
- h.-f. coaxial cannula
- h.-f. regulator

high-frequency
- h.-f. jet ventilator
- h.-f. miniature probe
- h.-f. miniprobe
- h.-f. tweezer-type epilator
- h.-f. ultrasound biomicroscope

high-humidity
- h.-h. face mask
- h.-h. tracheostomy collar
- h.-h. tracheostomy mask
- h.-h. tracheostomy shield

Highlighter low-vision aid

Highlight spectral indirect ophthalmoscope

high-output extended aerosol respiratory therapy

high-pass filter

high-performance liquid chromatograph

high-pressure
- h.-p. Blue Max balloon
- h.-p. liquid chromatograph
- h.-p. mercury arc lamp

high-purity germanium detector

high-resolution
- h.-r. brain SPECT system
- h.-r. fan-beam collimator
- h.-r. linear array transducer
- h.-r. multileaf collimator
- h.-r. probe
- h.-r. real-time scanner

high-sensitivity collimator

high-speed
- h.-s. air drill
- h.-s. dermabrader
- h.-s. diamond wheel bur
- h.-s. drill
- h.-s. electrical tissue morcellator
- h.-s. gradient coil
- h.-s. microdrill
- h.-s. rotation dynamic angioplasty catheter
- h.-s. tungsten carbide bur
- h.-s. two-grit bur

high-torque
- h.-t. bur
- h.-t. wire

High-Vision surgical telescope

high-voltage
    h.-v. electron microscope
    h.-v. generator
    h.-v. pulsed current (HVPC)
    h.-v. transformer
high-volume evacuator
HIHA tendon implant
Hilal
    H. coil
    H. embolization apparatus
    H. microcoil
    H. modified headhunter catheter
hilar clamp
Hildebrandt uterine hemostatic forceps
Hildreth
    H. coagulator
    H. electrocautery
    H. electrode
    H. ocular cautery
    H. transilluminator
Hildyard nasal forceps
Hilgenreiner brace
Hilger facial nerve stimulator
Hilight Advantage System CT scanner
Hill
    H. Air-Drop HA90C table
    H. Air-Flex table
    H. nasal raspatory
    H. rectal retractor
Hill-Bosworth saw
Hill-Ferguson rectal retractor
Hillis
    H. eyelid retractor
    H. fetal stethoscope
    H. perforator
    H. refractor
HiLo
    H. BodyTable
    H. MultiPro table
    H. PowerTilt massage table
    H. PowerTilt table
Hi-Lo
    H.-L. Evac endotracheal tube
    H.-L. Jet tracheal tube
Hi-Loo Power lift
Hilsinger tonsillar knife
Hilton self-retaining sutureless infusion
    cannula
Himalaya dressing forceps
Himmelstein
    H. pulmonary valvulotome
    H. sternal retractor

Hinderer
    H. cartilage forceps
    H. malar prosthesis
hindfoot orthosis
Hind Site anal retractor
hinge
    h. articulator
    Camber axis h. (CAH)
    Compass Universal h.
    Dee elbow h.
    elbow h.
    Lacey rotating h.
    offset h.
    Weser dental h.
hinged
    h. articulated fixator
    h. articulator
    h. cast
    h. constrained knee prosthesis
    h. great toe replacement prosthesis
    h. implant
    h. Thomas splint
    h. total knee prosthesis
hinged-leaflet vascular prosthesis
hingeless heart valve prosthesis
Hingson-Edwards caudal needle
Hingson-Ferguson spinal needle
Hinkle-James rectal speculum
Hinz tongs
hip
    anthropometric total h.
    h. arthroplasty gouge
    h. disarticulation prosthesis
    h. distractor
    h. endoprosthesis
    Gemini h.
    h. guidance orthosis
    Gustilo-Kyle total h.
    Howmedica PCA textured h.
    Link anatomical h.
    PCA total h.
    Precision Osteolock total h.
    h. shell implant
    h. skid
    h. spica cast
    h. spica dressing
HIPciser abduction splint
Hi-Per Flex exchange guidewire
hipGRIP pelvic positioning system
hip-knee-ankle orthosis
hip-knee orthosis
Hiploc compression hip screw

NOTES

H

Hipokrat bimodular shoulder system
Hippel trephine
Hippocrates bandage
Hipp & Sohn dental scissors
hipRAP pelvic positioning system
Hircoe denture base material
HiRider motorized lift wheelchair
Hirji-Callandar grid
Hirsch
> H. hypophyseal punch
> H. hypophysis punch forceps
> H. mucosal clamp

Hirschberg electromagnet magnet
Hirschman
> H. anoscope
> H. anoscope rectal speculum
> H. hemorrhoidal forceps
> H. hooked cannula
> H. iris hook
> H. iris spatula
> H. jeweler's forceps
> H. lens forceps
> H. lens manipulator
> H. lens spatula
> H. nasoendoscope
> H. pile clamp
> H. proctoscope
> H. retractor

Hirschman-Martin proctoscope
Hirschowitz
> H. gastroduodenal fiberscope
> H. gastroscope

Hirschtick utility shoulder splint
Hirst
> H. obstetrical forceps
> H. placental forceps
> H. spore trap

Hirst-Emmet
> H.-E. obstetrical forceps
> H.-E. placental forceps

His bundle catheter
Hi-seat Artherapedic hip chair
Hishida pine-needle sound
HiSonic ultrasonic bone conduction hearing device
HiSpeed
> H. Advantage CT scanner
> H. Advantage helical scanner

Hi-Star midfield MRI system
Histoacryl glue
Histofreezer cryosurgical system
Hitachi
> H. Altaire open MRI system
> H. automated chemistry analyzer
> H. convex-convex biplane probe
> H. convex ultrasound probe
> H. CT scanner
> H. EUB-515C ultrasound console

> H. EUB-series diagnostic ultrasound
> H. EUB-405 ultrasound scanner
> H. EUB-405 ultrasound system
> H. fingertip ultrasound probe
> H. H-series electron microscope
> H. linear ultrasound probe
> H. MR scanner
> H. open MRI system
> H. PCT-3600W PET scanner
> H. SPECT 2000H-40 gamma camera
> H. transrectal ultrasound probe
> H. transvaginal ultrasound probe
> H. UB 420 digital ultrasound system
> H. U-series spectrophotometer

hitch
> ankle h.
> girth h.

Hitchcock stereotactic immobilization frame
HiTec insufflator
Hite-Rite stadiometer
Hi-Top
> H.-T. foot/ankle brace
> H.-T. II CAM Walker boot
> H.-T. shoe

Hi-Torque
> H.-T. Balance middleweight guidewire
> H.-T. Cross-It guidewire
> H.-T. Flex-T guidewire
> H.-T. Floppy guide catheter
> H.-T. Floppy II guidewire
> H.-T. Intermediate guidewire
> H.-T. Memcore guidewire
> H.-T. Spartacore guidewire
> H.-T. Steel core guidewire
> H.-T. Supra Core guidewire
> H.-T. Wiggle guidewire

Hitselberger-McElveen neural dissector
Hittenberger prosthesis
Hix-Fix fracture fixation system
Hixon-Oldfather prediction table
HK
> heat killed
> HK binder
> HK Breast/Torso garment
> HK pad
> HK sheet

HmX hematology flow cytometer
Hobbs
> H. dilatation balloon catheter
> H. needle
> H. polypectomy snare
> H. sheath brush
> H. stent set
> H. stone basket

hockey-stick
  h.-s. catheter
  h.-s. electrosurgical probe
Hockin lucite ovoid
Hodge
  H. obstetrical forceps
  H. pessary
Hodgen
  H. apparatus
  H. hip splint
  H. leg splint
Hodlick needle holder
hoe
  Hough h.
  Hough-Saunders stapes h.
  Joe's h.
  Nordent h.
  Sloane LASEK micro h.
  stapes h.
Hoefer GS 300 laser densitometer
Hoefflin suture passer
Hoek-Bowen cement removal system
Hoen
  H. alligator forceps
  H. bayonet forceps
  H. dressing forceps
  H. dural separator
  H. grasping forceps
  H. hemilaminectomy retractor
  H. hemostatic forceps
  H. intervertebral disc rongeur
  H. laminar gouge
  H. laminectomy rongeur
  H. laminectomy scissors
  H. nerve hook
  H. periosteal elevator
  H. periosteal raspatory
  H. pituitary rongeur
  H. scalp forceps
  H. scalp retractor
  H. skull plate
  H. tissue forceps
  H. ventricular cannula
  H. ventricular needle
Hoffer
  H. corneal marker
  H. forward-cutting knife cannula
  H. ridged intraocular lens
  H. ridged lens implant
Hoffman/Buratto LASIK marker
Hoffman II Compact external fixation system

Hoffmann
  H. apex fixation pin
  H. ear punch forceps
  H. ear rongeur
  H. external fixation device
  H. external fixator
  H. eye implant
  H. II compact external fixation component
  H. ligament clamp
  H. scleral fixation pick
  H. traction device
  H. transfixion pin
Hoffmann-Osher-Hopkins plaster knife
Hoffmann-Pollock forceps
Hoffmann-Vidal external fixation device
Hoffrel transesophageal probe
Hoff towel clamp
Hofmeister
  H. drainage bag
  H. endometrial biopsy curette
Hogness box
Hohmann
  H. bone lever
  H. clamp
  H. osteotome
  H. retractor
Hohmann-Aldinger bone lever
Hohn
  H. catheter
  H. vessel dilator
hoist
  Temco h.
Hoist 4400 exercise machine
Hoke
  H. lumbar brace
  H. lumbar corset
  H. osteotome
  H. spoon
Hoke-Martin tractor
Hoke-Roberts spoon
Holcombe gastric tourniquet
Hold-and-Hold positioner
Holden uterine curette
holder
  A1-Askari needle h.
  Abbey needle h.
  Adson dural needle h.
  Aesculap needle h.
  Alabama-Green eye needle h.
  Alabama needle h.
  Allen well leg h.

NOTES

H

439

holder *(continued)*

Alvarado surgical knee h.
Anchor needle h.
Andrews rigid chest support h.
Anis-Barraquer needle h.
Anis needle h.
Anspach leg h.
APC foot and leg h.
Arruga eye h.
Arruga needle h.
arthroscopic ankle h.
arthroscopic leg h.
Aslan needle h.
Axhausen needle h.
Azar needle h.
baby Barraquer needle h.
baby Crile needle h.
baby Crile-Wood needle h.
Bard leg bag h.
Barraquer curved h.
Barraquer needle h.
Barraquer-Troutman needle h.
Baumgartner needle h.
Baum-Metzenbaum sternal needle h.
Baum needle h.
bayonet needle h.
Bechert-Sinskey needle h.
Berry sternal needle h.
Bethea sheet h.
Bihrle dorsal clamp-T-C needle h.
Bihrle T-C needle h.
Birks Mark II micro cross-
  action h.
Birks Mark II needle h.
Björk-Shiley heart valve h.
bladebreaker h.
Blair-Brown needle h.
Bodkin thread h.
bone-graft h.
Bookler swivel-ball laparoscopic
  instrument h.
boomerang needle h.
Bovie h.
Boyce needle h.
Boynton needle h.
Bozeman-Finochietto needle h.
Bozeman needle h.
Bozeman-Wertheim needle h.
Bumgardner dental h.
Bunt forceps h.
Carb-Bite needle h.
Castroviejo-Barraquer needle h.
Castroviejo blade h.
Castroviejo-Kalt needle h.
Castroviejo needle h.
Castroviejo razor h.
Catalano needle h.
catheter guide h.
catheter leg tube h.

catheter tube h.
catheter waist tube h.
Cath-Secure catheter h.
Cath-Secure dual-tab h.
CBI stereotactic head h.
Cherf leg h.
Circon leg h.
clamp h.
Cohan needle h.
Colles needle h.
Collier needle h.
Collins leg h.
Converse needle h.
Cooley Vital microvascular
  needle h.
Corboy needle h.
Cottle needle h.
Crile-Murray needle h.
Crile needle h.
Crile-Wood needle h.
Crile-Wood Vital needle h.
Crockard suction tube h.
Dainer-Kaupp needle h.
Dale drainage bulb and G-tube h.
Dale Foley catheter legband h.
Dale gastrostomy tube h.
Dale nasal dressing h.
Dale tapeless wound dressing h.
Dale tracheostomy tube h.
Dean knife h.
DeBakey needle h.
DeBakey Vital needle h.
Dees h.
DeMartel-Wolfson h.
Derf needle h.
Derf Vital needle h.
Derlacki ossicle h.
DeRoyal catheter tube h.
Diamond-Jaw needle h.
Doyen needle h.
Drews needle h.
Drummond hook h.
Dubecq-Princeteau angulating
  needle h.
Eber h.
Eiselsberg-Mathieu needle h.
Elliot femoral condyle h.
Ellis needle h.
Endo-Assist endoscopic needle h.
Ermold needle h.
E-series needle h.
eye needle h.
Ferguson bone h.
Ferris-Smith needle h.
Finochietto needle h.
Foley catheter h.
foot h.
French-eye Vital needle h.
French needle h.

Fukushima-Giannotta needle h.
Furacin gauze h.
Gambro dialyzer h.
Gardner needle h.
GHM KLE II x-ray film h.
Gifford needle h.
Gillies needle h.
Gillquist-Oretorp-Stille needle h.
goniotomy needle h.
Grant needle h.
Green eye needle h.
Grieshaber needle h.
Hagedorn needle h.
Hagfer needle h.
Halsey Vital needle h.
Halsey-Webster needle h.
Hampton needle h.
Hannover needle h.
head h.
Heaney Vital needle h.
Hegar-Mayo-Seeley needle h.
Hegar-Olsen needle h.
Hodlick needle h.
Hosel needle h.
House-Urban temporal bone h.
Huang vein h.
Hufnagel-Ryder needle h.
Hyde needle h.
Ilg needle h.
intracardiac needle h.
I-tech needle h.
Ivy needle h.
Jacobson spring-handled needle h.
Jacobson-Vital needle h.
Jaffe needle h.
Jako laryngeal needle h.
Jameson needle h.
Jannetta bayonet needle h.
Jannetta bayonet-shaped needle h.
Jannetta needle h.
Jarcho tenaculum h.
Jarit forceps h.
Jarit microsurgical needle h.
Jarit sternal needle h.
Jarit wire h.
Johnson prostatic needle h.
Jones IMA needle h.
Jones needle h.
Jordan-Caparosa h.
Juers-Derlacki Universal head h.
Julian needle h.
Kalman needle h.

Kalt-Arruga needle h.
Kalt eye needle h.
Kalt-Vital needle h.
Keeler-Catford micro jaws
 needle h.
Kilner needle h.
Knolle needle h.
Langenbeck needle h.
laser Heaney needle h.
laser Julian needle h.
leg h.
Lenny Johnson surgical-assist
 knee h.
Lewy chest h.
Lewy laryngoscope h.
Lichtenberg needle h.
limb h.
Lindley needle h.
lion jaw bone h.
Lundia dialyzer h.
Malis needle h.
Margraf beam aligning film h.
Marquette 3-channel laser h.
Masing needle h.
Mason leg h.
Masson-Luethy needle h.
Masson-Mayo-Hegar needle h.
Masson needle h.
Masson-Vital needle h.
mat h.
Mathieu needle h.
Mathieu-Olsen needle h.
Mathieu-Stille needle h.
Mayo-Hegar curved-jaw needle h.
Mayo needle h.
McAllister needle h.
McIntyre fish-hook needle h.
McPherson microsurgery eye
 needle h.
Metzenbaum needle h.
Micra needle h.
microneedle h.
microsurgical needle h.
microvascular needle h.
Millin boomerang needle h.
Mills microvascular needle h.
Miltex Crile needle h.
mirror h.
Murray h.
nasal dressing h.
needle h.
Neivert needle h.

NOTES

H

441

holder *(continued)*
Neo-Fit neonatal endotracheal
  tube h.
Neumann razor blade fragment h.
neurosurgical needle h.
New Orleans needle h.
O'Gawa needle h.
Okmian microneedle h.
Olson-Hegar extra-delicate needle h.
Olympic needle h.
Osher needle h.
OSI arthroscopic well-leg leg h.
Paparella monkey-head h.
Paton eye needle h.
Pilling needle h.
pin h.
Pittman needle h.
3-point head h.
Portmann speculum h.
Posilok instrument h.
Potts-Smith needle h.
press plate needle h.
prostatic needle h.
prosthetic valve h.
Punctur-Guard Revolution safety
  needle h.
Quinn h.
Ravich needle h.
razor blade h.
Reill needle h.
Reverdin h.
Rhoton bayonet needle h.
Rhoton microneedle h.
Rica forceps h.
Rinn XCP film h.
Rochester needle h.
Rogers needle h.
Rubio needle h.
Ryder needle h.
Sarot needle h.
Sarot-Vital needle h.
Scabbard needle h.
Scanlan microneedle h.
Schaefer sponge h.
Schlein shoulder h.
Shea speculum h.
Sheehan-Gillies needle h.
sheet h.
Silber microneedle h.
Sims sponge h.
Sinskey needle h.
speculum h.
spring-handled needle h.
spring needle h.
Stanzel needle h.
Steinmann h.
Stenstrom nerve h.
Stephenson needle h.
sterile forceps h.

sternal needle h.
Stevens needle h.
Stevenson needle h.
Stille-French cardiovascular
  needle h.
Storz needle h.
Stratte needle h.
suction tube h.
Sugita head h.
Surcan knee h.
Surcan leg h.
SurgAssist surgical leg h.
suture h.
Swan eye needle h.
Swiss blade h.
swivel joint suture h.
tapered-spring needle h.
Taylor catheter h.
TC needle h.
temporal bone h.
tenaculum h.
Tennant needle h.
Thomas endotracheal tube h.
thumb-ring needle h.
Tilderquist needle h.
Toennis needle h.
Tomac vest-style h.
Torres needle h.
tracheostomy tube h.
TRAKE-fit tracheostomy tube h.
trochanter h.
Troutman-Barraquer needle h.
Troutman needle h.
Tru-Cut biopsy needle h.
Turner-Warwick needle h.
Twisk needle h.
Universal head h.
Universal speculum h.
Vacutainer h.
vascular needle h.
VBH head h.
Vickers needle h.
Vital-Baumgartner needle h.
Vital-Castroviejo eye needle h.
Vital-Cooley French-eye needle h.
Vital-Cooley general tissue h.
Vital-Cooley intracardiac needle h.
Vital-Cooley microvascular
  needle h.
Vital-Cooley neurosurgical needle h.
Vital-Crile-Wood needle h.
Vital-DeBakey cardiovascular
  needle h.
Vital-Derf eye needle h.
Vital-Finochietto needle h.
Vital French eye-needle h.
Vital-Halsey eye-needle h.
Vital-Heaney needle h.

Vital-Jacobson spring-handled
needle h.
Vital-Julian needle h.
Vital-Kalt eye needle h.
Vital-Masson needle h.
Vital-Mayo-Hegar needle h.
Vital microsurgery needle h.
Vital microvascular needle h.
Vital-Mills vascular needle h.
Vital-Neivert needle h.
Vital neurosurgical needle h.
Vital-New Orleans needle h.
Vital-Olsen-Hegar needle h.
Vital-Rochester needle h.
Vital-Ryder needle h.
Vital-Sarot needle h.
Vital-Stratte needle h.
Vital-Wangensteen needle h.
Vital-Webster needle h.
V. Mueller laser Rhoton
microneedle h.
V. Mueller-Vital laser Heaney
needle h.
V. Mueller-Vital laser Julian
needle h.
Vogel-Bale-Hohner head h.
Wangensteen needle h.
Wangensteen-Vital needle h.
washer h.
Watanabe pin h.
Watson heart value h.
Web needle h.
Webster-Halsey needle h.
Webster-Kleinert needle h.
Webster needle h.
Webster-Vital needle h.
Wehbe arm h.
Weisenbach sterile forceps h.
well-leg h.
Wertheim needle h.
Williams Uni-Quad leg h.
Wister forceps h.
Wolf-Castroviejo needle h.
Worcester instrument h.
Yasargil bayonet needle h.
Yasargil microneedle h.
Young boomerang needle h.
Young-Hryntschak boomerang
needle h.
Young-Millin boomerang needle h.
Young needle h.

Zollinger leg h.
Zweifel needle h.
holding
  h. forceps
  h. mitt
2-hole
  2-h. miniplate
  2-h. plate
3-hole
  3-h. aspiration cannula
  3-h. plate
4-hole anteromedial Alta straight plate
6-hole mandibular plate
7-hole plate
Holinger
  H. anterior commissure
    laryngoscope
  H. applicator
  H. bronchoscopic magnet
  H. bronchoscopic telescope
  H. cannula
  H. curved scissors
  H. endoscopic magnet
  H. hook-on folding laryngoscope
  H. hourglass anterior commissure
    laryngoscope
  H. infant bougie
  H. infant bronchoscope
  H. infant esophageal speculum
  H. infant esophagoscope
  H. laryngeal dissector
  H. modified Jackson laryngoscope
  H. needle
  H. open-end aspirating tube
  H. slotted laryngoscope
  H. specimen forceps
  H. ventilating fiberoptic
    bronchoscope
Holinger-Benjamin laser diverticuloscope
Holinger-Garfield laryngoscope
Holinger-Hurst bougie
Holinger-Jackson bronchoscope
Holladay posterior capsular polisher
Hollander clogs
Hollenback carver
HolliGard seal closed stoma pouch
Hollister
  H. adhesive
  H. bridge suture bolster
  H. circumcision device
  H. clamp
  H. collecting device

NOTES

H

Hollister *(continued)*
    H. colostomy bag
    H. colostomy irrigator
    H. disposable convex insert
    H. drainable fecal collector
    H. drainage bag
    H. external catheter
    H. First Choice pouch
    H. Flextend skin barrier
    H. Hot/Ice knee blanket
    H. irrigator drain
    H. laryngoscope
    H. medical adhesive bandage
    H. replacement filters pouch cover
    H. self-adhesive catheter
    H. urostomy bag
    H. wound exudate absorber
hollow
    h. chisel
    h. fiber (HF)
    h. fiber dialyzer
    h. mill
    h. needle
    h. Silastic disc heart valve
    h. sphere prosthesis
    h. visceral tonometer
hollow-sphere orbital implant
Holman
    H. flushing apparatus
    H. lung retractor
Holman-Mathieu salpingography cannula
Holmes
    H. cartilage gouge
    H. chisel
    H. fixation forceps
    H. nasopharyngoscope
    H. scissors
holmium
    h. laser
    h. laser lithotripter
holmium:YAG laser
holmium:yttrium-aluminum-garnet laser
holmium:yttrium-argon-garnet laser
Holofax Oxford retroillumination cataract camera
Hologic
    H. EP 2000 electrophysiology imaging system
    H. 1000 QDR dual-energy absorptiometer
    H. QDR-series densitometer
    H. QDR 1000W dual-energy x-ray absorptiometry scanner
Holscher nerve retractor
Holter
    H. connector
    H. distal atrial catheter
    H. distal catheter passer
    H. distal peritoneal catheter

    H. elliptical valve
    H. external drainage system
    H. high-pressure valve
    H. hydrocephalus shunt system
    H. in-line shunt filter
    H. introducer
    H. lumboperitoneal catheter
    H. medium-pressure valve
    H. mini-elliptical valve
    H. monitor
    H. pump
    H. shunt
    H. straight valve
    H. ventricular catheter
    H. ventriculostomy reservoir
Holter-Hausner
    H.-H. catheter
    H.-H. valve
Holter-Rickham ventriculostomy reservoir
Holter-Salmon-Rickham ventriculostomy reservoir
Holter-Selker ventriculostomy reservoir
Holth
    H. corneoscleral punch
    H. cystotome
    H. punch forceps
    H. scleral punch
    H. sclerectomy punch
Holth-Rubin punch
Holt self-retaining catheter
Holtz endometrial curette
Holzbach
    H. abdominal retractor
    H. hysterectomy forceps
Holzheimer
    H. automatic skin retractor
    H. mastoid retractor
HomeCare Simplimatt Plus Zoned foam mattress
Homecraft Folding EasiReach reacher
HomeKair bed
Homepump infusion system
Homer
    H. localizaton needle
    H. Mammalok breast localization needle
Homerlok needle
Homestretch lumbar traction
HomeTrac
    H. cervical traction
    H. cervical traction unit
home uterine activity monitor (HUAM)
Homiak radium colpostat
HomMed monitoring system
Homochron monitor
homogeneous screen
homogenizer
    Polytron PT 3000 h.

Potter-Elvehjem h.
Wheaton tissue h.

homograft

CryoLife h.
denatured h.
h. implant
h. prosthesis

homonuclear spin system

Honan

H. balloon
H. cuff
H. manometer
H. sphygmometer

Honeywell recorder

hood

Disposa-Hood disposable infant
  oxygen h.
H. dissector
H. electrodermatome
H. Laboratories Eccovision acoustic
  rhinometer
laminar flow h.
H. manual dermatome
Olympic Oxyhood oxygen h.
H. stoma stent
surgical h.
H. truss

Hood-Graves vaginal speculum

Hood-Westaby T-Y stent

hook

Abramson h.
Adson angular h.
Adson blunt dissecting h.
Adson brain h.
Adson dissecting h.
Adson dural h.
Adson sharp h.
Allport h.
Amenabar discission h.
anchor h.
Anderson suture pusher and
  double h.
Andre h.
h. approximator
Arruga extraction h.
Ashbell h.
attic h.
Aufranc h.
Azar lens h.
ball nerve h.
Bane h.
Barr crypt h.

Barr rectal fistular h.
Barton double h.
Bellucci h.
Berens scleral h.
Bethune nerve h.
bifid h.
Billeau ear h.
Birks Mark II h.
Blair palate h.
h. blocker
blunt dissecting h.
blunt nerve h.
boat h.
Bobechko sliding barrel h.
Boettcher tonsillar h.
bone h.
Bonn micro iris h.
Bonn microiris h.
Bose tracheostomy h.
Boyes-Goodfellow h.
Bozeman h.
Braun decapitation h.
Braun obstetrical h.
Brimfield cannulated grasping h.
Brown h.
Bryant mitral h.
Buck h.
Burch h.
button h.
buttressed h.
canted finger h.
Carroll bone h.
Carroll skin h.
Caspar h.
Catalano muscle h.
caudal h.
cautery h.
C-D h.
Chavasse squint h.
Chavasse strabismus h.
Chernov tracheostomy h.
Clayman iris h.
cleft palate sharp h.
Cloward cautery h.
Cloward dural h.
coarctation h.
Cohen maxillary fixation h.
cold knife h.
Collier-Martin h.
Colver examining h.
Colver retractor h.
compression h.

NOTES

H

445

hook *(continued)*

Converse skin h.
corkscrew dural h.
corneal h.
Cotrel-Dubousset h.
Cottle angled skin h.
Cottle double h.
Cottle-Joseph double h.
Cottle nasal h.
Cottle skin h.
Cottle tenaculum h.
cranial Jacobs h.
Crawford h.
Crile nerve h.
crochet h.
crural h.
crypt h.
Culler rectus muscle h.
Cushing dural h.
Cushing gasserian ganglion h.
Cushing nerve h.
cystic h.
Daily fixation h.
Dandy nerve h.
Davis h.
Day ear h.
DeBakey valve h.
DePuy Isola h.
DePuy Moss Miami h.
destructive obstetrical h.
Dingman zygomatic h.
dissecting h.
h. dissector
distraction h.
h. distractor
Dohlman incus h.
double-pronged Cottle h.
double-pronged Fomon h.
double-tenaculum h.
Doyen rib h.
Drews-Sato suture-pickup h.
Drummond h.
Dudley rectal h.
Dudley tenaculum h.
dural h.
ear h.
Edwards-Levine h.
Edwards rectal h.
Effler-Groves h.
h. electrode
Emmet h.
expressor h.
h. expressor
extraction h.
Feaster lens h.
fenestration h.
Ferszt dissecting h.
fibroid h.
finger h.

Fink oblique muscle h.
Finsen tracheal h.
Finsen wound h.
Fisch dural h.
fistula h.
fixation twist h.
flat tenotomy h.
Fomon nasal h.
footplate h.
h. forceps
Frazier cordotomy h.
Frazier dural h.
Frazier nerve h.
Frazier skin h.
Freer skin h.
Fresnel manipulating h.
Fukasaku pupil snapper h.
Galand lens manipulating h.
Gam-Mer nerve h.
Gass muscle h.
Gass retinal detachment h.
Gillies h.
Gillies bone h.
Gillies-Converse skin h.
Gillies dural h.
Gillies nasal h.
Gillies skin h.
Gillies zygomatic h.
goiter h.
Goldman Universal nerve h.
Goodhill h.
Graefe iris h.
Graefe strabismus h.
Graether mushroom h.
Graham blunt h.
Graham dural h.
Graham muscle h.
Graham nerve h.
Green muscle h.
Green strabismus h.
Gross ear h.
Guthrie fixation h.
Guthrie iris h.
Guthrie skin h.
Gwathmey h.
Gynex angle h.
Gynex iris h.
Hall modified Moe h.
Hamilton-Forewater amniotomy h.
Hardesty tendon h.
Hardesty tenotomy h.
Harrington pedicle h.
Harris-Sinskey microlens h.
Haven skin graft h.
Hebra h.
Helvestoon h.
H. hemi-harness shoulder
   immobilizer
Henton tonsillar suture h.

Hirschman iris h.
Hoen nerve h.
Hosmer Dorrance h.
House crural h.
House incus h.
House oval-window h.
House plate h.
House strut h.
House tragus h.
Hunkeler ball-point h.
h. impactor
instant skin h.
intermediate C-D h.
intracapsular lens expressor h.
intraocular h.
iris h.
irrigating iris h.
IUD remover h.
Jackson tracheal h.
Jacobs cranial h.
Jacobson blunt h.
Jaeger strabismus h.
Jaffe iris h.
Jaffe lens-manipulating h.
Jaffe-Maltzman h.
Jaffe microlens h.
Jako fine ball-tip h.
Jako-Kleinsasser ball-tip h.
Jameson muscle h.
Jameson strabismus h.
Jannetta h.
Jardine h.
Jarit bone h.
Jarit palate h.
jaw h.
Johnson skin h.
Jordan h.
Joseph nasal h.
Joseph single-prong h.
Joseph skin h.
Joseph tenaculum h.
Juers h.
Katena boat h.
Keene compression h.
Kelly uterine tenaculum h.
Kelman irrigation h.
Kelman manipulator h.
Kennerdell-Maroon h.
Kennerdell-Maroon-Jameson h.
Kennerdell muscle h.
Kennerdell nerve h.
Kilner goiter h.

Kilner skin h.
Kimball nephrostomy h.
Kirby double-fixation muscle h.
Klapp tendon h.
Kleinert-Kutz skin h.
Kleinsasser h.
Klemme dural h.
Klintskog amniotomy h.
Knapp iris h.
h. knife
Kratz iris push-pull h.
Krayenbuehl dural h.
Krayenbuehl nerve h.
Krayenbuehl vessel h.
Kuglen manipulating iris h.
Küntscher nail-extracting h.
Lahey Clinic dural h.
Lambotte bone h.
laminar C-D h.
Lange fistular h.
Lange plastic surgery h.
Laqua black line retinal h.
large ball nerve h.
Leader iris h.
Leader vas h.
Leatherman alar h.
Leatherman compression h.
Leinbach olecranon h.
lens h.
Levy-Kuglen iris h.
Lewicky microlens h.
Lillie attic h.
Lillie ear h.
Linton vein h.
Loughnane prostatic h.
Lucae h.
lyre-shaped finger h.
Madden sympathectomy h.
Magielski h.
Maidera-Stern suture h.
Malgaigne patellar h.
Malis nerve h.
h. manipulator
Manson double-ended strabismus h.
Martin rectal h.
Maumenee iris h.
Mayo fibroid h.
McIntyre irrigating iris h.
McMahon nephrostomy h.
McReynolds lid-retracting h.
Meyerding skin h.
Microlens h.

NOTES

H

447

hook *(continued)*

Miltex Cottle double h.
Miltex Wiener corneal h.
Miya h.
Moe alar h.
Morgenstein h.
Morrison skin h.
Moss h.
Muelly h.
multispan fracture h.
Murphy ball-end h.
muscle h.
Neivert nasal polyp h.
nerve h.
neutral h.
Newell nucleus h.
Newhart h.
New tracheostomy h.
New tracheotomy h.
Nova jaw h.
Nugent iris h.
oblique muscle h.
O'Brien rib h.
obstetrical decapitating h.
Ochsner h.
O'Connor flat tenotomy h.
O'Connor muscle h.
Oesch h.
ophthalmic h.
Osher irrigating implant h.
Pajot decapitating h.
palate h.
Paul tendon h.
PCL-oriented placement marking h.
pear-shaped nerve h.
pediatric C-D h.
pediatric TSRH h.
pedicle h.
pedicle C-D h.
Penn swivel h.
Pickrell h.
Pitie-Salpetriere saphenous vein h.
plain ear h.
Praeger iris h.
Pratt crypt h.
Pratt cystic h.
Pratt rectal h.
Pucci-Seed h.
h. pusher
Rainin iris h.
Rainin lens h.
Ramsbotham decapitating h.
Rappazzo iris h.
recession ophthalmic muscle h.
rectal h.
resection ophthalmic double h.
retinal detachment h.
h. retractor
retractor h.

Rhoton nerve h.
Rica cerumen h.
Richards bone h.
Rogozinski h.
Rolf muscle h.
Rollet lacrimal sac h.
Rollet strabismus h.
Rosser crypt h.
h. rotary scissors
Russian four-pronged fixation h.
Sachs dural h.
Sadler bone h.
Saunders-Paparella stapes h.
Scanlan micronerve h.
Scanlan microvessel h.
Scheer h.
Schnitman skin h.
Schuknecht stapes h.
Schwartz cervical tenaculum h.
scleral h.
scleral twist fixation h.
Scobee oblique muscle h.
Scoville blunt h.
Scoville curved nerve h.
Scoville dural h.
Scoville retractor h.
Searcy fixation h.
Selby II h.
Selverstone cordotomy h.
Shambaugh endaural h.
Shambaugh fistula h.
Shambaugh microscopic h.
sharp h.
Sharpley h.
Shea fenestration h.
Shea fistular h.
Shea oblique h.
Shea stapes h.
Sheets iris h.
Shepard reversed iris h.
side-opening laminar h.
Simon fistula h.
Sinskey iris h.
Sinskey lens-manipulating h.
Sinskey microlens h.
Sisson spring h.
skin h.
sliding barrel h.
Sluder sphenoidal h.
Smellie obstetrical h.
SMIC cerumen h.
Smith expressor h.
Smith lid-retracting h.
Smithwick h.
Smithwick ganglion h.
Smithwick nerve h.
Smithwick sympathectomy h.
spatula h.
h. spatula

Speare dural h.
Speer suture h.
split-finger h.
spring h.
square-ended h.
squint h.
Stallard scleral h.
Stamler sideport fixation h.
stapes h.
Starion thermal cautery h.
Stevens muscle h.
Stevens tenotomy h.
Stewart crypt h.
Stewart rectal h.
Stille coarctation h.
St. Martin-Franceschetti cataract h.
Storz iris h.
strabismus h.
straight nerve h.
Strandell-Stille tendon h.
Strully dural twist h.
strut bar h.
Suraci elevator h.
suture h.
sympathectomy h.
Tauber ligature h.
tenaculum h.
tendon h.
Tennant anchor lens-insertion h.
Tennant iris h.
tenotomy h.
Toennis dural h.
Tomas iris h.
Tomas suture h.
tonsil h.
Torchia-Kuglen h.
Torchia lens h.
tracheal h.
tracheostomy h.
tracheotomy h.
triple h.
TSRH buttressed laminar h.
TSRH circular laminar h.
TSRH pedicle h.
tubal h.
twist fixation h.
Tyrrell h.
Tyrrell skin h.
UCLA CAPP TD h.
University of Kansas h.
up-angled h.
vas h.

Visitec angled lens h.
Visitec corneal suture
    manipulating h.
Visitec double iris h.
Visitec straight lens h.
V. Mueller blunt h.
Volkmann bone h.
Volkmann vas h.
von Graefe muscle h.
von Graefe strabismus h.
von Szulec h.
Wagener h.
Walsh h.
Weary nerve h.
Welch Allyn rectal h.
Wiener corneal h.
Wiener scleral h.
Wiener suture h.
Wilder foreign body h.
Wilder lens h.
Y h.
Yankauer h.
Yasargil spring h.
Zaufel-Jansen ear h.
Zielke bifid h.
Zoellner h.
zygoma h.
Zylik-Joseph h.
hooked
    h. catheter
    h. intramedullary nail
    h. knife
    h. needle
hook-rod
    Cotrel-Dubousset h.-r.
    Isola h.-r.
    TSRH h.-r.
hook-type dermal curette
hookwire needle
Hooper pediatric scissors
Hoopes corneal marker
Hope
    H. processor
    H. resuscitation bag
    H. resuscitator
Hopener clamp
Hopkins
    H. aortic forceps
    H. aortic occlusion clamp
    H. arthroscope
    H. dilator
    H. direct-vision telescope

NOTES

H

Hopkins *(continued)*
    H. forward-oblique telescope
    H. Hospital periosteal raspatory
    H. hysterectomy clamp
    H. II rod lens
    H. lateral telescope
    H. nasal endoscopy telescope
    H. pediatric telescope
    H. Percuflex drainage catheter
    H. plaster knife
    H. retrospective telescope
    H. rod
    H. rod lens telescope
    H. sigmoidoscope
    H. tympanoscope
Hopkins-Cushing periosteal elevator
Hopp
    H. anterior commissure
      laryngoscope blade
    H. laryngoscope
Hopp-Morrison laryngoscope
Horgan
    H. center blade
    H. retractor
Horgan-Coryllos-Moure rib shears
Horgan-Wells rib shears
Horico
    H. diamond instrument
    H. disc
Horizon
    H. AutoAdjust CPAP system
    H. LT nasal CPAP system
    H. LX scanner
    H. phacoemulsification system
    H. prostatic stent
    H. surgical ligating and marking
      clip
horizontal
    h. drain attachment device
    h. flexible bar retractor
    h. pull headgear
    h. ring curette
    h. tube attachment device
1-horn bridge
Horn endo-otoprobe laser
horopter
    Vieth-Mueller h.
horseshoe
    h. headrest
    h. heel pad
    h. magnet
    h. tourniquet
horseshoe-shaped pad
Horsley
    H. bone cutter
    H. bone-cutting forceps
    H. bone wax
    H. cranial bone rongeur
    H. dural knife

    H. dural separator
    H. elevator
    H. spine cutter
    H. suture
    H. trephine
Horsley-Clarke stereotactic frame
Horsley-Stille
    H.-S. bone-cutting forceps
    H.-S. rib shears forceps
hose
    Juzo h.
    TED h.
    thromboembolic disease h.
Hosel
    H. needle holder
    H. retractor
Hosemann
    H. choledochus forceps
    H. choledochus knife
Hosford
    H. double-ended lacrimal dilator
    H. foreign body spud
    H. meibomian gland expressor
Hosford-Hicks
    H.-H. needle
    H.-H. transfer forceps
hosiery
    Spa Ready-To-Wear gradient
      pressure therapy h.
    Spa SoftBasics gradient pressure
      therapy h.
    Spa UltraSilk Sheers gradient
      pressure therapy h.
Hoskins
    H. beaked Colibri forceps
    H. fine straight forceps
    H. fixation forceps
    H. microstraight forceps
    H. nylon suture laser
    H. razor fragment blade
    H. suture forceps
Hoskins-Barkan goniotomy infant lens
Hoskins-Castroviejo corneal scissors
Hoskins-Colibri forceps
Hoskins-Dallas intraocular lens-inserting
  forceps
Hoskins-Drake implant
Hoskins-Luntz forceps
Hoskins-Skeleton
    H.-S. fine forceps
    H.-S. grooved broad-tipped forceps
Hoskins-Westcott tenotomy scissors
Hosmer
    H. above-knee rotator
    H. Dorrance hook
    H. single-axis locking knee
    H. voluntary control four-bar knee
      orthosis
    H. WALK prosthesis

H. weight-activated locking knee prosthesis
Hosmer-Dorrance 4-bar knee mechanism
Hosokawa E-Spart analyzer
Hospidex microtiter plate
hospital
  h. bed
  Texas Scottish Rite H. (TSRH)
Hossli suction tube
hot
  h. biopsy forceps
  h. cathode x-ray tube
  h. flexible forceps
  h. knife
  h. moist pack
  h. pad
  h. quartz lamp
  h. salt sterilizer
  H. Sampler disposable hot biopsy forceps
  h. water bottle
  h. wet pack
  h. wire anemometer
HotBlade
  Patton H.
Hotchkiss ear suction tube
Hot/Ice
  H. cold therapy cooler
  H. System III knee blanket
Hotline fluid-warming device
Hotmitt
  Champ arthritis H.
Hotsy high-temperature cautery
Hottentot apron
hot-tip laser
hot-tipped catheter
hot-wire
  h.-w. pneumotachometer
  h.-w. respirometer
Hotz ear probe
Hough
  H. anterior crurotomy nipper
  H. bed
  H. chisel
  H. crurotomy saw
  H. curette
  H. drape
  H. drum scraper
  H. fascial knife
  H. gouge
  H. hoe
  H. incision knife

H. oval-window excavator
H. scissors
H. spatula
H. spatula elevator
H. stapedectomy footplate pick
H. stapedial footplate auger
H. Teflon cutter
H. whirlybird
H. whirlybird excavator
H. whirlybird knife
Hough-Boucheron ear speculum
Hough-Cadogan suction tube
Hough-Derlacki mobilizer
Hough-Powell digitizer
Hough-Rosen knife
Hough-Saunders
  H.-S. excavator
  H.-S. stapes hoe
Houghton rongeur
Hough-Wullstein crurotomy saw bur
Hounsfield unit
24-hour ambulatory electrocardiographic recorder
hourglass
  h. anterior commissure laryngoscope
  h. dressing
Hourin tonsillar needle
House
  H. adapter
  H. alligator crimper forceps
  H. alligator grasping forceps
  H. alligator scissors
  H. alligator strut forceps
  H. bur
  H. calipers strut
  H. chisel
  H. crural hook
  H. cup forceps
  H. detachable blade
  H. dissector
  H. ear curette
  H. ear elevator
  H. ear forceps
  H. ear knife
  H. ear separator
  H. endaural elevator
  H. endolymphatic shunt
  H. excavator
  H. Gelfoam press
  H. Gelfoam pressure forceps
  H. grading system
  H. grasping forceps

NOTES

H

House *(continued)*
- H. handheld double-end retractor
- H. implant
- H. incudostapedial joint knife
- H. incus hook
- H. knife blade
- H. lacrimal dilator
- H. lancet knife
- H. malleus nipper
- H. measuring rod
- H. middle ear mirror
- H. miniature forceps
- H. myringoplasty knife
- H. myringotomy knife
- H. myringotomy knife handle
- H. neurovascular clip
- H. obtuse pick
- H. ophthalmic blade
- H. oval-cup forceps
- H. oval-window hook
- H. oval-window pick
- H. piston
- H. piston prosthesis
- H. piston wire
- H. plate hook
- H. pressure forceps
- H. and Pulec otic-periotic shunt
- H. round knife
- H. sickle knife
- H. stapes curette
- H. stapes elevator
- H. stapes needle
- H. stapes speculum
- H. strut calipers
- H. strut forceps
- H. strut guide
- H. strut hook
- H. strut pick
- H. sucker irrigator
- H. suction tube
- H. tantalum prosthesis
- H. tapping hammer
- H. Teflon-coated elevator
- H. Teflon cutting block
- H. tragus hook
- H. T-tube irrigator
- H. tympanoplasty curette
- H. tympanoplasty knife
- H. wire guide
- H. wire loop
- H. wire stapes prosthesis

House-Barbara
- H.-B. pick
- H.-B. shattering needle

House-Baron suction tube
House-Bellucci alligator scissors
House-Bellucci-Shambaugh alligator scissors
House-Billeau ear loop

House-Buck curette
Housecall transtelephonic ICD monitoring system
House-Crabtree dissector
House-Delrin cutting block
House-Derlacki chisel
House-Dieter
- H.-D. eye forceps
- H.-D. malleus nipper

House-Hough excavator
House-Paparella stapes curette
Housepian
- H. aneurysm clip
- H. clip-applying forceps
- H. sellar punch

Houser
- H. cul-de-sac irrigator tube
- H. silicone T-tube

House-Radpour
- H.-R. suction irrigator
- H.-R. suction tube

House-Rosen
- H.-R. knife
- H.-R. needle

House-Saunders middle ear curette
House-Sheehy knife curette
House-Stevenson
- H.-S. suction irrigator
- H.-S. suction tube

House-Urban
- H.-U. marker
- H.-U. microsurgery cine camera
- H.-U. middle fossa retractor
- H.-U. temporal bone holder
- H.-U. tube
- H.-U. UEM-100 cine camera
- H.-U. vacuum rotary dissector

House-Urban-Pentax camera
House-Urban-Stille camera
House-Wullstein
- H.-W. alligator forceps
- H.-W. cup ear forceps
- H.-W. perforating bur

Houspian clip-applying forceps
Housset-Debray gastroscope
Houston
- H. halo
- H. halo cervical traction
- H. nasal osteotome

Houtz endometrial curette
Hoverbed bed
Hoveround HVR 100 wheelchair
Howard
- H. closing forceps
- H. corneal abrader
- H. Jones needle
- H. spinal curette
- H. spiral stone dislodger
- H. stone basket

H. tonsillar forceps
H. tonsil-ligating forceps
Howard-DeBakey aortic aneurysm clamp
Howard-Flaherty spiral stone dislodger
Howard-Schatz laser
Howarth nasal raspatory
Howell
H. biliary aspiration needle
H. biliary introducer brush
H. biopsy aspiration needle
H. rotatable BII papillotome
H. rotatable BII sphincterotome
Howland lock
Howmedica
H. Centrax head replacement
H. cerclage
H. Duracon implant
H. hip fracture stem
H. HNR system
H. Kinematic II knee prosthesis
H. Microfixation System drill bit
H. Microfixation System forceps
H. Monotube
H. monotube external rotator
H. Osteonics bone cement
H. PCA textured hip
H. pediatric osteotomy system
H. Simplex P cement
H. total ankle system
H. Unitrax hip fracture system
H. Universal compression screw
Howorth
H. elevator
H. osteotome
H. prosthesis
H. toothed retractor
Howse-Coventry hip prosthesis
Howtek Scanmaster DX scanner
Hoxworth
H. clip
H. forceps
Hoya
H. AR-570 autorefractor
H. HDR objective refractometer
H. MRM objective refractometer
Ho:YAG laser
Hoyer
H. lift
H. snare

Hoyt
H. deep-surgery forceps
H. hemostatic forceps
Hoytenberger tissue forceps
HP
Hewlett-Packard
HP M1350A fetal monitor
HP MIDA
HP OmniPlane TEE imaging transducer
HP Sonos 2500 cardiac/vascular diagnostic ultrasound
HP Sonos ultrasound imaging system
HP1035 gel heel protector
HPC guidewire
HPS II total hip prosthesis
Hruby
H. contact implant
H. contact lens
H. laser
Hryntschak catheter
H-series electron microscope
HSG
hysterosalpingogram
HSG catheter
H-shaped plate
HSS total condylar knee prosthesis
HTO
high tibial osteotomy
HTO fixator
HTO wedge tissue allograft
HTR
hard tissue replacement
HTR polymer
HTR-MFI
hard tissue replacement-malleable facial implant
HTR-MFI chin implant
HTR-MFI malar implant
HTR-MFI onlay facial augmentation implant
HTR-MFI paranasal implant
HTR-MFI premaxillary implant
HTR-MFI ramus implant
HTR-MFI straight implant
H-TRON plus V100 insulin infusion pump
HTR-PMI
hard tissue replacement-patient matched implant
HTR-PMI implant

NOTES

H

HUAM
  home uterine activity monitor
Huang
  H. Universal arm retractor
  H. vein holder
Hubbard
  H. airplane vent tube
  H. bolt
  H. corneoscleral forceps
  H. electrode
  H. hydrotherapy tank
  H. plate
  H. retractor
Hubbard-Nylok bolt
Hubell meatoscope
Huber
  H. forceps handle
  H. point needle
  H. probe
HubGuard IV cushion pad
Hub saw
Huco diamond knife
Hudgins salpingography cannula
Hudson
  H. adapter
  H. All-Clear nasal cannula
  H. bone drill
  H. bone retractor
  H. brace bur
  H. brain forceps
  H. cerebellar attachment
  H. cerebellar extension
  H. clamp
  H. conical bur
  H. cranial bur
  H. cranial drill
  H. cranial forceps
  H. dressing forceps
  H. Hydro-Float cushion
  H. Lifesaver resuscitator
  H. Multi-Vent
  H. rongeur forceps
  H. shank
  H. tissue forceps
  H. TLSO brace
  H. T Up-Draft II disposable
    nebulizer
  H. type oxygen mask
Hudson-Ewald tissue forceps
Hudson-Jones knee cage brace
Huegli
  H. meatoscope
  H. meatotome
Hueter
  H. bandage
  H. perineal dressing
Huey scissors

Huffman
  H. infant vaginal speculum
  H. infant vaginoscope
**Huffman-Graves adolescent vaginal
  speculum**
Huffman-Huber
  H.-H. infant urethrotome
  H.-H. infant vaginoscope
Hufford esophagoscope
Hufnagel
  H. aortic clamp
  H. commissurotomy knife
  H. implant
  H. low-profile heart prosthesis
  H. mitral valve forceps
  H. prosthetic valve
Hufnagel-Kay heart valve
Hufnagel-Ryder needle holder
Hu-Friedy
  H.-F. dental bur
  H.-F. elevator
  H.-F. PermaSharp suture
  H.-F. suction tip aspirator
Huger diamond-back nasal scissors
Hugg-L-O pillow
Hughes
  H. eye implant
  H. fulguration electrode
Hugly aspirating tube
HUI
  Harris uterine injector
  HUI catheter
  HUI Mini-Flex
  HUI Mini-Flex uterine injector
Huibregtse biliary stent
Huibregtse-Katon
  H.-K. ERCP catheter
  H.-K. needle knife
  H.-K. papillotome
  H.-K. sphincterotome
Hulbert
  H. electrosurgical knife
  H. endo-electrode set
Hulka
  H. clip
  H. clip applier
  H. clip forceps
  H. tenaculum forceps
  H. uterine cannula
  H. uterine manipulator
  H. uterine tenaculum
Hulka-Clemens clip
Hulka-Kenwick
  H.-K. uterine-elevating forceps
  H.-K. uterine elevator
Hulten-Stille cannula
Humagen
  H. blastomere biopsy micropipet
  H. polar body biopsy micropipet

human
- h. allograft tissue
- h. glucose monitoring (HGN)

HumatroPen injection device
Humby knife
Hume aortic clamp
humeral
- h. cutting guide
- h. head depressor
- h. impactor
- h. reamer
- h. retractor
- h. saw

HUMI
- Harris-Kronner uterine manipulator-injector
- HUMI cannula
- HUMI uterine manipulator

HumidAire heated humidifier
HumidFilter heat and moisture exchanger
humidifier
- Bard-Parker U-Mid/Lo h.
- Bemis air h.
- Bennett Cascade II Servo controlled heated h.
- bubble h.
- cold-mist h.
- Fisher & Paykel HC-series heated h.
- HumidAire heated h.
- hygroscopic condenser h. (HCH)
- jet h.
- Mistogen passover h.
- MRT tidal h.
- Oasis h.
- OEM 503 h.
- Ohio Bubble h.
- passover h.
- Respironics Oasis h.
- room h.
- Sullivan HumidAire heated h.
- Whisper Mist cool mist h.

Humid-Vent Port 1 elbow connector
Hummer
- H. microdebrider
- H. V Sputter coater

Hummingbird wand
hump
- h. forceps
- h. gouge

Humphrey
- H. Atlas Eclipse corneal topography system
- H. automatic keratometer
- H. automatic refractor
- H. B-scan
- H. coronary sinus-sucker suction tube
- H. lens analyzer
- H. Mastervue corneal topography system
- H. perimeter
- H. retinal imager
- H. visual field analyzer

Humphries
- H. aortic aneurysm clamp
- H. reverse-curve aortic clamp

Humphriss binocular balance
Hundley knee knife
Hunkeler
- H. ball-point hook
- H. frown incision marker
- H. intraocular lens
- H. lightweight intraocular lens implant

Hunsaker
- H. jet ventilation tube
- H. Mon-Jet tube anesthesia system

Hunstad
- H. Handle flow control
- H. infusion needle
- H. Quik-Clik device
- H. tumescent anesthesia system

Hunt
- H. angiographic trocar
- H. angled serrated ring forceps
- H. arachnoid dissector
- H. bipolar forceps
- H. bladder retractor
- H. chalazion forceps
- H. chalazion scissors
- H. colostomy clamp
- H. grasping forceps
- H. metal sound
- H. needle
- H. organizer
- H. tumor forceps
- H. vessel forceps

Hunter
- H. balloon
- H. open cord tendon implant

NOTES

H

455

Hunter *(continued)*
    H. 1-piece all-PMMA intraocular lens
    H. separator
    H. splinter forceps
    H. tendon prosthesis
    H. tendon rod
    H. uterine curette
Hunter-Satinsky clamp
Hunter-Sessions
    H.-S. balloon
    H.-S. vena cava-occluding balloon catheter
Hunt-Lawrence pouch
Huntleigh
    H. Diagnostics Inc. (HDI)
    H. Fetal Dopplex II FD2+ monitor
    H. mattress
Hunt-Reich secondary cannula
Hunt-Yasargil pituitary forceps
Hupp tracheal retractor
Hurd
    H. bipolar diathermy electrode
    H. bone-cutting forceps
    H. bone forceps
    H. pillar retractor
    H. septal bone-cutting forceps
    H. septal elevator
    H. septum-cutting forceps
    H. suture needle
    H. tonsillar dissector
    H. tonsillar pillar retractor
    H. turbinate electrode
Hurd-Morrison dissector
Hurdner tissue forceps
Hurd-Weder tonsillar dissector
Hurson
    H. flexible pressure clamp
    H. flexible retractor
    H. flexible sliding clamp
Hurst
    H. bullet-tip esophageal dilator
    H. mercury-filled dilator
    H. mercury-filled esophageal bougie
Hurst-Maloney dilator
Hurst-Tucker pneumatic dilator
Hurteau forceps
Hurtig dilator
Hurwitt catheter
Hurwitz
    H. dialysis catheter
    H. esophageal clamp
    H. intestinal clamp
    H. thoracic trocar
Huse cannula
Husen button
Husk mastoid rongeur
Hustead epidural needle

Hutch evacuator
Hutchins biopsy needle
Hutchinson iris retractor
Huxley respirator
huygenian eyepiece
Huygens eyepiece
Huzly
    H. applicator
    H. aspirator
HV
    HV NightSplint splint
    HV SoftSplint splint
H. Vantage graft
HVF ventilator
HVPC
    high-voltage pulsed current
hyaluronic acid (HA)
Hyams scleral knife
Hybond-N filter
Hybond N+ nylon membrane
hybrid
    h. capture system
    h. fixation of hip replacement component
    h. graft
    h. PET/SPECT camera
    h. prosthesis
HybridFit
    H. total hip system
    H. total knee system
hybridization
    fluorescent in situ h.
HyCoSy catheter
hyCure
    h. collagen hemostatic wound dressing
    h. G hydrogel dressing
Hyde
    H. astigmatism ruler
    H. double-curved corneal forceps
    H. irrigating-aspirating cannula
    H. irrigator & aspirator unit
    H. needle holder
Hyde-Osher keratometric ruler
Hydra
    H. Vision
    H. Vision ES urology system
    H. Vision IV urology imaging system
    H. Vision Plus DR urological imaging system
    H. Vision Plus HP urological imaging system
HydraClearTM endoscopic cleansing system
HydraClense sitz bath
Hydracon contact lens
HydraCross TLC PTCA catheter

Hydradjust
    H. IV table
    H. urology system
Hydragran absorption dressing
Hydrajaw insert
Hydrasoft contact lens
Hydrasorb
    H. foam wound dressing
    H. Plus dressing
hydraulic
    h. capillary infusion system
    h. chamber
    h. hand dynamometer
    h. knee unit prosthesis
    h. vein stripper
Hydro
    H. Bonnet
    H. Plus coated guidewire
    H. Soothe recliner
    H. TherAblator ablator
hydroactive dressing
Hydro-Bell
    Hydro-Tone H.-B.
HydroBlade keratome
HydroBrader irrigating-aspirating dermabrader
HydroBrush keratome
Hydro-Cast
    H.-C. dental mold
    H.-C. reliner
HydroCath central venous catheter
hydrocephalus shunt
Hydrocoat hydrophilic coating
hydrocollator
    H. heating unit
    h. pack
    H. pad
    H. steam pack
hydrocolloid occlusive dressing
Hydrocol sacral wound dressing
Hydrocurve lens
hydrodelineation cannula
HydroDerm transparent dressing
hydrodissection
    Akahoshi ophthalmic h.
    h. cannula
hydrodissector
    cortical cleaving h.
    Mectra h.
    Nezhat-Dorsey trumpet valve h.
    Pearce nucleus h.
    trumpet valve h.

hydrodynamic thrombectomy system
Hydro-Ease
    H.-E. II gel flotation mattress overlay
    H.-E. I water flotation mattress overlay
Hydrofera Blue PVA dressing
Hydroflex
    H. II intraocular lens
    H. penile semirigid implant
    H. sphincter
HydroFlex irrigation system
hydrofloat cushion
Hydrofloss electronic oral irrigator
hydrogel
    h. intraocular lens
    h. plug
    h. sheet
    Stericare glycerin h.
    h. wound dressing
Hydrogel-coated PTCA balloon catheter
Hydrojette aspirator
hydrokeratome
    Visijet h.
Hydrokinetic Vichy shower
Hydrolene polymer
Hydrolyser
    H. microcatheter
    H. thrombectomy catheter
hydromassage table
Hydromer
    H. coated bipolar coagulation probe
    H. coated polyurethane stent
    H. grafted catheter
Hydron
    H. burn bandage
    H. lens
Hydronol hydrophilic guidewire
hydrophilic
    h. contact lens
    h. dilator
    h. polymer-coated steerable guidewire
    h. polyurethane foam dressing
    h. tent
hydrophilic-coated
    h.-c. guide wire
    h.-c. guiding catheter
hydrophobic barrier pen
hydrophone
    Imotec needle h.
HydroPlus stent

NOTES

H

hydropolymer pad
hydrosector
    Reddick-Saye h.
Hydrosight lens
Hydro-Splint II splint
hydrostatic
    h. bag
    h. balloon
    h. balloon catheter
    h. bed
    h. dilator
    h. dissector
HydroSurg laparoscopic irrigator
hydrotherapy tub
HydroThermAblator endometrial
  ablation system
Hydro-Tone Hydro-Bell
Hydrotrack underwater treadmill
Hydroview
    H. foldable IOL
    H. lens
Hydrovisage full-face hot/cold compress
Hydroxial hip prosthesis
hydroxyapatite
    h. adhesive
    h. bead
    h. coated implant
    h. implant
    Interpore 200 porous h.
    LPPS h.
    h. ocular implant
    h. ossicular prosthesis
    porous block h.
hydroxyapatite-coated stem
HyFil hydrogel dressing
Hyfrecator
    Birtcher H.
    H. coagulator
    Hall-Fish H.
Hyfrecutter
Hygene semen collection kit
HygieniKit breast milk collection system
hygroscopic
    h. condenser humidifier (HCH)
    h. heat and moisture exchanger
Hylamer
    H. acetabular liner
    H. orthopaedic bearing polymer
Hylashield
Hylasine viscoelastic material
Hylinks clip
Hylin rasp
Hymes
    H. double-lumen catheter
    H. meatal clamp
Hymes-Timberlake electrode
Hymlek portable chest tube
Hypafix retention tape
Hypan tent

hyperalimentation catheter
hyperbaric
    h. bed
    h. boot
    h. chamber
hyperbolic glasses
hyperextension
    h. brace
    cruciform anterior spinal h.
    (CASH)
    h. fracture frame
Hyperex thoracic orthosis
Hyperflex
    H. flexible guidewire
    H. tracheostomy tube
Hypergel hydrogel wound dressing
Hyperion
    H. LTK laser
    H. wound gel dressing
Hyper-Oxy portable hyperbaric chamber
HyperPACS system
Hypertie bandage
Hypobaric
    H. transfemoral system
    H. transtibial system
hypodermic needle
hypophysectomy forceps
hypophysial curette
Hypospray jet injection needle
Hypotherm Gel Kap
hypothermia
    h. blanket
    h. mattress
    h. oxygen warmer
Hyrax appliance
Hysorb wound dressing
hysterectomy
    h. clamp
    h. forceps
    h. kit
    h. retractor
hysterofiberscope
    Olympus flexible h.
hysteroflator
    Hamou h.
hysterosalpingogram (HSG)
hysterosalpingography catheter
hysteroscope
    ACMI h.
    ACMI Micro-H h.
    Amsco h.
    Baggish h.
    Baloser h.
    Circon ACMI h.
    contact h.
    diagnostic h.
    Elmed h.
    examining h.
    fiberoptic h.

flexible h.
Fujinon flexible h.
Galileo rigid h.
Hamou h.
Karl Storz 15 French flexible h.
Liesegang LM-Flex 7 flexible h.
MicroSpan h.
Olympus h.
OPERA Star SL h.
Scopemaster contact h.
h. sheath

Storz h.
Valle h.
Van Der Pas h.
hysteroscopic insufflator
Hysteroser contact hysteroscopy system
Hysto-vac drain
Hy-Tape
  H.-T. latex-free surgical tape
  H.-T. waterproof adhesive tape
Hy-Tec Plus Automated EIA system
HyTek guidewire

NOTES

H

I&A
  irrigating-aspirating
  irrigation-aspiration
  irrigation and aspiration
    I&A coaxial cannula
    I&A kit
    I&A machine
    I&A system
    I&A unit
IAB
  intraaortic balloon
    IAB catheter
IABP
  intraaortic balloon pump
    Bard TransAct IABP
Ialo photocoagulator
IBD-Check ELISA test kit
I-beam
    I-b. cement punch
    I-b. hemiarthroplasty hip prosthesis
    Jergesen I-b.
    I-b. press-fit punch
IBF
  Insall-Burstein-Freeman
    IBF knee instrument
    IBF total knee instrumentation
IBM
    IBM field-cycling research
    relaxometer
    IBM NMR spectrometer
iBOT wheelchair
IC
  intensive care
    IC bed
Icarex 25 Med mirror reflex lens camera
I-Cath
    Firlit-Sugar intermittent catheter I-C.
ICD
  implantable cardioverter-defibrillator
    Cadence biphasic ICD
    dual-chamber ICD
    Guardian ICD
    Telectronics Guardian ATP II ICD
    transthoracically implanted ICD
    Ventritex Cadence ICD
    Vitatron Diamond ICD
ice
    i. bag
    i. clot evacuator
    Liquid I.
    Sealed I.
    I. Wedge hot/cold therapy wrap
I.C.E. Down cold pack

Iceflex Endurance suction suspension sleeve
ICE-Magic pain reduction kit
Iceman
    I. cold therapy pad
    I. continuous cold therapy unit
Iceross
    I. Comfort Plus silicone gel liner
    I. sleeve
ice-tong calipers
Icex
    I. 4-hole lock
    I. socket
Icofly infusion needle
Icon foot prosthesis
ICP
  intracranial pressure
    ICP catheter
    ICP Express digital monitor
    ICP monitoring line
ICP-T fiberoptic ICP monitoring catheter
ICR
  intrastromal corneal ring
    KeraVision ICR
ICV
  intracerebroventricular
    ICV reservoir
ICV-10 ventilator
IDC
  interlocking detachable coil
Ideal
    I. cardiac device
    I. tourniquet
Idecap dialyzer
Identifit hip prosthesis
Identity ADx pacemaker
IDI
    Instituto Dermopatico dell'Immacolata
    IDI corneoscope
IDIS
  intraarterial digital subtraction
    IDIS angiography system
I-Flow nerve block infusion kit
Igaki-Tamai stent
Iglesias
    I. continuous-flow resectoscope
    I. dilator
    I. electrode
    I. evacuator
    I. fiberoptic resectoscope
    I. microlens resectoscope
Igloo Heatshield system
Ikeda capsulorrhexis forceps
IKI catgut suture

I-knife
Alcon I-k.
Ikuta
I. clamp approximator
I. fixation device
IL

IL 1640 blood/gas electrolyte
system
IL MED laser
ILA stapler
IL-282 CO-oximeter
ileoneobladder
Hautmann i.
W-shaped i.
ileostomy
i. appliance
i. bag
Ile-Sorb absorbent gel packet
iLEX stomal seal
Ilfeld
I. brace
I. splint
Ilg
I. capsular forceps
I. insertion forceps
I. needle
I. needle holder
I. probe
iliac
i. artery stent
i. clamp
i. forceps
i. graft separator
i. screw
Iliff
I. blepharochalasis forceps
I. clamp
I. lacrimal probe
I. lacrimal trephine
Iliff-Park speculum
Iliff-Wright fascia needle
iliosacral
i. and iliac fixation construct
i. screw
Ilizarov
I. circular external fixator
I. distractor
I. external ring fixator
I. fixation device
I. frame
I. hybrid fixator
I. limb-lengthening system
I. ring
I. screw
Illi
I. intracranial fixation device
I. intracranial pressure monitoring
device
Illinois needle

Illiterate E chart
Illouz
I. modified tip
I. standard tip
I. suction cannula
Illumena injector system
Illumen guiding catheter
Illumina Pro series laparoscopic laser
illuminated
i. probe
i. suction needle
i. vaginal speculum
illuminating stylet
illuminator
Barkan i.
Britetrac i.
Cogent XL i.
DyoBrite i.
fiberoptic surgical field i.
intramedullary i.
Light Commander xenon i.
Luxo surgical i.
Mammo Mask i.
Novar oral i.
Pelosi i.
Pilling fiberoptic i.
slit i.
suspended operating i.
XL i.
I.L.Med instrument
Il Med laser
Ilopan disposable syringe
ILUS
intraluminal ultrasound
ILUS catheter
IM
intramedullary
IM Jaws alligator forceps
IM nail
IM tendon stripper
IMA
inferior mesenteric artery
intermetatarsal angle
internal mammary artery
IMA graft
IMA retractor
IMA scissors
image
I. custom external breast prosthesis
i. intensifier
i. intensifier tube
i. Orthicon tube
i. processing unit
Image3 disposable face mask
Imagecath
I. angioscope
I. rapid exchange angioscope
ImageChecker CT LN-1000 system
ImageNet image digitizing system

imager
    DentaScan i.
    Digirad 2020tc i.
    digital slit-lamp i.
    Drystar dry i.
    flat-panel megavoltage i.
    GE Signa Genesis MR i.
    GE Signa Horizon EchoSpeed
      MR i.
    Hewlett-Packard color flow i.
    Humphrey retinal i.
    I. II angiographic catheter
    Infinion 0.6T magnetic resonance i.
    Integris V3000 i.
    Intera I/T interventional magnetic
      resonance i.
    Kodak 1200 Digital Science
      medical i.
    laser i.
    Magnetom SP MRI i.
    NeuroScan 3D i.
    OIS digital slit-lamp i.
    Signa i.
    Sonata i.
    Sonos 2000-series, 5000-series
      ultrasound i.
    Tesla Signa magnetic resonance i.
    I. Torque selective catheter
Image-View system
imaging
    blood flow i.
    Bucky high-contrast i.
    cine magnetic resonance i.
    color-flow Doppler real-time 2-D
      blood flow i.
    Color Power Angio i.
    Computer Technology and I. (CTI)
    Dent-X digital i.
    diffusion-weighted MR i.
    3-dimensional fast spin-echo
      magnetic resonance i.
    3-dimensional fast spin-echo
      magnetic resonance i.
    Discovery LS fusion i.
    Doppler transesophageal color
      flow i.
    dynamic contrast-enhanced magnetic
      resonance i.
    Dynamic Optical Breast I. (DOBI)
    echoplanar magnetic resonance i.
    endorectal coil magnetic
      resonance i.

    endorectal surface coil MR i.
    Epistar magnetic resonance i.
    Exceltech i.
    fast-imaging steady precession
      sequence 3-dimensional magnetic
      resonance i.
    Integris cardiovascular i.
    LaparoScan laparoscopic
      ultrasonic i.
    Lunar Artoscan M-series magnetic
      resonance i.
    Magnes magnetic source i.
    magnetic resonance i. (MRI)
    magnetic source i.
    MedMorph III patient video i.
    molecular coincidence detection i.
    phased-array body coil MR i.
    Philips Orthoralix i.
    radionucleotide i.
    Resurface laser resurfacing i.
    SieScape i.
    Tissue Specific i.
    transesophageal color flow
      Doppler i.
    Ultrafast magnetic resonance i.
imaging-angioplasty balloon catheter
Imagyn
    I. microlaparoscope
    I. surgical stapler
Imatron
    I. C-150XL ultrafast CT scanner
    I. electron beam tomography
      scanner
    I. Fastrac C-100 cine x-ray CT
      scanner
    I. system
imbedded microtransducer
Imbibe bone marrow aspiration syringe
**Imcor No-Touch implant placement
system**
Imed
    I. Gemini PC-2 volumetric pump
    I. infusion pump
IM/EM
    intramedullary/extramedullary
    IM/EM tibial resection guide
    IM/EM tibial resection stylus
Imex
    I. antepartum monitor
    I. Pocket-Dop OB Doppler
    I. scleral implant
Imexlab vascular diagnostic system

NOTES

Imhoff tank
IMMA lens
ImmEdge pen
immediate
    I. Implant Impression system
    I. Impression implant
    I. Load implant
    i. postoperative prosthesis (IPOP)
    I. Response Mobile Analysis
      (IRMA)
Immergut
    I. suction-coagulation tube
    I. suction tube
immersible video camera
Immix bioabsorbable implant
immobilization jacket
immobilizer
    Angle-Iron skull i.
    AP-PA skull i.
    arm and shoulder i.
    Breg slingshot arm and shoulder i.
    Circumstraint infant i.
    Comfort wrist i.
    cross-table leg i.
    dual leg i.
    Ezy Wrap shoulder i.
    Hook hemi-harness shoulder i.
    knee i.
    leg i.
    long leg i.
    Olympic Neostraint i.
    Pedi-Wrap i.
    QuickCast wrist i.
    shoulder abduction i.
    SpeedBlocks head i.
    sternal occipital mandibular i.
      (SOMI)
    sternooccipitomanubrial i.
    Tab-Strap knee i.
    tomographic skull i.
    Trimline knee i.
    i. vascular control instrument
    Velpeau shoulder i.
    Watco 2001 knee i.
    Westfield-style acromioclavicular i.
    Zinco Gunslinger II shoulder i.
immobilizing bandage
Immulite Dynamic Duo analyzer
Immune Cell Function assay kit
immunoadsorption column
immunocytometer
immunomagnetic bead
immunonephelometer
    BNA-100-Behring Diagnostics i.
immunostainer
    Shandon Candenza i.
    Ventana 320 automated i.
immunoturbidimetry analyzer
Imotec needle hydrophone

IMP
    Innovative Medical Products
    IMP bone screw targeter
    IMP Femur finder
    IMP Steri-Clamp clamp
    IMP surgical leg pedestal
    IMP turnstile casting stand
    IMP Universal lateral positioner
Impac PDQ abutment
impact
    I. balloon dilatation catheter
    I. drug and alcohol testing system
    i. glove
    I. lithotripter
    i. mitt
    I. modular porous prosthesis
    I. modular total hip system
impactor
    Bio-Moore II stem i.
    bone graft i.
    Cloward bone graft i.
    Cloward dowel i.
    Cohort spinal i.
    Dawson-Yuhl i.
    electromechanical i.
    femoral i.
    hook i.
    humeral i.
    Küntscher i.
    lateral gutter i.
    Moe i.
    mushroom i.
    orthopaedic i.
    i. plate
    Pollock wimp wire i.
    Raylor bone i.
    i. rod
    rotating arm i.
    shell i.
    Smith-Petersen i.
    Universal acetabular graft i.
    vertebral body i.
impactor-extractor
    Fox i.-e.
ImPad inflation pad
Impax PACS system
IMP-Capello
    I.-C. arm support
    I.-C. slimline abduction pillow
impedance
    i. electrode
    i. phlebograph
    i. threshold valve
Imperator handpiece
Imperatori laryngeal forceps
Imperial alloy
impermeable dressing
Imperson catheter

impervious
  i. stockinette
  i. U-sheet sheet
Impex
  I. aspiration & injection needle
  I. diamond radial keratotomy knife
Impex/Lerner foldable lens removing set
Impingement-Free tibial guide
impingement rod
ImplaMed
  I. gold screw
  I. implant system
implant
  AART calf i.
  AART chin i.
  AART gluteal i.
  AART malar i.
  AART pectoralis i.
  acorn-shaped eye i.
  acrylic conformer eye i.
  acrylic ocular i.
  Acticon neosphincter i.
  adjustable breast i.
  Advanta facial i.
  AdVent i.
  Aequalis humeral head i.
  afterloading i.
  alar-columellar i.
  Allen-Braley lens i.
  Allen ePTFE ocular i.
  Allen Supramid i.
  Alpar intraocular lens i.
  Alpha I penile i.
  Amelogen dental i.
  AMO scleral i.
  anterior chamber acrylic i.
  AO/ASIF orthopaedic i.
  Appolionio eye lens i.
  Arenberg-Denver inner-ear valve i.
  Arion i.
  Arnett Lefort i.
  Arroyo i.
  Arruga eye i.
  Arruga-Moura-Brazil orbital i.
  articulated chin i.
  artificial joint i.
  Ashworth-Blatt i.
  A-type dental i.
  Avanta soft skeletal i.
  Azar Tripod eye i.
  Baerveldt glaucoma drainage i.

  Baerveldt seton i.
  BAK/C cervical interbody fusion i.
  BAK/Proximity interbody fusion i.
  Balnetar i.
  Bannon-Klein i.
  Bard collagen Contigent i.
  Barkan infant lens i.
  Barraquer i.
  Bechert intraocular lens i.
  Becker expandable i.
  Beekhuis-Supramid mentoplasty augmentation i.
  Berens conical eye i.
  Berens orbital i.
  Berens pyramidal eye i.
  Berens-Rosa scleral i.
  Berens sphere eye i.
  Bicon dental i.
  Bietti eye i.
  bifocal lens i.
  bilumen mammary i.
  Binder Submalar facial i.
  Binkhorst collar stud lens i.
  Binkhorst eye i.
  Binkhorst lens i.
  Binkhorst 4-loop iris-fixated i.
  Biocare dental i.
  Biocell anatomical reconstructive mammary i.
  Biocell breast i.
  Biocell RTV saline-filled mammary i.
  Biocell textured breast i.
  Bioceram 2-stage series II endosteal dental i.
  Biocoral i.
  Biodel i.
  BioDimensional saline-filled i.
  Bio-eye hydroxyapatite ocular i.
  Biofix biodegradable i.
  BioHorizon i.
  Biomatrix ocular i.
  Biomet Repicci II unicompartment i.
  Bionx SmartNail bioresorbable i.
  bioresorbable orbital i.
  BioSorb FX dental i.
  Bio-Vent i.
  Biovert ceramic i.
  blade endosteal i.
  blade-form i.
  Blair-Brown i.

NOTES

implant *(continued)*
    i. blank
    Boberg-Ans lens i.
    Bonaccolto eye i.
    Bonaccolto orbital i.
    BoneSource i.
    Bosker transmandibular i.
    bovine collagen i.
    Boyd orbital i.
    Brånemark endosteal i.
    Braun i.
    Brawner orbital i.
    breast i.
    Brink PeriPyriform i.
    Brown-Dohlman Silastic corneal i.
    build-up eye i.
    Bunker i.
    calcar replacement i.
    Calcitek i.
    calcium phosphate ceramic i.
    candle vaginal cesium i.
    carbon i.
    Cardona focalizing fundus lens i.
    Cardona goniofocalizing i.
    carpal lunate i.
    Carrion-Small penile i.
    cartilage i.
    Castroviejo acrylic eye i.
    Celestin i.
    celluloid i.
    ceramic endosteal i.
    ceramometal i.
    Charnley i.
    Chatzidakis i.
    chessboard i.
    chin i.
    Choyce Mark VIII eye i.
    Christensen TMJ i.
    chromium-cobalt alloy i.
    Clarion cochlear i.
    Clarion Multi-Strategy cochlear i.
    Clayman lens i.
    cobalt-chromium coated i.
    cobalt-chromium-molybdenum alloy
      metal i.
    cobalt-chromium-tungsten-nickel
      alloy i.
    Coburn Mark IX eye i.
    cochlear i.
    Codere-Durette orbital floor i.
    Codere orbital floor i.
    collagen i.
    i. collar
    collared Press-Fit femoral stem i.
    columellar i.
    Combi-40 cochlear i.
    Compliant pre-stress bone i.
    condylar i.
    Conform Binder submalar facial i.

conical eye i.
contact shell i.
Contigen Bard collagen i.
Contour Profile natural saline
  breast i.
Contour Profile silicone breast i.
conventional reform eye i.
conventional shell-type eye i.
Cooper i.
Corail Corail HA-coated femoral i.
Corail HA-coated stem hip i.
Core-Vent dental i.
corneal i.
cosmetic contact shell i.
i. cover screw
Cox-Uphoff i.
Cronin mammary i.
Cryo-Barrages vitreous i.
CUI columellar i.
CUI dorsal i.
CUI malar i.
CUI rhinoplasty i.
curl-back shell eye i.
curvilinear chin i.
Custodis i.
custom-contoured i.
Cutler eye i.
Cutter i.
cylinder-type i.
3D Accuscan facial i.
Dacron i.
Dacron-backed i.
Dannheim eye i.
DeBakey i.
defibrillator i.
Deflux system i.
de la Cruz stapes i.
dental i.
Dentsply i.
DePuy orthopaedic i.
Dermostat orbital i.
DeWecker eye i.
3DKnee total knee i.
Doherty spherical eye i.
Donnheim i.
dorsal columellar i.
double-lumen breast i.
double-plate Molteno i.
double-stem i.
Dow Corning i.
Dragstedt i.
D-shaped i.
Duracon knee i.
Dura II concealable penile i.
dural i.
durapatite i.
Duros leuprolide i.
Dynaflex penile i.
Ehmke platinum Teflon i.

i. elastomer shell
electrical i.
endodontic endosteal i.
endo-osseous dental i.
EndoPearl bioabsorbable ACL i.
Endopore i.
endosseous HA i.
endosteal i.
epilepsy i.
ePTFE i.
Esser i.
esthetic Taylor mandibular angle i.
Ethrone i.
E-type dental i.
Evolve orthopaedic i.
Ewing eye i.
expandable breast i.
expanded polytetrafluoroethylene i.
extended anatomical high-profile
  malar i.
extraoral bone-anchored i.
eye spherical i.
fascia lata i.
feathered extended malar i.
Ferguson i.
Fibrel gelatin matrix i.
Fine magnetic i.
finger joint i.
Finney penile i.
fixed-bearing knee i.
fixed mandibular i.
Flatt i.
Flexblock cranial i.
flexible digital i.
flexible Dualens i.
flexible rod penile i.
Flexi-Flate penile i.
Flexi-Rod II penile i.
Flowers dorsal nasal i.
Flowers Extended Tear Trough i.
Flowers Mandibular Glove i.
Flowers Tear Trough i.
Fox eyelid i.
Fox spherical eye i.
free i.
freestanding i.
Frialoc transgingival threaded
  dental i.
Friatec i.
front build-up i.
Fyodorov type I, II lens i.
Galin intraocular lens i.

gel-filled i.
Gelfilm retinal i.
GEO Structure spinal i.
Gillies i.
Glasgold Wafer chin i.
glass sphere eye i.
gold eyelid load i.
Goldmann multimirror lens i.
gonioscopic i.
Gore-Tex nasal i.
Gore-Tex SAM facial i.
Gore-Tex vascular i.
Gott i.
great toe i.
Greissinger multi-axis joint i.
grooved silicone i.
Guist sphere eye i.
HA-coated hip i.
HA-coated Micro-Vent i.
HA-coated root-form dental i.
Haik eye i.
haptic area i.
hard tissue replacement-malleable
  facial i. (HTR-MFI)
hard tissue replacement-patient
  matched i. (HTR-PMI)
Harris i.
Harrison i.
Hartley i.
HA-threaded hexlock i.
helicoid endosteal i.
hemi-interpositional i.
hemisphere eye i.
Herrick silicone lacrimal i.
heterograft i.
hex i.
Heyer-Schulte breast i.
Heyer-Schulte lens i.
Heyer-Schulte rhinoplasty i.
HIHA tendon i.
hinged i.
hip shell i.
Hoffer ridged lens i.
Hoffmann eye i.
hollow-sphere orbital i.
homograft i.
Hoskins-Drake i.
House i.
Howmedica Duracon i.
Hruby contact i.
HTR-MFI chin i.
HTR-MFI malar i.

NOTES

implant *(continued)*

HTR-MFI onlay facial augmentation i.
HTR-MFI paranasal i.
HTR-MFI premaxillary i.
HTR-MFI ramus i.
HTR-MFI straight i.
HTR-PMI i.
Hufnagel i.
Hughes eye i.
Hunkeler lightweight intraocular lens i.
Hunter open cord tendon i.
Hydroflex penile semirigid i.
hydroxyapatite i.
hydroxyapatite coated i.
hydroxyapatite ocular i.
Imex scleral i.
Immediate Impression i.
Immediate Load i.
Immix bioabsorbable i.
Implantech Binder i.
Implantech conform binder submalar facial i.
Implantech Flowers i.
Implantech Mittelman i.
Implantech Terino i.
Imtec premounted threaded i.
IMZ endosteal i.
inlay i.
I. Innovations titanium screw
Insall-Burstein intracondylar total knee i.
Intacs corneal ring i.
Integral Omniloc i.
Intermedics intraocular lens i.
Interpore osteointegrated i.
interstitial i.
intracochlear i.
intraocular lens i.
intraorbital i.
Iovision i.
Iowa orbital i.
ITI-Bonefit endosseous i.
ITI dental i.
Ivalon lucite orbital eye i.
Ivalon sponge eye i.
Jardon-Straith chin i.
Jardon-Straith nasal i.
joint i.
Jonas i.
Jordan eye i.
K i.
Kalix flat foot i.
Keragen i.
Kerato-Gel i.
Kerato-Lens i.
Kinetik great toe i.
King orbital i.

Klockner i.
Koenig total great toe i.
Koeppe intraocular lens i.
Kratz i.
Kratz-Sinskey intraocular lens i.
Krause-Wolfe i.
Kryptok bifocal lens i.
Lacey total knee i.
LaminOss i.
Landegger orbital i.
LaPorta great toe i.
Lash-Loeffler penile i.
Lawrence first metatarsophalangeal joint i.
Lemoine orbital i.
lens i.
Levitt eye i.
Lifecath peritoneal i.
Lincoff scleral sponge i.
Linkow blade i.
Little intraocular lens i.
Liverpool elbow i.
4-loop iris clip i.
4-loop iris fixated i.
Loptex laser intraocular lens i.
low-profile breast i.
lucite sphere i.
Luhr i.
lumbar anterior root stimulator i.
lunate i.
Lyda-Ivalon-Lucite i.
MacIntosh i.
magnetic eye i.
malar i.
malleable facial i.
mammary i.
Marlex mesh i.
McCannel i.
McCutchen hip i.
McGhan breast i.
McGhan eye i.
McGhan facial i.
Medallion intraocular lens i.
MedDev gold eyelid i.
Medical Optics intraocular lens i.
Medical Workshop intraocular lens i.
Medicornea Kratz intraocular lens i.
Medpor biomaterial i.
Medpor facial i.
Medpor malar i.
Medpor Quad motility i.
Medpor reconstructive i.
Melauskas acrylic orbital i.
Meme mammary i.
Meniscus Arrow i.
Mentor malleable semirigid penile i.

I

Mentor Siltex i.
Mentor Spectrum breast i.
meridional i.
Mersilene i.
metacarpophalangeal i.
metal-backed acetabular
  component i.
metal hemi-toe i.
metal orthopaedic i.
methyl methacrylate beads i.
methyl methacrylate eye i.
Mettelman prejowl chin i.
Micro-Vent i.
middle ear i.
Millen otologic i.
Mini-Matic i.
MIS dental i.
Mittelman Pre Jowl-Chin i.
3M mammary i.
mobile-bearing knee i.
modular i.
Molteno double-plate i.
Molteno glaucoma double-plate i.
Molteno glaucoma single-plate i.
Moss Miami load-sharing spinal i.
Muhlberger orbital i.
multichannel cochlear i.
Naden-Rieth i.
nasal dorsal i.
nasal shell i.
needle endosteal i.
NeuFlex metacarpophalangeal
  joint i.
NeuroControl Freehand i.
NexGen knee i.
Nexus i.
Niebauer-Cutter i.
Nobel Biocare dental i.
Nobelpharma i.
Nocito i.
NovaGold breast i.
NovaSaline inflatable breast i.
Nucleus 22 cochlear i.
Nucleus 24 multichannel auditory
  brainstem i.
Octa-Hex i.
Oculo-Plastik ePTFE ocular i.
Ollier-Thiersch i.
O'Malley self-adhering lens i.
Omniloc dental i.
onlay i.
Ophtec occlusion i.

optic i.
oral i.
orbital floor i.
Organon percutaneous E2 i.
orthopaedic i.
orthotic attachment i.
Osseodent dental i.
osseointegrated oral i.
Osseotite 2-stage procedure i.
osseous i.
OsteoGen HA dental i.
Osteogen resorbable osteogenic
  bone-filling i.
Osteonics-HA coated femoral i.
Osteoplate i.
Padgett i.
Panje i.
Paragon Complete i.
Paragon SwissPlus i.
Partnership i.
Pasqualini i.
patch i.
patella-resurfacing i.
patient-matched i.
peanut eye i.
Pearce vaulted-Y lens i.
pectoralis muscle i.
pedicle i.
penile i.
percutaneous dorsal column
  stimulator i.
Periotest i.
Permacol permanent surgical i.
PermaRidge i.
PhacoFlex II foldable intraocular
  lens i.
Phystan i.
piggyback i.
pin i.
Pisces i.
planoconvex eye i.
plastic sphere eye i.
Platina intraocular lens i.
platinum eyelid i.
Plexiglas eye i.
PMI i.
PMMA i.
Polaris adjustable spinal cage i.
polyethylene sphere i.
polyglycolide i.
polylactide i.
polymer tooth replica i.

NOTES

implant *(continued)*
    polymethyl methacrylate i.
    Polystan i.
    polytetrafluoroethylene i.
    polyurethane-coated silicone
      breast i.
    polyvinyl sponge i.
    Porex Medpor i.
    Porex paranasal i.
    Porex PHA i.
    porous polyethylene i.
    posterior chamber lens i.
    Precision-Cosmet intraocular lens i.
    Press-Fit i.
    Primus flexible great toe i.
    processed carbon i.
    ProOsteon synthetic bone i.
    Proplast preformed facial i.
    Proplast-Teflon disc i.
    Protek joint i.
    PTFE-containing i.
    pyramidal eye i.
    Radin-Rosenthal i.
    radiocarpal i.
    Radovan breast i.
    ramus blade i.
    ramus endosteal i.
    Rastelli i.
    Rayner-Choyce eye i.
    reform eye i.
    Repicci II unicompartment i.
    Repiphysis pediatric bone
      replacement i.
    Restore bone i.
    Restore orthobiologic soft-tissue i.
    retinal Gelfilm i.
    ReUnite hammertoe i.
    Reuter bobbin i.
    Reverdin i.
    reverse-shape i.
    rHead radial i.
    rhinoplasty i.
    Ridley anterior chamber lens i.
    Ridley Mark II lens i.
    Rizzo dorsal i.
    Roberts dental i.
    Rodin orbital i.
    root-form dental i.
    Rosa-Berens orbital i.
    Ruedemann eye i.
    Ruiz plano fundal lens i.
    saline-filled anatomical breast i.
    SAM facial i.
    Sargon i.
    Sauerbruch i.
    Schepens hollow hemisphere i.
    Schocket tube i.
    Schwaber otologic i.
    scleral i.

scleral buckle eye i.
screw-type i.
Screw-Vent i.
Seeburger i.
seed i.
self-tapping screw-type i.
semishell eye i.
Septopal i.
serrefine i.
Severin i.
Sgarlato hammertoe i.
shelf-type i.
shell eye i.
Shepard intraocular lens i.
SHIP hammertoe i.
Shirakabe nasal i.
Sichel movable orbital i.
Sichi i.
Silastic chin i.
Silastic corneal eye i.
Silastic Cronin i.
Silastic eye i.
Silastic finger i.
Silastic Gel-filled testicular i.
Silastic midfacial malar i.
Silastic penile i.
Silastic rhinoplasty i.
Silastic scleral buckle i.
Silastic scleral buckler eye i.
Silastic silicone rubber i.
Silastic subdermal i.
Silastic toe i.
silicone buckling i.
silicone button eye i.
silicone elastomer rubber ball i.
silicone-filled anatomical breast i.
silicone-filled mammary i.
silicone-filled round breast i.
silicone-gel breast i.
silicone meshed motility i.
silicone MP i.
silicone nasal strut i.
silicone pad eye i.
silicone rod i.
silicone sleeve eye i.
silicone sponge i.
silicone strip eye i.
silicone textured mammary i.
silicone tire eye i.
Siloxane i.
Siltex mammary i.
Simcoe-AMO eye i.
Simcoe intraocular lens i.
single-channel cochlear i.
single-stage screw i.
single-tooth subperiosteal i.
Sinskey lens i.
Sinterlock i.
i. site dilator

Sled i.
sleeve i.
i. sleeve
Small-Carrion Silastic rod for
  penile i.
SmartScrew bioabsorbable i.
Smith orbital floor i.
Snellen conventional reform eye i.
Snellen reform i.
SoftForm facial i.
soft silicone sphere i.
solid silicone buttock i.
solid silicone with Supramid
  mesh i.
Spectra-System i.
Spectrum breast i.
Spectrum Designs facial i.
spherical eye i.
Sphero Flex i.
spiral endosteal i.
Spline Twist microtextured
  titanium i.
split-thickness i.
i. sponge
sponge i.
stainless steel i.
Star-Lock Press-Fit cylinder i.
Startanius blade i.
Star/Vent 1-stage dental screw i.
Steri-Oss endosteal dental i.
Stimoceiver i.
Stone eye i.
Straith chin i.
Straith nasal i.
Strampelli i.
S-type dental i.
subdermal i.
submucosal i.
subperiosteal i.
SuperCat self-tapping i.
superficial i.
I. Support Systems titanium screw
Supramid i.
Supramid-Allen i.
Surgicel i.
Surgitek Flexi-Flate II penile i.
Surgitek mammary i.
Sustain HA-coated threaded i.
Sustain hydroxyapatite biointegrated
  dental i.
Sutter hinged great toe i.
Swanson carpal lunate i.

Swanson finger joint i.
Swanson great toe i.
Swanson metacarpophalangeal i.
Swanson radial head i.
Swanson radiocarpal i.
Swanson Silastic i.
Swanson small joint i.
Swanson titanium carpal
  scaphoid i.
Swanson trapezium i.
Swanson ulnar head i.
Swanson wrist joint i.
Swede-Vent TL self-tapping
  external hex i.
Swiss MP joint i.
Syed-Neblett i.
Syed template i.
Symphonix Vibrant Soundbridge i.
System-S soft skeletal i.
Szulc orbital i.
tantalum mesh eye i.
tapered Micro-Vent i.
Taper-Lock external hex i.
Taylor lateral mandibular angle i.
Tear-Trough i.
Techmedica i.
Teflon mesh i.
Teflon orbital floor i.
temporomandibular joint i.
tendon i.
Tennant Anchorflex lens i.
Tensilon i.
Terino anatomical chin i.
testicular i.
Tevdek i.
TG Osseotite single-stage
  procedure i.
TheraSeed therapeutic i.
thick-walled Dacron-backed i.
Thiersch i.
ThreadLoc i.
Tibon anterior cervical fusion i.
TiMesh patient-configured titanium
  craniomaxillofacial i.
TiOblast dental i.
tire eye i.
Tissue Tak arthroscopic i.
titanium alloy i.
titanium plasma-sprayed dental i.
Titan penile i.
TiUnite dental i.

NOTES

implant *(continued)*
  Tobin anatomical malar
    prosthetic i.
  tobramycin-impregnated PMMA i.
  total top i.
  Townley i.
  transmandibular i.
  transosseous i.
  transosteal pin i.
  trapezium i.
  trial i.
  Trilucent breast i.
  triple-lumen i.
  Troncoso gonioscopic lens i.
  Troutman eye i.
  T-type dental i.
  tunneled eye i.
  Twist MTX i.
  Ultex lens i.
  unicompartmental knee i.
  Unilab Surgibone surgical i.
  ureteral i.
  Uribe orbital i.
  Usher Marlex mesh i.
  U-type dental i.
  VA magnetic orbital i.
  Varigray i.
  Varilux lens i.
  Virilis I, II penile i.
  Vitallium eye i.
  Vitrasert intraocular ganciclovir i.
  Vivosil i.
  VoCoM thyroplasty i.
  Volk conoid i.
  Walter Reed i.
  WasherLoc i.
  Weber hip i.
  Weck-Cel i.
  Weil i.
  Weil-modified Swanson i.
  Wheeler spherical eye i.
  wire mesh eye i.
  Wolf i.
  Zeichner i.
  Zenoderm dural i.
  Zest subperiosteal i.
  Zoladex i.
  Zyderm I or II collagen i.
  Zyplast injectable collagen i.
implantable
  i. access catheter
  i. access port
  i. artificial heart
  i. atrial defibrillator
  i. automatic cardioverter-defibrillator
  i. cardioverter-defibrillator (ICD)
  i. cardioverter defibrillator
  i. cardioverter-defibrillator catheter
  i. electrode

  i. infusion port
  i. neural stimulator
  i. osmotic pump
  i. pacemaker
  i. pulse generator
  i. silicone microballoon
  i. vascular access device
  i. venous access device (IVAD)
  i. ventricular assist device (IVAD)
**Implantaid Di-Lock cardiac lead
  introducer**
implantation forceps
Implantech
  I. Binder implant
  I. conform binder submalar facial
    implant
  I. Flowers implant
  I. Mittelman implant
  I. moulage kit
  I. SE-100 smoke aspiration tip
  I. Terino implant
implanted
  i. infusion pump
  i. NCP generator
implanter
  Geuder i.
  Wallner interstitial prostate i.
implant-retained denture
implant-supported
  i.-s. fixed prosthesis
  i.-s. overdenture
Implast bone cement
Implatome dental tomography system
Implens intraocular lens
Impra
  I. bypass graft
  I. Carboflo ePTFE vascular graft
  I. collagen-impregnated Dacron
    prosthesis
  I. Flex vascular graft
  I. microporous PTFE vascular graft
  I. peritoneal catheter
impregnated
  i. dressing
  i. electrode
Impregum impression material
impression
  i. material syringe
  i. mattress
  i. tonometer
Impress Softpatch incontinence pad
IMProv cement
ImPulse
  I. Elite electronic oxygen
    conserving device
  I. Select oxygen conserving device
impulse inertial exercise trainer
IMSC five-hole nail
IMSI-Metripond operating room table

IMT
    inspiratory muscle training
    integrated massage therapy
Imtec
    I. BioBarrier membrane
    I. premounted threaded implant
IMx PSA system
IMZ endosteal implant
in
    I. Charge diabetes control system
    i. situ valve scissors
    i. situ venous valve scissors
    i. vitro fertilization micropipette
    i. vivo generator
    i. vivo image-guided H-magnetic
      resonance spectroscopy
    i. vivo optical spectroscopy
      (INVOS)
Inaba and Ezaki dissector
inactive electrode
Inamura
    I. Race chopper
    I. small incision capsulorrhexis
      forceps
INCA
    infant nasal CPAP assembly
    INCA infant CPAP system
incandescent
    i. endoscope lamp
    i. sheath
Incardia valve system
InCare
    I. brace
    I. pelvic floor therapy office
      system
Incavo wire passer
Incenti-neb nebulizer
incentive
    i. inspirometer
    i. spirometer
In-Ceram
    I.-C. Alumina bonding
    I.-C. Cerestore bonding
    I.-C. Dicor bonding
    I.-C. Empress bonding
    I.-C. Fortress bonding
    I.-C. Optec bonding
    I.-C. Spinell bonding
Incert bioabsorbable implantable sponge
Incise
    I. drape
    I. pouch

incision
    i. dilator
    i. knife
    limbal relaxing i. (LRI)
    i. retractor
    i. spreader
Incisor arthroscopic blade
incisor-mandibular plane angulator
Inclan graft
inclination guidewire
inclinometer
    analog electronic i.
    electronic i.
Incono bag
incontinence
    i. clamp
    i. ring
incubator
    double-walled i.
    Forma water-jacketed i.
    Giraffe i.
    Ohmeda Care-Plus i.
incudostapedial joint knife
incus replacement prosthesis
indentation tonometer
indenter
    diamond pyramid i.
independent jaw chuck
Indermil tissue adhesive
index
    Gradient I. (GRIN)
indexed splint
Index Knobber II massage tool
Indiana
    I. reamer
    I. tome carpal tunnel release
      system
Indian club needle
India rubber suture
indicator
    AccuAngle i.
    Berens-Tolman ocular
      hypertension i.
    finger i.
    fundamental frequency i.
    Neesone root canal depth i.
    ocular hypertension i.
    Pio root canal depth i.
    SPI-Lite sleep position i.
indifferent electrode

NOTES

Indigo
    I. diffuser fiber
    I. LaserOptic treatment system
indirect laser ophthalmoscope
indocyanine green angiogram
Indomitable scanner
Indong Oh prosthesis
InDuct
    I. breast aspirator
    I. breast microcatheter
Industrial Work brace
indwelling
    i. cannula
    i. catheter
    i. Foley catheter
    i. nonvascular shunt
    i. stent
    i. subclavian catheter
    i. transcutaneous vascular access device
    i. ureteral stent
Inerpan flexible burn dressing
inertial suction sampler
In-Exsufflator
    CoughAssist I.-E.
infant
    i. abdominal retractor
    i. abduction splint
    i. Ambu resuscitator
    i. biopsy forceps
    i. dilator
    i. esophagoscope
    I. 450 EV foot/ankle controller
    i. eyelid retractor
    i. female/male catheter
    I. Flow nasal CPAP system
    i. Karickhoff laser lens
    i. laryngoscope
    i. 3-mirror laser lens
    i. mucus extractor
    i. nasal cannula assembly
    i. nasal CPAP assembly (INCA)
    i. passive mitt
    I. PRAFO 450 heel connector
    i. rib retractor
    i. rib shears
    I. Star high-frequency ventilator
    i. telescope
    i. urethrotome
    i. urethrotome blade
    i. ventilation monitor
infantometer
    Infantrac i.
    Measure Mat i.
Infantrac infantometer
In-Fast
    I.-F. bone screw system
    I.-F. cystourethropexy
    I.-F. female sling system

inferior
    i. mesenteric artery (IMA)
    i. vena cava (IVC)
    i. vena caval catheter
    i. vena caval clip
    i. vena caval umbrella filter
InFerno moist heat therapy
infiltration cannula
infiltrator
    Klein i.
    I. local drug delivery device
Infinion 0.6T magnetic resonance imager
Infiniti
    I. catheter
    I. vision system
Infinity
    I. modular hip prosthesis
    I. sensor
    I. stirrups
InFix interbody fusion system
inflatable
    i. bone tamp
    i. carrot finger orthosis
    i. elbow splint
    i. Foley bag catheter
    i. mammary prosthesis
    i. Mentor penile prosthesis
    i. penile prosthesis
    i. thoracic lumbosacral orthosis
    i. tourniquet cuff
    i. tracheal tube cuff
inflated balloon
inflator
    Bonney retrograde i.
    Encore i.
    LeVeen i.
    Ogden-Senturia eustachian i.
    rapid cuff i.
inflow
    i. cannula
    i. coronary stent
InfraGuide
    I. delivery system
    Heraeus LaserSonics I.
infrared
    i. applicator
    i. camera
    i. coagulator
    i. laser-Doppler flowmeter
    i. light-emitting diode
    i. liver scanner
    i. optometer
    i. ray photocoagulator
    i. thermometer
infrared-beam diode laser
Infrasonic QIGong 5.5 pain management device
Infrasonics ventilator

Infumed pump
infundibular
    i. forceps
    i. punch
InfuO.R. drug delivery pump
Infusaid
    I. catheter
    I. Infuse-a-Port
    I. infusion pump
    I. needle
InfusaSleeve
    I. II catheter
    Kaplan-Simpson I.
    LocalMed I.
Infuse-A-Cath catheter
Infuse-a-Port
    I.-a.-P. catheter
    Infusaid I.-a.-P.
    I.-a.-P. port
    I.-a.-P. pump
    I.-a.-P. vascular access system
Infuse bone graft
infuser
    Abbott LifeCare PCA Plus II i.
    Anne anesthesia i.
    Baxter i.
    Critikon pressure i.
    Dento-Infuser i.
    Ethox Surgi-Press pressure i.
    Heart pillow i.
    MicroFuse i.
    Ohio pressure i.
    Paragon i.
    Parker micropump insulin i.
    PCA i.
    PCA Plus II i.
    Single-Day Baxter i.
    Surgi-Press pressure i.
    Travenol i.
    Tycos pressure i.
    UROS i.
Infuset GP syringe
infusion
    i. cannula
    i. catheter
    i. device
    i. handpiece
    i. port
    i. pump
    i. sleeve
    i. suction vitreous cutter
    i. tube

Infu-Surg pressure infuser bag
Ingals
    I. antral cannula
    I. flexible silver cannula
    I. nasal speculum
    I. rectal injection cannula
Inge
    I. lamina spreader
    I. laminectomy retractor
Ingersoll
    I. adenoid curette
    I. tonsillar needle
Ingold M-series glass electrode pH
  monitor
Ingraham-Fowler
    I.-F. clip
    I.-F. clip-applying forceps
    I.-F. tantalum clip
Ingraham skull punch
Ingram
    I. bicycle seat
    I. catheter
    I. trocar
ingress/egress cannula
inguinal truss
inhalation
    i. breath unit
    i. cannula
inhalator
    Oxy-Quik Mark IV oxygen i.
Inhale deep lung delivery system
inhaler
    Ace i.
    AeroChamber bronchial i.
    AeroChamber metered-dose i.
    AeroDose i.
    Aerosol Cloud Enhancer i.
    AERx electronic i.
    AERx i.
    breath-operated i.
    Chiesi powder i.
    Diskhaler i.
    dry-powder i.
    Easi-Breathe i.
    Henderson-Haggard i.
    Inhalet i.
    InspirEase i.
    Junker i.
    metered-dose i. (MDI)
    metered solution i.
    Nebuhaler i.
    OptiHaler metered-dose i.

NOTES

inhaler *(continued)*
    Orion i.
    Oxford miniature vaporizer i.
    Rondo i.
    Rotahaler i.
    Schimelbusch i.
    Spinhaler Turbo-Inhaler i.
    Spiral Mark V portable ultrasonic
      drug i.
    Turbuhaler i.
    ultrasonic i.
Inhalet inhaler
inherent filter
inhibited
    dual-mode, ventricular i. (DVI)
InjecAid system
InjectaFLOW injection needle
Injectate probe
injection
    i. cannula
    i. catheter
    i. electrode catheter
    i. gold probe
    i. needle
    I. Superview Speedband ligator
Injectoflex respirator jet
injector
    Amplatz i.
    Angiomat angiographic i.
    Bioject jet i.
    Cordis i.
    Dermo-Jet high-pressure i.
    Dyonics syringe i.
    EpiE-Z Pen epinephrine i.
    EZ-Ject i.
    E-Z 'Jector i.
    Fujinon variceal i.
    GenJect i.
    Gentle Jet pediatric i.
    Harris uterine i. (HUI)
    Hercules power i.
    HUI Mini-Flex uterine i.
    Injex needle-free i.
    Lakatos Teflon i.
    Lumin laparoscopic uterine
      manipulator i.
    Marcon-Haber i.
    Mark V Plus i.
    Medi-Jector i.
    Medrad contrast medium i.
    Medrad Mark IV angiographic i.
    Medrad power angiographic i.
    Miller ratchet i.
    Mill-Rose esophageal i.
    Mini-Flex flexible Harris uterine i.
    modified Mark IV R-wave-triggered
      power i.
    MR-compatible power i.
    NordiPen i.

    NovolinPen i.
    Olympus 13 L i.
    Optistat handheld power i.
    Peninject 2.25 i.
    PercuPump disposable syringe
      and i.
    power i.
    pressure i.
    Robinject needle i.
    Rowden uterine manipulator i.
    Spectris power i.
    Syrijet Mark II needleless i.
    Taveras i.
    Teflon i.
    Tubex i.
    uterine i.
    Virag i.
InjecTx
    I. cystoscope
    I. transurethral injection device
    I. unit
Injex
    I. disposable needle
    I. needle-free injector
    I. needle-free injector system
ink
    Bonney blue i.
inlay
    i. bone graft
    i. implant
inlet
    Berry rotating i.
    Fish i.
    i. forceps
in-line
    i.-l. blood gas monitor
    i.-l. trap
    i.-l. venous pressure monitor
Inmed whistle tip urethral catheter
inner
    i. heel wedge
    i. lip plate
InnerDyne trocar
Inner Lok ankle brace
innerspring
    Nylex II Convoluted i.
InnerVasc vascular access device
Innervision
    I. MR scanner
    I. ventricular catheter
Innoboot night splint
Innoflex variable stiffness colonoscope
Innomed
    I. arthroplasty measuring system
    I. Assistant Free surgical
      instrument
    I. bone curette
    I. Ortho rongeur

Innova
- I. feminine incontinence treatment system
- I. pelvic floor stimulator

Innovasive Devices ROC XS suture anchor

Innovative
- I. Medical Products (IMP)
- I. Medical Products Steri-Clamp clamp

InnovaTome microkeratome device

Innovator Holter system

Innsbruck electrode

Inokucki vascular stapler

inorganic dental cement

Inoue
- I. balloon catheter
- I. self-guiding balloon

INOvent delivery system

InPath cervical cancer screening system

Inpersol peritoneal dialysis set

InPouch TV subculture kit

Input percutaneous sheath introducer

Inrad HiLiter ultrasound-enhanced stylet

Inronail
- I. fingernail prosthesis
- I. toenail prosthesis

Inro surgical nail splint

Insall-Burstein
- I.-B. II modular knee system
- I.-B. intracondylar total knee implant
- I.-B. posterior stabilizer

Insall-Burstein-Freeman (IBF)
- I.-B.-F. total knee instrumentation

insemination
- i. dish
- intrauterine i. (IUI)

inseminator

insert
- articular i.
- A-Trac i.
- Durasul acetabular i.
- Endostat calibration pod i.
- FemSoft continence i.
- FemSoft urethral i.
- Fogarty i.
- Fogarty-Hydragrip i.
- Gel Sole shoe i.
- Hapad felt shoe i.
- Hollister disposable convex i.
- Hydrajaw i.
- Johnson & Johnson PFC cruciate-substituting i.
- Orthex Relievers shoe i.
- Poly-Dial i.
- POWERPoint orthotic shoe i.
- P.R. heat moldable i.
- Profix confirming tibial i.
- Reliance urinary control i.
- retainer i.
- Roho solid seat i.
- Softjaw i.
- S-ROM Poly-Dial i.
- Sur-Fit disposable convex i.
- urinary control urethral i.
- Warm'N'Form i.

inserter
- AMO-PhacoFlex lens i.
- BioStinger Hornet meniscal fixation i.
- deluxe FIN pin i.
- diaphragm i.
- Dilamezinsert i.
- Ernest-McDonald soft intraocular lens i.
- Hess Memory Lens i.
- Kirschner wire i.
- Lehner II i.
- Lens-Eze i.
- Mport lens i.
- Nichamin II lens i.
- Prodigy lens i.
- Robinson-Moon prosthesis i.
- Shaffner orthopaedic i.
- SmartNeedle i.
- Storz i.
- Tytan tube i.

insertion forceps

inside-the-needle infusion catheter

Insight
- I. 40000 endoscope
- I. knee positioning and alignment system

InSight manometry system

insole
- Anti-Shox gel i.
- Come-Orthotic sports replacement i.
- Comf-Orthotic 3/4 length i.
- Comf-Orthotic sports i.
- Darco moldable i.
- Diab-A-Foot rocker i.
- Diab-A-Pad i.

NOTES

insole *(continued)*
    Diab-A-Sole i.
    Diabetic Diagnostic I.
    D-Soles i.
    Emed i.
    Ever-Flex i.
    FlatFoot i.
    Flexi-Therm diabetic diagnostic i.
    Hapad metatarsal i.
    Kinetic Wedge molded i.
    moldable i.
    Orthex reliever i.
    Plexidure i.
    Poron 400 i.
    PPT MXL soft molded i.
    PPT Plastazote i.
    PPT RX firm molded i.
    PumpPals i.
    Sherform silicone i.
    silicone i.
    Spenco i.
    S-Soles i.
    TechnoGel i.
    Viscoped i.
InSound XT
InSpectra tissue spectrometer
inspirator
inspiratory muscle training (IMT)
InspirEase inhaler
inspirometer
    incentive i.
Inspiron
    I. inspiratory training device
    I. Instromedix computer
Inspirx incentive spirometer
Insta-Mold
    I.-M. ear protection device
    I.-M. silicone ear impression
    material
Insta-Nerve device
instant
    i. cold pack
    i. fever tester thermometer
    I. Response technology generator
    i. skin hook
Insta-Pulse heart rate monitor
Insta-Putty silicone earplug
InstaScan scanner
Instat
    I. MCH microfibrillar collagen
    hemostat
InstaTrak
    I. system
    I. System image-guided surgery
Instead feminine protection cup
InStent
    I. CardioCoil stent
    I. CarotidCoil stent

institute
    Cancer and Blood I. (CBI)
    Texas Heart I. (THI)
Instituto Dermopatico dell'Immacolata (IDI)
INSTRA-mate instrument-holding spring
Instron machine
instrument
    Abradabloc dermabrasion i.
    Accurate Surgical and
    Scientific I.'s (ASSI)
    AccuSharp i.
    Activator adjusting i.
    Acufex arthroscopic i.
    Acufex MosaicPlasty i.
    American Hydron i.
    arterial oscillator endarterectomy i.
    Arthrotek Ellipticut hand i.
    ASSI S&T microsurgical i.
    Atlas orthogonal percussion i.
    Austin middle ear i.
    Auto Ref-keratometer i.
    AxyaWeld i.
    Ayerst i.
    BabyBeat ultrasound i.
    Backlund stereotactic i.
    Bard BladderScan bladder
    volume i.
    bibeveled cutting i.
    Biomer microsuturing i.
    Biophysic Ophthascan S i.
    BirdBeak orthopaedic grasper i.
    Blue Dolphin denture i.
    bone abduction i.
    Bone Grafter i.
    BOSS surgical i.
    Britetrac fiberoptic i.
    Carl Zeiss i.
    Carter Tubal Assistant surgical i.
    cervical range-of-motion i.
    Cheshire-Poole-Yankauer suction i.
    chiropractic adjusting i.
    Clarke stereotactic i.
    CLICKline surgical i.
    Cobb spinal i.
    i. coding tape
    cold conization i.
    Collis TDR i.
    conization i.
    contour-facilitating i.
    Cooley neonatal i.
    Cooley neonatal i.
    Crit-Line whole blood diagnostic i.
    cryosurgical i.
    currycomb i.
    CVIS imaging catheter i.
    Daisy I&A i.
    Daniel EndoForehead i.
    DePuy Keystone graft i.

Dilamezinsert surgical i.
Disk-Criminator discrimination i.
Dix double-ended i.
DORC surgical i.
Dualine digital hearing i.
Duette double lumen ERCP i.
Dwyer i.
Dyonics arthroscopic i.
EarCheck Pro i.
Eckardt backflush i.
Eckardt Heme-Stopper i.
Electro Surgical I.'s (ESI)
EndoDissect i.
Endoflex endoscopy i.
Endo Grasp i.
EndoMax advanced laparoscopic i.
EndoShears i.
endosonography i.
Endo Stitch i.
Endotrac endoscopy i.
EndoWrist i.
ESI Lite-Pipe fiberoptic i.
falloposcope endoscopic i.
FirstStep tibial osteotomy i.
Fleming conization i.
Friatec manual arthroscopy i.
gnathologic i.
Godina vessel-fixation i.
GPX rotary i.
Graefe i.
graft measuring i.
GripTrack hand i.
Guilford-Wright middle ear i.
guillotine vitrectomy i.
HandPort laparoscopic i.
HBT Sleuth hydrogen breath test instrument
Horico diamond i.
IBF knee i.
I.L.Med i.
immobilizer vascular control i.
Innomed Assistant Free surgical i.
Iolab titanium i.
IOS immunodiagnostic testing i.
ISI laparoscopic i.
Isse Endo Brow i.
ITD-FG dental diamond i.
Johnson Endobag i.
Jordan middle ear i.
Jordan strut-measuring i.
Karl Ilg i.
Keeler cryosurgical i.

Kerato-Kontours i.
Kimberley diamond i.
Kirschner surgical i.
Kitner blunt dissecting i.
knot-tying i.
Koh ultramicro i.
Kos middle ear i.
Krwawicz cataract cryosurgical i.
K x-ray fluorescence i.
Ladmore plastic filling i.
LapTie endoscopic knot-tying i.
LaserTweezers optical trapping i.
ligature-passing i.
I. Makar biodegradable interference screw
Malis bipolar i.
Matsuda titanium surgical i.
McCabe measuring i.
McCall i.
McGee middle ear i.
mechanical radial-scanning i.
3M filling i.
Micro-Aire pneumatic power i.
Micro Diamond-Point microsurgery i.
MicroFrance minimally invasive surgical i.
Micromedics surgical i.
MicroXcisor ethmoid bone cutting i.
Midas Rex pneumatic i.
Millet neurological test i.
Miracompo filling i.
Mitek SuperAnchor i.
Mity Roto rotary i.
M4 Kerr Safety Hedstrom i.
Monarch II bleaching i.
myoma fixation i.
Neuro-Trace i.
Newport medical i.
Nicolet Compass electromyography i.
Nordent filling i.
Nucleotome Endoflex i.
Obwegeser orthognathic surgery i.
OPG-Gee i.
Ortho-Athrex i.
OrthoVise orthopaedic i.
pencil-grip i.
Pen-Probe i.
Plastibell compression i.
plugging i.

NOTES

instrument *(continued)*
  point-search i.
  PolyTome i.
  ProLine endoscopic i.
  PROloop i.
  Purstring disposable i.
  Quantec endodontic i.
  Quinton suction biopsy i.
  Radionics bipolar i.
  reciprocal planing i.
  reduction i.
  Reichert Ultramatic Rx Master
    Phoroptor refracting i.
  RE-New laparoscopic i.
  Retinomax refractometry i.
  i. retrieval container
  RingLoc i.
  Rizzuti-Bonaccolto i.
  Rizzuti-Fleischer i.
  Rizzuti-Kayser-Fleischer i.
  Rizzuti-Lowe i.
  Rizzuti-Maxwell i.
  Rizzuti-Soemmering i.
  Rosenberg gynecomastia
    dissection i.
  Rosen middle ear i.
  rotary cutting i.
  Ruggles neurosurgical i.
  Rumex titanium i.
  Safco diamond i.
  Salinger reduction i.
  Scheer middle ear i.
  Schneider PTCA i.
  Schuknecht middle ear i.
  Semmes-Weinstein monofilament i.
  Sensonic plaque removal i.
  Shea middle ear i.
  Siemens custom tinnitus control i.
  single-beveled cutting i.
  single-plane i.
  single-reference-point i.
  slotted i.
  small-diameter endosonographic i.
  Smith-Miller-Patch cryosurgical i.
  Snowden-Pencer laparoscopic
    cholecystectomy i.
  Sofamor spinal i.
  solid-state i.
  spark-gap i.
  SpeedReducer i.
  spinal adjusting i.
  Splintrex i.
  spring loaded biopsy i.
  i. stabilizer pad
  Steele filling i.
  stereotaxic i.
  strut measuring i.
  Surgi-Tron thoracoscopic i.
  SutureLasso orthopaedic i.

  Tardy Microbur i.
  Tessier craniofacial i.
  test handle i.
  Thomas Kapsule i.
  time domain reflectometry i.
  Todd-Wells stereotaxic i.
  ultrasonic bone-cutting i.
  Unfolder Silver implantation i.
  Unitech i.
  United States Catheter & I.'s
    (USCI)
  Valleylab laparoscopic i.
  VAPORbar i.
  VAPORloop i.
  Vibrasonic hearing i.
  Vilmann-Hancke biopsy handle i.
  Wallach minifreezer cryosurgical i.
  Wiet graft measuring i.
  Wigand endoscopic i.
  Wright-Guilford middle ear i.
  XP peritympanic hearing i.
  XQ video i.
  Zetafuge centrifuge i.
instrumentation
  Advanced Breast Biopsy I. (ABBI)
  anterior distraction i.
  AO fixateur interne i.
  AO notched i.
  ArthroPlastics ankle i.
  Baxter V. Mueller laparoscopic i.
  biofeedback i.
  Bio-Moore II i.
  Caspar anterior i.
  CD i.
  Claris titanium spinal i.
  compression U-rod i.
  Cotrel-Dubousset pedicle screw i.
  Cotrel-Dubousset pedicular i.
  Cotrel-Dubousset spinal i.
  craniofacial i.
  distraction i.
  Dwyer i.
  Edwards i.
  EEG and PSG i.
  EndoMax endoscopic i.
  halo-Ilizarov distraction i.
  Harms-Moss anterior thoracic i.
  Harrington distraction i.
  Harrington rod i.
  Harrington spinal i.
  IBF total knee i.
  Insall-Burstein-Freeman total knee i.
  InSurg laparoscopic i.
  interspinous segmental spinal i.
  Kambin i.
  Kambin-Gellman i.
  Kaneda anterior spinal i.
  Kostuik-Harrington spinal i.
  Louis i.

L-rod i.
lumbosacral spine transpedicular i.
Luque semirigid segmental spinal i.
MIDA CoroNet i.
Midas Rex i.
modular i.
Moss Miami spinal i.
Mueller laparoscopic i.
Passport i.
posterior distraction i.
posterior hook-rod spinal i.
Putti-Platt/Bankart i.
sacral spine modular i.
sacral spine Universal i.
segmental spinal i.
Smith-Richards i.
Steffee spinal i.
Stryker power i.
Tacit craniofacial i.
Zielke pedicular i.
InstruWipes surgical sponge
insufflation
i. device
i. needle
insufflator
Bonney i.
Buckstein colonic i.
colonic i.
Dench i.
DyoPneumatic i.
Eder i.
gas i.
HiTec i.
hysteroscopic i.
Kelly i.
Kidde tubal i.
laparoscopic i.
Medicam 900 i.
Milex vaginal i.
Neal i.
Op-Pneu CO_2 i.
Pneumomat laparoscopic i.
Semm Pelvi-Pneu i.
Sieger i.
Snowden-Pencer i.
Stille i.
Storz Laparoflator i.
variable-flow i.
Venturi i.
Weber colonic i.
Wisap i.

Insuflon
I. infusion set
I. insulin delivery device
insulated
i. bayonet forceps
i. curved scissors
i. electrode needle
i. gate field-effect transistor
i. knife handle
i. monopolar forceps
i. straight scissors
i. tissue forceps
insulin infusion pump
InsulScan insulation testing system
Insul-Sheath vaginal speculum sheath
InSurg
I. common bile duct basket
I. laparoscopic instrumentation
I. LapTie needle driver suturing
device
InSync
I. cardiac resynchronization therapy
I. cardiac stimulator
I. ICD system
inSync miniform
Insyte AutoGuard catheter
In-Tac bone anchoring system
Intacs
I. corneal ring implant
I. intrastromal corneal ring
Intact
I. bioprosthetic valve
I. catheter
I. porcine bioprosthesis
I. xenograft valve
**Intagortor MS-126 Foot Circulation
machine**
**Intec AID cardioverter-defibrillator
generator**
Integra
I. artificial skin
I. II balloon
I. catheter
I. dermal regeneration template
I. tissue expander
integral
I. distal centralizer
I. hip system
I. Interlok femoral prosthesis
I. Omniloc implant
i. spinal angulator
i. uniformity scintillation camera

NOTES

481

integrated
- i. ankle orthotic ankle joint
- i. electromyography
- i. headholder
- i. massage therapy (IMT)
- i. sideport access portal

Integriderm mattress

Integris
- I. cardiovascular imaging
- I. V3000 imager

Integrity
- I. acetabular cup
- I. ADx pacemaker
- I. AFx AutoCapture
- I. AFx DR AutoCapture pacing system
- I. AFx pacemaker
- I. neutral liner
- I. shell

InteguDerm dressing

Intelect
- I. Legend Combo stimulator
- I. 600MP microcurrent stimulator

IntelliCath pulmonary artery catheter

Intelligent dressing

Intelliject pump

IntelliJet arthroscopic fluid management system

intensified
- I. Radiographic Imaging System (IRIS)
- i. radiographic imaging system scanner

intensifier
- C-arm image i.
- image i.
- OEC-Diasonics mobile C-arm image i.

intensifying screen

intensive care (IC)

Inteq
- I. small joint suturing system
- I. TFC repair kit

Inter
- I. Fix RP threaded spinal fusion cage device
- I. Fix threaded spinal fusion cage

Interad whole body CT scanner

Intera I/T interventional magnetic resonance imager

Interax total knee system

interbody
- i. fusion rasp
- i. graft tamp

intercalary allograft

intercardiac sucker

Interceed absorbable adhesion barrier

Intercept
- I. esophageal internal MR microcoil
- I. internal microcoil
- I. urethral internal MR coil
- I. Vascular guidewire

Interceptor M3 triple-channel, solid-state monitor

interchangeable
- i. vein stripper
- i. vein stripper olive

intercostal
- i. catheter
- i. drain
- i. trocar

interdental splint

interdigitating coil stent

interface
- I. arterial blood filter
- Monarch Mini Mask nasal i.
- PressureWire i.
- Quicknet monitor i.
- ShearGuard low-friction i.

interference
- i. barrier filter
- i. screw

interferential
- i. stimulator
- i. therapy

interferometer
- Fizeau-Tolansky i.

Interfit-Pharmacea Intermedic intraocular lens

Interflux intraocular lens

interfragmentary
- i. lag screw
- i. plate

InterGard
- I. heparin vascular graft
- I. knitted collagen
- I. knitted collagen hemostatic material

interimplant papillary template

interlaminar clamp

Interlink
- I. injection cap
- I. lever lock cannula
- I. threaded lock cannula
- I. vial access cannula

interlocking
- i. detachable coil (IDC)
- i. sound

Interlok femoral component

INtermate
- Baxter I.

intermaxillary wire

intermediate
- i. C-D hook
- i. splint

I

Intermedics
I. atrial antitachycardia pacemaker
I. Cyberlith X multiprogrammable pacemaker
I. intraocular lens implant
I. intraocular tonometer
I. lens
I. lithium-powered pacemaker
I. Marathon dual-chamber rate-responsive pacemaker
I. natural hip system
I. Natural-Knee knee prosthesis
I. phaco I&A unit
I. Quantum unipolar pacemaker
I. RES-Q implantable cardioverter-defibrillator
I. Stride pacemaker
I. Thinlith II pacemaker
intermetatarsal angle (IMA)
intermittent
i. demand flow machine
i. extremity pump
i. flow machine
i. pneumatic compression boot
internal
i. biliary stent
i. ear prosthesis
i. fiberoptic cable
i. fixation device
i. fixation spring
i. hex-thread connection
i. mammary artery (IMA)
i. mammary artery catheter
i. monitor
i. nucleus hydrodelineation needle
i. Reed switch
i. tibial torsion brace
i. ureteral stent
internal/external catheter
International
I. Biomedical Mode 745-100 microcapillary infusion system
I. compression system
Cox Uphoff I. (CUI)
I. standard goniometer
I. 10-20 system
interne
AO fixateur i.
Inter-Op acetabular shell
interosseous wire
Interpore
I. bone replacement material

I. ceramic material
I. graft
I. hydroxyapatite
I. IMZ implant system
I. osteointegrated implant
I. 200 porous hydroxyapatite
Interpret ultrasound catheter
interrogation device
interrupted pledgeted suture
Interseal acetabular cup
intersegmental table
Intersept cardiotomy reservoir
Interson biopsy needle guide
Intersorb
I. absorptive burn pad
I. fine mesh gauze
I. 6-ply absorbent roll stretch gauze
I. wide mesh gauze
interspace
i. shaper
i. width marker
I. YAG laser lens
Interspec
I. Apogee CX 100 ultrasound
I. XL ultrasound
interspinous
i. cable
i. segmental spinal instrumentation
Interstate spatula
InterStim therapy
interstitial
i. implant
i. probe
Intertach pacemaker
Intertech
I. anesthesia breathing circuit
I. Mapleson D nonrebreathing circuit
I. nonrebreathing modified Jackson-Rees circuit
I. Perkin-Elmer gas sampling line
Intertherapy intravascular ultrasound
Intertron therapy microprocessor
intervener
Love-Gruenwald i.
interventional catheter
intervertebral
i. curette
i. disc forceps
i. disc rongeur
i. spreader

NOTES

Interzeag bowl perimeter
intestinal
- i. anastomosis clamp
- i. anastomosis forceps
- i. bag
- i. clamp
- i. closing forceps
- i. decompression trocar
- i. holding forceps
- i. occlusion clamp
- i. occlusion retractor
- i. plication needle
- i. resection clamp
- i. ring clamp
- i. tissue forceps

in-the-ear (ITE)
- i.-t.-e. hearing aid
- i.-t.-e. listening device

Intimax
- I. arterial embolectomy catheter
- I. biliary catheter
- I. cholangiography catheter
- I. occlusion catheter
- I. vascular catheter

intraaortic
- i. balloon (IAB)
- i. balloon assist device
- i. balloon catheter
- i. balloon pump (IABP)
- i. counterpulsation balloon

IntraArc 9963 arthroscopic power system
intraarterial
- i. cannula
- i. digital subtraction (IDIS)

Intrabeam intraoperative radiotherapy system
intracapsular
- i. lens expressor
- i. lens expressor hook
- i. lens forceps
- i. lens loop

intracardiac
- i. accelerometer
- i. cannula
- i. catheter
- i. needle holder
- i. patch
- i. retractor
- i. shunt
- i. sucker
- i. sucker guard
- i. suction tube
- i. sump tube

Intracath catheter
intracavitary
- i. afterloading applicator
- i. probe

Intracell
- I. mechanical muscle device
- I. myofascial trigger-point device
- I. Sprinter stick

intracerebral depth electrode
intracerebroventricular (ICV)
intracervical bag
intracochlear implant
IntraCoil
- I. endoprosthesis
- I. self-expanding peripheral stent

Intracone intramedullary reamer
intracorneal lens
intracoronal retainer
intracoronary
- i. Doppler flow wire
- i. guiding catheter
- i. perfusion catheter
- i. stent
- i. vascular ultrasound (IVUS)

intracranial
- i. pressure (ICP)
- i. pressure catheter
- i. pressure monitor
- i. pressure monitor screw

IntraDop
- I. intraoperative Doppler
- I. probe

Intraducer
- I. peritoneal cannula
- I. peritoneal catheter

intraductal
- i. imaging catheter
- i. ultrasound
- i. ultrasound probe

intradural retractor
Intradyn tear-away introducer sheath
IntraEAR Round Window E Catheter
Intrafix tibial fastener
Intraflex
- I. intramedullary pin
- I. intramedullary pin extractor

intragastric
- i. balloon
- i. cannula
- i. continuous pH-meter meter

IntraLase FS laser
intraligamentary syringe
intraluminal
- i. probe
- i. reference electrode
- i. Safe-Steer guidewire system
- i. stapler
- i. stripper
- i. suture
- i. ultrasound (ILUS)

intrameatal electrode
Intramed angioscopic valvulotome

Intramedic PE-50 polyethylene tubing
intramedullary (IM)
- i. alignment rod
- i. bar
- i. broach
- i. brush
- i. canal plug
- i. catheter
- i. drill
- i. fixation device
- i. guide
- i. illuminator
- i. pin
- i. reamer
- i. Rush rod
- i. skeletal kinetic distractor (ISKD)
- i. skeletal kinetic distractor nail
- i. supracondylar multihole nail

intramedullary/extramedullary (IM/EM)
Intran
- I. intrauterine pressure measurement catheter
- I. Plus catheter

intranasal
- i. bivalve splint
- i. hammer

intraocular
- i. balloon
- i. hook
- i. irrigating forceps
- i. lens (IOL)
- i. lens cannula
- i. lens dialer
- i. lens folder
- i. lens forceps
- i. lens glide
- i. lens implant
- i. tension recorder

Intra-Op autotransfusion system
intraoperative
- i. gamma probe
- i. ultrasonic probe

IntraOptics
- I. intraocular lens
- I. lensometer

intraoral
- i. fracture appliance
- i. stent
- i. titanium mandibular distraction device

intraorbital implant
intraosseous needle

intrapartum monitor
intraperitoneal onlay mesh
intrapleural
- i. catheter
- i. sealed drainage unit

intraportal endovascular ultrasonography
Intra-Prostatic stent
Intrascan ultrasound
intrascapular roll
Intrasil catheter
IntraSite
- I. gel Applipak
- I. gel wound dressing

IntraSonix Tulip laser device
Intrasound
IntraSpectra tissue spectrometer
IntraStent
- I. DoubleStent biliary endoprosthesis
- I. DoubleStrut biliary endoprosthesis

intrastromal corneal ring (ICR)
intrathoracic forceps
intraurethral
- i. coil
- i. prostatic bridge catheter

intrauterine
- i. balloon cannula
- i. catheter (IUC)
- i. device (IUD)
- i. insemination (IUI)
- i. insemination cannula
- i. insemination catheter
- i. pessary
- i. pressure catheter
- i. pressure monitor

intravaginal ring
intravascular (IV)
- i. accurate control (IVAC)
- i. catheter electrode
- i. oxygenator
- i. stent
- i. ultrasound catheter

intravenous (IV)
- i. accurate control device
- i. needle
- i. pacing catheter
- i. Soluset
- i. ultrasound catheter

intravenous-enhanced MRI
intraventricular (IV, IVT)
- i. pressure monitoring catheter

NOTES

485

intravitreal
i. cryoprobe
i. laser
Intrel 3 spinal cord stimulation system
Intrepid
I. balloon catheter
I. percutaneous transluminal coronary angioplasty catheter
I. PTCA catheter
intrinsic transverse connector
Introcan Safety IV catheter
Intro Deuce double-lumen introducer
introducer
ACS percutaneous i.
Allen spherical eye i.
Atkinson i.
Avanti i.
Balkin Up & Over i.
Cardak percutaneous catheter i.
Carter spherical eye i.
catheter i.
Check-Flo i.
Cholangiocath i.
Ciaglia percutaneous tracheostomy i.
Cook micropuncture i.
Cook Peel-Away i.
Cope-Saddekni i.
Czaja-McCaffrey rigid stent i.
Davol pacemaker i.
Desilets i.
Desilets-Hoffman pacemaker i.
Dumon-Gilliard prosthesis i.
Embryon GIFT i.
Encapsulon sheath i.
endolymphatic shunt tube i.
Eric Lloyd i.
Eschmann endotracheal tube i.
Fast-Cath Duo hemostasis i.
Fast-Cath Trio hemostasis i.
FasTrac i.
Goodhill strut i.
gum elastic bougie i.
i. gun
Hedwig i.
Hemaquet i.
H-H shunt i.
Holter i.
Implantaid Di-Lock cardiac lead i.
Input percutaneous sheath i.
Intro Deuce double-lumen i.
Introsyte Autoguard shielded i.
Littleford Spector i.
Littleford-Spector i.
Maryfield i.
Micropuncture Peel-Away i.
Morgan vent tube i.
Neuroguide peel-away catheter i.
Nottingham i.

PD Access peel-away needle i.
Peel-Away i.
Pennine-O'Neil urinary catheter i.
percutaneous i.
pull-apart i.
Razi cannula i.
Richardson polyethylene tube i.
SafeSheath CSG i.
SafeSheath Long i.
i. sheath
silicone i.
sphere i.
split-sheath i.
stent i.
Super Arrow-Flex transseptal sheath i.
SupraFoley suprapubic i.
Swartz SL Series Fast-Cath i.
Taut percutaneous i.
Terumo Radiofocus i.
Tuohy-Borst i.
UMI transseptal Cath-Seal catheter i.
USCI i.
ventricular catheter i.
Weaver trocar i.
Wellwood-Ferguson i.
introducing forceps
Introl bladder neck support prosthesis
Intron A multidose pen
Introsyte Autoguard shielded introducer
intubation laryngoscope
Invacare
I. alternating pressure mattress
I. APM mattress
I. Comfort-Mate extra cushion
I. padded shower chair
I. Venture II HomeFill complete home oxygen system
I. vinyl transfer bench
I. wheelchair
invaginator
Lempert i.
invalid
i. chair
i. cushion
i. ring
InVance male sling system
inverted
i. buttoned device
i. cone bur
i. U-pouch ileal reservoir
inverter
Baladi i.
Barrett appendix i.
Damian i.
Mayo-Boldt i.
I. vitrectomy system
Invertrac equipment

Investa suture
INVOS
  in vivo optical spectroscopy
    INVOS 2100-series, 3100-series
      cerebral oximeter
INX stainless steel stent
Inyo nail
Ioban
  I. antimicrobial incise drape
  I. 2 incise film
  I. 2 iodophor cesarean sheet
Iocare titanium needle
iodine
  i. catgut suture
  i. cup
iodized surgical gut suture
iodochromic catgut suture
Iodoflex
  I. absorptive dressing
  I. solid gel pad
iodoform gauze
iodoform-impregnated plastic sheet
iodophor-impregnated adhesive wrap
Iodosorb absorptive dressing
Iogel intraocular lens
IOL
  intraocular lens
    AC IOL
    accommodative IOL
    IOL dialer
    Hydroview foldable IOL
    Kearney side-notch IOL
    MemoryLens IOL
    Staar low-diopter IOL
    Staar toric IOL
Iolab
  I. Azar intraocular lens
  I. I&A photocoagulator
  I. irrigating needle
  I. taper-cut needle
  I. taper-point needle
  I. titanium instrument
  I. titanium needle
Iomed Phoresor electrode
iON
  i. intraoperative navigation system
ion
  i. chromatograph
  i. laser
  i. pump
Ionalyzer ion measurement system

Ionescu-Shiley
  I.-S. aortic valve prosthesis
  I.-S. artificial cardiac valve
  I.-S. pericardial patch
  I.-S. pericardial valve
  I.-S. pericardial xenograft
  I.-S. vascular graft
  I.-S. xenograft
Ionescu tri-leaflet valve
ionization counter
ionizer
  Mavello water i.
ion-selective electrode
ion-sensitive field-effect transistor
ion-specific field effect transducer
Iontopatch transdermal drug delivery
  system
Iontophor drug delivery system
iontophoresis
  Dynaphor i.
  i. electrode
iontophoretic applicator
Ioptex
  I. intraocular lens
  I. TabOptic lens
IOS immunodiagnostic testing
  instrument
Iotec trocar
Iovision implant
Iowa
  I. membrane forceps
  I. orbital implant
  I. Precoat total hip prosthesis
  I. pudendal needle guide
  I. State fixation forceps
  I. stem
  I. total hip prosthesis
  I. trumpet
  I. trumpet needle guide
  I. University periosteal elevator
Iowa-Mengert membrane forceps
Ipas
  I. flexible cannula
  I. syringe
Ipco-Partridge defibrillator
I-Plant brachytherapy seed
I-plate
  Syracuse anterior I.-p.
I-Plus humeral brace
Ipomax knee orthosis

NOTES

IPOP
    immediate postoperative prosthesis
    IPOP cast dressing
ipos
    i. arch support system
    i. forefoot relief orthosis
    i. heel relief orthosis
    i. heel relief shoe
IQ nasal mask
Irby head frame
Irene lens
Irex Exemplar ultrasound
iridectomy scissors
Iriderm
    I. Apex 800 diode laser
    I. DioLite 532 laser
iridium
    i. needle
    i. prosthesis
iridocapsular intraocular lens
iridocapsulotomy scissors
iridodialysis spatula
iridotomy scissors
IRIS
    Intensified Radiographic Imaging System
    IsoStents for Restenosis Intervention
        Study
        IRIS coronary stent
        IRIS 10,000 overlay
iris
    i. bipolar forceps
    i. claw lens
    i. expressor
    i. forceps
    i. hook
    i. hook cannula
    i. knife
    i. lens manipulator
    i. microforceps
    i. needle
    I. Oculight SLx MicroPulse laser
    I. pressure-reduction mattress
    i. repositor
    i. retractor
    i. scanner
    i. scissors
    i. spatula
    i. speculum
    i. suture microforceps
    i. tissue forceps
iriscorder
    i.'s portable infrared video
        pupillography system
    i. recorder
iris-supported intraocular lens
IRMA
    Immediate Response Mobile Analysis
    IRMA SL blood analysis system

IRMA SL blood gas analysis
    system
iron
    Böhler i.
    I. Intern retractor
    Jewett bending i.
    i. lung
    Lusskin subungual hematoma i.
    Pineda LASIK Flap I.
Irox endocardial pacing lead
irradiation
    local i. (LX)
irradiator
    portable blood i.
Irri-Cath suction system
irrigating
    i. cannula
    i. catheter
    i. Connor wand
    i. cystotome
    i. dialer
    i. iris hook
    i. lens loop
    i. lens manipulator
    i. mushroom retractor
    i. needle
    i. notched spatula
    i. probe
    i. pupil expander
    i. sheath
    i. tip
    i. uterine curette
    i. vectis loop
irrigating-aspirating (I&A)
    i.-a. cannula
    i.-a. vectis
irrigation
    i. and aspiration (I&A)
    i. cannula
    i. catheter
    Endo-AID suction i.
irrigation-aspiration (I&A)
    i.-a. handpiece
irrigator
    anterior chamber i.
    antral i.
    Barraquer i.
    Baumrucker clamp i.
    Bishop-Harman anterior chamber i.
    Carabelli i.
    DeVilbiss eye i.
    Endo-Flo i.
    endoscopic i.
    eye i.
    Fink cul-de-sac i.
    Fisch bone drill i.
    Fluvog i.
    Fox hydrostatic i.
    Gibson anterior chamber i.

Goldstein anterior chamber i.
Gum Machine oral i.
Hartstein i.
Hollister colostomy i.
House-Radpour suction i.
House-Stevenson suction i.
House sucker i.
House T-tube i.
Hydrofloss electronic oral i.
HydroSurg laparoscopic i.
Irrijet i.
Kelman i.
Kemp i.
laser-assisted intrastromal
  keratomileusis flap i.
LASIK flap i.
Lukens double-channel i.
LySonix Delta Tip i.
McKenna Tide-Ur-Ator i.
Moncrieff anterior chamber i.
nasal i.
Nezhat i.
olive-tipped i.
Ortholav pulsed i.
Perio Pik i.
Perry ostomy i.
Pro Pulse i.
Radpour i.
Radpour-House suction i.
Randolph i.
Rollet anterior chamber i.
Shambaugh i.
Shea i.
sinus i.
Sterling-Sylva i.
Stropko i.
Stryker suction i.
suction i.
SurgiLav Plus i.
Sylva anterior chamber i.
Thornwald antral i.
Valentine i.
Vidaurri LASIK flap i.
Water Pik i.
Wells i.
Younge i.
Zimmer suction i.
Irrigo syringe
Irrijet
  I. DS irrigation system
  I. irrigator
Irrivac syringe

Irvine
  I. corneal scissors
  I. I&A unit
  I. probe-pointed scissors
  I. Scientific Embryo Freeze Media
    kit
  I. Scientific Embryo Thaw Media
    kit
  I. viable organ-tissue transport
    system
**IS1000 gel documentation imaging
  system**
Isaacs endometrial cell sampler
ISAH stereotactic immobilizing mask
I-S artificial cardiac valve
Isberg scleral plug
Isch-Dish
  I.-D. CFT pressure-relieving seat
    surface
  I.-D. cushion
  I.-D. Plus cushion
ischial
  i. containment socket
  i. weightbearing brace
  i. weightbearing prosthesis
iseikonic lens
Iselin forceps
Ishihara
  I. I-Temp cautery
  I. IV slit lamp
  I. pseudoisochromatic plate
  I. test chart
ISI laparoscopic instrument
ISKD
  intramedullary skeletal kinetic distractor
  ISKD internal limb lengthening
    system
Isobar
  I. barostat distension device
  I. TTL posterior spinal system
Isobex dynamometer
Isocam SPECT imaging system
Iso-C-arm
  Siremobil I.-C.-a.
Isocon camera
isodiametric bipolar screw-in lead
isoelastic
  i. pelvic prosthesis
  i. rip clamp
Isoflex
  I. bed

NOTES

Isoflex *(continued)*
   I. mattress
   I. portable pressure relief system
Isoflow pump
isokinetic
   i. cycloergometer
   i. Unex III exerciser
Isola
   I. hook-rod
   I. spinal instrumentation system
   I. vertebral screw
   I. wire
isolation
   i. bag
   i. face mask
   i. forceps
Isolator
   I. blood culture system
   I. lysis-centrifugation tube
isolator
   ankle i.
   Vickers i.
isolette
   Airshields i.
Isolex 300i magnetic stem cell selection system
IsoMed
   I. constant-flow infusion system
   I. implantable drug pump
Isomet
   I. low-speed saw
   I. Plus precision saw
Isometer
   I. bone graft placement site detector
   tension I.
isometric strain gauge
Isoprene plastic splint
Iso-Quadron exerciser
Isosal syringe
Isosleeve needle delivery system
Isostar iodine-125 brachytherapy seed
IsoStents for Restenosis Intervention Study (IRIS)
Isotac pilot wire
Isotechnologies B-200 back testing and rehabilitation system
Iso-Thermex 16-channel electronic thermometer
Isotoner glove
isotonic machine
isotope calibrator
isotopic pulse generator pacemaker
Isovis wound protector
Israel
   I. Benzedrine vaporizer
   I. blunt rake retractor
   I. camera
   I. nasal rasp

   I. suction tube
   I. tongue depressor
   I. tonsillar dissector
Isse Endo Brow instrument
i-STAT handheld analyzer
Itard catheter
ITC radiopaque balloon catheter
ITD-FG dental diamond instrument
ITE
   in-the-ear
   ITE listening device
I-tech
   I-t. cannula
   I-t. intraocular foreign body forceps
   I-t. needle holder
   I-t. splinter forceps
   I-t. tying forceps
I-tech-Castroviejo bladebreaker
ITI
   I. dental implant
   I. dental implant system
ITI-Bonefit endosseous implant
Ito
   I. laser pen
   I. needle
Itrel
   I. II, III spinal cord stimulation system
   I. II quadripolar pulse generator
   I. programmed transmitter-receiver
IUC
   intrauterine catheter
IUD
   intrauterine device
   ParaGard T380 copper IUD
   IUD remover hook
IUI
   intrauterine insemination
   IUI catheter
   IUI disposable cannula
IV
   intravascular
   intravenous
   intraventricular
   IV catheter
   IV needle
IVAC
   intravascular accurate control
   IVAC device
   IVAC 831 drip controller
   IVAC needleless IV system
   IVAC Temp Plus II thermometer
   IVAC ventilator
   IVAC volumetric infusion pump
IVAD
   implantable venous access device
   implantable ventricular assist device
Ivalon
   I. compressed patch graft

I. dressing
I. embolic sponge
I. foam
I. lucite orbital eye implant
I. prosthesis
I. sponge
I. sponge eye implant
I. suture
I. wire coil
Ivan
I. laryngeal applicator
I. nasopharyngeal applicator
IVC
inferior vena cava
IVEC-10 neurotransmitter analyzer
Ives
I. anoscope
I. rectal speculum
Ives-Fansler anoscope
I.V. House wound cover

Ivinsco cervical dilator
Ivocryl resin
Ivory rubber dam clamp
IVT
intraventricular
IVT percutaneous catheter
introducer sheath
IVUS
intracoronary vascular ultrasound
IVUS catheter
Ivy
I. loop
I. mastoid rongeur
I. needle holder
I. wire
Iwabuchi clip
iWALKfree crutch
Iwashi clamp approximator
Iwata-Ricky gonioscopic lens

NOTES

J

J board
J exchange guidewire
J exchange wire
J guidewire
J needle
J orthogonal electrode
J pad
J retention wire
J Rosen guidewire
J stent

Jabaley scissors
Jabaley-Stille scissors
Jaboulay button
Jace

J. continuous passive motion ankle system
J. hand continuous passive motion unit
J. knee brace
J. shoulder exerciser
J. W550 continuous passive motion wrist device

JACE-Stim

J.-S. electrical stimulator
J.-S. electrotherapy unit

jacket

body j.
Bonchek-Shiley cardiac j.
Boston soft body j.
Calot j.
cervicothoracic j.
cuirass j.
Daily cooling j.
Frejka j.
immobilization j.
Kydex body j.
Lexan j.
low-profile plastic body j.
Medtronic cardiac cooling j.
Minerva plastic back j.
Orfizip body j.
Orthoplast j.
plaster-of-Paris j.
Prenyl j.
Radix-Raney j.
Raney j.
Risser wedging j.
Royalite body j.
Sayre j.
Vitrathene j.
Von Lackum transection shift j.
Willock respiratory j.
Wilmington plastic j.

Jack Frost hot/cold pack

Jackman

J. coronary sinus electrode catheter
J. orthogonal catheter

Jackson

J. alligator grasping forceps
J. anterior commissure laryngoscope
J. approximation forceps
J. aspirating tube
J. biopsy forceps
J. bite block
J. bone clamp
J. bone-extension clamp
J. bone-holding clamp
J. broad staple forceps
J. bronchial dilator
J. button forceps
J. cane-shaped tracheal tube
J. conventional foreign body forceps
J. costophrenic bronchoscope
J. cross-action forceps
J. cylindrical-object forceps
J. double-concave rat-tooth forceps
J. double-prong forceps
J. down-jaw forceps
J. dressing forceps
J. dull-pointed forceps
J. endoscopic forceps
J. esophageal dilator
J. esophageal scissors
J. esophageal shears
J. esophagoscope
J. fenestrated forceps
J. fenestrated peanut-grasping forceps
J. fiberoptic slide laryngoscope
J. flexible upper lobe bronchus forceps
J. forward-grasping forceps
J. full-lumen bronchoscope
J. globular object forceps
J. head-holding forceps
J. hemostatic forceps
J. hollow-object forceps
J. imaging table
J. infant biopsy forceps
J. intervertebral disc rongeur
J. lacrimal intubation set
J. laryngeal applicator
J. laryngeal applicator forceps
J. laryngeal atomizer
J. laryngeal basket forceps
J. laryngeal-dressing forceps
J. laryngeal-grasping forceps
J. laryngeal punch forceps

Jackson · Jacobson

Jackson *(continued)*
- J. laryngeal ring-rotation forceps
- J. laryngeal scissors
- J. laryngectomy tube
- J. laryngofissure forceps
- J. laryngostat
- J. magnification ruler set
- J. open-end aspirating tube
- J. papilloma forceps
- J. perichondrial elevator
- J. pin-bending costophrenic forceps
- J. punch
- J. punch forceps
- J. radiopaque bougie
- J. ring-jaw forceps
- J. ring-rotation forceps
- J. rod
- J. self-retaining goiter retractor
- J. sharp-pointed rotation forceps
- J. side-curved forceps
- J. silver tracheostomy tube
- J. sister-hook forceps
- J. sliding laryngoscope
- J. spinal surgery table
- J. sponge carrier
- J. square punch tip
- J. staging system
- J. standard laryngoscope
- J. steel-stem woven filiform bougie
- J. tendon-seizing forceps
- J. tracheal bistoury
- J. tracheal bistoury knife
- J. tracheal bougie
- J. tracheal dilator
- J. tracheal hemostat
- J. tracheal hemostatic forceps
- J. tracheal hook
- J. tracheal retractor
- J. tracheal scalpel
- J. tracheal tenaculum
- J. tracheal tube
- J. tracheoscope
- J. tracheotomic bistoury
- J. triangular brass dilator
- J. triangular-punch forceps
- J. tunneler
- J. turbinate scissors
- J. vaginal retractor
- J. vaginal speculum
- J. velvet-eye aspirating tube
- J. warning stop tube

Jackson-Moore shears
Jackson-Mosher cardiospasm dilator
Jackson-Plummer dilator
Jackson-Pratt
- J.-P. bifurcated drain extension
- J.-P. catheter
- J.-P. dissector
- J.-P. flat drain
- J.-P. Gold wound drain
- J.-P. Hemaduct drain
- J.-P. hysterectomy kit
- J.-P. large-volume round silicone drain kit
- J.-P. large-volume suction reservoir
- J.-P. PVC kit
- J.-P. round PVC drain
- J.-P. silicone flat drain
- J.-P. silicone round drain
- J.-P. suction drain
- J.-P. suction tube
- J.-P. T-tube drain

Jackson-Rees
- J.-R. apparatus
- J.-R. circuit
- J.-R. endotracheal tube

Jackson-Trousseau dilator
Jacobaeus thoracoscope
Jacobaeus-Unverricht thoracoscope
Jacob capsular fragment forceps
Jacobs
- J. biopsy forceps
- J. capsular fragment forceps
- J. chuck adapter
- J. chuck drill
- J. clamp
- J. cranial hook
- J. distraction rod
- J. locking hook spinal rod
- J. snap-lock chuck
- J. T-handle chuck
- J. uterine tenaculum
- J. vulsellum
- J. vulsellum forceps

Jacobsen template
Jacobson
- J. bayonet-shaped scissors
- J. bipolar forceps
- J. bladder retractor
- J. blood vessel probe
- J. blunt hook
- J. bulldog clamp
- J. counter-pressure elevator
- J. curette
- J. dressing forceps
- J. endarterectomy spatula
- J. fork
- J. goiter retractor
- J. hemostatic forceps
- J. microscissors
- J. mosquito forceps
- J. spring-handled needle holder
- J. spring-handled scissors
- J. suture pusher
- J. vas deferens probe
- J. vessel clamp
- J. vessel knife

494

J. vessel probe
J. vessel punch
Jacobson-Potts vessel clamp
Jacobson-Vital needle holder
Jacobs-Palmer laparoscope
Jacob-Swan
    J.-S. gonioprism
    J.-S. gonioscope
    J.-S. gonioscopic prism
    J.-S. goniotomy pliers
Jacobus mammotome
Jacoby heel splint
Jacques
    J. catheter
    J. gastric tube
Jade
    J. Audio-Starr hearing aid
    J. II SSI pacemaker
Jaeger
    J. acuity card
    J. eye chart
    J. keratome
    J. keratome knife
    J. LE3000 treadmill
    J. lid retractor
    J. metal lid plate
    J. reading chart
    J. strabismus hook
Jaeger-Whiteley catheter
Jaffe
    J. blepharoplasty laser
    J. Cilco lens
    J. eyelid speculum
    J. intraocular spatula
    J. iris hook
    J. lens-manipulating hook
    J. lens spatula
    J. microlens hook
    J. needle holder
    J. 1-piece all-PMMA intraocular lens
    J. suturing forceps
    J. tying forceps
    J. wire lid retractor
Jaffe-Bechert nucleus rotator
Jaffe capsulorrhexis forceps
Jaffe-Givner lid retractor
Jaffe-Maltzman
    J.-M. hook
    J.-M. lens manipulator
Jager meniscal forceps
Jagwire guidewire

Jahnke anastomosis clamp
Jahnke-Barron heart support net
Jahnke-Cook-Seeley clamp
jail
    stent j.
JainSuture/VesiBand organizer
Jako
    J. clamp
    J. facial nerve monitor
    J. fine ball-tip hook
    J. knot pusher
    J. laryngeal forceps
    J. laryngeal knife
    J. laryngeal mirror
    J. laryngeal needle holder
    J. laryngeal probe
    J. laryngeal suction tube
    J. laryngoscope
    J. laser aspirating tube
    J. laser retractor
    J. laser trocar
    J. microlaryngeal cup forceps
    J. microlaryngeal grasping forceps
    J. microlaryngeal scissors
    J. microlaryngoscope
    J. suction-irrigator
    J. suction tube
    J. transilluminator
Jako-Cherry laryngoscope
Jako-Kleinsasser
    J.-K. ball-tip hook
    J.-K. knife
    J.-K. microforceps
    J.-K. microscissors
Jako-Pilling laryngoscope
Jalaguier-Reverdin needle
Jamar
    J. hydraulic hand dynamometer
    J. hydraulic pinch gauge
James
    J. lumbar peritoneal catheter
    J. wound-approximation forceps
Jameson
    J. eye calipers
    J. facelift scissors
    J. muscle clamp
    J. muscle hook
    J. muscle recession forceps
    J. needle holder
    J. strabismus forceps
    J. strabismus hook

J

NOTES

Jameson *(continued)*
J. strabismus needle
J. tracheal muscle forceps
Jameson-Metzenbaum scissors
Jameson-Werber scissors
Jamshidi-Kormed bone marrow biopsy needle
Jamshidi liver biopsy needle
Janacek reimplantation set
Janelli clip
Janes
J. fracture appliance
J. fracture frame
Janet bladder swab
Janeway
J. gastroscope
J. sphygmomanometer
Jannetta
J. alligator grasping forceps
J. aneurysm neck dissector
J. angular elevator
J. angular knife
J. bayonet forceps
J. bayonet needle holder
J. bayonet scissors
J. bayonet-shaped needle holder
J. bayonet-shaped scissors
J. double-pronged fork
J. duckbill elevator
J. hook
J. microbayonet forceps
J. needle holder
J. posterior fossa retractor
J. probe
J. sterilizing rack
Jannetta-Kurze dissecting scissors
Jansen
J. bayonet dressing forceps
J. bayonet ear forceps
J. bayonet nasal forceps
J. bayonet rongeur
J. bone curette
J. bone rongeur
J. clamp
J. dissecting forceps
J. dressing forceps
J. ear rongeur
J. mastoid raspatory
J. mastoid retractor
J. monopolar forceps
J. mouthgag
J. nasal-dressing forceps
J. periosteotome
J. scalp retractor
J. thumb forceps
Jansen-Anderson intrauterine catheter
Jansen-Cottle rongeur
Jansen-Gifford mastoid retractor
Jansen-Gruenwald forceps

Jansen-Middleton
J.-M. nasal-cutting forceps
J.-M. punch forceps
J.-M. rongeur
J.-M. scissors
J.-M. septal forceps
J.-M. septal punch
J.-M. septotomy forceps
J.-M. septum-cutting forceps
Jansen-Mueller forceps
Jansen-Newhart mastoid probe
Jansen-Sluder mouthgag
Jansen-Struyken septal forceps
Jansen-Wagner mastoid retractor
Jansen-Zaufel rongeur
Japanese
J. Bruening anastigmatic aural magnifier
J. erection ring
J. fingertrap
J. Medical Supply (JMS)
J. suction tip
Japonicum laminaria
Jaquet apparatus
jar
bubble j.
GasPak j.
Jarabak arch wire
Jarabak-type archwire
Jarcho
J. pressometer
J. self-retaining uterine cannula
J. tenaculum forceps
J. tenaculum holder
J. uterine tenaculum
Jardine hook
Jardon eye shield
Jardon-Straith
J.-S. chin implant
J.-S. nasal implant
Jarell forceps
Jarit
J. air injection cannula
J. anterior resection clamp
J. bipolar coagulator
J. bladebreaker
J. bone hook
J. brain forceps
J. cartilage clamp
J. comedo extractor
J. cross-action retractor
J. disposable trocar
J. dissecting scissors
J. endarterectomy scissors
J. finger goniometer
J. flat-tip scissors
J. forceps holder
J. hand surgery osteotome
J. intestinal clamp

J. lacrimal cannula
J. lower lateral scissors
J. mallet
J. meniscal clamp
J. microstitch scissors
J. microsurgery scissors
J. microsurgical needle holder
J. microsuture tying forceps
J. mosquito forceps
J. palate hook
J. P.E.E.R. retractor
J. periosteal elevator
J. peripheral vascular scissors
J. pin cutter
J. plaster knife
J. plaster shears
J. 3-prong cast spreader
J. renal sinus retractor
J. reverse adenoid curette
J. rotator
J. Rotator endoscope
J. spring-wire retractor
J. sterilizer forceps
J. sternal needle holder
J. stitch scissors
J. tendon-pulling forceps
J. tube-occluding forceps
J. tuning fork
J. utility shears
J. wire holder
J. wire-pulling forceps
Jarit-Allis tissue forceps
Jarit-Crafoord forceps
Jarit-Dandy forceps
Jarit-Deaver retractor
Jarit-Graves vaginal speculum
Jarit-Kerrison rongeur
Jarit-Liston bone-cutting forceps
Jarit-Mason cast breaker
Jarit-Pederson vaginal speculum
Jarit-Poole abdominal suction tube
Jarit-Ruskin rongeur
Jarit-Yankauer suction tube
Jarvik-7, -8, 2000 artificial heart
Jarvis
J. hemorrhoidal forceps
J. pile clamp
J. snare
JAS
joint activated system
JAS elbow device
Jasbee esophagoscope

Jasin Frontal Ostent stent
Jatene arterial switch valve
Jatene-Macchi prosthetic valve
Javal
J. keratometer
J. ophthalmometer
Javerts
J. placental forceps
J. polyp forceps
Javid
J. bypass clamp
J. bypass tube
J. carotid clamp
J. carotid shunt
J. catheter
J. shunt clamp
jaw
j. exerciser
j. forceps
j. hook
j. rongeur
j. spreader
Y j.'s
Jawz disposable biopsy forceps
Jay
J. Care wheelchair seating system
J. J2 wheelchair
J. Rave cushion
J. Triad cushion
J. Xtreme cushion
Jayco H2 lactose breath analyzer
Jayles forceps
Jazbi tonsillar dissector
Jeb graft
Jefferson self-retaining retractor
Jeffrey introducer set
Jehle coronary perfusion catheter
jejunal feeding tube
jejunoileal shunt
jejunostomy
j. catheter
needle catheter j.
percutaneous endoscopic j.
j. tube
Jelco
J. intravenous catheter
J. intravenous stylet
J. needle
Jelenko
J. arch bar
J. facial fracture appliance

NOTES

Jelenko *(continued)*
    J. pliers
    J. splint
Jelm 2-way catheter
Jelonet dressing
JEM-100B, 100S electron microscope
Jena colposcope
Jena-Schiotz tonometer
Jenkins chisel
Jennings Loktite mouthgag
Jennings-Skillern mouthgag
Jenning-Streifeneder gastroscope
Jenny mammary prosthesis
Jensen
    J. capsular polisher
    J. capsular scratcher
    J. intraocular lens forceps
    J. lens-inserting forceps
Jensen-Thomas
    J.-T. I&A cannula
    J.-T. irrigating-aspirating cannula
Jentzer trephine
Jerald forceps
Jergensen reamer
Jergensen-Trinkle reamer
Jergesen I-beam
jerkin plethysmograph
Jervey
    J. capsular fragment forceps
    J. iris forceps
Jesberg
    J. aspirating tube
    J. grasping forceps
    J. infant bronchoscope
    J. laryngectomy clamp
    J. oval esophagoscope
    J. upper esophagoscope
Jesco scissors
jet
    j. humidifier
    Injectoflex respirator j.
    j. nebulizer
    Riwomat respirator j.
    J. shield
    j. stylet
    J. Vac cement dispenser
Jet-Air splint
Jetco spray cannula
Jeter
    J. lag screw
    J. position screw
Jettmobile
    Tumble Forms J.
Jewel
    J. AF implantable cardioverter-
      defibrillator
    J. AF implantable cardioverter
      defibrillator system
    J. AF implantable defibrillator

    J. atrial fibrillation dual chamber
      device
    J. pacer-cardioverter-defibrillator
    J. PCD
    J. programmable cardioverter-
      defibrillator
jeweler's
    j. bipolar forceps
    j. pickup forceps
    j. tweezers
Jewett
    J. bar
    J. bending iron
    J. bone chip packer
    J. bone extractor
    J. contraflexion brace
    J. contraflexion orthosis
    J. double-angled osteotomy plate
    J. driver
    J. electrode
    J. fracture appliance
    J. frame
    J. gouge
    J. hip nail
    J. hyperextension brace
    J. nail
    J. pickup screw
    J. postfusion brace
    J. postfusion orthosis
    J. prosthesis
    J. slotted plate
    J. socket reamer
    J. thoracolumbosacral orthosis
    J. urethral sound
    J. uterine dilator
    J. uterine sound
Jewett-Benjamin
    J.-B. cervical brace
    J.-B. cervical orthosis
JFET
    junction field-effect transistor
J-FX bipolar head
J-Glas Prefabs orthotic
Jiffy tube
jig
    Ace-Hershey halo j.
    chamfer j.
    Charnley tibial onlay j.
    cutting j.
    extramedullary tibial alignment j.
    fixation j.
    Osteonics j.
    Plexiglas j.
    precompression j.
jigsaw blade
Jimmie
    half J.
Jimmy
    J. dislodger

J. dissector
J. John colonic irrigation system
Jinotti
J. closed suctioning system
J. dual-purpose catheter
J & J
Johnson & Johnson
JL4
Judkins left 4
JL4 catheter
JL5 catheter
JL catheter
J-loop
J.-l. electrode
J.-l. posterior chamber intraocular
lens
J-Maxx stent
JMS
Japanese Medical Supply
JMS fistula needle
JMS injection needle
J-needle
J.-n. laparoscopic suturing needle
Unimar J.-n.
Joal lens
Jobert de Lamballe suture
Jobskin pressure garment
Jobson-Horne
J.-H. cotton applicator
J.-H. probe
Jobson-Pynchon tongue depressor
Jobst
J. air band
J. appliance
J. athrombic pump system
J. athrombotic pump
J. extremity pump
J. facelift dressing
J. glove
J. mammary support dressing
J. postoperative air boot
J. pressure garment
J. prosthesis
J. sleeve
J. UlcerCare dressing
J. Vairox support stocking
J. VPGS stocking
Jobstens neurostimulator
Jobst-Stride support stocking
Jobst-Stridette support stocking
**Jocath Maestro coronary balloon
catheter**

Joel scanning electron microscope
Joe's
J. hoe
J. hoe retractor
Jography angiographic catheter
Joguide
J. coronary guiding catheter
J. guiding catheter
Johannson
J. hip nail
J. lag screw
Johannson-Stille
J.-S. cystotomy trocar
J.-S. lag screw
John
J. A. Tucker mediastinoscope
J. Bunn Mini-Mist nebulizer
J. Green calipers
J. Green pendulum scalpel
J. Weiss forceps
Johns
J. Hopkins bulldog clamp
J. Hopkins coarctation clamp
J. Hopkins forceps
J. Hopkins gallbladder forceps
J. Hopkins gallbladder retractor
J. Hopkins gall duct forceps
J. Hopkins hemostatic forceps
J. Hopkins modified Potts clamp
J. Hopkins occluding forceps
J. Hopkins serrefine forceps
J. Hopkins stone basket
Johnson
J. brain tumor forceps
J. canaliculus wire
J. cervical thoracic orthosis
J. cheek retractor
J. coagulation suction tube
J. dental band
J. double cannula
J. Endobag instrument
J. erysiphake
J. evisceration knife
J. gauze sponge
J. hook retractor
J. intestinal tube
Johnson & J. (J & J)
J. & Johnson Band-Aid sterile
drape
J. & Johnson biliary stent
J. & Johnson coronary stent
J. & Johnson dressing

NOTES

Johnson *(continued)*
    J. & Johnson gauze sponge
    J. & Johnson hemopump
    J. & Johnson non-stick pad
    J. & Johnson PFC cruciate-
    substituting insert
    J. & Johnson PFC Sigma system
    J. & Johnson saliva ejector
    J. & Johnson tourniquet
    J. & Johnson waterproof tape
    J. Kydex chairback orthosis
    J. prostatic needle holder
    J. ptosis forceps
    J. ptosis knife
    J. screwdriver
    J. skin hook
    J. spatula
    J. stone dislodger
    J. swab sampler
    J. thoracic forceps
    J. total hip stabilization orthosis
    J. twin-wire appliance
    J. ureteral stone basket
    J. ventriculogram retractor
Johnson-Bell erysiphake
Johnson-Kerrison punch
Johnson-Tooke corneal knife
Johnston
    J. clamp
    J. fixation ring
    J. gastrostomy plug
    J. infant dilator
    J. LASIK flap applanator
joint
    j. activated system (JAS)
    artificial hip j.
    Ascension MCP total j.
    Ascension PIP total j.
    j. cinch
    CUI j.
    Delrin j.
    distal radioulnar j. (DRUJ)
    j. distraction cuff
    Fillauer dorsiflexion assist ankle j.
    Fillauer PDC ankle j.
    Gaffney j.
    gliding hinge j.
    Greissinger multi-axis j.
    j. implant
    integrated ankle orthotic ankle j.
    Klenzak double-channeled ankle j.
    Klenzak knee j.
    Metasul j.
    Ottoback 3R65 children's hydraulic
    knee j.
    Perlstein j.
    Scotty stainless ankle j.
    Tamarack flexure j.

    temporomandibular j. (TMJ)
    T rotating j.
Joint-Jack finger splint
Jo-Kath catheter
joker
    j. dissector
    j. elevator
Jolly uterine dilator
Jomed stent
Jometrics SmartWire pressure guidewire
Jonas
    J. implant
    J. penile prosthesis
Jonas-Graves vaginal speculum
Jonathan Livingston Seagull patella
prosthesis
Jonell
    J. countertraction finger splint
    J. thumb splint
Jones
    J. abduction frame
    J. adenoid curette
    J. arm splint
    J. brace
    J. cervical knife
    J. dissecting scissors
    J. dressing
    J. forearm splint
    J. hemostatic forceps
    J. IMA diamond knife
    J. IMA epicardial retractor
    J. IMA forceps
    J. IMA kit
    J. IMA needle holder
    J. IMA scissors
    J. keratome
    J. lacrimal canaliculus dilator
    J. metacarpal splint
    J. nasal splint
    J. needle holder
    J. pin
    J. punctum dilator
    J. Pyrex tube
    J. suspension traction
    J. tear duct tube
    J. thoracic clamp
    J. towel clamp
    J. towel forceps
    J. traction splint
Jonesco
    J. bone wire guide
    J. wire suture needle
Joplin
    J. bone-holding forceps
    J. tendon passer
    J. tendon stripper
    J. toe prosthesis
Jordan
    J. canal elevator

J. canal incision knife
J. capsular knife
J. eye implant
J. hook
J. middle ear instrument
J. needle
J. perforating bur
J. stapedectomy knife
J. strut forceps
J. strut-measuring instrument
J. wire loop dilator
Jordan-Caparosa holder
Jordan-Day
J.-D. cutting bur
J.-D. dermatome
J.-D. drill
J.-D. fenestration bur
J.-D. polishing bur
Jordan-Hermann chisel
Jordan-Rosen
J.-R. curette
J.-R. elevator
Jorgenson
J. dissecting scissors
J. gallbladder scissors
J. retractor
J. thoracic scissors
Joseph
J. angular knife
J. antral perforator
J. bayonet saw
J. bistoury knife
J. button-end knife
J. cervical knife
J. chisel
J. double-edged knife
J. guard
J. measuring ruler
J. nasal brace
J. nasal elevator
J. nasal hook
J. nasal knife
J. nasal rasp
J. nasal raspatory
J. nasal saw
J. nasal scissors
J. nasal splint
J. periosteal elevator
J. periosteal raspatory
J. periosteotome
J. punch
J. saw guide

J. saw protector
J. septal bar
J. septal clamp
J. septal fracture appliance
J. septal frame
J. septal splint
J. serrated scissors
J. single-prong hook
J. skin hook
J. skin hook retractor
J. tenaculum hook
J. wound retractor
Josephberg probe
Joseph-Farrior saw
Joseph-Killian septal elevator
Joseph-Maltz
J.-M. angular nasal saw
J.-M. knife
J.-M. scissors
Josephson
J. quadpolar mapping electrode
J. quadripolar catheter
Joseph-Stille saw
Joseph-Verner
J.-V. raspatory
J.-V. saw
Jostent
J. bifurcation stent
J. coronary stent
J. Flex stent
J. Flex Supreme system
J. peripheral stent
J. Plus stent
J. SelfX endoscopic stent
J. side branch stent
Jostra
J. arterial blood filter
J. cardiotomy reservoir
J. catheter
joule counter
Jousto dropfoot skid orthosis
Joyce-Loebl Magiscan image analysis system
Joystick retractor
J-periosteal elevator
JR catheter
JR5 catheter
JR4 catheter
J-scope esophagoscope
J-shaped
J-s. endoscope
J-s. I&A cannula

NOTES

J

J-shaped *(continued)*
    J-s. pacemaker electrode
    J-s. tube
JSM-6400 scanning electron microscope
JS Quick-fill system
J-tipped guidewire
Jubileum 2.0 gastroesophageal pH probe
Judd
    J. cannula
    J. clamp
    J. cystoscope
    J. strabismus forceps
    J. suture forceps
    J. trocar
    J. urethroscope
Judd-Allis
    J.-A. clamp
    J.-A. intestinal forceps
    J.-A. intestinal retractor
    J.-A. tissue forceps
Judd-DeMartel gallbladder forceps
Judd-Mason
    J.-M. bladder retractor
    J.-M. prostatic retractor
Judet
    J. dissector
    J. hip prosthesis
    J. impactor for acetabular component
    J. impactor for acetabular cup
    J. strut
Judkins
    J. coronary catheter
    J. curve LAD catheter
    J. curve LCX catheter
    J. curve STD catheter
    J. 4 diagnostic catheter
    J. guiding catheter
    J. left 4 (JL4)
    J. left 4 catheter
    J. left coronary catheter
    J. pigtail catheter
    J. right catheter
    J. right coronary catheter
    J. torque-control catheter
    J. USCI catheter
Judson-Smith manipulator
Juers
    J. crimper forceps
    J. ear curette

    J. hook
    J. lingual forceps
    J. wire crimper
Juers-Derlacki Universal head holder
Juers-Lempert
    J.-L. endaural rongeur
    J.-L. rongeur forceps
Juevenelle clamp
jugular
    right internal j. (RIJ)
jugular venous catheter
Julian
    J. cystoresectoscope
    J. needle holder
    J. splenorenal forceps
    J. thoracic artery forceps
Julian-Damian thoracic forceps
Julian-Fildes clamp
junctional pacemaker
junction field-effect transistor (JFET)
Jung
    J. Autostainer XL
    J. CV 5000 Robotic Coverslipper
    J. microtome knife
Junior Tompkins portable aspirator
Junker inhaler
Junod boot
Jurasz laryngeal forceps
Jurgan
    J. pin
    J. pin ball
    J. pin protector
JustVision diagnostic ultrasound scanner
Jutte tube
Jux-A-Cisor exerciser
Juzo
    J. hose
    J. Patellaligner brace
    J. shrinker
    J. stocking
Juzo-Hostess
    J.-H. compression stocking
    J.-H. two-way stretch compression stocking
J-Vac
    J-V. bulb suction reservoir
    J-V. catheter
    J-V. closed wound drainage system
    J-V. drain
J-wire
    safety J-w.

K

K blade
K dissector sponge
K implant
K pack
K pad
K reamer
K root canal file
K stylet
K wire driver
K x-ray fluorescence instrument

K-2000 surgical saw blade
K9 Scooter
KAAT II Plus intraaortic balloon pump
Kader

K. fishhook needle
K. gastrostomy
K. intestinal spatula

Kadesky forceps
Kadir Hi-Torque guidewire
Kaessman handpiece
Kaessmann nail
KAFO

knee-ankle-foot orthosis
Generation II KAFO
KAFO prosthesis

Kahler

K. bronchial biopsy forceps
K. bronchoscopic forceps
K. bronchus-grasping forceps
K. double-action tip
K. laryngeal biopsy forceps
K. polyp forceps

Kahn

K. scissors
K. tenaculum forceps
K. traction tenaculum
K. uterine dilator
K. uterine trigger cannula

Kahn-Graves vaginal speculum
Kahre-Williger periosteal elevator
Kairos pacemaker
Kaiser speculum
Kalamarides dural retractor
Kal-Dermic suture
Kaleidoscope chair
Kalginate calcium alginate wound dressing
Kalinowski

K. ear speculum
K. perforator
K. rasp

Kalinowski-Verner

K.-V. ear speculum
K.-V. rasp

Kalish Duredge wire extractor
Kalix flat foot implant
Kalk

K. electrode
K. esophagoscope
K. palpitation probe

Kallassy

K. ankle brace
K. ankle support
K. orthosis

Kall modification of Silverman needle
Kallmorgen vaginal spatula
Kalman

K. filter
K. needle holder
K. occluding forceps
K. tube-occluding forceps

Kalos pacemaker
Kalt

K. capsular forceps
K. corneal needle
K. eye needle
K. eye needle holder
K. eye spoon
K. needle holder clamp
K. vein needle

Kalt-Arruga needle holder
Kaltenborn-Evjenth Concept Wedge mobilization wedge
Kaltostat

K. calcium sodium alginate wound dressing
K. Fortex dressing
K. hydrofiber wound packing
K. rope
K. wound packing material

Kalt-Vital needle holder
Kambin-Gellman instrumentation
Kambin instrumentation
Kamdar microscissors
Kamerling

K. Capsular 90 lens
K. 1-piece all-PMMA intraocular lens

Kaminsky

K. catheter
K. stent

Kammann ophthalmic speculum
Kamppeter anomaloscope
Kam Super Sucker
Kanavel

K. apparatus

K

Kanavel *(continued)*
    K. brain-exploring cannula
    K. cock-up splint
    K. conductor
    K. table
Kanavel-Senn retractor
Kandel stereotactic apparatus
Kane
    K. obstetrical clamp
    K. umbilical cord clamp
Kaneda
    K. anterior scoliosis system
    K. anterior spinal instrumentation
    K. anterior spine stabilizing device
    K. distraction device
    K. distractor
    K. rod
kangaroo
    K. feeding pump
    K. silicone gastrostomy feeding tube
    k. tendon suture
Kangnian acupuncture needle
Kangoo
    K. Jumps exercise boot
    K. Thera-P bar
Kansas
    K. City band truss
    K. University corneal forceps
Kantor
    K. circumcision clamp
    K. forceps
Kantor-Berci video laryngoscope
Kantrowitz
    K. dressing forceps
    K. hemostatic clamp
    K. pacemaker
    K. thoracic clamp
    K. thoracic forceps
    K. tissue forceps
Kap
    Hypotherm Gel K.
    Kold K.
Kaplan
    K. PenduLaser laser
    K. resectoscope
    K. tracheostomy needle
Kaplan-Simpson InfusaSleeve
Kapp
    K. clip
    K. forceps
    K. microarterial clamp
    K. microclamp
    K. Surgical Instrument prosthetic knee
    K. Surgical Instrument total hip calipers
    K. Surgical Instrument total knee retractor

Kappa DR 400-series pacemaker
Kapp-Beck
    K.-B. bronchial clamp
    K.-B. coarctation clamp
    K.-B. colon clamp
    K.-B. forceps
Kapp-Beck-Thomson clamp
Kaprelian easy-access tweezers (KEAT)
Kaps operating microscope
Kara
    K. cataract-aspirating cannula
    K. cataract needle
    K. erysiphake
Karakashian-Barraquer scissors
Karamar-Mailatt tarsorrhaphy clamp
Karaya
    K. adhesive ileostomy appliance
    K. dressing
    K. electrode
    K. seal ileostomy stomal bag
    K. self-adhesive conductive material
Karickhoff
    K. diagnostic lens
    K. double cannula
    K. keratoscope
    K. laser lens
Karl
    K. Ilg instrument
    K. Storz Calcutript endoscope
    K. Storz coagulator
    K. Storz flexible endoscope
    K. Storz flexible ureteropyeloscope
    K. Storz 15 French flexible hysteroscope
    K. Storz lithotripter
    K. Storz-Lutzeyer lithotripter
    K. Storz pediatric bronchoscopy system
Karlin
    K. crank frame retractor
    K. microknife
Karman cannula
Karmen catheter
Karmody
    K. vascular spring retractor
    K. venous scissors
Karolinska-Stille punch
Karp
    K. aortic punch
    K. aortic punch forceps
Karras angiography needle
Kartchner carotid artery clamp
Kartch pigtail probe
Kartush
    K. insulated retractor
    K. stimulus dissection elevator
    K. tympanic membrane patcher
Karwetsky U-bow activator
Kasai peritoneal venous shunt

Kasdan retractor
Kashiwabara laryngeal mirror
Kaslow gastrointestinal tube
Kaster mitral valve prosthesis
kastRAP wrap
Kataya seal closed stoma pouch
Katena
- K. boat hook
- K. cannula
- K. double-edged sapphire blade
- K. forceps
- K. iris spatula
- K. Quick Switch I/A system
- K. ring
- K. scleral shield
- K. speculum
- K. spoon and spatula
- K. trephine

Katena-Barron trephine
Kato-Asch coaxial needle
Katon catheter
Katsch chisel
Katzeff cartilage scissors
Katzen
- K. flap unzipper
- K. infusion wire
- K. long balloon dilatation catheter

Katzenstein rectal cannula
Katzin
- K. corneal transplant scissors
- K. trephine

Katzin-Barraquer
- K.-B. Colibri forceps
- K.-B. corneal forceps

Katzin-Long balloon
Katzin-Troutman scissors
Kaufer type II retractor
Kaufman
- K. adapter
- K. catheter
- K. clip applier
- K. ENT forceps
- K. III anti-incontinence prosthesis
- K. II vitrector
- K. incontinence device
- K. kidney clamp
- K. male urinary incontinence prosthesis
- K. type II retractor
- K. vitrector
- K. vitreophage

KaVo
- K. dental handpiece
- K. oral surgery system

Kawasumi infusion set
Kay
- K. aortic anastomosis clamp
- K. rhinolaryngeal stroboscope

Kaycel towel
Kay-Cross suction tip suction tube
Kaye
- K. blepharoplasty scissors
- K. facelift scissors
- K. fine dissecting scissors
- K. Kinder chair
- K. tamponade balloon

Kay-Lambert clamp
Kayser-Fleischer ring
Kay-Shiley
- K.-S. disc valve prosthesis
- K.-S. heart valve

Kay-Suzuki
- K.-S. heart valve
- K.-S. prosthesis

Kazanjian
- K. action-type osteotome
- K. bone-cutting forceps
- K. cutting forceps
- K. guide
- K. nasal forceps
- K. nasal hump forceps
- K. nasal splint
- K. scissors
- K. tooth button

Kazanjian-Cottle forceps
Kazanjian-Goldman rongeur
K-Blade microsurgical blade
KBM
- KBM absorbent gauze
- KBM gauze swab

K/B prosthesis
KC1 Delta coagulation analyzer
K-Centrum anterior spinous fixation system
KDC-Healthdyne nonfluorescent spotlight
KD chin prosthesis
KDF-2.3
- K. intrauterine insemination cannula
- K. intrauterine insemination catheter

Keane Mobility bed
Kean-M-4 occluder

K

NOTES

Kearney
- K. side-notch intraocular lens
- K. side-notch IOL

Kearns
- K. bag catheter
- K. bladder dilator

KEAT
- Kaprelian easy-access tweezers

Kebab graft

K-edge filter

keel
- Deltafit k.
- McNaught k.
- Montgomery laryngeal k.
- k. stent

Keeler
- K. camera
- K. cryoextractor
- K. cryophake
- K. cryophake unit
- K. cryosurgical instrument
- K. cryosurgical unit
- K. extended round tip forceps
- K. fiberoptic headlight
- K. intraocular foreign body grasping forceps
- K. intravitreal scissors
- K. lamp
- K. lancet tip
- K. lightsource stand
- K. loupe mounting system
- K. Magnalite fiberoptic headlamp
- K. microscissors
- K. micro spear tip
- K. ophthalmoscope
- K. panoramic lens
- K. panoramic loupe
- K. panoramic surgical telescope
- K. pantoscope
- K. prism
- K. prosthesis
- K. Pulsair noncontact tonometer
- K. puncture tip
- K. razor tip
- K. retinoscope
- K. retractable blade
- K. round tip
- K. ruby knife
- K. spotlight lens loupe
- K. Tearscope
- K. triple-facet tip
- K. ultrasonic cataract removal lancet
- K. video headlamp
- K. wide-angle lens loupe

Keeler-Amoils
- K.-A. curved cataract probe
- K.-A. glaucoma probe
- K.-A. long-shank retinal probe
- K.-A. ophthalmic cryosystem
- K.-A. ophthalmic Machemer retinal probe
- K.-A. ophthalmic vitreous probe

Keeler-Amoils-Machemer retinal probe

Keeler-Catford micro jaws needle holder

Keeler-Fison tissue retractor

Keeler-Galilean surgical loupe

Keeler-Keislar lacrimal cannula

Keeler-Konan Specular microscope

Keeler-Meyer diamond knife

Keeler-Pierse eye speculum

Keeler-Rodger iris retractor

Keeley vein stripper

Keene
- K. compression hook
- K. obturator

Keen Edge disposable biopsy forceps

Keener-Arlt lens loop

keeper
- line k.
- Nelson line k.

Keer aneurysm clip

Kees clip applier

Kegel
- K. exerciser
- K. perineometer

Kehr
- K. gallbladder tube
- K. T-tube

Keisler lacrimal cannula

Keith
- K. abdominal needle
- K. drain

Keithley clamp kit

Keitzer infant urethrotome

Keizer-Lancaster
- K.-L. eye speculum
- K.-L. lid retractor

Keizer lid retractor

Kelikian foot dressing

Kellan
- K. capsular sparing system
- K. hydrodissection cannula
- K. sutureless incision blade

Keller-Blake leg splint

Keller cephalometric device

Kelley-Goerss Compass stereotactic system

Kelling gastroscope

Kellman-Elschnig spatula

Kellogg tongue depressor

Kelly
- K. abdominal retractor
- K. arterial forceps
- K. clamp
- K. curette
- K. cystoscope

K. direct-vision adenotome
K. dressing forceps
K. endoscope
K. fistular scissors
K. hemostat
K. hemostatic forceps
K. inflatable T-tube
K. insufflator
K. intestinal needle
K. orifice dilator
K. ovum forceps
K. placental forceps
K. polypus forceps
K. proctoscope
K. punch
K. rectal speculum
K. sigmoidoscope
K. sphincter dilator
K. sphincteroscope
K. stereotactic system
K. tissue forceps
K. tube
K. urethral forceps
K. uterine dilator
K. uterine scissors
K. uterine tenaculum
K. uterine tenaculum hook
K. vulsellum
Kelly-Descemet membrane punch
Kelly-Gray
K.-G. uterine curette
K.-G. uterine forceps
Kelly-Murphy forceps
Kelly-Rankin forceps
Kelly-Sims vaginal retractor
Kelly-Wick vascular tunneler
Kelman
K. air cystotome
K. aspirator
K. Cry-O-Cadet
K. cryoextractor
K. cryophake
K. cryosurgical unit
K. cyclodialysis cannula
K. cystotome
K. cystotome knife
K. dipstick
K. double-bladed cystotome
K. flexible tripod lens
K. I&A unit
K. II 3-point fixation rigid tripod
  intraocular lens

K. implantation forceps
K. intraocular forceps
K. iris retractor
K. irrigating handpiece
K. irrigation hook
K. irrigator
K. irrigator forceps
K. knife cystotome
K. manipulator hook
K. Multiflex II intraocular lens
K. needle
K. Omnifit intraocular lens
K. PC 27LB CapSul lens
K. phacoemulsifier
K. Quadraflex intraocular lens
K. S-flex intraocular lens
K. tip
Kelman-Cavitron I&A unit
Kelman-McPherson
K.-M. corneal forceps
K.-M. suture forceps
K.-M. tissue forceps
K.-M. tying forceps
Kelocote sheeting
Kelsey
K. pile clamp
K. unloading exercise therapy
Kelsey-Fry bone awl
Kelvin Sensor pacemaker
Kempf internal screw fixation
Kemp irrigator
Ken
K. driver
K. drive sleeve
K. screwdriver
K. sliding nail
Kendall
K. A-V impulse system
K. compression stocking
K. endotracheal tube cuff
K. McGaw Intelligent pump
K. sequential compression device
K. Ventex wound dressing system
Kenna knee scale
Kennedy
K. bar
K. LAD
K. ligament augmentation device
K. sinus pack
K. spillproof cup
K. vulsellum forceps
Kennedy-Cornwell bladder evacuator

K

NOTES

Kennerdell
  K. bayonet forceps
  K. medial orbital retractor
  K. muscle hook
  K. nerve hook
  K. spatula
Kennerdell-Maroon
  K.-M. dissector
  K.-M. duckbill elevator
  K.-M. hook
  K.-M. orbital retractor
  K.-M. probe
Kennerdell-Maroon-Jameson hook
Kennett tenaculum
Kenny crutch
Kenny-Howard splint
Kensey
  K. atherectomy catheter
  K. dynamic angioplasty catheter
Kent forceps
Kenwood
  K. finger cot
  K. laparotomy sponge
Keofeed
  K. feeding tube
  K. II enteral feeding pump
  K. infusion pump
  K. tube
Keolar implant material
Keracor laser
KeraCorneoScope scope
Keragen implant
Kerascan
keratectomy scissors
Kerato-Gel implant
keratographer
  Keravue k.
keratoiridoscope
Kerato-Kontours instrument
Kerato-Lens implant
Keratolux fixation device
keratome
  Agnew k.
  Atkinson k.
  Bard-Parker k.
  Beaver blade k.
  Berens partial k.
  k. blade
  Castro-Martinez k.
  Castroviejo angled k.
  Czermak k.
  Daily k.
  Draeger modified k.
  filamentary k.
  Fuchs lancet-type k.
  k. guard
  Guyton-Lundsgaard k.
  Hansen k.
  HydroBlade k.

  HydroBrush k.
  Jaeger k.
  Jones k.
  Kirby k.
  Kirby-Duredge k.
  Lancaster k.
  Landolt k.
  Lichtenberg k.
  Martinez k.
  Martinez-Castro k.
  McCaslin wave-edge k.
  McReynolds k.
  McReynolds-Castroviejo k.
  McReynolds pterygium k.
  Rowland k.
  SatinSlit k.
  Storz k.
  Storz-Duredge k.
  Thomas k.
  Tri-Beeled trapezoidal k.
  UniShaper single-use k.
  Wiener k.
keratometer
  Autoref k.
  Bausch & Lomb manual k.
  Canon autorefraction k.
  Haag-Streit k.
  Helmholtz k.
  Humphrey automatic k.
  Javal k.
  k. lens
  Marco manual k.
  Osher surgical k.
  Storz k.
  surgical k.
  Terry k.
  Topcon k.
Keratom excimer laser system
keratomileusis
  laser-assisted intrastromal k.
   (LASIK)
  laser-assisted in situ k. (LASIK)
  laser subepithelial k. (LASEK)
keratoplasty
  laser thermal k. (LTK)
  k. scissors
keratoprosthesis
  Eckardt temporary k.
  Lander wide-field temporary k.
  PHEMA core-and-skirt k.
keratoscope
  Karickhoff k.
  Klein self-luminous k.
  Placido k.
  Polack k.
  Van Loenen operating k.
  wire-loop k.
keratotomy
  radial k. (RK)

keratotomy forceps
KeraVision
   K. ICR
   K. Intacs intracorneal ring
Keravue keratographer
Kerboull acetabular reinforcement
  device
Kerlix
   K. bandage roll
   K. cast pad
   K. cast padding
   K. disposable laparotomy sponge
   K. dressing
   K. gauze bandage
   K. packing sponge
   K. super sponge
   K. wrap
Kern
   K. bone-holding clamp
   K. bone-holding forceps
Kernan-Jackson coagulating
  bronchoscope
Kerner dental mirror
Kern-Lane bone-holding forceps
Kerpel bone curette
Kerr
   K. abduction splint
   K. clip applier
   K. electro-torque drill
   K. Endopost
   K. hand drill
   K. K-Flex file
   K. M4 safety handpiece
Kerrison
   K. bone punch
   K. cervical rongeur
   K. forceps
   K. laminectomy punch
   K. lumbar rongeur
   K. mastoid rongeur
   K. microrongeur
   K. retractor
Kerrison-Costen rongeur
Kerrison-Ferris Smith rongeur
Kerrison-Jacoby punch
Kerrison-Morgenstein rongeur
Kerrison-Rhoton sellar punch
Kerrison-Schwartz rongeur
Kerrison-Spurling rongeur
Kershner
   K. LASIK flap forceps

   K. one-step micro capsulorrhexis
    forceps
   K. reversible eyelid speculum
Kersting colostomy clamp
Kesilar cannula
Kesling
   K. appliance
   K. tooth-spacing spring
Kessel osteotomy plate
Kessler
   K. external fixator
   K. metacarpal distractor
   K. podiatry rasp
   K. prosthesis
   K. stitch
   K. traction frame
Kessler-Kleinert suture
Kestler ambulatory head tractor
Ketac
   K. Fil cement
   K. liner
   K. Silver cement
Keuch pupil dilator
Kevlar glove
Kevorkian
   K. endocervical curette
   K. endometrial curette
   K. uterine biopsy forceps
Kevorkian-Younge
   K.-Y. cervical biopsy forceps
   K.-Y. endocervical biopsy curette
   K.-Y. uterine applicator
   K.-Y. uterine biopsy forceps
   K.-Y. uterine curette
key
   Allen hex k.
   Ambu ResCue k.
   K. periosteal elevator
   K. rasp
keyboard
   ErgoLogic k.
   Kinesis k.
keyed
   k. filling device
   k. supracondylar plate
Keyes
   K. bone-splitting chisel
   K. cutaneous biopsy punch
   K. cutaneous trephine
   K. dermatologic punch
   K. lithotrite

NOTES

Keyes (*continued*)
   K. skin punch
   K. vulvar punch
Keyes-Ultzmann-Luer cannula
keyhole punch
KeyMed
   K. automatic reprocessor
   K. dilator
   K. disposable variceal injection
     needle
   K. esophageal tube
   K. fiberoptic scope
Keys-Briston type spline
Keys-Kirschner traction bow
keystone
   k. last
   K. PF analyzer
   K. Plus oxygenator concentrator
   K. splint
Kezerian
   K. chisel
   K. curette
   K. gouge
K-file
   nitinol K-f.
K-Fix fixator
K-Flexofile
   K.-F. Batt tip
   K.-F. file
K-Gar umbilical clamp
Khan-Jaeger clamp
Khodadad
   K. clamp
   K. clip
   K. microclamp
   K. microclip forceps
Khosia cautery
Khouri
   K. hydrodissection cannula
   K. phacofragmentation system
kick bucket
Kicker
   K. Pavlik harness
   K. Pavlik harness brace
Kidd
   K. cystoscope
   K. U-tube tube
Kidde
   K. nebulizer
   K. tourniquet
   K. tubal insufflator
   K. uterine cannula
Kid-Dee-Lite orthosis
Kidde-Robbins tourniquet
Kid-Kart wheelchair
kidney
   Ask-Upmark k.
   k. elevating forceps
   k. internal splint

   k. internal stent
   k. pedicle clamp
   k. pedicle forceps
   k. retractor
   k. stone basket
   k. stone forceps
   k. suturing needle
Kido suprapubic trocar
Kiefer clamp
Kiel graft
Kiene bone tamp
Kifa
   K. clip
   K. green, grey, red, yellow
     catheter
Killearn rongeur
killed
   heat k. (HK)
Killey molar retractor
Killian
   K. antral cannula
   K. antrum cannula
   K. cutting forceps tip
   K. dissector
   K. double-articulated forceps tip
   K. frontal sinus chisel
   K. gouge
   K. laryngeal spatula
   K. nasal cannula
   K. nasal speculum
   K. probe
   K. rectal speculum
   K. septal compression forceps
   K. septal elevator
   K. septal speculum
   K. suspension gallows
   K. tonsillar knife
   K. tube
Killian-Claus chisel
Killian-Eichen cannula
Killian-Halle nasal speculum
Killian-Jameson forceps
Killian-King goiter retractor
Killian-Lynch suspension laryngoscope
Killian-Reinhard chisel
Killip wire
Kilner
   K. chisel
   K. elevator
   K. goiter hook
   K. malar lever
   K. mouthgag
   K. nasal retractor
   K. needle holder
   K. skin hook
   K. skin hook retractor
   K. suture carrier
Kilner-Dott mouthgag
Kilpatrick retractor

Kilp lens
KilRoid single-handed ligator
Kimball
  K. catheter
  K. nephrostomy hook
Kimberley diamond instrument
Kimpton vein spreader
Kim-Ray
  K.-R. Greenfield antiembolus filter
  K.-R. Greenfield vena caval filter
Kimura
  K. cartilage graft
  K. platinum spatula
Kimwipes absorbent wipes
KinAir
  K. III, TC low-air-loss bed
  K. IV mattress
Kinamed Exact-Fit ATH system
Kin-Con
  K.-C. device
  K.-C. isokinetic exercise system
Kinder
  K. chair
  K. Design pedodontic forceps
  K. Incontinence Supplies (KINS)
Kindt
  K. arterial clamp
  K. carotid clamp
KineMatch patellofemoral replacement
Kinematic
  K. facebow
  K. II rotating-hinge total knee
  system
Kinemax
  K. Plus total knee system
  K. removable fixation peg
  K. spacer
Kinemetric guide system
kinesiological electromyogram
Kinesio Tex tape
Kinesis keyboard
kinestatic charge detector
kinesthesiometer
Kinetec
  K. clubfoot CPM exerciser
  K. ECT system
  K. hip CPM machine
kinetic
  k. continuous passive motion
  device
  K. Dual-Channel ultrasound unit
  k. rehabilitation device

  K. Wedge molded insole
  K. Wedge orthotic
Kinetik
  K. great toe implant
  K. great toe implant system
Kinetix ventilation monitor
**Kinetron muscle strengthening
  apparatus**
King
  K. adenoidal punch
  K. cardiac bioptome
  K. cervical brace
  K. clamp
  K. connector adapter
  K. corneal trephine
  K. double-umbrella closure system
  K. guiding catheter
  K. of Hearts Express II cardiac
  event recorder
  K. of Hearts Holter monitor
  K. interlocking device
  K. multipurpose coronary graft
  catheter
  K. orbital implant
  K. self-retaining goiter retractor
  K. suture needle
  K. tissue forceps
  K. wound forceps
King-Hurd
  K.-H. retractor
  K.-H. tonsillar dissector
King-Prince
  K.-P. knife
  K.-P. muscle forceps
  K.-P. recession forceps
Kingsley
  K. grasping forceps
  K. orthodontic plate
  K. splint
  K. Steplite foot
kink-resistant peritoneal catheter
KINS
  Kinder Incontinence Supplies
  KINS all-in-1 cotton brief
  KINS draw sheet
  KINS fitted mattress protector
  KINS pull-on waterproof bloomer
Kinsella-Buie lung clamp
Kinsella periosteal elevator
Kinsey atherectomy catheter
Kip laser

NOTES

Kirby
K. angulated iris spatula
K. capsular forceps
K. cataract knife
K. corneoscleral forceps
K. curved zonular separator
K. cylindrical zonular separator
K. double-ball separator
K. double-fixation muscle hook
K. eye tissue forceps
K. fixation forceps
K. flat zonular separator
K. hook expressor
K. intracapsular lens expressor
K. intracapsular lens forceps
K. intracapsular lens loop
K. intracapsular lens spoon
K. intraocular lens loop
K. iris forceps
K. keratome
K. lens dislocator
K. lens forceps
K. lid retractor
K. refractor
K. scissors
Kirby-Arthus fixation forceps
Kirby-Bracken iris forceps
Kirby-Duredge
K.-D. keratome
K.-D. knife
Kirchner retractor
Kirk
K. bone hammer
K. mallet
K. orthopaedic hammer
Kirkheim-Storz urethrotome
Kirkland
K. cement
K. cement dressing
K. curette
K. knife
K. periodontal pack
K. retractor
Kirklin
K. atrial retractor
K. fence
K. sternal awl
Kirkpatrick tonsillar forceps
Kirmisson
K. periosteal elevator
K. periosteal raspatory
Kirschenbaum
K. foot positioner
K. retractor
Kirsch laser
Kirschner
K. abdominal retractor
K. bone drill
K. boring wire

K. extension bow
K. femoral canal plug
K. guiding probe
K. hip replacement system
K. II-C shoulder system
K. integrated shoulder system
K. interlocking intramedullary nail
K. Medical Dimension hip replacement
K. Modular IIC shoulder prosthesis
K. pin fixation
K. skeletal traction
K. surgical instrument
K. suture
K. total shoulder prosthesis
K. traction apparatus
K. traction bow nut
K. Universal self-centering captive-head bipolar component
K. wire
K. wire cutter
K. wire drill
K. wire fixation
K. wire inserter
K. wire pin
K. wire splint
K. wire spreader
K. wire tightener
K. wire traction
K. wire traction bow
K. wire tractor
Kirschner-Balfour abdominal retractor
Kirschner-Ullrich forceps
Kirwan
K. bipolar coagulator
K. bipolar electrosurgical forceps
K. coaptation ophthalmic bipolar forceps
K. cranioblade
K. jeweler's ophthalmic bipolar forceps
Kirwan-Adson ophthalmic bipolar forceps
Kirwan-Nadler coaptation ophthalmic bipolar forceps
Kirwan-Tenzel ophthalmic bipolar forceps
Kishi lens
Kish urethral catheter
kissing
k. balloon
k. stent
Kistner
K. plastic tracheostomy tube
K. probe
K. tracheal button
kit
ABI Prism dye terminator cycle sequencing ready reaction k.

Active Free beta-hCG ELISA
test k.
Adjust-A-Flow colostomy
irrigation k.
AeroGear asthma action k.
Amelogen Lite k.
Amelogen UltraLite k.
Amelogen Universal k.
Amplicor HIV-1 test k.
Amplicor PCR k.
Amplicor tissue typing k.
anterior cervical fusion k.
Apdyne phenol applicator k.
Aptima Combo 2 assay k.
Arrow pneumothorax k.
Auto D-dimer assay k.
Avesta procedure k.
Bard Sequence II Plus incontinent
skin care k.
Bard-Steigmann-Goff variceal
ligation k.
Bergland-Warshawski phaco/cortex
adapter k.
Bindazyme ELISA k.
Biosearch jejunostomy k.
BiPort hemostasis introducer
sheath k.
Boehringer k.
Brimms Quik-Fix denture repair k.
Burnett Pap smear k.
BVI neurosurgical dissection k.
"cake mix" k.
Carey-Coons biliary
endoprosthesis k.
carpal tunnel release relief k.
Cartmill feeding tube k.
Ceramco porcelain k.
Circulon System Step 1, 2 venous
ulcer k.
CloseSure procedure k.
Cloward posterior lumbar interbody
fusion k.
Codman IMA k.
Codman internal mammary
artery k.
Coloscreen VPI test k.
Concept CTS Relief k.
Confide HIV test k.
Cordis lead conversion k.
Core-Assure k.
Core-Assure bone biopsy k.
Crystar porcelain k.

CTS relief k.
Dentifix denture repair k.
diabetic orthosis k.
Diethrich coronary artery bypass k.
disposable airway k.
Dover midstream urine
collection k.
Dynacor enema cleansing k.
DynaPak electrode k.
Elastafit tubing k.
Enemette enema cleansing k.
Etch-Master k.
Exerball k.
Extended Wear self-adhering
urinary external catheter starter k.
Extract-N-Amp blood PCR k.
FastRNA, Green k.
Fillauer Scottish Rite orthosis k.
Flexiflo Inverta-PEG gastrostomy k.
Flexiflo Lap G laparoscopic
gastrostomy k.
Flexiflo Lap J laparoscopic
jejunostomy k.
Flexiflo over-the-guidewire
gastrostomy k.
Fluorognost HIV-1 IFA assay k.
Fome-Cuf laser k.
Freedom T-tap leg bag k.
Fresenius Euro-Collins k.
gastrostomy catheter k.
GeneAmp RNA PCR k.
GenProbe collection k.
Gentle Touch colostomy/ileostomy
postoperative k.
Gentle Touch urostomy
postoperative k.
Gore Eze-Sit valvulotome k.
Hall Osteon irrigation k.
Handi-Cath catheter k.
HerpeSelect test k.
Heyer-Schulte PVC k.
Heyer-Schulte silicone k.
Hygene semen collection k.
hysterectomy k.
I&A k.
IBD-Check ELISA test k.
ICE-Magic pain reduction k.
I-Flow nerve block infusion k.
Immune Cell Function assay k.
Implantech moulage k.
InPouch TV subculture k.
Inteq TFC repair k.

K

NOTES

kit *(continued)*
    Irvine Scientific Embryo Freeze Media k.
    Irvine Scientific Embryo Thaw Media k.
    Jackson-Pratt hysterectomy k.
    Jackson-Pratt large-volume round silicone drain k.
    Jackson-Pratt PVC k.
    Jones IMA k.
    Keithley clamp k.
    KLS-Martin modular neuro k.
    Ko-Lec-Pac urinary collection k.
    Lacrimedics Lacrimal Occlusion Starter k.
    Laitinen high-precision stereotactic-assisted radiation therapy k.
    Laitinen percutaneous tumor biopsy k.
    Laserscope discography k.
    Lingeman k.
    lumbar interbody fusion k.
    Lymwrap lymphedema bandaging k.
    Malis brain retractor k.
    Mallinckrodt ultra tag labeling k.
    Marlen biliary drainage k.
    Massachusetts Vision k.
    Matritech NMP22 test k.
    McGhan fill k.
    MediCordz tubing k.
    Medi-Jector Choice needle-free syringe k.
    Medscand Pap smear k.
    MERmaid k.
    Metra PS procedure k.
    Micro E irrigation k.
    Moss G-tube PEG k.
    No Pour Pak II suction catheter k.
    Oncor ApopTaq k.
    One Time dressing k.
    Ortho diaphragm k.
    OsteoSet resorbable bead k.
    ototome irrigation k.
    Otovent autoinflation k.
    Ott-Mayo channel sampling k.
    OvuStick ovulation test k.
    Panda NCJ k.
    pelvic reconstruction k.
    Percufix catheter cuff k.
    percutaneous access k. (PAK)
    Per-fit percutaneous tracheostomy k.
    Perry Noz-Stop k.
    Persona monitoring k.
    Pleurx catheter drainage k.
    Preci-Vertix k.
    Prep-IM k.
    Protocult stool collection k.
    Pro-Vent arterial blood sampling k.
    Pro-Vent Plus arterial blood sampling k.
    Pulsator dry heparin arterial blood gas k.
    Pulse-Pak infusion k.
    Qiagen RNeasy Mini k.
    QIAmp tissue k.
    Quanta Lite ANA ELISA test k.
    Quick-Sil starter k.
    Radiofocus introducer B k.
    radioimmunoassay k.
    RNeasy Mini k.
    Rosenberg meniscal repair k.
    Russell gastrostomy k.
    Sacks-Vine gastrostomy k.
    sensory stimulation k.
    Set-Op myringotomy k.
    Shiley distention k.
    shunt k.
    Sims Per-fit percutaneous tracheostomy k.
    stereotactic-assisted radiation therapy k.
    Stomate low-profile gastrostomy k.
    Straith nasal splint k.
    Tacticon peripheral neuropathy k.
    Tisseel VH k.
    Toomey syringe k.
    Tri-Port hemostasis introducer sheath k.
    UMI amniocentesis k.
    UniPort hemostasis introducer sheath k.
    Unna-Flex Plus venous ulcer k.
    Varioligator k.
    Vaxcel Mini-Stick vascular entry k.
    Versa-PEG gastrostomy k.
    Vesica percutaneous bladder neck suspension k.
    Wilson-Cook feeding tube k.
    Wood colonic k.
    Wound-Evac k.
    Xomed sinus irrigation k.
    You-Bend hemodialysis catheterization k.

Kitchen postpartum gauze packer

Kitner
    K. blunt dissecting instrument
    K. clamp
    K. dissecting scissors
    K. goiter forceps
    K. retractor
    K. thyroid-packing forceps

Kittner dissector
Kiwi OmniCup
Kiwisch bandage
Kjelland
    K. blade
    K. obstetrical forceps

Kjelland-Barton forceps
Kjelland-Luikart obstetrical forceps
Klaar headlight
Klaff septal speculum
Klammt elastic open activator
Klapp tendon hook
Klatskin liver biopsy needle
Klauber band setter
Klause antral punch
Klause-Carmody antral punch
Klearway appliance
Klebanoff
  K. bougie
  K. common duct sound
  K. gallstone scoop
Kleegman
  K. cannula
  K. dilator
Kleen-Needle system
KleenSpec
  K. disposable anoscope
  K. disposable laryngoscope
  K. disposable vaginal speculum
  K. fiberoptic disposable
    sigmoidoscope
  K. forceps
  K. otoscope adapter
Kleer base plate
Kleesattel
  K. elevator
  K. raspatory
Klein
  K. cannula tip
  K. curved cannula
  K. 1-hole infiltrator tip
  K. infiltration needle
  K. infiltrator
  K. multihole infiltrator tip
  K. pump
  K. punch
  K. self-luminous keratoscope
  K. transseptal introducer sheath
  K. ventilation tube
Klein-Delrin Luer-Lok handle
Kleinert-Kutz
  K.-K. bone cutter
  K.-K. bone-cutting forceps
  K.-K. bone file
  K.-K. bone rongeur
  K.-K. clamp
  K.-K. clamp approximator
  K.-K. dissector

  K.-K. elevator
  K.-K. hook retractor
  K.-K. microclip
  K.-K. rasp
  K.-K. rongeur forceps
  K.-K. skin hook
  K.-K. synovectomy rongeur
  K.-K. tendon forceps
  K.-K. tendon-passing forceps
  K.-K. tendon retriever
  K.-K. tendon-retrieving forceps
Kleinert-Ragnell retractor
Kleinert splint
Kleinsasser
  K. anterior commissure
    laryngoscope
  K. hook
  K. knife
  K. lens loop
  K. microlaryngeal scissors
  K. operating laryngoscope
  K. probe
  K. retractor
Kleinsasser-Riecker laryngoscope
Kleinschmidt appendectomy clamp
Klemme
  K. appendectomy retractor
  K. dural hook
  K. gasserian ganglion retractor
  K. laminectomy retractor
Klenzak
  K. brace
  K. double-channeled ankle joint
  K. double-upright splint
  K. knee joint
Kleppinger bipolar forceps
Klevas clamp
KLI
  KLI bipolar forceps
  KLI laprocator laparoscope
  KLI monopolar forceps
Klima needle
Klima-Rosegger sternal needle
Kliners alar retractor
Kling
  K. adhesive dressing
  K. fluff roll
  K. gauze
  K. gauze bandage
  K. gauze dressing
  K. sponge
Klinikum-Berlin tubing clamp

K

NOTES

515

Klinkenbergh-Loth scissors
Klintmalm clamp
Klintskog amniotomy hook
Klippel retractor
Klockner implant
Kloehn
K. facebow
K. headgear
Klondike bed
Kloti vitreous cutter
KLS
KLS Centre-Drive screw
KLS Centre-Drive screwdriver
KLS-Martin
KLS-M. Centre-Drive screw
KLS-M. modular neuro kit
KLS-M. modular osteosynthesis
system
Klutch denture adhesive
Klute clamp
KM-1 breast pump
KMC femoral stem prosthesis
KMP fenestrated femoral stem
KM-series shell
KMW/PC femoral prosthesis
Knapp
K. blade
K. cataract knife
K. cataract spoon
K. cyclodialysis spatula
K. cystotome
K. eye speculum
K. iris hook
K. iris knife
K. iris knife needle
K. iris probe
K. iris repositor
K. iris scissors
K. iris spatula
K. lacrimal sac retractor
K. lens loop
K. lens scoop
K. lens spoon
K. refractor
K. strabismus scissors
K. trachoma forceps
Knapp-Culler speculum
Knapp-Luer trachoma forceps
Knead-A-Ball
K.-A.-B. hand exerciser
K.-A.-B. therapy balloon
knee
Anatomic Modular K. (AMK)
k. arthrography bolster
k. bolster
k. brace splint
k. cage brace
Endo-Model total hinge k.
k. extension orthosis

GeoFlex k.
Gustilo-Kyle total k.
Hosmer single-axis locking k.
k. immobilizer
k. immobilizer splint
Kapp Surgical Instrument
prosthetic k.
Link Endo-Model rotational k.
Mauch Swing and Stance
hydraulic k.
k. MD brace
Miller-Galante unicompartmental k.
Noiles posterior stabilized k.
Noiles rotating hinge k.
Otto Bock modular rotary
hydraulic k.
Otto Bock Safety constant-
friction k.
PCA k.
PCA revision total k.
PCA unicompartmental k.
K. Pillo pillow
pneumatic 4-bar k.
PolymerFriction total k.
k. positioner
Press-Fit condylar total k.
k. rest
k. retractor
self-aligning k.
K. Signature system
single-axis friction k.
single-axis locking k.
Stanmore total k.
Total Knee 2100 prosthetic k.
Ultimate k.
variable-axis k.
k. wedge
weight-activated locking k.
(WALK)
knee-ankle-foot orthosis (KAFO)
knee-ankle orthosis
knee-bearing prosthesis
Kneed-It knee guard
kneeguard
KneeRAP compressive wrap
KneeThing exerciser
3DKnee total knee implant
knife
Abraham tonsillar k.
ACL graft k.
Adson dural k.
Agnew canaliculus k.
AK diamond k.
Alcon A-OK phacoemulsification
slit k.
Alcon A-OK ShortCut k.
Alcon crescent k.
Aleman meniscotomy k.
Alexander otoplasty k.

Alio MICS k.
Allen-Barkan k.
Allen-Hanbury k.
amputation k.
Anderson double-end k.
anterior crurotomy k.
arachnoid k.
Arenberg endolymphatic sac k.
Arthro-Lok k.
arthroscopic k.
arthroscopy k.
ASICO diamond k.
Atkins tonsillar k.
Austin dental k.
Austin dissection k.
Austin sickle k.
Auth k.
Ayre cone k.
Ayre-Scott cervical cone k.
Backhaus cervical k.
backward-cutting k.
Bailey-Glover-O'Neill
  commissurotomy k.
Bailey-Morse mitral k.
Bailey round k.
Ballenger cartilage k.
Ballenger mucosal k.
Ballenger nasal swivel k.
Ballenger septal k.
Bard-Parker k.
Barkan goniotomy k.
Barker Vacu-tome suction k.
Baron ear k.
Barraquer corneal k.
Barraquer keratoplasty k.
Barrett uterine k.
bayonet k.
Beard lid k.
Beaver k.
Beaver blade cataract k.
Beaver blade discission k.
Beaver cataract k.
Beaver ear k.
Beaver goniotomy needle k.
Beaver tonsillar k.
Beaver Xstar k.
Beck tonsillar k.
Beer canaliculus k.
Beer cataract k.
Bellucci lancet k.
Berens cataract k.
Berens glaucoma k.

Berens iris k.
Berens keratoplasty k.
Berens ptosis k.
Berens sclerotomy k.
Bickle microsurgical k.
Bircher cartilage k.
Bishop-Harman k.
bistoury k.
blade k.
k. blade
bladebreaker k.
Blair-Brown skin graft k.
Blair cleft palate k.
Blake gingivectomy k.
Blount k.
Bock k.
Bodenham-Blair skin graft k.
Bodenham-Humby k.
Bodian discission k.
Bonta mastectomy k.
Bosher commissurotomy k.
Bowman discission k.
Bowman eye k.
Braithwaite skin graft k.
Brock mitral valve k.
Brock pulmonary valve k.
Brophy bistoury k.
Brophy cleft palate k.
Brown-Blair skin graft k.
Brown cleft palate k.
Buck myringotomy k.
Bucy cordotomy k.
Burford-Lebsche sternal k.
button-end k.
Caltagirone skin graft k.
Canad meniscal k.
canal k.
canaliculus k.
Canfield tonsillar k.
k. cannula cystotome
capsular k.
capsulotomy k.
Carter septal k.
cartilage k.
cast k.
Castroviejo discission k.
Castroviejo ophthalmic k.
Castroviejo twin k.
Castroviejo-Wheeler discission k.
cataract k.
Catlin amputation k.
Cave cartilage k.

K

NOTES

knife *(continued)*
Celita Elite k.
Celita Sapphire k.
cervical cone k.
chalazion k.
circle k.
clasp k.
ClearCut dual-bevel line k.
ClearCut ophthalmic dual bevel k.
ClearCut SatinSlit k.
Clearpath corneal diamond k.
Cobbett skin graft k.
cold k.
cold coning k.
Collin amputation k.
Collings electrosurgery k.
Colver tonsillar k.
commissurotomy k.
Concept arthroscopic k.
Converse nasal k.
cordotomy k.
corneal k.
cornea-splitting k.
Cornman dissecting k.
Cottle nasal k.
Crescent plaster k.
Crile cleft palate k.
Crile gasserian ganglion k.
Cronin cleft palate k.
Cronin palate k.
Crosby k.
Culbertson canal k.
Curdy sclerotome k.
Cushing dural hook k.
Cusick goniotomy k.
k. cystotome
Davidoff cordotomy k.
Daviel chalazion k.
Day tonsillar k.
Dean iris k.
Dean tonsillar k.
DeLee laparotrachelotomy k.
Dench ear k.
DePalma k.
Derlacki capsular k.
Derra commissurotomy k.
Derra guillotine k.
D'Errico laminar k.
Desmarres iris k.
Desmarres paracentesis k.
Deutschman cataract k.
Devonshire k.
DGH-KOI diamond k.
Diamatrix trapezoidal diamond k.
diamond blade k.
diamond-dusted k.
diamond micrometer k.
diamond phaco k.
Diamontek k.

diathermy k.
discission k.
dissection k.
dissector k.
k. dissector
double-edged sickle k.
double-ended flap k.
Douglas tonsillar k.
Down epiphyseal k.
Downing cartilage k.
drum elevator k.
Dupuytren k.
ear furuncle k.
EdgeAhead IOL k.
EdgeAhead MVR k.
EG-series clear corneal k.
k. electrode
Elschnig cataract k.
Elschnig corneal k.
Elschnig pterygium k.
Endopath EZ45 No k.
epiretinal delamination diamond k.
Esmarch plaster k.
eye k.
EZ45 No K.
facial nerve k.
Farrior otoplasty k.
Farrior septal cartilage stripper k.
Farrior sickle k.
Farrior triangular k.
Feaster Accura diamond k.
Feaster radial keratotomy k.
Feaster RK diamond k.
Feather clear cornea k.
Ferris-Robb tonsillar k.
Fisher tonsillar k.
flap k.
Fletcher tonsillar k.
Foerster capsulotomy k.
Fomon double-edge k.
k. and fork
Frazier cordotomy k.
Frazier pituitary capsulectomy k.
Freedom k.
Freer nasal submucous k.
Freer septal k.
Freiberg cartilage k.
Freiberg meniscectomy k.
Friesner ear k.
gamma k.
Gerzog ear k.
Gill corneal k.
Gill-Hess k.
Gill iris k.
Gill pop-up arcuate diamond k.
Gillquist-Oretorp-Stille k.
Gill-Welsh k.
gingivectomy k.
Girard-Swan k.

Goldman-Fox k.
Goldman guillotine nerve k.
goniopuncture k.
goniotomy k.
Goodhill k.
Goodyear tonsillar k.
Goulian k.
Graefe cataract k.
Graefe cystotome k.
Graefe iris k.
Graf cervical cordotomy k.
Green cataract k.
Green corneal k.
Grieshaber ruby k.
Grieshaber Ultrasharp k.
Groff electrosurgical k.
Grover meniscus k.
Guilford-Wright crurotomy k.
Guilford-Wright double-edged k.
Guilford-Wright elevator k.
Guilford-Wright flap k.
Guilford-Wright incudostapedial k.
Guilford-Wright roller k.
guillotine k.
Guy tenotomy k.
Guyton-Lundsgaard cataract k.
Haab after-cataract k.
Haab eye k.
Haab scleral resection k.
Halle dural k.
Halle trigeminus k.
k. handle
Harrison capsular k.
Harrison myringoplasty k.
Harrison-Shea k.
Harris tonsillar k.
Hartmann k.
Herbert sclerotomy k.
Hilsinger tonsillar k.
Hoffmann-Osher-Hopkins plaster k.
hook k.
hooked k.
Hopkins plaster k.
Horsley dural k.
Hosemann choledochus k.
hot k.
Hough fascial k.
Hough incision k.
Hough-Rosen k.
Hough whirlybird k.
House ear k.
House incudostapedial joint k.

House lancet k.
House myringoplasty k.
House myringotomy k.
House-Rosen k.
House round k.
House sickle k.
House tympanoplasty k.
Huco diamond k.
Hufnagel commissurotomy k.
Huibregtse-Katon needle k.
Hulbert electrosurgical k.
Humby k.
Hundley knee k.
Hyams scleral k.
Impex diamond radial
  keratotomy k.
incision k.
incudostapedial joint k.
iris k.
Jackson tracheal bistoury k.
Jacobson vessel k.
Jaeger keratome k.
Jako-Kleinsasser k.
Jako laryngeal k.
Jannetta angular k.
Jarit plaster k.
Johnson evisceration k.
Johnson ptosis k.
Johnson-Tooke corneal k.
Jones cervical k.
Jones IMA diamond k.
Jordan canal incision k.
Jordan capsular k.
Jordan stapedectomy k.
Joseph angular k.
Joseph bistoury k.
Joseph button-end k.
Joseph cervical k.
Joseph double-edged k.
Joseph-Maltz k.
Joseph nasal k.
Jung microtome k.
Keeler-Meyer diamond k.
Keeler ruby k.
Kelman cystotome k.
Killian tonsillar k.
King-Prince k.
Kirby cataract k.
Kirby-Duredge k.
Kirkland k.
Kleinsasser k.
Knapp cataract k.

K

NOTES

knife *(continued)*

Knapp iris k.
Korte plaster k.
Kreissl meatotomy k.
Krull acetabular k.
Kyle crypt k.
Ladd k.
laminar k.
Lancaster k.
Lance k.
lancet k.
Landolt eye k.
Lange blade k.
Lange cartilage k.
Langenbeck flap k.
Langenbeck resection k.
Langerman angled tunnel k.
Lang eye k.
Lanigan cartilage k.
laryngeal k.
Laseredge microsurgical k.
Lebsche sternal k.
Lee cartilage k.
Lee-Cohen k.
Leksell gamma k.
Leland-Jones tonsillar k.
Leland tonsillar k.
Lempert k.
ligamentum teres k.
Lillie tonsillar k.
Lindvall meniscectomy k.
Lindvall-Stille meniscal k.
Lipschiff k.
Lister k.
Liston amputation k.
Liston phalangeal k.
Lorez PC/TC ultra-sharp k.
Lothrop tonsillar k.
Lowe-Breck cartilage k.
Lowell glaucoma k.
Lowe microtome k.
Lucae ear perforation k.
Lundsgaard k.
Lundsgaard-Burch k.
Lynch obtuse-angle laryngeal k.
Lynch tonsillar k.
MacCallum k.
Machemer scleral k.
MacKenty cleft palate k.
Magielski bayonet canal k.
Maltz button-end k.
Maltz cartilage k.
Mandelbaum ear k.
Marcks k.
Martinez corneal dissector k.
Maumenee goniotomy k.
Mayo k.
McCabe canal k.
McCaslin k.

McGee tympanoplasty k.
McHugh facial nerve k.
McHugh-Farrior canal k.
McHugh flap k.
McKeever cartilage k.
McMurray tenotomy k.
McPherson-Wheeler eye k.
McPherson-Ziegler microiris k.
McReynolds-Castroviejo
  pterygium k.
McReynolds pterygium k.
Mead lancet k.
meniscal k.
meniscectomy k.
Mercer cartilage k.
Merrifield k.
Metzenbaum septal k.
Meyer Swiss diamond lancet k.
Meyer Swiss diamond wedge k.
Meyhöffer eye k.
Micra k.
Midas Rex k.
Millette tonsillar k.
Millette-Tyding k.
Miltex ligature k.
Mitchell cartilage k.
Monahan-Lewis k.
Moncorps k.
Moorehead ear k.
Morgenstein periosteal k.
Moritz-Schmidt k.
Murphy plaster k.
Myocure k.
myringoplasty k.
myringotomy k.
nasal k.
k. needle
Neff meniscal k.
Neivert tonsillar k.
Neoflex bendable k.
Newman uterine k.
Niche k.
Niedner commissurotomy k.
Nordent periodontic k.
Nunez-Nunez mitral stenosis k.
OIU cold k.
Olivecrona trigeminal k.
Olk membrane peeler k.
Optima diamond k.
Orandi k.
Oretorp retractable k.
orthopaedic k.
Osher diamond k.
Osher micrometer cataract k.
Pace hysterectomy k.
Page tonsillar k.
Paparella canal k.
Paparella-House k.
Paparella incudostapedial joint k.

Paparella sickle k.
paracentesis k.
Parasmillie k.
Parker serrated discission k.
Parker tenotomy k.
Paton corneal k.
Paufique corneal k.
Paufique-Duredge k.
Paufique graft k.
Paufique keratoplasty k.
Phaco-4 diamond k.
plaster k.
platelet-shaped k.
Politzer angular ear k.
Politzer paracentesis k.
Politzer-Ralks k.
Pope rectal k.
Potter modified k.
Potter sickle k.
Potts expansile k.
pterygium k.
ptosis k.
pull k.
Questus Leading Edge sheathed
  arthroscopy k.
radial keratotomy k.
Ralks reversible k.
Rayport dural k.
razor blade k.
Reese ptosis k.
Rehne skin graft k.
Reiner plaster k.
retrograde k.
retrograde-cutting hook-shaped k.
Rhein Advantage diamond k.
Rhein clear-cornea diamond k.
Rica trigeminal k.
Ridlon plaster k.
Rish cartilage k.
Rizzuti-Spizziri cannula k.
Robb tonsillar k.
Robertson tonsillar k.
Robinson flap k.
Rochester mitral stenosis k.
rocker k.
Roentgen k.
Roger septal k.
roller k.
Rosen cartilage k.
Rosen ear incision k.
round ruby k.
Royce bayonet ear k.

ruby diamond k.
Ryerson tenotome k.
Salenius meniscal k.
sapphire k.
Sarot k.
SatinCrescent implant k.
SatinShortCut implant k.
SatinSlit implant k.
Sato corneal k.
scarifier k.
Schanz k.
Scheer elevator k.
Scheie goniopuncture k.
Scheie goniotomy k.
Scholl meniscal k.
Schuknecht roller k.
Schuknecht sickle k.
Schultze embryotomy k.
Schwartz cordotomy k.
scleral resection k.
sculp k.
Seiler tonsillar k.
self-fixating sideport diamond k.
Sellor mitral valve k.
semilunar cartilage k.
septal k.
serrated fine-cutting k.
Sexton ear k.
Shaffer modification of Barkan k.
Shambaugh k.
Shambaugh-Lempert k.
Sharpoint k.
Shea incision k.
Sheehy canal k.
Sheehy-House k.
Sheehy myringotomy k.
Sheehy round k.
Sherman k.
ShortCut A-OK small-incision k.
Shorti limbal relaxing inciusion
  diamond k.
Sichel iris k.
sickle k.
Silver k.
Silverstein round k.
Silverstein sickle k.
Simon fistula k.
Simons cleft palate k.
Sims k.
skiving k.
slit blade k.
Sluder k.

NOTES

521

knife *(continued)*
SMIC sternal k.
Smillie meniscal cartilage k.
Smith cartilage k.
Smith cataract k.
Smith cordotomy k.
Smith-Fisher cataract k.
Smith-Green cataract k.
Speed-Sprague k.
Spizziri cannula k.
k. spud
stapedectomy k.
Stealth DBO free-hand diamond k.
Stecher arachnoid k.
Step-Knife diamond blade k.
1-step limbar relaxing incision
  diamond k.
sternal k.
Stewart cartilage k.
stiletto k.
stitch-removing k.
Stiwer furuncle k.
Storz-Duredge steel cataract k.
Storz folding-handle ear k.
Storz sheath-handle ear k.
straight tympanoplasty k.
Strayer meniscal k.
Stryker cartilage k.
Stryker-School meniscal k.
Suker spatula k.
Sur-Cut guillotine k.
Swan discission k.
Swan spade-type needle k.
Swets goniotomy k.
swift-cut phaco incision k.
swivel k.
sword k.
Tabb double-ended flap k.
Tabb ear k.
Tabb myringoplasty k.
Taylor k.
tendon k.
teres k.
testing drum k.
thermal k.
Thiersch skin graft k.
Thornton ophthalmic triple
  micrometer k.
Thornton T-incision diamond k.
Tiemann-Meals tenolysis k.
Tobold laryngeal k.
Toennis dural k.
tonsil k.
Tooke corneal k.
Tooke iris k.
Tooke-Johnson corneal k.
Torchia corneal k.
trifacet k.
trigeminal k.

triple-edge diamond-blade k.
triple-lumen needle k.
Troilius capsulotomy k.
Troutman corneal k.
Troutman-Tooke corneal k.
Tubby tenotomy k.
Tweedy canaliculus k.
twin k.
Tydings tonsillar k.
tympanoplasty k.
Ullrich fistula k.
Ullrich uterine k.
UltraCision ultrasonic k.
Unicat k.
Unigraft k.
Unitome k.
upward-cutting triangular k.
Vacu-tome k.
Vannas abscess k.
Vaughan abscess k.
vessel k.
Vic hair transplant k.
Vic Vallis running hair k.
Virchow brain k.
Virchow cartilage k.
Virchow skin graft k.
Visitec circular k.
Visitec crescent k.
Visitec EdgeAhead phaco slit k.
Visitec stiletto k.
V-lance k.
von Graefe k.
Wagner k.
Walb k.
Wallace-Maloney k.
Walton ear k.
Watson skin graft k.
wave-edge k.
Weber canaliculus k.
Weber iris k.
Webster skin graft k.
Weck k.
Wheeler discission k.
Wheeler iris k.
Wheeler malleable-shape k.
Wilder cystotome k.
Williams cartilage k.
Woodruff spatula k.
Wright-Guilford double-edged k.
Wright-Guilford elevator k.
Wright-Guilford flap k.
Wright-Guilford incudostapedial k.
Wright-Guilford roller k.
Wullstein double-edged k.
X-Acto utility k.
XKnife k.
Yamanda k.
Yasargil arachnoid k.
Yund ligamentum teres k.

ZAP diamond k.
Ziegler iris k.
Knight
K. biopsy needle
K. brace
K. nasal-cutting forceps
K. nasal scissors
K. nasal septum-cutting forceps
K. polyp forceps
K. septal forceps
K. septum-cutting forceps
K. turbinate forceps
Knighton-Crawford forceps
Knighton hemilaminectomy self-retaining retractor
Knighton-Kerrison punch
Knight-Sluder nasal forceps
KnightStar
K. 330 bi-level ventilator
K. 335 respiratory support system
Knight-Taylor
K.-T. brace
K.-T. and Williams spinal orthosis
Knit
Koper K.
Knit-Rite suspension sleeve
knitted
k. Dacron
k. Dacron velour graft
k. graft
k. prosthesis
k. sewing ring
k. Teflon prosthesis
k. vascular prosthesis
Knobble massager
Knoche tube
Knodt distraction rod
Knolle
K. anterior chamber irrigating cannula
K. capsular polisher
K. capsular scraper
K. capsular scratcher
K. dipstick
K. lens cortex spatula
K. lens gauge
K. lens implantation forceps
K. lens nucleus spatula
K. lens speculum
K. needle holder

Knolle-Kelman
K.-K. cannulated cystotome
K.-K. sharp cystotome
Knolle-Pearce
K.-P. cannula
K.-P. irrigating lens loop
K.-P. vectis
Knolle-Shepard lens-holding forceps
Knolle-Volker lens-holding forceps
knot
k. pusher
k. tier
knotting forceps
knot-tying
k.-t. forceps
k.-t. instrument
Knowles
K. bandage scissors
K. hip pin
knuckle-bender splint
knurled handle
Knutsson
K. penile clamp
K. urethrography clamp
Knuttsen bending film
Koagamin dressing
Koala
K. clamp
K. intrauterine pressure catheter
Kobak needle
Kobayashi
K. retractor
K. vacuum extractor
Koby cataract forceps
Koch
K. chopper
K. limbal relaxing incision marker
K. nucleus hydrolysis needle
K. phaco manipulator
Kocher
K. arterial forceps
K. artery forceps
K. bladder retractor
K. bladder spatula
K. blade retractor
K. bone retractor
K. brain spoon
K. bronchocele sound
K. depressor
K. gallbladder retractor
K. goiter director
K. goiter dissector

NOTES

K

523

Kocher *(continued)*
- K. grooved director
- K. hemostat
- K. hemostatic forceps
- K. intestinal clamp
- K. kidney-elevating forceps
- K. Micro-Line intestinal forceps
- K. periosteal dissector
- K. periosteal elevator
- K. probe
- K. raspatory
- K. self-retaining goiter retractor

Kocher-Crotti self-retaining goiter retractor
Kocher-Langenbeck retractor
Kocher-Ochsner hemostatic forceps
Kocher-Wagner retractor
Koch-Julian sphincterotome
Koch-Mason dressing
Koch-Minami ophthalmic chopper
Koch-Salz nucleus splitter
Kock
- K. ileal reservoir
- K. nipple
- K. nipple valve

Kodak
- K. 1200 Digital Science medical imager
- K. Ektachem autoanalyzer
- K. XAR-5 x-ray film
- K. XRP-1 x-ray film

Kodel
- K. polyester elbow protector
- K. sling

Kodex drill
Koeberlé forceps
Koehler illumination system
Koenig
- K. elevator
- K. graft
- K. grooved director
- K. metatarsal broach
- K. MPJ implant and arthroplasty system
- K. MPJ prosthesis
- K. nail-splitting scissors
- K. probe
- K. rasp
- K. tonsillar swab
- K. total great toe implant
- K. vascular forceps
- K. vein retractor

Koenig-Stille scissors
Koeppe
- K. diagnostic lens
- K. goniolens
- K. gonioscopic lens
- K. intraocular lens implant
- K. lamp

Koerte
- K. gallstone forceps
- K. retractor

Koffler-Hajek
- K.-H. laminectomy rongeur
- K.-H. sphenoidal punch

Koffler-Lillie septal forceps
Koffler septal forceps
Kogan
- K. endocervical speculum
- K. endospeculum
- K. endospeculum forceps
- K. urethra speculum

Koh
- K. colpotomizer system
- K. ultramicro instrument

Kohlman urethral dilator
Kohn needle
KoKo
- K. Mate spirometer
- K. Moe filter
- K. Rhythm PC-Based ECG
- K. Trek spirometer

Kokowicz raspatory
Kolb
- K. bronchial forceps
- K. trocar

Kold
- K. Kap
- K. Kompress cold pack
- K. Wrap
- K. Wrap cold compression bandage

Ko-Lec-Pac urinary collection kit
Koln clip
Kolodny
- K. clamp
- K. forceps

Koman-Nair iris repositor
Komet XK-95 surgical drill system
Komform coated gauze dressing
Konan SP8000 noncontact specular microscope
Koneg retractor
Konica KFDR-S laser film scanner
Konig bar chart
Konigsberg
- K. 5-channel solid-state catheter
- K. microtransducer

Kontack temporary crown
Kontron
- K. electrode
- K. intraaortic balloon catheter
- K. TFT 45.6 rotor

Koo foldable intraocular lens cutter
Kooijman eye model
Kool Kit cold therapy pack
Koontz hernia needle
Kopan breast lesion localization needle
Koper Knit

Kopetzky sinus bur
Korex cork sheet
Kormed disposable liver biopsy needle
Korn Cage knee brace
koroscope
Koros EndoMax scissors
Korotkoff sound
Korte
    K. abdominal spatula
    K. gallstone forceps
    K. plaster knife
    K. retractor
Korte-Wagner retractor
Korth ureterotome
Kos
    K. attic cannula
    K. chisel
    K. crimper forceps
    K. curette
    K. ear suction tube
    K. elevator
    K. middle ear instrument
    K. pick
Koslowski
    K. hip nail
    K. microforceps
Kostuik
    K. internal spine fixation system
    K. rod
    K. screw
Kostuik-Harrington
    K.-H. anterior distraction system
    K.-H. spinal instrumentation
Kowa
    K. angiographic camera
    K. fluorescein system
    K. FM-500 laser flare meter
    K. fundus camera
    K. hand camera
    K. laser flare-cell photometer
    K. Optimed slit lamp
    K. PRO II retinal camera
    K. RC-XV fundus camera
Kowa-Optimed camera
Koylon foam rubber dressing
Kozlinski retractor
K-Pratt dilator
Krackow
    K. HTO blade staple
    K. suture
Kraff
    K. capsular polisher

    K. capsule polisher curette
    K. cortex cannula
    K. hyperopic fixation ring
    K. intraocular utility forceps
    K. lens-inserting forceps
    K. limbal relaxing incision marker
    K. nucleus lens loop
    K. nucleus splitter
    K. suturing forceps
    K. tying forceps
Kraff-Osher lens forceps
Kraff-Utrata
    K.-U. capsulorrhexis forceps
    K.-U. intraocular utility forceps
    K.-U. tear capsulotomy forceps
Krahn exophthalmometer
Krakau tonometer
Kramer
    K. direct-vision telescope
    K. ear speculum
    K. forceps
    K. operating laryngoscope
Kramer-Collins Spore trap
Kramp scissors
Krasky retractor
Krasnov lens
Kratz
    K. aspirating speculum
    K. capsular scraper
    K. capsular scratcher
    K. cystotome
    K. diamond-dusted needle
    K. elliptical-style lens
    K. implant
    K. iris push-pull hook
    K. lens-inserting forceps
    K. modified J-loop intraocular lens
    K. polisher
    K. posterior chamber intraocular lens
Kratz-Barraquer wire speculum
Kratz-Jensen
    K.-J. capsular scratcher
    K.-J. polisher
Kratz-Johnson modified J-loop intraocular lens
Kratz-Sinskey intraocular lens implant
Krause
    K. angular oval punch
    K. antral trocar
    K. arm rest
    K. biopsy forceps

NOTES

Krause *(continued)*
  K. ear polyp snare
  K. esophagoscopy forceps
  K. laryngeal snare
  K. nasal polyp snare
  K. nasal snare cannula
  K. oval punch tip
  K. punch forceps
  K. punch forceps tip
  K. square-basket tip
  K. Universal forceps
Krause-Davis spatula
Krause-Wolfe
  K.-W. graft
  K.-W. implant
  K.-W. prosthesis
Krayenbuehl
  K. dural hook
  K. nerve hook
  K. vessel hook
Kraylex odor barrier
Krego elevator
Kreiger-Spitznas vibrating scissors
Kreischer bone chisel
Kreiselman
  K. infant warmer
  K. resuscitation unit
Kreissl meatotomy knife
Kremer
  K. excimer laser
  K. fixation forceps
  K. 2-point fixation forceps
  K. triple-optical zone corneal
    marker
Krentz
  K. gastroscope
  K. photogastroscope
Kretschmer retractor
Kretz Combison 330 ultrasound scanner
Kreuscher semilunar cartilage scissors
Kreutzmann
  K. cannula
  K. trocar
Krieger wide-field fundus lens
Krinkle gauze roll
Krinsky-Prince accommodation ruler
Kristeller
  K. vaginal retractor
  K. vaginal speculum
Kristiansen eyelet lag screw
Kritzinger-Updegraff
  K.-U. elevator
  K.-U. manipulator
Krogh apparatus spirometer
Krol esophageal dilator
Krol-Koski tracheal dilator
Kromayer lamp

Kron
  K. bile duct dilator
  K. bile duct probe
Kronecker aneurysm needle
Kronendonk pin
Kronfeld
  K. eyelid retractor
  K. micropin forceps
  K. pin
  K. refractor
  K. surface electrode
  K. suturing forceps
Krönlein-Berke retractor
Krönlein hemostatic forceps
Kronner
  K. external fixation device
  K. Manipujector manipulator
Krosnick vesicourethral suspension clamp
Krueger instrument stop
Krukenberg
  K. pigment spindle forceps
  K. sponge
Krull acetabular knife
Krumeich-Barraquer
  K.-B. lasitome
  K.-B. microkeratome
Krumeich stereoscope
Krupin-Denver eye valve
Krupin eye disc
Krwawicz
  K. cataract cryosurgical instrument
  K. cataract extractor
KryMed
  K. cryopexy unit
  K. 300 probe
Kryptok bifocal lens implant
krypton red laser
K/S-Allis forceps
KSK articulator
K-Sponge
  K-S. hydrocellulose sponge
  K-S. spear
KT1000, 2000 knee ligament arthrometer
KT1000/S knee ligament arthrometer
KTK laminaria tent
KTP
  potassium titanyl phosphate
    KTP laser
    KTP laser probe
KTP/532
    KTP/532 surgical laser
    KTP/532 surgical laser system
KTP/Nd:YAG
    KTP/Nd:YAG laser
    KTP/Nd:YAG XP surgical laser
      system
KTP/YAG laser

Kudo elbow prosthesis
Kugel
    K. hernia patch
    K. mesh
Kuglen
    K. angled lens manipulator
    K. irrigating lens manipulator
    K. lens retractor
    K. manipulating iris hook
    K. pusher
    K. refractor
    K. straight lens manipulator
Kuhlman
    K. cervical brace
    K. cervical traction device
Kuhn
    K. endotracheal tube
    K. mask
Kuhn-Bolger
    K.-B. angled curette
    K.-B. seeker
Kuhnt
    K. capsular forceps
    K. corneal scarifier
    K. fixation forceps
    K. gouge
Kulvin-Kalt
    K.-K. iris forceps
    K.-K. mules
Kulzer inlay system
Kummel intestinal spatula
Kumpe catheter
Kundin wound measurement gauge
Küntscher
    K. cloverleaf nail
    K. drill
    K. extractor
    K. femur guide pin
    K. finisher
    K. hammer
    K. impactor
    K. intramedullary nail
    K. nail driver
    K. nail-extracting hook
    K. traction device
Küntscher-Hudson brace
Kunzli orthopaedic sports shoe
Kurer anchor
Kurlander orthopaedic wrench
Kurosaka interference-fit screw
Kurtin
    K. handpiece

    K. planing dermabrasion brush
    K. vein stripper
    K. wire brush
Kurz
    K. pulsation orthodontic headgear
    K. tube
Kurze
    K. dissecting scissors
    K. dissector
    K. microbiopsy forceps
    K. micrograsping forceps
    K. microscissors
    K. pickup forceps
    K. suction-irrigator
    K. suction tube
Kurzweil reading machine
Kusch'kin Ace wheelchair
Kushner-Tandatnick endometrial biopsy curette
Kuske breast template
Kuslich
    Bagby and K. (BAK)
Küstner
    K. suture
    K. tenaculum
    K. uterine tenaculum forceps
Kuttner
    K. dissector
    K. wound stretcher
Kutzmann clamp
Kuyper-Murphy sternal retractor
Kwapis
    K. interdental forceps
    K. ligature carrier
    K. subcondylar retractor
Kwik
    K. Board IV and arterial line stabilizer
    K. wax
Kwik-Skan monitor
Kwitko
    K. conjunctival spreader
    K. lens spatula
Kydex
    K. body jacket
    K. brace
Kyle
    K. applicator
    K. crypt knife
    K. nasal speculum
kyphosis brace
KyphX inflatable bone tamp

K

NOTES

527

KY pliers

LA4072 low-air-loss overlay
lab
    Orthopedic Casting L. (OCL)
Labcor Synergy valve
laboratory
    Advanced Technology L.'s (ATL)
    l. automation system
    University of California
      Berkeley L. (UCBL)
Laborde
    L. forceps
    L. tracheal dilator
Labotech embryo transfer catheter
Labpette FX pipette
Labtician oval sleeve
Labtron stethoscope
labyrinth curette
LaCarrere
    L. electrode
    L. electrodiaphake
lace
    Shoe Curl no-tie shoe l.
    spyrolace shoe l.
lace-on brace
L.A. cervical orthosis
Lacey
    L. prosthesis
    L. rotating hinge
    L. total knee implant
lacidem suture
Lack tongue retractor
Lacor tube
lacquer
    Penlac nail l.
LacriCath lacrimal duct catheter
lacrimal
    l. apparatus
    l. awl
    l. balloon catheter
    l. canaliculus dilator
    l. duct probe
    l. duct T-tube
    l. intubation probe
    l. irrigating cannula
    l. needle
    l. osteotome
    l. probe
    l. sac bur
    l. sac chisel
    l. sac gouge
    l. sac retractor
    l. sac rongeur
    l. sound
    l. stent
    l. trephine

Lacrimedics Lacrimal Occlusion Starter kit
Lact-Aid STARTrainer nursing system
Lactina Select breast pump
Lactomer
    L. absorbable subcuticular skin staple
    L. copolymer absorbable stapler
LactoSorb
    L. anterior cruciate ligament crosspin system
    L. resorbable craniomaxillofacial fixation
LAD
    ligament augmentation device
    Kennedy LAD
LADARVision excimer laser
Ladd
    L. calipers
    L. elevator
    L. fiberoptic system
    L. intracranial pressure monitor
    L. intracranial pressure sensor
    L. knife
    L. lid clamp
    L. raspatory
ladder
    finger l.
    shoulder l.
Ladmore plastic filling instrument
Lady & Sir Dignity Plus pant
LAE cast
Laerdal
    L. compact suction unit
    L. infant resuscitator
Lafayette skinfold calipers
LaForce
    L. adenotome
    L. adenotome blade
    L. golf-club knife spud
    L. hemostatic tonsillectome
LaForce-Grieshaber adenotome
LaForce-Stevenson adenotome
LaForce-Storz adenotome
lag
    l. screw
    l. screw plate
LAGB
    Lap-Band adjustable gastric banding
    LAGB system
Lagleyze needle
Lagrange
    L. eye scissors
    L. sclerectomy scissors
Lagrange-Letoumel hip prosthesis

L

Lahey
- L. arterial forceps
- L. bag
- L. bronchial clamp
- L. Carb-Edge scissors
- L. catheter
- L. clamp
- L. Clinic dural hook
- L. Clinic nerve root retractor
- L. Clinic skull trephine
- L. Clinic spinal fusion gouge
- L. Clinic thin osteotome
- L. delicate scissors
- L. dissecting forceps
- L. dissecting scissors
- L. drain
- L. gall duct forceps
- L. goiter retractor
- L. goiter-seizing forceps
- L. goiter tenaculum
- L. goiter vulsellum forceps
- L. hemostat
- L. hemostatic forceps
- L. ligature carrier
- L. ligature passer
- L. lock arterial forceps
- L. needle
- L. operating scissors
- L. thoracic clamp
- L. thoracic forceps
- L. thyroid retractor
- L. thyroid scissors
- L. thyroid tenaculum forceps
- L. thyroid traction vulsellum forceps
- L. Y-tube tube

Lahey-Babcock forceps
Lahey-Sweet dissecting forceps
Laidley double-catheterizing cystoscope
Laing
- L. concentric hip cup
- L. osteotomy plate

Laird spatula
LAIS
- Laser Advanced Interventional Systems
- LAIS excimer laser
- LAIS laser energy percutaneous coronary catheter

Laitinen
- L. CT guidance system
- L. high-precision stereotactic-assisted radiation therapy kit
- L. percutaneous tumor biopsy kit
- L. stereotactic head frame

Lajeune hemostatic forceps
Lakatos Teflon injector
Lakeside
- L. cotton roll
- L. nasal scissors

Lalonde
- L. bone clamp
- L. delicate hook forceps
- L. dynamic compression bone clamp
- L. tendon approximator

Lamb cannula
Lambda
- L. Omni Stanicor pacemaker
- L. Physik EMG 103 laser
- L. Plus PDL1, PDL2 photodynamic laser

lambdoidal suture
Lambert
- L. aortic clamp
- L. chalazion forceps

Lambert-Berry rib raspatory
Lambert-Heiman scissors
Lambert-Kay
- L.-K. anastomosis forceps
- L.-K. aortic clamp
- L.-K. vascular clamp

Lambert-Lowman
- L.-L. bone clamp
- L.-L. chisel

Lambone demineralized laminar bone
Lambotte
- L. bone chisel
- L. bone-holding clamp
- L. bone-holding forceps
- L. bone hook
- L. elevator
- L. exhaust system
- L. fibular forceps
- L. osteotome
- L. rib raspatory

Lambotte-Henderson osteotome
Lambrinudi splint
lamellar blade
lamina
- EpiFilm otologic l.
- l. spreader

laminar
- l. air flow unit
- l. C-D hook
- l. dissector
- l. elevator
- l. flow hood
- l. flow system
- l. knife

laminaria
- l. cervical tent
- Dilapan l.
- Japonicum l.
- l. seaweed obstetrical cervical dilator

laminectomy
- l. blade
- l. chisel

l. frame
l. rongeur
l. self-retaining retractor
l. wedge sponge
Laminex needle
LaminOss implant
Lamis
L. Autofuse infusion pump
L. infusion system
L. patellar clamp
Lamitrode surgical lead
Lamont
L. elevator
L. nasal rasp
L. nasal saw
lamp
Aero-Kromayer l.
Alzheimer l.
Bausch-Lomb-Thorpe slit l.
Bausch & Lomb-Thorpe slit l.
Binner head l.
Birch l.
Birch-Hirschfeld l.
black light l.
BQ 900 slit l.
Campbell slit l.
carbon arc l.
Circline magnifier l.
Coburn-Rodenstock slit l.
Coherent LaserLink slit l.
Davis l.
Duke-Elder l.
Eldridge-Green l.
examining l.
Finsen l.
fluorescent l.
gas discharge l.
Grafco perineal l.
Gullstrand slit l.
Haag-Streit slit l.
Hague cataract l.
halogen l.
head l.
Heine HSL 100 handheld slit l.
high-pressure mercury arc l.
hot quartz l.
incandescent endoscope l.
Ishihara IV slit l.
Keeler l.
Koeppe l.
Kowa Optimed slit l.
Kromayer l.

LaserLink slit l.
Marco slit l.
mercury arc l.
mercury vapor l.
Nightingale examining l.
Nikon zoom photo slit l.
Nitra l.
Posner slit l.
quartz l.
Quick-Lite l.
Reichert slit l.
Rodenstock slit l.
Rusch laryngoscope l.
Rycroft l.
sigmoidoscope replacement l.
slit l.
Specular reflex slit l.
Thorpe slit l.
Topcon SL-E series slit l.
tungsten-halogen l.
ultraviolet l.
Universal Mack l.
Universal slit l.
Uviolite l.
VG slit l.
V-slit l.
Wood l.
xenon arc l.
xenon flash l.
Zeiss carbon arc slit l.
Lancaster
L. eye magnet
L. eye speculum
L. keratome
L. knife
L. lid speculum
L. ocular transilluminator
L. red-green screen
L. sclerotome
Lancaster-O'Connor
L.-O. forceps
L.-O. speculum
lance
L. knife
Rolf l.
Lanceford prosthesis
lancet
l. blade
Cleanlet l.
Keeler ultrasonic cataract
removal l.
l. knife

L

NOTES

lancet *(continued)*
    L. laser device
    Lipectron ultrasonic l.
    Meyer Swiss diamond knife l.
    Microlance blood l.
    Microlet Vaculance l.
    Pharmacia l.
    Phazet l.
    Surelite blood l.
    suture l.
    l. suture
    Swan l.
lancet-shaped
    l.-s. biopsy forceps
    l.-s. electrode
Landau
    L. dilator
    L. speculum
    L. trocar
    L. vaginal retractor
Landegger orbital implant
Landers
    L. biconcave lens
    L. contact lens
    L. irrigating vitrectomy ring
    L. vitrectomy lens forceps
Landers-Foulks
    L.-F. prosthesis
    L.-F. temporary keratoprosthesis
    lens
Lander wide-field temporary
   keratoprosthesis
Landmark midline catheter
Landolt
    L. C acuity chart
    L. cannula
    L. C ring
    L. enucleation scissors
    L. eye knife
    L. keratome
    L. pituitary speculum
    L. spreader
    L. spreading forceps
Landon
    L. colpostat
    L. forceps
    L. narrow-bladed retractor
Landry
    L. vein light
    L. vein light venoscope
Lane
    L. bone-holding clamp
    L. bone-holding forceps
    L. bone lever
    L. bone screw
    L. cleft palate needle
    L. dissector
    L. fasciatome
    L. fracture plate

    L. gastroenterostomy clamp
    L. gastrointestinal forceps
    L. intestinal clamp
    L. intestinal forceps
    L. mouthgag
    L. periosteal elevator
    L. periosteal raspatory
    L. rectal catheter
    L. retractor
    L. screwdriver
    L. screw-holding forceps
    L. suturing needle
    L. tissue forceps
    L. towel clamp
    L. ureteral meatotomy electrode
Lanex medium screen
Lang
    L. dissector
    L. eye knife
    L. eye scoop
    L. eye speculum
    L. iris forceps
    L. suture
Lange
    L. antral punch
    L. approximation forceps
    L. blade
    L. blade knife
    L. bone elevator
    L. bone retractor
    L. cartilage knife
    L. fistular hook
    L. plastic surgery hook
    L. skinfold calipers
Lange-Converse nasal root rongeur
Lange-Hohmann
    L.-H. bone lever
    L.-H. bone retractor
Langenbeck
    L. bone-holding forceps
    L. flap knife
    L. metacarpal amputation saw
    L. needle holder
    L. periosteal elevator
    L. periosteal rasp
    L. periosteal retractor
    L. resection knife
Langenbeck-Cushing vein retractor
Langenbeck-Green retractor
Langenbeck-Mannerfelt retractor
Langenbeck-O'Brien raspatory
Langerman angled tunnel knife
Langinate impression material
language acquisition device
Lanigan cartilage knife
Lanz
    L. low-pressure cuff endotracheal
    tube

L. pressure regulating valve
L. tracheostomy tube
lap
l. pad
L. Sac
l. tape
LAP-13 Ranfac cholangiographic catheter
laparator
Weck high-flow l.
Laparocam
Storz L.
Laparofan
L. pneumoperitoneum device
L. smoke evacuator
Laparolift system
Laparomed
L. cholangiogram vacuum system
L. suture-applier device
LaparoSAC
L. obturator
L. trocar
LaparoScan laparoscopic ultrasonic imaging
laparoscope
ACMI l.
ACMI transvaginal hydro l.
American Medical Source l.
AMS autoclavable l.
Aslan l.
Cabot Medical Corporation diagnostic/operating l.
Circon ACMI diagnostic l.
Cuda l.
Cuda l.
Daniel double-punch laser l.
0-degree l.
3-dimensional l.
3Dscope l.
Dyonics rod lens l.
Eder l.
Elmed diagnostic/operating l.
flexible video l.
Frangenheim l.
Fujinon diagnostic l.
Fujinon flexible fiberoptic l.
Fujinon operating l.
Hasson l.
Jacobs-Palmer l.
KLI laprocator l.
Marlow Surgical Technologies, Inc. diagnostic/operating l.

Menghini-Wildhirt l.
MiniSite l.
offset operating l.
Olympus diagnostic l.
Polaris l.
Richard Wolf Medical Instruments diagnostic/operating l.
Ruddock l.
Sharplav l.
Solos endoscopy diagnostic l.
Stoltz l.
Storz diagnostic/operating l.
Surgiview multi-use l.
USA Series Distortion-Free Hydro l.
Weerda l.
Wildhirt l.
Wisap diagnostic/operating l.
Ziskie operating l.
laparoscopic
l. Allis clamp
l. cannula
l. cholangiography catheter
l. Doppler probe
l. forceps
l. grasper
l. insufflator
l. laser
l. manipulator system
l. needle driver
l. pneumodissector
l. probe
l. retraction system
l. scissors
l. sleeve
l. trocar
l. ultrasound probe
laparoscopy
ACMI transvaginal hydro l.
LaparoSonic coagulating shears
Laparostat
Olsen self-retaining L.
laparotomy
l. sponge
l. sponge ring
Laparo Vac I&A system
Lap-Bag specimen retrieval pouch
Lap-Band adjustable gastric banding (LAGB)
Lapides
L. catheter
L. collecting bag

NOTES

Lapides *(continued)*
    L. ileostomy bag
    L. needle
Lapidus alternating air-pressure mattress
Laplace
    L. forceps
    L. liver retractor
LaPorta great toe implant
Lapras catheter
Lapra-Ty absorbable suture clip
Lapro-Clip ligating clip
Lapro-Flex laparoscopic retractor
Lapro-Loop device
LapSac collection sack
Lapse monitor
LapTie endoscopic knot-tying instrument
LapTop cushion
Lapwall
    L. laparotomy sponge
    L. wound protector
Laqua black line retinal hook
Lar-A-Jext laryngectomy tube
Lardennois button
Laredo-Bard needle
Lares dental handpiece
large
    l. antral cannula
    l. ball nerve hook
    extra l. (XL)
    l. field-of-view gamma camera
    l. loop excision of transformation zone (LLETZ)
    l. loop excision of transition zone (LLETZ)
    l. nail spicule bur
large-base quad cane
large-bore
    l.-b. angiocatheter
    l.-b. bile duct endoprosthesis
    l.-b. cannula
    l.-b. catheter
    l.-b. chest tube
    l.-b. heat probe
    l.-b. imaging system scanner
    l.-b. magnet
    l.-b. slotted aspirating needle
large-caliber chest tube
large-channel
    l.-c. endoscope
    l.-c. therapeutic duodenoscope
large-loop electrode
large-lumen catheter
large-tip electrode
large-volume round silicone drain
LaRivetti-Levinson intraluminal shunt
LaRocca nasolacrimal tube
LaRoe undermining forceps

Larrey
    L. bandage
    L. dressing
Larry
    L. rectal director
    L. rectal probe
Larsen
    L. tendon forceps
    L. tendon-holding forceps
laryngeal
    l. applicator
    l. applicator forceps
    l. atomizer
    l. basket forceps
    l. biopsy forceps
    l. bronchial grasping forceps
    l. cannula
    l. curette forceps
    l. dilator
    l. dissector
    l. grasping forceps
    l. knife
    l. mask
    l. mirror
    l. probe
    l. punch forceps
    l. retractor
    l. rotation forceps
    l. saw
    l. scissors
    l. snare
    l. sponging forceps
    l. stent
    l. syringe
    l. trocar
laryngectomy clamp
laryngofissure
    l. forceps
    l. retractor
Laryngoflex reinforced tracheostomy tube
laryngonasopharyngoscope
    Berci-Ward l.
laryngopharyngoscope
    Berci-Ward l.
    Proctor l.
    Stuckrad magnifying l.
laryngoscope
    adult l.
    adult reverse-bevel l.
    Albert-Andrews l.
    Andrews infant l.
    anterior commissure l.
    Atkins-Tucker shadow-free l.
    baby Miller l.
    Benjamin binocular slimline l.
    Benjamin-Lindholm microsuspension l.
    Benjamin pediatric operating l.

Bizzarri-Giuffrida l.
l. blade
Briggs l.
Broyles anterior commissure l.
Broyles optical l.
Broyles wasp-waist l.
Bullard intubating l.
Burton l.
Chevalier Jackson l.
commissure l.
Dedo l.
Dedo-Jako l.
Dedo-Pilling l.
direct l.
ESI l.
fiberoptic slide l.
Fink l.
Finnoff l.
Flagg l.
Flexiblade l.
Foregger l.
Fragen l.
Guedel l.
Haslinger l.
Holinger anterior commissure l.
Holinger-Garfield l.
Holinger hook-on folding l.
Holinger hourglass anterior
  commissure l.
Holinger modified Jackson l.
Holinger slotted l.
Hollister l.
Hopp l.
Hopp-Morrison l.
hourglass anterior commissure l.
infant l.
intubation l.
Jackson anterior commissure l.
Jackson fiberoptic slide l.
Jackson sliding l.
Jackson standard l.
Jako l.
Jako-Cherry l.
Jako-Pilling l.
Kantor-Berci video l.
Killian-Lynch suspension l.
KleenSpec disposable l.
Kleinsasser anterior commissure l.
Kleinsasser operating l.
Kleinsasser-Riecker l.
Kramer operating l.
laser l.

Lewy anterior commissure l.
Lewy suspension l.
Lindholm operating l.
Lundy l.
Lynch suspension l.
Machida fiberoptic l.
MacIntosh l.
Magill l.
Mantel l.
Miller l.
mirror l.
Negus l.
Olympus ENF-P-series l.
optical l.
Ossoff-Karlan-Dedo l.
Ossoff-Karlan-Jako l.
Ossoff-Karlan laser l.
pediatric l.
pencil-handled l.
Polio l.
l. profilometer
reverse-bevel l.
Rica anesthetic l.
Rica anterior commissure l.
Rica infant l.
Riecker-Kleinsasser l.
Roberts self-retaining l.
Rusch l.
Sanders intubation l.
self-retaining l.
shadow-free l.
Shapshay-Healy operating l.
Shapshay-Healy phonatory l.
Siker mirror l.
sliding l.
slotted l.
SMIC anterior commisure l.
standard Jackson l.
Stange l.
Storz anterior commissure l.
Storz-Riecker l.
straight-blade l.
suspension l.
Tucker anterior commissure l.
Tucker-Holinger l.
Tucker-Jako l.
Tucker mid-lighted optic slide l.
Tucker slotted l.
wasp-waist l.
Weerda l.
Welch Allyn l.
Wisconsin l.

L

NOTES

laryngoscope *(continued)*
    Wis-Foregger l.
    Wis-Hipple l.
    Yankauer l.
laryngostat
    Jackson l.
    Lewy l.
    Priest wasp-waist l.
    Proctor l.
    Proctor-Hellens l.
    Roman l.
laryngostroboscope
    Nagashima LS-3 l.
larynx
    American artificial l.
    artificial l.
    Bivona Optivox artificial
      electronic l.
    Cooper-Rand intraoral artificial l.
    electronic artificial l.
    external auditory l.
    Nu-Vois artificial l.
    Optivox artificial electronic l.
    SolaTone artificial l.
    Xomed intraoral artificial l.
Lasag contact lens
Laschal suture scissors
LaseAway
    L. ruby laser system
    L. ruby Nd:YAG laser
    L. Smooth Touch laser
LASEK
    laser subepithelial keratomileusis
LASER
    light activation by stimulated emission of
    radiation
laser
    AccuLase excimer l.
    AcuBlade robotic l.
    acupuncture l.
    l. adapter
    ADDStat l.
    L. Advanced Interventional Systems
      (LAIS)
    Aesculap argon ophthalmic l.
    Aesculap Meditec excimer l.
    Albarran l.
    alexandrite DP l.
    AlexLAZR l.
    AMO YAG 100 l.
    Apex Plus excimer l.
    Apogee 9300/6200 alexandrite l.
    Apogee hair removal l.
    Aramis l.
    ArF excimer l.
    argon l.
    argon blue l.
    argon fluoride l.
    argon green l.

argon ion l.
argon krypton l.
argon pump dye l.
argon-pumped dye l.
argon-pumped tunable dye l.
ArthroGuide carbon dioxide l.
ArthroProbe l.
Articu-Lase l.
atheroblation l.
Athos l.
Aura desktop l.
Aurora diode l.
Aurora HL l.
Axcis percutaneous myocardial
    revascularization l.
l. balloon
balloon-centered argon l.
biocavity l.
Biophysic Medical YAG l.
Britt argon pulsed ion l.
Britt BL-12 l.
Britt krypton l.
Britt pulsed argon l.
Candela l.
Candela C-beam l.
Candela MOL Lasertripter l.
Candela pulsed dye l.
Candela ScleroLaser l.
carbon dioxide l.
Cardona l.
Carl Zeiss YAG l.
Cavitron l.
CB Diode/532 l.
C-beam l.
CB Erbium/2.94 l.
Centauri Er:YAG l.
char-free carbon dioxide l.
Chromaser dermatology l.
l. CHRP rigid fiberscope system
Chrys surgical CO_2 l.
Cilco argon l.
Cilco Frigitronics l.
Cilco Hoffer Laseridge l.
Cilco krypton l.
Cilco Lasertek argon l.
Cilco YAG l.
ClearView CO_2 l.
CO_2 l.
CO_3 l.
Coherent carbon dioxide l.
Coherent CO_2 surgical l.
Coherent EPIC l.
Coherent Medical YAG l.
Coherent Novus Omni
    multiwavelength l.
Coherent Selecta 7000 l.
Coherent UltraPulse 5000C l.
cold beam l.
Colpolase l.

continuous-wave argon l.
continuous-wave diode l.
cool l.
CoolGlide l.
cool-tip l.
CoolTouch Nd:YAG l.
Cooper argon l.
Cooper LaserSonics l.
CooperVision YAG l.
copper bromide l.
copper vapor pulsed l.
CO_2 Sharplan l.
CrTmEr:YAG l.
Crystalase Erbium2 l.
CTE:YAG l.
CVX-300 excimer l.
Cynosure l.
Depilase l.
Dermablate skin rejuvenation l.
Derma 20 Er:YAG l.
Derma-K CO_2 l.
Derma-K Er:YAG l.
DermaLase l.
DIAGNOdent dental l.
l. digitizer
l. diode
diode pumped Nd:YAG l.
DioLite 532 l.
Diomed surgical diode l.
l. Doppler flowmeter
l. Doppler perfusion monitor
l. Doppler velocimeter
Dornier Medilas H
  holmium:YAG l.
Dynatronics Model 1620 l.
EC-5000 excimer l.
Eclipse holmium l.
Eclipse TMR holmium l.
EndoLase l.
endoscopic l.
Epic l.
EpiLaser hair removal l.
Epistar diode l.
erbium CrystaLase l.
erbium Renaissance l.
erbium:YAG infrared l.
ErCr:YAG l.
Er:glass dermatologic l.
Er:YAG l.
EsteLux dermatological l.
esthetic CO_2 l.
Evergreen Lasertek l.

ExciMed UV200 excimer l.
excimer l.
l. extensometer
FCP2 l.
FeatherTouch CO_2 l.
l. fiber
l. fiber director
l. fiberendoscope
FiberLase l.
l. flare meter
flashlamp pulsed Nd:YAG l.
Flexlase 600 l.
fluorescence-guided "smart" l.
Fotona Novalis Er:YAG l.
Fotona Novalis R ruby l.
frequency doubled
  neodymium:yttrium-aluminum-
  garnet l.
l. fume absorber
GaAs l.
gallium-aluminum-arsenide l.
gallium-arsenide l.
gas l.
Genesis 2000 carbon dioxide l.
GentleLASE l.
GentleLASE Plus l.
Gherini-Kauffman endo-otoprobe l.
Gish micro YAG l.
Gold portable CO_2 l.
green l.
GyneLase diode l.
l. Heaney needle holder
Heart Laser 2 CO_2 l.
helium-cadmium diagnostic l.
helium-neon l.
HeNe l.
Heraeus LaserSonics l.
HF infrared l.
HGM argon green l.
HGM intravitreal l.
HGM ophthalmic l.
HGM Spectrum K1 krypton yellow
  & green l.
high-energy l.
holmium l.
holmium:YAG l.
holmium:yttrium-aluminum-garnet l.
holmium:yttrium-argon-garnet l.
Horn endo-otoprobe l.
Hoskins nylon suture l.
hot-tip l.
Howard-Schatz l.

L

NOTES

laser *(continued)*
Ho:YAG l.
Hruby l.
Hyperion LTK l.
L. I bubble system
Illumina Pro series laparoscopic l.
IL MED l.
Il Med l.
l. imager
infrared-beam diode l.
IntraLase FS l.
intravitreal l.
ion l.
Iriderm Apex 800 diode l.
Iriderm DioLite 532 l.
Iris Oculight SLx MicroPulse l.
Jaffe blepharoplasty l.
l. Julian needle holder
Kaplan PenduLaser l.
Keracor l.
Kip l.
Kirsch l.
Kremer excimer l.
krypton red l.
KTP l.
KTP/Nd:YAG l.
KTP/532 surgical l.
KTP/YAG l.
LADARVision excimer l.
LAIS excimer l.
Lambda Physik EMG 103 l.
Lambda Plus PDL1, PDL2 photodynamic l.
L. Lancet laser
laparoscopic l.
l. laryngoscope
LaseAway ruby Nd:YAG l.
LaseAway Smooth Touch l.
Laserex Era 4106 YAG l.
LaserHarmonic l.
Laser Lancet l.
Laserscope KTP/532 l.
LaserSecure skin resurfacing l.
LaserSonics Paragon l.
LaserSonics SurgiBlade l.
Lasertek YAG l.
Lassag Micropter II l.
Lastec System angioplasty l.
Lateralase l.
lateral-firing l.
Lightstic fiberoptic l.
liquid organic dye l.
Lithognost flash-lamp pulsed dye l.
l. lithotripter
low-energy l.
LPK-80 II argon l.
Lumonics YAG l.
Luxar NovaPulse CO_2 l.
Lyra l.

MedArt 470 l.
Medilas fiberTome l.
Medilas Nd:YAG surgical l.
MeDioStar hair removal l.
Meditech l.
MedLite Q-Switched neodymium-doped yttrium-aluminum-garnet l.
MedLite Q-Switched YAG l.
Mel 60 excimer l.
Mel 70 flying spot l.
Merimack 1040 CO_2 l.
l. microlaryngeal cup forceps
l. microlaryngeal grasping forceps
Microlase transpupillary diode l.
Microlight 830 low-level l.
MicroProbe ophthalmic l.
l. microscope
microsecond pulsed flashlamp-pumped dye l.
midinfrared l.
mid-infrared pulsed l.
Mira AGL-400 l.
l. mirror
Mochida CO_2 Medi-Laser l.
mode-locked l.
Moeller l.
molectron l.
MultiLase D copper vapor l.
MultiLase Nd:YAG surgical l.
Myriadlase Side-Fire l.
Nanolas Nd:YAG l.
NaturaLase erbium l.
NaturaLase Er:YAG l.
Nd:YAG l.
Nd:YLF l.
neodymium l.
neodymium-doped yttrium-aluminum-garnet l.
neodymium:YAG l.
neodymium:yttrium-aluminum-garnet l.
neodymium:yttrium-lithium-fluoride photodisruptive l.
Neurolase microsurgical CO_2 l.
Nidek EC-series excimer l.
NovaLine excimer l.
NovaLine Litho-S DUV excimer l.
NovaPulse CO_2 l.
Novascan scanning headpiece l.
Novatec Lightblade l.
Novulase 660 l.
Novus Omni multiwavelength l.
OcuLight SL diode l.
OcuLight SLx ophthalmic l.
oculocutaneous l.
OmniMed argon-fluoride excimer l.
OmniPulse holmium l.
OmniPulse-Max holmium l.
Ophthalas argon l.

Ophthalas krypton l.
Opmilas 144 surgical l.
l. optometer
orange dye l.
orthogonal l.
OtoLam l.
l. ovary forceps
Palomar E2000 l.
Palomar EsteLux l.
Palomar SLP1000 l.
Paragon l.
PBI Medical copper vapor l.
PBI MultiLase D copper vapor l.
PC EDO ophthalmic office l.
Pegasus Nd:YAG surgical l.
Pegasus-PIV l.
PhotoDerm HR l.
photodisrupting l.
PhotoGenica VLS pulsed dye l.
PhotoGenica V-Star l.
Photon l.
PhotoPoint l.
photovaporizing l.
Polaris 1.32 Nd:YAG l.
Polytec LaseAway Q-switched
  ruby l.
potassium titanyl phosphate l.
Prima KTP/532 l.
l. probe
Prolase II lateral firing Nd:YAG l.
Prostalase l.
ProYellow+ vascular treatment l.
pulsed dye l.
pulsed metal vapor l.
pulsed tunable dye l.
pulsed yellow dye l.
PulseMaster l.
Pulsolith coumarin pulsed-dye l.
pumped dye l.
Q-LAS 0 YAG l.
QS alexandrite l.
Q-switched alexandrite l.
Q-switched Er:YAG l.
Q-switched Nd:YAG l.
Q-switched neodymium:YAG l.
Q-switched neodymium:yttrium
  aluminum-garnet l.
Q-switched ruby l.
Q-YAG 5 l.
red l.
red-beam l.
Reichel-Mainster retina l.

Renaissance erbium l.
RevitaLase erbium cosmetic l.
rhodamine l.
l. rod
rotational ablation l.
ruby l.
RubyStar tattoo removal l.
l. scalpel
scanning excimer l.
ScleroLaser l.
ScleroPLUS LongPulse dye l.
Selecta 7000 glaucoma l.
Sharplan argon l.
Sharplan CO_2 l.
Sharplan Medilas Nd:YAG
  surgical l.
Sharplan SilkTouch flashscan
  surgical l.
SharpLase Nd:YAG l.
SideFire l.
Silhouette endoscopic l.
Silk L.
SilkLaser l.
Site argon l.
Skinlight erbium yttrium-aluminum-
  garnet l.
Skinlight Er:YAG l.
SLT CL MD/Dual Contact l.
SLT Contact MTRL l.
SmartEpil l.
Smoothbeam dermatologic l.
SoftLight l.
Spectranetics CVX-300 excimer l.
Spectra-Physics argon l.
Spectra-Physics microsurgical l.
spectroscopy-directed l.
Spectrum K1 l.
Spectrum Q-switched ruby l.
SPTL vascular lesion l.
Star S3 ActiveTrak Excimer l.
Star X carbon dioxide l.
STATLase-SDL diode l.
Staurenghi 230 scanning l.
stereotaxic l.
Storz l.
l. subepithelial keratomileusis
  (LASEK)
Summit Excimed UV 200 l.
Summit Omnimed excimer l.
Summit SVS Apex Plus excimer l.
SurgiBlade l.
Surgica K6 l.

L

NOTES

laser *(continued)*
  surgical l.
  Surgicenter 40 CO_2 l.
  Surgilase CO_2 l.
  Surgilase 150 high-powered CO_2 l.
  Surgilase Nd:YAG l.
  SurgiLight OptiVision YAG l.
  Surgipulse XJ 150 CO_2 l.
  SVS Apex Plus excimer l.
  Tactilaze angioplasty l.
  Takata l.
  l. taper
  TEC 2100 positioning l.
  TE MOO mode beam l.
  THC:YAG l.
  l. thermal keratoplasty (LTK)
  thulium-holmium-chromium:yttrium-aluminum-garnet l.
  thulium-holmium:YAG l.
  Topaz CO_2 l.
  tracker-assisted PRK l.
  transpupillary l.
  Trimedyne holmium l.
  TruPulse CO_2 l.
  tunable pulsed dye l.
  L. Tweezers
  UltraFine erbium l.
  UltraLine l.
  UltraPulse 5000C CO_2 l.
  UltraPulse surgical l.
  ultraviolet l.
  Urolase CO_2 l.
  Vbeam l.
  Veinlase captured-pulse l.
  VersaLight l.
  VersaPulse cosmetic holmium l.
  VersaPulse Select l.
  Viridis l.
  Visulas argon l.
  Visulas Nd:YAG l.
  Visulas YAG l.
  Visx 2020 excimer l.
  Visx Star S2 excimer l.
  V-Star l.
  Waterlase Millennium l.
  Wild l.
  Xanar 20 Ambulase CO_2 l.
  XeCl excimer l.
  xenon-chloride excimer l.
  Xtrac excimer l.
  YAG l.
  yttrium-aluminum-garnet l.
  Zeiss H l.
  Zeiss Opmilas surgical l.
  Zeiss Visulas 690s l.
  Zyoptix l.
laser-adjustable lens

laser-assisted
  l.-a. intrastromal keratomileusis (LASIK)
  l.-a. intrastromal keratomileusis aspiration spoon
  l.-a. intrastromal keratomileusis cannula
  l.-a. intrastromal keratomileusis flap irrigator
  l.-a. in situ keratomileusis (LASIK)
Laserdish
  L. electrode
  L. pacing lead
laser-Doppler
  l.-D. flowmetry probe
  l.-D. Periflux PF-3 probe
  l.-D. spectroscopy
Laseredge microsurgical knife
Laserex Era 4106 YAG laser
Laserflo
  L. blood perfusion monitor
  L. BPM^2 laser Doppler monitor
Laserflow Doppler probe
LaserHarmonic laser
Laseridge Optics lens
laser-induced
  l.-i. thermography (LITT)
  l.-i. thermotherapy (LITT)
  l.-i. thermotherapy applicator
laserlight-induced fluorescence endoscopy (LIFE)
LaserLink slit lamp
Laseroptic treatment system
LaserPen device
LaserScan LSX excimer laser system
Laserscope
  L. discography kit
  L. disposable Endostat fiber
  L. KTP/532 laser
LaserSecure skin resurfacing laser
LaserSonics
  L. EndoBlade
  L. Nd:YAG LaserBlade scalpel
  L. Paragon laser
  L. SurgiBlade laser
Lasertek YAG laser
Laser-Trach endotracheal tube
Lasertubus endotracheal tube
LaserTweezers optical trapping instrument
Lasette laser finger perforator
Lash-Loeffler penile implant
LASIK
  laser-assisted intrastromal keratomileusis
  laser-assisted in situ keratomileusis
  LASIK aspiration spoon
  LASIK eye guard
  LASIK flap irrigator
  LASIK flap manipulator

LASIK Lindstrom irrigating cannula
LASIK spear
lasitome
Krumeich-Barraquer l.
Lassag Micropter II laser
lasso
L. circular mapping catheter
lens l.
l. snare
last
bunion l.
keystone l.
Lastec System angioplasty laser
lata
Fascian human fascia l.
Suspend Tutoplast processed
fascia l.
Tutoplast fascia l.
latent pacemaker
lateral
l. guide pin
l. gutter impactor
l. hand positioner
l. lumbar support
l. microlens telescope
l. osteotome
l. positioner
l. screw
l. skull block
l. trap suture
l. vaginal retractor
l. wall retractor
Lateralase laser
lateral-firing laser
latex
l. bag
l. balloon
l. catheter
l. drain
l. O band
l. rubber tourniquet strap
l. sponge graft
l. wheelchair cushion
LaTeX device
Latham
L. appliance
L. bowl
Lathbury cotton applicator
**lathe-cut polymethyl methacrylate
intraocular lens**
Latis catheter
LaTIS intravascular laser system

Latrobe soft palate retractor
Latson multipurpose catheter
Lattimer Silastic testicular prosthesis
Laufe
L. aspirating curette
L. cervical dilator
L. divergent outlet forceps
L. obstetrical forceps
L. portable uterine evacuator
L. uterine polyp forceps
Laufe-Barton-Kjelland obstetrical forceps
**Laufe-Barton-Kjelland-Piper obstetrical
forceps**
Laufe-Barton obstetrical forceps
Laufe-Novak gynecologic curette
Laufe-Piper
L.-P. obstetrical forceps
L.-P. uterine polyp forceps
Laufe-Randall gynecologic curette
Laufman forceps
**Laurens-Alcatel nuclear powered
pacemaker**
Laurer forceps
Laurus needle driver
Lavacuator gastric evacuator
lavage
Easi-Lav gastric l.
Hi Speed Pulse l.
l. needle
pulsatile jet l.
Pulsavac l.
pulse l.
Simpulse pulsing l.
Tum-E-Vac gastric l.
Laval advancement forceps
LaVeen helical stripper
Lawford speculum
Lawrence
L. Add-A-Cath
L. deep forceps
L. first metatarsophalangeal joint
implant
L. hemostatic forceps
Lawrie modified circumflex scissors
Lawson-Thornton plate
Lawton
L. corneal scissors
L. forceps
Lawton-Balfour self-retaining retractor
Lawton-Schubert biopsy forceps
Lawton-Wittner cervical biopsy forceps
Layden infant lens

L

NOTES

4-layer bandage
Layman tongue depressor
Lazar microsuction forceps
LB 9501 luminometer
L buttress plate
L-Cath peripherally inserted neonatal catheter
LCS
    low-contact stress
        LCS mobile bearing knee system
        LCS total knee system
LC strip
LDS
    ligate-divide-staple
        LDS clip
        LDS clip applier
Le
    L. Bag urinary pouch
    L. Blond R diamond dental bur
    L. Fort follower
    L. Grand-Gullstrand eye model
lead
    Accufix pacemaker l.
    active fixation l.
    active fixation pacemaker l.
    Aescula left ventricular l.
    AngeFix l.
    AngeFlex defibrillation l.
    AngePass defibrillation l.
    l. apron
    barbed epicardial pacing l.
    Biotronik l.
    bipolar pacing l.
    l. block
    l. bra
    brain l.
    Cadence TVL nonthoracotomy l.
    capped l.
    CAPSure EPI pacing l.
    CAPSure Fix pacing l.
    CAPSure SP Novus pacing l.
    CAPSure SP pacing l.
    CAPSure VDD pacing l.
    CAPSure Z Novus pacing l.
    Cardifix EZ endocardial pacing l.
    Cordis pacing l.
    CPI endocardial defibrillation rate-sensing pacing l.
    CPI Endotak SQ electrode l.
    CPI porous tined-tip bipolar pacing l.
    CPI Sentra endocardial l.
    CPI Sweet Tip l.
    dual coil transvenous l.
    dual octapolar l.
    dual quadrapolar l.
    Easytrak coronary venous l.
    Ela ventricular pacing l.
    endocardial balloon l.

endocardial bipolar pacemaker l.
endocardial cardiac l.
endocardial screw-in l.
Endotak C transvenous l.
Endotak C tripolar pacing/sensing/defibrillation l.
Endotak DSP l.
Endotak Endurance EZ l.
Endotak Endurance RX l.
Endotak Reliance defibrillator l.
epicardial l.
l. eye shield
Fast-Pass endocardial l.
finned pacemaker l.
fishhook l.
floating l.
Frank XYZ orthogonal l.
Guidant l.
l. hand
Irox endocardial pacing l.
isodiametric bipolar screw-in l.
Lamitrode surgical l.
Laserdish pacing l.
left ventricular transvenous l.
Lewis l.
limb l.
l. locking device
Medtronic CapSure SP Novus pacing l.
Medtronic CapSure VDD pacing l.
Medtronic CapSure Z Novus pacing l.
Medtronic Spirit l.
Medtronic Spring l.
Medtronic Transvene endocardial l.
modified chest l.
myocardial l.
Nehb D l.
nonintegrated transvenous defibrillation l.
nonintegrated tripolar l.
octapolar l.
Oscor atrial l.
Oscor pacing l.
Osypka atrial l.
over-the-wire pacing l.
Pacesetter Tendril DX steroid-eluting active-fixation pacing l.
l. pellet marker
permanent cardiac pacing l.
Permathane l.
l. pin
Pisces-Sigma l.
Pisces Z Quad low-impedance l.
l. plate
Polyrox fractal l.
precordial l.
Retrox Fractal active fixation l.
scalar l.

screw-in pacemaker l.
screw-on l.
segmented ring tripolar l.
silicone l.
single-pass l.
Stela electrode l.
l. suture
Sweet Tip bipolar l.
Telectronics Accufix pacing l.
temporary pervenous l.
Tendril l.
Tendril DX implantable pacing l.
Tendril SDX active-fixation l.
ThinLine EZ bipolar cardiac
  pacing l.
transcutaneous l.
Transvene-RV l.
transvenous defibrillator l.
tripolar l.
2-turn epicardial l.
3-turn epicardial l.
Unipass endocardial pacing l.
VDD pacing l.
**Leadbetter-Politano ureteral implant
  prosthesis**
Leadcare handheld blood lead analyzer
Leader
L. iris hook
L. vas hook
L. vas isolation forceps
Leader-Kohlman dilator
lead-filled mallet
lead-rubber apron
lead-shot tie suture
leaf
l. gauge
l. splint
leaflet retractor
leaf-spring brace
Leahey
L. chalazion forceps
L. clamp
L. marginal chalazion forceps
L. suture forceps
Leake Dacron mandible prosthesis
Leander
L. chiropractic table
L. motorized flexion table
LEAP
Lewis expandable adjustable prosthesis
LEAP balloon

LEAP collimator
LEAP system
Leasure
L. aspirator
L. nasal forceps
L. round punch tip
L. tracheal retractor
L. tuning fork
Lea's vaginal shield
Lea Symbol chart
leather
L. antegrade valvulotome
l. orthosis
L. retrograde valvulotome
Leather-Karmody in situ valve scissors
Leatherman
L. alar hook
L. compression hook
L. trochanteric retractor
Leaver sclerotomy forceps
LeBag reservoir
Lebensohn chart
Lebsche
L. forceps
L. raspatory
L. rongeur
L. saw guide
L. sternal chisel
L. sternal knife
L. sternal punch
L. sternal shears
L. wire saw
LeCocq brace
Lectromed urinary investigation system
LED
light-emitting diode
Ledor pigtail catheter
Ledraplastic exercise ball
Lee
L. bracket
L. bronchus clamp
L. cartilage knife
L. cryoprobe
L. diamond bur
L. double-ended retractor
L. graft
L. lingual button
L. microvascular clamp
L. needle
L. orthodontic resin
L. & Westcott needle
Lee-Ahn sinus injection needle sheath

L

NOTES

leeches
  Biopharm l.
Lee-Cohen
  L.-C. knife
  L.-C. septal elevator
Leeds-Keio ligament prosthesis
Leeds-Northrup Speedomax recorder
Lee-Fischer plastic bracket
LEEP
  loop electrosurgical excision procedure
  LEEP active loop electrode
  LEEP system
  LEEP system 1000 workstation
Lees
  L. arterial forceps
  L. bronchus clamp
  L. nontraumatic forceps
  L. vascular clamp
  L. wedge resection clamp
LeeSpec speculum
Leff
  L. alloy
  L. stethoscope
Lefferts
  L. bone-cutting forceps
  L. rib shears
  L. rib spreader
LeFort
  L. dilator
  L. filiform
  L. filiform bougie
  L. filiform guide
  L. male urethral catheter
  L. speculum
  L. suture
  L. urethral sound
  L. urethral ultrasound
  L. uterine sound
left
  l. coronary catheter
  l. heart catheter
  l. internal mammary artery (LIMA)
  Judkins l. 4 (JL4)
  l. Judkins catheter
  l. long leg brace
  l. ventricular (LV)
  l. ventricular assist device (LVAD)
  l. ventricular assist system (LVAS)
  l. ventricular bypass pump
  l. ventricular sump catheter
  l. ventricular transvenous lead
left-handed cornea scissors
leg
  l. bag strap
  l. brace
  l. holder
  l. immobilizer
  l. positioner
  l. sling

Legacy phacoemulsifier
Legasus Sport CPM device
Legend pacemaker
Legen self-retaining retractor
3-legged cage heart valve
Leggiero hydrophilic-coated
  microcatheter
legging
  traction l.
Legg osteotome
legholder
  Bickel l.
  lithotomy l.
  Low Profile l.
  Prep-Assist l.
  Surbaugh l.
leg-holding device
Legueu
  L. bladder retractor
  L. kidney retractor
  L. spatula
Lehman
  L. aortographic catheter
  L. pancreatic manometry catheter
  L. ventriculography catheter
Lehner
  L. II inserter
  L. II loader
Lehnhardt Universal cap
Leibinger
  L. 3-D bone plate
  L. E-Z flap
  L. locking system
  L. Micro Dynamic mesh
  L. Micro Plus plate
  L. Micro Plus screw
  L. Micro System drill bit
  L. Micro System plate cutter
  L. Micro System plate-holding
  forceps
  L. miniplate system
  L. mini Würzburg plate
  L. Mini Würzburg screw
  L. plating system
  L. Profyle hand system
  L. titanium mini Würzburg implant
  system
  L. titanium Würzburg mandibular
  reconstruction system
  L. Würzburg plate
  L. Würzburg screw
Leica
  L. M680 surgical microscope
  L. vibrating knife microtome
Leicaflex camera
Leigh capsular forceps
Leighton needle
Leinbach
  L. head and neck endoprosthesis

L. head and neck total hip prosthesis
L. olecranon hook
L. olecranon screw
L. osteotome
Leios pacemaker
Leisegang colposcope
Leiske intraocular lens
Leiter tube
Leitz
L. image analysis system
L. microscope
L. 1600 Saw microtome
Leivers
L. blade
L. mouthgag
Lejeune
L. cotton applicator
L. thoracic forceps
Leksell
L. arc
L. bone rongeur
L. cardiovascular rongeur
L. D-shaped stereotactic frame
L. gamma knife
L. grooved director
L. laminectomy rongeur
L. Model G stereotactic frame
L. punch
L. rongeur forceps
L. selector
L. stereotactic device
L. stereotactic gamma unit
L. stereotactic system
L. sternal approximator
L. sternal spreader
L. trephine
Leksell-Elekta stereotactic frame
Leksell-Stille thoracic rongeur
Leland
L. refractor
L. tonsillar knife
Leland-Jones
L.-J. forceps
L.-J. tonsillar knife
L.-J. vascular clamp
Lell
L. bite block
L. esophagoscope
L. laryngofissure saw
L. tracheal tube

LEMA
lower extremity mobility aid
LEMA strap
LeMaitre biliary catheter
LeMaitre-Bookwalter dilator
Lembert suture
Lem-Blay circumcision clamp
Lemmon
L. blade
L. intimal dissector
L. needle
L. rib contractor
L. self-retaining sternal retractor
L. sternal approximator
L. sternal elevator
L. sternal spreader
Lemmon-Russian forceps
Lemoine
L. forceps
L. orbital implant
L. serrefine
Lemoine-Searcy
L.-S. anchor
L.-S. fixation anchor loop
L.-S. fixation anchor loupe
Lemole
L. atrial valve self-retaining retractor
L. mitral valve retractor
lemon-squeezer obstetrical elevator
Lempert
L. bone curette
L. bone rongeur
L. diamond-dust polishing bur
L. endaural curette
L. endaural retractor
L. endaural rongeur
L. endaural speculum
L. excavator
L. fenestration bur
L. fine curette
L. heavy elevator
L. invaginator
L. knife
L. malleus cutter
L. malleus nipper
L. malleus punch
L. narrow elevator
L. perforator
L. periosteal elevator
L. retractor

L

NOTES

Lempert *(continued)*
    L. rongeur forceps
    L. rongeur headrest
**Lempert-Beckman-Colver endaural
  speculum**
Lempert-Colver
    L.-C. endaural speculum
    L.-C. retractor
Lempert-Juers rongeur
Lempert-Storz
    L.-S. lens
    L.-S. lens loop
    L.-S. loupe
Lempka vein stripper
Lems lens
Lenard ray tube
Lenbach hip system
Lennarson tube
**Lenny Johnson surgical-assist knee
  holder**
Lenox
    L. bucket
    L. Hill Spectralite knee brace
lens
    Abraham contact l.
    Abraham iridectomy laser l.
    Abraham iridectomy YAG laser l.
    Abraham peripheral button
      iridotomy l.
    Accuflex intraocular l.
    AccuGel l.
    AC intraocular l.
    acrylic l.
    AcrySof foldable intraocular l.
    AcrySof single-piece intraocular l.
    Acuflex intraocular l.
    Acuvue bifocal l.
    Acuvue disposable contact l.
    Acuvue Etafilcon A l.
    Additions multifocal soft
      progressive l.
    Advent Flurofocon contact l.
    Albarran l.
    Alcon intraocular l.
    Alcon MA 60 BM l.
    Alien WildEyes l.
    Allen-Braley intraocular l.
    Allergan-Simcoe C-loop
      intraocular l.
    all-in-the-bag intraocular l.
    all-PMMA one-piece C-loop
      intraocular l.
    Amercal intraocular l.
    Amercal-Shepard intraocular l.
    American Medical Optics Baron l.
    AMO Advent contact l.
    AMO Array foldable intraocular l.
    AMO Phacoflex II foldable
      intraocular l.

    AMO Sensar intraocular l.
    AMO Ultraviolet-Absorbing l.
    AMO ultraviolet-absorbing l.
    Amsoft l.
    Anis staple l.
    anterior chamber intraocular l.
    Aquaflex contact l.
    Aquasight l.
    Arnott 1-piece all-PMMA
      intraocular l.
    Array foldable intraocular l.
    Artisan phakic intraocular l.
    aspheric l.
    aspherical ophthalmoscopic l.
    aspheric cataract l.
    auxiliary l.
    Azar Mark II intraocular l.
    bag-fixated intraocular l.
    Bagolini l.
    Baikoff l.
    bandage contact l.
    bandage soft contact l.
    Barkan gonioscopic l.
    Barkan infant l.
    Barkan operating l.
    Baron intraocular l.
    Barraquer J-loop intraocular l.
    Barrett hydrogel intraocular l.
    Bausch & Lomb Optima l.
    Bausch & Lomb Softlens 66
      contact l.
    Bausch & Lomb Surgical
      L161U l.
    Bechert 1-piece all-PMMA
      intraocular l.
    biconcave contact l.
    biconvex intraocular l.
    bicylindrical l.
    Bietti l.
    bifocal intracorneal l.
    Binkhorst l.
    Binkhorst collar stud intraocular l.
    Binkhorst-Fyodorov l.
    Binkhorst 2-loop intraocular l.
    Binkhorst mustache lens
      intraocular l.
    BioComFold foldable intraocular l.
    BioCurve Gold toric contact l.
    biomicroscopic indirect l.
    Bi-Soft l.
    bispherical l.
    Blaydes angled l.
    Bloodshot WildEyes l.
    Blumenthal intraocular l.
    Boberg l.
    Boberg-Ans intraocular l.
    Boston Envision l.
    Boston scleral l.
    Bowling l.

Boys-Smith laser l.
Burian-Allen contact l.
Byrne expulsive hemorrhage l.
Capsulform l.
Cardona fiberoptic diagnostic l.
Carl Zeiss l.
cast-molded PMMA intraocular l.
catadioptric l.
CeeOn Edge foldable l.
CeeOn heparinized intraocular l.
Centra-Flex l.
CGI-1 contact l.
Charles contact l.
Charles intraocular l.
Charles irrigating l.
Chiroflex C11UB l.
Choyce Mark intraocular l.
Choyce-Tennant l.
Ciba Soft l.
Ciba Thin l.
Cilco intraocular l.
Cilco-Kelman Multiflex all-PMMA
  intraocular l.
Cilco MonoFlex PMMA l.
Cilco Optiflex intraocular l.
Cilco posterior chamber
  intraocular l.
Cilco-Simcoe II l.
Cilco Slant l.
Cilco-Sonometrics l.
ClariFlex foldable intraocular l.
clariVit Central Mag vitrectomy l.
clariVit Wide Angle vitrectomy l.
Clayman intraocular l.
C-loop posterior chamber l.
closed-loop intraocular l.
Coburn equiconvex l.
Coburn intraocular l.
Coburn Optical Industries-Feaster
  intraocular l.
Coburn-Storz intraocular l.
Cogan-Boberg-Ans l.
Collamer intraocular l.
L. Comfort ultrasound cleaning and
  disinfecting system
compressible acrylic intraocular l.
compression-molded PMMA
  intraocular l.
condensing l.
CooperVision-Cilco Novaflex
  anterior chamber intraocular l.
CooperVision PMMA-ACL Flex l.

Copeland anterior chamber
  intraocular l.
Copeland radial loop intraocular l.
Copeland radial panchamber UV l.
coquille plano l.
crimped toric l.
Crookes l.
crystalline l.
CSI l.
cylindrical l.
Darin l.
diopter l.
direct gonioscopic l.
disc lens intraocular l.
dispersing l.
Donnheim l.
Drews l.
Dulaney intraocular implant l.
Duragel l.
Durasoft 2 contact l.
Durasoft toric l.
Edge III hydrogel contact l.
Emcee l.
Emery l.
endocapsular artificial l.
l. enucleation scoop
Envision l.
Epstein collar stud acrylic l.
Epstein posterior chamber
  intraocular l.
ERG-Jet disposable contact l.
Eschenback Optik l.
etafilcon A disposable contact l.
European in-the-bag l.
l. expressor
extended-wear soft contact l.
EZ.1 multifocal contact l.
EZVue violet haptic intraocular l.
Falcon l.
Feaster Dualens intraocular l.
Feaster dual-placement intraocular l.
Fechtner intraocular l.
fiberoptic l.
Flexcon l.
flexible fluoropolymer contact l.
flexible loop anterior chamber
  intraocular l.
flexible loop posterior chamber
  intraocular l.
Flexlens l.
F/M base curve contact l.
Focus Night & Day contact l.

L

NOTES

lens *(continued)*
    foldable intraocular l.
    folding l.
    3-footed lens intraocular l.
    FormFlex formocresal l.
    FormFlex intraocular l.
    formocresol l.
    foroblique l.
    Fresnel l.
    Friedman handheld Hruby l.
    fundal contact l.
    fundal laser l.
    fundus contact l.
    fundus focalizing l.
    fundus laser l.
    fused bifocal l.
    Fyodorov 4-loop iris clip
      intraocular l.
    Fyodorov type I, II intraocular l.
    Galand disc l.
    Galand in-the-bag l.
    Galin intraocular implant l.
    Genesis l.
    Gentex PDQ polycarbonate l.
    Gill intraocular implant l.
    Gilmore intraocular implant l.
    l. glide cutter
    glued-on hard contact l.
    Goldmann macular contact l.
    Goldmann 3-mirror gonioscopy l.
    Goldmann multimirror l.
    goniolens l.
    gonioscopic l.
    Gould intraocular implant l.
    gradient index l.
    GRIN l.
    Gullstrand l.
    handheld Hruby l.
    haptic area l.
    haptic-fixated intraocular l.
    haptic plate l.
    hard contact l.
    Harris modified J-loop
      intraocular l.
    Harris rigid quadriped intraocular l.
    Hart pediatric 3-mirror l.
    Hersbury anterior chamber
      intraocular l.
    Hoffer ridged intraocular l.
    l. hook
    Hopkins II rod l.
    Hoskins-Barkan goniotomy infant l.
    Hruby contact l.
    Hunkeler intraocular l.
    Hunter 1-piece all-PMMA
      intraocular l.
    Hydracon contact l.
    Hydrasoft contact l.
    Hydrocurve l.
    Hydroflex II intraocular l.
    hydrogel intraocular l.
    Hydron l.
    hydrophilic contact l.
    Hydrosight l.
    Hydroview l.
    IMMA l.
    l. implant
    l. implantation forceps
    Implens intraocular l.
    infant Karickhoff laser l.
    infant 3-mirror laser l.
    Interfit-Pharmacea Intermedic
      intraocular l.
    Interflux intraocular l.
    Intermedics l.
    Interspace YAG laser l.
    intracorneal l.
    intraocular l. (IOL)
    IntraOptics intraocular l.
    Iogel intraocular l.
    Iolab Azar intraocular l.
    Ioptex intraocular l.
    Ioptex TabOptic l.
    Irene l.
    iridocapsular intraocular l.
    iris claw l.
    iris-supported intraocular l.
    iseikonic l.
    Iwata-Ricky gonioscopic l.
    Jaffe Cilco l.
    Jaffe 1-piece all-PMMA
      intraocular l.
    J-loop posterior chamber
      intraocular l.
    Joal l.
    Kamerling Capsular 90 l.
    Kamerling 1-piece all-PMMA
      intraocular l.
    Karickhoff diagnostic l.
    Karickhoff laser l.
    Kearney side-notch intraocular l.
    Keeler panoramic l.
    Kelman flexible tripod l.
    Kelman II 3-point fixation rigid
      tripod intraocular l.
    Kelman Multiflex II intraocular l.
    Kelman Omnifit intraocular l.
    Kelman PC 27LB CapSul l.
    Kelman Quadraflex intraocular l.
    Kelman S-flex intraocular l.
    keratometer l.
    Kilp l.
    Kishi l.
    Koeppe diagnostic l.
    Koeppe gonioscopic l.
    Krasnov l.
    Kratz elliptical-style l.

Kratz-Johnson modified J-loop
  intraocular l.
Kratz modified J-loop intraocular l.
Kratz posterior chamber
  intraocular l.
Krieger wide-field fundus l.
Landers biconcave l.
Landers contact l.
Landers-Foulks temporary
  keratoprosthesis l.
Lasag contact l.
laser-adjustable l.
Laseridge Optics l.
l. lasso
lathe-cut polymethyl methacrylate
  intraocular l.
Layden infant l.
Leiske intraocular l.
Lempert-Storz l.
Lems l.
Lester notch intraocular l.
Levick 1-piece all-PMMA
  intraocular l.
Lewicky intraocular l.
Lieb-Guerry cataract implant l.
Lindstrom Centrex l.
Lindstrom modified J-loop, three-
  piece reverse PMMA optic
  intraocular l.
Liteflex l.
Little-Arnott tripod intraocular l.
long-wearing contact l.
l. loop
l. loop forceps
l. loupe
Lovac fundal contact l.
Lovac gonioscopic l.
Lovac 6-mirror gonioscopic l.
low-vacuum contact l.
Lynell intraocular l.
Machemer flat l.
Machemer infusion contact l.
Machemer magnifying vitrectomy l.
macular contact l.
Mainster-HM retinal laser l.
Mainster retinal laser l.
Mainster-S retinal laser l.
Mainster Ultra Field PRP laser l.
Mainster-WF retinal laser l.
Mainster wide-field l.
Maltese cross l.
Mandelkorn suture lysis l.

l. manipulator
March laser l.
Marco trial l. (MTL)
Mark IX l.
Mazzocco silicone intraocular l.
McGhan l.
McLean prismatic fundus laser l.
Meditech bandage contact l.
Mehta intraocular l.
MemoryLens foldable intraocular l.
meniscal posterior concave
  intraocular l.
Mentor ORC MemoryLens l.
meter l.
MiniQuad XL l.
3M intraocular l.
3-mirror contact l.
4-mirror goniolens l.
3-mirror intraocular l.
l. mitral heart valve
modified C-loop intraocular l.
modified J-loop, posterior chamber
  intraocular l.
Momosi spider lens intraocular l.
Monoflex l.
Morgan therapeutic l.
Multi-Optics l.
multiple-piece intraocular l.
narrow l.
Neolens l.
New Orleans l.
NewVues l.
Nikon aspheric l.
Nikon SMZ 2T magnifying l.
Nokrome bifocal l.
Nova Aid l.
Nova Curve l.
Novaflex intraocular l.
Nova Soft II l.
NuVita l.
NuVue l.
objective l.
Oculaid l.
ocular Gamboscope l.
O'Malley-Pearce-Luma l.
Omnifit intraocular l.
omnifocal l.
open l.
open-loop intraocular l.
Ophtec Co. l.
Optical Radiation intraocular l.
2-Optifit toric l.

L

NOTES

lens *(continued)*
    Optiflex intraocular l.
    Optima contact l.
    Opti-Vu l.
    Opt-Visor l.
    ORC posterior chamber
      intraocular l.
    orthoscopic l.
    O'Shea l.
    Osher-Fresnel intraocular l.
    Osher pan-fundus l.
    Osher surgical posterior pole l.
    Packard intraocular l.
    Palmer l.
    Palmer-Buono contact l.
    panchamber UV l.
    Pannu II intraocular l.
    PanoView Optics l.
    parfocal defraction l.
    PBII blue loop l.
    Pearce-Keates bifocal intraocular l.
    Pearce posterior chamber
      intraocular l.
    Pearce Tripod intraocular l.
    pediatric 3-mirror laser l.
    Permalens l.
    Perspex CQ intraocular l.
    Perspex CQ-Shearing-Simcoe-
      Sinskey l.
    Peyman-Green vitrectomy l.
    Peyman-Tennant-Green l.
    Peyman wide-field l.
    Phakic 6 l.
    Pharmacia Intermedics ophthalmics
      intraocular l.
    Pharmacia Visco J-loop l.
    3-piece acrylic intraocular l.
    3-piece modified J-loop
      intraocular l.
    3-piece silicone intraocular l.
    piggyback contact l.
    plano l.
    planoconcave l.
    planoconvex l.
    planoconvex nonridge l.
    Platina clip l.
    plus power l.
    PMMA hard contact l.
    PMMA intraocular l.
    Pointer 1-piece all-PMMA
      intraocular l.
    3-point fixation intraocular l.
    4-point fixation intraocular l.
    polypropylene intraocular l.
    Posner diagnostic l.
    posterior chamber intraocular l.
    posterior convex intraocular l.
    Precision Cosmet l.
    prismatic contact l.

    prismatic gonioscopic l.
    Prokop intraocular l.
    prosthetic l.
    punctal l.
    l. pusher
    QuadPediatric fundus l.
    Rappazzo intraocular l.
    Rayner l.
    Rayner-Choyce intraocular l.
    Red Reflex Lens Systems l.
    retroscopic l.
    reverse intraocular l.
    Revolution l.
    rigid gas-permeable contact l.
    rigid intraocular l.
    Ritch contact l.
    Ritch nylon suture laser l.
    Ritch trabeculoplasty laser l.
    Rodenstock panfundus l.
    Rohm and Haas PMMA
      intraocular l.
    Roussel-Fankhauser contact l.
    Ruiz fundal contact l.
    Ruiz fundal laser l.
    Ruiz plano fundal l.
    Sableflex anterior chamber
      intraocular l.
    sapphire l.
    SaturEyes contact l.
    Sauflon PW hydrophilic contact l.
    Schachar l.
    Scharff l.
    SeeQuence disposable contact l.
    self-stabilizing vitrectomy l.
    semiflexible intraocular l.
    semirigid intraocular l.
    Sensar acrylic intraocular l.
    Sensar foldable acrylic posterior
      chamber intraocular l.
    Sensar OptiEdge acrylic
      intraocular l.
    Severin multiple closed-loop
      intraocular l.
    Shah-Shah intraocular l.
    Shearing J-Loop intraocular l.
    Shearing posterior chamber
      intraocular l.
    Shearing S-style anterior chamber
      intraocular l.
    Sheets closed-loop posterior
      chamber intraocular l.
    Shepard flexible anterior chamber
      intraocular l.
    Shepard Universal intraocular l.
    short C-loop intraocular l.
    Siepser intraocular l.
    Signet Optical l.
    silica contact l.
    silicone elastomer l.

Silsoft extended wear contact l.
silvered contact l.
Simcoe C-loop intraocular l.
SingleStitch PhacoFlex l.
Sinskey J-loop intraocular l.
Slant haptic intraocular l.
Slimfit l.
Smith intraocular implant l.
Snellen soft contact l.
Soflens contact l.
SoFlex l.
soft contact l.
soft intraocular l.
SoftSITE high add aspheric multifocal contact l.
Sola Optical USA Spectralite high-index l.
Sola VIP l.
Sovereign bifocal l.
l. spatula
Spectralite Transitions l.
spherocylindrical l.
l. spoon
Staar foldable intraocular l.
Staar implantable contact l.
Staar toric l.
Stableflex l.
Stankiewicz iris clip intraocular l.
Stokes l.
Strampelli l.
Super Field NC slit lamp l.
Supramid l.
Surefit intraocular l.
Surevue contact l.
Surgidev Leiske anterior chamber intraocular l.
Sutherland l.
Tano double-mirror peripheral vitrectomy l.
Tennant Anchorflex anterior chamber intraocular l.
Thorpe gonioprism l.
Thorpe 4-mirror goniolaser l.
Thorpe 4-mirror vitreous-fundus l.
Tillyer bifocal l.
T-lens therapeutic contact l.
Tolentino prism l.
Tolentino vitrectomy l.
Topcon aspheric l.
toric contact l.
toric intraocular l.
Touchlite zoom l.

tripod intraocular l.
Trokel l.
Trokel-Peyman laser l.
Troncoso tubular l.
Trupower aspherical l.
Ultex l.
UltraCon RGP contact l.
UltraCon rigid gas permeable contact l.
Ultra view SP slit lamp l.
ultraviolet-blocking intraocular l.
uniplanar intraocular l.
Univision low-vision microscopic l.
Urrets-Zavalia retinal surgical l.
uvea-fixated intraocular l.
uvea-supported intraocular l.
Uvex l.
UVR-absorbing intraocular l.
Varigray l.
Varilux Infinity l.
Varilux Plus l.
Viscolens l.
Visiontech l.
Visitec l.
Volk conoid l.
Volk high-resolution aspherical l.
Volk panretinal l.
Volk QuadrAspheric fundus l.
Volk SuperField NC l.
Volk SuperPupil XL l.
Volk Super Quad 160 l.
Wang l.
Weber-Elschnig l.
Wesley-Jessen l.
Wild l.
Wise iridotomy laser l.
Wise sphincterotomy laser l.
Worst gonioprism contact l.
Worst iris claw l.
Worst lobster-claw l.
Worst Medallion l.
Yalon intraocular l.
Yannuzzi fundus laser l.
Youens l.
Zeiss aspheric l.
Ziski iris clip intraocular l.
Zoeffle soft intraocular l.

LensCheck Advanced Logic lensometer
lensed fiber-tip laser delivery catheter
Lens-Eze inserter
Lensmeter 701 lensometer

NOTES

lensometer
- Allergan-Humphrey l.
- AMO l.
- Carl Zeiss l.
- Coburn l.
- Hardy l.
- IntraOptics l.
- LensCheck Advanced Logic l.
- Lensmeter 701 l.
- Marco l.
- Reichert l.
- Reichert-Lenschek advanced logic l.
- Topcon LM P5 digital l.

lens-threading forceps
Lente silver nitrate probe
Lent photolaparoscope
Lentulo spiral drill
Leo
- L. Bathlifter
- L. Schwartz sponge-holding forceps

Leon
- L. cobra cannula
- L. cobra tip

Leonard
- L. catheter
- L. forceps

Leone expansion screw
LePad breast exam training pad
Lepley-Ernst tracheal tube
Leptos pacemaker
Lere bone mill
Leriche
- L. hemostatic forceps
- L. spatula
- L. tissue forceps

Lerman
- L. hinge brace
- L. noninvasive halo
- L. SHO
- L. shoulder holster orthosis

Lermoyez nasal punch
LeRoy
- L. clip-applying forceps
- L. infant scalp clip
- L. ventricular catheter

LeRoy-Raney scalp clip
Leslie Parachute stone retrieval device
L'Esperance
- L. erysiphake
- L. needle

Lester
- L. A. Dine camera
- L. fixation forceps
- L. Jones tube
- L. lens manipulator
- L. muscle forceps
- L. notch intraocular lens

Lester-Burch eye speculum

Letournel
- L. acetabular fracture bone plate
- L. guideline

leucocyte detection strip
LEUHR
- low-energy ultra-high resolution
- LEUHR fan-beam collimator

leukocyte
- l. automatic recognition computer
- l. reduction filter

LeukoNet filter
Leukopore tape
leukoscope
Leukos pacemaker
Leukotape P sports tape
leukotome
- Bailey l.
- Dorsey transorbital l.
- Freeman transorbital l.
- Lewis l.
- Lours l.
- Love l.
- McKenzie l.
- Nosik transorbital l.
- Tworek transorbital l.

Leukotrap red cell storage system
Leung endoscopic nasal biliary drainage set
Leur-par collimator
Leurs nasal rasp
Leusch atraumatic obturator
Levant stone dislodger
LeVasseur-Merrill retractor
levator snare
LeVeen
- L. ascites shunt
- L. catheter
- L. dialysis shunt
- L. inflation syringe
- L. inflator
- L. inflator with pressure gauge
- L. needle electrode
- L. peritoneal shunt
- L. peritoneovenous shunt
- L. plaque cracker
- L. plaque-cracker
- L. valve

level
- L. Anchorage system
- L. I normothermic irrigating system
- L. One normothermic IV fluid set

Levenson tissue forceps
lever
- Alexander bone l.
- Bennett bone l.
- bone l.
- Bristow l.
- Buck-Gramcko bone l.
- Charnley femoral l.

Cottle bone l.
Hohmann-Aldinger bone l.
Hohmann bone l.
Kilner malar l.
Lane bone l.
Lange-Hohmann bone l.
Murphy bone l.
Norrbacka-Stille l.
l. pessary
Sellheim obstetrical l.
Torpin obstetrical l.
Wagner bone l.
Watson-Jones bone l.

Levick 1-piece all-PMMA intraocular lens

Levin

L. drill guide
L. duodenal tube
L. thermocouple cordotomy electrode
L. tube catheter

Levin-Davol tube

Levine

L. curetting spud
L. foreign body spud

Levinthal surgery retractor

Levis arm splint

Levitt eye implant

Levora fixation forceps

Levret forceps

Levy

L. articulating retractor
L. perineal retractor
L. & Rappel foot orthosis

Levy-Kuglen

L.-K. iris hook
L.-K. lens manipulator

Levy-Okun stripper

Lewicky

L. capsular scraper
L. cortex extractor
L. formed cystotome
L. intraocular lens
L. IOL spatula
L. microlens hook
L. needle
L. self-retaining chamber maintainer
L. threaded infusion cannula

Lewin

L. baseball finger splint
L. bone-holding clamp
L. bone-holding forceps

L. bunion dissector
L. elevator
L. sesamoidectomy dissector
L. spinal-perforating forceps

Lewin-Stern

L.-S. finger splint
L.-S. thumb splint

Lewis

L. dental mirror
L. expandable adjustable prosthesis (LEAP)
L. expandable adjustable prosthesis system
L. hemostat
L. intramedullary device
L. laryngectomy tube
L. lead
L. lens loop
L. lens scoop
L. leukotome
L. mouthgag
L. nail
L. nasal rasp
L. Pair-Pak needle
L. periosteal elevator
L. recording cystometer
L. retractor
L. septal forceps
L. suspension device
L. tongue depressor
L. tonsillar hemostatic forceps
L. tonsillar screw
L. tonsillar snare
L. ureteral stone isolation forceps
L. vertical slot bracket

Lewis-Leigh positive-pressure nonrebreathing valve

Lewis-Resnik punch

Lewkowitz

L. lithotomy forceps
L. ovum forceps
L. placental forceps

Lewy

L. anterior commissure laryngoscope
L. chest holder
L. laryngoscope holder
L. laryngostat
L. suspension apparatus
L. suspension device
L. suspension laryngoscope

L

NOTES

Lewy *(continued)*
    L. Teflon glycerine-mixture injection needle
    L. Teflon glycerine-mixture syringe
Lewy-Holinger Teflon injection needle
Lewy-Rubin Teflon glycerine-mixture injection needle
Lexan jacket
Lexer
    L. chisel
    L. Durotip dissecting scissors
    L. gouge
    L. osteotome
    L. tissue forceps
Lex-Ton lumbar laminectomy frame
Leycom volume conductance catheter
Leydig drain
Leyla
    L. flexible arm
    L. self-retaining brain retractor
    L. self-retaining tractor bar
Leyla-Yasargil self-retaining retractor
Leyro-Diaz thoracic forceps
Lezinski Flex-HA PORP ossicular chain prosthesis
Lezius suction tube
L-F Uniflex diathermy electrosurgical unit
LGM filter
L-hook electrosurgical probe
Libbe lower bowel evacuation device
Liberator Universal locking stylet
Liberte coronary stent
Liberty
    L. electrical stimulator
    L. One splint
    L. spinal system
    L. thumb brace
Lichtenberg
    L. corneal trephine
    L. keratome
    L. needle holder
Lichtwicz
    L. abdominal trocar
    L. antral cannula
    L. antral needle
    L. antral trocar
Lichtwicz-Bier antral needle
Licox brain tissue oxygen monitoring system
lid
    l. clamp
    l. everter
    l. expressor
    l. forceps
    l. plate
    l. retractor
    l. scalpel
    l. speculum

Liddicoat aortic valve retractor
Liddle aortic clamp
LidFix speculum
Lidge cement gun
Lido
    L. Active Multijoint system
    L. Lift
    L. Multi Joint II isokinetic dynamometer
    L. Passive Multijoint system
    L. WorkSet work simulator
Lidoback isokinetic dynamometry system
Lido-Pen auto-injector
Liebel-Flarsheim CT 9000 contrast delivery system
Lieberman
    L. abrader
    L. aspirating speculum
    L. fragmentor
    L. K-Wire speculum
    L. MicroFinger manipulator
    L. phaco crusher
    L. proctoscope
    L. sigmoidoscope
    L. suturing forceps
    L. tying forceps
Lieberman-Pollock double corneal forceps
Lieb-Guerry
    L.-G. cataract implant lens
    L.-G. forceps
Liebreich probe
Lieppman
    L. microcystitome
    L. sharp cystotome
    L. spatula
Liesegang LM-Flex 7 flexible hysteroscope
LIFE
    laserlight-induced fluorescence endoscopy
Life
    L. Liner stick-resistant and cut-resistant glove
    L. Pack 5 cardiac monitor
    L. Suit
    L. White Light bronchoscope
Life-Air 1000 hypothermic therapy system
Lifecare ventilator
Lifecath
    L. catheter
    L. peritoneal implant
LifeCell AlloDerm acellular dermal graft
Lifecore Restore wide diameter implant system

LifeJet high-flow chronic dialysis catheter
Lifeline electrode
Life-Lok clamp
LIFE-Lung fluorescence endoscopy system
Lifemask infant resuscitator
Lifemed
    L. blood tubing
    L. cannula
    L. catheter
    L. heterologous heart valve
LifeNest portable seating system
Lifepak
    L. defibrillator
    L. 5, 7 monitor
Lifepath AAA endovascular graft system
LifePort
    L. endotracheal tube
    L. endotracheal tube adapter
Lifesaver disposable resuscitator
lifesaving tube
LifeScan blood glucose monitoring system
Lifescope 12 bedside monitor
LifeShirt
    L. continuous ambulatory monitor
    L. system
LifeSite hemodialysis access system
Lifestream
    L. centrifugal pump
    L. coronary dilation catheter
Lifestride treadmill
Life-Tech flowmeter
LifeVest wearable defibrillator
lift
    Adjust-A-Lift heel l.
    BTE dynamic l.
    EasyPivot patient l.
    Grice l.
    heel l.
    Hi-Loo Power l.
    Hoyer l.
    Lido L.
    pneumatic chair l.
    Porto-Lift l.
    Sabina l.
    shoe l.
    Vander-Lift l.
LiftALERT electronic device
lift/commode

lifter
    Gulani ophthalmic edge l.
    Seibel LASIK flap l.
    tissue l.
    waltzing areolar l.
    Yasargil tissue l.
LiF thermoluminescence dosimeter
LiftMate patient transfer device
LiftStation lifting assessment system
Ligaclip
    L. endoscopic clip
    L. MCA multiple-clip applier
    L. surgical clip
ligament
    anterior cruciate l. (ACL)
    l. augmentation device (LAD)
    l. button
    l. chisel probe
    l. clamp
    Dacron mesh synthetic l.
    Zenotech synthetic l.
ligament-grasping forceps
ligamentum
    l. flavum forceps
    l. teres knife
Ligamentus Ankle orthosis
Ligapak suture
Lig-A-Ring separator
LigaSure vessel sealing system
ligate-divide-staple (LDS)
ligating and dividing stapler
ligation device
ligator
    Arrequi laparoscopic knot pusher l.
    Barron hemorrhoidal l.
    Centrix PDQ l.
    Clarke-Reich l.
    endoscopic band l.
    Friction-fit adapter from Stiegmann-Goff endoscopic l.
    Hashizume endoscopic l.
    hemorrhoidal l.
    Injection Superview Speedband l.
    KilRoid single-handed l.
    Lurz-Goltner l.
    McGivney hemorrhoidal l.
    Microvasive Speedband Superview l.
    multiple band l.
    Preston-Hopkins l.
    RapidFire multiple band l.
    rubber band l.

L

NOTES

ligator *(continued)*
  Rudd l.
  Saeed Six-Shooter multiband l.
  Salvatore umbilical cord l.
  Sanford l.
  Scanlan l.
  4,6,10 Shooter Saeed multiband l.
  Speedband multiple-band l.
  Stiegmann-Goff Clearvue
    endoscopic l.
  Tucker hemorrhoidal l.
  Twist-Mate l.
ligature
  l. cannula
  l. carrier
  Desault l.
  l. director
  l. forceps
  l. guide
  l. needle
  l. passer
  Potts l.
  l. scissors
  Speedband l.
  Surgiwip suture l.
  Tahoe Surgical Instruments l.
  l. tie wire
  l. tucker
ligature-carrying forceps
ligatureless bracket
ligature-locking pliers
ligature-passing instrument
light
  l. activation by stimulated emission
    of radiation (LASER)
  Amsco l.
  Barkan l.
  l. carrier
  Castle surgical l.
  Chick surgical l.
  Clar head l.
  Co-Axa l.
  cobalt blue l.
  Cogent l.
  L. Commander xenon illuminator
  CoolSpot l.
  l. cross-slot screwdriver
  dermatologic ultraviolet l.
  EfosLite curing l.
  floor-standing surgical l.
  Floxite mirror l.
  fluorescent pulsed l. (FPL)
  Fotofil l.
  Fragen laryngoscope fiberoptic l.
  Gass neurosurgical l.
  L. headrest
  Landry vein l.
  Lumiwand l.
  Maglite l.

  l. monitoring probe
  Murphy l.
  Optilux 501 curing l.
  overhead l.
  l. pen
  l. pipe
  l. pipette
  Prolite fluorescent pulsed l.
  pulsed l.
  Ringlite fiberoptic l.
  Solar Beam medical examination l.
  L. Talker
  ultraviolet l.
  ViziLite disposable l.
  l. wire appliance
  Witt dental l.
  Wood l.
Lightblade
  Novatec L.
light-curing resin
lighted
  l. retractor
  l. speculum
  l. stent
  l. stylet
light-emitting diode (LED)
Lighthouse ETDRS acuity chart
Lightning high-speed vitrectomy
  handpiece
LighTouch Neonate thermometer
LightRing balloon catheter
LightSheer laser hair removal system
LightSpeed
  L. multidetector CT scanner
  L. QX/i CT scanner
  L. Ultra CT scanner
Lightstic
  CardioFocus L.
  L. fiberoptic laser
Light-Veley
  L.-V. bur
  L.-V. cranial drill
  L.-V. headrest
LightWare retractor
LightWear headlight
Ligmajet syringe
Liguory endoscopic nasal biliary drain
Liko Golvo lift system
Liks Russian disc rotation heart valve
Lilienthal
  L. probe
  L. rib guillotine
  L. rib spreader
Lilienthal-Sauerbruch
  L.-S. retractor
  L.-S. rib spreader
Lillehei
  L. pacemaker

L. retractor
L. valve-grasping forceps
Lillehei-Cruz-Kaster valve prosthesis
Lillehei-Kaster pivoting-disc prosthetic mitral valve
Lillehei-Warden catheter
Lillie
L. antral trocar
L. attic cannula
L. attic hook
L. ear hook
L. frontal sinus probe
L. gouge
L. intestinal forceps
L. nasal speculum
L. rectus tendon clamp
L. retractor
L. rongeur
L. tissue-holding forceps
L. tonsillar knife
L. tonsillar scissors
Lillie-Killian septal forceps
Lilliput neonatal oxygenator
LIMA
left internal mammary artery
LIMA-Lift spreading system
LimaLoop shoe system
LIMAvator chest wall retractor
limb
l. gym
l. holder
l. lead
limbal
l. relaxing incision (LRI)
l. relaxing incision diamond blade
l. relaxing incision marker
limited-contact dynamic compression plate
limiter
Becker 655 motion control l.
LINAC
linear accelerator
LINAC gantry
Varian LINAC
LINAC-based radiosurgical system
Linatrix suture
Lin clamp
Lincoff
L. design of Storz scleral buckling balloon catheter
L. lens sponge
L. scleral sponge implant

L. sponge implant material
L. sponge rod
Lincoln-Metzenbaum scissors
Lincoln pediatric scissors
Lindbergh pump
Linde
L. cryogenic probe
L. cryoprobe
Lindemann
L. bone cutter
L. bur
L. self-retaining uterine vacuum cannula
L. transfusion needle
Lindemann-Silverstein Arrow ventilation tube
Lindholm
L. microlaryngoscope
L. operating laryngoscope
L. tracheal tube
Lindholm-Stille elevator
Lindley
L. needle holder
L. scissors
Lindner
L. anastomosis clamp
L. corneoscleral suture
L. cyclodialysis spatula
L. cyclodialysis spoon
Lindo-Levian dental elevator
Lindorf
L. lag screw
L. position screw
Lindsay-Rea forceps
Lindstrom
L. arcuate incision marker
L. astigmatic marker
L. Centrex lens
L. LASIK flap roller
L. lens-insertion forceps
L. modified J-loop, three-piece reverse PMMA optic intraocular lens
L. Star nucleus manipulator
L. Trident ophthalmic splitter
Lindstrom-Chu aspirating speculum
Lindvall meniscectomy knife
Lindvall-Stille meniscal knife
line
Arrow PICC l.
arterial l.
Hickman l.

L

NOTES

557

line *(continued)*
    ICP monitoring l.
    Intertech Perkin-Elmer gas
      sampling l.
    l. keeper
    oxygen supply l.
    PICC l.
    Wackenheim clivus canal l.
linear
    l. accelerator (LINAC)
    l. accelerator system
    l. accelerator unit
    l. actuator
    l. array echoendoscope
    l. array hydrophone assembly
    l. array transducer
    l. array ultrasound probe
    l. convex array scanner
    l. hearing aid
    L. hip stem
    l. inline ligature carrier
    L. KGT tonometer
    l. 35-MHz transducer
    l. potentiometer
    l. scissor punch
    l. stapler
    l. stapling device
    L. total hip system
    l. transducer
Lineback adenoidal punch
linen suture
liner
    Accents permanent lash l.
    Ardee denture l.
    cast l.
    Cavitec cavity l.
    Cavoline cavity l.
    Copalite cavity l.
    DePuy acetabular l.
    Dignity Plus l.
    elevated rim acetabular l.
    Enduron acetabular l.
    Fillauer prosthesis l.
    Fillauer silicone suspension l.
    Gore cast l.
    Gore-Tex waterproof cast l.
    grommet bone l.
    Hylamer acetabular l.
    Iceross Comfort Plus silicone
      gel l.
    Integrity neutral l.
    Ketac l.
    Maramed ThermoFlex l.
    OrthoGel l.
    Ortho-Wick foam l.
    pantaloon l.
    polyethylene l.
    Polysorb l.
    Procel cast l.

    provisional l.
    Pulpdent cavity l.
    rubber bite l.
    Silosheath gel l.
    splint l.
    TEC l.
    Teflon l.
    Tempo denture l.
    ThermoFlex l.
    Tubulitec cavity l.
    UHMWPe ball l.
Lingeman
    L. kit
    L. 3-in-1 procedure drape
    L. TUR drape
lingoscope
lingual
    l. arch
    l. bar
    l. cortical plate
    l. forceps
    l. spatula
    l. wire
link
    L. acetabular cage
    L. anatomical hip
    L. approximator
    L. Ellis external minifixator
    L. Endo-Model rotational knee
    L. Lubinus AP hip system
    L. Lubinus SP II total hip
      replacement system
    L. microporous hip stem
    L. MP hip noncemented
      reconstruction prosthesis
    L. Saddle Prosthesis Endo-Model
      hip replacement system
    L. stack split splint
    L. toe splint
    Waldmar l.
Linkow
    L. blade implant
    L. dental implant material
Link-Plus retention pin
Linnartz
    L. forceps
    L. intestinal clamp
    L. stomach clamp
Linn-Graefe iris forceps
Linson electronic cell counter
lint-free sponge
Linton
    L. elastic stocking
    L. esophageal tube
    L. splanchnic retractor
    L. tourniquet
    L. vein hook
    L. vein stripper
Linton-Blakemore needle

Linton-Nachlas tube
Lintro-Scan scanner
Linvatec
    L. arthroscopic infusion pump
    L. bioabsorbable interference screw
    L. cannula
    L. cannulated interference screw
    L. driver
    L. meniscal BioStinger anchor
      suture
    L. microdebrider
    L. wrist arthroscopy traction tower
Linvotec microdebrider
Linx
    L. extension wire
    L. guidewire extension
Linx-EZ cardiac device
lion
    l. forceps
    L. hearing aid
    l. jaw bone holder
    l. jaw tenaculum
lion-head clamp
LionHeart
    L. catheter
    L. ventricular assist system
lion-jaw
    l.-j. bone-holding forceps
    l.-j. clamp
Lion's
    L. Claw grasper
    L. Paw grasper
Liotta-BioImplant LPB prosthetic valve
Liotta total artificial heart
lip
    l. clamp
    l. retractor
    l. traction bow
Lipectron
    L. ultrasonic lancet
    L. ultrasonic scalpel
Lipisorb dressing
Lipo-Medi girdle
Lipoprint cholesterol subfraction test
    system
Liposorber cholesterol filter
liposuction
    B.U.S. Endotron-Lipectron
      ultrasonic l.
Lipovacutainer cannister
Lipowitz metal
Lippes loop intrauterine device

Lippman hip prosthesis
Lippy modified prosthesis
Lipschiff knife
Lipschwitz needle
Lipscomb-Anderson drill guide
Lipshultz epididymovasostomy
    microdissection scissors
LiquiBand topical skin tissue adhesive
liquid
    L. Embolic system
    L. Ice
    l. organic dye laser
    l. scintillation spectrometer
    l. scintillation spectrophotometer
    l. vitreous-aspirating cannula
Liquiderm
    L. liquid adhesive
    L. liquid healing bandage
Lisco sponge
Liss
    L. CES device
    L. locking distal femoral plate
Listening Glass hearing aid
Lister
    L. bandage
    L. bandage scissors
    L. conjunctival forceps
    L. dressing
    L. knife
    L. lens manipulator
    L. mules
Lister-Burch eye speculum
List needle
Liston
    L. amputation knife
    L. bone-cutting forceps
    L. phalangeal knife
    L. plaster-of-Paris scissors
    L. shears
    L. splint
Liston-Key bone-cutting forceps
Liston-Key-Horsley
    L.-K.-H. forceps
    L.-K.-H. rib shears
Liston-Littauer
    L.-L. bone-cutting forceps
    L.-L. rongeur
Liston-Luer-Whiting rongeur
Liston-Ruskin shears
Liston-Stille bone-cutting forceps
LiteAire disposable dual-valved holding
    chamber

L

NOTES

Lite blade
Liteflex lens
Lite-Gait partial weight-bearing gait
  therapy device
LiteNest portable seating system
Lite-Pipe
  Millard L.-P.
lithium
  l. iodine battery
  l. pacemaker
lithium-powered pacemaker
LithoCatch stone retrieval device
LithoCath immobilization device
LithoClast
  L. ballistic energy generator
  L. lithotripter
Lithognost flash-lamp pulsed dye laser
Lithospec lithotripter
Lithostar
  L. lithotripsy unit
  L. Plus lithotripter
lithotomy
  l. forceps
  l. legholder
lithotripsy table
lithotripter, lithotriptor
  l. basket
  Breakstone l.
  Calcusplit pneumatic l.
  Calcutript electrohydraulic l.
  Candela laser l.
  Circon ACMI l.
  Compact S l.
  Diasonics Therasonic l.
  Direx Tripter l.
  Direx Tripter X-1 l.
  DoLi S l.
  Dormia gallstone l.
  Dormia waterbath l.
  Dornier compact l.
  Dornier Compact S l.
  Dornier Epos Ultra l.
  Dornier extracorporeal shock
    wave l.
  Dornier HM-series l.
  Dornier MPL 9000 gallstone l.
  Edap LT.2 l.
  electrohydraulic l.
  electromagnetic l.
  extracorporeal piezoelectric l.
  extracorporeal shock wave l.
  gallstone l.
  holmium laser l.
  Impact l.
  Karl Storz l.
  Karl Storz-Lutzeyer l.
  laser l.
  LithoClast l.
  Lithospec l.

Lithostar Plus l.
manual l.
Medispec Econolith spark plug l.
Medstone extracorporeal shock-
  wave l.
Modulith SL 20 l.
MonoLith single-piece mechanical l.
Northgate SD-3 dual-purpose l.
Pentax l.
percutaneous ultrasonic l.
piezoelectric shock wave l.
Piezolith l.
pneumoballistic l.
l. probe
Pulsolith laser l.
second generation l.
shock wave l.
Sonolith Praktis l.
Sonotrode l.
Storz Monolith l.
Swiss LithoClast l.
Therasonics l.
third generation l.
tubeless l.
ultrasonic l.
water cushion l.
lithotriptoscope
  Ravich l.
lithotrite
  Alcock l.
  Bigelow l.
  Hendrickson l.
  Keyes l.
  Löwenstein l.
  Lowsley l.
  Marmite l.
  Ravich l.
  Reliquet l.
  Teale gorget l.
  Wolf l.
Lithovac Master suction and aspiration
system
LITT
  laser-induced thermography
  laser-induced thermotherapy
  LITT applicator
Littauer
  L. bone-cutting forceps
  L. ciliary forceps
  L. dissecting scissors
  L. ear-dressing forceps
  L. ear polyp forceps
  L. nasal-dressing forceps
  L. rongeur
  L. suture scissors
Littauer-Liston bone-cutting forceps
Littauer-West
  L.-W. cutting forceps
  L.-W. rongeur

Littell cannula
Little
  L. cargo vest
  L. intraocular lens implant
  L. Ones pediatric urine collector
  L. Ones Sur-Fit pediatric belt
  L. retractor
Little-Arnott tripod intraocular lens
Littleford Spector introducer
Littleford-Spector introducer
Littler
  L. dissecting scissors
  L. suture-carrying scissors
Littlewood tissue forceps
Littmann
  L. defibrillation pad
  L. ECG electrode
  L. galilean magnification changer
Litton dental handpiece
Litvak-Pereyra ligature needle
Litwak
  L. cannula
  L. clamp
  L. mitral valve scissors
Litwin scissors
liver
  l. biopsy needle
  l. coil
  HepatAssist bioartificial l.
  l. retractor
Livermore trocar
Livernois
  L. lens-holding forceps
  L. pickup and folding forceps
Livernois-McDonald forceps
Liverpool
  L. elbow implant
  L. knee prosthesis
  L. radial head replacement
Livewire
  L. Duo-Decapolar catheter
  L. TC ablation catheter
  L. TC Compass ablation catheter
Living Air XL-15 unit
Livingston
  L. forceps
  L. intramedullary bar
  L. peribulbar wedge
Lixiscope
  L. inspection device
  L. pocket-size x-ray imaging
  system

LKB/Wallach 1277 automatic gamma counter
LLETZ
  large loop excision of transformation
  zone
  large loop excision of transition zone
  LLETZ loop electrode
Llobera fixation forceps
Llorente dissecting forceps
Lloyd
  L. adapter
  L. bronchial catheter
  L. chiropractic table
  L. double catheter
  L. esophagoscopic catheter
  L. flexion/distraction table
  L. nail driver
  L. nail extractor
Lloyd-Davies
  L.-D. clamp
  L.-D. occlusion forceps
  L.-D. rectal scissors
  L.-D. sigmoidoscope
  L.-D. stirrups
LMA-Unique disposable laryngeal mask
  airway
L'Nard
  L. boot
  L. long opponens hand and wrist
  orthosis
  L. Multi-Podus orthosis
  L. thoracolumbosacral orthosis
Lo
  L. Bak spinal support
  L. Rider prosthetic foot
loader
  Lehner II l.
  Nichamin II ophthalmic l.
lobectomy
  l. forceps
  l. scissors
lobe-grasping forceps
lobe-holding forceps
Lobenstein-Tarnier forceps
lobotomy
  l. electrode
  l. needle
lobster-tail catheter
local
  l. gradient coil
  l. irradiation (LX)
Localisa cardiac navigation system

L

NOTES

localizer
Berman l.
FlashPoint optical l.
Risser l.
Roper-Hall l.
Suetens-Gybels-Vandermeulen
angiographic l.

localizing
l. electrode
l. probe

LocalMed
L. catheter infusion sleeve
L. InfusaSleeve

locator
Berman l.
Berman foreign body l.
Bronson-Turner foreign body l.
foreign body l.
Gill-Thomas l.
Neosono MC apex l.
Neuro-Pulse nerve l.
Odontometer electronic apex l.
Porex nerve l.
Root ZX apex l.
Roper-Hall foreign body l.
saddle l.
Staodyn Insight point l.
Sweet l.
ToDyeFor root canal l.

Loc guidewire extension

lock
L. Clamshell device
English l.
French l.
heparin l.
Howland l.
Icex 4-hole l.
Luer cannula l.
l. needle
Össur VariLock modular socket l.
pivot l.
sliding l.

Locke
L. bone clamp
L. clamp

Lockhart-Mummery
L.-M. probe
L.-M. retractor

lock-in amplifier

locking
Anatomic Medullary L. (AML)
l. clamp
l. device
l. nut
l. peg
l. prosthesis
l. reconstruction plate
l. screw
l. stylet

LockJaw
L. arch bar
L. dental bonding arch

Lockwood
L. clamp
L. intestinal forceps
L. tissue forceps

Lockwood-Allis
L.-A. intestinal forceps
L.-A. tissue forceps

Loc-Light lumbar support belt

Loewi suspension device

Lofberg
L. thyroid retractor
L. vaginal speculum

Lofric disposable urethral catheter

Lofstrand
L. brace
L. crutch

log
Fin & Flipper exercise l.

Logan
L. dissector
L. lacrimal sac self-retaining
retractor
L. lip traction bow
L. periosteal elevator

LogiCal pressure transducer system

logMAR chart

Lok-it screwdriver

Lok-Mesh bonding base

Lok-screw double-slot screwdriver

lollipop stick

Lombard-Beyer
L.-B. forceps
L.-B. rongeur

Lombard-Boise mastoid rongeur

Lombard rongeur

Lombart
L. radioscope
L. tonometer

Londermann corneal trephine

London
L. College foil carrier
L. narrow-bladed retractor
L. tissue forceps

Lone Star retractor

long
l. above-elbow cast
l. arm navicular cast
l. arm splint
L. Beach stereotactic robot
l. below-elbow cast
L. Brite Tip guiding catheter
l. double upright brace
L. Island College Hospital
placental forceps
l. leg brace
l. leg cylinder cast

l. leg immobilizer
l. leg plaster cast
l. leg posterior molded splint
l. leg splint
l. leg walking cast
l. nail-mounted drill guide
l. needle
l. scalpel
L. Skinny over-the-wire balloon
catheter
l. taper shaft Glidewire
l. tissue forceps
Long45 endocutter
long-bore collimator
Longdwel
L. catheter needle
L. Teflon catheter
Longevity V-Lign hip prosthesis
long-handle offset gouge
Longmire-Mueller curved valvulotome
Longmire-Storm clamp
Longmire valvulotome
long-term
l.-t. ambulatory physiologic
surveillance monitor
l.-t. internal jugular catheter
long-wearing contact lens
Lonnecken tube
Look
L. capsular polisher
L. cortex extractor
L. cystotome
L. I&A coaxial cannula
L. irrigating lens loop
L. irrigating vectis
L. micropuncture device
L. retrobulbar needle
L. suture
loop
Adler tripronged lens l.
Amenabar lens l.
2-angled polypropylene l.
Atwood l.
Aus-Jena-Gullstrand lens l.
Axenfeld nerve l.
l. ball electrode
Beck twisted wire snare l.
Beebe lens l.
Berens lens l.
Berger l.
Berget lens l.
Billeau ear l.

Billeau-House ear l.
bipolar cutting l.
bipolar urological l.
Blair-Ivy l.
Bunnell finger l.
Callahan lens l.
Cannon endarterectomy l.
Castroviejo lens l.
Clayman-Knolle irrigating lens l.
cutting l.
Diaflex retrieval l.
Duncan l.
ear l.
l. electrode
l. electrosurgical excision procedure
(LEEP)
Elschnig-Weber l.
finger l.
Flynn lens l.
foreign body l.
FormFlex lens l.
Gerdy interatrial l.
Gills-Welsh-Morrison lens l.
Gill-Welsh lens l.
Greenwald cutting l.
l. & hook strapping
House-Billeau ear l.
House wire l.
intracapsular lens l.
irrigating lens l.
irrigating vectis l.
Ivy l.
Keener-Arlt lens l.
Kirby intracapsular lens l.
Kirby intraocular lens l.
Kleinsasser lens l.
Knapp lens l.
Knolle-Pearce irrigating lens l.
Kraff nucleus lens l.
Lemoine-Searcy fixation anchor l.
Lempert-Storz lens l.
lens l.
Lewis lens l.
Look irrigating lens l.
McKenzie leukotomy l.
Medevice surgical l.
Meyer temporal l.
l. monitor
nucleus delivery l.
nucleus removal l.
nylon l.
Oculus lens l.

L

NOTES

loop *(continued)*
    Olympus resectoscope l.
    Pearce-Knolle irrigating lens l.
    physiologic endometrial
      ablation/resection l. (PEARL)
    pressure length l.
    Ransford l.
    l. retractor
    Retract-O-Tape surgical vessel l.
    retrieval l.
    l. scaler
    l. scissors
    l. shunt
    Simcoe double-end lens l.
    Simcoe II posterior chamber
      nucleus delivery l.
    Simcoe nucleus lens l.
    Snellen lens l.
    soft wire l.
    spring wire l.
    Stierlen lens l.
    Storz Universal lens l.
    Surg-I-Loop silicone l.
    Surgitite ligating l.
    Teflon Silastic l.
    tenaculum hook l.
    toe l.
    Torchia vectis l.
    tri-pronged l.
    unipolar cutting l.
    UreSil radiopaque silicone-band
      vessel l.
    vaginal speculum l.
    vascular l.
    vectis l.
    Vedder l.
    vessel l.
    Visitec nucleus removal l.
    V. Mueller vascular l.
    Ward-Lempert lens l.
    Weber-Elschnig lens l.
    Weber lens l.
    Wilder lens l.
    wire l.
    Zein l.

4-loop
    4-l. iris clip implant
    4-l. iris fixated implant

Loopuyt needle

loose
    l. body grasper
    l. body suction forceps

Lopez enteral valve
Lopez-Reinke tonsillar dissector
Lo-Por
    L.-P. tracheal tube
    L.-P. vascular graft

LoPresti
    L. fiberoptic esophagoscope
    L. panendoscope
Lo-Profile
    L.-P. II steerable dilatation catheter
    L.-P. tracheostomy tube
    L.-P. urostomy pouch
Loptex laser intraocular lens implant
Lorad
    L. M-IV mammography system
    L. Selenia full-field digital
      mammography system
Lord
    L. cup
    L. total hip prosthesis
Lordan chalazion forceps
Lord-Blakemore tube
Lordex lumbar spine system
Lordoticiser exerciser
Lore
    L. subglottic forceps
    L. suction tube
Lore-Lawrence tracheotomy tube
Lorenz
    L. Blue multi-vector external
      distraction device
    L. brace
    L. chisel
    L. gauze packer
    L. Micro-Power dense bone drilling
      and cutting system
    L. osteosynthesis system
    L. PC/TC scissors
    L. plating system
    L. reamer
    L. screw
    L. SMO prosthesis
    L. titanium screws and plate
Lorez PC/TC ultra-sharp knife
lorgnette occluder
Lorie
    L. antral trephine
    L. cheek retractor
Loring ophthalmoscope
Lorna-Edna
    L.-E. towel clamp
    L.-E. towel forceps
Lorna non-perforating towel clamp
Loth-Kirschner drill
Lothrop
    L. dissector
    L. hemostat
    L. ligature forceps
    L. tonsillar knife
    L. tonsillar retractor
    L. uvular retractor
Lo-Trau side-cutting needle
Lottes
    L. pin

L. reamer
L. triflange intramedullary nail
Loughnane prostatic hook
Louis instrumentation
Louisville elevator
Lounsbury placental curette
loupe
Arlt lens l.
Bausch & Lomb Duoloupe lens l.
binocular l.
Callahan lens l.
Castroviejo lens l.
Codman magnifying l.
corneal monocular l.
Daviel lens l.
Elschnig-Weber l.
fiberoptic l.
Galilean l.
Gullstrand lens l.
Gullstrand-Zeiss lens l.
Keeler-Galilean surgical l.
Keeler panoramic l.
Keeler spotlight lens l.
Keeler wide-angle lens l.
Lemoine-Searcy fixation anchor l.
Lempert-Storz l.
lens l.
Magill magnifying l.
l. magnification
Magni-Focuser lens l.
magnifying l.
Mark II Magni-Focuser l.
May hook-on lens l.
microloupe l.
monocular l.
New Orleans lens l.
ocular Gamboscope l.
Ono l.
operating l.
Opticaid lens l.
Opt-Visor l.
panoramic l.
prism l.
surgical l.
Troutman lens l.
Wilder l.
Zeiss-Gullstrand l.
Zeiss lens l.
Zeiss operating field l.
Lours leukotome
Loute wire tightener

Lovac
L. fundal contact lens
L. gonioscopic lens
L. 6-mirror gonioscopic lens
Love
L. leukotome
L. nasal splint
L. nasopharyngeal retractor
L. nerve root retractor
L. pituitary rongeur
L. uvula retractor
Love-Adson periosteal elevator
Love-Gruenwald
L.-G. alligator forceps
L.-G. cranial rongeur
L.-G. intervener
L.-G. intervertebral disc rongeur
L.-G. laminectomy rongeur
L.-G. pituitary forceps
L.-G. pituitary rongeur
Lovejoy retractor
Love-Kerrison
L.-K. rongeur
L.-K. rongeur forceps
Lovelace
L. bladder forceps
L. gallbladder traction forceps
L. hemostatic forceps
L. lung-grasping forceps
L. thyroid-traction vulsellum forceps
L. tissue forceps
L. traction lung forceps
L. traction tissue forceps
Loversan infusion set
Lovitt-Uhler postfusion brace
low
l. impedance thermocouple
L. Profile legholder
L. Profile PMV 2001 purple tracheostomy
L. Profile walker
low-air-loss
l.-a.-l. bed
l.-a.-l. mattress
Löw-Beer forceps
low-compliance balloon
low-contact
l.-c. dynamic compression plate
l.-c. stress (LCS)
l.-c. stress plate

L

NOTES

LowDye
 L. strapping
 L. taping
Lowe-Breck cartilage knife
Lowell
 L. glaucoma knife
 L. pleural needle
Lowe microtome knife
Löwenberg forceps
low-energy
 l.-e. laser
 l.-e. ultra-high resolution (LEUHR)
 l.-e. ultra high-resolution fan-beam
  collimator
Löwenstein lithotrite
lower
 l. extremity mobility aid (LEMA)
 l. extremity mobility aid strap
 l. gall duct forceps
 l. lateral forceps
 l. limb prosthesis
Lowette needle
Lowette-Verner needle
low-field MR scanner
low-flow
 l.-f. circuit
 l.-f. regulator
low-flux cuprammonium dialyzer
Lowis
 L. intervertebral disc forceps
 L. periosteal elevator
Lowman
 L. bone-holding clamp
 L. bone-holding forceps
 L. chisel
 L. hand retractor
 L. rongeur
Lowman-Gerster bone clamp
Lowman-Hoglund
 L.-H. chisel
 L.-H. clamp
Lown cardioverter
low-pass filter
low-pressure
 l.-p. plasma-sprayed (LPPS)
 l.-p. voice prosthesis
low-profile
 l.-p. angioplasty balloon
 l.-p. balloon-positioning catheter
 l.-p. breast implant
 l.-p. mitral heart valve
 l.-p. plastic body jacket
 l.-p. prosthesis
 l.-p. R-K marker
low-quarter Blucher shoe
low-resistance rolling seal spirometer
Lowsley
 L. grasping forceps
 L. hemostat

 L. lithotrite
 L. prostate retractor
 L. prostatic forceps
 L. prostatic tractor
 L. retractor with hand-sutured
  closure
 L. ribbon-gut needle
 L. stone crusher
 L. suprapubic tractor
 L. urethroscope
Lowsley-Luc forceps
Lowsley-Peterson
 L.-P. cystoscope
 L.-P. endoscope
low-speed
 l.-s. Christmas tree diamond bur
 l.-s. rotation angioplasty catheter
 l.-s. tapered carbide bur
low-vacuum contact lens
low-viscosity bone cement
low-vision aid
LPK-80 II argon laser
L-plate
 L-p. plate
 Synthes mini L-p.
LPPS
 low-pressure plasma-sprayed
 LPPS hydroxyapatite
 LPPS hydroxyapatite adhesive
LRI
 limbal relaxing incision
 LRI diamond blade
 LRI marker
L-rod
 L-r. implant material
 L-r. instrumentation
 Luque L-r.
LSC 7000 curved array transducer
L-shaped
 L-s. aneurysm clip
 L-s. cautery
 L-s. elevator
 L-s. miniplate
 L-s. plate
LSI
 LSI Gold self-adhesive electrode
 LSI Silver self-adhesive electrode
LSK One microkeratome
**LSM-2100C Eye Bank specular
 microscope**
LSU reciprocation-gait orthosis
LT-cage lumbar tapered fusion device
L.T. Jones tear duct tube
LTK
 laser thermal keratoplasty
LTV800 ventilator
LTX PTCA catheter
Lubafax dressing

Lubinus
L. acetabular component
L. AP hip system
L. knee prosthesis
L. SP II hip stem
L. SP II hip system

Lübke uterine vacuum cannula
Lubri-Flex ureteral stent
Lubriglide coated guidewire
Luc
L. ethmoidal forceps
L. nasal-cutting forceps
L. septal forceps
L. septum-cutting forceps

Lucae
L. bayonet
L. bayonet dressing forceps
L. bayonet ear forceps
L. bayonet tissue forceps
L. dissecting forceps
L. ear perforation knife
L. ear probe
L. ear speculum
L. eustachian catheter
L. hook
L. mastoid mallet

Lucas
L. alveolar curette
L. chisel
L. gouge

Lucchese mitral valve dilator
lucite sphere implant
Luck
L. bone drill
L. bone saw
L. fasciatome

Luck-Bishop saw
Lu corneal marker
Ludwig
L. middle ear applicator
L. sinus applicator

Luedde exophthalmometer
Luer
L. bone curette
L. bone rongeur
L. cannula lock
L. connection
L. connector
L. curette forceps
L. double-ended tracheal retractor
L. eye speculum
L. hemorrhoidal forceps

L. lock fitting
L. mallet
L. needle
positioner L.
L. retractor
L. rongeur forceps
L. scoop
L. speaking tube
L. S-shaped retractor
L. suction cannula adapter
L. syringe
L. thoracic rongeur
L. tracheal cannula
L. tracheal tube

Luer-Friedman bone rongeur
Luer-Hartmann rongeur
Luer-Koerte gallstone scoop
Luer-Liston-Wheeling rongeur
Luer-Lok
L.-L. adapter
L.-L. B-D syringe
L.-L. jet ventilator connector
L.-L. male adapter plug
L.-L. needle
L.-L. port
L.-L. stopcock

Luer-Stille rongeur
Luer-Whiting
L.-W. forceps
L.-W. rongeur
L.-W. rongeur forceps

Luetje stimulating dissector
Luhr
L. fixation plate
L. implant
L. implant screw
L. mandibular plate
L. maxillofacial fixation system
L. MCS bone plate
L. microbone plate
L. microfixation cranial plate
L. microfixation system
L. microfixation system drill bit
L. microfixation system plate cutter
L. microfixation system plate-
holding forceps
L. microfixation system pliers
L. microplate
L. minifixation bone plate
L. miniplate
L. MRS system
L. pan fixation system

L

NOTES

Luhr *(continued)*
    L. pan plate
    L. Vitallium micromesh plate
    L. Vitallium screw
Luikart-Bill
    L.-B. forceps
    L.-B. traction handle
Luikart forceps
Luikart-Kjelland obstetrical forceps
Luikart-McLane obstetrical forceps
Luikart-Simpson obstetrical forceps
Lukens
    L. aspirator
    L. bone wax dressing
    L. cannula
    L. catgut suture
    L. collecting tube
    L. collector
    L. double-channel irrigator
    L. double-ended tracheal retractor
    L. epiglottic retractor
    L. needle
    L. orthodontic band
    L. thymus retractor
    L. trap
Lulu clamp
Luma cervical imaging system
Lumaguide infusion catheter
lumbar
    l. anterior root stimulator implant
    l. aortography needle
    l. corset
    l. external drainage system
    l. interbody fusion cage
    l. interbody fusion kit
    l. intersomatic fusion expandable
    cage
    l. orthosis
    l. pedicle screw
    l. port
    l. puncture needle
    l. retractor
    l. roll
Lumbard airway
lumbosacral
    l. corset
    l. fusion elevator
    l. orthosis
    l. spine transpedicular
    instrumentation
    l. support pelvic traction
lumbotomy retractor
lumbrical bar
Lumelec pacing catheter
lumen
    l. cannula
    l. finder
Lumenator injectable guidewire
LuMend Frontrunner CTO catheter

4-lumen polyvinyl manometric catheter
Lumex
    L. lightweight wheelchair
    L. Preferred Care recliner
    L. shower bed
    L. shower stretcher
    L. Tilt-in-Space reclining
    wheelchair
    L. walker
Lumi alloy
Lumina
    L. guidewire
    L. operating telescope
    L. rod lens arthroscope
luminal stent
Lumina-SL telescope
Luminexx biliary stent
Lumin laparoscopic uterine manipulator
    injector
luminometer
    LB 9501 l.
Lumiscan scanner
Lumisys scanner
Lumiwand light
Lumix dental x-ray unit
Lumonics YAG laser
Lunar
    L. Artoscan M-series magnetic
    resonance imaging
    L. DPX densitometer
    L. DPX dual-energy absorptiometer
    L. DPX total-body scanner
    L. Expert densitometer
lunate
    l. implant
    l. prosthesis
Lunax boot
Lund-Dodick punch
Lunderquist
    L. catheter
    L. coat hanger wire
    L. extra-stiff wire guide
    L. guidewire
Lunderquist-Ring torque wire guide
Lundholm
    L. plate
    L. screw
Lundia dialyzer holder
Lundsgaard
    L. blade
    L. knife
    L. rasp
    L. sclerotome
Lundsgaard-Burch
    L.-B. corneal rasp
    L.-B. knife
    L.-B. sclerotome
Lundy
    L. fascial needle

L. laryngoscope
L. tubing hand-roller
Lundy-Irving caudal needle
Luneau retinoscopy rack
lung
artificial l.
l. dissecting scissors
l. exclusion clamp
l. forceps
l. imaging fluorescence endoscope
iron l.
membrane artificial l.
l. retractor
l. tissue forceps
lung-grasping forceps
Luntz-Dodick punch
Luomanen oral airway
Luongo
L. curette
L. hand retractor
L. needle
L. septal elevator
L. sphenoid irrigating cannula
Luque
L. cerclage wire
L. fixation device
L. II plate
L. II screw
L. L-rod
L. rectangle
L. rod
L. semirigid segmental spinal
    instrumentation
L. sublaminar wire
Lurz-Goltner ligator
Lusskin
L. bone drill
L. subungual hematoma iron
Luther-Peter
L.-P. lid everter
L.-P. lid retractor
Lutz
L. automatic reprocessor
L. septal forceps
Luxar
L. NovaPulse CO_2 laser
L. Silhouette noninvasive body
    appearance equipment
Luxation patellar saw
Luxator extractor
Lux culture dish

Luxo
L. illuminated magnifier
L. surgical illuminator
Luxtec
L. fiberoptic system
L. illuminated surgical telescope
L. surgical telescope
Luys separator
LV
left ventricular
LV apex cannula
LVAD
left ventricular assist device
vented-electric HeartMate LVAD
LVAS
left ventricular assist system
LVAS implantable pump
LX
local irradiation
LX 20 laser system
LX needle
Lyda-Ivalon-Lucite implant
Lyman-Smith
L.-S. toe drop brace
L.-S. tractor
Lymphapress compression pump
LymphoScan nuclear imaging system
Lymwrap lymphedema bandaging kit
Lynch
L. blunt dissector
L. cup-shaped curette forceps
L. curette
L. electrode
L. laryngeal dissector
L. laryngeal forceps
L. laryngeal knife handle
L. mucosa separator plate
L. obtuse-angle laryngeal knife
L. scissors
L. septal splint
L. spatula
L. suspension apparatus
L. suspension laryngoscope
L. tonsillar dissector
L. tonsillar knife
Lynco
L. biomechanical orthotic system
L. foot orthosis
Lynell intraocular lens
Lynx
L. orthosis
L. OTW catheter

L

NOTES

Lyodura dura mater graft
LYOfoam A, C, T water resistant
  dressing
Lyon
  L. forceps
  L. ring
  L. tube
lyophilized graft
Lyra
  L. implantable cardioverter-
    defibrillator
  L. laser

Lyrelle patch
lyre-shaped finger hook
LySonix
  L. 250 aspirator
  L. Delta Tip irrigator
  L. TTD cannula system
Lyster water bag
Lyte Fit orthotic
Lytle metacarpal splint

3M

3M Clean Seals waterproof bandage
3M Coban LF self-adherent wrap
3M drape
3M filling instrument
3M intraocular lens
3M limb isolation bag
3M mammary implant
3M matrix tape
3M Microdon dressing
3M Micropore surgical tape
3M microvascular anastomotic coupling device
3M No Sting barrier film
3M Reston self-adhering foam roll
3M scanner
3M small aperture Steri-Drape drape
3M SoftCloth adhesive wound dressing
3M Tegaderm HP high MVTR transparent dressing
3M Tegaderm transparent dressing with absorbent pad
3M Tegapore wound contact material
3M Tegasorb hydrocolloid dressing
3M Vi-drape

M4

M4 Kerr Safety Hedstrom instrument
M4 rigid fixation system
M4 safety handpiece

M2a-taper metal-on-metal hip system prosthesis

MAC

multiaccess catheter
MAC cervical collar

Macaluso stent remover

MacAusland

M. bone mallet
M. chisel
M. dissector
M. finishing-ball reamer
M. finishing-cup reamer
M. hip skid
M. muscle retractor

MacAusland-Kelly retractor
Macbeth ColorChecker
MacCallum knife
MacCarty forceps
MacDonald

M. dissector

M. gastric clamp
M. periosteal elevator

Macewen

M. drill
M. saw

Macey tendon carrier

MacGregor

M. conjunctival forceps
M. mules
M. osteotome

MA 53 2-channel audiometer

Machat

M. adjustable aspirating wire speculum
M. double-ended marker
M. superior flap LASIK marker

Machemer

M. calipers
M. diamond-dust-coated foreign body forceps
M. diamond-dusted forceps
M. flat lens
M. infusion contact lens
M. magnifying vitrectomy lens
M. scleral knife
M. VISC vitrector
M. vitreous cutter

Machida

M. fiberoptic laryngoscope
M. flexible endoscope
M. light source connector
M. nasolaryngoscope

machine

Accuray Neurotron 1000 m.
Acoma portable x-ray m.
Aestiva/5 MRI anesthesia m.
AK-10 dialysis m.
Aloka echocardiograph m.
Aquatic Bike aquatic therapy m.
Berkeley suction m.
Biodex isokinetic testing m.
B-mode ultrasound m.
Borazon blade cutting m.
Brown-Bovari m.
Burdick Eclipse ECG m.
bypass m.
CamStar 8-way cervical exercise m.
cardiopulmonary bypass m.
Cavitron m.
Cavitron-Kelman phacoemulsification m.
Century heart lung m.
cobalt megavoltage m.
Cobe-Stockert heart-lung m.

M

machine *(continued)*
constant passive-motion m.
cooling m.
Corometrics Aloka ultrasound m.
Corometrics Model 900SC in-office
mammography m.
CPM m.
Crafoord-Senning heart-lung m.
Danniflex CPM m.
demand flow m.
DermaScan m.
Diapulse m.
Diapulse electromagnetic therapy m.
2-dimensional ultrasound m.
Drake-Willock dialysis m.
endoscopic sewing m.
Endotek m.
Epilatron hair-removal m.
Exerstrider m.
Faxitron x-ray m.
F&F m.
Finapres Dinamap blood
pressure m.
focused, segmented, ultrasound m.
Fresenius dialysis m.
Gambro AK10 m.
General Electric Pass-C
echocardiograph m.
G5 massage and percussion m.
HemoTec ACT m.
Hewlett-Packard Echo-Doppler m.
Hicor angiography m.
Hoist 4400 exercise m.
I&A m.
Instron m.
Intagortor MS-126 Foot
Circulation m.
intermittent demand flow m.
intermittent flow m.
isotonic m.
Kinetec hip CPM m.
Kurzweil reading m.
Mayo-Gibbon heart-lung m.
Med-Fit Senior Circuit m.
Medicamat ultrasound-assisted
lipoplasty m.
MedX functional testing m.
MedX knee m.
MedX Mark II lumbar
extension m.
MedX stretch m.
MegaPeel microdermabrasion m.
megavoltage m.
Morwel ultrasound-assisted
lipoplasty m.
Narco esophageal motility m.
Narkomed anesthesia m.
NervePace nerve conduction
testing m.

neutron therapy m.
NightBird nasal CPAP m.
Orthion traction m.
Orthopantomograph-series panoramic
x-ray m.
OssaTron orthopaedic shockwave
treatment m.
OsteoPower drilling and cutting m.
Panelipse panoramic x-ray m.
Panex-E panoramic x-ray m.
Panorex panoramic x-ray m.
PC-1000 panoramic x-ray m.
Philips ultrasound m.
Portadial kidney m.
Primus prostate m.
Respironics CPAP m.
Respitrace m.
Rife m.
Rotograph Plus dental
radiography m.
SDU-400 EchoView ultrasound m.
Sebbin ultrasound-assisted
lipoplasty m.
Senographe 2000D
mammography m.
Siemens Hicor angiography m.
SMEI ultrasound-assisted
lipoplasty m.
Stat Scrub handwasher m.
Status-X m.
Surgitron ultrasound-assisted
lipoplasty m.
Swing exerciser m.
TENS m.
Toshiba echocardiography m.
Toshiba electrocardiography m.
transcutaneous electrical nerve
stimulation m.
Vasa Trainer exercise m.
VersaClimber exercise m.
Visual-Tech m.
Water Bike aquatic therapy m.
Wikco ankle m.
Machlett collimator
Macima reusable underpad
MacIntosh
M. blocker
M. fiberoptic laryngoscope blade
M. implant
M. laryngoscope
M. tibial plateau prosthesis
Maciol suture needle set
Mack
M. ear plug
M. lingual tonsillar tonsillectome
M. serrefine
M. tonometer

MacKay
- M. contour self-retaining retractor
- M. nasal splint

MacKay-Marg tonometer

MacKenty
- M. cleft palate knife
- M. laryngectomy tube
- M. periosteal elevator
- M. scissors
- M. septal elevator
- M. sphenoidal punch
- M. tissue forceps

MacKenty-Converse periosteal elevator

Mackenzie polygraph

Mackinnon-Dellon Disc-Criminator

Mackler intraluminal tube

MacKool capsular retractor

Mackray short-cuffed endobronchial tube

Mack's earplug

Maclaren mobile buggy

Maclay tonsillar scissors

Mac-Lee enema bag

Mac-Loc Ultrathane Cope nephroureterectomy stent

Macmed pediatric intramedullary nail

MacNab-English shoulder prosthesis

MacNamara cataract spoon

Macon Hospital speculum

MacQuigg-Mixter forceps

MacRae flap flipper

Macro-5 camera

Macroduct system

Macrofit hip prosthesis

Macroplastique implantable device

MacroPore OS reconstruction system

Macropro Beta-Glucan gel dressing

MacroSorb
- M. PowerBath
- M. PowerPen
- M. PS macroporous protective sheet
- M. StarBurst surgical screw
- M. surgical screwdriver

macular contact lens

Macula retinoscope

MaculoScope

MacVicar double-end strabismus retractor

MAC-Vu electrocardiograph

MadaJet XL jet-injection anesthesia system

Madayag biopsy needle

Maddacare child bath seat

Maddacrawler prone support walker

Maddapult Asissto-Seat

Madden
- M. dissector
- M. forceps
- M. intestinal clamp
- M. ligature carrier
- M. sympathectomy hook

Madden-Potts
- M.-P. intestinal forceps
- M.-P. tissue forceps

Maddox
- M. caudal needle
- M. cheiroscope
- M. LASIK spatula
- M. prism
- M. rod
- M. rod occluder

Madlab conjunctival retractor

Madoff suction tube

madreporic
- m. coral
- m. hip prosthesis

Madsen OB822 clinical audiometer

Maestro
- M. implantable cardiac pacemaker
- M. MRI system

MAFO
- molded ankle-foot orthosis
- MAFO cane

Magellan monitor

Magerl
- M. hook-plate system
- M. plate-screw system

Maggi disposable biopsy needle guide

Magic
- M. microcatheter
- M. Torque guidewire
- M. Wallstent stent
- M. Wand vibrator

Magicap
- Coltene M.

MagicFil dual-curing compomer

Magic-Wall stent

Magielski
- M. bayonet canal knife
- M. coagulating forceps
- M. coagulation cautery
- M. coagulator
- M. elevator

M

NOTES

m. resonance imaging-guided
 focused ultrasound sector
 transducer
m. resonance imaging scan
m. resonance neurography (MRN)
m. resonance spectroscopy
m. retriever
m. shielded cabin
m. source imaging
m. stimulator
m. support belt
M. Surgery system
m. wrap
magnetically activated cell sorter
magnetoencephalography (MEG)
Magnetom
M. Open MRI system
M. SP MRI imager
M. Symphony whole-body scanner
magnetometer probe
Magnetrode cervical unit
Magnetron MRI system
magnet-tipped flexible catheter
Magnex
M. Alpha MR system
M. magnet
M. MR scanner
MagneZorb magnetic heel cushion
magnification
loupe m.
magnifier
anastigmatic aural m.
aural m.
Bruening Japanese anastigmatic
 aural m.
Bruening-Storz anastigmatic
 aural m.
Japanese Bruening anastigmatic
 aural m.
Luxo illuminated m.
Optelec Passport m.
Storz-Bruening anastigmatic
 aural m.
Magni-Focuser lens loupe
magnifying
m. colonoscope
m. glasses
m. loupe
Magni-Viewer
PC M.-V.
Magnum
M. bariatric bed

M. chisel
M. curette
M. guidewire
M. 101 Plus table
M. stimulator
M. wire
Magnum-Meier system
Magnuson
M. abduction humeral splint
M. circular twin saw
M. double counter-rotating saw
M. single circular saw
M. strut
M. twist drill
M. valve prosthesis
Magovern-Cromie ball-cage prosthetic
valve
Magovern heart valve
Magrina-Bookwalter
M.-B. vaginal Deaver blade
M.-B. vaginal retractor
Magstim 200 stimulator
Maguire-Harvey vitreous cutter
Mahnstrom cup
Mahoney
M. dilator
M. intranasal antral speculum
Mahorner
M. dilator
M. thyroid retractor
Mahurkar
M. dual-lumen femoral dialysis
 catheter
M. fistular needle
Maico Gamma hearing aid
Maico-MA 20 audiometer
Maidera-Stern suture hook
Maier
M. dressing forceps
M. polyp forceps
M. sponge forceps
M. uterine forceps
Mailler
M. colon forceps
M. cut-off forceps
M. intestinal forceps
M. rectal forceps
main
m. pancreatic duct (MPD)
m. pancreatic duct stent
Maine gonioscope

M

NOTES

575

Maingot
- M. clamp
- M. gallbladder tube
- M. hysterectomy forceps

Mainstay
- M. soft tissue anchor
- M. urologic soft tissue anchor

Mainster
- M. retinal laser lens
- M. Ultra Field PRP laser lens
- M. wide-field lens

Mainster-HM retinal laser lens
Mainster-S retinal laser lens
Mainster-WF retinal laser lens
maintainer
- anterior chamber m.
- Blumenthal anterior chamber m.
- filter m.
- Lewicky self-retaining chamber m.
- self-retaining chamber m.

Mainz
- M. pouch
- M. pouch urinary reservoir

Maisonneuve
- M. bandage
- M. urethrotome

Maison retractor
Majewski nasal curette
Major amblyoscope
Makar coagulator
maker
- Diamond pocket m.

Maki scissors
Maklakoff tonometer
Makler
- M. cannula
- M. insemination device
- M. reusable semen analysis chamber
- M. sperm counting device

Mako shaver blade
Mala-paedic shoe
malar
- m. implant
- m. periosteum-SMAS flap fixation suture

Malcolm-Lynn
- M.-L. C-RXF cervical retractor frame
- M.-L. radiolucent spinal retraction system

Malcolm-Rand
- M.-R. carbon-composite headholder
- M.-R. cranial x-ray frame
- M.-R. radiolucent headrest and retraction system

male
- m. compression girdle

- m. urinal
- m. washer

Malecot
- M. nephrostomy catheter
- M. nephrostomy tube
- M. self-retaining urethral catheter
- M. Silastic catheter
- M. suprapubic cystostomy catheter
- M. 2-wing catheter
- M. 4-wing catheter
- M. 2-wing drain
- M. 4-wing drain

Malette-Spencer coronary cannula
malformation
- arteriovenous m. (AVM)

Malgaigne
- M. apparatus
- M. clamp
- M. patellar hook

Malibu cervical orthosis
Malik cystic duct catheter clamp
Maliniac
- M. nasal brace
- M. nasal rasp
- M. nasal retractor

Malis
- M. angled bayonet forceps
- M. bipolar coagulating/cutting system
- M. bipolar coagulation forceps
- M. bipolar coagulator
- M. bipolar cutting forceps
- M. bipolar instrument
- M. bipolar irrigating forceps
- M. bipolar microcoagulator
- M. brain retractor kit
- M. cerebellar retractor
- M. cerebral retractor
- M. clip applier
- M. CMC-III electrosurgical system
- M. CMC-II PC bipolar coagulator
- M. cup forceps
- M. curette
- M. dissector
- M. electrocoagulation unit
- M. elevator
- M. hinge clamp
- M. irrigating forceps stylet
- M. irrigation tubing set
- M. jeweler's bipolar forceps
- M. ligature passer
- M. needle holder
- M. nerve hook
- M. neurosurgical scissors
- M. solid state coagulator
- M. titanium microsurgical forceps

Malis-Frazier suction tube

Malis-Jensen
  M.-J. bipolar forceps
  M.-J. microbipolar forceps
Malith pacemaker
malleable
  m. blade
  m. blade retractor
  m. copper retractor
  m. facial implant
  m. metal finger splint
  m. microsurgical suction device
  m. multipore suction tube
  m. passing needle
  m. probe
  m. prosthesis
  m. retractor blade
  m. retractor system
  m. ribbon retractor
  m. spatula
  m. stainless steel retractor
  m. stylet
  m. sucker
malleolar gel sleeve
Malleoloc anatomic ankle orthosis
Malleo-med soft ankle support
MalleoTrain ankle support
mallet
  Bakelite m.
  Bergman m.
  Blount nylon m.
  bone m.
  Boxwood m.
  brass m.
  Brown m.
  Carroll aluminum m.
  cervical m.
  Chandler m.
  Children's Hospital m.
  copper m.
  Cottle m.
  Crane m.
  Doyen bone m.
  fiber m.
  Gerzog bone m.
  Hajek m.
  hard m.
  Heath m.
  Henning m.
  Hibbs m.
  Jarit m.
  Kirk m.
  lead-filled m.

  Lucae mastoid m.
  Luer m.
  MacAusland bone m.
  Mead m.
  Meyerding m.
  No Bounce m.
  nylon face m.
  nylon head m.
  Ombrédanne m.
  polyethylene-faced m.
  Ralks m.
  Rica bone m.
  Richards combination m.
  Rissler m.
  Rush m.
  slotted m.
  SMIC surgical m.
  Smith-Petersen m.
  standard pattern m.
  Steinbach m.
  Stille m.
  surgical m.
  Swanson m.
  White m.
malleus
  m. cutter
  m. forceps
  m. nipper
malleus-footplate assembly
malleus-incus prosthesis
malleus-stapes assembly
Mallinckrodt
  M. angiographic catheter
  M. endotracheal tube
  M. Hi-Care pulmonary hygiene system
  M. Laser-Flex tube
  M. scanner
  M. sensor system
  M. ultra tag labeling kit
  M. vertebral catheter
Mallory-Head
  M.-H. Interlok calcar trimmer
  M.-H. Interlok primary femoral component
  M.-H. Interlok rasp
  M.-H. Interlok reamer
  M.-H. modular acetabular template
  M.-H. modular calcar system
  M.-H. porous primary femoral prosthesis
Mallory RM-1 cell pacemaker

NOTES

M

Malm-Himmelstein pulmonary valvulotome
Maloney
    M. catheter
    M. mercury-filled esophageal dilator
    M. no-hole lens manipulator
    M. nucleus rotator
    M. tapered mercury-filled esophageal bougie
    M. tapered-tip dilator
Maloney-Hurst dilator
Maloney-type bougie
malsensing pacemaker
Malstrm-Westman cannula
Malström
    M. cup
    M. vacuum extractor
Malteno valve
Maltese cross lens
Maltz
    M. bayonet saw
    M. button-end knife
    M. cartilage knife
    M. nasal rasp
    M. needle
    M. retractor
Maltz-Anderson nasal rasp
Maltz-Lipsett nasal rasp
Maltzman needle
Malvern analyzer
Mammalok Ultra repositionable breast localization needle
mammary
    m. implant
    m. prosthesis
    m. support dressing
Mammatech breast prosthesis
Mammex TR computer-aided mammography diagnosis system
mammographic view box
Mammo-Lume
    M.-L. imaging system
    M.-L. view box
Mammo Mask illuminator
Mammomat C3 mammography system
mammometer
Mammopatch gel self adhesive
MammoReader computer-aided detection system
Mammoscan digital imaging system
MammoSite
    M. radiation therapy system
    M. RTS
MammoSpot spot cone
Mammotest
    M. Plus breast biopsy system
    M. Select breast biopsy system
mammotome
    M. core biopsy device

    Jacobus m.
    Rogers m.
    M. ultrasound biopsy system
Mammoviewer viewer
Mamtat probe
Manan cutting needle
Manashil sialography catheter
Manche
    M. LASIK forceps
    M. LASIK speculum
Manchester
    M. knee replacement
    M. LDR implant system
    M. nasal osteotome
    M. ovoid
Manchu cotton dressing
Mancke flex-rigid gastroscope
Mancusi-Ungaro scissors
Mandelbaum
    M. cannula
    M. catheter
    M. ear knife
Mandelkorn suture lysis lens
mandibular
    m. advancement appliance
    m. advancement device
    m. angle fracture intraoral open reduction microplate
    m. arch bar
    m. body retractor
    m. bridging plate
    M. Excursiometer
    m. mesh
    m. miniplate
    m. orthopaedic repositioning appliance
    m. overdenture
    m. positioning device
    m. prosthesis
    m. sheet
    m. staple bone plate
mandrel
    m. graft
    steam-shaping m.
mandrin dilator
Man facelift expander
Mangat curvilinear chin prosthesis
Mangoldt epithelial graft
Mangum knot pusher
Manhattan
    M. Eye & Ear corneal dissector
    M. Eye & Ear probe
    M. Eye & Ear spatula
    M. Eye & Ear suturing forceps
ManHood absorbent pouch
Mani cerebral catheter
manifold
    M. II slot-blot apparatus

Morse m.
3-stopcock m.
manipulation board
manipulator
  Akahoshi nucleus m.
  Barrett flange lens m.
  button-tip m.
  ClearView uterine m.
  4-degree-of freedom m.
  Drysdale nucleus m.
  Feaster lens m.
  Friedman lens m.
  Grieshaber three-function m.
  Grieshaber two-function m.
  Guimaraes implantable contact
    lens m.
  Harris-Kronner uterine m.
  Hasson uterine m.
  Hirschman lens m.
  hook m.
  Hulka uterine m.
  HUMI uterine m.
  iris lens m.
  irrigating lens m.
  Jaffe-Maltzman lens m.
  Judson-Smith m.
  Koch phaco m.
  Kritzinger-Updegraff m.
  Kronner Manipujector m.
  Kuglen angled lens m.
  Kuglen irrigating lens m.
  Kuglen straight lens m.
  LASIK flap m.
  lens m.
  Lester lens m.
  Levy-Kuglen lens m.
  Lieberman MicroFinger m.
  Lindstrom Star nucleus m.
  Lister lens m.
  Maloney no-hole lens m.
  McIntyre irrigating iris m.
  Microbeam m.
  multi-coordinate m.
  Multi Koordinaten m.
  Osher nucleus lens m.
  Pelosi uterine m.
  Rappazzo intraocular m.
  RUMI uterine m.
  Sinskey lens m.
  Smith-Leiske lens m.
  Universal phaco m.
  uterine m.

  Valchev uterine m.
  Vico angled m.
  Visitec Vico m.
  Wan sideport nucleus m.
  Zinnanti uterine m. (ZUMI)
manipulator-injector
  Harris-Kronner uterine m.-i.
    (HUMI)
Mannerfelt
  M. chisel
  M. gouge
  M. raspatory
  M. retractor
Mann forceps
Manning
  M. forceps
  M. retractor
Mannis
  M. suture
  M. suture probe
manometer
  aneroid m.
  catheter-tipped m.
  Dinamap ultrasound blood
    pressure m.
  Honan m.
  Mercury Medical airway
    pressure m.
  Tycos m.
  Validyne m.
  ventilator pressure m.
manometer-tipped catheter
manometric
  m. catheter
  m. sensor
manometry system
manoptoscope
Mansfield
  M. Atri-Pace 1 catheter
  M. balloon
  M. balloon dilatation catheter
  M. bioptome
  M. forceps
  M. orthogonal electrode catheter
  M. Polaris electrode
  M. Scientific dilatation balloon
    catheter
**Mansfield-Webster deflectable curved
  catheter**
Manson-Aebli corneal section scissors
Manson double-ended strabismus hook
Mansson urinary pouch

NOTES

Mantel laryngoscope
Mantisol drain
Mantis retrograde forceps
Mantoux needle
Mantz rectal dilator
manual
    m. dermatome
    m. dermatome brush
    m. dermatome thickness gauge
    m. esthesiometer
    m. lithotripter
    m. osteotome
    m. resuscitation bag
ManuTrain wrist support
many-tailed
    m.-t. bandage
    m.-t. dressing
MAPcath stylet
Maple Leaf orthosis
Mapper hemostasis EP mapping sheath
mapping
    m. catheter
MAPwire J-tip guidewire
Maquet operating table
Maramed
    M. Miami fracture brace system
    M. ThermoFlex liner
Marathon guiding catheter
Marax dilator
Marbach episiotomy scissors
Marble bone pin
March
    M. laser lens
    M. laser sclerostomy needle
Marchac forehead template
Marchal interventional sialendoscope
March-Barton forceps
Marcks knife
Marco
    M. ARK-2000 refractor
    M. chart projector
    M. lensometer
    M. manual keratometer
    M. prism exophthalmometer
    M. radius gauge
    M. slit lamp
    M. SurgiScope 3 operating
    microscope
    M. trial lens (MTL)
Marcon colon decompression set
Marcon-Haber injector
Marcuse
    M. forceps
    M. tube clamp
Mardis
    M. firm stent with HydroPlus
    coating
    M. soft stent
Mardis-Dangler ureteral stent

Marena Comfortwear compression
    garment
MA-1 respirator
Marex MRI system
marginal
    m. chalazion forceps
    m. clamp
Margolis appliance
Margraf beam aligning film holder
Margulies
    M. coil
    M. intrauterine device
Marici bronchoscope
Marino
    M. rotatable transsphenoidal
    enucleator
    M. transsphenoidal curette
Marin reamer
Marion
    M. drain
    M. oxygen resuscitation system
    M. screw
Marion-Reverdin needle
Mark
    M. II Chandler total knee retractor
    M. II distal femur distractor
    M. II femoral component extractor
    M. III halo system
    M. II Kodros radiolucent awl
    M. II lateral collateral ligament
    retractor
    M. II Magni-Focuser loupe
    M. II modular weighted retractor
    M. II Sorrells hip arthroplasty
    retractor system
    M. II Stubbs short-prong collateral
    ligament retractor
    M. II Stulberg hip positioner
    M. II tibial component extractor
    M. II wide PCL knee retractor
    M. II Wixson hip positioner
    M. IV breathing pacemaker
    M. IV Moss decompression-feeding
    catheter
    M. IX lens
    M. VII cooling vest
    M. V Plus injector
Markell
    M. brace boot
    M. Mobility Health clogs
    M. Mobility Shoes
    M. open-toe shoe
    M. tarso medius straight shoe
    M. tarso pronator outflare shoe
marker
    Accu-line surgical m.
    Akura partial-depth astigmatic
    keratotomy m.
    Amsler scleral m.

Anastomark coronary artery bypass graft m.
Arrowsmith corneal m.
astigmatic m.
Berkeley optic zone m.
biprong muscle m.
Bores optic zone m.
Bores radial m.
Brems astigmatism m.
Castroviejo corneal transplant m.
Castroviejo scleral m.
m. catheter
Chayet corneal m.
Codman m.
corneal m.
Deblasio LASIK m.
Dell astigmatism m.
Desmarres m.
Dulaney LASIK m.
facelift flap m.
Fechtner trabeculectomy m.
Feldman radial keratotomy m.
fiducial m.
fine-line tissue m.
Fine toric/limbal relaxing incision m.
Fink biprong m.
Fink muscle m.
Freeman cookie cutter areola m.
Friedlander m.
Fukuyama limbal relaxing incision m.
Gass scleral m.
Geggel corneal transplant m.
Gel Mark Ultra biopsy site m.
Gonin m.
Green corneal m.
Green optical crater m.
Hoffer corneal m.
Hoffman/Buratto LASIK m.
Hoopes corneal m.
House-Urban m.
Hunkeler frown incision m.
interspace width m.
Koch limbal relaxing incision m.
Kraff limbal relaxing incision m.
Kremer triple-optical zone corneal m.
lead pellet m.
limbal relaxing incision m.
Lindstrom arcuate incision m.
Lindstrom astigmatic m.

low-profile R-K m.
LRI m.
Lu corneal m.
Machat double-ended m.
Machat superior flap LASIK m.
Matos laser axis m.
McDonald optic zone m.
Mendez corneal m.
metallic skin m.
Mickey and Minnie surgical m.
MicroMark tissue m.
Nano ophthalmic arcuate m.
Neuhann glaucoma m.
Neumann double corneal m.
Neumann-Shepard corneal m.
Nordan-Ruiz trapezoidal m.
O'Brien m.
O'Connor m.
ocular m.
Oshar-Neumann 8-line corneal m.
Perone LASIK m.
Pinnacle R/O II radiopaque m.
Probst Smiley[2] LASIK m.
radial keratotomy m.
radiopaque gold m.
retroreflective m.
RK m.
roentgenographic opaque m.
round optical zone m.
Ruiz adjustable m.
Ruiz-Shepard m.
Saunders-Paparella m.
scleral m.
Shepard optical center m.
Simcoe corneal m.
Sitzmarks radiopaque m.
skin m.
Skin Skribe m.
SklarScribe skin m.
Soll suture and incision m.
Squeeze-Mark surgical m.
Storz radial incision m.
tantalum-ball m.
tape m.
Thornton corneal m.
Thornton 360-degree arcuate keratotomy m.
Thornton low-profile radial m.
Thurmond pachymeter m.
T-incision m.
TLS surgical m.
trephine m.

M

NOTES

581

marker *(continued)*
  vein graft ring m.
  Visitec RK zone m.
  Vismark surgical skin m.
  window rasp m.
  Zaldivar limbal relaxing
    incision m.
Markham biopsy needle
**Markham-Meyerding hemilaminectomy
  retractor**
marking
  m. pen
  m. scissors
Markley
  M. orthodontic wire
  M. retention pin
  M. retractor
Markwalder
  M. bone rongeur
  M. rib forceps
  M. rib rongeur
Marlen
  M. biliary drainage kit
  M. colostomy appliance
  M. ileostomy bag
  M. leg bag
  M. SkinShield adhesive skin barrier
  M. UltraLite one-piece convex
    disposable system
Marlex
  M. band
  M. bandage
  M. mesh
  M. mesh graft
  M. mesh implant
  M. mesh prosthesis
  M. mesh snare
  M. methyl methacrylate prosthesis
  M. methyl methacrylate sandwich
  M. PerFix plug
  M. suture
Marlin
  M. cervical collar
  M. cervical orthosis
  M. thoracic catheter
Marlow
  M. disposable cannula
  M. disposable trocar
  M. Primus handle
  M. Primus shaft
  M. Primus tip
  M. Surgical Technologies, Inc.
    diagnostic/operating laparoscope
Marmite lithotrite
Marmor modular knee prosthesis
maroon
  M. lip curette
  m. spoon
Maroon-Jannetta dissector

Marqez-Gomez conjunctival graft
Marquardt bone rongeur
Marquest Respirgard II nebulizer
Marquette
  M. Case-12 electrocardiographic
    system
  M. 3-channel laser holder
  M. electrocardiograph
  M. 8000 Holter monitor
  M. Responder 1500 multifunctional
    defibrillator
  M. treadmill
Marritt dilator
Marrs intrauterine catheter
MARS
  modular acetabular reconstruction system
  Modular Acetabular Revision System
  MARS acetabular reconstructive
    system
  MARS revision acetabular
    component
Marshall V-suture
Marshik
  M. tonsillar forceps
  M. tonsil-seizing forceps
Marstock apparatus
Marsupial
  M. belt
  M. pouch
Martel
  M. conductor
  M. intestinal clamp
Marten hair eye brush
Martin
  M. abdominal retractor
  M. ballpoint scissors
  M. bandage
  M. bipolar coagulation forceps
  M. blade
  M. bur
  M. cartilage chisel
  M. cartilage clamp
  M. cartilage forceps
  M. cartilage scissors
  M. cheek retractor
  M. dermal curette
  M. diamond wire cutter
  M. endarterectomy stripper
  M. hip gouge
  M. laryngectomy tube
  M. lip retractor
  M. meniscal forceps
  M. muscle clamp
  M. nasopharyngeal biopsy forceps
  M. nerve root retractor
  M. palate retractor
  M. pelvimeter
  M. rectal hook
  M. rectal hook retractor

M. rectal speculum
M. rubber dressing
M. snare
M. Surefit lens pusher
M. tenaculum
M. throat scissors
M. thumb forceps
M. tissue forceps
M. tracheostomy tube
M. uterine fistula probe
M. uterine needle
M. uterine sound
M. uterine tenaculum forceps
M. vaginal retractor
M. vaginal speculum
M. Vigorimeter
Martinez
M. corneal dissector knife
M. corneal transplant centering ring
M. corneal trephine blade
M. disposable corneal trephine
M. double-ended corneal dissector
M. keratome
M. scleral centering ring
M. Universal interstitial template
Martinez-Castro keratome
Martini bone curette
Martius graft
Marx
M. bridging plate system
M. needle
Maryan biopsy punch forceps
Maryfield introducer
Mary Jane breast pump
Maryland
M. bridge
M. forceps
M. monopolar electrosurgical dissector
Masciuli silicone sponge
Mascot indirect ophthalmoscope
Masimo
M. Set oximeter sensor
M. Set pulse oximeter
Masing needle holder
mask
Accurox m.
Aclaim nasal m.
Advantage 1000 CBA-RCA gas m.
AeroChamber face m.
AirSep ultimate nasal m.
Aquaplast m.

Armstrong CPR m.
Bili m.
BioMask m.
bridgeless m.
cold compress m.
Comfort Classic nasal m.
contour deluxe nasal m.
convolution m.
CP2 Inflat-A-Mask inflatable sinus m.
DreamSeal m.
EndoShield m.
face m.
Finney m.
GoldSeal nasal m.
Hans Rudolph full face m.
high-humidity face m.
high-humidity tracheostomy m.
Hudson type oxygen m.
Image3 disposable face m.
IQ nasal m.
ISAH stereotactic immobilizing m.
isolation face m.
Kuhn m.
laryngeal m.
Mirage full-face m.
Mirage nasal m.
mouth m.
nasal m.
Nic the Asthmatic Dragon aerosol m.
nonrebreathing m.
OEM Venturi MixOMask m.
open face m.
Orfit m.
oxygen m.
partial rebreathing m.
Patil-Syracuse m.
Pegaus FLO_2 m.
PEP m.
Petit facial m.
Phantom nasal m.
RBS face m.
rebreathing m.
Rendell-Baker Soucek face m.
reservoir face m.
Respironics nasal m.
Rudolph m.
SealEasy resuscitation m.
sinus m.
SoftFit ultra nasal CPAP m.
SOMNOmask sleep apnea m.

M

NOTES

mask *(continued)*
    surgical m.
    Swiss Therapy eye m.
    Ultimate nasal m.
    ventilated m.
    Venturi m.
    Weinmann SomnoMask m.
Masket
    M. forceps
    M. phaco spatula
Mason
    M. leg holder
    M. splint
    M. suction tube
    M. tonsil suction dissector
    M. vascular clamp
Mason-Allen
    M.-A. hand splint
    M.-A. snare
Mason-Auvard weighted vaginal speculum
Mason-Judd
    M.-J. bladder retractor
    M.-J. self-retaining retractor
Mason-Likar 12-lead EKG system
Mason-School aspirating needle
mass
    m. flow anemometer
    M. Isotopomer Distribution Analysis (MIDA)
    m. spectrometer
    m. spectrophotometer
Massachusetts Vision kit
Massageboard board
massager
    Body Belt body m.
    Cryocup ice m.
    G5 Vibracare m.
    Knobble m.
    Morfam m.
    Original Backnobber muscle m.
    Silhouette m.
    Vibracare m.
Massage Time Pro hydromassage table
Masselon
    M. glasses
    M. spectacles
Masseran trepan bur
Massie
    M. driver
    M. extractor
    M. II plate
    M. nail assembly
    M. screwdriver
    M. sliding nail
    M. sliding nail tube
Massiot polytome
Masson
    M. fascial needle
    M. fascial stripper
    M. fasciatome
    M. needle holder
Masson-Luethy needle holder
Masson-Mayo-Hegar needle holder
Masson-Vital needle holder
MAST
    military antishock trousers
    MAST pants
    MAST suit
    MAST trousers
mastectomy skin flap retractor
Mastel
    M. compass-guided arcuate keratotomy system
    M. diamond compass
    M. trifaceted diamond blade
master
    m. cement
    M. Flow Pumpette
    M. Flow Pumpette pump
    NeuroCom Balance M.
    Pro Balance M.
    M. screwdriver
    Smart Balance M.
    M. step foot prosthesis
Masterbrace 3 functional ACL knee brace
MasterCraft hearing aid
MasterFlex pump
Masterpiece Jupiter ionizer alkaliner
Masters intestinal clamp
Masterson
    M. hysterectomy forceps
    M. pelvic clamp
Masters-Schwartz
    M.-S. intestinal clamp
    M.-S. liver clamp
Master-Stim interferential stimulator
masticatory apparatus
Mastin
    M. goiter forceps
    M. muscle clamp
    M. muscle forceps
Mastisol liquid adhesive
mastoid
    m. bur
    m. catheter
    m. chisel
    m. curette
    m. dressing
    m. gouge
    m. probe
    m. rongeur
    m. searcher
    m. self-retaining retractor
    m. suction tube

mastopexy form
Masy angioscope
mat
    Dermafit massage m.
    Harris footprint m.
    m. holder
    Scoot-Gard m.
    Secur-Its silicon cushion m.
    silicone-spiked m.
    sting m.
Matas vessel band
Matchett-Brown
    M.-B. hip endoprosthesis
    M.-B. prosthesis
    M.-B. stem rasp
mater
    Tutoplast dura m.
material
    ACCO impression m.
    AccuGel impression m.
    Accu-Mix impression m.
    acrylic implant m.
    Acuflex impression m.
    Adaptic II dental restorative m.
    Agarloid impression m.
    Algee impression m.
    alginate impression m.
    Algitec impression m.
    allogeneic lyophilized bone graft
      implant m.
    alloplastic graft m.
    Aneuroplast acrylic m.
    Apligraf skin graft m.
    Apligraf venous ulcer graft m.
    Aquasil Smart Wetting
      impression m.
    Astron investment m.
    AudiSil silicone ear mold m.
    Augmen bone-grafting m.
    Aurovest investment m.
    Avitene collagen hemostatic m.
    Avitene hemostatic m.
    Biobrane/HF graft m.
    bioceramic implant m.
    biocompatible spacing m.
    Bioglass bone substitute m.
    Biograft bovine heterograft m.
    BioMend periodontal m.
    Bio-Oss bone graft m.
    Bio-Oss collagen hemostatic m.
    Bioplastique nasal augmentation m.
    Biovert implant m.

    Bonaccolto monoplex orbital
      implant m.
    bone implant m.
    bone substitute m. (BSM)
    bucrylate collagen hemostatic m.
    Carboplast II thermoplastic
      composite sheet m.
    Carbo-Zinc skin barrier m.
    Castorit investment m.
    Celestin graft m.
    Cellolite m.
    Co-Cr-Mo alloy prosthesis m.
    Codman cranioplastic m.
    Coe impression m.
    collagen hemostatic m.
    Collagraft bone graft matrix m.
    Collastat collagen hemostatic m.
    Coltene impression m.
    Coltex impression m.
    CompaFill MH dental
      restorative m.
    CompaLay dental restorative m.
    CompaMolar dental restorative m.
    Contigen Bard collagen
      hemostatic m.
    Contigen implant collagen
      hemostatic m.
    corundum ceramic implant m.
    cranioplastic acrylic m.
    Cristobalite investment m.
    Crossfire polyethylene bearing m.
    cyanoacrylate fixed orbital silicone
      sleds implant m.
    Dentemp filling m.
    Dentloid impression m.
    Dermalogen m.
    Derma-Sil impression m.
    DermAssist wound filling m.
    Dermatell hydrocolloid dressing m.
    Dermostat eye implant m.
    DiamondLite restorative m.
    DualMesh m.
    Durafill dental restorative m.
    durapatite bone replacement m.
    Dur-A-Sil ear impression m.
    Edwards Teflon intracardiac patch
      implant m.
    Elgiloy clip m.
    Embarc bone repair m.
    EndoAvitene collagen hemostatic m.
    Endur bonding m.
    Epicel skin graft m.

M

NOTES

material *(continued)*
   Epigrip m.
   Estilux dental restorative m.
   Evazote cushioning m.
   Flexistone impression m.
   FlowGel barrier m.
   Fotofil dental restorative m.
   Frosted Flex earmold m.
   G-C Vest investment m.
   glycolide trimethylene carbonate m.
   gold weight and wire spring
     implant m.
   Gore cast liner m.
   Gore subcutaneous augmentation m.
   Gore-Tex alloplastic m.
   Gore-Tex periodontal m.
   Gore-Tex regenerative m.
   Graflex m.
   Grafton bone grafting m.
   Gypsona rapid-setting cast m.
   Hand-Aid strapping m.
   Hapex bioactive m.
   Hapset bone graft plaster m.
   Healos bone graft substitute m.
   heavy-gauge suture m.
   Hedrocel bone substitute m.
   Hemopad collagen hemostatic m.
   Hemotene collagen hemostatic m.
   Hircoe denture base m.
   Hylasine viscoelastic m.
   Impregum impression m.
   Insta-Mold silicone ear
     impression m.
   InterGard knitted collagen
     hemostatic m.
   Interpore bone replacement m.
   Interpore ceramic m.
   Kaltostat wound packing m.
   Karaya self-adhesive conductive m.
   Keolar implant m.
   Langinate impression m.
   Lincoff sponge implant m.
   Linkow dental implant m.
   L-rod implant m.
   MediFlex earmold m.
   Medpor allograft m.
   Medpor alloplastic m.
   Medpor block facial structure
     building m.
   methyl methacrylate implant m.
   3M Tegapore wound contact m.
   Multidex wound-filling m.
   MycroMesh graft m.
   NeoDura tissue m.
   Omega splinting m.
   Omniflex impression m.
   Opotow filling m.
   Opteform allograft m.
   Optison contrast m.

OrthoDyn bone substitute m.
Orthofit 9001 orthotic m.
Orthoglass splint m.
Ortho-Jel impression m.
Osteogenics BoneSource synthetic
  bone replacement m.
OsteoGraf bone grafting m.
OsteoGraf/D bone grafting m.
OsteoGraf/LD bone grafting m.
OsteoGraf/N-Block grafting m.
Palfique Estelite tooth shade
  resin m.
Paradentine dental restorative m.
paraffin implant m.
Pearlon impression m.
Pe-lite m.
PerioGlas m.
Perma-Cryl denture base m.
PermaMesh m.
PermaSoft reline m.
Permatone denture m.
Platorit investment m.
Poloxamer 407 barrier m.
polyether implant m.
polyethylene implant m.
polyurethane implant m.
Polyviolene polyester suture m.
PolyWic wound filling m.
Porites coral m.
Porocoat m.
precollagenous filamentous m.
ProOsteon implant graft m.
Proplast I, II porous implant m.
Protegen m.
Provit filling m.
Ramitec bite registration m.
Rema-Exakt investment m.
Reprodent acrylic tooth m.
Scialom dental implant m.
Scutan temporary splint m.
SeamGuard staple line
  reinforcement m.
Septosil impression m.
ShearBan orthotic m.
shell implant m.
ShowerSafe protector m.
Sili-Gel impression m.
SiloLiner interface m.
Silon silicone thermoplastic
  splinting m.
Small-Carrion penile implant m.
solid silicone exoplant implant m.
Spitz-Holter valve implant m.
sponge silicone implant m.
SR-Isosit dental restorative m.
SR-Ivocap denture m.
SR-Ivolen impression m.
SR-Ivoseal impression m.
Stellite ring m.

subcutaneous augmentation m. (SAM)
Surgamid polyamide suture m.
Surgical Nu-Knit collagen hemostatic m.
Surgicel collagen hemostatic m.
Surgicel Nu-Knit absorbable hemostatic m.
Thoralon implant m.
Tissucol fibrin adhesive m.
titanium implant m.
transcatheter umbrella implant m.
Triangle gelatin-sealed sling m.
Tru-Chrome band m.
tunnel-type implant m.
twisted cotton nonabsorbable surgical suture m.
Unigraft bone graft m.
Unilab Surgibone collagen hemostatic m.
Vitallium implant m.
Wirosol investment m.
Wirovest investment m.
Xcelon nylon balloon m.
Zyclast collagen hemostatic m.
Zyderm I or II collagen hemostatic m.

Mathews
M. drill point
M. hand drill
M. load drill
M. osteotome
M. rectal speculum

Mathieu
M. double-ended retractor
M. foreign body forceps
M. needle
M. needle holder
M. pliers
M. raspatory
M. tongue forceps
M. urethral forceps

Mathieu-Horton-Devine flip-flap
Mathieu-Olsen needle holder
Mathieu-Stille needle holder
Mathrop hemostat
Mathys prosthesis
Matos laser axis marker
Matritech NMP22 test kit
matrix
Accor dental m.
AlloGro demineralized bone m.

Aquasorb Border gel m.
m. band
demineralized bone m. (DBM)
DuraGen absorbable dural graft m.
Dynafill graft biomedium mineralized bone m.
FortaFlex bioengineered collagen m.
m. Grafton putty
OrCel bilayered cellular m.
Osteovit bone m.
PermaMesh hydroxyapatite woven sheet m.
m. retainer
Walser m.

Matroc femoral head
Matrol femoral head prosthesis
MatScan system
Matson
M. raspatory
M. rib elevator
M. rib stripper

Matson-Alexander
M.-A. raspatory
M.-A. rib elevator
M.-A. rib stripper

Matson-Mead
M.-M. apicolysis retractor
M.-M. periosteum stripper

Matson-Plenk raspatory
Matsuda titanium surgical instrument
matte black forceps
Matthew
M. cross-leg clamp
M. forceps

matting
Dycem roll m.

Mattis corneal scissors
Mattison-Upshaw retractor
Mattox aortic clamp
Mattox-Potts scissors
mattress
AccuMax self-adjusting pressure management m.
Air-O-Ease static air flotation m.
Air-O-Pad air m.
Airsoft replacement m.
Akros extended-care m.
AkroTech m.
apnea alarm m.
Babytherm IC gel m.
Bedge antireflux m.
Bio Core therapeutic m.

M

NOTES

mattress *(continued)*
Bio Gard Plus m.
Clinisert m.
Comfort nylon m.
convoluted foam m.
Critical Care m.
D.A.D. m.
DeCube therapeutic m.
Dermasoft m.
Dräger thermal gel m.
DynaGuard APM alternating pressure m.
dynamic flotation m.
Econo-Float water flotation m.
eggcrate m.
FirstStep m.
FlairCair m.
foam cube m.
Geo-Matt m.
HomeCare Simplimatt Plus Zoned foam m.
Huntleigh m.
hypothermia m.
Impression m.
Integriderm m.
Invacare alternating pressure m.
Invacare APM m.
Iris pressure-reduction m.
Isoflex m.
KinAir IV m.
Lapidus alternating air-pressure m.
low-air-loss m.
MaxiFloat DFP+/DXP+ pressure reduction m.
MaxiFloat DFP, EF, LFP pressure-reduction m.
Medisupra m.
Medline Aero-Flow II air m.
Medline deluxe air m.
Medline Saf-T-Side m.
microAir Turn-Q Plus m.
Neuropedic multidensity m.
NewLife therapeutic m.
Nirvana pressure-reducing m.
OptiMax Supreme pressure-reduction m.
Orthoderm convertible II m.
overlay m.
Phoenix PX 115 Powerloft series II alternating air flotation m.
Pneu-Care Plus m.
pressure m.
PressureGuard IV alternating-pressure m.
ProForm maxim-VE pressure-reduction m.
Q-Star IV pressure-relief m.
Q-Star Voyager pressure-reduction m.

Rik Defender prevention m.
Roho m.
SeCure therapeutic m.
Silhouette therapeutic m.
Sof-Care m.
Sofflex m.
Sof-Matt pressure reducing m.
SPR.Plus II m.
static air m.
Stop-Leak gel flotation m.
Tempur-Med hospital m.
Tempur-Pedic pressure-relieving Swedish m.
Tempur-Plus m.
TheraKair air pulsation m.
TheraRest m.
TriFloat Plus pressure-reduction m.
UltraForm therapeutic m.
Unitek I decubitus m.

Mattrix spinal cord stimulation system
Maturna bra system
Matzenauer vaginal speculum
Mauch
M. double-sheathed plastic wash pipe
M. GaitMaster system
M. Swing and Stance hydraulic knee

Mauermayer
M. resectoscope
M. stone punch

Maumenee
M. capsular forceps
M. corneal forceps
M. cross-action capsular forceps
M. erysiphake
M. goniotomy cannula
M. goniotomy knife
M. iris hook
M. straight-action capsular forceps
M. Suregrip forceps
M. tissue forceps
M. vitreous-aspirating needle
M. vitreous sweep spatula

Maumenee-Barraquer vitreous sweep spatula
Maumenee-Colibri corneal forceps
Maumenee-Park
M.-P. erysiphake
M.-P. eye speculum

Maunder oral screw mouthgag
Maunoir iris scissors
Mavello water ionizer
Maverick
M. balloon dilatation catheter
M. Monorail balloon catheter

Max
M. FiberScan laser system
M. Fine scissors

M. Fine tying forceps
M. Force balloon dilatation catheter
M. Force TTS biliary balloon
dilatation catheter
M. Plus MR scanner
M. ventilator
Maxair Autohaler
Maxam suture
MaxBloc bite block
MaxCast
M. cast
M. fiberglass casting tape
Maxenon Xi 300 xenon light source
MaxiCare adult disposable undergarment
Maxi-Driver driver
MaxiFloat
M. DFP+/DXP+ pressure reduction mattress
M. DFP, EF, LFP pressure-reduction mattress
M. wheelchair cushion
MaxiFlo breathable underpad
Maxi LD PTA dilatation catheter
Maxilift Combi patient lifting system
Maxilith
M. pacemaker
M. pacemaker pulse generator
maxillary
m. arch bar
m. disimpaction forceps
m. fracture forceps
m. prosthesis
m. removable implant-retained denture
m. sinus cannula
m. splint
maxillofacial
m. bone screw
m. osteotome
Maxillume 250 watt quartz halogen light source
Maxim
M. modular knee system
M. revision knee system
Maxima
M. Forte blood oxygenator
M. II TENS unit
M. II transcutaneous electrical nerve stimulator
M. Plus plasma resistant fiber oxygenator

Maxi-Myst
M.-M. nebulizer system
M.-M. vaporizer
Max-I-Probe
M.-I.-P. endodontic irrigation syringe
M.-I.-P. irrigation probe
Maxon
M. absorbable suture
M. polyglyconate monofilament suture
Maxone I.V. fluid/blood warmer
Maxorb alginate wound dressing
Max-Relax pillow
Maxum
M. Carr-Locke angled forceps
M. reusable endoscopic forceps
Maxwell
M. coil
M. 3D field simulator
Maxxum balloon catheter
Maxxus orthopaedic latex surgical glove
May
M. anatomical bone plate
M. hook-on lens loupe
M. kidney clamp
M. ophthalmoscope
Maydl pessary
Mayer
M. forceps
M. nasal splint
M. orthotic
M. pessary
M. speculum
Mayfield
M. aneurysm clamp
M. aneurysm forceps
M. bayonet osteotome
M. CIS-RE aneurysm clip
M. clip applicator
M. fixation frame
M. head clamp
M. head rest
M. malleable brain spatula
M. miniature clip applier
M. pediatric horseshoe headrest
M. pediatric horseshoe pad
M. radiolucent base unit
M. radiolucent headholder
M. radiolucent headrest
M. retractor
M. skull clamp adapter

M

NOTES

Mayfield (*continued*)
M. skull clamp pin
M. skull-pin headholder
M. spinal curette
M. surgical headrest system
M. swivel horseshoe headrest
M. temporary aneurysm clip applier
M. three-pin skull clamp
M. tic headholder
Mayfield/Acciss stereotactic workstation
Mayfield-Kees
M.-K. clip
M.-K. headholder
M.-K. headrest
M.-K. skull fixation apparatus
M.-K. table attachment
Mayo
M. abdominal retractor
M. bone-cutting forceps
M. catgut needle
M. clamp
M. common duct probe
M. common duct scoop
M. coronary perfusion cannula
M. coronary perfusion tip
M. curved scissors
M. cystic duct scoop
M. external vein stripper
M. fibroid hook
M. gallbladder scoop
M. gall duct scoop
M. gallstone scoop
M. goiter ligature carrier
M. hemostat
M. instrument table
M. intestinal needle
M. kidney clamp
M. kidney pedicle forceps
M. kidney stone probe
M. knife
M. linen suture
M. long dissecting scissors
M. needle holder
M. operating scissors
M. round blade scissors
M. semiconstrained elbow prosthesis
M. stand
M. straight scissors
M. tissue forceps
M. total ankle prosthesis
M. trocar-point needle
M. ureter isolation forceps
M. uterine probe
M. uterine scissors
M. vessel clamp
Mayo-Adams self-retaining appendectomy retractor

Mayo-Boldt inverter
Mayo-Collins
M.-C. appendectomy retractor
M.-C. double-ended retractor
M.-C. mastoid retractor
Mayo-Gibbon heart-lung machine
Mayo-Guyon
M.-G. kidney clamp
M.-G. vessel clamp
Mayo-Harrington
M.-H. dissecting scissors
M.-H. forceps
Mayo-Hegar curved-jaw needle holder
Mayo-Lexer scissors
Mayo-Lovelace
M.-L. abdominal retractor
M.-L. spur crusher
M.-L. spur crushing clamp
Mayo-Myers external vein stripper
Mayo-New scissors
Mayo-Noble dissecting scissors
Mayo-Ochsner
M.-O. cannula
M.-O. forceps
M.-O. trocar
Mayo-Potts dissecting scissors
Mayo-Robson
M.-R. gallstone scoop
M.-R. gastrointestinal forceps
M.-R. intestinal clamp
Mayo-Russian gastrointestinal forceps
Mayo-Simpson retractor
Mayo-Sims dissecting scissors
Mayo-Stille operating scissors
Mazlin intrauterine device
Mazzariello-Caprini
M.-C. stone forceps
M.-C. stone forceps sterilizing case
Mazzocco
M. flexible lens forceps
M. silicone intraocular lens
MBE
medium below-elbow
MBE cast
MBF3 infrared laser-Doppler flowmeter
M-brace corneal trephine
MBS snap-on orthotic
McAllister
M. needle holder
M. scissors
MCAS
modular clip application system
McAtee
M. apparatus
M. olecranon compression screw device
McBratney aspirating speculum
McBride
M. cup

M. femoral prosthesis
M. pin
M. plate
M. tripod pin traction
McBride-Moore prosthesis
McBurney
M. fenestrated retractor
M. thyroid retractor
McCabe
M. antral retractor
M. canal knife
M. crurotomy saw
M. crus guide fork
M. facial nerve dissector
M. flap knife dissector
M. measuring instrument
M. parotidectomy retractor
M. perforation rasp
M. posterior fossa retractor
McCabe-Farrior rasp
McCaffrey positioner
McCain
M. TMJ arthroscopic system
M. TMJ cannula
M. TMJ curette
M. TMJ forceps
McCall instrument
McCannel
M. implant
M. ocular pressure reducer
M. suture
McCarthy
M. bladder evacuator
M. catheter
M. coagulation electrode
M. continuous-flow resectoscope
M. diathermic knife electrode
M. endoscope
M. foroblique operating telescope
M. foroblique panendoscope
cystoscope
M. fulgurating electrode
M. infant electrotome
M. loop operating electrode
M. microlens resectoscope
M. miniature electrotome
M. miniature loop electrode
M. miniature resectoscope
M. miniature telescope
M. multiple resectoscope
M. panendoscope

M. punctate electrotome
M. visual hemostatic forceps
McCarthy-Alcock forceps
McCarthy-Campbell miniature
cystoscope
McCaskey
M. antral catheter
M. antral curette
M. sphenoid cannula
McCaslin
M. knife
M. needle
M. wave-edge keratome
McClamary elevator
McCleery-Miller
M.-M. intestinal anastomosis clamp
M.-M. locking device
McClintock
M. placental forceps
M. uterine forceps
McClure iris scissors
McCollough
M. elevator
M. internal tibial torsion brace
M. osteotome
M. rasp
M. tying forceps
McConnell
M. orthopaedic headrest
M. shoulder positioner
McCool capsule retractor
McCoy
M. laryngoscope blade
M. septal forceps
M. septum-cutting forceps
McCrea
M. cystoscope
M. dilator
M. infant sound
McCullough
M. externofrontal retractor
M. hysterectomy clamp
M. strabismus forceps
M. suture-tying forceps
M. suturing forceps
McCurdy staphylorrhaphy needle
McCutchen
M. hip implant
M. SLT hip prosthesis
McDavid
M. ankle guard

M

NOTES

McDavid (*continued*)
M. hinged knee guard
M. knee brace
McDermott
M. clip
M. extractor
M. Surgiclip
McDonald
M. bone plate
M. cerclage
M. dissector
M. expressor
M. gastric clamp
M. lens-folding forceps
M. optic zone marker
McDougal prostatectomy clamp
McDowell
M. mouthgag
M. needle
McElroy curette
McElveen-Hitselberger neural dissector
McFadden
M. cross-legged clip
M. Surgiclip
M. Vari-Angle aneurysm clip
M. Vari-Angle clip applier
McFadden-Kees clip
McFarland tibial graft
McGannon
M. iris retractor
M. lens forceps
M. refractor
McGaw
M. plastic bottle
M. skinfold calipers
M. tape measure
M. volumetric pump
McGee
M. canal elevator
M. ear piston prosthesis
M. footplate pick
M. middle ear instrument
M. oval-window rasp
M. platinum/stainless steel piston
M. prosthesis needle
M. rasp
M. splint
M. tympanoplasty knife
M. wire-closure forceps
M. wire crimper
M. wire-crimping forceps
McGee-Caparosa wire crimper
McGee-Paparella wire-crimping forceps
McGee-Priest
M.-P. wire-closure forceps
M.-P. wire crimper
McGee-Priest-Paparella forceps
McGehee elbow prosthesis

McGhan
M. breast implant
M. breast prosthesis
M. eye implant
M. facial implant
M. fill kit
M. lens
M. plastic surgical needle
M. tissue expander
McGill
M. forceps
M. neurological percussor
M. retractor
McGinnis balloon system
McGivney
M. hemorrhoidal forceps
M. hemorrhoidal ligator
McGlamry elevator
McGoey-Evans acetabular cup
McGoey Vitallium punch
McGoon
M. cannula
M. coronary perfusion catheter
McGovern nipple
McGowan-Keeley tube
McGowan needle
McGravey tissue forceps
McGregor
M. conjunctival forceps
M. needle
McGuire
M. clamp
M. conformer
M. corneal scissors
M. I&A system
M. marginal chalazion forceps
M. pelvic positioner
M. rib spreader
M. tendon tucker
McHenry tonsillar forceps
McHugh
M. facial nerve knife
M. flap knife
M. oval speculum
McHugh-Farrior canal knife
McIlwain tissue chopper
McIndoe
M. bone-cutting forceps
M. diathermy forceps
M. dissecting forceps
M. dressing forceps
M. elevator
M. nasal chisel
M. rasp
M. raspatory
M. retractor
M. rongeur forceps
M. scissors
McIntire splint

McIntosh
- M. double-lumen hemodialysis catheter
- M. suture-holding forceps

McIntyre
- M. anterior chamber cannula
- M. coaxial cannula
- M. coaxial I&A system
- M. fish-hook needle holder
- M. guarded cystotome
- M. I&A needle
- M. infusion handpiece
- M. infusion set
- M. irrigating iris hook
- M. irrigating iris manipulator
- M. irrigating spatula
- M. irrigation-aspiration needle
- M. lacrimal cannula
- M. microhook
- M. nylon cannula connector
- M. reverse cystotome
- M. suture tamper
- M. truncated cone

McIntyre-Binkhorst irrigating cannula
McIver nephrostomy catheter
McIvor mouthgag
McKay ear forceps
McKee
- M. brace
- M. femoral prosthesis
- M. speculum
- M. table
- M. totally constrained elbow prosthesis
- M. tri-fin nail

McKee-Farrar
- M.-F. acetabular cup
- M.-F. hip prosthesis

McKeever
- M. cartilage knife
- M. patellar cap prosthesis

McKenna
- M. Tide-Ur-Ator evacuator
- M. Tide-Ur-Ator irrigator

McKenzie
- M. AirBack support
- M. cervical roll
- M. clamp
- M. clip-applying forceps
- M. cranial drill
- M. enlarging bur
- M. hemostasis clip

- M. leukotome
- M. leukotomy loop
- M. lumbar roll
- M. night roll
- M. perforating twist drill
- M. silver brain clip
- M. V-clip

McKerman-Adson forceps
McKerman-Potts forceps
McKernan-Adson forceps
McKernan forceps
McKernan-Potts forceps
McKesson
- M. mouthgag
- M. mouth probe
- M. pneumothorax apparatus
- M. suction bottle unit

McKinley EpM pump
McKinney
- M. eye speculum
- M. fixation ring

McKissock keyhole areolar template
McLane
- M. obstetrical forceps
- M. pile forceps

McLane-Luikart obstetrical forceps
McLane-Tucker-Kjelland forceps
McLane-Tucker-Luikart forceps
McLane-Tucker obstetrical forceps
McLaughlin
- M. carpal scaphoid screw
- M. hip plate
- M. laser mirror
- M. laser vaginal measuring rod
- M. nail
- M. osteosynthesis device
- M. quartz rod
- M. speculum

McLean
- M. capsular forceps
- M. capsulotomy scissors
- M. clamp
- M. muscle-recession forceps
- M. ophthalmic forceps
- M. prismatic fundus laser lens
- M. suture
- M. tonometer

McLearie bone forceps
McLeod padded clavicular splint
McMahon nephrostomy hook
McMaster bone graft
McMurray tenotomy knife

M

NOTES

McMurtry-Schlesinger shunt tube
McNaught
- M. keel
- M. prosthesis

McNealey-Glassman
- M.-G. clamp
- M.-G. visceral retainer

McNealey-Glassman-Mixter
- M.-G.-M. clamp
- M.-G.-M. forceps

McNealey visceral retractor
McNealy-Glassman-Babcock forceps
McNeill-Goldmann
- M.-G. blepharostat
- M.-G. blepharostat ring
- M.-G. corneal transplant ring
- M.-G. scleral ring

McNutt
- M. driver
- M. extractor

MCP finger joint prosthesis
McPherson
- M. angled forceps
- M. bent forceps
- M. corneal forceps
- M. corneal section scissors
- M. eye speculum
- M. iris spatula
- M. irrigating forceps
- M. lens forceps
- M. microbipolar forceps
- M. microconjunctival scissors
- M. microcorneal forceps
- M. microiris forceps
- M. microsurgery eye needle holder
- M. microsuture forceps
- M. microtenotomy scissors
- M. straight bipolar forceps
- M. suture-tying forceps
- M. trabeculotome
- M. tying iris forceps

McPherson-Castroviejo
- M.-C. corneal section scissors
- M.-C. forceps
- M.-C. microcorneal scissors

McPherson-Pierse
- M.-P. microcorneal forceps
- M.-P. microsuturing forceps

McPherson-Vannas iris scissors
McPherson-Westcott
- M.-W. conjunctival scissors
- M.-W. stitch scissors

McPherson-Wheeler
- M.-W. blade
- M.-W. eye knife

McPherson-Ziegler microiris knife
McQueen vitreous forceps

McQuigg
- M. clamp
- M. forceps

McQuigg-Mixter bronchial forceps
McReynolds
- M. driver
- M. extractor
- M. eye spatula
- M. keratome
- M. lid-retracting hook
- M. pterygium keratome
- M. pterygium knife
- M. pterygium scissors

McReynolds-Castroviejo
- M.-C. keratome
- M.-C. pterygium knife

McShirley amalgamator
McSpadden compactor
M-cup vacuum extraction device
McWhinnie
- M. electrode
- M. tonsillar dissector

McWhorter
- M. hemostat
- M. tonsillar forceps

MD-111 bone allograft
MD 16 hemocytometer
MDI
- metered-dose inhaler

MDILog electronic monitor
MDS
- microdebrider system
- MDS microdebrider
- MDS Truspot articulating film

Meacham-Scoville forceps
Mead
- M. bone rongeur
- M. bridge/crown remover
- M. dental rongeur
- M. Johnson tube
- M. lancet knife
- M. mallet
- M. periosteal elevator

Meadox
- M. Dacron mesh
- M. Dardik Biograft
- M. graft sizer
- M. ICP monitor
- M. Microvel arterial graft
- M. Microvel double-velour Dacron graft
- M. Surgimed catheter
- M. Surgimed Doppler probe
- M. Teflon felt pledget
- M. vascular graft
- M. woven velour prosthesis

Meadox-Cooley woven low-porosity prosthesis

measure
  M. Mat infantometer
  McGaw tape m.
measurement
measurer
  Bunnell digital exertion m.
measuring
  m. gauge
  m. guide
  m. hat
  m. rod
Measuroll suture
meat
  m. forceps
  m. hook retractor
meatal
  m. clamp
  m. dilator
  m. sound
meatoscope
  Hubell m.
  Huegli m.
meatotome
  Bunge ureteral m.
  Ellik m.
  Huegli m.
  Riba electrical ureteral m.
meatotomy
  m. electrode
  m. scissors
mechanical
  m. articulated arm
  m. device
  m. finger
  m. finger forceps
  m. joint apparatus
  m. longitudinal echoendoscope
  m. percussor
  m. prosthesis
  m. radial-scanning instrument
  m. respirator
  m. rotating probe
  m. separator
  m. stapler
  m. ventilator
  m. vitrector
mechanically assisted respirator
mechanic's
  m. pin
  m. waste dressing

mechanism
  adjustable leg and ankle
    repositioning m. (ALARM)
  4-bar linkage prosthetic knee m.
  central extensor m.
  Hosmer-Dorrance 4-bar knee m.
  MicroStable liner locking m.
  Noiles rotating-hinge knee m.
  patient-operated selector m.
  sunburst m.
  terminal extensor m.
mechanized scissors
Meckel rod
Mecon-I hearing aid
meconium aspirator
Mecring acetabluar prosthesis
Mectra
  M. hydrodissector
  M. I&A system
  M. tissue sample retainer
Medallion
  M. intraocular lens implant
  M. lens expressor
Medamicus Axia RSN guidewire
  introducer safety needle
Medarmor puncture-resistant glove
MedArt 470 laser
Medasonics transcranial Doppler
MedCam Pro Plus video camera
Med-Co flexible catheter
Medcomp catheter
Medcor pacemaker
Meddars cardiac catheterization analysis
  system
MedDev gold eyelid implant
Medela
  M. Apgar timer
  M. Dominant vacuum delivery
    pump
  M. manual breast pump
  M. membrane regulator
Medelec
  M. DMG 50 Teflon-coated
    monopolar electrode
  M. five-channel neurophysiological
    device
Medelec-Van Gogh
  electroencephalographic recording
  system
Medevice
  M. surgical loop
  M. surgical paws

M

NOTES

Medex
  M. Protege 3010 syringe infusion pump
  M. Secure system
  M. transducer
Med-Fit
  M.-F. cranial-sacral table
  M.-F. Senior Circuit machine
Medfusion 1001, 2001 syringe infusion pump
MedGem calorimeter
Medgraphics
  M. body plethysmograph
MedGraphics
  M. CPE 2000 electronically braked bicycle
  M. CPX/D metabolic cart
  M. diffusion analyzer
Medi
  M. Plus compression stocking
  M. vascular stocking
Medi-aire
  Bard M.-a.
medial
  m. bicortical screw
  m. heel-and-sole wedge
  m. heel wedge
  m. sole wedge
  m. unicortical screw
mediaometer
mediastinal
  m. cannula
  m. catheter
  m. drain
  m. sump filter
  m. tube
mediastinoscope
  Carlens m.
  Freiburg m.
  Goldberg MPC m.
  John A. Tucker m.
MediBag
  Ambu M.
Medi-Band bandage
Medi-Breather IPPB device
MedicAIR spirometer
medical
  m. adhesive remover
  m. air compressor
  m. cyclotron
  M. Design brace
  M. Dynamics 5990 needle arthroscope
  m. gas analyzer
  M. genuine sheepskin pad
  m. implant system (MIS)
  M. Intelligence BodyFix device
  M. Management System (MMS)
  M. Marketing Group (MMG)

M. Optics intraocular lens implant
M. Professionals in Medicine (MPM)
M. Resources hydrophilic wound dressing
St. Jude M. (SJM)
M. Workshop intraocular lens implant
M. Z post surgery garment
Medicam
  M. camera
  M. 900 insufflator
  M. light source
Medicamat
  M. ultrasound-assisted lipoplasty machine
  M. ultrasound device
Medici aerosol adhesive tape remover dressing
medicinal nebulizer
medicine
  Medical Professionals in M. (MPM)
MediClenze therapy system
Medicon
  M. contractor
  M. rib retractor
  M. rib spreader
  M. ultrasonic liposuction device
  M. wire-twister forceps
Medicon-Jackson rectal forceps
Medicon-Packer mosquito forceps
Medicopaste bandage
MediCordz tubing kit
Medicornea Kratz intraocular lens implant
Medi-cult blastocyst thawing pack
Medicus bed
Medicut
  M. cannula
  M. catheter
  M. intravenous needle
Medi-Duct ocular fluid management system
Medifil collagen hemostatic wound dressing
Mediflex
  M. Gazayerli retractor
  M. MD-7 endoscopic video system
  M. retractor
MediFlex
  M. earmold material
Mediflex-Bookler device
Mediflow
  M. waterbase pillow
  M. Waterpillow
Mediform dural graft
Medi-graft vascular prosthesis

Medi-Ject needle-free insulin injection system
Medi-Jector
 M.-J. adapter
 M.-J. Choice needle-free syringe kit
 M.-J. injector
Medilas
 M. fiberTome laser
 M. Nd:YAG surgical laser
Medilog ambulatory ECG recorder
MedImage scanner
Medi-Mist nebulizer
Medina tube
Meding
 M. tonsil enucleator tonometer
 M. tonsil enucleator tonsillectome
Medinol
 M. NIRside slotted stent
 M. NIR stent
MeDioStar hair removal laser
Med-I-Pad (MIP)
 M.-I.-P. underpad
Medipatch Gel Z self adhesive
Mediplex with Safetac dressing
Medipore
 M. dressing cover
 M. Dress-it dressing
 M. H soft cloth surgical tape
MediPort infusion vascular access device
Medi-Quet tourniquet
Medi-Rip dressing
MediRule measuring device
Medisense Pen 2 blood glucose meter
Mediskin
 M. hemostatic sponge
 M. porcine biological wound dressing
Medis off-line quantitative coronary angiogram
Medison
 M. 3D/4D ultrasound
 M. scanner
Medisorb drug delivery system
MediSpacer
 AirLife M.
Medispec Econolith spark plug lithotripter
Medi-Stim stimulator
Medi-Strumpf stocking
Medisupra mattress

Medisystems fistula needle
Meditape tape
meditation bench
Meditech
 M. bandage contact lens
 M. laser
Medi-Tech
 M.-T. arterial dilatation catheter
 M.-T. bipolar probe
 M.-T. catheter system
 M.-T. fascial dilator
 M.-T. flexible stiffening cannula
 M.-T. guidewire
 M.-T. IVC filter
 M.-T. occlusion balloon catheter
 M.-T. sheath
 M.-T. steerable catheter
 M.-T. stone basket
 M.-T. wire
Medi-Tech-Mansfield dilating catheter
Medi-Trace electrode
Meditrode iontophoresis Transvene electrode
medium below-elbow (MBE)
MediVators DSD-91P endoscope reprocessor
Mediven lymphedema sleeve
Medivent
 M. self-expanding coronary stent
 M. vascular stent
Mediwrap blanket
MedJet microkeratome
Medline
 M. Aero-Flow II air mattress
 M. Alpha subacute care bed
 M. deluxe air mattress
 M. Derma-Gel dressing
 M. gauze sponge
 M. gel/foam wheelchair cushion
 M. Lap-pal safety cushion
 M. lateral stabilizer
 M. packing strip
 M. positioner
 M. roll
 M. Saf-T-Side mattress
 M. wedge
MedLite
 M. Q-Switched neodymium-doped yttrium-aluminum-garnet laser
 M. Q-Switched YAG laser
Medmetric KT1000/S knee laxity arthrometer

M

NOTES

Medmont M600 perimeter
MedMorph III patient video imaging
Med-Neb respirator
Mednext bone dissecting system
Medoc-Celestin
    M.-C. endoprosthesis prosthesis
    M.-C. tube
Medoff sliding femoral fracture plate
Medos
    M. mechanical circulatory support
    system
    M. valve
Medos-Hakim valve
Medox Dacron mesh
Medpacific LD 5000 Laser-Doppler
  perfusion monitor
Medpor
    M. allograft material
    M. alloplastic material
    M. biomaterial implant
    M. biomaterial wedge
    M. block facial structure building
    material
    M. coated tear drain
    M. facial implant
    M. malar implant
    M. Quad motility implant
    M. reconstructive implant
Medrad
    M. angiographic catheter
    M. contrast medium injector
    M. Mark IV angiographic injector
    M. MRInnervu endorectal colon
    probe
    M. power angiographic injector
Medrafil wire suture
Medscand
    M. cervical spatula
    M. Cytobrush Plus cell collector
    M. cytology brush
    M. endometrial brush
    M. Pap smear kit
MedSelect-R X system
Meds eye protector
Medspec MR imaging system
Medstone
    M. extracorporeal shock-wave
    lithotripter
    M. IRIS system
    M. STS lithotripsy system
    M. STS shockwave generator
Medtel pacemaker
Medtronic
    M. Activa tremor-control therapy
    M. Activitrax rate-responsive
    unipolar ventricular pacemaker
    M. AneuRx stent graft
    M. automated coagulation timer
    M. AVE S660 coronary stent

M. AVE stent system
M. balloon catheter
M. Bestent stent
M. Bio-Pump
M. bipolar pacemaker
M. Bridge X3 renal stent system
M. CapSure SP Novus pacing lead
M. CapSure VDD pacing lead
M. CapSure Z Novus pacing lead
M. cardiac cooling jacket
M. Cardiorhythm Atakr generator
M. Chardack pacemaker
M. ClearCut 2 handpiece
M. corkscrew electrode pacemaker
M. demand pacemaker
M. Elite II pacemaker
M. external cardioverter-defibrillator
M. external tachyarrhythmia control
device
M. Freestyle stentless valve
M. Gem automatic implantable
defibrillator
M. Gem III implantable
cardioverter-defibrillator
M. GFX 2 coronary stent system
M. GuardWire Plus system
M. Hancock II bioprosthesis
M. Hancock II tissue valve
M. Hemopump system
M. Intact bioprosthetic valve
M. Intact porcine bioprosthesis
M. Interactive Tachycardia
Terminating system
M. Interstim sacral nerve
stimulation system
M. interventional vascular stent
M. Jewel AF implantable
cardioverter-defibrillator
M. Jewel ICD device
M. Jewel Plus Active Can
defibrillator
M. Kappa DR 400-series
pacemaker
M. Micro Jewel II implantable
cardioverter-defibrillator
M. MiniMed 508 insulin pump
M. Minix pacemaker
M. Mosaic heart valve
M. Octopus 2 tissue stabilizer
M. Pacette pacemaker
M. prosthetic valve
M. pulse generator
M. Pulsor Intrasound system
M. radiofrequency receiver
M. RF 5998 pacemaker
M. spinal cord stimulation system
M. Spirit lead
M. SPO pacemaker
M. SP 502 pacemaker

M. Spring lead
M. S-series small vessel stent
M. Symbios pacemaker
M. SynchroMed implantable infusion pump
M. temporary pacemaker
M. Thera DR pacemaker
M. Thera "i-series" cardiac pacemaker
M. Transvene endocardial lead
M. tremor control therapy device
M. Zuma guiding catheter
Medtronic-Alcatel pacemaker
Medtronic-Byrel-SX pacemaker
Medtronic-Hall
M.-H. heart valve prosthesis
M.-H. monocuspid tilting-disc valve
M.-H. prosthetic heart valve
M.-H. tilting-disc valve prosthesis
Medtronic-Laurens-Alcatel pacemaker
Medtronics Sequestra 1000 autotransfusion system
Medtronic-Zyrel pacemaker
medullary
m. canal reamer
m. nail
m. pin
m. rod
Medwatch telemetry system
Med-Wick
M.-W. medication delivery system
M.-W. nasal pack
MedX
M. camera
M. functional testing machine
M. knee machine
M. Mark II lumbar extension machine
M. physical therapy device
M. scanner
M. stretch machine
Meek
M. pelvic traction belt
M. snare
Meeker
M. deep-surgery forceps
M. gallbladder forceps
M. gallstone clamp
M. hemostatic forceps
M. intestinal forceps

M. monopolar electrosurgical dissector
M. right-angle clamp
Meek-style clavicular strap
Meek-Wall
M.-W. dermatome
M.-W. microdermatome
Meerschaum probe
Mefilm dressing
Mefix adhesive tape
MEG
magnetoencephalography
MEG head-based coordinate system
MEG sensor
Mega
M. Peel resurfacing system
M. Tilt and Turn bed
Mega-Air bed
MegaDyne
M. all-in-1 hand control
M. arthroscopic hook electrode
M. cautery
M. electrocautery pencil
M. E-Z clean cautery tip
MegaDyne/Fann E-Z clean laparoscopic electrode
MegaFlo infusion set
MegaLink biliary stent
MegaPeel microdermabrasion machine
Megarcart electrocardiograph
MegaSonics PTCA catheter
Megasource penile prosthesis
megavoltage
m. CT scanner
m. machine
Megazinc Pink adhesive tape
Mehta intraocular lens
meibomian
m. expressor forceps
m. gland expressor
Meier magnum system
Meigs
M. endometrial curette
M. hemostat
M. retractor
M. suture
M. uterine curette
Mel
M. 60 excimer laser
M. 70 flying spot laser
Melauskas acrylic orbital implant

M

NOTES

**Melker emergency cricothyrotomy
catheter**
Meller
M. cyclodialysis spatula
M. lacrimal sac retractor
Mellinger
M. eye speculum
M. fenestrated blades speculum
M. magnet
Mellinger-Axenfeld eye speculum
Melmed blood freezing bag
Melotte metal
Melt elevator
Meltzer
M. adenoid punch
M. nasopharyngoscope
M. tonsillar punch
membrane
m. artificial lung
barrier m.
BioBarrier m.
BioGen nonporous barrier m.
Bio-Gide bilayer m.
BioMend absorbable collagen m.
Biopore m.
collagen m.
CytoFlex m.
m. delamination wedge
Duralon-UV nylon m.
DuraMatrix collagen dura
substitute m.
ePTFE augmentation m.
m. forceps
GeneScreen Plus nylon m.
Gore Resolut Adapt
regenerative m.
Gore-Tex surgical m.
HA m.
Hemophan m.
Hybond N+ nylon m.
Imtec BioBarrier m.
MSI nylon m.
OsseoQuest regenerative m.
m. oxygenator
m. peeler
m. peeler cutter (MPC)
m. perforator
polysulfone m.
Preclude pericardial m.
Preclude peritoneal m.
Preclude spinal m.
Regentex GBR-200 m.
Seprafilm bioresorbable m.
silicone m.
sodium hyaluronate-based
bioresorbable m.
m. tack
TefGen-FD guided tissue
regeneration m.

TissueMend fiber m.
ultrafiltration m.
Viresolve ultrafiltration m.
membrane-puncturing forceps
Meme
M. breast prosthesis
M. mammary implant
Memokath catheter
memory
M. basket
m. board
m. catheter
m. exercise card
M. II cushion
m. splint
MemoryLens
M. foldable intraocular lens
M. IOL
MemoryTrace
M. AT
M. AT ambulatory cardiac monitor
Memotherm
Bard M.
M. colorectal stent
M. endoscopic biliary stent
M. Flexx biliary stent
M. nitinol self-expandable stent
Mendel ligature forceps
Mendez
M. astigmatism dial
M. corneal marker
M. cystotome
M. degree calipers
M. degree gauge
M. multi-purpose LASIK forceps
M. ultrasonic cystotome
Mendez-Schubert aortic punch
Menge pessary
Mengert membrane-puncturing forceps
Menghini
M. cannula
M. liver biopsy needle
Menghini-type coring bevel
Menghini-Wildhirt
M.-W. laparoscope
M.-W. peritoneoscope
Meniett low-pressure pulse generator
meniscal
m. basket forceps
m. clamp
m. curette
m. cutter
m. hook scissors
m. knife
m. mirror
m. posterior concave intraocular
lens
m. repair needle
m. retractor

m. spoon
m. staple
m. suture grabber
meniscectomy
m. blade
m. electrode
m. knife
m. probe
m. scissors
meniscotome
m. blade
Bowen-Grover m.
Dyonics m.
Grover m.
Ruuska m.
Smillie m.
Meniscus
M. Arrow implant
M. Mender II system
Menlo Care catheter
Mentanium vitreoretinal instrument set
Mentor
M. absorbent pouch
M. Alpha 1 inflatable penile prosthesis
M. biliary stent
M. bladder pacemaker
M. breast prosthesis
M. B-VAT II monitor
M. B-VAT visual acuity chart
M. cinch bladder neck suspension anchor system
M. continent urinary coudé catheter
M. Contour Genesis system
M. Contour Genesis ultrasonic lipoplasty system
M. deluxe leg bag strap
M. Exeter ophthalmoscope
M. female self-catheter
M. Foley catheter
M. GFS penile prosthesis
M. IPP penile prosthesis
M. malleable penile prosthesis
M. malleable semirigid penile implant
M. Mark II penile prosthesis
M. ORC MemoryLens lens
M. saline-filled testicular prosthesis
M. Self-Cath penile prosthesis
M. Self-Cath soft catheter
M. Siltex implant
M. Spectrum breast implant

M. Spectrum contour expander
M. Spectrum mammary prosthesis
M. Tele-Cath ileal conduit sampling catheter
M. tissue expander
M. Wet-Field cautery
M. Wet-Field cordless coagulator
M. Wet-Field eraser
Mentor-Maumenee Suregrip forceps
Mentor-UroSan external catheter
Menuet Compact primary urodynamic nerve fiber analyzer
Mepiform self-adherent silicone dressing
Mepilex foam dressing
Mepitel
M. contact-layer wound dressing
M. nonadherent silicone dressing
Mepore absorptive dressing
Mercator atrial high-density array catheter
Mercedes
M. tip
M. tip cannula
Mercer cartilage knife
Mercier
M. catheter
M. sound
Merck respirator
mercury
m. arc lamp
m. cell-powered pacemaker
M. Medical airway pressure manometer
m. vapor lamp
mercury-filled
m.-f. dilator
m.-f. esophageal bougie
mercury-in-rubber strain gauge plethysmograph
mercury-in-Silastic strain gauge
mercury-weighted
m.-w. dilator
m.-w. rubber bougie
Meridian
M. intersegmental table
M. pacemaker
M. ST femoral implant component
M. TMZF femoral component
meridional
m. implant
m. refractometer
Merimack 1040 CO_2 laser

M

NOTES

Merit-B periodontal probe
Merlin
    M. arthroscopy blade
    M. bendable blade
    M. stone forceps
Merlis obstetrical excavator
MERmaid kit
Mermoud nonpenetrating glaucoma forceps
Merocel
    M. epistaxis packing
    M. sponge
    M. surgical spear
    M. tampon
MeroGel
    M. dressing
    M. nasal packing
    M. stent
Merriam forceps
Merrifield knife
Merrill-Levassier retractor
Merrimack laser adapter
Merry Walker
Mershon band pusher
Mersilene
    M. band
    M. braided nonabsorbable suture
    M. gauze hammock
    M. graft
    M. implant
    M. Kessler stitch
    M. mesh
    M. mesh sling
    M. tape
Mersilk suture
Merthiolate
    M. dressing
    M. swab
Mertz keratoscopy ring
Merz
    M. aortic punch
    M. hysterectomy forceps
Merz-Vienna nasal speculum
Mesalt sodium chloride-impregnated dressing
mesh
    Auto Suture surgical m.
    Bard Composix m.
    Bard Marlex m.
    Bard Sperma-Tex preshaped m.
    Bard Visilex m.
    Brennen biosynthetic surgical m.
    Composix E/X hernia m.
    craniomaxillofacial m.
    Dacron m.
    Dexon m.
    Dexon surgically knitted m.
    DualMesh hernia m.
    Dumbach mini m.

Dumbach regular m.
Dumbach titanium m.
Ethicon m.
flared patch m.
FortaGen m.
m. graft
m. graft dermatome
Herniamesh surgical m.
Hexcelite m.
intraperitoneal onlay m.
Kugel m.
Leibinger Micro Dynamic m.
mandibular m.
Marlex m.
Meadox Dacron m.
Medox Dacron m.
Mersilene m.
metallic m.
mixed m.
m. myringotomy tube
Parietex composite m.
Permacol m.
PermaMesh m.
polyamide m.
polyglactin m.
polyglycolic acid m.
polypropylene m.
polytetrafluoroethylene m.
Prolene m.
PTFE m.
ridge-form m.
sintered titanium m.
skin graft expander m.
Sperma-Tex preshaped m.
stainless steel m.
m. stent
m. stent prosthesis
Supramid polyamide m.
surgical m.
Surgipro m.
Surgipro prolene m.
SurgiSis m.
SynMesh m.
synthetic m.
tantalum m.
Teflon m.
ThermoFX m.
TiMesh cranial m.
TiMesh orbital m.
TiMesh titanium m.
titanium m.
Trelex natural m.
Visilex m.
mesher
    Brenner m.
    Collin m.
    skin graft m.
    Tanner m.
    Zimmer skin graft m.

Meshgraft skin expander
mesocaval
    m. H-graft shunt
    m. shunt
Messerklinger
    M. endoscope
    M. sinus endoscopy set
Messing root canal gun
Meta
    M. DDDR pacemaker
    M. II pacemaker
    M. MV cardiac pacemaker
    M. rate-responsive pacemaker
metabolator
    Sanborn m.
metabolic
    m. cart
    m. heat load stimulator
metacarpal
    m. broach
    m. double-ended retractor
    m. saw
    m. splint
metacarpophalangeal
    m. implant
    m. prosthesis
MetaFluor system
metal
    m. adapter
    m. ball-tip catheter
    m. bucket-handle prosthesis
    m. cannula
    Co-Cr-W-Ni alloy implant m.
    m. femoral head prosthesis
    m. Fox shield
    Hedrocel trabecular m.
    m. hemi-toe implant
    m. hybrid orthosis
    Lipowitz m.
    Melotte m.
    m. needle
    m. orthopaedic implant
    m. pin
    m. reconstruction plate
    m. ruler
    m. scleral shield
    m. sewing ring
    m. splint
    m. tongue depressor
    M. Z stent
metal-augmented polymer stent

metal-backed
    m.-b. acetabular component implant
    m.-b. socket
metal-ball tip cannula
metal-coated stent
Metalift crown and bridge removal
  system
Metaline dressing
metallic
    m. biliary endoprosthesis
    m. cage
    m. clip
    m. mesh
    m. needle
    m. screw
    m. skin marker
    m. staple
    m. stent
    m. suture
metallic-tip catheter
Metallograft
    titanium alloy M.
metal-on-metal articulating intervertebral
  disc prosthesis
Metaport catheter
Metasul
    M. hip joint component
    M. hip prosthesis
    M. joint
    M. metal-on-metal hip prosthesis
      system
metatarsal
    m. cookie
    m. stem broach
metatarsophalangeal endoprosthesis
metatarsus adductus/varus (MTA)
Metavox hearing aid
Metcalf spring drop brace
Metcher eye speculum
Metcoff pediatric biopsy needle
meter
    Aleo m.
    analog rate m.
    Astech peak flow m.
    AsthmaCheck peak flow m.
    AvocetPT rapid prothrombin
      time m.
    CentriFlow mass flow m.
    Chemstrip MatchMaker blood
      glucose m.
    Cybex finger-clip pulse m.
    ExacTech blood glucose m.

M

NOTES

meter *(continued)*
    exposure m.
    Fisher Accumet pH m.
    galvanic skin response m.
    Gammex RMI DAP m.
    Guyton-Minkowski potential
      acuity m.
    intragastric continuous pH-meter m.
    Kowa FM-500 laser flare m.
    laser flare m.
    m. lens
    Medisense Pen 2 blood glucose m.
    Narkotest m.
    One-Touch blood glucose m.
    OxiFlow m.
    oxygen saturation m.
    peak flow m. (PFM)
    Periflux PF 1 D blood-flow m.
    pH m.
    photovolt pH m.
    potential acuity m.
    reciprocal ohm m.
    Roentgen m.
    sound level m.
    Supreme II blood glucose m.
    SureStep glucose m.
    Synectics 6000 digital pH m.
    Universal ventilation m. (UVM)
    Venturi m.
    Wright peak flow m.
    Youlten nasal inspiratory peak
      flow m.
metered-dose inhaler (MDI)
metered solution inhaler
Metermatic nasal nebulizer
methacrylate
    polymethyl m. (PMMA)
methyl
    m. cyanoacrylate glue
    m. methacrylate bead
    m. methacrylate beads implant
    m. methacrylate block
    m. methacrylate cement adhesive
    m. methacrylate cranioplasty plug
    m. methacrylate ear stent
    m. methacrylate eye implant
    m. methacrylate graft
    m. methacrylate implant material
    m. methacrylate spacer
methylacrylate
Metico forceps
MetraGrasp ligament grasper
MetraPass suture passer
Metra PS procedure kit
Metras bronchial catheter
MetraTie knot pusher
Metrecom digitizer
metric ophthalmoscope
MetriTray system soaking tray

Metrix
    M. atrial defibrillation system
    M. implantable atrioverter
metrizamide-filled balloon
MetroFlex endoscopic cart
metronoscope
Metron Plus dispenser
METRx system
Mettelman prejowl chin implant
Mettler
    M. Dia-Sonic electrosurgical unit
    M. electrotherapy
Mett tube
Metzbaum
    M. curved operating scissors
    M. operating scissors
Metzelder modification activator
Metzel-Wittmoser forceps
Metzenbaum
    M. chisel
    M. delicate scissors
    M. dissecting scissors
    M. gouge
    M. needle holder
    M. operating scissors
    M. septal knife
    M. tonsillar forceps
Metzenbaum-Lipsett scissors
Metzenbaum-Tydings forceps
Meurig Williams spinal fusion plate
Mevatron 74 linear accelerator
Mewi-5 side-hole infusion catheter
Mewissen infusion catheter
Meyer
    M. biliary retractor
    M. cervical orthosis
    M. cyclodiathermy needle
    M. olive-tipped vein stripper
    M. spiral vein stripper
    M. Swiss diamond knife lancet
    M. Swiss diamond lancet knife
    M. Swiss diamond wedge knife
    M. temporal loop
Meyerding
    M. bone graft
    M. bone skid
    M. chisel
    M. curved gouge
    M. finger retractor
    M. hip bone skid
    M. hip skid
    M. laminectomy blade
    M. laminectomy retractor
    M. mallet
    M. osteotome
    M. prosthesis
    M. retractor blade
    M. saw-toothed curette

M. self-retaining laminectomy retractor
M. shoulder skid
M. skin hook
Meyerding-Deaver retractor
Meyer-Schwickerath coagulator
Meyhöffer
    M. bone curette
    M. chalazion curette
    M. eye knife
MF heel protector
MG
    Miller-Galante
    MG II total hip system
    MG II total knee system
MGH
    MGH knee prosthesis
    MGH osteotome
    MGH periosteal elevator
    MGH uterine vulsellum forceps
    MGH vulsellum
MGM glenoidal punch
MHS modular hip screw system
MI34 diagnostic tympanometer
Miami
    M. Acute Care cervical collar
    M. Acute Care cervical traction
    M. cervical fracture brace
    M. J cervical collar
    M. J collar cervical traction
    M. TLSO scoliosis brace
MIBB
    minimally invasive breast biopsy
    MIBB breast biopsy system
MIC
    minimal inhibitory concentration
    MIC bolus gastrostomy tube
    MIC gastroenteric tube
    MIC jejunal tube
    MIC jejunostomy tube
    MIC Thermal Option biopsy forceps
mica
    m. spectacles
    M. 3x sleeve
Michel
    M. aortic clamp
    M. clip-applying forceps
    M. clip-removing forceps
    M. pick
    M. rhinoscopic mirror
    M. scalp clip

M. skin clip
M. suture clip
M. tissue forceps
Michele trephine
Michelson infant bronchoscope
Michelson-Sequoia air drill
Michel-Wachtenfeldt clip
Michigan University intestinal forceps
Mick
    M. afterloading needle
    M. prostate template
    M. seed applicator
    M. TP-200 applicator
Mic-Key
    M.-K. button gastrostomy device
    M.-K. G gastrostomy tube
    M.-K. J gastrostomy tube
Mickey and Minnie surgical marker
Micor catheter
Micra
    M. knife
    M. needle holder
Micrins
    M. forceps
    M. microsurgical suture
micro
    M. Delta system
    M. Diamond-Point microsurgery instrument
    M. DiaryCard
    M. E irrigation kit
    M. Jewel II implantable cardioverter-defibrillator
    M. Link endoscope fiber
    M. Minix pacemaker
    M. Mist disposable nebulizer
    M. One pneumatonometer
    M. Plus plating system
    M. Plus screw
    M. Plus spirometer
    M. punctum plug
    m. round-tip needle
    M. series wire driver
    m. tissue forceps
Micro-6 ureteroscope
Micro-Aire
    M.-A. bur
    M.-A. drill
    M.-A. oscillating bone saw
    M.-A. osteotome
    M.-A. pneumatic power instrument
    M.-A. pulse lavage system

M

NOTES

MicroAire
    M. carpal tunnel release system
    M. power-assisted lipoplasty device
MicroAir nebulizer
microAir Turn-Q Plus mattress
microanalyzer
    electronic m.
    electron probe x-ray m.
microaspirator
    Ergo m.
microballoon
    implantable silicone m.
    Rand m.
Microbeam
    M. manipulator
    M. micromanipulator
microbipolar forceps
microblade
    Beaver m.
    Sharptome m.
Microblator ArthroWands
Microbrush
microcalipers
    Storz m.
Microcap handheld capnograph
microcarrier
    CultiSpher-G m.
    CultiSpher macroporous gel m.
microcatheter
    Cardima Pathfinder m.
    Cardima Revelation Tx m.
    coaxial m.
    Excel-14 m.
    Excelsior 1018 m.
    Hydrolyser m.
    InDuct breast m.
    Leggiero hydrophilic-coated m.
    Magic m.
    Pathfinder mapping m.
    Prowler m.
    Rebar-18 m.
    Renegade m.
    Revelation Tx m.
    Terumo SP hydrophilic-coated m.
    Therastream m.
    Tracker-10 m.
    Transit m.
    UltraLite flow-directed m.
MicroCell chamber
microcentrifuge
    Compac m.
    MicroPrep 2 m.
MicroChoice electric powered surgical system
microclamp
    disposable m.
    Kapp m.
    Khodadad m.

microclip
    m. applying forceps
    Heifitz m.
    Kleinert-Kutz m.
    Williams m.
    Yasargil m.
    Zylik m.
microcoagulator
    Malis bipolar m.
    Polar-Mate bipolar m.
MicroCO carbon monoxide monitor
microcoil
    endothelin-1 m.
    Hilal m.
    Intercept esophageal internal MR m.
    Intercept internal m.
    platinum m.
microcolpohysteroflator
    Hamou m.
microcomputer upper limb exerciser (MULE)
microconnector
    titanium m.
microcurette
    Accurette m.
    HemoCue m.
    Rhoton m.
    Ruggles m.
microcystitome
    Lieppman m.
microdebrider
    Hummer m.
    Linvatec m.
    Linvotec m.
    MDS m.
    Radnoid m.
    m. system (MDS)
    Wizard m.
MicroDelivery Peel pump
microdensitometer
    Vickers M85a m.
microdermabrader
    Pelle Peel m.
    SkinMaster MD7 m.
microdermatome
    Meek-Wall m.
microdialysis catheter
MicroDigitrapper apnea recorder
MicroDigitrapper-HR fingertrap
MicroDigitrapper-S
    M.-S apnea screening device
    M.-S fingertrap
MicroDigitrapper-V fingertrap
microdilution system
microdissecting forceps
microdissection
    Piezo power m.

microdissector
  Crockard m.
  Fukushima m.
  Hardy m.
  Rhoton m.
  Yasargil m.
Microdon dressing
Microdose Cath
microdrill
  high-speed m.
  Shea m.
microelectrode
  Eppendorf m.
  tungsten m.
microendoscope
  Omegascope OM2/070 flexible m.
  ophthalmic laser m.
  Toshiba m.
microendoscopic test card
MicroEnhancer UL micropigmentation device
MicroFet2 muscle testing device
MicroFET isometric force dynamometer
microfibrillar
  m. collagen
  m. collagen hemostat
Microfil silicone-rubber injection compound
microfilter
  Minnpure m.
Microflo test strip
MicroFlow phacoemulsification needle
Microfoam
  M. conformable foam elastic tape
  M. dressing
  M. surgical tape
microforceps
  Adson m.
  Anis m.
  Birks-Mathelone m.
  Collis m.
  DORC m.
  iris m.
  iris suture m.
  Jako-Kleinsasser m.
  Koslowski m.
  Nicola m.
  Rhoton m.
  Scanlan m.
  V. Mueller laser Rhoton m.
  Yasargil m.

MicroFrance
  M. minimally invasive surgical instrument
  M. pediatric backbiter
Microfuge tube
MicroFuse infuser
MicroGas monitor
Microgel surface-enhanced ventilation tube
Microglass pH electrode
Micro-Glide corneal suture
Micro-Guide catheter
MicroGuide microelectrode recording system
microguidewire
  Transcend m.
Microgyn II urinary incontinence device
Micro-Halogen otoscope
microhandpiece
MicroHartzler ACS balloon catheter system
microhemostat
  O'Brien-Storz m.
microhook
  Bonn m.
  McIntyre m.
  Shambaugh-Derlacki m.
  Simcoe m.
microhysteroflator
  Hamou m.
microhysteroscope
  Hamou contact m.
Micro-Imager high-resolution digital camera
microimpactor
  Codman m.
microimplant
  Artecoll injectable m.
  Bioplastique injectable m.
  silicone m.
microincision
  m. cataract surgery (MICS)
microirrigator
Microjet-based cutting and debriding device
Microjet Quark portable pump
micro-jewelers monopolar forceps
microkeratome
  Amadeus m.
  Barraquer m.
  Barraquer-Carriazo m.
  Barraquer-Krumeich-Swinger m.

M

NOTES

microkeratome *(continued)*
    BD K-3000 m.
    BKS m.
    Carriazo-Barraquer m.
    Chiron ACS m.
    FLAPmaker disposable m.
    Hansatome m.
    Krumeich-Barraquer m.
    LSK One m.
    MedJet m.
    ML m.
    ML m.
    One disposable m.
    Ruiz m.
    Summit Krumeich-Barraquer m.
microknife
    Karlin m.
Microknit vascular graft
Microlance blood lancet
MicroLap
    M. endoscope
    M. Gold microlaparoscopy system
microlaparoscope
    Imagyn m.
    Pixie m.
microlaryngeal
    m. endotracheal tube
    m. grasping forceps
    m. laser probe
    m. scissors
microlaryngoscope
    Abramson-Dedo m.
    anterior commissure m.
    Dedo-Jako m.
    Fragen anterior commissure m.
    Jako m.
    Lindholm m.
Microlase
    M. transpupillary diode
    M. transpupillary diode laser
Microlens
    M. cystourethroscope
    M. direct-vision telescope
    M. foroblique telescope
    M. hook
    M. urethroscope
Microlet
    M. electrode needle
    M. Vaculance
    M. Vaculance lancet
Microlight 830 low-level laser
Micro-Line arterial forceps
Microlith
    M. pacemaker pulse generator
    M. P pacemaker
Microloc
    M. knee prosthesis
    M. knee system

MicroLoop
    M. II spirometer
    M. ML3535 spirometer
microloupe loupe
microlumbar discectomy retractor
MicroLux video camera system
Microlyzer Gas analyzer
micromanipulator
    Microbeam m.
    MicroSpot m.
    self-centering m.
    UniMax 2000 laser m.
micromanometer
    m. catheter
    m. catheter system
micromanometer-tipped catheter
MicroMark tissue marker
MicroMax
    M. centrifuge
    M. drill system
    M. speed drill
MicroMed DeBakey ventricular assist device
Micromedics surgical instrument
micromesh
    m. cushioned abrasive
    m. sheeting
micrometer
    ultrasonic m.
MicroMewi multiple side-hole infusion catheter
Micro-Mill knee instrument system
micromirror
    Silverstein m.
MicroMirror gold sensor
MicroMite anchor suture
micromultileaf collimator
micron
    M. bobbin ventilation tube
    m. needle
    M. Res-Q implantable cardioverter-defibrillator
micronebulizer
    Bird m.
microneedle
    Colorado m.
    m. holder
Microny
    M. K SR
    M. KSR pacemaker
    M. SR+ cardiac pacemaker
    M. SR+ single-chamber, rate-responsive pulse generator
Micro-One dissecting forceps
Micropach 200P notebook corneal pachymeter
MicroPeel Plus system
microphone
    hearing aid m.

2-microphone acoustical rhinometer
MicroPhor iontophoretic drug delivery
   system
microphthalmoscope
micropipet
> Humagen blastomere biopsy m.
> Humagen polar body biopsy m.

micropipette
> in vitro fertilization m.

micropituitary rongeur
Microplaner blade
microplate
> C-shaped m.
> m. fixation
> Luhr m.
> mandibular angle fracture intraoral
>   open reduction m.
> m. reader

MicroPlex coil system
micropoint
> m. needle

MicroPoint suture scissors
Micropore
> M. surgical tape
> M. surgical tape dressing

MicroPrep 2 microcentrifuge
MicroProbe
> Endo Optics M.
> M. ophthalmic laser
> M. ophthalmic laser endoscope

microprocessor
> Intertron therapy m.

Micro-Pulsar TENS unit
micropuncture
> m. introducer needle
> m. needle
> M. Peel-Away introducer

microrasp
> Scanlan m.

microraspatory
> Yasargil m.

microreciprocating saw
microrongeur
> Kerrison m.

microruler
> Stecher m.

microsagittal saw
microscalpel
> Oasis feather m.

microscanner
> pQCT m.

microscissors
> Collis m.
> curved spring-handled m.
> DORC m.
> Gill-Welsh-Vannas angled m.
> Jacobson m.
> Jako-Kleinsasser m.
> Kamdar m.
> Keeler m.
> Kurze m.
> Rhoton m.
> Scanlan m.
> Shutt m.
> straight m.
> straight spring-handled m.
> Twisk m.
> V. Mueller laser Rhoton m.
> Yasargil m.

microscope
> Accu-Scope m.
> acoustic m.
> analytical electron m.
> Beckerscope binocular m.
> BHTU m.
> Bio-Optics specular m.
> Bitumi monobjective m.
> cine m.
> Cohan-Barraquer m.
> confocal m.
> conventional transmission
>   electron m.
> CooperVision m.
> corneal m.
> Czapski m.
> DigiScope handheld USB m.
> EIE 150F operating m.
> electron m.
> Elmiskop 101 electron m.
> endothelial specular m.
> epi-illuminated m.
> Fiberlite m.
> fiberoptic m.
> Galilean m.
> Hallpike-Blackmore ear m.
> Heyer-Schulte m.
> high-voltage electron m.
> Hitachi H-series electron m.
> H-series electron m.
> JEM-100B, 100S electron m.
> Joel scanning electron m.
> JSM-6400 scanning electron m.
> Kaps operating m.

M

NOTES

microscope *(continued)*
Keeler-Konan Specular m.
Konan SP8000 noncontact
specular m.
laser m.
Leica M680 surgical m.
Leitz m.
LSM-2100C Eye Bank specular m.
Marco SurgiScope 3 operating m.
Moller m.
multimode imaging confocal
optical m.
Olympus BHT-2 m.
Olympus CBK fluorescence m.
OM 2000 operating m.
operating m. (OM)
OPMI Pro magis surgical m.
OPMI Visu 200 m.
Optiphot-2UD m.
Optique m.
Philips CM-200 electron m.
pneumatic m.
projection x-ray m.
Project Research Ophthalmic
specular m.
Pro-Koester wide-field SCM m.
Protégé Plus m.
real-time confocal scanning
laser m.
Rheinberg m.
scanning electron m.
scanning laser acoustic m.
scanning slit confocal m.
scanning transmission electron m.
scanning tunneling m.
Seiler MC-M900 surgical m.
slit-lamp m.
SMZ-1 m.
SMZ zoom stereo m.
stereoscopic m.
Storz m.
surgical m.
tandem scanning confocal m.
Tomey ConfoScan confocal
microscope Model P4 m.
Topcon SP-series non-contact
specular m.
transmission electron m.
Urban m.
Varimic 900 m.
video specular m.
Weck m.
Wild M 690 operating m.
x-ray tomographic m.
Zeiss Axioskop m.
Zeiss-Barraquer cine m.
Zeiss-Contraves operating m.
Zeiss IDO3 phase-contrast m.
Zeiss-Jena surgical m.

Zeiss operating m.
Zeiss OPMI Mdo ophthalmic
surgical m.
Zeiss OPMI Pro magis m.
microscopic scissors
microscrew
Barouk m.
MicroSeal
M. nebulizer
M. phaco handpiece
Storz M.
microsecond pulsed flashlamp-pumped
dye laser
Microsect
M. curette
M. shaver
microserrefine
Storz m.
MicroShape keratome system
Micro-Sharp blade
microshaver
Micros infusion system
MicroSkin ostomy pouch
microslide
ColorFrost m.
ColorMark m.
MicroSmooth probe
Microsnap hemostatic forceps
microsnare
Amplatz gooseneck m.
Microsoftrac catheter
Micro-Soft Stream side-hole infusion
catheter
Microson hearing aid
MicroSpan
M. capnometer
M. hysteroscope
M. microhysteroscopy system
M. minihysteroscopy system
M. sheath
microspatula
Osher malleable m.
microspectroscope
microspectroscopy
Fourier transform infrared m.
microsphere
Embosphere m.
magnetic m.
paramagnetic m.
Microspike
M. approximator
M. approximator clamp
microsponge
Alcon m.
M. delivery system
Teardrop m.
M. Teardrop sponge
Weck-Cel m.
MicroSpot micromanipulator

Micross
    M. dilatation catheter
    M. SL balloon
MicroStable liner locking mechanism
microstaple
    Barouk m.
Microstar dialysis system
microstat
    Endo-Suction sinus m.
    M. handpiece
    M. ultrasonic nebulizer
Microstent II coronary stent
MicroStim 100 TENS device
microstomia prevention appliance
microsurgery
    robot-assisted m. (RAMS)
microsurgical
    m. grasping forceps
    m. needle holder
    m. retractor
    m. scissors
    m. tying forceps
microsuture
    Sharpoint m.
microsyringe
MicroTach
    M. pneumotach
    M. pneumotachometer
Microtaze microwave coagulator
Microtek
    M. cupped forceps
    M. Heine otoscope
    M. ScanMaker 9600XL scanner
    M. scissors
MicroTeq portable belt
Microthin P2 pacemaker
MicroTip phaco tip
microtip pressure transducer
microtitration plate reader
microtome
    Cryo-Cut m.
    Leica vibrating knife m.
    Leitz 1600 Saw m.
    Stadie-Riggs m.
microtonometer
    Computon m.
microtransducer
    m. catheter
    imbedded m.
    Konigsberg m.
Microtron accelerator
Micro-Two forceps

microtying forceps
MicroTymp2 handheld tympanometer
MicroVac catheter
microvascular
    m. anastomotic coupler system
    m. clamp
    m. clamp-applying forceps
    m. clip
    m. modified Alm retractor
    m. needle holder
    m. scissors
    m. tying forceps
Microvasive
    M. balloon retrieval catheter
    M. biliary stent system
    M. controlled radial expansion esophageal dilator
    M. disposable alligator-shaped forceps
    M. Glidewire
    M. papillotome
    M. radial jaw biopsy forceps
    M. retrieval balloon
    M. Rigiflex balloon catheter
    M. Rigiflex balloon dilator
    M. Rigiflex through-the-scope balloon
    M. Rigiflex TTS balloon
    M. sclerotherapy needle
    M. Speedband Superview ligator
    M. stent
    M. stiff piano wire guidewire
    M. Ultraflex esophageal stent system
    M. ultratome
MicroVein vascular system
Microvel
    M. double velour graft
    M. prosthesis
Microvena
    M. Amplatz Goose Neck snare
    M. Das Angel Wings occluder
Micro-Vent implant
MicroVent ventilator
MicroView sheath-based IVUS catheter
Microvit
    M. probe
    M. scissors
    M. vitrectomy cutter
    M. vitrectomy probe
    M. vitrector
microvitrectomy system (MVS)

M

NOTES

microvitreoretinal blade
Microvolt T-wave alternans device
Microwec scissors
Microwell washer
MicroWrist robotic surgical system
MicroXcisor ethmoid bone cutting
  instrument
Micro-Z neuromuscular stimulator
MICS
  microincision cataract surgery
micturition bag
MIDA
  Mass Isotopomer Distribution Analysis
    MIDA CoroNet instrumentation
    HP MIDA
Midas
  M. Rex craniotome
  M. Rex drill
  M. Rex instrumentation
  M. Rex instrumentation system
  M. Rex knife
  M. Rex pneumatic instrument
midcavity forceps
middle
  m. ear forceps
  m. ear implant
  m. ear prosthesis
Middledorpf
  M. retractor
  M. splint
Middlesex-Pointe retractor
Middleton
  M. adenoid curette
  M. rongeur
midgastric electrode
midinfrared laser
mid-infrared pulsed laser
Midland tilt table
Midline Hi-Lo Mat platform
Midmark 413 power female procedure
  chair
midoccipital electrode
Mighty Bite Zimmon lateral biopsy cup
  forceps
MightyLite headlamp
Mignon cataract extractor
Mijnhard electrical cycloergometer
Mikaelsson catheter
Mikros pacemaker
Mikro-Tip
  M.-T. angiocatheter
  M.-T. micromanometer-tipped
    catheter
  M.-T. pressure transducer catheter
Mikulicz
  M. abdominal retractor
  M. crusher
  M. drain
  M. liver retractor

M. pad
M. peritoneal clamp
M. peritoneal forceps
M. spatula
M. sponge
M. tonsillar forceps
Mikulicz-Radecki
  M.-R. clamp
  M.-R. drain
Milan uterine curette
Milch resection plate
Miles
  M. antral curette
  M. bone chisel
  M. Encore QA glucometer
  M. punch biopsy forceps
  M. rectal clamp
  M. retractor
  M. skin clip
  M. Teflon clip
Milette-Tyding dissector
Milewski driver
Milex
  M. forceps
  M. Jel-Jector vaginal applicator
  M. pessary
  M. retractor
  M. spatula
  M. vaginal insufflator
military antishock trousers (MAST)
mill
  hollow m.
  Lere bone m.
  OrthoBlend powered bone m.
Millar
  M. catheter tip pressure transducer
  M. Doppler catheter
  M. micromanometer catheter
  M. Mikro-Tip catheter pressure
    transducer
  M. pigtail angiographic catheter
  M. urodynamic catheter
Millard
  M. clamp
  M. Lite-Pipe
  M. mouthgag
Millenia
  M. balloon catheter
  M. balloon dilatation catheter
  M. percutaneous transluminal
    coronary angioplasty catheter
Millenium Lightning vitrectomy cutter
Millennium
  M. CX microsurgical system
  M. LX microsurgical system
  M. oxygen concentrator
Millen otologic implant
Mille Pattes screw

Miller
- M. articulating paper forceps
- M. bayonet forceps
- M. bone file
- M. bougie
- M. bracket positioner
- M. curette
- M. cystoscope
- M. dental elevator
- M. dilator
- M. dissecting scissors
- M. endotracheal tube
- M. fiberoptic laryngoscope blade
- M. laryngoscope
- M. operating scissors
- M. rasp
- M. ratchet injector
- M. rectal forceps
- M. rectal scissors
- M. retractor
- M. septostomy catheter
- M. stent
- M. tonsillar dissector
- M. vaginal speculum

Miller-Abbott double-lumen intestinal tube
Miller-Apexo elevator
Miller-Galante (MG)
- M.-G. hip prosthesis
- M.-G. I condylar total knee system
- M.-G. revision knee system
- M.-G. total knee system
- M.-G. unicompartmental knee

Miller-Senn double-ended retractor
Millesi scissors
Millet
- M. needle
- M. neurological test instrument
- M. test hammer

Millette tonsillar knife
Millette-Tyding knife
Millex
- M. GS-series filter
- M. GV-series filter

Millie female urinal
Milligan
- M. double-ended dissector
- M. self-retaining retractor
- M. speculum

Milliknit
- M. arterial prosthesis
- M. Dacron prosthesis

- M. graft
- M. vascular graft prosthesis

Millin
- M. bladder neck spreader
- M. bladder spatula
- M. boomerang needle holder
- M. capsular forceps
- M. clamp
- M. ligature-guiding forceps
- M. prostatectomy forceps
- M. retropublic bladder retractor
- M. self-retaining retractor
- M. suction tube
- M. T-shaped forceps

Millin-Bacon
- M.-B. bladder neck spreader
- M.-B. bladder self-retaining retractor
- M.-B. retropubic prostatectomy retractor

milliner's needle
millinery bag
Millipore
- M. suture
- M. ultrafree-CL centrifugal filter

Milli-Q water purification system
Mill-Rose
- M.-R. cytology brush
- M.-R. esophageal injector
- M.-R. flexible endoscopic overtube
- M.-R. RiteBite biopsy forceps
- M.-R. spiral stone basket
- M.-R. SureBite biopsy forceps
- M.-R. tube

Mills
- M. circumflex scissors
- M. coronary endarterectomy set
- M. coronary endarterectomy spatula
- M. dressing
- M. Glucometer II glucometer
- M. microvascular needle holder
- M. operative peripheral angioplasty catheter
- M. tissue forceps
- M. valvulotome

Milroy-Piper suction tube
Milteck scissors
Miltex
- M. bone saw
- M. Cottle double hook
- M. Cottle retractor
- M. Cottle skin elevator

M

NOTES

Miltex *(continued)*
    M. Crile needle holder
    M. Cushing bayonet forceps
    M. disposable biopsy punch
    M. gun
    M. ligature knife
    M. nail nipper
    M. pump
    M. rib spreader
    M. Wiener corneal hook
    M. wire twister
Milwaukee
    M. scoliosis brace
    M. scoliosis orthosis
    M. snare
Mi-Mark endocervical curette set
Mimix bone replacement system
MindSet toe splint
Miner osteotome
Minerva
    M. cast
    M. cervicothoracic orthosis
    M. collar
    M. neurosurgical robot
    M. plastic back jacket
    M. robot
**Mingograf 62 6-channel
electrocardiograph**
Mingograph
    Siemens M.
mini
    m. applier
    M. Crown stent
    m. lag screw
    m. vessel clamp
miniature
    m. blade
    m. bulldog clamp
    m. centrifugal fast analyzer
    m. probe
miniaturized ultrasound catheter probe
Mini-Bag Plus container
miniballoon
minibasket
    Shutt m.
miniBIRD position tracker
miniblade
    Beaver m.
Miniblaster
    Deldent M.
miniclip
    Stangel fallopian tube m.
minicoil
MiniCorr pulse oximeter
Minidop ES-100VX Pocket Doppler
mini-echo sounder
Mini-Fibralux pocket otoscope

minifixator
    Link Ellis external m.
    Pennig m.
Mini-Flex
    M.-F. flexible Harris uterine
     injector
    HUI M.-F.
miniforceps
miniform
    inSync m.
Miniguard
    M. adhesive patch
    M. stress incontinence device
MiniHEART low-flow nebulizer
Minilith
    M. pacemaker
    M. pacemaker pulse generator
Minilux pocket otoscope
minimagnet
    Hamblin m.
minimal inhibitory concentration (MIC)
minimallet
    Gam-Mer m.
**minimally invasive breast biopsy
(MIBB)**
Mini-Matic implant
Minimax 200 watt light source
MiniMed
    M. continuous glucose monitoring
     system
    M. III infusion pump
MiniMedBall hand exerciser
Mini-Motionlogger Actigraph
Mini-Neb nebulizer
miniosteotome
    Gam-Mer m.
MiniOX
    M. IA oxygen analyzer
    M. I, II, III, 100-IV oxygen
     monitor
    M. V pulse oximeter
miniplate
    2-hole m.
    L-shaped m.
    Luhr m.
    mandibular m.
    m. strut
    titanium m.
    Vitallium m.
minipouch
    Premier drainable m.
    Sur-Fit m.
miniprobe
    high-frequency m.
Mini-Profile dilatation catheter
minipump
    Alzer osmotic m.
    osmotic m.
MiniQuad XL lens

MiniQuick
    Genotropin M.
miniretractor
    R-Med m.
miniscope
    Candela m.
MiniSite laparoscope
Minispace IUI catheter
ministaple
    Bio-R-Sorb resorbable poly-L-lactic
    acid m.
    Richards m.
Mini-Stick
    Vaxcel M.-S.
MiniStim TENS unit
Mini-tip culturette
Mini-Wright peak flowmeter
Minix pacemaker
Minneapolis hip prosthesis
Minnesota
    M. impedance cardiograph
    M. retractor
    M. thermal disc temperature testing
    device
    M. tube
Minnpure microfilter
Minos air drill
Minuet DDD pacemaker
MIP
    Med-I-Pad
    MIP anatomic overlay
    MIP reusable cover
**Mipron digital computer-assisted
    calipers**
Mira
    M. AGL-400 laser
    M. cautery
    M. coagulator
    M. diathermy
    M. drill
    M. electrocautery
    M. encircling element
    M. endovitreal cryopencil
    M. femoral head reamer
    M. photocoagulator
    M. silicone rod
Mira-Charnley reamer
Miracompo filling instrument
Mirage
    M. full-face mask
    M. guidewire
    M. nasal mask

    M. nasal ventilation mask system
    M. over-the-wire balloon catheter
    M. spinal system
    M. top-tightening spinal system
Miralene suture
Miralva applicator
Mirasorb sponge
mirror
    Apfelbaum m.
    Articu-Lase laser m.
    bayonet transsphenoidal m.
    Buckingham m.
    m. cannula
    contact lens training m.
    curved laryngeal m.
    DenLite illuminated handheld m.
    fiberoptic lighted m.
    Grafco head m.
    Grafco laryngeal m.
    Hardy transsphenoidal m.
    head m.
    m. holder
    House middle ear m.
    Jako laryngeal m.
    Kashiwabara laryngeal m.
    Kerner dental m.
    laryngeal m.
    m. laryngoscope
    laser m.
    Lewis dental m.
    McLaughlin laser m.
    meniscal m.
    Michel rhinoscopic m.
    Neovision micro m.
    Oliair mouth m.
    Olyco mouth m.
    Olympia mouth m.
    Poh mouth m.
    polygon m.
    rhinoscopic m.
    SMIC mouth m.
    Stiwer laryngeal m.
    straight laryngeal m.
    straight magnifying m.
3-mirror
    3-m. contact lens
    3-m. intraocular lens
4-mirror
    4-m. goniolens
    4-m. goniolens lens
mirror-based reflective optics

M

NOTES

MIS
    medical implant system
    multiport illumination system
        MIS dental implant
Mischler-Pudenz shunt
Mischler shunt
Misdome-Frank curette
Mishima-Hedbys attachment pacemeter
Mishler
    M. dual-chamber valve
    M. flushing valve
Miskimon cerebellar self-retaining
    retractor
Missouri catheter
Misstique female external urinary
    collector
Mistogen
    M. nebulizer
    M. passover humidifier
mist tent
Misty-Neb nebulizer
Mitamura fine ceramic heart valve
Mitchel-Adam clamp
Mitchel aortotomy clamp
Mitchell
    M. cartilage knife
    M. osteotome
    M. stone basket
    M. ureteral stone dislodger
    M. viscoelastic removal I&A tip
Mitchell-Diamond biopsy forceps
Mitek
    M. absorbable bone anchor
    M. anchor appliance
    M. bone anchor
    M. Fastin threaded anchor
    M. GII Easy anchor
    M. GII suture anchor
    M. GII suture anchor system
    M. GL anchor
    M. Knotless anchor
    M. Ligament anchor
    M. Micro anchor
    M. Micro QuickAnchor
    M. Mini GII anchor
    M. Mini GLS anchor
    M. Mini QuickAnchor
    M. Panalok anchor
    M. QuickAnchor device
    M. rotator cuff anchor
    M. SuperAnchor instrument
    M. Tacit threaded anchor
    M. Vapr tissue removal system
Mithoefer-Jansen mouthgag
Mitraflex
    M. sterile spyrosorbent multilayer
        wound dressing
    M. wound dressing

mitral
    m. valve dilator
    m. valve retractor
Mitrathane wound dressing
Mitroflow
    M. pericardial prosthetic valve
    M. PeriPatch cylinder
    M. Synergy PC aortic heart valve
    M. Synergy PC stented pericardial
        bioprosthesis
Mitsubishi
    M. angioscope
    M. angioscopic catheter
mitt
    holding m.
    impact m.
    infant passive m.
    motion control m.
    paraffin m.
Mittelman Pre Jowl-Chin implant
Mittlemeir ceramic hip prosthesis
Mitutoyo Digimatic calipers
Mity
    M. engine H-file
    M. Gates Glidden file
    M. Hedström file
    M. Roto rotary instrument
    M. spreader
    M. Turbo File file
Mityvac
    M. cup vacuum extractor cup
    M. extractor
    M. obstetric vacuum extractor cup
    M. Super M cup
    M. vacuum delivery system
    M. vacuum extractor cup
    M. vacuum pump
mixed mesh
mixer/blender
    Aladdin m.
Mixter
    M. arterial forceps
    M. artery forceps
    M. baby hemostatic forceps
    M. brain biopsy punch
    M. common duct probe
    M. Dilaprobe probe
    M. dilating probe
    M. dissector
    M. gallbladder forceps
    M. gall duct probe
    M. gallstone forceps
    M. hemostat
    M. irrigating probe
    M. mosquito forceps
    M. operating scissors
    M. pediatric hemostatic forceps
    M. thoracic clamp

M. thoracic forceps
M. tube
Mixter-McQuigg forceps
Mixter-O'Shaughnessy
M.-O. dissecting forceps
M.-O. hemostatic forceps
Mixter-Paul
M.-P. arterial forceps
M.-P. hemostatic forceps
Mixtner catheter
Miya
M. hook
M. hook ligature carrier
Miyajima LASIK calipers
Miyoshi ophthalmic chopper
Mizuho surgical Doppler
Mizutani laminaria tent
Mizzy needle
MKG knee support
MKII automated scanner
MK IV ophthalmoscope
MKM AutoPilot stereotactic system
MKS II knee brace
ML
ML eye spear
ML microkeratome
Mladick
M. concave cannula
M. convex cannula
MLR+ camera
MLS small cannulated cancellous screw system
MM-6000 colposcope
MMG
Medical Marketing Group
MMG Easycath catheter
MMG Golden-Drain
MMG Ready Cath catheter
MMG/O'Neil sterile-field urinary catheter system
M-mode sector transducer
MMS
Medical Management System
MMS low-profile acetabular cup
MMS-10 tympanic displacement analyzer
Moberg
M. bone plate
M. chisel
M. forceps
M. osteotome
M. retractor

Moberg-Stille
M.-S. forceps
M.-S. retractor
Mobetron
M. intraoperative radiation therapy treatment system
M. mobile, self-shielded electron accelerator
mobile
m. air chair
m. electroconvulsive therapy apparatus
m. spiral computed tomography scanner
mobile-bearing knee implant
Mobilimb CPM device
mobilizer
Derlacki ear m.
Hough-Derlacki m.
Therabite m.
Mobils Professionals pedorthic footwear
Mobin-Uddin
M.-U. sieve
M.-U. umbrella vena caval filter
Moblvac suction unit
Mochida CO_2 Medi-Laser laser
model
Gullstrand 6-surface eye m.
Kooijman eye m.
Le Grand-Gullstrand eye m.
tube observation m. (TOM)
modeling carver
mode-locked laser
modified
m. chest lead
m. C-loop haptic
m. C-loop intraocular lens
m. Grace plate
m. Harrington rod
m. J-loop haptic
m. J-loop, posterior chamber intraocular lens
m. Mark IV R-wave-triggered power injector
m. Moore hip locking prosthesis
m. nasal trumpet
m. Oppenheimer splint
m. Rashkind PDA occluder
m. Robert Jones dressing
m. sclerectomy punch
m. spatula needle
m. sternal retractor

M

NOTES

modified *(continued)*
    m. suction tube
    m. Younge forceps
    m. zinc oxide-eugenol cement
    m. Z-stent
Modny
    M. drill
    M. guide
    M. pin
Modulap probe
modular
    m. acetabular reconstruction system (MARS)
    M. Acetabular Revision System (MARS)
    m. Austin Moore hip prosthesis
    m. calcar replacement stem
    m. clip application system (MCAS)
    m. head
    m. head remover
    m. implant
    m. instrumentation
    M. One pneumatonometer
    m. S-ROM total hip system
    m. stent graft
    m. total hip prosthesis
    Universal m. (UM)
modulator
    Tei-Shin spring m.
module
    A-Lastic m.
    AutoSPECT processing m.
    Capnostat Mainstream carbon dioxide m.
    CUSA electrosurgical m. (CEM)
    Datex-Ohmeda S/5 oxygen saturation m.
    dialysate preparation m.
    Peak gait m.
    SAM m.
Modulith SL 20 lithotripter
Modulock posterior spinal fixation device
Modulus CD anesthesia system
Moe
    M. alar hook
    M. bone curette
    M. gouge
    M. impactor
    M. intertrochanteric plate
    M. modified Harrington rod
    M. nail
    M. osteotome
    M. subcutaneous rod
Moehle
    M. cannula
    M. corneal forceps
Moeller laser
Moeltgen flexometer

Moersch
    M. bronchoscope
    M. bronchoscopic forceps
    M. cardiospasm dilator
    M. electrode
Moffat-Robinson bone pate collector
Mogen circumcision clamp
Mohr
    M. endoscopic scissors
    M. finger splint
    M. pinchcock clamp
MoistAir humidifying chamber
moistened fine-mesh gauze dressing
moist interactive dressing
moisture
    m. chamber
    m. exchanger
    m. vapor permeable (MVP)
moisture-retentive dressing
Mojave cataract extraction system
molar bracket
mold
    acrylic m.
    Altchek vaginal m.
    Aquaplast m.
    Biothotic orthotic m.
    Counsellor vaginal m.
    Hydro-Cast dental m.
    Silastic m.
    silicone m.
    sodium alginate wool m.
    Swyrls swim m.
    Teflon m.
    vaginal m.
moldable insole
molded
    m. ankle-foot orthosis (MAFO)
    m. ankle-foot orthosis cane
molding sock
Mold-In-Place back support
molectron laser
molecular
    m. coincidence detection imaging
    m. recognition unit (MRU)
    m. sieve
molecule
    Sonic Hedgehog signaling m.
moleskin
    m. bandage
    m. padding
    m. traction hitch dressing
Molestick padding
Molina
    M. mandibular distractor
    M. needle catheter
Moller microscope
Mollison
    M. mastoid rongeur
    M. self-retaining retractor

Molnar disc
Molt
- M. curette
- M. dissector
- M. mouthgag
- M. No. 4 elevator
- M. pedicle forceps
- M. periosteal elevator

Molteno
- M. double-plate implant
- M. glaucoma double-plate implant
- M. glaucoma single-plate implant
- M. implant glaucoma drainage device
- M. seton
- M. shunt tube
- M. valve

Moltz-Storz tonsillectome
molybdenum
- m. anode
- m. rotating-anode x-ray tube
- m. target tube

molybdenum-99 generator
molybdenum-technetium generator
Momberg tourniquet
Momentum pacemaker
Momma-Too Maternity Support
Momosi spider lens intraocular lens
Monaco broach
Monaghan
- M. respirator
- M. 300 ventilator

Monahan-Lewis knife
Monaldi drain
Monarch
- M. II bleaching instrument
- M. II IOL delivery system
- M. knee brace
- M. Mini Mask nasal interface
- M. transshaping gastrostomy tube

Monark
- M. bicycle
- M. bicycle ergometer
- M. Rehab Trainer

Mon-a-Therm 6510 two-channel thermometer
Moncorps knife
Moncrieff
- M. anterior chamber irrigating cannula
- M. anterior chamber irrigator

monitor
- Accucap CO_2/O_2 m.
- Accu-Chek blood glucose m.
- Accu-Chek Easy blood glucose m.
- Accu-Chek II Freedom blood glucose m.
- Accu-Chek InstantPlus blood glucose m.
- Accucom cardiac output m.
- AccuGuide injection m.
- Accutorr A1 blood pressure m.
- Accutorr Plus blood pressure m.
- Accutracker ambulatory blood pressure m.
- Accutracker II ambulatory blood pressure m.
- actocardiotocograph fetal m.
- Aequitron apnea m.
- aerosol inhalation m.
- Aesculap-Spiegelberg brain pressure m.
- AlphaCare m.
- AM1 asthma m.
- Ami infant apnea m.
- antepartum m.
- APM-2000 vital signs m.
- apnea m.
- AR+ portable heart m.
- Arrhythmia Net m.
- Arvee model 2400 infant apnea m.
- Baby Dopplex 3000 antepartum fetal m.
- Bear NUM-1 tidal volume m.
- Bedfont carbon monoxide m.
- bedside m.
- BellyBeats fetal Doppler m.
- Biocon impedance plethysmography cardiac output m.
- Biotrack coagulation m.
- BioTrainer exercise m.
- BladderScan m.
- blood perfusion m. (BPM)
- Brackmann facial nerve m.
- BreathCO breathe carbon monoxide m.
- Browne UroBreeze urodynamics m.
- Camino fiberoptic ICP m.
- Camino intracranial pressure m.
- Camino OLM intracranial pressure m.
- Camino postcraniotomy subdural pressure m.

NOTES

619

monitor *(continued)*

Capintec Generation II Vest m.
Capnocheck II handheld
   CO_2/SpO_2 m.
Capnogard capnograph m.
carbon monoxide m.
cardiac m.
cardiac/apnea m.
CardioBeeper CB-12L cardiac m.
CardioDiary heart m.
Cardioguard 4000
   electrocardiographic m.
Cardiotach heart rate m.
cardiovascular m.
CareLink cardiac m.
Cenflex central station m.
cerebral function m.
Chronicle implantable
   hemodynamic m.
Clear-Plan Easy fertility m.
CoaguChek Pro DM
   coagulation m.
Codman ICP m.
Colin ambulatory BP m.
Colin STBP-780 stress test blood
   pressure m.
Commucor A+V Patient m.
Companion 2 blood glucose m.
Contimed II pelvic floor
   muscle m.
Corometrics fetal apnea m.
Corometrics maternal m.
Cortexplorer cerebral blood
   flow m.
CO Sleuth carbon monoxide m.
CO_2SMO Plus continuous
   noninvasive respiratory profile m.
Cricket pulse oximetry m.
Criticare $ETCO_2/SpO_2$ m.
Criticare 506N2 vital signs m.
Criticare 507-series noninvasive
   blood pressure m.
Criticare 8100 vital signs m.
Datascope Accutor bedside m.
DeltaTrac II metabolic m.
DeVilbiss Mini-Dop fetal m.
DeVilbiss OB-Dop fetal m.
Digital Response HbA1c patient m.
Digitrapper Mark III sleep m.
Dinamap Plus vital signs m.
Dinamap Pro 100 vital signs m.
Doppler blood flow m.
Doppler Cavin m.
Doppler ultrasonic fetal heart m.
Doptone fetal m.
dosimetrist radiation beam m.
Duet glucose control m.
DynaPulse 5000A 24-hour
   ambulatory blood pressure m.

EarCheck m.
EcoCheck oxygen m.
EC50 Toxco breath carbon
   monoxide m.
EdenTec 2000W in-home
   cardiorespiratory m.
electrocardiographic
   transtelephonic m.
Endotek OM-3 Urodata m.
Endotek UDS-1000 m.
endotracheal cardiac output m.
Engstrom multigas m.
Escort 300A defibrillator/pacer m.
external m.
Fetal Dopplex II FD2+ m.
fetal heart rate m.
FetalPulse Plus m.
Fetasonde fetal m.
Finapres blood pressure m.
Flo-Stat fluid m.
FreeDop Doppler m.
Gastrolyzer breath hydrogen m.
Glucometer DEX blood glucose m.
GlucoScan 2000 m.
GlucoWatch bloodless glucose m.
Healthdyne apnea m.
HeartCard m.
Heart Rate 1-2-3 m.
HemoMatic blood collection m.
HemoSonic m.
HemoTec activated clotting
   time m.
Holter m.
home uterine activity m. (HUAM)
Homochron m.
HP M1350A fetal m.
Huntleigh Fetal Dopplex II
   FD2+ m.
ICP Express digital m.
Imex antepartum m.
infant ventilation m.
Ingold M-series glass electrode
   pH m.
in-line blood gas m.
in-line venous pressure m.
Insta-Pulse heart rate m.
Interceptor M3 triple-channel, solid-
   state m.
internal m.
intracranial pressure m.
intrapartum m.
intrauterine pressure m.
Jako facial nerve m.
Kinetix ventilation m.
King of Hearts Holter m.
Kwik-Skan m.
Ladd intracranial pressure m.
Lapse m.
laser Doppler perfusion m.

Laserflo blood perfusion m.
Laserflo BPM^2 laser Doppler m.
Life Pack 5 cardiac m.
Lifepak 5, 7 m.
Lifescope 12 bedside m.
LifeShirt continuous ambulatory m.
long-term ambulatory physiologic
 surveillance m.
loop m.
Magellan m.
Marquette 8000 Holter m.
M. Master monitor support
MDILog electronic m.
Meadox ICP m.
Medpacific LD 5000 Laser-Doppler
 perfusion m.
MemoryTrace AT ambulatory
 cardiac m.
Mentor B-VAT II m.
MicroCO carbon monoxide m.
MicroGas m.
MiniOX I, II, III, 100-IV
 oxygen m.
MonitorMate m.
Moor MBF3D m.
Mortara ELI 100 12-lead m.
MRL blood pressure m.
MRM-2 oxygen consumption m.
Multinex ID gas m.
Myotone EMG m.
MyoTRac2 EMG m.
Myotrace neuromuscular block m.
Nazorcap capnographic
 respiratory m.
N-Cat N-500 blood pressure m.
Nellcor Nl0 ETCO$_2$/SpO$_2$ m.
Nellcor Symphony N-series
 noninvasive blood pressure m.
neonatal m.
Neotrak 515A neonatal m.
Neotrend blood gas m.
nerve-integrity m.
Nerve Integrity Monitor-2 m.
Neurosign 100 nerve m.
NICO cardiopulmonary m.
Nicolet nerve integrity m.
nocturnal penile tumescence m.
noise level m.
noninvasive m.
noninvasive continuous cardiac
 output m.
NOxBox II nitric oxide m.

NOxBox Plus m.
Ohio Vortex respiration m.
Ohmeda 5250 respiratory gas m.
Omega 5600 noninvasive blood
 pressure m.
Omron Hem-601 automatic digital
 wrist blood pressure m.
Omron/Marshall 97 automatic
 oscillometric digital blood
 pressure m.
oscillometric blood pressure m.
Oxisensor fetal oxygen
 saturation m.
Oxy-Holter m.
Paratrend 7 continuous blood
 gas m.
Passport bedside m.
patient dose m.
perfusion m.
Pick and Go m.
picture-in-picture m.
Pocket-Dop 3 fetal heart rate m.
Polarus Vantage XL heart rate m.
Polar Vantage XL heart rate m.
Polar wrist m.
portable sleep m.
Porta-Resp m.
Press-Mate model 8800T blood
 pressure m.
Pressore m.
PressureSense m.
Pressurometer blood pressure m.
ProDynamic m.
Propaq Encore vital signs m.
Proview eye pressure m.
PSC fertility m.
PulseCO hemodynamic m.
Pulse Pro heart rate m.
Puritan Bennett 7250 metabolic m.
Q-Trak IAQ m.
QuietTrak ambulatory blood
 pressure m.
Quik Connect fetal m.
radiation beam m.
Rascal II anesthetic m.
Respiradyne respiratory m.
respiratory function m.
Respitrace m.
RhythmScan m.
RigiScan penile tumescence and
 rigidity m.

M

NOTES

monitor *(continued)*
>Rossmax automatic wristwatch blood pressure m.
>Scholar II vital sign m.
>Seer cardiac m.
>SentiLite neurological m.
>Sentinel-4 neurological m.
>Silverstein facial nerve m.
>sleep apnea m.
>Sonicaid Axis m.
>Sonicaid Team system 8000 fetal m.
>SpaceLabs Holter m.
>Stat-Temp II liquid crystal temperature m.
>Steritek ICP mini m.
>SureStep glucose m.
>Surveyor m.
>TC CO$_2$ m.
>TempTrac temperature m.
>Terumo Doppler fetal heart rate m.
>Thermograph temperature m.
>TINA m.
>Toitu cardiovascular m.
>tonometric blood pressure m.
>Tracer Blood Glucose m.
>Tramscope 12 m.
>transcutaneous m.
>transcutaneous carbon dioxide m.
>transcutaneous oxygen m.
>Transonic laser Doppler perfusion m.
>transtelephonic exercise m.
>Tri-Met apnea m.
>ultrasound m.
>uterine activity m.
>VAMOS anesthetic gas m.
>Vantage Performance m.
>Vasotrax BP m.
>VentCheck handheld respiratory m.
>ventricular arrhythmia m.
>Ventrix fiberoptic intracranial m.
>Verner-Smith m.
>VEST ambulatory ventricular function m.
>video m.
>ViewSite video m.
>Vip Bird infant/pediatric volume m.
>virtual labor m.
>Vitalograph aerosol inhalation m.
>Vitalograph BreathCO m.
>V5M transesophageal echocardiographic m.
>Wakeling fetal heart m.
>WinABP ambulatory blood pressure m.
>Xomed-Treace nerve integrity m.

monitoring
>active electrode m. (AEM)
>cardiac transplant m. (CTM)
>human glucose m. (HGN)
>m. probe

MonitorMate
>M. ergonomic monitor positioning control system
>M. monitor

MoniTorr
>M. ICP CSF drainage and monitoring system
>M. ICP lumbar catheter
>M. ICP ventricular catheter

Moniz carotid siphon
Monk hip prosthesis
Monks malar elevator
monoballoon
monoblock femoral component
monocortical screw
Monocryl poliglecaprone suture
monocular
>m. bandage
>m. eye dressing
>m. indirect ophthalmoscope
>m. loupe
>m. patch

Monod punch forceps
monofilament
>m. absorbable suture
>m. clear suture
>m. green suture
>m. nylon suture
>m. polypropylene suture
>Semmes-Weinstein nylon m.
>m. skin suture
>m. snare wire
>SofTip m.
>m. steel suture
>m. wire suture

Monofixateur external fixator
Monoflex lens
monofoil catheter
Monograms suture
Monogram total knee instrument system
Monoject
>M. bone marrow aspirator
>M. hypodermic needle

Monojector fingerstick device
MonoLith single-piece mechanical lithotripter
Monolyth oxygenator
monomer filter
monoplace chamber
monopolar
>m. cautery
>m. coagulating forceps
>m. diathermy forceps

m. electrocautery
m. forceps
m. insulated forceps
m. loop electrode
m. temporary electrode
m. tissue forceps
Monopty needle
Monorail
M. angioplasty catheter
M. guide wire
M. imaging catheter
Niroyal Elite M.
M. Piccolino catheter
M. Speedy balloon
Monoscopy locking trocar
Monosof suture
Monostrut cardiac valve prosthesis
Monosyn suture
Monotube
M. external fixator system
Howmedica M.
Monreal reflex hammer
Montague
M. abrader
M. proctoscope
M. sigmoidoscope
Montando tube
Montefiore tracheal tube
Montenovesi
M. cranial forceps
M. cranial rongeur
Montgomery
M. esophageal tube
M. laryngeal keel
M. laryngeal stent
M. Safe-T-Tube
M. salivary bypass tube
M. speaking valve
M. Stomeasure device
M. strap
M. strap dressing
M. thyroplasty implant system
M. tracheal cannula
M. tracheal fenestrator
M. tracheal T-tube
M. tracheal tube
M. tracheostomy
M. vaginal speculum
Montgomery-Bernstine speculum
Montgomery-Lofgren tapered Safe-T-Tube tube

Monticelli-Spinelli
M.-S. circular external fixation system
M.-S. distractor
M.-S. frame
Montreal positioner
Montrose dressing applicator
Moody fixation forceps
Moolgaoker forceps
Moon
M. Boot
M. Boot brace
M. rectal retractor
M. Walker
Moon-Robinson stapes prosthesis
Moonwalker weightbearing system
Moore
M. adjustable nail
M. blade plate
M. bone drill
M. bone elevator
M. bone reamer
M. bone retractor
M. direction finder
M. disc
M. driver
M. femoral neck prosthesis
M. fixation pin
M. gallbladder spoon
M. gall duct scoop
M. gallstone scoop
M. hip endoprosthesis
M. hollow chisel
M. hooked extractor
M. lens-inserting forceps
M. nail extractor
M. nail set
M. osteotome
M. prosthesis extractor
M. prosthesis-mortising chisel
M. raspatory
M. sliding nail plate
M. spinal fusion gouge
M. stem rasp
M. template
M. thoracoscope
M. tracheostomy button
M. tube
Moore-Blount
M.-B. driver
M.-B. extractor

M

NOTES

Moore-Blount *(continued)*
    M.-B. plate
    M.-B. screwdriver
Moorehead
    M. cheek retractor
    M. dental retractor
    M. dissector
    M. ear knife
    M. elevator
    M. lid clamp
    M. periosteotome
Moore-Troutman corneal scissors
Moore-Wilson hyperopic conformer
Moorfields
    M. curette
    M. cystotome
Moor MBF3D monitor
Moran-Karaya
    M.-K. disc
    M.-K. ring
    M.-K. sheet
morcellator
    Cook tissue m.
    DIVA laparoscopic m.
    electric tissue m.
    electromechanical m.
    FemRx laparoscopic m.
    Gynecare X-Tract tissue m.
    high-speed electrical tissue m.
    motorized m.
    OPERA Star m.
    rotating m.
    Semm m.
    Steiner electromechanical m.
    tissue m.
morcellizer
    Rubin septal m.
    Yarmo m.
Morch
    M. respirator
    M. swivel adapter
    M. swivel tracheostomy tube
    M. ventilator
More-Flow catheter
Moren-Moretz vena caval clip
Moreno gastroenterostomy clamp
Moretsky LASIK hinge protector
  fixation ring
Moretz
    M. prosthesis
    M. Tiny Tytan ventilation tube
    M. Tytan ventilation tube
Morfam massager
Morgan
    M. proctoscope
    M. therapeutic lens
    M. vent tube introducer
Morgan-Boehm proctoscope

Morganstern
    M. aspiration/injection system
    M. continuous-flow operating
      cystoscope
Morgenstein
    M. blunt forceps
    M. gouge
    M. hook
    M. periosteal knife
    M. spatula
Morgenstein-Kerrison rongeur
Moria
    M. obturator
    M. speculum
    M. trephine
Moria-France dacryocystorhinostomy
  clamp
Moritz-Schmidt
    M.-S. knife
    M.-S. laryngeal forceps
Morpho exerciser
Morrell crown remover
Morris
    M. aortic clamp
    M. biphase apparatus
    M. biphase screw
    M. cannula
    M. forceps
    M. mitral valve spreader
    M. Silastic thoracic drain
    M. splint
    M. thoracic catheter
Morrison-Hurd
    M.-H. pillar retractor
    M.-H. tonsillar dissector
Morrison skin hook
Morrissey Gigli-saw guide
Morrow-Brown needle
Morscher titanium anterior cervical
  plate
Morsch-Retec respirator
Morse
    M. backward-cutting aortic scissors
    M. blade
    M. manifold
    M. modified Finochietto retractor
    M. sternal retractor
    M. sternal spreader
    M. suction tube
    M. taper
    M. taper stem
    M. towel clip
    M. valve retractor
Morse-Andrews suction tube
Morse-Ferguson suction tube
Morson
    M. forceps
    M. trocar
Mortara ELI 100 12-lead monitor

mortising chisel
Morton
    M. bandage
    M. ophthalmoscope
    M. stone dislodger
    M. toe support
Mortson V-shaped clip
Morwel
    M. cannula
    M. silhouette suction apparatus
    M. ultrasound-assisted lipoplasty
      machine
Mosaic
    M. cardiac bioprosthesis
    M. porcine bioprosthetic heart
      valve
Mose concentric ring
Moseley
    M. fasciatome
    M. glenoid rim prosthesis
Mosher
    M. bag
    M. dilator
    M. drain
    M. esophagoscope
    M. ethmoid curette
    M. ethmoid punch forceps
    M. intubation tube
    M. Life Saver antichoke suction
      device
    M. lifesaver retractor
    M. life-saving tracheal suction tube
    M. nasal speculum
    M. strip
    M. urethral speculum
mosquito
    m. clamp
    m. hemostat
    m. hemostatic clamp
    m. hemostatic forceps
    m. lid clamp
Moss
    M. balloon triple-lumen gastrostomy
      tube
    M. cage
    M. decompression feeding catheter
    M. feeding tube
    M. fixation system
    M. gastric decompression tube
    M. gastrostomy tube
    M. G-tube PEG kit
    M. hook

    M. Mark IV tube
    M. Miami load-sharing spinal
      implant
    M. Miami polyaxial screw
    M. Miami spinal instrumentation
    M. nasal tube
    M. rod
    M. Suction Buster catheter
    M. T-anchor needle
    M. T-anchor needle introducer gun
Mossbauer spectrometer
Moss-Harms basket
Mosso sphygmomanometer
Motech cage
mother-baby endoscope
mother-daughter endoscope
mother-in-law grasper
Mother Jones dressing
Mother-To-Be abdominal support
motion
    continuous passive m. (CPM)
    controlled ankle m. (CAM)
    m. control mitt
motion-compensating format converter
Motivator FTR2000 exerciser
motorized
    m. meniscal shaver
    m. morcellator
    m. transducer pullback device
Moto-tool
    Dremel M.-t.
MotoVate rehabilitation system
Mot-R-Pak vitrectomy system
Mott
    M. double-ended retractor
    M. raspatory
Mottgen goniometer
Moule screw pin
Moult
    M. curette
    M. mouth prop
Moulton lacrimal duct tube
Mount intervertebral disc forceps
Mount-Mayfield aneurysmal forceps
Mount-Olivecrona
    M.-O. clip applier
    M.-O. forceps
Mouradian
    M. humeral fixation system
    M. humeral rod
Moure-Coryllos rib shears
Moure esophagoscope

M

NOTES

Mouse
   M. Nest mouse rest
   NoHands M.
MouseMitt Keyboarders wrist support
mouse-tooth
   m.-t. clamp
   m.-t. forceps
Mousseau-Barbin esophageal tube
moustache dressing
mouth
   m. gag frame
   m. mask
mouthgag
   Boettcher-Jennings m.
   Boyle-Davis m.
   Brophy m.
   Brown-Davis m.
   Brown-Fillebrown-Whitehead m.
   Brown-Whitehead m.
   Collis m.
   Crowe-Davis m.
   Dann-Jennings m.
   Davis-Crowe m.
   Denhardt m.
   Dingman m.
   Dingman-Denhardt m.
   Dott m.
   Dott-Kilner m.
   Doyen m.
   Doyen-Collin m.
   Ferguson m.
   Ferguson-Ackland m.
   Hayton-Williams m.
   Heister m.
   Hewitt m.
   Hibbs m.
   Jansen m.
   Jansen-Sluder m.
   Jennings Loktite m.
   Jennings-Skillern m.
   Kilner m.
   Kilner-Dott m.
   Lane m.
   Leivers m.
   Lewis m.
   Maunder oral screw m.
   McDowell m.
   McIvor m.
   McKesson m.
   Millard m.
   Mithoefer-Jansen m.
   Molt m.
   Negus m.
   Newkirk m.
   oral screw m.
   oral speculum m.
   palate-type m.
   Proetz m.
   Proetz-Jansen m.
   Pynchon m.
   Rabbit m.
   Ralks-Davis m.
   Rew-Wyly m.
   Roser m.
   Roser-Koenig m.
   Seeman-Seiffert m.
   side m.
   Sluder-Ferguson m.
   Sluder-Jansen m.
   Sydenham m.
   Thackray m.
   Trousseau m.
   Wesson m.
   Whitehead m.
   Whitehead-Jennings m.
   Wolf Loktite m.
mouthguard
   Oxyguard oxygenating m.
mouthpiece
   E-Z-Guard m.
   EZ Splint m.
   EZ Splint PM m.
   SafeTway m.
   Weidmann Spirette m.
movable-core guidewire
Movin' Step Gait cushion
Moxa heat therapy
Moynihan
   M. bile duct probe
   M. clip
   M. gallstone probe
   M. gallstone scoop
   M. intestinal forceps
   M. kidney pedicle forceps
   M. respirator
   M. speculum
   M. towel clamp
   M. towel forceps
Moynihan-Navratil forceps
M-Pact
   M-P. cast cutter
   M-P. cast spreader
   M-P. flexible orthotic
MPC
   membrane peeler cutter
   MPC automated intravitreal scissors
   MPC coagulation forceps
MPD
   main pancreatic duct
   MPD stent
MPL
   MPL aspirating syringe
   MPL dental needle
   MPL Hypo intraosseous needle
MPM
   Medical Professionals in Medicine
   MPM conductive hydrogel pad

MPM conductive hydrogel wound dressing
MPM GelPad dressing
MPM hydrogel dressing
MPM I multi-parameter monitoring system
MPM multilayer dressing
MPM Regenecare wound care gel dressing
MPO Active walking Multi Podus boot
Mport
    M. foldable lens placement system
    M. lens inserter
mPower PET scanner
MPR drain catheter
MR
    magnetic resonance
    MR 290 humidification chamber
    MR imaging system
    MR proton spectroscopy
    MR simulator
MR-compatible power injector
MReye filter
MRI
    magnetic resonance imaging
    cine MRI
    dynamic contrast-enhanced MRI
    endorectal coil MRI
    enhanced MRI
    Excelart short-bore MRI
    MRI extremity coil
    Fonar 360-degree MRI
    functional MRI
    Gyroscan superconducting MRI
    intravenous-enhanced MRI
    multiplanar MRI
    proton-density-weighted MRI
    MRI scan
    Siemens Vision MRI
    surface-coil MRI
    ThromboScan MRI
    Ultrafast MRI
MRL
    MRL blood pressure monitor
    MRL oximeter
MRM-2 oxygen consumption monitor
MRN
    magnetic resonance neurography
Mr. PainAway Health-Up TENS unit
MRT tidal humidifier
MRU
    molecular recognition unit

MS Classique balloon dilatation catheter
MSI nylon membrane
MSM-BMS coronary stent
MSM-CIS system
MST cryoprobe
Mt.
    Mt. Clemens Hospital clip applier
    Mt. Sinai skull clamp pin
MTA
    metatarsus adductus/varus
    MTA brace
    MTA headlamp
MTC Ventcontrol ventricular catheter
M-TEC 2000 surgical system
MTL
    Marco trial lens
    MTL trial frame
MTM 2 bur
MTS electrohydraulic piston
Mucat cervical sampler
Muck tonsillar forceps
mucoadhesive
    bioerodible m. (BEMA)
mucosal
    m. elevator
    m. separator plate
mucotome
    Castroviejo-Steinhauser m.
    Norelco m.
Mueller
    M. alkaline battery cautery
    M. aortic clamp
    M. bronchial clamp
    M. bur
    M. catheter
    M. coronary perfusion cannula
    M. curette
    M. Currentrol cautery
    M. electric corneal trephine
    M. electrocautery
    M. electronic tonometer
    M. eye shield
    M. eye speculum
    M. fixation device
    M. forceps
    M. giant eye magnet
    M. lacrimal sac retractor
    M. laparoscopic instrumentation
    M. needle
    M. pediatric clamp
    M. refractor

M

NOTES

Mueller *(continued)*
    M. saw
    M. suction tube
    M. telescope
    M. tongue blade
    M. total hip prosthesis
    M. Ultralite brace
    M. vena caval clamp
Mueller-Balfour self-retaining retractor
Mueller-Charnley total hip prosthesis
Mueller-Frazier suction tube
Mueller-Hinton-supplemented agar plate
Mueller-LaForce adenotome
Mueller-Markham patent ductus forceps
Mueller-Poole suction tube
Mueller-Pynchon suction tube
Mueller-type
    M.-t. acetabular cup
    M.-t. femoral head replacement
Mueller-Yankauer suction tube
Muelly hook
Muenster cast
Muer anoscope
Mufson-Cushing retractor
Muhlberger orbital implant
Mui
    M. Scientific 6-channel esophageal pressure probe
    M. Scientific pressurized capillary infusion system
Muir
    M. hemorrhoidal forceps
    M. rectal cautery clamp
    M. rectal speculum
Muirhead-Little pelvic rest tractor
Muirhead pelvic rest
Muldoon
    M. lid retractor
    M. meibomian forceps
    M. tube
MULE
    microcomputer upper limb exerciser
    MULE upper limb exerciser
mules
    Bishop-Harman m.
    Colibri m.
    Gill-Hess m.
    Graefe m.
    Halsted m.
    Heath m.
    Kulvin-Kalt m.
    Lister m.
    MacGregor m.
    Paton-Berens m.
    M. prosthesis
    M. scoop
    M. vitreous sphere
Mulholland growth guidance system

Mullan
    M. percutaneous trigeminal ganglion microcompression set
    M. trigeminal ganglion microcompression set
    M. wire
Muller acetabular roof reinforcement ring
Mulligan
    M. anastomosis clamp
    M. cervical biopsy punch
    M. dissector
    M. Silastic prosthesis
Mullins
    M. blade
    M. sheath system
    M. tongue depressor
    M. transseptal catheter
    M. transseptal catheterization sheath
MultAport cannula
Multi
    M. Dopplex II Doppler
    M. Koordinaten manipulator
    M. Podus foot system
multiaccess catheter (MAC)
multiaxial screw
multiaxis foot
Multibite multiple sample biopsy forceps
MultiBoot
    M. Basic flexion boot
    M. orthosis
multicellular stent
multichannel
    m. analyzer
    m. cochlear implant
    m. signal averager
Multiclip disposable ligating clip device
multi-coordinate manipulator
Multicor
    M. Gamma pacemaker
    M. II cardiac pacemaker
multicoupled loop-gap resonator
multicrystal gamma camera
multidetector
    m. CT
    m. CT scanner
    m. system
Multidex
    M. maltodextrin wound dressing
    M. wound-filling material
multidimensional
    m. analysis
    M. Scalogram analysis
    M. Voice Program 4305
multidirectional distractor
MultiDop XS system
multielectrode
    m. basket catheter

m. impedance catheter
m. probe
multifilament steel suture
multifire
m. clip applicator
M. Endo GIA stapling device
M. Endo hernia clip applier
M. GIA-series stapler
M. TA-series stapler
M. VersaTack stapler
Multi-Fit Luer-Lok control tonsillar syringe
multiflanged Portnoy catheter
MultiGuide mandibular distractor
multihole collimator
multi-incision 10-facet diamond blade
MultiLase
M. D copper vapor laser
M. Nd:YAG surgical laser
multilead electrode
multileaf collimator
MultiLight system
Multi-Link
M.-L. Duet coronary stent balloon
M.-L. OTW Ultra coronary stent
M.-L. Penta coronary stent balloon
M.-L. Pixel coronary stent system
M.-L. RX Ultra coronary stent
M.-L. Tetra coronary stent
M.-L. Tristar coronary stent
M.-L. Zeta coronary stent balloon
Multilith pacemaker
Multiload Cu-375 intrauterine device
Multilok hand operating table
multilumen
m. manometric catheter
m. probe
Multi-Med triple-lumen infusion catheter
multimode imaging confocal optical microscope
Multinex ID gas monitor
Multi-Optics lens
MultiPad absorptive dressing
multiparameter sensor
multiparticle cyclotron
multiplanar
m. mandibular distractor
m. MRI
m. transducer
multiplane
m. intracavitary probe
m. scanner

multiple
m. automated sample harvester
m. band ligator
M. Parameter telemetry device
m. pinhole occluder
multiple-piece intraocular lens
multiple-point electrode
Multi-Ply reusable electrode
Multi-Podus foot orthosis
Multipoise headrest
multipolar
m. bipolar cup
m. catheter
m. electrode catheter
m. impedance catheter
multiport illumination system (MIS)
Multi-Pro 2000 biopsy needle
multiprogrammable
m. dual-chamber cardiac pulse generator
m. pacemaker
m. pulse generator
MultiPro table
Multipulse
M. 1000 compression pump
M. laser system
multipurpose
m. ball electrode
m. breathing circuit
Multipurpose-SM catheter
multirod collimator
multiscope
roaming optical access m. (ROAM)
Multiseal cap
multisensor catheter
multisensory structured light range digitizer scanner
multi-sideport catheter
multislice CT scanner
multispan fracture hook
Multispatula cervical sampling device
MultiSPIRO
M. Clear Advantage pulmonary function filter
M. system
Multistim electrode catheter
Multistix Pro urinalysis test strip
multistrand suture
MultiVac vacuum
multivane intensity modulation compensator

M

NOTES

Multi-Vent
    Hudson M.-V.
multiwire
    m. gamma camera
    m. proportional chamber
Mumford Gigli-saw guide
Munchen endometrial biopsy curette
Mundie placental forceps
Munich-Crosstreet anoscope
Munro
    M. brain scissors
    M. self-retaining retractor
Muraco vaporizer
Murdock eye speculum
Murdock-Wiener eye speculum
Murdoon eye speculum
Murless
    M. fetal head extractor
    M. head extractor forceps
    M. head retractor
Murphy
    M. ball-end hook
    M. ball reamer
    M. bone lever
    M. bone skid
    M. brace
    M. chisel
    M. common duct dilator
    M. gallbladder retractor
    M. gouge
    M. intestinal needle
    M. light
    M. osteotome
    M. plaster knife
    M. punch
    M. rake retractor
    M. ring finger splint
    M. scissors
    M. sling
    M. tonsillar forceps
Murphy-Balfour
    M.-B. center blade
    M.-B. retractor
Murphy-Johnson anastomosis button
Murphy-Lane
    M.-L. bone elevator
    M.-L. bone skid
Murphy-Péan hemostatic forceps
MurphyScope neurologic device
Murray
    M. forceps
    M. holder
    M. knee prosthesis
Murray-Jones arm splint
Murray-Thomas arm splint
Murtagh self-retaining infant scalp
    retractor
muscle
    m. biopsy clamp

    m. clamp
    m. forceps
    m. hook
    M. Jack orthopaedic retractor
Museholdt nasal-dressing forceps
Museux
    M. tenaculum
    M. tenaculum forceps
    M. uterine forceps
    M. vulsellum forceps
Museux-Collins uterine vulsellum
    forceps
Musgrave pedobarograph
mushroom
    m. catheter
    m. impactor
mushroom-shaped walker glide
Musial tissue forceps
Musken tonometer
muslin dressing
Mussen frame
mustache dressing
Mustang steerable guidewire
Mustarde
    M. awl
    M. forceps
MVP
    moisture vapor permeable
    SiteGuard MVP
MVR blade
MVS
    microvitrectomy system
    MVS cannula
    MVS phacoemulsifier
MVV ventilator
MX2-300 xenon quality light source
MycroMesh
    M. biomaterial
    M. graft material
    M. Plus biomaterial
myelography needle
Myelo-Nate
    M.-N. lumbar puncture set
    M.-N. needle
Myerson
    M. antral trocar
    M. biting punch
    M. biting tip
    M. bronchial forceps
    M. electrode
    M. laryngeal forceps
    M. laryngectomy saw
    M. resin
    M. wash tube
Myerson-Moncrieff cannula
Mylar catheter
Myles
    M. antral curette
    M. guillotine

M. guillotine adenotome
M. guillotine tonsillectome
M. hemorrhoidal clamp
M. hemorrhoidal forceps
M. nasal forceps
M. nasal punch
M. nasal speculum
M. sinus cannula
M. tonsillectome snare
Myles-Ray speculum
Mynol endodontic cement
Myobock artificial hand
myocardial
    m. clamp
    m. dilator
    m. electrode
    m. lead
Myocardial Protection system
myochronoscope
Myocure
    M. blade
    M. blade scalpel
    M. knife
    M. phacoblade
MyoDac 2 EMG
myodynamometer
myoelectric prosthesis
Myoexcorciser II, III portable EMG device
Myograph 2000 neuromuscular function analyzer
Myogyn II stimulator
myokinesimeter
myoma fixation instrument
myomatome
    Segond m.

myometer
Myopulse muscle stimulator
MyoScan sensor
myoscope
MyoSight dedicated nuclear cardiology camera system
MyoSIGHT nuclear cardiology camera
myosthenometer
Myosynchron muscle stimulator
Myotest train-of-four nerve stimulator
MYOtherm XP cardioplegia delivery system
Myotone EMG monitor
MyoTRac2 EMG monitor
MyoTRac biofeedback incontinence training device
Myotrace
    M. neuromuscular block monitor
    M. Plus electromyography unit
Myowire II cardiac electrode
Myriadlase Side-Fire laser
myringoplasty knife
myringotome
    barbed m.
    Buck m.
    Rica m.
    SMIC m.
myringotomy
    m. blade
    m. drain tube
    m. knife
    m. knife blade
Myrtle leaf probe
Mystic balloon catheter

M

NOTES

Nabatoff vein stripper
Nabors probe
Nachlas gastrointestinal tube
Nachlas-Linton
    N.-L. esophagogastric balloon
      tamponade device
    N.-L. tube
Naclerio diaphragm retractor
Nada-Chair Back-Up portable back
  sling
Naden-Rieth
    N.-R. implant
    N.-R. prosthesis
Nadler
    N. bipolar coaptation forceps
    N. superior radial scissors
Naegele obstetrical forceps
Naeser laser home treatment program
  for the hand
Nagahara
    N. karate chopper
    N. ophthalmic quick chopper
    N. phaco chopper
Nagaraja endoscopic nasal biliary drain
Nagashima
    N. antroscope trocar
    N. electrogustometer
    N. LS-3 laryngostroboscope
    N. right-angle antroscope
Nagel anomaloscope
Nager
    N. palatal needle
    N. tonsillar needle
Nagielski needle
nail
    Albizzia n.
    antegrade compression n.
    AO slotted medullary n.
    Augustine boat n.
    Baumer locking n.
    Bickel intramedullary n.
    Biomet ankle arthrodesis n.
    blind medullary n.
    boat n.
    Böhler hip n.
    Brooker double-locking unreamed
      tibial n.
    Brooker-Wills n.
    cannulated n.
    Capener n.
    Chandler unreamed interlocking
      tibial n.
    closed Küntscher n.
    cloverleaf n.
    crutch and belt femoral closed n.

Curry hip n.
Delitala T-nail n.
Delta Recon n.
Delta reconstruction n.
diamond n.
double-ended n.
n. drill
elastic stable intramedullary n.
Ender n.
Fixion IM n.
Fixion interlocking medullary
  proximal femoral n.
4-flanged n.
flexible intramedullary n.
fluted Sampson n.
fluted titanium n.
Gamma trochanteric locking n.
Gissane spike n.
Grosse-Kempf femoral n.
Grosse-Kempf locking n.
Grosse-Kempf tibial n.
Hahn bone n.
half-and-half n.
Hansen-Street self-broaching n.
Hansen-Street solid
  intramedullary n.
Harris condylocephalic n.
Harris medullary n.
hooked intramedullary n.
IM n.
IMSC five-hole n.
intramedullary skeletal kinetic
  distractor n.
intramedullary supracondylar
  multihole n.
Inyo n.
Jewett n.
Jewett hip n.
Johannson hip n.
Kaessmann n.
Ken sliding n.
Kirschner interlocking
  intramedullary n.
Koslowski hip n.
Küntscher cloverleaf n.
Küntscher intramedullary n.
Lewis n.
Lottes triflange intramedullary n.
Macmed pediatric intramedullary n.
Massie sliding n.
McKee tri-fin n.
McLaughlin n.
medullary n.
Moe n.
Moore adjustable n.

nail *(continued)*
  Neufeld n.
  n. nipper
  noncannulated n.
  Nylok self-locking n.
  Nystroem hip n.
  Nystroem-Stille hip n.
  OEC-Kuntscher Interlocking Pathfinder n.
  Orthofix intramedullary n.
  OrthoSorb pin n.
  Palmer bone n.
  Peterson n.
  Pidcock n.
  n. plate
  Pugh self-adjusting n.
  Recon reconstruction n.
  retrograde compression n.
  ReVision n.
  RT n.
  Rush intramedullary n.
  Russell-Taylor Delta tibial n.
  Russell-Taylor interlocking medullary n.
  Rydell n.
  Sampson fluted n.
  Schneider intramedullary n.
  n. scissors
  Seidel humeral locking n.
  Sirus intramedullary n.
  Slocum-Smith-Petersen n.
  slotted n.
  Smillie n.
  Smith-Petersen cannulated n.
  Smith-Petersen femoral neck n.
  Smith-Petersen transarticular n.
  spring-loaded n.
  S.S.T. orthopaedic n.
  Staples osteotomy n.
  Steinmann extension n.
  supracondylar n.
  Sven Johansson femoral neck n.
  Synthes titanium elastic n.
  Temple University n.
  Terry n.
  Thatcher n.
  Thornton n.
  Tiemann n.
  titanium elastic n.
  TriGen intramedullary n.
  True/Flex intramedullary n.
  Uniflex intramedullary n.
  Vector intertrochanteric n.
  Venable-Stuck n.
  Vesely n.
  Vesely-Street n.
  Vitallium n.
  V-medullary n.
  Watson-Jones n.

  Williams interlocking Y n.
  Z-fixation n.
  Zickel n.
nail-cutting forceps
nail-extracting forceps
nail-pulling forceps
Najo head wedge
Nakamura brace
Nakao
  N. Ejector biopsy forceps
  N. QuickTrap trap
Nakayama
  N. clamp
  N. microvascular stapler
  N. ring
  N. staple
Na-K exchange pump
Nalebuff-Goldman strut
Nalgene capsule filter
Namic
  N. angiographic syringe
  N. catheter
  N. localization needle
Nanoduct neonatal sweat analysis system
Nanolas Nd:YAG laser
Nano ophthalmic arcuate marker
Nanos 1 pacemaker
NanoWalker robot
napkin ring calcar allograft
Naraghi-DeCoster reduction clamp
Narco
  N. Biosystems rectilinear recorder
  N. esophageal motility machine
Narcomatic flowmeter
Narkomed anesthesia machine
Narkotest meter
narrow
  n. AO dynamic compression plate
  n. lens
narrow-base quad cane
NarrowFlex
  N. intraaortic balloon catheter
  N. Universal IAB catheter
nasal
  n. alligator forceps
  n. aspirator
  n. bivalve speculum
  n. cannula
  n. catheter
  n. chisel
  n. CPAP system
  n. curette
  n. cutting forceps
  n. dilator
  n. dorsal implant
  n. dressing forceps
  n. dressing holder
  n. gouge

n. hump-cutting forceps
n. irrigator
n. knife
n. mask
n. osteotome
n. pack
n. packing
n. packing forceps
n. polyp forceps
n. probe
n. prongs
n. prosthesis
n. punch
n. rasp
n. retractor
n. saw
n. scissors
n. septal forceps
n. shell implant
n. snare
n. snare cannula
n. snare wire
n. splint
n. suction bulb
n. suction tube
n. tampon
n. tamponade
n. tampon sponge
n. tenaculum
n. trumpet
nasal-tip dressing
Nasa-Spec nasal speculum
Nash needle
Nashold
N. biopsy needle
N. TC electrode
nasobiliary
n. catheter
n. drain
n. tube
nasocystic
n. catheter
n. drain
n. drainage tube
nasoendoscope
Hirschman n.
nasoendotracheal tube
nasoenteric feeding tube
nasofrontal suture
nasogastric (NG)
n. feeding tube
nasojejunal feeding tube

nasolacrimal duct probe
nasolaryngoscope
Machida n.
nasometer
nasopancreatic catheter
nasopharyngeal
n. biopsy forceps
n. fiberscope
n. speculum
nasopharyngeoscope
DuraView OL-1 flexible n.
nasopharyngolaryngofiberscope
Pentax n.
nasopharyngolaryngoscope
flexible n.
nasopharyngoscope
Broyles n.
Holmes n.
Meltzer n.
National n.
Smith & Nephew ENT n.
Naso-Tamp nasal packing sponge
nasotracheal catheter
nasovesicular catheter
Natchez Mobil-Trac system
Nathan pacemaker
Nathanson liver retractor
National
N. all-metric transilluminator
N. cautery
N. cautery electrode
N. coagulator
N. ear speculum
N. electricator
N. general purpose cystoscope
N. Graves vaginal speculum
N. Institutes of Health (NIH)
N. nasopharyngoscope
N. opal glass transilluminator
N. proctoscope
natural
n. pacemaker
N. Profile abutment system
n. suture
NaturaLase
N. erbium laser
N. Er:YAG laser
natural-feel breast prosthesis
Natural-Hip
N.-H. prosthesis
N.-H. titanium hip stem
Natural-Knee II system

NOTES

635

Natural-Lok
    N.-L. acetabular cup
    N.-L. acetabular cup prosthesis
Nature Boy & Girl diaper
Natvig wire-twister forceps
Naugh os calcis apparatus
Naugle orbitometer exophthalmometer
Nauth traction device
NavAblator catheter
Navarre
    N. interventional radiology device
    N. Universal drainage catheter
navicular screw
navigator
    N. flexible endoscope
    Hemi-Arc surgical n.
Navigus
    N. cranial electrode system
    N. trajectory guide
Naviport
    N. deflectable-tip guiding catheter
    N. hollow-lumen guiding catheter
NaviPro Image-Free navigation system
Navi-Star
    N.-S. ablation catheter
    N.-S. Biosense Webster mapping
      catheter
    N.-S. electrophysiology catheter
**Navitrack computer-assisted navigation
  system**
Navius stent
Navratil
    N. retractor
    N. stirrups
**Nazorcap capnographic respiratory
  monitor**
NBIH cardiac device
NC
    noncompliant
    NC Bandit PTCA catheter
    NC Big Ranger OTW balloon
      catheter
    NC Cobra balloon
N-Cat N-500 blood pressure monitor
NCC Hi-Lo Jet endotracheal tube
NC-stat nerve conduction system
NDM adhesive wound dressing
NDSB occlusion balloon catheter
Nd:YAG
    Nd:YAG laser
    Nd:YAG laser catheter
Nd:YLF laser
Neal
    N. catheter
    N. fallopian cannula
    N. insufflator
near-infrared (NIR)
    n.-i. electronic endoscope
    n.-i. spectroscope

Nearly Me breast form
Nebauer ophthalmoendoscope
NEB total hip prosthesis
Nebuhaler inhaler
nebulizer
    Acorn II n.
    AeroEclipse breath-actuated n.
    Aeroneb portable n.
    AeroSonic ultrasonic n.
    AeroTech II n.
    air-powered n.
    Babbington n.
    Bestneb n.
    bulb-operated n.
    Centimist n.
    Compu-Neb ultrasonic n.
    Dench n.
    DeVilbiss Pulmo-Aide n.
    DuraNeb portable n.
    Fisons n.
    G5 Mist-Ease n.
    handheld n.
    Heart n.
    Hudson T Up-Draft II
      disposable n.
    Incenti-neb n.
    jet n.
    John Bunn Mini-Mist n.
    Kidde n.
    Marquest Respirgard II n.
    medicinal n.
    Medi-Mist n.
    Metermatic nasal n.
    MicroAir , n.
    Micro Mist disposable n.
    MicroSeal n.
    Microstat ultrasonic n.
    MiniHEART low-flow n.
    Mini-Neb n.
    Mistogen n.
    Misty-Neb n.
    NE-C21 CompAir Elite n.
    Omron compressor n.
    penicillin n.
    PermaNeb n.
    Proneb Ultra n.
    Pulmo-Aide n.
    PulmoMate n.
    PulmoSonic ultrasonic n.
    Raindrop medication n.
    Respirgard II n.
    Schuco 2000 n.
    Selrodo n.
    Shuco-Myst n.
    side-arm n.
    SideStream n.
    small-volume n.
    Sonix 2000 ultrasonic n.
    spinning disc n.

Tote-A-Neb n.
Tracheolife HME oxygen port n.
Twin Jet n.
Ultra-Neb 99 ultrasonic n.
ultrasonic n.
UniHeart n.
updraft n.
VixOne n.
NE-C21 CompAir Elite nebulizer
Necelon surgical glove
neck
n. rest
n. retractor
n. roll
n. support
Neckcare pillow
Neck-Hugger cervical support pillow
Neck-Roll aromatherapy hot/cold pack
Necktrac traction device
Nec Loc cervical collar
needle
Abrams biopsy n.
abscission n.
AccuCore biopsy n.
Accuject dental n.
Ackerman n.
Acland n.
AcuMaster acupuncture n.
Adair-Veress n.
Addix n.
Adson aneurysm n.
Adson-Murphy trocar point n.
Adson scalp n.
Adson suture n.
advancement n.
Agnew tattooing n.
Agricola tattooing n.
Ailee n.
air aspirator n.
Albarran-Reverdin n.
Alcon irrigating n.
Alcon reverse-cutting n.
Alcon spatula n.
Alcon taper-cut n.
Alcon taper-point n.
Aldrete n.
Alexander tonsillar n.
Altmann n.
Amersham CDCS A-type n.
Amplatz angiography n.
Amsler aqueous transplant n.
Anchor surgical n.

aneurysm n.
angiography n.
angular n.
antral trocar n.
aortic air aspirator n.
aortic root perfusion n.
aortography n.
aqueous transplant n.
arachnophlebectomy n.
Arkan sharpening-stone n.
Arrow-Fischell EVAN n.
arterial n.
arteriography n.
Articulator injection n.
ASAP channel-cut automated
   biopsy n.
ASAP PinPoint guiding
   introducer n.
ASAP prostate biopsy n.
asia-med acupuncture n.
aspirating n.
Atkinson retrobulbar n.
Atkinson single-bevel blunt-tip n.
Atkinson tip peribulbar n.
Atraloc n.
atraumatic n.
atraumatic suture n.
Austin n.
automated biopsy n.
Autovac n.
AV fistula n.
Babcock n.
Backlund spiral biopsy n.
Bailey fontonal n.
Baldwin perineum n.
Ballade n.
Barbara n.
Bard biopsy n.
Bard Biopty cut n.
Barker spinal anesthesia n.
Barraquer-Vogt n.
Barrett hebosteotomy n.
Bauer Temno biopsy n.
BD bone marrow biopsy n.
BD Safety-Gard n.
BD SafetyGlide shielding
   hypodermic n.
B-D spinal n.
Beath n.
Bengash n.
Berbecker n.
Bergeret-Reverdin n.

N

NOTES

needle *(continued)*
Berges-Reverdin n.
beveled n.
Beyer paracentesis n.
bicurved n.
Biegeleisen n.
Bier lumbar puncture n.
Bierman n.
biopsy n.
Biopty-Cut biopsy n.
bipolar n.
Birtcher electrosurgical n.
Black-Decker n.
Blackmon n.
Blair-Brown n.
bleeding n.
blunt n.
blunt-end n.
bone marrow biopsy n.
Bonney n.
boomerang bladder n.
Bovie n.
Bowman cataract n.
Bowman discission n.
Bowman iris n.
Bowman stop n.
brain biopsy n.
Braun n.
breast localization n.
BRK-series transseptal n.
Brockenbrough transseptal n.
Brophy n.
Brophy-Deschamps n.
Brown cleft palate n.
Brown-Sanders fascial n.
Brown staphylorrhaphy n.
Brughleman n.
Brunner ligature n.
Buerger prostatic n.
Buncke quartz n.
Bunnell tendon n.
Burr butterfly n.
butterfly n.
Calhoun n.
Calhoun-Hagler lens n.
Calhoun-Merz n.
Campbell ventricular n.
cardioplegic n.
Cardiopoint cardiac surgery n.
Carlens n.
carotid angiogram n.
carpular n.
Carroll n.
Castroviejo vitreous-aspirating n.
cataract n.
cataract aspirating n.
catgut n.
n. catheter jejunostomy
caudal n.

cesium n.
Charles flute n.
Charles vacuuming n.
Charlton antral n.
Chiba biopsy n.
Chiba eye n.
Chiba transhepatic
  cholangiography n.
Child-Phillips intestinal plication n.
Cibis ski n.
CIF n.
CIF-4 n.
Clagett n.
Clas von Eichen n.
Cleasby spatulated n.
cleft palate n.
Cloquet n.
coaxial sheath cut biopsy n.
Cobb-Ragde n.
Colapinto transjugular n.
Colorado microdissection n.
Colts cutting n.
Colver tonsillar n.
concentric n.
Concept Multi-Liner lining n.
Concept suturing n.
cone biopsy n.
cone ventricular n.
Conrad-Crosby bone marrow
  biopsy n.
Continental n.
Control Release pop-off n.
Cook endomyocardial n.
Cook Longdwel n.
Cook percutaneous entry n.
Cook trocar n.
Cooley aortic vent n.
Cooley ventricular n.
Cooper chemopallidectomy n.
Cooper ligature n.
Cooper pallidectomy n.
CooperVision irrigating n.
CooperVision spatulated n.
Cope pleural biopsy n.
Cope thoracentesis n.
copper-clad steel n.
Core aspiration/injection n.
Core CO_2 insufflation n.
corneal suture n.
Costen iris n.
couching n.
Cournand arteriography n.
Cournand-Grino n.
Cournand-Potts n.
Craig biopsy n.
Crawford epidural n.
Crawford fascial n.
Crosby biopsy n.
Crown n.

CryoNeedles n.
CT1 n.
C-type acupuncture n.
CU-8 n.
Culp biopsy n.
Curran knife n.
Curry cerebral n.
CUSALap ultrasonic accessory n.
Cushing ventricular n.
cut biopsy n.
cut taper n.
cutting n.
cyclodiathermy n.
dacryocystorhinostomy n.
Daily cataract n.
Daiwa dental n.
Damshek n.
Dandy-Cairns brain n.
Dandy-Cairns ventricular n.
Dandy ventricular n.
Davis knife n.
Davis tonsillar n.
Dean antral n.
Dean iris n.
Dean knife n.
debridement n.
Dees renal n.
Dees suture n.
Deknatel K-needle n.
Denis Browne cleft palate n.
DermX cosmetic surgery n.
D'Errico ventricular n.
Deschamps ligature n.
desiccation n.
Desmarres paracentesis n.
Devonshire n.
diamond-point suture n.
Diamond SharpPoint n.
diathermy n.
Dieckmann intraosseous n.
Dingman malleable passing n.
discission n.
discographic n.
disposable acupuncture n.
disposable aspiration n.
disposable biopsy n.
disposable concentric n.
disposable injection n.
disposable suturing n.
Dispos-A-Ture single-use surgical n.
n. dissector
Dix n.

DLP cardioplegic n.
DN acupuncture n.
docking n.
Docktor n.
Dorsey n.
Dos Santos lumbar aortography n.
double-barreled n.
double-hub emulsifying n.
double-lumen n.
Douglas suture n.
Doyen n.
Drews cataract n.
Drews lavage n.
n. driver
D-Tach removable n.
dural n.
Durham n.
Durrani dorsal vein complex
  ligation n.
Dyonics n.
East-Grinstead n.
Echo-Coat ultrasound biopsy n.
echogenic n.
Eclipse blood collection n.
egress n.
n. electrode
electrosurgical n.
electrosurgical probe n.
Elschnig extrusion n.
Emmet n.
Empire n.
Endopath Ultra Veress n.
n. endosteal implant
Entree disposable CO_2
  insufflation n.
epilation n.
Epstein n.
ergonomic vascular access n.
  (EVAN)
Erosa disposable hypodermic n.
Espocan combined spinal/epidural n.
Ethicon BV-75-3 n.
Ethicon ST-4 straight taper-point n.
Ethicon TG Plus n.
Ethicon TGW n.
Ethiguard n.
Euro-Med FNA-21 aspiration n.
EUSN-1 EchoTip n.
eXcel-DR disposable/reusable
  Glasser laparoscopic n.
eXcel-DR pneumothorax n.
exploring n.

NOTES

needle *(continued)*
    extended n.
    ExtraSafe butterfly infusion n.
    extrusion n.
    eyed suture n.
    eyeless n.
    eyeless atraumatic suture n.
    E-Z-EM cut biopsy n.
    Falk n.
    fascial n.
    Federspiel n.
    Feild-Lee biopsy n.
    Fein n.
    Ferguson round-body n.
    Ferguson suture n.
    Ferris disposable bone marrow aspiration n.
    filiform steel n.
    fine intestinal n.
    Finochietto n.
    Fischer pneumothorax n.
    Fisher eye n.
    fishhook n.
    fistula n.
    flat spatula n.
    flexible aspiration n.
    flexible biopsy n.
    flexible injection n.
    Floyd pneumothorax n.
    flute n.
    Foltz n.
    foreign body n.
    Frackelton fascial n.
    Framer tendon-passing n.
    Francke n.
    Frankfeldt hemorrhoidal n.
    Franklin liver puncture n.
    Franklin-Silverman prostatic biopsy n.
    Franseen n.
    Franseen liver biopsy n.
    Frazier ventricular n.
    Frederick pneumothorax n.
    Freeman pudendal n.
    French-eye n.
    French spring-eye n.
    Fritz vitreous transplant n.
    front wall n.
    Gallini bone marrow aspiration n.
    ganglion injection n.
    Gardner n.
    gastrointestinal n.
    general closure n.
    Geuder corneal n.
    Geuder keratoplasty n.
    Gill n.
    Gillmore n.
    GIP/Medi-Globe prototype n.
    Girard anterior chamber n.
    Girard cataract-aspirating n.
    Girard-Swan n.
    gold n.
    Goldbacher rectal n.
    Goldenberg Snarecoil bone marrow biopsy n.
    Goldmann knife n.
    Gordh n.
    Gorsch n.
    Graefe iris n.
    GraNee n.
    Grantham lobotomy n.
    Greene n.
    Greenfield n.
    Greenwald n.
    Grice suture n.
    Grieshaber corneal n.
    Grieshaber iris n.
    Gripper n.
    GS-9 n.
    Gynex extended-reach n.
    Haab knife n.
    Hagedorn operation suture n.
    half-intensity n.
    Halle septal n.
    Halsey n.
    hammer-type acupuncture n.
    harelip n.
    Harken heart n.
    Harlow Wood spinal biopsy n.
    Harvard n.
    Haverhill n.
    Hawkeye suture n.
    Hawkins-Akins n.
    Hawkins breast localization n.
    Hearn n.
    heart n.
    Hegar n.
    Hegar-Baumgartner n.
    Hemoject n.
    hemorrhoidal n.
    Henton suture n.
    Henton tonsillar n.
    heparin-flushing n.
    Hessburg lacrimal n.
    Hey-Groves n.
    Heyner double n.
    Hingson-Edwards caudal n.
    Hingson-Ferguson spinal n.
    Hobbs n.
    Hoen ventricular n.
    n. holder
    n. holder clamp
    Holinger n.
    hollow n.
    Homer localizaton n.
    Homerlok n.
    Homer Mammalok breast localization n.

hooked n.
hookwire n.
Hosford-Hicks n.
Hourin tonsillar n.
House-Barbara shattering n.
House-Rosen n.
House stapes n.
Howard Jones n.
Howell biliary aspiration n.
Howell biopsy aspiration n.
Huber point n.
Hunstad infusion n.
Hunt n.
Hurd suture n.
Hustead epidural n.
Hutchins biopsy n.
hypodermic n.
Hypospray jet injection n.
Icofly infusion n.
Ilg n.
Iliff-Wright fascia n.
Illinois n.
illuminated suction n.
Impex aspiration & injection n.
Indian club n.
Infusaid n.
Ingersoll tonsillar n.
InjectaFLOW injection n.
injection n.
Injex disposable n.
insufflation n.
insulated electrode n.
internal nucleus hydrodelineation n.
intestinal plication n.
intraosseous n.
intravenous n.
Iocare titanium n.
Iolab irrigating n.
Iolab taper-cut n.
Iolab taper-point n.
Iolab titanium n.
iridium n.
iris n.
irrigating n.
Ito n.
IV n.
J n.
Jalaguier-Reverdin n.
Jameson strabismus n.
Jamshidi-Kormed bone marrow
  biopsy n.
Jamshidi liver biopsy n.

Jelco n.
JMS fistula n.
JMS injection n.
J-needle laparoscopic suturing n.
Jonesco wire suture n.
Jordan n.
Kader fishhook n.
Kall modification of Silverman n.
Kalt corneal n.
Kalt eye n.
Kalt vein n.
Kangnian acupuncture n.
Kaplan tracheostomy n.
Kara cataract n.
Karras angiography n.
Kato-Asch coaxial n.
Keith abdominal n.
Kelly intestinal n.
Kelman n.
KeyMed disposable variceal
  injection n.
kidney suturing n.
King suture n.
Klatskin liver biopsy n.
Klein infiltration n.
Klima n.
Klima-Rosegger sternal n.
Knapp iris knife n.
knife n.
Knight biopsy n.
Kobak n.
Koch nucleus hydrolysis n.
Kohn n.
Koontz hernia n.
Kopan breast lesion localization n.
Kormed disposable liver biopsy n.
Kratz diamond-dusted n.
Kronecker aneurysm n.
lacrimal n.
Lagleyze n.
Lahey n.
Laminex n.
Lane cleft palate n.
Lane suturing n.
Lapides n.
Laredo-Bard n.
large-bore slotted aspirating n.
lavage n.
Lee n.
Lee & Westcott n.
Leighton n.
Lemmon n.

N

NOTES

needle *(continued)*

L'Esperance n.
Lewicky n.
Lewis Pair-Pak n.
Lewy-Holinger Teflon injection n.
Lewy-Rubin Teflon glycerine-
 mixture injection n.
Lewy Teflon glycerine-mixture
 injection n.
Lichtwicz antral n.
Lichtwicz-Bier antral n.
ligature n.
Lindemann transfusion n.
Linton-Blakemore n.
Lipschwitz n.
List n.
Litvak-Pereyra ligature n.
liver biopsy n.
lobotomy n.
lock n.
long n.
Longdwel catheter n.
Look retrobulbar n.
Loopuyt n.
Lo-Trau side-cutting n.
Lowell pleural n.
Lowette n.
Lowette-Verner n.
Lowsley ribbon-gut n.
Luer n.
Luer-Lok n.
Lukens n.
lumbar aortography n.
lumbar puncture n.
Lundy fascial n.
Lundy-Irving caudal n.
Luongo n.
LX n.
Madayag biopsy n.
Maddox caudal n.
Magielski n.
Mahurkar fistular n.
malleable passing n.
Maltz n.
Maltzman n.
Mammalok Ultra repositionable
 breast localization n.
Manan cutting n.
Mantoux n.
March laser sclerostomy n.
Marion-Reverdin n.
Markham biopsy n.
Martin uterine n.
Marx n.
Mason-School aspirating n.
Masson fascial n.
Mathieu n.
Maumenee vitreous-aspirating n.
Mayo catgut n.

Mayo intestinal n.
Mayo trocar-point n.
McCaslin n.
McCurdy staphylorrhaphy n.
McDowell n.
McGee prosthesis n.
McGhan plastic surgical n.
McGowan n.
McGregor n.
McIntyre I&A n.
McIntyre irrigation-aspiration n.
Medamicus Axia RSN guidewire
 introducer safety n.
Medicut intravenous n.
Medisystems fistula n.
Menghini liver biopsy n.
meniscal repair n.
metal n.
metallic n.
Metcoff pediatric biopsy n.
Meyer cyclodiathermy n.
Mick afterloading n.
MicroFlow phacoemulsification n.
Microlet electrode n.
micron n.
micropoint n.
micropuncture n.
micropuncture introducer n.
micro round-tip n.
Microvasive sclerotherapy n.
Millet n.
milliner's n.
Mizzy n.
modified spatula n.
Monoject hypodermic n.
Monopty n.
Morrow-Brown n.
Moss T-anchor n.
MPL dental n.
MPL Hypo intraosseous n.
Mueller n.
Multi-Pro 2000 biopsy n.
Murphy intestinal n.
myelography n.
Myelo-Nate n.
Nager palatal n.
Nager tonsillar n.
Nagielski n.
Namic localization n.
Nash n.
Nashold biopsy n.
Nelson ligature n.
neurography n.
neurosurgical suture n.
Neville ascending aorta air vent n.
Newman rectal injection n.
New oral n.
Nichols-Deschamps-Navratil
 ligature n.

Noci stimuli n.
NoKor n.
noncoring Huber n.
noncutting suture n.
nonferromagnetic n.
Nordenstrom Rotex II biopsy n.
Nottingham colposuspension n.
nucleus hydrolysis n.
Oaks double n.
O'Brien airway n.
obstetrical block anesthesia n.
Ochsner n.
Oldfield n.
olive-tipped n.
Olympus NM-K-series
  sclerotherapy n.
Olympus NM-L-series n.
OmniTip side-firing laser n.
Op-Pneu laparoscopy n.
optical n.
Optivis Surgalloy n.
osen n.
Osgood n.
Osterballe precision n.
Ostycut bone biopsy n.
Overholt rib n.
Pace ventricular n.
Page n.
Palmer-Drapier n.
palpating n.
Pannett n.
Paparella straight n.
paracentesis n.
paracervical nerve block n.
paraPRO paracentesis n.
Parhad n.
Parhad-Poppen n.
Parker n.
Parker-Pearson n.
Payr vein n.
PC-7 n.
pediatric biopsy n.
Pencan spinal n.
Penfield biopsy n.
PercuCut cut-biopsy n.
PercuGuide n.
percutaneous n.
percutaneous access n.
percutaneous cutting n.
Pereyra n.
peribulbar n.
pericardiocentesis n.

permanent n.
Permark micropigmentation n.
Pharmaseal n.
pilot n.
Pischel n.
Pitkin spinal n.
plain eye n.
pleural biopsy n.
plication n.
Plum-Blossom acupuncture n.
Pneumo-Matic insufflation n.
pneumoperitoneum n.
pneumothoracic injection n.
polypropylene n.
polytef-sheathed n.
pop-off n.
Poppen ventricular n.
positioning n.
postmortem suture n.
Potocky n.
Potter n.
Potts n.
Potts-Cournand angiography n.
PrecisionGlide n.
precision lancet cutting n.
Presbyterian Hospital ventricular n.
Pricker n.
n. probe
probe n.
ProBloc insulated regional block n.
Promex biopsy n.
prostatic biopsy n.
Protect Point n.
PS-2 n.
pudendal block anesthesia n.
Pulec n.
puncture n.
puncture-tip n.
Punctur-Guard n.
Quantico n.
Quick-Core biopsy n.
Quincke Babcock n.
Quincke spinal n.
radium n.
Radpour n.
Ranfac soft-tissue n.
Rashkind septostomy n.
razor-tip n.
RCB biopsy n.
retrobulbar n.
Retter aneurysm n.
Reverdin suture n.

N

NOTES

needle *(continued)*
   reverse-cutting n.
   Rhoton straight point n.
   ribbon gut n.
   Rica aneurysm n.
   Rica cerebral angiography
    puncture n.
   Rica suturing n.
   Rider-Moeller n.
   Riedel corneal n.
   Riley arterial n.
   Ring drainage catheter n.
   Riza-Ribe n.
   Robb n.
   Roberts n.
   Robinson-Smith n.
   Rochester aortic vent n.
   Rochester-Meeker n.
   Rolf lance n.
   root n.
   Rösch-Uchida n.
   Rosenthal aspiration n.
   Roser n.
   Ross n.
   Rotex II biopsy n.
   Rotunda perineum n.
   round body n.
   Rubin n.
   Rubin-Arnold n.
   Ruskin antral trocar n.
   Ruskin sphenopalatine ganglion n.
   Rutner biopsy n.
   Rycroft n.
   Sabreloc spatula n.
   Sachs n.
   SafeTap tapered spinal n.
   Safety AV fistula n.
   Sahli n.
   Salah sternal puncture n.
   SampleMaster biopsy n.
   Sanders-Brown n.
   Sanders-Brown-Shaw aneurysm n.
   Sarot n.
   Sato cataract n.
   Saunders cataract n.
   Saunders-Paparella n.
   Savariaud-Reverdin n.
   scalpene n.
   scalp vein n.
   Schanz n.
   Schecter-Bryant aortic vent n.
   Scheer n.
   Scheie cataract-aspirating n.
   Schmieden n.
   Schmieden-Dick n.
   Schuknecht n.
   Schutt n.
   scleral spatula n.
   sclerostomy n.

sclerotherapy n.
Scoville ventricular n.
screw-tipped intraosseous n.
Sedan-Nashold n.
Seirin acupuncture n.
Seldinger arterial n.
Seldinger gastrostomy n.
self-aspirating cut-biopsy n.
septal n.
Septoject n.
Seraflo AV fistular n.
seton n.
Seven-Star Plum Blossom
  acupuncture n.
Shambaugh palpating n.
Sharpoint Ultra-Guide ophthalmic n.
shattering n.
Sheldon-Spatz vertebral
  arteriogram n.
Sheldon-Swann n.
Shirodkar aneurysm n.
Shirodkar cervical n.
short n.
sialography n.
side-cutting spatulated n.
4-sided cutting n.
side-flattened n.
sidewall holed n.
silver n.
Silverman biopsy n.
Silverman-Boeker n.
Simcoe anterior chamber
  receiving n.
Simcoe II PC aspirating n.
Simcoe irrigating n.
Simcoe suture n.
Simmonds cricothyrotomy n.
Sims abdominal n.
Singer n.
single-wall n.
Site I&A n.
ski n.
Skinny Chiba n.
Sklar ligature n.
slotted n.
Sluder n.
small-bore n.
small-caliber n.
SMIC suture n.
Smiley-Williams arteriography n.
Snarecoil bone marrow biopsy n.
Solitaire n.
SonoVu US aspiration n.
n. spatula
spatula split n.
spatulated n.
spatulated half-circle n.
sphenopalatine ganglion n.
spinal n.

Spinelli biopsy n.
spoon n.
n. spoon
spring-eye n.
spring-hook wire n.
spring-loaded biopsy n.
Sprotte epidural n.
Sprotte spinal n.
spud n.
n. spud
stab n.
Stallerpointe n.
Stamey n.
standard n.
stapes n.
staphylorrhaphy n.
steel-winged butterfly n.
Steis bone marrow transplant n.
StereoGuide n.
stereotactic breast biopsy n.
sternal puncture n.
Stifcore transbronchial aspiration n.
Stille-Mayo-Hegar n.
Stille-Seldinger n.
Stimuplex block n.
Stocker cyclodiathermy puncture n.
stop n.
Storz aspiration biopsy n.
Storz flexible injection n.
strabismus n.
straight suturing n.
Strasbourg-Fairfax in vitro
  fertilization n.
Straus curved retrobulbar n.
Sturmdorf cervical n.
Sturmdorf pedicle n.
Stylus suture n.
Subco n.
subconjunctival n.
suction biopsy n.
Sudan n.
Sulze diamond-point n.
Surecan safety Huber n.
Sure-Cut biopsy n.
Suresharp blood collecting n.
Suresharp dental n.
Sur-Fast n.
Surgicraft suture n.
Surgimedics TMP air aspirator n.
Surgineedle pneumoperitoneum n.
Sutton biopsy n.
suture n.

suturing n.
swaged n.
swaged-on n.
Swan n.
Swedgeon already-threaded n.
Symmonds n.
Szabo-Berci n.
taper n.
Tapercut n.
tapered n.
taper-point suture n.
tattooing n.
Tauber n.
tax double n.
Teflon-coated hollow-bore n.
Teflon-coated stimulation n.
Teflon-covered n.
Teflon glycerine-mixture
  injection n.
Tek-Pro n.
Temno biopsy n.
Temno II cutting n.
tendon n.
Terry-Mayo n.
Terumo AV fistula n.
Terumo dental n.
Terumo hypodermic n.
Tew n.
thermistor n.
n. thermocouple
THI n.
thin acupuncture n.
thin-walled n.
Thomas n.
thoracentesis n.
Thornton retrobulbar n.
threaded eye n.
through-the-scope injection n.
Ticsay transpubic n.
tie-on n.
tissue desiccation n.
titanium alloy n.
Titus venoclysis n.
Tocantins bone marrow biopsy n.
Todd eye cautery n.
Torrington French spring n.
transaxillary n.
transjugular n.
translocation n.
transpubic n.
Travenol Tru-Cut biopsy n.
Travert n.

N

NOTES

needle *(continued)*
n. trephination system
trocar n.
n. trocar
Troutman n.
Tru-Cut biopsy n.
Trupp ventricular n.
Tru Taper Ethalloy n.
tungsten microdissection n.
Tuohy lumbar aortography n.
Tuohy-Schliff n.
Tuohy spinal n.
Turkel liver biopsy n.
Turkel sternal n.
Turner biopsy n.
Turner-Warwick urethroplasty n.
Tworek bone marrow-aspirating n.
Ultra-Core biopsy n.
ultrasonic irrigating n.
Ultra-vue amniocentesis n.
Unimar J n.
University of Illinois biopsy n.
University of Illinois marrow n.
University of Illinois sternal
puncture n.
Updegraff cleft palate n.
Updegraff staphylorrhaphy n.
urethroplasty n.
uterine n.
Vacutainer n.
Vacutainer Safety-Gard n.
vacuuming n.
Variject n.
vascular access n.
Vastack n.
Veenema-Gusberg prostatic
biopsy n.
Veirs n.
Venaflo n.
venipuncture n.
venous n.
ventricular n.
Verbrugge n.
Veress-Frangenheim n.
Veress pneumoperitoneum n.
Veress spring-loaded laparoscopic n.
Vicat n.
Viers n.
Viking n.
Vim n.
Vim-Silverman biopsy n.
Virginia n.
Visi-Black surgical n.
Visitec retrobulbar n.
vitreous aspirating n.
vitreous transplant n.
V. Mueller paracervical nerve
block n.
V. Mueller pudendal nerve
block n.
Vogt-Barraquer corneal n.
Voorhees n.
Walker tonsillar n.
Wang n.
Wangensteen intestinal n.
Wannagat injection n.
Ward French n.
Ward French-eye n.
Waterfield n.
Watson-Williams n.
wedge-line n.
Weeks n.
Weiss n.
Weiss fixed wing epidural n.
Welsh olive-tipped n.
Wergeland double n.
Wertheim-Navratil n.
Westcott n.
Westcott biopsy n.
Westerman-Jensen n.
whirlybird n.
Whitacre spinal n.
Wiener eye n.
Williams cystoscopic n.
Williamson biopsy n.
winged steel n.
Wolf antral n.
Wood aortography n.
Wooten eye n.
Worst n.
Wright-Crawford n.
Wright fascia n.
Wright ophthalmic n.
Yale Luer-Lok n.
Yang n.
Yankauer septal n.
Yankauer suture n.
Yueh centesis disposable
catheter n.
Zavala lung biopsy n.
Ziegler iris n.
Zoellner n.
**NeedleBuster transdermal drug delivery
system**
Needle-Ease device
needleholder
Denis Browne n.
needle-holder forceps
needle-knife
n.-k. fistulotome
n.-k. papillotome
n.-k. wire
needle-nose
n.-n. pliers
n.-n. rongeur
n.-n. vise-grip pliers

needlepoint
  n. cautery
  n. electrocautery
Needle-Pro needle protection device
needlescope device
Needlescoper endoscope
needle-tipped sphincterotome
Neer
  N. I, II, III shoulder prosthesis
  N. II total knee system
Neesone root canal depth indicator
Neff
  N. femorotibial nail system
  N. meniscal knife
  N. percutaneous access set
negative
  n. eyepiece
Negus
  N. bronchoscope
  N. laryngoscope
  N. ligature pusher
  N. mouthgag
  N. telescope
  N. tonsillar forceps
Negus-Broyles bronchoscope
Negus-Green forceps
Nehb D lead
Neider valvulotome
Neil-Moore
  N.-M. meatotomy electrode
  N.-M. perforator drill
Neiman nasal splint
Neisser syringe
Neitz CT-R cataract camera
Neivert
  N. chisel
  N. dissector
  N. double-ended retractor
  N. knife guide
  N. nasal polyp hook
  N. needle holder
  N. osteotome
  N. rocking gouge
  N. tonsillar knife
Neivert-Anderson osteotome
Neivert-Eves
  N.-E. tonsillar snare
  N.-E. tonsillar wire
Nek-L-O
  N.-L.-O. hot & cold pillow
  N.-L.-O. orthopaedic support

Nélaton
  N. bullet probe
  N. rubber tube drain
  N. urethral catheter
Nellcor
  N. Durasensor adult oxygen transducer
  N. FS-series oximeter sensor
  N. Nl0 $ETCO_2/SpO_2$ monitor
  N. N-series fetal oxygen saturation monitoring system
  N. OxiFirst fetal oxygen saturation monitoring system
  N. Puritan Bennett 840 ventilator system
  N. Symphony N-series noninvasive blood pressure monitor
Nellcor-Puritan Bennett 840 ventilator system
Nelson
  N. empyema trocar
  N. ligature needle
  N. line keeper
  N. lobectomy scissors
  N. lung-dissecting scissors
  N. lung forceps
  N. rib spreader
  N. rib stripper
  N. self-retaining rib retractor
  N. thoracic trocar
  N. tissue forceps
Nelson-Bethune shears
Nelson-Martin forceps
Nelson-Metzenbaum scissors
Nelson-Patterson empyema trocar
Nelson-Roberts stripper
Nelson-Vital dissecting scissors
Nemdi tweezer epilation device
NeoControl pelvic floor therapy system
NeoDerm dressing
NeoDura tissue material
neodymium-doped yttrium-aluminum-garnet laser
neodymium laser
neodymium:YAG laser
neodymium:yttrium-aluminum-garnet laser
neodymium:yttrium-lithium-fluoride photodisruptive laser
Neo-Fit neonatal endotracheal tube holder
Neoflex bendable knife

N

NOTES

Neoguard percussor
NeoKnife cautery
NeoLead
    Neotech N.
Neolens lens
Neolyte laser indirect ophthalmoscope
Neomed electrocautery
neonatal
    n. monitor
    n. vascular clamp
    N. Y TrachCare catheter
NeoNaze nasal function restoration
  device
Neoplex catheter
Neoplush foam
neoprene
    n. ankle support
    n. back support
    n. dressing
    n. elbow sleeve
    n. glove
    n. hinged-knee brace
    n. Osgood-Schlatter knee brace
    n. wrist brace
    n. wrist orthosis
    n. wrist strap
NeoProbe
    N. gamma detection probe
    N. radioactivity detector
Neo-Sert umbilical vessel catheter
Neos M pacemaker
Neosonic piezo ultrasonic unit
Neosono MC apex locator
neosphincter
    Acticon n.
Neotech NeoLead
Neo-Therm neonatal skin temperature
  probe
Neotrak 515A neonatal monitor
Neotrend
    N. blood gas monitor
    N. system
Neotrode II neonatal electrode
NeoV0$_2$R volume control resuscitator
Neovent ventilator
Neovision micro mirror
nephelometer
nephrolithotomy forceps
NephroMax nephrostomy balloon
  catheter
nephroscope
    Cabot n.
    Storz n.
Nephross dialyzer
nephrostomy
    n. catheter
    Cope loop n.
    n. tube
nephroureteral stent

nerve
    n. cuff
    n. fiber analyzer
    N. Fiber Analyzer laser
    ophthalmoscope
    n. hook
    N. Integrity Monitor-2 monitor
    n. retractor
    n. root laminectomy dissector
    n. root retractor
    n. separator spatula
    n. stimulation therapy (NST)
    n. stimulator
nerve-integrity monitor
NervePace nerve conduction testing
  machine
Nesbit
    N. cystoscope
    N. electrode
    N. electrotome
    N. hemostatic bag
    N. removable partial denture
    N. resectoscope
    N. tonsillar snare
nested trocar
Nestor guiding catheter
net
    Jahnke-Barron heart support n.
    Roth polyp retrieval n.
    Tubegauz elastic n.
    ureteric retrieval n.
Netra intravascular ultrasound
Netterville double-ended elevator
Nettleship
    N. canaliculus dilator
    N. iris repositor
Nettleship-Wilder lacrimal dilator
Neubauer
    N. foreign body forceps
    N. hemocytometer
    N. lancet cannula
    N. vitreous micro-extractor forceps
Neubeiser adjustable forearm splint
Neuber bone tube
Neubuser tube-seizing forceps
Neufeld
    N. cast
    N. driver
    N. femoral nail plate
    N. nail
    N. pin
    N. screw
    N. traction
    N. tractor
NeuFlex metacarpophalangeal joint
  implant
Neuhann
    N. cystotome
    N. glaucoma marker

Neumann
- N. calipers block
- N. depth gauge
- N. double corneal marker
- N. razor blade fragment holder
- N. scissors

Neumann-Shepard corneal marker
Neurairtome drill
neural
- n. dissector
- n. prosthesis

Neuray neurosurgical strip
Neuro
- N. Navigational flexible endoscope
- N. N-50 lesion generator
- N. Stim 2000 Mk$_1$ stimulator
- N. Vasx interventional device

Neuro-Aide testing device
NeuroAvitene applicator
NeuroCol neurosurgical sponge
NeuroCom Balance Master
NeuroControl Freehand implant
NeuroCybernetic prosthesis
NeuroDrape surgical drape
neuroendoscope
- Chavantes-Zamorano n.
- Neuroview n.

Neurofax electroencephalograph
NeuroFocus scanned focal point scanner
Neuroform microdelivery stent system
Neurogard TCD system
neurography
- magnetic resonance n. (MRN)
- n. needle

Neuroguard transcranial Doppler
Neuroguide
- N. optical handpiece
- N. peel-away catheter introducer
- N. suction-irrigation adapter
- N. Visicath viewing catheter

Neurolase microsurgical CO$_2$ laser
NeuroLink II EEG data acquisition system
Neurolite SPECT perfusion scanner
neurological
- N. Institute periosteal elevator
- n. percussion hammer
- n. percussor
- n. tuning fork

NeuroMate stereotactic robot
Neuromed Octrode implantable pain management device

Neuromeet
- N. nerve approximator
- N. Universal soft tissue approximator

neurometer device
Neuromod TENS unit
neuromuscular
- n. electronic stimulator (NMES)
- n. III stimulator

Neuropak 8 system
Neuropath biofeedback device
Neuropedic multidensity mattress
Neuroperfusion pump
NeuroPlan CRW stereotactic system
Neuroprobe 500 pain management system
NeuroPro rigid fixation system
Neuro-Pulse
- N.-P. nerve locator
- N.-P. TENS unit

NeuroScan 3D imager
NeuroSector ultrasound system
NeuroShield filter system
Neurosign 100 nerve monitor
NeuroStation frameless system
Neurostat Mark II cryoanalgesia system
NeuroStim TENS unit
neurostimulator
- BioTENS n.
- Grass n.
- Jobstens n.
- percutaneous epidural n.
- Staodyne EMS+2 n.

neurosurgical
- n. bur
- n. cottonoid
- n. dissector
- n. dressing forceps
- n. headrest
- n. ligature forceps
- n. needle holder
- n. pledget
- n. scissors
- n. suction forceps
- n. suture
- n. suture needle
- n. tissue forceps

Neurotips neurological examination pin
neurotome
- Bradford enucleation n.

Neurotone biofeedback device
Neuro-Trace instrument

N

NOTES

Neurotrac II neurological monitoring
system
Neurotrend continuous multiparameter
system
neurovascular
 n. forceps
 n. scissors
Neuroview
 N. integrated visualization system
 N. neuroendoscope
NeuroVision
 N. intraoperative nerve guidance
 system
 N. System
neurSector scanner
neutral
 n. density filter
 n. electrode
 n. hook
 n. position splint
Neutrocim dental cement
neutron therapy machine
Neuwirth-Palmer forceps
Nevada gonioscope
Neville
 N. ascending aorta air vent needle
 N. stent
 N. tracheal reconstruction prosthesis
 N. tracheobronchial prosthesis
Neville-Barnes forceps
Nevins
 N. dressing forceps
 N. tissue forceps
Nevyas
 N. double sharp cystotome
 N. drape retractor
 N. lens forceps
New
 N. Beginnings GelShapes silicone
 gel sheeting
 N. biopsy forceps
 N. England Baptist acetabular cup
 N. England scoliosis brace
 N. Glucorder analyzer
 N. Jersey hemiarthroplasty
 prosthesis
 N. Jersey-LCS shoulder prosthesis
 N. Jersey-LCS total knee prosthesis
 N. Luer-type speaking tube
 N. Mind Set toe splint
 N. oral needle
 N. Orleans corneal cutting block
 N. Orleans endarterectomy stripper
 N. Orleans Eye & Ear fixation
 forceps
 N. Orleans lens
 N. Orleans lens loupe
 N. Orleans needle holder
 N. Skimmer blade

N. speaking tube
N. suture scissors
N. tenaculum
N. tissue forceps
N. tracheal retractor
N. tracheostomy hook
N. tracheotomy hook
N. ultra-thick powder-free latex
 surgical glove
N. Vision magnification system
N. Weavenit Dacron prosthesis
N. Yorker guidewire
N. York erysiphake
N. York Eye and Ear cannula
N. York Eye and Ear Hospital
 fixation forceps
N. York glass suction tube
N. York Hospital electrode
N. York Hospital retractor
N. York Orthopedic front-opening
 orthosis
newborn eyelid retractor
Newell
 N. lid retractor
 N. nucleus hook
Newhart-Casselberry snare
Newhart hook
Newhart-Smith cup
Newington orthotic
Newkirk mouthgag
New-Lambotte osteotome
NewLife
 N. Elite oxygen concentrator
 N. therapeutic mattress
 N. therapeutic surface
Newman
 N. proctoscope
 N. rectal injection needle
 N. tenaculum
 N. toenail plate
 N. uterine knife
 N. uterine tenaculum forceps
Newport
 N. cartilage gouge
 N. collar
 N. E100M ventilator
 N. HT50 ventilator
 N. MC total hip orthosis
 N. medical instrument
 N. Wave VM200 ventilator
Newsom side port nucleus cracker
NewTom scanner
Newton LLT guidewire
Newton-Morgan retractor
Newvicon
 N. camera tube
 N. vacuum chamber pickup tube
NewVues lens
Nexacryl tissue adhesive

Nexerciser Plus exercise system
NexFlex
    N. total hip system
    N. total knee system
NexGen
    N. complete knee replacement
    N. knee implant
    N. offset stem extension
NexStent carotid stent
NexTemp Precision Phase Change thermometer
Nextep
    N. Contour lower-leg walker
    N. knee brace
    N. Silhouette lower-leg walker
Nexus
    N. coronary stent
    N. hip prosthesis
    N. implant
    N. 2 linear ablation catheter
    N. wheelchair seating system
Ney articulator
Nezhat-Dorsey
    N.-D. hydrodissection pump
    N.-D. suction-irrigator
    N.-D. trumpet valve
    N.-D. trumpet valve hydrodissector
Nezhat irrigator
NG
    nasogastric
    NG feeding tube
    NG strip nasal tube fastener
NHS-activated HiTrap affinity column
Niagara temporary dialysis catheter
Niamtu video imaging system
Nibbler laparoscopic probe
Niblitt dissector
Nic the Asthmatic Dragon aerosol mask
Nicati foreign body spud
N'ice Stretch night splint
Nichamin
    N. fixation ring
    N. hydrodissection cannula
    N. II lens inserter
    N. II ophthalmic loader
    N. LASIK irrigating cannula
    N. quick chopper
    N. triple chopper
    N. vertical chopper
Niche knife

Nichols
    N. aortic clamp
    N. infundibulectomy rongeur
    N. nasal siphon
Nichols-Deschamps-Navratil ligature needle
Nichols-Jehle coronary multihead catheter
Nickell cystoscope adapter
Nickelplast blank
nickel-titanium file
Nickerson Biggy vial
NICO cardiopulmonary monitor
Nicola
    N. forceps
    N. gouge
    N. microforceps
    N. pituitary rongeur
    N. rasp
    N. raspatory
    N. tendon clamp
Nicolet
    N. Biomedical UltraSom NT polysomnography system
    N. Compass electromyography instrument
    N. Elite obstetrical Doppler
    N. nerve integrity monitor
    N. NIM-2
    N. NMR spectrometer
    N. Pathfinder I recording device
    N. SM-300 stimulator
    N. Viking Iie EMG
    N. Viking II electrophysiologic system
Nicoll
    N. bone graft
    N. plate
    N. tendon prosthesis
Nidek
    N. AR-2000 objective automatic refractor
    N. 3Dx camera
    N. EchoScan
    N. EC-series excimer laser
    N. MK-2000 keratome system
Niebauer
    N. finger joint replacement prosthesis
    N. trapezium replacement prosthesis
Niebauer-Cutter implant

N

NOTES

Niedner
> N. anastomosis clamp
> N. commissurotomy knife
> N. dissecting forceps
> N. pulmonic clamp

Niehaber prosthesis

night
> n. drainage bag
> n. drain bottle
> N. Preservers underpad

NightBird nasal CPAP machine
Nightimer carpal tunnel support
Nightingale examining lamp
NightOwl pocket polygraph
NIH
> National Institutes of Health
> NIH left ventriculography catheter
> NIH mitral valve forceps

Nihon-Kohden electroencephalograph
Nihon tocodynamometer
Nikon
> N. aspheric lens
> N. FS-3 photo slit lamp biomicroscope
> N. microprocessor-controlled camera
> N. Retinomax K-Plus autorefractor
> N. Retinopan fundus camera
> N. SMZ 2T magnifying lens
> N. zoom photo slit lamp

Nilsson-Stille abortion suction tube
Nilsson suction tube
NIM-2
> Nicolet NIM-2

Nimbus Hemopump cardiac assist device
Niplette device
nipper
> anterior crurotomy n.
> cuticle n.
> Dieter n.
> Dieter-House n.
> English anvil nail n.
> Hough anterior crurotomy n.
> House-Dieter malleus n.
> House malleus n.
> Lempert malleus n.
> malleus n.
> Miltex nail n.
> nail n.
> Rica malleus head n.
> SMIC malleus head n.
> Tabb crural n.
> Turnbull nail n.
> Wister n.

nipple
> Kock n.
> McGovern n.

NIR
> near-infrared

NIR ON Ranger premounted stent
NIR Primo balloon expandable stent
NIR Primo Monorail stent system
NIR stent
NIR with SOX over-the-wire coronary stent

NIRflex coronary stent
Niro
> N. arch bar
> N. bone-cutting forceps
> N. wire-twister forceps
> N. wire-twisting forceps

Niroyal
> N. Advance balloon expandable stent
> N. Elite Monorail

Nirvana pressure-reducing mattress
Nisbet
> N. eye forceps
> N. fixation forceps

Nishimoto Sangyo scanner
Nishizaki-Wakabayashi suction tube
Nissen
> N. cystic forceps
> N. gall duct forceps
> N. hassux forceps
> N. rib spreader
> N. suture

Nite
> N. Train'r bedwetting alarm
> N. Train'r DVC bedwetting alarm

nitinol
> n. guidewire
> n. K-file
> n. mesh-covered frame
> n. mesh stent
> n. self-expanding coil stent
> n. shape-memory alloy wire
> n. snare
> n. Strecker stent
> n. subglottic stenosis stent
> n. thermal memory stent
> n. U-clip

Ni-Ti Shape Memory alloy compression stapler
Nitra lamp
nitric oxide analyzer
nitrile glove
nitrogen-phosphorus detector
Nitro wheelchair
NLite laser collagen replenishment system
NMES
> neuromuscular electronic stimulator

NMR
> nuclear magnetic resonance
> NMR LipoProfile device

NMR probe circuit
NMR spectrometer

No
N. Bounce mallet
N. Pour Pak II suction catheter kit
N. Sting barrier film
Nobel Biocare dental implant
Nobelpharma
N. gold prosthetic retaining screw
N. implant
N. implant system
Nobetec dental cement
Nobis aortic occluder
Noble
N. iris forceps
N. scissors
Noblock retractor
Noci stimuli needle
Nocito implant
N₂O cryosurgical unit
nocturnal penile tumescence monitor
Nogenol dental cement
NoHands Mouse
Noiles
N. posterior stabilized knee
N. posterior stabilized knee prosthesis
N. rotating hinge knee
N. rotating-hinge knee mechanism
N. rotating-hinge total knee prosthesis
noise
n. level monitor
n. reduction device
N. Stik II pediatric hearing screener
NoKor needle
Nokrome bifocal lens
Noland-Budd cervical curette
Nolan system collimator mounted contact shield
No-Lok compression screw
nomogram
Casebeer-Lindstrom n.
Nomos
N. multiprogrammable R-wave inhibited demand pacemaker
N. stereotactic system
nonabsorbable
n. surgical suture
n. suture

nonadherent foam
nonadhesive dressing
non-arcon articulator
noncannulated nail
non-child-resistant container
noncompetitive pacemaker
noncompliant (NC)
n. balloon
nonconductive guidewire
noncontact tonometer
noncoring Huber needle
noncrushing
n. anterior resection clamp
n. bowel clamp
n. common duct forceps
n. gastroenterostomy clamp
n. gastrointestinal clamp
n. intestinal clamp
n. intestinal forceps
n. liver-holding clamp
n. pickup forceps
n. tissue-holding forceps
n. vascular clamp
noncutting suture needle
nondetachable
n. endovascular balloon
n. occlusive balloon
nonenclosed magnet
nonfenestrated
n. forceps
n. Moore-type femoral stem
nonferromagnetic
n. clip
n. MR-compatible frame
n. needle
n. positioning device
nonflotation catheter
nonhinged knee prosthesis
Nonin Onyx pulse oximeter
nonintegrated
n. transvenous defibrillation lead
n. tripolar lead
noninterfering separator
noninvasive
n. continuous cardiac output monitor
n. immobilization device
n. monitor
n. paddle
n. temporary pacemaker
non-irrigating
nonlatex dental dam

N

NOTES

nonmagnetic
n. dressing forceps
n. tissue forceps
nonmetallic cage
nonocclusive dressing
nonperforating
n. towel clamp
n. towel forceps
nonpneumatic tourniquet
nonporous-coated endoprosthesis
nonrebreathing
n. mask
n. valve
nonrigid endoscope
nonslipping forceps
NonSpil drug delivery system
nonthoracotomy
n. defibrillation lead system
n. lead implantable cardioverter-defibrillator
n. system antitachycardia device
nontoothed forceps
nontraumatizing
n. catheter
n. visceral forceps
nonweightbearing brace
nonwoven sponge
Noon
N. AV fistula clamp
N. AV fistular tunneler
N. modified vascular access tunneler
NoProfile
N. balloon
N. balloon catheter
Norco ulnar deviation support
Norcross periosteal elevator
Nordan-Colibri forceps
Nordan-Ruiz trapezoidal marker
Nordan tying forceps
Nordenstrom Rotex II biopsy needle
Nordent
N. amalgam condenser
N. bone chisel
N. bone curette
N. bone file
N. burnisher
N. carver
N. excavator
N. explorer
N. filling instrument
N. hatchet
N. hoe
N. margin trimmer
N. oral surgery elevator
N. periodontic knife
N. scaler
Nordent-Ochsenbein periodontic chisel

NordiCare
N. Back Therapy system
N. Enabler exerciser
N. Strider exerciser
NordicTrack ski exerciser
NordiPen injector
Nord orthodontic plate
Nordotrack motion EMG
No-React
N.-R. pericardial patch
N.-R. Pneumo-Pledgets staple-line seal
Norelco mucotome
Norfolk intrauterine aspiration catheter
Norian SRS cement
Norland
N. digital oscilloscope
N. pQCT XCT2000 scanner
N. XR26 bone densitometer
Norman
N. tibial bolt
N. tibial pin
Normlgel protective wound dressing
Norport pump
Norrbacka bone elevator
Norrbacka-Stille lever
Norris
N. button
N. sponge forceps
Northbent suture scissors
Northgate SD-3 dual-purpose lithotripter
North-South retractor
Northville brace
Norton
N. adjustable cup reamer
N. ball reamer
N. endotracheal tube
N. flow-directed Swan-Ganz thermodilution catheter
Norwegian system
Norwood
N. forceps
N. rectal snare
nose
n. cone
n. guard splint
Nosik transorbital leukotome
notcher device
notchplasty blade
Noto
N. dressing forceps
N. ovum forceps
N. polypus forceps
N. sponge forceps
No-Touch delivery system
Nott-Gutmann vaginal speculum
Nottingham
N. colposuspension needle
N. introducer

N. One-Step tapered dilator
N. ureteral dilator
Nott vaginal speculum
Nounton blade
Nourse bladder syringe
NouveauDerm socks
Nova
N. Aid lens
N. Celltrak 12 hematology analyzer
N. Curve lens
N. II pacemaker
N. jaw hook
N. Microsonics Image Vue system
N. MR pacemaker
N. Soft II lens
N. thermodilution catheter
NovaBone
N. bone graft
NovaBone-C/M
NovaBone-C/M bone graft
NovaBone-C/M synthetic bone graft
particulate
NovaCath multilumen infusion catheter
Novack special extraction set
Novacor
N. Diasys left ventricular assist
device
N. left ventricular assist system
Novafil suture
Novaflex intraocular lens
NovaGel silicone gel sheeting
NovaGold breast implant
Novak
N. fixation forceps
N. uterine biopsy curette
Novak-Schoeckaert endometrial curette
NovaLine
N. excimer laser
N. excimer laser system
N. Litho-S DUV excimer laser
Novametrix
N. combination O_2/CO_2 sensor
N. pulse oximeter
N. Tidal Wave Sp handheld
capnograph/pulse oximeter
NovaPulse
N. CO_2 laser
N. laser system
Novar oral illuminator
NovaSaline inflatable breast implant
Novascan scanning headpiece laser
Novastent stent

NovaSure
N. ablator
N. endometrial ablation system
Novatec
N. Lightblade
N. Lightblade laser
Novex wedged wheelchair cushion
NovolinPen injector
Novoste
N. Beta-Cath system
N. catheter
Novulase 660 laser
Novus
N. hydrocephalic valve
N. LC threaded interbody fusion
cage
N. Medical image card
N. Omni multiwavelength laser
N. Omni 2000 photocoagulator
N. Verdi diode-pumped green
photocoagulator
NOxBox
N. II nitric oxide monitor
N. Plus monitor
Noyes
N. chalazion punch
N. ear forceps
N. iridectomy scissors
N. iris scissors
N. nasal-dressing forceps
N. nasal forceps
N. rongeur
N. speculum
Noyes-Shambaugh scissors
Nozovent anti-snoring device
NP-3S auto chart projector
**NPB-series handheld capnograph/pulse
oximeter**
NS2000 bipolar generator system
NST
nerve stimulation therapy
ReliefBand NST
N-Terface contact-layer wound dressing
Nu
N. Gauze dressing
N. Gauze sponge
**Nu-Abrasion microdermabrasion
handpiece**
**Nu-Brede packing and debridement
sponge**
nubular blade

NOTES

N

nuclear
n. magnetic resonance (NMR)
n. magnetic resonance spectrometer
n. medicine camera
n. probe
n. scanner
n. stent
nuclear-powered pacemaker
Nucleotome
N. Endoflex instrument
N. Flex II cutting probe
N. Micro I probe
Nucletron
N. applicator
N. simulator
nucleus
N. 22 cochlear implant
N. 24 Contour cochlear implant system
n. cracker
n. delivery cannula
n. delivery loop
n. erysiphake
n. expressor
n. hydrolysis needle
N. 24 multichannel auditory brainstem implant
n. removal loop
n. rotator
n. spatula
Nu-Comfort colostomy appliance
Nu-Derm foam island dressing
Nu-Form truss
Nu-Gel wound dressing
Nugent
N. erysiphake
N. fixation forceps
N. iris hook
N. rectus forceps
N. soft cataract aspirator
N. superior rectus forceps
N. utility forceps
Nugent-Gradle stitch scissors
Nugent-Green-Dimitry erysiphake
Nugowski forceps
Nu-Hope
N.-H. adhesive
N.-H. adhesive waterproof skin barrier
N.-H. drainable urinary pouch
N.-H. hole cutter
N.-H. skin barrier strip
N.-H. urine collection bottle
Nu-Knit
N.-K. absorbable hemostat
Surgicel N.-K.
NuKo knee orthosis
Numby Stuff electrode

NuMED
N. intracoronary Doppler catheter
N. single balloon
Nunc cryotube
Nunez
N. aortic clamp
N. auricular clamp
N. sternal approximator
N. ventricular ventilation tube
Nunez-Nunez mitral stenosis knife
Nuport PEG tube
NuPulse device
Nurolon suture
Nussbaum
N. bracelet
N. intestinal clamp
N. intestinal forceps
NuStep
N. exerciser
N. total body recumbent stepper
nut
n. alignment guide
Close Encounter n.
Kirschner traction bow n.
locking n.
nylon n.
sleeved n.
Stable-Lok n.
Nu-Thor thoracostomy device
Nu-Tip laparoscopic scissors
NutraCol hydrocolloid wound dressing
NutraDress zinc-saline dressing
NutraFil hydrophilic B dressing
NutraGauze hydrophilic wound dressing
Nu-Trake
N.-T. cricothyrotomy device
N.-T. Weiss emergency airway system
NutraStat calcium alginate wound dressing
NutraVue hydrogel dressing
Nutricath silicone elastomer catheter
nutrition
total parenteral n. (TPN)
Nutromat Pad S feeding pump
Nuttall retractor
Nuva-Lite ultraviolet activator
Nuvaring contraceptive vaginal ring
NuVasc stent graft
Nuvaseal resin
Nuva-Tach resin
Nuvistor electronic tonometer
NuVita lens
Nuvo barrier film
Nu-Vois artificial larynx
Nuvolase 660 laser system
NuVue lens
Nuwave TENS
Nuway in-the-ear hearing aid

Nu-wrap roll dressing
Nyboer esophageal electrode
Nycore angiography pigtail catheter
Nyhus-Nelson
    N.-N. gastric decompression tube
    N.-N. jejunal feeding tube
Nyhus-Potts intestinal forceps
Nykanen RF perforation catheter
Nylatex
    N. strap
    N. wrap
Nylex II Convoluted innerspring
Nylok
    N. bolt
    N. self-locking nail
nylon
    n. catheter
    n. face mallet
    n. head mallet
    n. loop
    n. monofilament suture

    n. nut
    n. retention suture
    Rica n.
    n. 66 suture
nystagmus
    n. bulb
    n. glasses
Nystar Plus electronystagmogram
Nystroem
    N. abdominal suction tube
    N. hip nail
    N. nail driver
    N. retractor
    N. tumor forceps
Nystroem-Stille
    N.-S. driver
    N.-S. hip nail
    N.-S. retractor
Nytone enuretic alarm
NYU-Hosmer electric elbow and
    prehension actuator

NOTES

N

OAdjuster knee brace
O₂ Advantage oxygen conserver
Oaks
    O. double needle
    O. double straight cannula
oardlike retractor
Oasis
    O. collagen plug
    O. feather microscalpel
    O. guiding/pushing catheter
    O. humidifier
    O. sheet introducer system
    O. thrombectomy catheter
    O. wound dressing
OAsys brace
OATS
    Osteochondral Autograft Transfer System
OB-10 Comfort bite block
Obagi Blue Peel
O'Beirne sphincter tube
Oberhill
    O. obstetrical forceps
    O. self-retaining retractor
Ober tendon passer
Oberto mouth prop
obese walker
OB Gees maternity orthotic
objective lens
oblique
    o. bandage
    o. hand positioner
    o. muscle hook
    o. prism
oblique-viewing
    o.-v. echoendoscope
    o.-v. endoscope
O'Brien
    O. airway needle
    O. fixation forceps
    O. foreign body spud
    O. marker
    O. phrenic retractor
    O. rib hook
    O. rib retractor
    O. rongeur
    O. spatula
    O. stitch scissors
    O. suture scissors
    O. tissue forceps
O'Brien-Elschnig forceps
O'Brien-Mayo scissors
O'Brien-Storz microhemostat
Obstbaum
    O. lens spatula
    O. synechia spatula

obstetrical
    o. block anesthesia needle
    o. decapitating embryotome
    o. decapitating hook
    o. forceps
    o. retractor
    o. spoon
obstructed shunt tube
OBT
    Olivier-Bertrand-Tipal
    OBT frame
Obtura II gutta percha system
obturator
    Alcock o.
    Alcock-Timberlake o.
    o. appliance
    Arrow sheath o.
    blunt o.
    blunt-tip o.
    cannulated o.
    coagulating suction cannula o.
    convex o.
    Cripps o.
    distending o.
    double-catheterizing sheath and o.
    Endopath Optiview laparoscopic o.
    Endotrac o.
    Frazier suction tube o.
    Hemaflex PTCA sheath with o.
    Keene o.
    LaparoSAC o.
    Leusch atraumatic o.
    Moria o.
    Optiview optical surgical o.
    palatal o.
    Rumel tourniquet-eyed o.
    sheath and o.
    Thal-Mantel o.
    Thermafil Plus o.
    Thora-Port o.
    Timberlake o.
    tourniquet-eyed o.
    ureteral catheter o.
    visual o.
Obus back support
OB-View workstation
Obwegeser
    O. awl
    O. channel retractor
    O. orthognathic surgery instrument
    O. periosteal retractor
    O. splitting chisel
Obwegeser-Dalpont internal screw
    fixation

O

occluder
Amplatzer o.
Amplatzer duct o.
Amplatzer septal o.
aortic o.
ASDOS umbrella o.
Bard clamshell septal o.
black/white o.
Brockenbrough curved-tip o.
catheter tip o.
clamshell double umbrella o.
clamshell septal o.
clip-on o.
Endofit vessel o.
Goffman o.
Halberg trial clip o.
Heifitz carotid o.
Helex septal o.
Kean-M-4 o.
lorgnette o.
Maddox rod o.
Microvena Das Angel Wings o.
modified Rashkind PDA o.
multiple pinhole o.
Nobis aortic o.
PFO-Star o.
pinhole o.
Plus punctal o.
Pram combination o.
radiolucent plastic o.
Rashkind double-disc umbrella o.
red lens o.
Rumison side port fixation o.
StarFlex o.
vessel o.
occluding
o. clamp
o. forceps
o. fracture frame
occlusal rest bar
occlusion
o. balloon
o. catheter
o. coil
occlusive
o. balloon
o. collodion dressing
o. moisture-retentive dressing
o. semipermeable dressing
occlusor
Elastoplast eye o.
Ochsner
O. aortic clamp
O. arterial clamp
O. artery clamp
O. ball-tipped scissors
O. cartilage forceps
O. diamond-edged scissors
O. flexible spiral gallstone probe

O. gallbladder trocar
O. gallbladder tube
O. gall duct probe
O. gallstone probe
O. hemostat
O. hemostatic forceps
O. hook
O. malleable retractor
O. needle
O. ribbon retractor
O. ring
O. scissors
O. spiral probe
O. thoracic clamp
O. thoracic trocar
O. tissue forceps
O. total enarterectomy set
O. vascular retractor
O. wire twister
Ochsner-DeBakey spur crusher
Ochsner-Dixon arterial forceps
Ochsner-Favaloro self-retaining retractor
Ochsner-Fenger gallstone probe
Ockerblad
O. forceps
O. kidney clamp
O. vessel clamp
OCL
Orthopedic Casting Lab
OCL PolyLite synthetic splinting system
OCL Splint Roll Contour splinting system
OCL volar splint
Ocoee scalp cleansing unit
O'Connor
O. abdominal retractor
O. biopsy forceps
O. double-edged curette
O. drape
O. eye forceps
O. finger cup
O. flat tenotomy hook
O. grasping forceps
O. hook punch
O. iris forceps
O. lid clamp
O. lid forceps
O. marker
O. muscle hook
O. operating arthroscope
O. rectal finger cot
O. scleral depressor
O. sheath
O. sponge forceps
O. vaginal retractor
O'Connor-Elschnig fixation forceps
O'Connor-O'Sullivan self-retaining vaginal retractor

octagon roll
Octa-Hex implant
octapolar
    o. catheter
    o. lead
Octopus
    O. 1-2-3 perimeter
    O. retractor
    O. 2, 2+, 3 tissue stabilization
    system
OctreoScan
    O. scanner
    O. system
Ocu-Guard ophthalmic wrap
Oculab Tono-Pen tonometer
Oculaid lens
ocular
    o. cautery
    o. cup
    o. Gamboscope lens
    o. Gamboscope loupe
    o. hypertension indicator
    o. marker
    o. pressure reducer
    o. prosthesis
Oculex drug delivery system
OcuLight
    O. GLx green laser
    photocoagulator
    O. SL diode laser
    O. SLx ophthalmic laser
oculocerebrovasculometer
oculocutaneous laser
oculography
    Binocular Infrared O. (BIRO)
oculogyric stimulator
Oculo-Plastik ePTFE ocular implant
oculoplasty corneal protector
oculoplethysmograph
Oculus
    O. lens loop
    O. trial frame
Ocumeter
    Timoptic O.
Ocuscan
    Sonometric O.
    O. 400 transducer
Ocutech Vision Enhancing system
ocutome
    Berkeley Bioengineering o.
    CooperVision series 10,000 o.
    disposable o.

    O. II fragmentation system
    o. probe
    STOO Series Ten Thousand o.
    O. vitrectomy unit
    o. vitrector
    o. vitreous blade
Odelca camera
O'Dell spicule forceps
Odland ankle prosthesis
Odman-Ledin catheter
O'Donoghue
    O. cartilage feeler
    O. cystourethroscope
    O. dressing
    O. knee splint
    O. probe
    O. stirrup splint
    O. suture passer
odontoid peg-grasping forceps
Odontometer electronic apex locator
odor-absorbent dressing
O'Dwyer tube
Odyssey phacoemulsification system
OEC
    OEC Dual-Op barrel/plate
    component
    OEC Mini 6600 imaging system
OEC-Diasonics
    OEC-D. 9400 fluoroscopy C-arm
    system
    OEC-D. mobile C-arm image
    intensifier
OEC-Kuntscher Interlocking Pathfinder
nail
OEC-series FluoroTrak navigation
system
OEM
    OEM 503 humidifier
    OEM Venturi MixOMask mask
Oertli wire lid retractor
Oesch
    O. hook
    O. stripper
Oettingen abdominal self-retaining
retractor
offset
    o. cane
    o. hand retractor
    o. hinge
    o. modified prosthesis
    o. operating laparoscope
    o. suspension feeder

O

NOTES

O'Gawa
- O. cataract-aspirating cannula
- O. irrigating cannula
- O. needle holder
- O. suture-fixation forceps
- O. suture forceps
- O. two-way I&A cannula

O'Gawa-Castroviejo tying forceps
O'Gawa tying forceps
Ogden
- O. Anchor soft tissue device
- O. plate
- O. soft tissue to bone anchor
- O. tissue reattachment mini system

Ogden-Senturia eustachian inflator
Ogee acetabular cup
Ogura
- O. cartilage forceps
- O. nasal saw
- O. tissue
- O. tissue forceps

O'Hanlon
- O. forceps
- O. intestinal clamp

O'Hanlon-Poole suction tube
O'Hara forceps
O'Harris-Petruso cup
Ohio
- O. bed
- O. Bubble humidifier
- O. critical care ventilator
- O. Hope resuscitator
- O. Nuclear Delta scanner
- O. pressure infuser
- O. safety trap overflow bottle
- O. Vortex respiration monitor
- O. warmer

Ohl periosteal elevator
Ohmeda
- O. Care-Plus incubator
- O. 9000 computer-cotrolled infusion pump
- O. continuous-vacuum regulator
- O. handheld pulse oximeter
- O. probe
- O. Rascal II Raman spectroscope
- O. 5250 respiratory gas monitor
- O. Sevotec 5 vaporizer
- O. thoracic suction regulator

ohmmeter
oiled
- o. silk dressing
- o. silk suture

ointment
- Carlesta o.
- Catrix o.
- Ethezyme papain-urea debriding o.
- Xenaderm o.

OIS
optical intrinsic signal
- OIS digital slit-lamp imager
- OIS image digitizing system

OIU
optical internal urethrotomy
- OIU cold knife

Oklahoma
- O. ankle joint orthosis
- O. ankle prosthesis
- O. City cable
- O. iris wire retractor

Okmian microneedle holder
Okonek-Yasargil tumor fork
Olbert
- O. balloon
- O. balloon catheter
- O. balloon dilator
- O. NoProfile balloon dilatation catheter

Oldberg
- O. brain retractor
- O. dissector
- O. elevator
- O. intervertebral disc forceps
- O. intervertebral disc rongeur
- O. laminectomy rongeur
- O. pituitary rongeur
- O. pituitary rongeur forceps
- O. straight retractor

Oldfield needle
Old Smoothie bur
Oleeva
- O. fabric sheeting
- O. scar sheeting

Olerud
- O. internal fixator
- O. PSF fixation system
- O. PSF rod
- O. PSF screw

Oliair
- O. articulator
- O. mouth mirror

OligoDetect system
oligonucleotide probe
olivary catheter
olive
- Eder-Puestow metal o.
- interchangeable vein stripper o.
- o. ring
- o. wire

Olivecrona
- O. aneurysm clamp
- O. aneurysm forceps
- O. angular scissors
- O. brain spatula
- O. brain spoon
- O. clip applier
- O. clip-applying/removing forceps

O. conchotome
O. dissector
O. dural scissors
O. endaural rongeur
O. guillotine scissors
O. rongeur forceps
O. silver clip
O. trigeminal knife
O. wire saw
Olivecrona-Gigli wire saw
Olivecrona-Stille dissector
Olivecrona-Toennis clip-applying forceps
Olivella-Garrigosa photocoagulator
Oliver scalp retractor
olive-tipped
o.-t. bougie
o.-t. cannula
o.-t. catheter
o.-t. dilator
o.-t. irrigator
o.-t. monopolar electrosurgical dissector
o.-t. needle
Welsh flat o.-t.
Olivier-Bertrand-Tipal (OBT)
O.-B.-T. frame
Olk
O. membrane peeler
O. membrane peeler knife
O. retinal spatula
O. vitreoretinal pick
O. vitreoretinal spatula
Ollier
O. graft
O. rake retractor
O. rasp
Ollier-Thiersch
O.-T. graft
O.-T. implant
Olsen
O. bayonet monopolar forceps
O. cholangiogram clamp
O. self-retaining Laparostat
Olshevsky tube
Olson
O. calibrated cornea trephine system
O. nucleus quick chopper
O. phaco chopper
Olson-Hegar extra-delicate needle holder

Olyco
O. articulator
O. mouth mirror
Olympia
O. articulator
O. mouth mirror
O. Vacpac support
Olympic
O. BiliLight
O. needle holder
O. Neostraint immobilizer
O. Oxyhood oxygen hood
Olympus
O. alligator-jaw endoscopic forceps
O. angioscope
O. basket-type endoscopic forceps
O. BF-series bronchoscope
O. BHT-2 microscope
O. CBK fluorescence microscope
O. CD-Z-series heat probe thermocoagulator
O. CF-20 fibercolonoscope
O. CF-HM-series magnifying colonoscope
O. CF-L-series flexible sigmoidoscope
O. CF-MB-series colonoscope
O. CF-OSF-series flexible sigmoidoscope
O. CF-PL-series colonoscope
O. CF-P-series colonoscope
O. CF-series colonofiberscope
O. CF-series colonoscope
O. CF-series flexible sigmoidoscope
O. CF-T-series colonoscope
O. CF-UM3 colonoscope
O. CF-UM-series echoendoscope
O. CF-UM20 ultrasonic endoscope
O. CF-VL-series colonoscope
O. CG-P-series colonofiberscope
O. CHF-BP30 endoscope
O. CHF-P-series choledochoscope
O. CHF-Q10 cholangioscope
O. CHF-series choledochoscope
O. clip-fixing device
O. CLV-series fiberoptic system
O. continuous-flow resectoscope
O. CV-series colonoscope
O. CYF-series OES cystofiberscope
O. diagnostic laparoscope
O. disposable cannula
O. disposable trocar

O

NOTES

Olympus *(continued)*

O. duodenofiberscope
O. endocamera
O. endoscopic ultrasound scanner
O. Endo-Therapy disposable biopsy forceps
O. ENF-P2 rhinolaryngoscope
O. ENF-P-series laryngoscope
O. esophagofiberscope
O. esophagoscope
O. EU-M-series endosonography image processor
O. Europe ETD automated endoscope washer
O. EU-series endoscope
O. EUS-series endoscope
O. EVIS Q-series endoscope
O. EW-series fiberoptic duodenoscope
O. FBK-series forceps
O. FB-series biopsy forceps
O. FG-series forceps
O. fiberoptic bronchoscope
O. fiberoptic scope
O. fiberoptic sigmoidoscope
O. flexible hysterofiberscope
O. forward-viewing endoscope
O. FS-K-series endoscopic suture-cutting forceps
O. FS-series endoscopic suture-cutting forceps
O. gastrocamera
O. gastrostomy
O. GF-series gastroscope
O. GF-UM30P echoendoscope
O. GF-UM-series echoendoscope
O. GF-UM-series endoscope
O. GIF-EUM-series echoendoscope
O. GIF-HM-series endoscope
O. GIF-J-series endoscope
O. GIF-K-series gastroscope
O. GIFK-XQ-series endoscope
O. GIF-Q-series endoscope
O. GIF-series gastroscope
O. GIF-T-series videoendoscope
O. GIF-XP-series endoscope
O. GIF-XQ-series flexible gastroscope
O. GIF-XV-series endoscope
O. grasping rat-tooth forceps
O. GTF-series gastroscope
O. heat probe
O. hot biopsy forceps
O. hysteroscope
O. II PTCA dilatation catheter
O. JF-series video duodenoscope
O. JF-T-series endoscope
O. JF-TV-series endoscope
O. JF-UM-series echoendoscope

O. JF-V-series video duodenoscope
O. JT-series video duodenoscope
O. light source connector
O. 13 L injector
O. magnetic extractor forceps
O. MAJ363 FNA needle system
O. MH-908 slim ultrasonic probe
O. neonatal cystoscope
O. NM-K-series sclerotherapy needle
O. NM-L-series needle
O. OES fiberscope
O. OES 4000 resectoscope
O. OES-series gastroscope
O. OM-1 endoscopic camera
O. One-Step Button gastrostomy tube
O. operating camera
O. OSF flexible sigmoidoscope
O. OSP fluorescence measuring system
O. OTV-S-series miniature camera
O. PCF-series pediatric colonoscope
O. pelican-type endoscopic forceps
O. PJF-series pediatric duodenoscope
O. P-series endoscope
O. PW-1L wash catheter
O. Q-series endoscope
O. rat-tooth endoscopic forceps
O. resectoscope loop
O. reusable oval cup forceps
O. SD-5L semicircular snare
O. shark-tooth endoscopic forceps
O. side-viewing endoscope
O. SIF-M-series video enteroscope
O. SIF-series video enteroscope
O. SIF-SW-series video enteroscope
O. SP-series image analyzer
O. S20-20R endoscope
O. SSIF-series video enteroscope
O. stone retrieval basket
O. TJF-series endoscope
O. transnasal fiberendoscope
O. 2T-2000 twin-channel therapeutic gastroscope
O. UES-series snare cautery device
O. ultrasonic esophagoprobe
O. ultrathin balloon-fitted ultrasound probe
O. UM-R-series miniature ultrasonic probe
O. UM-W-series endoscopic probe
O. URF-P2 translaparoscopic choledochofiberscope
O. video duodenoscope
O. video urology procedure system
O. VU-M-series echoendoscope
O. W-shaped endoscopic forceps

O. XCF-XK-series endoscope
O. XIF-UM-series echoendoscope
O. XK-series oblique-viewing flexible fiberscope
O. XMP-U2 catheter echoprobe
O. XP-series endoscope
O. XQ-series gastroscope
O. XSIF-series video enteroscope

OM
operating microscope
OM 2000 operating microscope
OM 4 ophthalmometer

O'Malley
O. jaw fracture splint
O. self-adhering lens implant
O. vitrector

O'Malley-Heintz
O.-H. infusion cannula
O.-H. vitreous cutter

O'Malley-Pearce-Luma lens
O'Malley-Skia transilluminator
Ombrédanne
O. forceps
O. mallet

Omed
O. bulldog vascular clamp
O. vented instrument guard

Omega
O. compression hip screw
O. CSI MR system
O. 5600 noninvasive blood pressure monitor
O. Plus compression hip system
O. splinting material

Omega21 expandable screw
Omega-NV balloon
OmegaPort access port
Omegascope OM2/070 flexible microendoscope
omental plug
Omiderm transparent adhesive film dressing
Ommaya
O. CSF reservoir
O. intraventricular reservoir system
O. reservoir device
O. shunt
O. ventricular reservoir

Omni
O. Bloc bite block
O. 1, 2 blood gas analyzer

O. catheter
O. flush catheter
O. infant heel warmer
O. knee brace
O. press
O. pretibial buttress
O. retractor
O. selective catheter
O. SST balloon

Omni-Atricor pacemaker
OmniBed
Giraffe O.

Omnicarbon
O. heart valve prosthesis
O. prosthetic heart valve

OmniCath atherectomy catheter
Omnicor pacemaker
OmniCup
Kiwi O.

Omni-Ectocor pacemaker
Omnifit
O. acetabular cup
O. HA femoral component
O. HA hip stem
O. HA hip system
O. intraocular lens
O. knee prosthesis
O. Plus hip system

Omnifix tape
Omniflex
O. balloon catheter
O. impression material
O. PTCA stent

Omni-Flexor wrist exerciser
Omni-Flow 4000 Plus medication management system
omnifocal lens
Omni-LapoTract support system
OmniLink biliary stent
Omniloc dental implant
OmniMed argon-fluoride excimer laser
OmniMedia XRS scanner
Omni-Orthocor pacemaker
Omni-Park speculum
OmniPhase penile prosthesis
OmniPlane TEE transducer
Omniport hand-assisted laparoscopic device
OmniPulse holmium laser
OmniPulse-Max holmium laser

O

NOTES

Omniscience
    O. single-leaflet cardiac valve
      prosthesis
    O. tilting-disc valve
Omnisense 7000S bone sonometer
Omnisil putty
Omni-Stanicor pacemaker
OmniStent stent
Omni-Theta pacemaker
OmniTip side-firing laser needle
Omnitone hearing aid
Omni-Tract
    O.-T. retractor system
    O.-T. vaginal retractor
Omni-Ventricor pacemaker
OmoTrain shoulder support
Omron
    O. compressor nebulizer
    O. Hem-601 automatic digital wrist
      blood pressure monitor
**Omron/Marshall 97 automatic
oscillometric digital blood pressure
monitor**
On2 lateral transfer device
On-Command catheter
Oncor ApopTaq kit
on-demand analgesia computer
One
    O. Action Stent Introduction
      System
    O. Disposable microkeratome
    O. Time dressing kit
    O. Touch Basic
    O. Touch basic glucometer
    O. Touch II hospital blood glucose
      monitoring system
O'Neill
    O. cardiac clamp
    O. cardiac surgical scissors
Oneseal reducer cap
One-Shot ablation device
One-Time disposable skin stapler
One-Touch
    O.-T. blood glucose meter
    O.-T. electrolysis unit
Ong capsulotomy scissors
**Onik-Cohen percutaneous access
catheter**
onlay implant
OnLine ABG monitoring system
Ono
    O. laryngobronchoscope atomizer
    O. loupe
On-Q
    O.-Q pain management system
    O.-Q pump
On-X bileaflet prosthetic heart valve
Onyx finger pulse oximeter
Onyx-R NiTi file

Opaca-Garcea ureteral catheter
Opart MRI imaging system
Opdima digital mammography system
open
    o. face mask
    o. lens
    o. magnet
    o. MRI system
opener
    Heister jaw o.
**OpenGene automated DNA sequencing
system**
open-loop
    o.-l. insulin delivery system
    o.-l. intraocular lens
Open Pivot heart valve
OpenSail coronary dilatation catheter
OPERA
    outpatient endometrial resection and
      ablation
    OPERA Star resectoscope
    OPERA Star SL hysteroscope
    OPERA system
operating
    O. Arm system
    o. loupe
    o. microscope (OM)
    o. platform
    o. scissors
OPG-Gee instrument
Ophtec
    O. Co. lens
    O. occlusion implant
Ophthalas
    O. argon laser
    O. krypton laser
ophthalmic
    o. blade
    o. calipers
    o. cautery electrode
    o. cup
    o. electrocautery
    o. endocoagulator
    o. endoscope
    o. hook
    o. laser microendoscope
    o. pick
    o. sable brush
    o. sponge
ophthalmodynamometer
    Bailliart o.
    Reichert o.
ophthalmoendoscope
    Nebauer o.
    Zylik o.
ophthalmometer
    American Optical o.
    AO o.
    Haag-Streit o.

Hertel o.
Javal o.
OM 4 o.
ophthalmoplethysmograph
ophthalmoscope
Alcon indirect o.
AO indirect o.
Bailliart o.
o. camera
confocal laser scanning o.
confocal scanning laser o.
Exeter o.
Fisons indirect binocular o.
Friedenwald o.
Ful-Vue o.
Grafco o.
Gullstrand o.
Halberg indirect o.
halogen coaxial o.
Helmholtz o.
Highlight spectral indirect o.
indirect laser o.
Keeler o.
Loring o.
Mascot indirect o.
May o.
Mentor Exeter o.
metric o.
MK IV o.
monocular indirect o.
Morton o.
Neolyte laser indirect o.
Nerve Fiber Analyzer laser o.
Panoramic 200 nonmydriatic o.
polarizing o.
Polle pod attachment for o.
Propper binocular indirect o.
Propper-Heine o.
Reichert binocular indirect o.
Reichert Ful-Vue binocular o.
Rodenstock scanning laser o.
scanner laser o.
scanning laser o.
Schepens o.
Schepens-Pomerantzeff o.
Schultz-Crock binocular o.
TopSS scanning laser o.
Vantage indirect o.
visuscope o.
Welch Allyn o.
Zeiss o.
Ophthalon suture

ophthalsonic pachymeter
Ophthascan
Alcon-Biophysic O.
O. S ultrasound
Ophthasonic Ultrasonic biometer
Ophthimus High-Pass Resolution
  perimeter
Ophtho-bur
Concept O.-b.
Opiela brace
OPMI
OPMI colposcope
OPMI microscopic drape
OPMI Pro magis surgical
  microscope
OPMI Visu 200 microscope
Opmilas
O. 144 Plus laser system
O. 144 surgical laser
Opotow filling material
Oppenheim
O. brace
O. spring wire splint
Oppenheimer knuckle-bender splint
Op-Pneu
O.-P. CO$_2$ insufflator
O.-P. laparoscopy needle
Oppociser hand exerciser
opponens splint
opposed loop-pair quadrature NMR coil
Opraflex
O. dressing
O. incise drape
Opsis DistalCam video system
OpSite
O. drape
O. Flexifix transparent film
  dressing
O. Flexigrid dressing
O. occlusive dressing
O. Plus wound dressing
Opta 5 catheter
Opteform allograft material
Optelec Passport magnifier
Op-Temp disposable electrocautery
Opteon femoral stem
Optetrak
O. comprehensive knee system
O. total knee system
Opthascan Mini-A scanner
Opticaid lens loupe

NOTES

O

optical
American O. (AO)
o. aspirating curette
o. biopsy forceps
O. Biopsy system
O. catheter
o. digitizer
o. Doppler velocimeter
o. esophagoscope
o. internal urethrotomy (OIU)
o. intrinsic signal (OIS)
o. laryngoscope
o. multichannel analyzer system
o. needle
o. pachometer
o. pachymeter
o. pedobarograph
O. Radiation intraocular lens
O. Tracking System (OTS)
o. ureterotome
optically transparent electrode
Opticath catheter
OptiChamber valved holding chamber
optic implant
Opticon catheter
optics
Allergan Medical O. (AMO)
American Medical O. (AMO)
Boutin o.
confocal o.
mirror-based reflective o.
SinuScope rigid rod lens o.
Wappler cystoscope with
microlens o.
Wappler resectoscope with
microlens o.
2-Optifit toric lens
Opti-Fix
O.-F. acetabular cup
O.-F. femoral component
O.-F. total hip system
Optiflex intraocular lens
Opti-Flow permanent dialysis catheter
OptiForm mitral valve
Opti-Gard eye protector
OptiHaler
O. drug delivery system
O. metered-dose inhaler
Optilume prostate balloon dilator
Optilux 501 curing light
Optima
O. contact lens
O. diamond knife
O. I MPI pacemaker
O. MPT-series III pacemaker
O. pulse generator
O. SPT pacemaker
**OptiMax Supreme pressure-reduction
mattress**

Optimaze surgical ablation system
Optimed glaucoma pressure regulator
optimizer
Sports Breather lung power o.
Optimum blade
Option hip system
Optiphot-2UD microscope
Opti-Plast XT balloon catheter
Optipore wound-cleaning sponge
Opti 1 portable pH/blood gas analyzer
Optipost
Opti-Pure system
Optique microscope
OptiQue sensing catheter
**Opti-Qvue CCO pulmonary artery
catheter system**
Optiscan 2000 scanner
Optiscope
O. angioscope
O. catheter
Optison contrast material
Optistar MR contrast delivery system
Optistat handheld power injector
Optiva IV catheter
Optiview
O. optical surgical obturator
O. trocar
Optivis Surgalloy needle
Optivox artificial electronic larynx
Opti-Vue plastic barrel
OptiVu HDVD system
Opti-Vu lens
optode
fluorescent o.
optoelectric measuring apparatus
optokinetic stimulator
optometer
infrared o.
laser o.
OptoTrak motion-analysis system
Opt-Visor
O.-V. lens
O.-V. loupe
Opus pacemaker
Oracle
O. Focus PTCA catheter
O. Focus ultrasound imaging
catheter
O. Megasonics catheter
O. Micro intravascular ultrasound
catheter
O. Micro Plus PTCA catheter
**Ora-Gard disposable intraoral bite
block**
oral
o. appliance
o. endoscope
o. endotracheal tube
o. esophageal tube

o. forceps
o. implant
o. pharyngeal airway
o. screw mouthgag
o. speculum mouthgag
o. surgery handpiece
Oral-B soft foam interdental brush
Oral-Cath catheter
Orandi knife
orange dye laser
Orascoptic
O. fiberoptic headlight
O. loupe extension
OraSure HIV-1 oral specimen collection device
Oratek
O. chisel
O. device
O. thermal shrinking probe
Orban curette
Orbasone system
orbicular retractor
Orbis prosthetic heart valve
Orbis-Sigma
O.-S. shunt
O.-S. valve
orbital
o. compressor
o. depressor
o. floor implant
o. floor prosthesis
o. retractor
O. shoulder stabilizer brace
Orbit blade
Orbiter treadmill
Orbix x-ray unit
Orbscan
O. corneal topography system
O. pachymeter
Orbus
O. coronary R stent
O. R stent SVS stent
Orca surgical blade
ORC-B Ranfac cholangiographic catheter
OrCel bilayered cellular matrix
orchidometer
punched-out o.
Test-Size o.
ORC posterior chamber intraocular lens

Oregon
O. prosthesis
O. tunneler
O'Reilly esophageal retractor
Orentreich punch
Oreopoulos-Zellerman catheter
Oretorp retractable knife
Orfit
O. mask
O. splint
Orfizip
O. body jacket
O. casting system
O. knee cast
Organdi blade
organic
o. dental cement
o. liquid scintillator
organizer
Hunt o.
JainSuture/VesiBand o.
Shelhigh suture o.
Organon percutaneous E2 implant
orgastic tube
OriGen Biomedical dual-lumen catheter
OriGHel hydrogel dressing
Origin
O. PDB 1000 balloon
O. tacker
O. trocar
Original
O. Backnobber massage tool
O. Backnobber muscle massager
O. Index Knobber II massage tool
O. Jacknobber massage tool
O. McKenzie CPM roll
O-ring
O-r. attachment
elastic O-r.
Orion
O. anterior cervical plate
O. balloon
O. cardiovascular information management system
O. continence system
O. inhaler
O. lumbar support
O. model AE-940 ion analyzer
O. pacemaker
O. plate and screw
Oris pin

NOTES

Orlando
- O. hip-knee-ankle-foot orthosis
- O. tibial plateau fracture bracing system

OrlandoTPFx bracing system

ORLAU
Orthotic Research and Locomotor Assessment Unit
- ORLAU swivel walker
- ORLAU swivel walker orthosis

Orley retractor

Orlon vascular prosthesis

Orlowski stent

Ormco
- O. appliance
- O. band scissors
- O. band setter
- O. ligature director
- O. orthodontic arch-expander
- O. orthodontic hemostat
- O. orthodontic pliers
- O. pin
- O. preformed band
- O. wire bracket

oroendotracheal tube

oroesophageal overtube

orogastric Ewald tube

oropharyngeal pack

orotome
Steinhauser o.

orotracheal tube

Orozco plate

Orr
- O. automatic reprocessor
- O. gall duct forceps

Orr-Buck extension tractor

Orthair oscillating saw

Orthairtome II drill

Orthawear antiembolism stocking

Orth-evac autotransfusion system

Orthex
- O. cannulated titanium bone screw
- O. reliever insole
- O. Relievers shoe insert

Orthicon camera

Orthion traction machine

Ortho
- O. All-Flex diaphragm
- O. Cytofluorograf 50-H flow cytometer
- O. diaphragm kit
- O. Dx electromedical stimulator
- O. rongeur

Ortho-Arch II orthotic

Ortho-Athrex instrument

Orthoband traction band

Ortho-Biotic recliner

OrthoBlast osteoconductive bioimplant paste

OrthoBlend powered bone mill

OrthoBone pillow

Ortho-Cel pad

Orthoceph
- O. OC100 cephalostat
- O. x-ray unit

Orthocomp cement

Orthocor II pacemaker

Orthoderm
- O. consummate air therapy bed
- O. convertible II mattress

Orthodoc presurgical planning system

orthodontic
- o. aligner
- o. angulator
- o. appliance
- o. band
- o. band driver
- o. band setter
- o. base plate
- o. bracket
- o. cement
- o. impression tray
- o. resin

OrthoDyn
- O. bone substitute
- O. bone substitute material

Ortho-evac
- O.-e. evacuator
- O.-e. postoperative autotransfusion system

Orthofeet-Gel footbed

Orthofit
- O. 9000 orthotic
- O. 9001 orthotic material

Orthofix
- O. Cervical-Stim stimulator
- O. external fixation device
- O. intramedullary nail
- O. ISKD system
- O. lengthening device
- O. M-100 distractor
- O. monolateral femoral external fixator
- O. pin
- O. prosthesis
- O. screw

Orthoflex
- O. dressing
- O. elastic plaster bandage

Ortho-Foam pad

OrthoFrame external fixation

Orthofuse implantable growth stimulator

OrthoGel liner

OrthoGen bone growth stimulator

Orthoglass splint material

orthognathic occlusal relator

orthogonal
    o. film
    o. laser
Ortho-Grip silicone rubber handle
OrthoGuard AB bone pin sleeve
Ortho-Ice Multipaks pack
Ortho-Jel impression material
Orthokinetics travel chair
OrthoKnit joint support
Ortho-last splint
Ortholav
    O. irrigation and suction device
    O. pulsed irrigator
    O. suction
Ortholign orthosis
Ortholoc Advantim revision knee
    system
OrthoLogic bone growth stimulator
Orthomatrix binder
Orthomedics
    O. brace
    O. Stretch and Heel splint
Orthomet
    O. Axiom total knee system
    O. Perfecta total hip system
Orthomite
    O. II adhesive
    O. resin
Ortho-Mold
    O.-M. spinal brace
    O.-M. splint
OrthoNail intramedullary fixation device
orthopaedic, orthopedic
    o. bone file
    o. broach
    o. bur
    o. depth gauge
    o. dynamometer
    o. elevator
    o. fixation device
    o. forceps
    o. goniometer
    o. gouge
    o. hammer
    o. hemostat
    o. impactor
    o. implant
    o. knife
    o. osteotome
    o. pin
    o. plate
    o. positioning seat

    o. rasp
    o. reamer
    o. rod
    o. rongeur
    o. scissors
    o. screw
    o. staple
    o. stockinette
    o. strap clavicle splint
    o. surgical pliers
    o. surgical stripper
    o. Universal drill
OrthoPak
    O. bone growth stimulator system
    O. II bone growth stimulator
Ortho-Pal body support
Orthopantomograph-series panoramic x-
    ray machine
orthopedic (*var. of* orthopaedic)
Orthopedic Casting Lab (OCL)
Orthopedic Systems, Inc. (OSI)
Orthoplast
    O. dressing
    O. fracture brace
    O. isoprene splint
    O. jacket
    O. slipper cast
Orthoptic
    O. eye patch
    O. Therapy amblyoscope
orthorhythmic pacemaker
orthoscopic lens
Orthoset
    O. cement
    O. radiopaque bone cement
    adhesive
orthosis
    AccuFlex dynamic elbow o.
    adjustable advanced reciprocating
    gait o.
    Advanced Reciprocating Gait O.
    (ARGO)
    Advance Dynamic ROM o.
    A-frame o.
    Aliplast custom molded foot o.
    Ambroise dynamic wrist o.
    ankle o. (AO)
    ankle-foot o. (AFO)
    Aspen cervical thoracic o.
    balanced forearm o. (BFO)
    balance padding o.
    bar-and-shoe o.

O

NOTES

orthosis *(continued)*
    Bauerfeind Malleolic ankle o.
    Beaufort seating o.
    Bebax o.
    Becker cranial remolding o.
    Bodi Dynamic o.
    Bodi knee extension o.
    Boston hip o.
    cable-twister o.
    calcaneal spur cookie o.
    Caligamed ankle o.
    Canadian serial knee o.
    CASH o.
    cervical o.
    cervicothoracic o.
    Comfy elbow o.
    Comfy knee o.
    copolymer ankle-foot o.
    Craig-Scott o.
    CranioCap craniofacial o.
    cruciform anterior spinal
      hyperextension o.
    Daytona cervical o.
    derotation o.
    Diabetic D-Sole foot o.
    dial-lock o.
    dual-photon electrospinal o.
    dynamic elbow o.
    dynamic knee o.
    dynamic wrist o.
    elbow-wrist-hand o.
    electrospinal o.
    Engen palmar finger o.
    external o.
    EZ arm abduction o.
    finger o.
    Flex Foam o.
    Foot Levelers o.
    Frejka o.
    Gator plastic o.
    Gillette joint o.
    GunSlinger shoulder o.
    G/W Heel Lift, Inc. o.
    hallux valgus o.
    halo cervical o.
    halo-vest o.
    Heelfit o.
    Herbst Cradle o.
    hindfoot o.
    hip guidance o.
    hip-knee o.
    hip-knee-ankle o.
    Hosmer voluntary control four-bar
      knee o.
    Hyperex thoracic o.
    inflatable carrot finger o.
    inflatable thoracic lumbosacral o.
    Ipomax knee o.
    ipos forefoot relief o.

    ipos heel relief o.
    Jewett-Benjamin cervical o.
    Jewett contraflexion o.
    Jewett postfusion o.
    Jewett thoracolumbosacral o.
    Johnson cervical thoracic o.
    Johnson Kydex chairback o.
    Johnson total hip stabilization o.
    Jousto dropfoot skid o.
    Kallassy o.
    Kid-Dee-Lite o.
    knee-ankle o.
    knee-ankle-foot o. (KAFO)
    knee extension o.
    Knight-Taylor and Williams
      spinal o.
    L.A. cervical o.
    leather o.
    Lerman shoulder holster o.
    Levy & Rappel foot o.
    Ligamentus Ankle o.
    L'Nard long opponens hand and
      wrist o.
    L'Nard Multi-Podus o.
    L'Nard thoracolumbosacral o.
    LSU reciprocation-gait o.
    lumbar o.
    lumbosacral o.
    Lynco foot o.
    Lynx o.
    Malibu cervical o.
    Malleoloc anatomic ankle o.
    Maple Leaf o.
    Marlin cervical o.
    metal hybrid o.
    Meyer cervical o.
    Milwaukee scoliosis o.
    Minerva cervicothoracic o.
    molded ankle-foot o. (MAFO)
    MultiBoot o.
    Multi-Podus foot o.
    neoprene wrist o.
    Newport MC total hip o.
    New York Orthopedic front-
      opening o.
    NuKo knee o.
    Oklahoma ankle joint o.
    Orlando hip-knee-ankle-foot o.
    ORLAU swivel walker o.
    Ortholign o.
    patellar tendon weightbearing
      brace o.
    pediatric pressure relief ankle
      foot o.
    pelvic stabilization o.
    Perlstein o.
    Phase II Multi-Podus foot o.
    Phelps o.
    plastic o.

Pneu-trac cervical traction o.
polypropylene glycol ankle-foot o.
polypropylene glycol
  thoracolumbosacral o.
posterior leaf-spring ankle-foot o.
pressure-relief ankle-foot o.
  (PRAFO)
Pro-glide o.
Progressive ankle o.
PSA thermoplastic o.
Pucci inflatable knee o.
Pucci pediatrics hand o.
Rancho Los Amigos o.
Rebel knee o.
reciprocating gait o.
resting o.
Rochester hip-knee-ankle-foot o.
Salera HKAFO o.
Scott-Craig o.
Scottish Rite hip o.
Seattle o.
Select joint o.
semirigid polypropylene ankle-
  foot o.
Shaeffer rigid o.
shoulder o.
shoulder-elbow-wrist-hand o.
shoulder holster o. (SHO)
single-photon electrospinal o.
Slim Option shoe o.
Sof Gel HeelCup o.
SofTec Lumbo o.
SOLEutions custom o.
SOMI o.
SportsFit thumb o.
Sport-Stirrup o.
standing frame o.
sterno-occipital-mandibular
  immobilization o.
supracondylar knee-ankle-foot o.
supramalleolar o.
Swede-O-Universal o.
Taylor thoracolumbosacral o.
Thera-Pos elbow o.
Thera-Pos knee o.
Thera-Soft hand/wrist o.
Theratotic firm foot o.
Theratotic soft foot o.
Thomas cervical collar o.
Thomas heel o.
thoracolumbar spinal o. (TLSO)
thoracolumbar standing o.

thoracolumbosacral spinal o.
Tib-Transformer o.
tone-reducing ankle-foot o.
  (TRAFO)
Toronto parapodium o.
TPE ankle-foot o.
TPE biomechanical foot o.
TRAFO o.
Transpire wrist o.
turnbuckle wrist o.
UCBL o.
Ultrabrace o.
VAPC dorsiflexion assist o.
Vari-Duct hip and knee o.
Viscoheel K, N o.
Viscoheel SofSpot o.
weight-relieving o.
Williams o.
wrist-driven prehension o.
Orthosleep pillow
OrthoSorb
  O. absorbable pin
  O. pin fixation
  O. pin nail
Orthoss resorbable bone void filler
Orthostar surgical table
Orthotech Performer knee brace
**Orthotec pressurized fluid irrigation
  system**
orthotic
  Amfit o.
  ankle-foot o.
  o. attachment implant
  BIOflex magnetic o.
  Biofoot o.
  BioSole-GEL o.
  Biothotic foot o.
  Blue Line o.
  Castaway o.
  CLC o.
  o. coiled spring twister
  cork, leather, and elastic o.
  DesignLine o.
  Diab-A-Thotics o.
  DressFlex o.
  DSIS o.
  D-Soles o.
  Extreme o.
  FirmFlex Plus custom o.
  Foot Levelers custom o.
  functional o.
  Golden Comfort o.

O

NOTES

orthotic *(continued)*
> Golden Fitness o.
> Healthflex o.
> Heel Spur Special o.
> J-Glas Prefabs o.
> Kinetic Wedge o.
> Lyte Fit o.
> Magnathotics o.
> Mayer o.
> MBS snap-on o.
> M-Pact flexible o.
> Newington o.
> OB Gees maternity o.
> Ortho-Arch II o.
> Orthofit 9000 o.
> OrthoVise o.
> ParFlex Plus o.
> Plastazote o.
> o. plate
> Polydor Preforms o.
> PRAFO adjustable o.
> ProLite Plus runner's o.
> ProThotics o.
> Pucci Air o.
> Rediform o.
> O. Research and Locomotor
>   Assessment Unit (ORLAU)
> Rohadur-Polydor o.
> Rohadur-Schaefer o.
> Rohadur-Whitman o.
> Sandalthotics o.
> Ser Form silicone o.
> Shoethotic o.
> SkiFlex Plus o.
> Slimthetics o.
> Soft Super Sport o.
> Soft Support Preforms o.
> soft-tissue Super Sport o.
> Sport Preforms o.
> Stratos o.
> Superform Contours o.
> Supralen cradle o.
> Supralen Schaefer o.
> Swiss Balance o.
> Theraform Selectives o.
> Thermo HK/Rohadur o.
> Thermo HK/Tepefom o.
> Thinline uncovered o.
> Tothonator o.
> UCOheal o.
> UCOlite o.
> UltraEnergy o.
> UltraStep o.
> Walk-Rite o.
> XO-soft-sole o.

orthotopic
> o. biventricular artificial heart
> o. univentricular artificial heart

Ortho Trac motorized traction unit

Orthotrac pneumatic vest
Orthotron exerciser
Ortho-Turn transfer aid
Ortho-Vent bandage
OrthoVise
> O. orthopaedic instrument
> O. orthotic

OrthoWedge healing shoe
Ortho-Wick foam liner
Ortho-Yomy facebow
OrthPAT autotransfusion system
Orton enamel cleaver
Ortopad orthoptic patch
Ortron modular femoral prosthesis
Ortved stone dislodger
OS-5/Plus 2 knee brace
Osada
> O. Beaver-XL handpiece unit
> O. saw

Osbon pressure-point tension ring
Osborne
> O. goniometer
> O. osteotomy plate
> O. punch

Oscar ultrasonic bone cement removal system
Osciflator balloon inflation syringe
oscillating
> o. grid
> o. saw
> O. Techniques for Isometric
>   Stabilization

oscillator
> Hayek o.

OscilloMate 930 blood pressure measurement system
oscillometric
> o. blood pressure cuff
> o. blood pressure monitor

oscilloscope
> cathode ray o.
> Norland digital o.
> single-channel electromyograph o.
> single-channel nonfade o.
> Tektronix digital o.

Oscor
> O. atrial lead
> O. pacemaker
> O. pacing lead

osen needle
Osgood needle
Oshar-Neumann 8-line corneal marker
O'Shaughnessy
> O. clamp
> O. pince

O'Shaughnessy artery forceps
O'Shea lens
Osher
> O. air-bubble removal cannula

O. bipolar coaptation forceps
O. capsular forceps
O. conjunctival forceps
O. corneal scissors
O. diamond knife
O. foreign body forceps
O. globe rotator
O. haptic forceps
O. internal calipers
O. iris retractor
O. irrigating implant hook
O. lens-vacuuming cannula
O. lid retractor
O. malleable microspatula
O. micrometer cataract knife
O. needle holder
O. nucleus lens manipulator
O. nucleus stab expressor
O. pan-fundus lens
O. superior rectus forceps
O. surgical keratometer
O. surgical posterior pole lens
Osher-Fresnel intraocular lens
Oshukova collapsible bougie guide
OSI
Orthopedic Systems, Inc.
OSI arthroscopic well-leg leg holder
OSI extremity elevator
OSI modular table system
OSI Well Leg Support
OSM2 in vitro oximeter
OSM3 Radiometer
Osmed hydrogel tissue expander
Osmette osmometer
OsmoCyte
O. island wound care dressing
O. PCA pillow wound dressing
O. pillow
osmometer
freezing point o.
Osmette o.
Vapro Vapor pressure o.
Osmo reverse-osmosis unit
osmotic minipump
OssaTron
O. extracorporeal shockwave system
O. orthopaedic shockwave treatment machine
OsseoCare
O. drill
O. drilling equipment

Osseodent
O. dental implant
O. surgical drill
OsseoFix implant system
osseointegrated oral implant
OsseoQuest regenerative membrane
Osseotite 2-stage procedure implant
osseous
o. coagulum trap
O. Coagulum Trap collecting system
o. implant
o. pin
ossicle
Tutoplast auditory o.
ossicle-holding
o.-h. clamp
o.-h. forceps
ossicular chain replacement prosthesis
Ossoff-Karlan
O.-K. laser forceps
O.-K. laser laryngoscope
O.-K. laser suction tube
O.-K. microlaryngeal laser probe
Ossoff-Karlan-Dedo laryngoscope
Ossoff-Karlan-Jako laryngoscope
Ossoff-Sisson surgical stent
Ossoinig ophthalmic shell
Ossur
O. pressure pad
O. VariLock modular socket lock
Ostalloy 202 alloy
Ostby dam frame
OsteoAnalyzer bone densitometer
OsteoArthritic knee brace
osteoarticular allograft
Osteobond
O. copolymer bone cement
O. vacuum mixing system
OsteoCap hip prosthesis
Osteochondral Autograft Transfer System (OATS)
Osteo-Clage cable system
osteoclast
Collin o.
Phelps-Gocht o.
Rizzoli o.
osteodistractor
Ace/Normed o.
OsteoDONTEX bone graft substitute
OsteoGen
O. bone graft

O

NOTES

OsteoGen *(continued)*
    O. HA dental implant
    O. implantable stimulator
OsteoGen-D bone stimulator
Osteogenics BoneSource synthetic bone replacement material
Osteogen resorbable osteogenic bone-filling implant
OsteoGraf
    O. binder
    O. bone grafting material
OsteoGraf/D bone grafting material
OsteoGraf/LD bone grafting material
OsteoGraf/N-Block grafting material
OsteoHarvester bone harvester
Osteolock
    O. HA femoral component
    O. hip prosthesis
    O. NP acetabular component
Osteomeasure computer-assisted image analyzer
osteomeatal stent
OsteoMed
    O. bioresorbable fixation system
    O. screw
osteomicrotome
    Tessier o.
Osteomin
    O. demineralized bone
    O. freeze dried bone
    O. Thermo-Ashed bone powder Pulvograft
Osteon
    O. bur
    O. drill
Osteonics
    O. acetabular dome hole plug
    O. jig
    O. Omnifit-C long stem system
    O. Omnifit-HA hip stem
    O. prosthesis
    O. reamer
    O. Scorpio posterior cruciate retaining total knee system
    O. spinal system
    O. total shoulder system
Osteonics-HA coated femoral implant
Osteopal
    O. G low-viscosity cement
    O. V vertebroplasty bone cement
Osteopatch test system
osteophyte elevator
Osteo-Pin pin
osteoplastic flap clamp
Osteoplate implant
OsteoPower drilling and cutting machine
OsteoSet
    O. bone filler

    O. bone graft substitute
    O. resorbable bead kit
OsteoStat
    O. disposable power tool
    O. single-use power surgical equipment
OsteoStim
    O. apparatus
    O. implantable bone grown stimulator
    O. traditional allograft
OsteoTite bone screw
osteotome
    Albee o.
    Alexander perforating o.
    Anderson-Neivert o.
    Andrews o.
    API V-notched o.
    Army o.
    arthroscopic o.
    Barsky nasal o.
    bayonet o.
    Blount scoliosis o.
    Bowen o.
    box o.
    Buck o.
    Burton o.
    Campbell o.
    Carroll o.
    Carroll-Legg o.
    Carroll-Smith-Petersen o.
    Chermel o.
    Cherry o.
    Cinelli o.
    Clayton o.
    Cloward spinal fusion o.
    Cobb o.
    Codman o.
    Converse o.
    Cook o.
    Cottle o.
    Crane o.
    Cross o.
    Dautrey-Munro o.
    Dawson-Yuhl o.
    Dingman o.
    disposable one-piece o.
    Dunn-Dautrey o.
    Epstein o.
    flexible blade o.
    Fomon o.
    Frazier o.
    French-pattern o.
    guarded o.
    Hardt-Delima o.
    Hendel guided o.
    hexagonal handle o.
    Hibbs o.
    Hohmann o.

Hoke o.
Houston nasal o.
Howorth o.
Jarit hand surgery o.
Kazanjian action-type o.
lacrimal o.
Lahey Clinic thin o.
Lambotte o.
Lambotte-Henderson o.
lateral o.
Legg o.
Leinbach o.
Lexer o.
MacGregor o.
Manchester nasal o.
manual o.
Mathews o.
maxillofacial o.
Mayfield bayonet o.
McCollough o.
Meyerding o.
MGH o.
Micro-Aire o.
Miner o.
Mitchell o.
Moberg o.
Moe o.
Moore o.
Murphy o.
nasal o.
Neivert o.
Neivert-Anderson o.
New-Lambotte o.
orthopaedic o.
osteotome o.
Padgett o.
Parkes lateral osteotomy o.
Parkes-Quisling o.
Peck o.
Read o.
Rhoton o.
Richards-Hibbs o.
Rish o.
Ristow o.
Rowland o.
Rubin o.
Sheehan o.
Silver nasal o.
sinus lift o.
slotting-bur o.
Smith-Petersen curved o.
Smith-Petersen straight o.

Stille o.
Stille-Stiwer o.
straight o.
Swanson o.
Tardy o.
Tessier o.
Toriumi o.
Ultra-Cut Hoke o.
Ultra-Cut Smith-Petersen o.
U.S. Army o.
Ward nasal o.
osteotomy
    Amstutz-Wilson o.
    high tibial o. (HTO)
    o. pin
OsteoView
    O. desktop hand x-ray system
    O. 2000 digital bone densitometer
Osteovit bone matrix
Osterballe precision needle
Ostic plaster dressing
ostium seeker
ostomy
    o. appliance
    o. bag
    O. Shadow Buddy
Ostreg spinal marker system
ostrum
    o. antral punch
    o. punch forceps
Ostrup vascularized rib graft
Ostycut bone biopsy needle
O'Sullivan
    O. self-retaining abdominal retractor
    O. vaginal retractor
O'Sullivan-O'Connor
    O.-O. self-retaining abdominal
      retractor
    O.-O. vaginal retractor
    O.-O. vaginal speculum
Oswestry-O'Brien spinal stapler
Osypka
    O. atrial lead
    O. Cereblate electrode
Otis
    O. anoscope
    O. bougie à boule
    O. bougie à boule dilator
    O. ureterotome
    O. urethral sound
    O. urethrotome
Oti Vac lighted suction unit

O

NOTES

otoabrader
    Dingman o.
Otocap
    O. myringotomy blade
    O. myringotomy scalpel
OtoClear disposable tip
OtoLam laser
otologic
    o. cup forceps
    o. scissors
OtoScan
    O. device
    O. ear aeration system
otoscope
    acoustic o.
    Advanced Beta 200 o.
    Alpha fiberoptic pocket o.
    Bruening pneumatic o.
    Brunton o.
    Earscope o.
    fiberoptic o.
    Grafco o.
    halogen o.
    Micro-Halogen o.
    Microtek Heine o.
    Mini-Fibralux pocket o.
    Minilux pocket o.
    pneumatic o.
    Politzer air-bag o.
    Rica pneumatic o.
    Riester o.
    Sabre all-in-1 deluxe o.
    Siegle antique pneumatic o.
    SMIC pneumatic o.
    surgical o.
    Toynbee o.
    video o.
    Welch Allyn dual-purpose o.
    Welch Allyn operating o.
    Wullstein ototympanoscope o.
Ototemp 3000 tympanic thermometer
ototome
    o. irrigation kit
    o. otological drill
Otovent autoinflation kit
Oto-Wick
    Pope O.-W.
OTS
    Optical Tracking System
    Radionics OTS
Ottenheimer common duct dilator
Ott insufflator filter tubing
Ott-Mayo channel sampling kit
Otto
    O. Bock 1D25 Dynamic Plus foot
    O. Bock electric hands prosthesis
    O. Bock Greissinger Plus foot
        prosthesis

O. Bock modular rotary hydraulic
    knee
O. Bock Safety constant-friction
    knee
O. tissue forceps
Ottoback 3R65 children's hydraulic
    knee joint
OTW
    over-the-wire
    OTW Lifestream coronary dilation
        catheter
    OTW Photon coronary dilation
        catheter
Oudin resonator
Oughterson forceps
Oulu neuronavigator system
Ousley insertion spatula
OutBound syringe
Outerbridge uterine dilator
outflow cannula
outlet
    o. cannula
    o. forceps
outpatient
    o. endometrial resection and
        ablation (OPERA)
    O. Endometrial Resection and
        Ablation System
output signal processor
outrigger
    o. splint
    o. wire
oval
    o. cup forceps
    o. cutting bur
    o. snare
    o. speculum
    o. window curette
oval-open esophagoscope
oval-window
    o.-w. excavator
    o.-w. piston evacuator
ovary forceps
Ovation
    O. falloposcopy system
    O. in-the-ear hearing aid
oven
    Coltene o.
    Thermoprep heating o.
over-bed table
overcouch tube
overdenture
    bar-supported o.
    implant-supported o.
    mandibular o.
    removable partial o.
overhead
    o. fracture frame

o. frame trapeze
o. light
Overholt
O. clip-applying forceps
O. dissecting forceps
O. periosteal elevator
O. rib needle
O. rib raspatory
O. rib spreader
Overholt-Finochietto rib spreader
Overholt-Geissendörfer arterial forceps
Overholt-Jackson bronchoscope
Overholt-Mixter dissecting forceps
overlapping pincer
overlay
Airdance pressure-reducing
mattress o.
Air-3787 static air mattress o.
Alamo alternating low-air-loss
mattress o.
Bi-Wave mattress o.
Bodyline sleeper mattress o.
BodyWrap premium o.
DeRoyal mattress o.
First Step Select low-air o.
Geo-Matt therapeutic foam o.
Hydro-Ease II gel flotation
mattress o.
Hydro-Ease I water flotation
mattress o.
IRIS 10,000 o.
LA4072 low-air-loss o.
o. mattress
MIP anatomic o.
Rik fluid o.
Span+Guard mattress o.
Stimulite honeycomb mattress o.
Tempur-Med hospital o.
Topper mattress o.
UltraForm mattress o.
Vari-Zone variable density
convoluted mattress o.
x-ray o.
oversensing pacemaker
over-shoulder strap
Overstreet polyp forceps
over-the-door traction unit
over-the-endoscope Witzel dilator
over-the-guidewire esophageal dilator
over-the-needle infusion catheter
over-the-wire (OTW)
o.-t.-w. pacing lead

o.-t.-w. probe
o.-t.-w. PTCA balloon catheter
overtube
flexible endoscopic o.
Mill-Rose flexible endoscopic o.
oroesophageal o.
split o.
Steigmann-Goff endoscopic
ligature o.
Williams varices injection o.
over-tying wire
Oves
O. cervical cap
O. fertility cap
ovoid
Delclos o.
Fleming o.
Fletcher-Suit tandem and o.
Hankins lucite o.
Hockin lucite o.
Manchester o.
ovum
o. curette
o. forceps
OvuStick ovulation test kit
Owatusi double catheter
Owen
O. balloon
O. cloth dressing
O. gauze dressing
O. hemostatic bag
O. Lo-Profile dilation catheter
O. nonadherent surgical dressing
Owens silk
oxalate
o. dentin bonding system
o. system
Oxford
O. fixator
O. laryngoscope blade
O. magnet
O. Medilog frequency-modulated
recorder
O. miniature vaporizer inhaler
O. nonkinking cuffed tube
O. prosthesis
O. 2-T large-bore imaging system
scanner
O. unicompartmental knee femoral
component
**OxiClip PC20 demand oxygen
conserver**

O

NOTES

oxide
    ethylene o. (ETO)
OxiFirst fetal monitoring system
OxiFlow meter
OxiLink oximetry probe cover
OxiMax pulse oximetry system
oximeter
    Accusat pulse o.
    American Optical o.
    AO o.
    Armstrong handheld pulse o.
    AutoCorr digital pulse o.
    BCI FingerPrint handheld pulse o.
    BCI 3301 handheld pulse o.
    Biox III ear o.
    CO$_2$SMO Plus! capnograph/pulse o.
    Cricket recording pulse o.
    Criticare pulse o.
    Critikon o.
    Datascope Accusat pulse o.
    Datex-Ohmeda 3800 pulse o.
    Digit finger o.
    ear o.
    FingerPrint handheld pulse o.
    handheld pulse o.
    Healthdyne pulse o.
    Hewlett-Packard ear o.
    INVOS 2100-series, 3100-series cerebral o.
    Masimo Set pulse o.
    MiniCorr pulse o.
    MiniOX V pulse o.
    MRL o.
    Nonin Onyx pulse o.
    Novametrix pulse o.
    Novametrix Tidal Wave Sp handheld capnograph/pulse o.
    NPB-series handheld capnograph/pulse o.
    Ohmeda handheld pulse o.
    Onyx finger pulse o.
    OSM2 in vitro o.
    Oximetrix 3 o.
    OxiScan pulse o.
    Oxypleth pulse o.
    Oxyrak pulse o.
    OxyShuttle pulse o.
    OxyTemp handheld pulse o.
    Oxytrak pulse o.
    Palco pulse o.
    PalmSAT o.
    pulse o.
    Radical pulse o.
    Respironics pulse o.
    Satellite Plus pulse o.
    Somanetics Invos 3100 cerebral o.
    SpotCheck+ handheld pulse o.
    Tidal Wave Sp capnometer/pulse o.
    tissue reflectance o.
    TuffSat handheld o.
    VitalSAT pulse o.
oximetric catheter
Oximetrix 3 oximeter
oximetry
    o. catheter
    o. sensor
Oxiplex/AP adhesion barrier
Oxiport blade
OxiScan pulse oximeter
Oxisensor
    O. fetal oxygen saturation monitor
    O. II adult oxygen transducer
    O. oxygen analyzer
Oxycel
    O. dressing
    O. gauze
Oxycure topical oxygen system
Oxydome oxygen therapy system
oxygen
    o. analyzer
    o. cannula support
    o. mask
    o. saturation meter
    o. supply line
    o. tank
    o. tent
oxygenation
    extracorporeal membrane o. (ECMO)
oxygenator
    Affinity NT o.
    Bentley o.
    Biocor 200 high-performance o.
    bubble o.
    Capiox hollow flow o.
    Cobe CML o.
    Cobe Optima hollow-fiber membrane o.
    DeBakey heart pump o.
    Digi-Dyne cardiopulmonary bypass o.
    disc o.
    extracorporeal membrane o.
    extracorporeal pump o.
    Gambro o.
    High Flex D 700 S bubble o.
    intravascular o.
    Lilliput neonatal o.
    Maxima Forte blood o.
    Maxima Plus plasma resistant fiber o.
    membrane o.
    Monolyth o.
    Oxyhood o.
    pump o.
    Sarns membrane o.
    Shiley o.
    SpiralGold o.

Oxyguard
    O. mouth block
    O. oxygenating mouthguard
Oxy-Holter monitor
Oxyhood
    O. oxygenator
    O. pressurizer
Oxylator EM-100 emergency
   resuscitation device
Oxylator-EM 100 resuscitation system
OxyLead interconnect cable
OxyLite oxygen conserving system
Oxymatic electronic oxygen conserver

Oxymizer device
Oxypleth pulse oximeter
Oxy-Quik Mark IV oxygen inhalator
oxyquinoline dressing
Oxyrak pulse oximeter
OxyShuttle pulse oximeter
OxyTemp handheld pulse oximeter
OxyTip sensor
Oxytrak pulse oximeter
Oxy-Ultra-Lite ambulatory oxygen
   system
Oyloidin suture

NOTES

O

PA

PA 120 Osypka radiofrequency probe
PA portal
PA Watch position-monitoring catheter

pace

p. card
P. hysterectomy knife
P. periosteal elevator
P. Plus System scanner
P. ventricular needle

Paceart complete pacemaker testing system

Pacefinder lead placement system

Pacel bipolar pacing catheter

pacemaker

AAI single-chamber p.
AAT p.
Accufix p.
Acculith p.
Activitrax II p.
Activitrax variable-rate p.
activity-guided p.
activity-sensing p.
Actros p.
AddVent atrioventricular p.
Aequitron p.
Affinity p.
AFx p.
AICD p.
AICD-B p.
AICD-BR p.
AID-B p.
Alcatel p.
American Optical Cardiocare p.
Amtech-Killeen p.
antitachycardia p.
AOO p.
Arco atomic p.
Arco lithium p.
artificial p.
Arzco p.
Astra p.
asynchronous mode p.
asynchronous ventricular VOO p.
atrial-based p.
atrial demand-inhibited p.
atrial demand-triggered p.
atrial-synchronous ventricular-inhibited p.
atrial synchronous ventricular-inhibited p.
atrial tracking p.
atrial triggered ventricular-inhibited p.
Atricor p.
atrioventricular junctional p.
atrioventricular sequential demand p.
Aurora dual-chamber p.
Autima II dual-chamber cardiac p.
Avius sequential p.
AV junctional p.
AV sequential p.
AV sequential demand p.
AV synchronous p.
Axios p.
Basix p.
bifocal demand p.
Biorate p.
Biotronik demand p.
bipolar p.
bladder p.
breathing p.
burst p.
Byrel SX/Versatrax p.
cardiac p.
Cardio-Control p.
Cardio-Pace Medical Durapulse p.
p. catheter
Chardack-Greatbatch Medtronic p.
Chorus DDD p.
Chorus RM rate-responsive dual-chamber p.
Chronocor IV external p.
Chronos p.
cilium p.
Circadia dual-chamber rate-adaptive p.
Classix p.
Command PS p.
committed-mode p.
Cook p.
Coratomic p.
Coratomic R-wave inhibited p.
Cordis Atricor p.
Cordis Chronocor IV p.
Cordis Ectocor p.
Cordis fixed-rate p.
Cordis Gemini cardiac p.
Cordis Multicor p.
Cordis Omni Stanicor Theta transvenous p.
Cordis Sequicor cardiac p.
Cordis Stanicor unipolar ventricular p.
Cordis Synchrocor p.
Cordis Ventricor p.

P

pacemaker *(continued)*

Cosmos II DDD p.
Cosmos pulse-generator p.
CPI Astra p.
CPI DDD p.
CPI Maxilith p.
CPI Microthin DI, DII lithium-
  powered programmable p.
CPI Minilith p.
CPI Ultra II p.
CPI Vigor p.
CPI Vista-T p.
cross-talk p.
Cyberlith demand p.
Cybertach antiarrhythmic p.
Daig screw-in lead p.
Dart p.
Dash single-chamber rate-adaptic p.
DDD p.
DDI mode p.
Delta TRS p.
demand cardiac p.
Dialog p.
Diamond II DDDR p.
Diamond II DDR p.
Discovery DDDR p.
Dromos p.
dual-chamber p.
dual-chamber Medtronic Kappa p.
dual-chamber rate-responsive p.
dual-sensing, dual-pacing, dual-
  mode p.
DVI p.
ECT p.
ectopic atrial p.
Ela Chorus DDD p.
Elecath p.
p. electrode
Electrodyne p.
Elema p.
Elgiloy lead-tip p.
Elite p.
Encor p.
Enterra p.
Entity p.
epicardial p.
Ergos O_2 dual-chamber rate-
  responsive p.
escape p.
external p.
external asynchronous p.
external demand p.
external transthoracic p.
fixed-rate p.
fixed-rate asynchronous atrial p.
fixed-rate asynchronous
  ventricular p.
Galaxy p.
GE p.

Gemini DDD p.
General Electric p.
Genisis dual-chamber p.
Guardian p.
Guidant CRM p.
heart p.
hermetically sealed p.
Identity ADx p.
implantable p.
Integrity ADx p.
Integrity AFx p.
Intermedics atrial antitachycardia p.
Intermedics Cyberlith X
  multiprogrammable p.
Intermedics lithium-powered p.
Intermedics Marathon dual-chamber
  rate-responsive p.
Intermedics Quantum unipolar p.
Intermedics Stride p.
Intermedics Thinlith II p.
Intertach p.
isotopic pulse generator p.
Jade II SSI p.
junctional p.
Kairos p.
Kalos p.
Kantrowitz p.
Kappa DR 400-series p.
Kelvin Sensor p.
Lambda Omni Stanicor p.
latent p.
Laurens-Alcatel nuclear powered p.
Legend p.
Leios p.
Leptos p.
Leukos p.
Lillehei p.
lithium p.
lithium-powered p.
Maestro implantable cardiac p.
Malith p.
Mallory RM-1 cell p.
malsensing p.
Mark IV breathing p.
Maxilith p.
Medcor p.
Medtel p.
Medtronic Activitrax rate-responsive
  unipolar ventricular p.
Medtronic-Alcatel p.
Medtronic bipolar p.
Medtronic-Byrel-SX p.
Medtronic Chardack p.
Medtronic corkscrew electrode p.
Medtronic demand p.
Medtronic Elite II p.
Medtronic Kappa DR 400-series p.
Medtronic-Laurens-Alcatel p.
Medtronic Minix p.

Medtronic Pacette p.
Medtronic RF 5998 p.
Medtronic SP 502 p.
Medtronic SPO p.
Medtronic Symbios p.
Medtronic temporary p.
Medtronic Thera DR p.
Medtronic Thera "i-series" cardiac p.
Medtronic-Zyrel p.
Mentor bladder p.
mercury cell-powered p.
Meridian p.
Meta DDDR p.
Meta II p.
Meta MV cardiac p.
Meta rate-responsive p.
Microlith P p.
Micro Minix p.
Microny KSR p.
Microny SR+ cardiac p.
Microthin P2 p.
Mikros p.
Minilith p.
Minix p.
Minuet DDD p.
Momentum p.
Multicor Gamma p.
Multicor II cardiac p.
Multilith p.
multiprogrammable p.
Nanos 1 p.
Nathan p.
natural p.
Neos M p.
Nomos multiprogrammable R-wave inhibited demand p.
noncompetitive p.
noninvasive temporary p.
Nova II p.
Nova MR p.
nuclear-powered p.
Omni-Atricor p.
Omnicor p.
Omni-Ectocor p.
Omni-Orthocor p.
Omni-Stanicor p.
Omni-Theta p.
Omni-Ventricor p.
Optima I MPI p.
Optima MPT-series III p.
Optima SPT p.

Opus p.
Orion p.
Orthocor II p.
orthorhythmic p.
Oscor p.
oversensing p.
Pacesetter Regency SC+ p.
Pacesetter Synchrony p.
Pacette p.
Paragon p.
Pasar tachycardia reversion p.
Pasys p.
PDx pacing and diagnostic p.
permanent myocardial p.
permanent rate-responsive p.
permanent transvenous p.
permanent transvenous demand p. (PTDP)
permanent ventricular p.
Permathane Pacesetter lead p.
Philos DR p.
Philos DR-T p.
Phoenix 2 p.
Phoenix single-chamber p.
Phymos 3D p.
physiologic p.
Pinnacle p.
PolyFlex implantable pacing lead p.
Precept DR p.
Prima p.
Prism-CL p.
Programalith AV p.
Programalith II, III p.
programmable p.
Prolith p.
Prolog p.
Pulsar DDD p.
Pulsar Max II p.
Pulsar NI implantable p.
P-wave-triggered ventricular p.
QT interval sensing p.
Quantum p.
radiofrequency p.
rate-modulated p.
rate-responsive p.
Reflex p.
Regency p.
Relay cardiac p.
rescuing p.
respiratory-dependent p.
reversion p.

NOTES

P

685

pacemaker *(continued)*
RS4 p.
R-synchronous VVT p.
Ruby II DDD p.
Savvi synchronous p.
Schaldach electrode p.
Schuletz p.
Seecor p.
Sensolog II, III p.
sensor-based single-chamber p.
Sensor Kelvin p.
sequential demand p.
Sequicor II, III p.
Shaldach p.
shifting p.
Siemens-Elema
  multiprogrammable p.
Siemens-Pacesetter p.
single-chamber p.
single-lead VDD p.
single-pass p.
sinus node p.
Sohes p.
Solar p.
Solis p.
Solus p.
Sorin p.
Spectraflex p.
Spectrax bipolar p.
Spectrax programmable
  Medtronic p.
Spectrax SX, SX-HT, SXT, VL,
  VM, VS p.
standby p.
Stanicor Gamma p.
Stanicor Lambda demand p.
Starr-Edwards p.
Starr-Edwards hermetically-sealed p.
Stride cardiac p.
Swing DR1 DDDR p.
Symbios p.
synchronous p.
synchronous burst p.
synchronous mode p.
Synchrony I, II p.
Synergyst DDD p.
Synergyst II p.
Syticon 5950 bipolar demand p.
tachycardia-terminating p.
Tachylog p.
Telectronics p.
temperature-sensing p.
temporary AV sequential p.
temporary transvenous p.
Thera DR p.
Thera-SR p.
Thermos p.
Thinlith II p.
tined lead p.

Topaz II SSIR p.
transcutaneous p.
transmural antitachycardia p.
transpericardial p.
transthoracic p.
transvenous ventricular demand p.
Trilogy DC+ p.
Trilogy SR+ single-chamber p.
Trios M p.
Triumph VR p.
Ultra p.
Unilith p.
unipolar p.
unipolar atrial p.
unipolar atrioventricular p.
unipolar sequential p.
Unity-C p.
Unity-C cardiac p.
Unity VDDR p.
USCI Vario permanent p.
variable rate p.
VAT p.
VDD p.
Ventak AICD p.
Ventak ECD p.
Ventricor p.
ventricular asynchronous p.
ventricular demand p.
ventricular demand-inhibited p.
ventricular demand-triggered p.
ventricular-suppressed p.
ventricular-triggered p.
Verity ADx p.
Versatrax cardiac p.
Versatrax II p.
Vicor p.
Vigor DDDR p.
Vigor DR p.
Vista p.
Vitatron Diamond II p.
Vivalith-10 p.
Vivatron p.
VVD mode p.
VVI/AAI p.
VVI bipolar Programalith p.
VVIR single-chamber rate-
  adaptive p.
VVI single-chamber p.
VVT p.
wandering atrial p.
Xomed dual-chamber p.
Xyrel p.
Zitron p.
Zoll NTP noninvasive p.
pacemeter
Haag-Streit p.
Mishima-Hedbys attachment p.
Paceport catheter
Pace-Potts forceps

pacer-cardioverter-defibrillator
    Jewel p.-c.-d.
Pacesetter
    P. APS
    P. knee brace
    P. Regency SC+ pacemaker
    P. Synchrony III pulse generator
    P. Synchrony pacemaker
    P. Tendril DX steroid-eluting
      active-fixation pacing lead
    P. Trilogy DR+ pulse generator
Pacette pacemaker
Pacewedge dual-pressure bipolar pacing
  catheter
PachKnife
    Corneo-Gage P.
pachometer
    optical p.
Pach-Pen
    P.-P. XL pachymeter
    P.-P. XL tonometer
pachymeter
    Advent p.
    Compuscan-P p.
    corneal p.
    Micropach 200P notebook
      corneal p.
    ophthalsonic p.
    optical p.
    Orbscan p.
    Pach-Pen XL p.
    Pocket p.
    Sonogage ultrasound p.
    Villasensor ultrasonic p.
Pachymetric analyzer
Pacific
    P. Coast flexible laminar bone
      strip
    P. Coast hearing aid
Pacifico
    P. cannula
    P. catheter
pacing
    p. catheter
    p. counter
    p. esophageal stethoscope
    p. wire
    p. wire electrode
pack
    Apollo Pak hot/cold knee p.
    Back-Ease aromatherapy hot/cold p.
    Barrier laparoscopy/LAVH p.

Baxter personal Von-Loc ice p.
BodyIce cold p.
ColdHot p.
Colpacs ice p.
cool p.
Cool Comfort cold p.
DynaHeat hot p.
EndoClip ML/Surgiport System p.
ErgoForm contoured cold p.
Expandacell nasal p.
Flents breast comfort p.
gauze p.
gel p.
Glacier P.
hot moist p.
hot wet p.
hydrocollator p.
Hydrocollator steam p.
I.C.E. Down cold p.
instant cold p.
Jack Frost hot/cold p.
K p.
Kennedy sinus p.
Kirkland periodontal p.
Kold Kompress cold p.
Kool Kit cold therapy p.
Medi-cult blastocyst thawing p.
Med-Wick nasal p.
nasal p.
Neck-Roll aromatherapy hot/cold p.
oropharyngeal p.
Ortho-Ice Multipaks p.
PCA periodontal p.
Peri-Cold p.
Peri-Gel p.
Peri-Warm p.
Polar P.
Rhino Rocket nasal p.
Slik-Pak nonstick nasal p.
Softouch cold/hot p.
Speedi-Pak sinus p.
Super Pak posterior nasal p.
TheraBeads microwaveable moist
  heat p.
Thera-Med cold p.
ThermalSoft hot & cold p.
Thermophore hot p.
Unna-Flex Plus venous ulcer
  convenience p.
Whitehall Glacier p.
Packard
    P. Auto-Gamma 5650 analyzer

NOTES

P

Packard *(continued)*
     P. intraocular lens
     P. radioimmunoassay system
packer
     Allport gauze p.
     amalgam p.
     Angell gauze p.
     August automatic gauze p.
     Balshi p.
     Bernay uterine gauze p.
     dental amalgam p.
     gauze p.
     Jewett bone chip p.
     Kitchen postpartum gauze p.
     Lorenz gauze p.
     P. mosquito forceps
     Ralks nasal gauze p.
     Torpin automatic uterine gauze p.
     P. tunnel silicone sponge
     P. Wick extrusion handpiece
     Woodson p.
packet
     Ile-Sorb absorbent gel p.
Packiam retractor
packing
     ENTaxis p.
     p. forceps
     Kaltostat hydrofiber wound p.
     Merocel epistaxis p.
     MeroGel nasal p.
     nasal p.
     SinuSeal resorbable nasal p.
     p. strip
     Weimert epistaxis p.
Pac-Kit Army-type tourniquet
Packo pars plana cannula
paclitaxel-coated coronary stent
PACS
     Picture Archiving and Communications
     System
     PathSpeed PACS
PAD
     pressure applied dressing
pad
     Action OR p.
     Airex balance p.
     AirLITE wheelchair support p.
     Akton p.
     Aquaflex ultrasound gel p.
     Attends p.
     Aware breast self-examination p.
     balance p.
     Bauerfeind silicone heel p.
     B-D Sensability breast self-
       examination p.
     Bovie grounding p.
     buttress p.
     Cairpad incontinence p.

CarraGauze hydrogel wound
  dressing p.
Charnley foam suture p.
Chaston eye p.
Chux incontinence p.
cold p.
Conform II w/heel-ease Nature
  Sleep pressure p.
convoluted mattress p.
CP2 Inflat-A-Wrap cold p.
Curity ABD p.
dancer p.
decubitus bed p.
Dignity Plus briefmates p.
disposable electrode p.
eggcrate mattress p.
Elasto-Gel pressure p.
p. electrode
electrode p.
Elta dermal sterile impregnated
  hydrogel gauze p.
EPI foam p.
EPIfoam adhesive foam p.
ESU dispersive p.
Etch-Master felt p.
eye p.
EZ hold adhesive catheter tube
  holder p.
flotation gel p.
fluid control trauma p.
Free & Active incontinence p.
gel p.
gelatin sponge p.
Gelfoam p.
Hapad longitudinal metatarsal
  arch p.
heat p.
HK p.
horseshoe heel p.
horseshoe-shaped p.
hot p.
HubGuard IV cushion p.
Hydrocollator p.
hydropolymer p.
Iceman cold therapy p.
ImPad inflation p.
Impress Softpatch incontinence p.
instrument stabilizer p.
Intersorb absorptive burn p.
Iodoflex solid gel p.
J p.
Johnson & Johnson non-stick p.
K p.
Kerlix cast p.
lap p.
LePad breast exam training p.
Littmann defibrillation p.
MagneCore magnetic therapy p.
magnetic mat p.

Mayfield pediatric horseshoe p.
Medical genuine sheepskin p.
Mikulicz p.
MPM conductive hydrogel p.
3M Tegaderm transparent dressing with absorbent p.
Ortho-Cel p.
Ortho-Foam p.
Össur pressure p.
Pedifix hammertoe p.
Pen/Alps distal p.
Presence bladder control p.
Pre-Vent boot style stirrup p.
Pre-Vent knee crutch p.
Pre-Vent OR table p.
Pro-Ophtha eye p.
Pro Peak decubitus p.
Protouch p.
Provide incontinence p.
Ray-Tec x-ray detectable lap p.
Relton frame p.
Roho Dry Flotation wheelchair p.
Roho heel p.
Scholl p.
second skin knee p.
sensor p.
Signa p.
Silipos digital p.
SofSeat pressure relief p.
Softeze self-adhering foam p.
Sof-Wick lap p.
SomaSensor p.
Staph-Chek p.
Steri-Pad gauze p.
Stimulite honeycomb seating p.
Super Eidersoft bed p.
Super-Plus Trimshield p.
Sure Sport p.
Telfa adhesive p.
Telfa gauze p.
Tempur-Med lumbar p.
Tempur-Med O.R. table p.
Tempur-Med stretch p.
TenderCloud pressure p.
Tendersorb ABD p.
TENS p.
T-Foam flotation p.
Thermophore moist heat p.
TopiFoam gel-backed self-adhering foam p.
UltraEase ultrasound p.
Vac-Pak p.

wheelchair p.
Zell p.
ZeroG pressure relief p.
Zimfoam p.

padded

p. aluminum splint
p. board splint
p. clamp
p. plywood splint

padding

cast p.
Delta-Rol cast p.
Kerlix cast p.
moleskin p.
Molestick p.
pressure relief p.
Profex cast p.
Protouch orthopaedic p.
QuickStick p.
Reston p.
Sifoam p.
Sof-Rol cast p.
Softexe non-adherent sub-bandage p.
splint p.
SurePress absorbent p.
Thero-Skin gel p.

paddle

compression p.
defibrillation p.
defibrillator p.
noninvasive p.
Rosen nucleus p.
spot compression p.

Padgett

P. baseline pinch gauge
P. dermatome blade
P. electrodermatome
P. endoscope
P. hydraulic hand dynamometer
P. implant
P. manual dermatome
P. mesh skin graft
P. osteotome
P. prosthesis
P. shark-mouth cannula

Padgett-Concorde suction cannula
Padgett-Hood dermatome
PadKit sample collection system
Padua bladder urinary pouch
Page

P. needle

NOTES

P

Page *(continued)*
    P. tonsillar forceps
    P. tonsillar knife
Pagedas
    P. retrieval pouch
    P. self-locking suture
Pagenstecher
    P. lens scoop
    P. linen thread suture
pain
    P. Care 3000 pain management
    device
    p. threshold gauge
PainBuster infusion delivery system
PainDoc computerized support system
Paine retinaculotome
PainPump pump
Pajot decapitating hook
PAK
    percutaneous access kit
Pak
    Akorn P.
    SCD MaleFactor P.
Pak-Its hydrogel gauze dressing
Palacos
    P. cement adhesive
    P. Radiopaque bone cement
Palamed
    P. bone cement
    P. G bone cement
palatal
    p. bar
    p. obturator
    p. prosthesis
palate
    p. hook
    p. retractor
palate-free activator
palate-type mouthgag
palatorrhaphy elevator
Palco pulse oximeter
Palex
    P. colostomy irrigation starter set
    P. expansion screw
Palfique Estelite tooth shade resin
    material
Palfyn suture
Pall
    P. Biomedical heat- and moisture-
    exchanging filter
    P. leukocyte removal filter
    P. PL-series leukocyte removal
    filter
    P. RC-series leukocyte removal
    filter
    P. transfusion filter
pallesthesiometer

Pallin
    P. lens spatula
    P. spring-assisted syringe
palmar
    p. clip
    p. plate
    p. wrist splint
Palmaz
    P. arterial stent
    P. balloon-expandable iliac stent
    P. biliary stent
    P. Corinthian transhepatic biliary
    stent
    P. Genesis transhepatic biliary stent
    P. vascular stent
Palmaz-Schatz
    P.-S. balloon-expandable stent
    P.-S. biliary stent
    P.-S. coronary stent
    P.-S. Crown balloon-expandable
    stent
PalmCups percussor
Palmer
    P. biopsy forceps
    P. bone nail
    P. cruciate ligament guide
    P. cutting forceps
    P. grasping forceps
    P. lens
    P. ovarian biopsy forceps
    P. uterine dilator
Palmer-Buono contact lens
Palmer-Drapier
    P.-D. forceps
    P.-D. needle
palm guard
PalmSAT oximeter
Palomar
    P. E2000 laser
    P. EsteLux laser
    P. SLP1000 laser
Palpagraph breast density mapping
    device
palpating needle
palpation probe
palpator
    Farrior blunt p.
Palumbo
    P. ankle stabilizer
    P. dynamic patellar brace
    P. knee brace
    P. patella tracker
    P. stabilizing knee brace
Pampéan vessel clamp
Panacryl absorbable suture
Panalok
    P. absorbable anchor
    P. absorbable suture

P. RC QuickAnchor Plus suture
anchor
Panasol II home phototherapy system
Panasonic hearing aid
pancake MRI magnet
panchamber UV lens
Pancoast suture
pancreatic
p. duct stent
p. endoprosthesis
pancreatoscope
ultra-thin p.
Pancretec pump
Panda
P. gastrostomy tube
P. nasoenteric feeding tube
P. NCJ kit
Panelipse panoramic x-ray machine
panendoscope
cap-fitted p.
p. electrode
flexible forward-viewing p.
foroblique p.
LoPresti p.
McCarthy p.
Stern-McCarthry p.
Storz p.
Wolf rigid p.
Panex-E panoramic x-ray machine
panfundoscope
Rodenstock p.
Pang
P. biopsy forceps
P. nasopharyngeal forceps
Panje
P. implant
P. tube
P. voice button
P. voice prosthesis
Panje-Shagets tracheoesophageal fistula
forceps
Pannett needle
panning dish
Pannu II intraocular lens
Pannu-Kratz-Barraquer speculum
Panogauze
P. dressing
P. hydrogel-impregnated gauze
Panomat infusion pump
Panoplex hydrogel wound dressing

Panoramic
P. 200 nonmydriatic
ophthalmoscope
P. 200 Ultra-Widefield ophthalmic
imaging device
panoramic loupe
Panorex panoramic x-ray machine
Panos G. Koutrouvelis, M.D.
stereotactic device
PanoView
P. arthroscope
P. arthroscopic system
P. Optics lens
P. rod-lens ureteroscope
pant
Conveen net p.
Dignity Plus regular p.
Lady & Sir Dignity Plus p.
MAST p.'s
Prevent Plus training p.
Promise washable knit p.
Sani-Garm waterproof p.
Simplicity contoured p.
Soft & Silent diaper p.
pantaloon
p. brace
p. liner
Panther catheter
pantoscope
Keeler p.
panty
compression p.
Free & Active incontinence p.
Panzer gallbladder scissors
Papanicolaou smear tray
Paparella
P. angled-ring curette
P. canal knife
P. catheter
P. duckbill elevator
P. fenestrometer
P. footplate pick
P. incudostapedial joint knife
P. mastoid curette
P. monkey-head holder
P. myringotomy tube
P. probe
P. rasp calipers
P. self-retaining retractor
P. sickle knife
P. stapes curette
P. straight needle

NOTES

P

Paparella *(continued)*
    P. tissue press
    P. type II ventilation tube
    P. wire-cutting scissors
Paparella-Frazier suction tube
Paparella-Hough excavator
Paparella-House
    P.-H. curette
    P.-H. knife
Paparella-Weitlaner retractor
Papercuff disposable blood pressure cuff
paper drape
Papette cervical cell collector
papilla drain
papilloma forceps
papillomatome
    Swenson p.
papillotome
    30-30 p.
    Accuratome precurved p.
    Apollo 3 triple-lumen p.
    Bard Companion p.
    Bilisystem wire-guided p.
    Companion p.
    Cremer-Ikeda p.
    double-lumen tapered-tip p.
    double-lumen wire-guided p.
    dual-lumen p.
    Erlangen p.
    Frimberger-Karpiel 12 o'clock p.
    Howell rotatable BII p.
    Huibregtse-Katon p.
    Microvasive p.
    needle-knife p.
    Piggyback needle-knife p.
    precut p.
    ProForma double-lumen p.
    shark fin p.
    Swenson p.
    Wilson-Cook p.
    Wiltek p.
    wire-guided p.
    Zimmon p.
papillotome/sphincterotome
    Soehendra BII p.
    Soehendra Precut p.
Papineau bone graft
Papnet computer-assisted Pap smear testing system
PapNet reader
papoose
    p. board
    p. board restraint
Pap-Perfect supply system
Pap Plus speculoscopy
Paquelin cautery
Parabath paraffin system

paracentesis
    p. knife
    p. needle
paracervical nerve block needle
Parachute stone retrieval device
Paracine dressing
Paradentine dental restorative material
Paradigm
    P. Dicon ocular blood flow analyzer
    P. insulin infusion pump
paraffin
    p. block
    p. dressing
    p. gauze
    p. graft
    p. implant material
    p. mitt
Parafil wax
ParaFlow right heart support system
ParaGard
    P. intrauterine device
    P. T380 copper IUD
Paragon
    P. amalgam
    P. ambulatory pump
    P. Champion stent
    P. Complete implant
    P. coronary stent
    P. infuser
    P. laser
    P. nitinol stent
    P. pacemaker
    P. single-stage dental implant system
    P. SwissPlus implant
Parahisian EP catheter
parallel
    p. flow dialyzer
    p. plate dialyzer
parallel-hole
    p.-h. collimator
    p.-h. medium sensitivity collimator
parallel-loop electrode
parallel-plate flow chamber
paramagnetic microsphere
Parama pulse wave generator
ParaMax
    P. angled driver
    P. cruciate guide system
parametrium
    p. clamp
    p. forceps
Parapost bur
paraPRO paracentesis needle
Parascan scanning device
Parasmillie knife
Parastep I system

Paratrend
    P. 7 continuous blood gas monitor
    P. 7 fiberoptic PCO_2 sensor
    P. 7 intravenous blood gas monitoring system
    P. 7+ sensor
ParCA catheter
PAR-C-Scan videokeratoscope
Parel-Crock vitreous cutter
Paré suture
ParFlex Plus orthotic
parfocal defraction lens
Parhad needle
Parhad-Poppen needle
Parham
    P. band
    P. support
Parham-Martin
    P.-M. band
    P.-M. bone-holding clamp
    P.-M. fracture apparatus
Pariefix mesh fixation
parietal shunt
Parietex composite mesh
Paris
    P. manual therapy table
    plaster of P.
    P. ultrasound system
Parisian Peel Prestige medical microdermabrasion system
Paritene mesh graft
Pari Vortex holding chamber
Park
    P. blade
    P. blade septostomy catheter
    P. eye speculum
    P. irrigating cannula
    P. lens implantation forceps
    P. Medical Systems scanner
    P. rectal spreader
Parker
    P. clamp
    P. double-ended retractor
    P. fixation forceps
    P. micropump insulin infuser
    P. needle
    P. serrated discission knife
    P. tenotomy knife
    P. thumb retractor
    P. tube

Parker-Bard
    P.-B. blade
    P.-B. handle
Parker-Glassman intestinal clamp set
Parker-Heath
    P.-H. anterior chamber syringe
    P.-H. cautery
    P.-H. electrocautery
    P.-H. piggyback
    P.-H. piggyback probe
Parker-Kerr
    P.-K. basting suture
    P.-K. forceps
    P.-K. intestinal clamp
Parker-Mott double-ended retractor
Parker-Pearson needle
Parkes
    P. hump gouge
    P. lateral osteotomy osteotome
    P. nasal rasp
    P. nasal retractor
Parkes-Quisling osteotome
Park-Guyton-Callahan eye speculum
Park-Guyton eye speculum
Park-Guyton-Maumenee speculum
Parkinson headholder
Park-Maumenee speculum
Park-O-Tron drill system
Parks
    P. anal retractor
    P. anal speculum
    P. bidirectional Doppler flowmeter
    P. ileoanal reservoir
    P. ileostomy pouch
Parma band
Parodi catheter
paronychia bur
parotidectomy retractor
parquetry set
Parr closed-irrigation system
Par scissors
Parsonnet
    P. aortic clamp
    P. coronary probe
    P. dilator
    P. epicardial retractor
    P. pulse generator pouch
partial
    p. lower denture
    p. ossicular reconstruction prosthesis (PORP)

NOTES

P

partial *(continued)*
    p. ossicular replacement prosthesis (PORP)
    p. rebreathing mask
    p. upper denture
partially-implantable catheter
partially-threaded pin
partial-occlusion
    p.-o. clamp
    p.-o. forceps
    p.-o. inferior vena caval clip
particulate
    NovaBone-C/M synthetic bone graft p.
    PerioGlas bone graft p.
    p. respirator
Partipilo clamp
Partnership implant
Partsch
    P. bone chisel
    P. bone gouge
Pasar tachycardia reversion pacemaker
Paschall orthopaedic grasping retractor
P.A.S. Port Fluoro-Free catheter
Pasqualini implant
PASS
    polyaxial spine system
    Encore PASS
Passage
    P. balloon dilation catheter
    P. exchange balloon
Passager
    P. endoprosthesis
    P. introducing sheath
    P. stent
Passarelli one-pass capsulorrhexis forceps
Passavant
    P. bar
    P. cushion
passer
    Arans pulley p.
    Batzdorf cervical wire p.
    Brand tendon p.
    Bunnell tendon p.
    Capio suture p.
    Carroll tendon p.
    Carter-Thomason suture p.
    Charnley wire p.
    Concept ACL/PCL graft p.
    Concept 2-pin p.
    Crile wire p.
    dermis-fat p.
    Dingman wire p.
    Ferszt ligature p.
    Framer tendon p.
    Gallie tendon p.
    Garrett vein p.
    Gore suture p.
    Hewson suture p.
    Hoefflin suture p.
    Holter distal catheter p.
    Incavo wire p.
    Joplin tendon p.
    Lahey ligature p.
    ligature p.
    Malis ligature p.
    MetraPass suture p.
    Ober tendon p.
    O'Donoghue suture p.
    2-pin p.
    Protect-a-Pass suture p.
    pulley p.
    Shuttle-Relay suture p.
    suture p.
    tendon p.
    Uni-Shunt catheter p.
    Wedeen wire p.
    wire p.
    Withers tendon p.
    Worm curving suture p.
    Yankauer ligature p.
passing forceps
passive
    p. motion device
    p. track detector
passively shimmed superconducting magnet
passover humidifier
Passow chisel
Passport
    P. bedside monitor
    P. instrumentation
PassPort trocar
Passy-Muir
    P.-M. speaking valve
    P.-M. tracheostomy speaking valve
    P.-M. valve (PMV)
    P.-M. ventilator connector
paste
    bismuth iodoform parafin p. (BIPP)
    Calcipulpe calcium hydroxide p.
    electrode p.
    OrthoBlast osteoconductive bioimplant p.
    polytef p.
Pastegraft
    Dembone demineralized cortical powder P.
Pasteur pipette
Pasys pacemaker
pat
patch
    AcuSeal cardiovascular p.
    Bard Composix Kugel hernia p.
    cardiac p.
    CardioFix p.
    CardioFix pericardium p.

CardioFix pericardium cardiovascular p.
Carrel p.
Chase cardiovascular p.
Composix Kugel hernia p.
Cosmo-TENS wireless p.
Dacron p.
defibrillator p.
Donaldson eye p.
Dura-Guard p.
Dymedix precision chin p.
p. electrode
epicardial p.
eye p.
glue p.
Gore-Tex cardiovascular p.
Gore-Tex soft tissue p.
p. graft
p. implant
intracardiac p.
Ionescu-Shiley pericardial p.
Kugel hernia p.
Lyrelle p.
Miniguard adhesive p.
monocular p.
No-React pericardial p.
Orthoptic eye p.
Ortopad orthoptic p.
pericardial p.
polypropylene intracardiac p.
polytef soft tissue p.
Prolene Hernia system p.
Pro-Ophtha eye p.
RapiSeal p.
Rutkow sutureless plug and p.
SaliCept oral p.
SJM pericardial p.
Snugfit eye p.
St. Jude Medical pericardial p.
subcutaneous polytef p.
Tanne corneal p.
Teflon intracardiac p.
Testoderm p.
Torpedo eye p.
transcatheter p.
Vascu-Guard bovine pericardial surgical p.
Vascu-Guard peripheral vascular p.
wicking glue p.

patcher

Kartush tympanic membrane p.

Xomed Kartush tympanic membrane p.

Patel intraocular magnet
Patellaligner knee brace
Patellamed knee support
patellar

p. aligner
p. band
P. Band knee protector
p. bone saw
p. brace
p. button
p. cement clamp
p. drill guide
p. planer bushing
p. reamer guide
p. resection guide
p. shaft reamer
p. tendon bearing (PTB)
p. tendon-bearing below-knee prosthesis
p. tendon weightbearing brace orthosis

patella-resurfacing implant
patella tracker
patent

p. ductus clamp
p. ductus forceps
p. ductus retractor
p. stent

Paterson

P. brain clip forceps
P. laryngeal cannula
P. laryngeal forceps
P. long-shank brain clip

Pathfinder

P. catheter
P. guidewire
P. mapping microcatheter
P. microcatheter system
P. wire

pathometer attachment
PathSpeed picture archiving communication system
patient

p. dose monitor
p. self-administration device

patient-controlled analgesia pump
PatientGuard underpad
patient-matched implant
patient-operated selector mechanism
Patil stereotactic system

NOTES

P

Patil-Syracuse mask
Paton
  P. anterior chamber lens implant forceps
  P. capsular forceps
  P. corneal dissector
  P. corneal forceps
  P. corneal knife
  P. corneal transplant forceps
  P. double spatula
  P. extra-delicate forceps
  P. eye needle holder
  P. eye shield
  P. see-through corneal trephine
  P. single spatula
  P. suturing forceps
  P. transplant spatula
  P. tying/stitch removal forceps
Paton-Berens mules
Patrick drill
Patten-Bottom-Perthes brace
pattern
  breast reduction p.
  Harrington-Flocks multiple p.
  p. matching card
  p. trephine
  p. umbilical scissors
Patterson
  P. bronchoscopic forceps
  P. empyema trocar
  P. specimen forceps
Patterson-Nelson empyema trocar
Patton
  P. bur
  P. cannula
  P. coaxial catheter set
  P. esophageal dilator
  P. HotBlade
  P. septal speculum
  P. vaginal speculum
PattStrap knee support
patty
  Cellolite p.
  Codman surgical p.
  cottonoid p.
Paufique
  P. blade
  P. corneal knife
  P. corneal trephine
  P. graft knife
  P. keratoplasty knife
  P. suturing forceps
Paufique-Duredge knife
Paul
  P. condom bag
  P. hemostatic bag
  P. intestinal drainage tube
  P. lacrimal sac retractor
  P. tendon hook

Paul-Mixter tube
Paulson
  P. infertility microtissue forceps
  P. infertility microtying forceps
  P. knee retractor
Paulus
  P. chin plate
  P. midfacial plate
  P. trocar system
Pautler infusion cannula
Pauwels fracture forceps
Pavenik monodisk device
Pavlik
  P. harness
  P. harness splint
Pavlo-Colibri corneal forceps
paws
  Medevice surgical p.
  Sil-Med instrument p.
Payne-Ochsner arterial forceps
Payne-Péan arterial forceps
Payne-Rankin arterial forceps
Payne retractor
Payr
  P. abdominal retractor
  P. gastrointestinal clamp
  P. grooved director
  P. probe
  P. pylorus clamp
  P. pylorus forceps
  P. resection clamp
  P. stomach clamp
  P. vein needle
Payr-Schmieden probe
PBI
  PBI Medical copper vapor laser
  PBI MultiLase D copper vapor laser
PBII blue loop lens
PBN hysterosalpingography catheter
PC
  PC EDO ophthalmic office laser
  PC EEA stapler
  PC Magni-Viewer
  PC Performer knee prosthesis
  PC shunt
PC-1000 panoramic x-ray machine
PC-7 needle
PCA
  porous-coated anatomic
  PCA acetabular cup
  PCA E-Series hip replacement
  PCA hip component
  PCA infuser
  PCA knee
  PCA modular total knee system
  PCA Peel
  PCA periodontal pack
  PCA Plus II infuser

PCA pump
PCA revision total knee
PCA total hip
PCA total hip stem
PCA unicompartmental knee

PCD

programmable cardioverter-defibrillator
Jewel PCD
PCD Transvene implantable
cardioverter-defibrillator

PCEEA stapler
PCL-oriented placement marking hook
PD

PD Access peel-away needle
introducer
PD copper band
PD crown post
PD dental wax
PD excavator
PD orthodontic wire
PD polishing strip
PD preformed crown
PD reamer
PD root canal post
PD SS matrix band

PDA umbrella
PDB preperitoneal distention balloon
**pDEXA x-ray peripheral bone
densitometer**
PDL intraligamentary syringe
PDS

polydioxanone suture
PDS II Endoloop suture
PDS Vicryl suture

PDT guidewire
PDx pacing and diagnostic pacemaker
PE

PE catheter
PE Plus II balloon dilatation
catheter

Peabody splint
Peacekeeper cannula
peacock dressing
peak

P. anterior compression plate
system
p. flow meter (PFM)
p. flow whistle
P. gait module

Péan

P. arterial forceps

P. hemostatic clamp
P. hemostatic forceps
P. hysterectomy clamp
P. hysterectomy forceps
P. intestinal clamp
P. intestinal forceps
P. scissors
P. sponge forceps

peanut

p. dissector sponge
p. eye implant
p. grasping forceps
P. Secto dissector
p. sponge-holding forceps

peanut-fenestrated forceps
peapod

p. chisel
p. intervertebral disc forceps
p. intervertebral disc rongeur

Pearce

P. coaxial I&A cannula
P. eye speculum
P. intraocular glide
P. nucleus hydrodissector
P. posterior chamber intraocular
lens
P. Tripod intraocular lens
P. vaulted-Y lens implant

Pearce-Keates bifocal intraocular lens
Pearce-Knolle irrigating lens loop
PEARL

physiologic endometrial
ablation/resection loop
PEARL technology

Pearlcast polymer plaster bandage
Pearlon impression material
Pearman

P. penile prosthesis
P. transurethral hemostatic bag

Pearsall

P. Chinese twisted suture
P. silk suture

pear-shaped

p.-s. bur
p.-s. extension tube
p.-s. fluted bag
p.-s. nerve hook

Pearson

P. attachment to Thomas frame
P. chisel
P. flexed-knee apparatus

NOTES

P

Pease
- P. bone drill
- P. reamer

Pease-Thomson traction bow
PeBA anchor
Peck
- P. chisel
- P. inlay wax
- P. osteotome
- P. rake retractor

Peck-Joseph scissors
pectoral catheter
pectoralis
- p. muscle implant
- p. retractor

Peczon
- P. I&A cannula
- P. I&A vectis

pedal-mode ergometer
Pedar in-shoe pressure measurement system
Pederson vaginal speculum
pedestal
- IMP surgical leg p.
- p. massage table
- surgical p.

Pedi
- P. Asta frameless air support therapy
- P. PEG tube

Pedia-Trake tube
pediatric
- p. abdominal retractor
- p. balloon catheter
- p. biopsy needle
- p. biplane TEE probe
- p. bridge
- p. bulldog clamp
- p. C-D hook
- p. circle
- p. circle system
- p. drainable pouch
- p. endoscope
- p. esophagoscope
- p. finger clip sensor
- p. Foley catheter
- p. forceps
- p. gastroscope
- p. laryngoscope
- p. lid speculum
- p. mastoid retractor blade
- p. 3-mirror laser lens
- P. Nutrition Surveillance System
- p. perineal retractor ring
- p. pigtail catheter
- p. pressure relief ankle foot orthosis
- p. rectal dilator
- p. retractor adjustable arm

- p. retractor malleable wire hand
- p. sandbag
- p. self-retaining retractor
- p. speculum
- p. telescope
- p. transfer pouch
- p. TSRH hook
- p. tube
- p. urostomy pouch
- p. vascular clamp

pedicle
- p. C-D hook
- p. clamp
- p. connector
- p. finder
- p. forceps
- p. hook
- p. implant
- p. plate
- p. screw
- p. screw construct
- p. sounder

Pedic sponge
Pedi-Cushions cushion
Pedifix hammertoe pad
PediKair pediatric low-air-loss bed
Pedilen polyurethane foam
Pediplast
- P. cushion
- P. moldable footcare compound

Pedi-Wrap immobilizer
pedobarograph
- Biokinetics p.
- Emed SF p.
- Musgrave p.
- optical p.
- Sheffield p.

pedometer
Pedors orthopaedic shoe
Peel
- Derma P.
- Obagi Blue P.
- P. Pak bag
- PCA P.

peel-away
- p.-a. banana catheter
- P.-a. introducer
- P.-a. sheath

peeler
- membrane p.
- Olk membrane p.

Peeler-Cutter vitrector
peel-off catheter
Peep
- P. valve
- P. ventilator

Peers towel clamp
Peeso reamer

Peet
- P. lighted splanchnic retractor
- P. mosquito forceps
- P. nasal rasp
- P. splinter forceps

Pee Wee low-profile gastrostomy tube

PEG

percutaneous endoscopic gastrostomy
- PEG bumper
- Gauderer-Ponsky PEG
- Ponsky-Gauderer type PEG
- PEG self-adhesive elastic dressing
- PEG tube

peg
- anchoring p.
- epithelial rete p.
- Fixion PF hip p.
- p. flap
- glenoid alignment p.
- Harrison-Nicolle polypropylene p.
- Kinemax removable fixation p.
- locking p.
- rete p.
- stringing p.

Pegasus
- P. Airwave pressure relief system
- P. Nd:YAG surgical laser

Pegasus-PIV laser

Pegasys electrosurgical generator

Pegaus FLO$_2$ mask

pegged tibial prosthesis

Peiper-Beyer bone rongeur

pelican biopsy forceps

Pe-lite material

Pelkmann
- P. foreign body forceps
- P. gallstone forceps
- P. sponge forceps
- P. uterine forceps

Pelle Peel microdermabrader

Pelli-Robson letter chart

Pelorus
- P. stereotactic frame
- P. surgical system

Pelosi
- P. fibrotome
- P. illuminator
- P. uterine manipulator

pelvic
- p. bench
- p. block
- p. clamp

- p. floor therapy system
- P. Organ Prolapse-Quantified system
- p. phased-array coil
- p. reconstruction kit
- p. reduction forceps
- p. snare
- p. stabilization orthosis
- p. tissue forceps
- p. traction belt

pelvimeter
- Baudelocque p.
- Briesky p.
- Collin p.
- Collyer p.
- DeLee p.
- Douglas measuring plate p.
- Hanley-McDermott p.
- Martin p.
- Rica p.
- Schneider p.
- Thole p.
- Thomas p.
- Thoms p.
- Williams internal p.

PelvX pessary

Pemberton
- P. forceps
- P. retractor
- P. sigmoid clamp
- P. spur-crushing clamp

Pemco
- P. cannula
- P. prosthetic valve
- P. retractor

pen
- EpiE-Z Pen-Jr. p.
- Genotropin p.
- gentian violet marking p.
- hydrophobic barrier p.
- ImmEdge p.
- Intron A multidose p.
- Ito laser p.
- light p.
- marking p.
- Pilot Spotlighter p.
- red-beam laser p.
- Seirin ProPoint acupuncture point-search p.
- skin marking p.
- Skin Skribe p.
- surgical marking p.

NOTES

P

pen *(continued)*
  Surgiscribe surgical marking p.
  Viomedex surgical marking p.
Pen/Alps distal pad
Penberthy double-action aspirator
Pencan spinal needle
pencil
  cataract p.
  p. cautery
  Cheshire electrosurgical p.
  ConMed electrosurgical p.
  p. Doppler probe
  p. drain
  p. electron beam
  electrosurgical p.
  glaucoma p.
  MegaDyne electrocautery p.
  PhD ergonomic pen and p.
  retinal detachment p.
  straight bipolar p.
  Valleylab p.
  vitreous p.
  Wallach cryosurgical p.
  Weck electrosurgery p.
pencil-grip instrument
pencil-handled laryngoscope
pencil-tip
  p.-t. cautery
  p.-t. drill
  p.-t. electrode
Penco Walker Sleds
Pendoppler ultrasonic fetal heart
  detector
Pendula cast cutter
pendulum scalpel
penetrating drill
Penetrator suture retriever
penetrometer
  Benoist p.
Penfield
  P. biopsy needle
  P. dissector
  P. retractor
  P. silver clip
  P. watchmaker suture forceps
penicillin nebulizer
penile
  p. Bio-Thesiometer
  p. clamp
  p. Doppler
  p. implant
  p. plethysmograph
Peninject 2.25 injector
Penlac nail lacquer
penlight
  Heine p.
  Welch Allyn halogen p.
Penlon
  P. Crystal laryngoscope blade

  P. infant resuscitator
  P. vaporizer
Penn
  P. finger drill
  P. pouch
  P. State total artificial heart
  P. State ventricular assist device
  P. swivel hook
  P. tuning fork
Penn-Anderson scleral fixation forceps
pennate suction catheter
Pennig
  P. dynamic wrist fixator
  P. minifixator
  P. minifixator device
Pennine
  P. leg bag
  P. Nélaton catheter
Pennine-O'Neil urinary catheter
  introducer
Pennington
  P. clamp
  P. hemorrhoidal forceps
  P. hemostatic forceps
  P. rectal speculum
  P. septal dissector
  P. septum elevator
  P. tissue forceps
  P. tissue-grasping forceps
Pennybacker rongeur
Pen-Probe instrument
PenRad mammography information
  system
Penrose
  P. drain
  P. sump drain
  P. tube
PentaCath catheter
Pentalumen catheter
PentaPace QRS catheter
Pentax
  P. bronchofiberscope
  P. bronchoscope
  P. choledochocystonephrofiberscope
  P. duodenoscope
  P. EC-series video endoscope
  P. EG-series video endoscope
  P. EG-2900 video gastroscope
  P. EndoNet
  P. EndoNet digital endoscope
  P. endoPRO system
  P. FC-series colonoscope
  P. FD-series duodenofiberscope
  P. FG-series ultrasound endoscope
  P. FG-series ultrasound
  gastrofiberscope
  P. FG-36UX scanning
  echoendoscope
  P. flexible endoscope

P. flexible sigmoidoscope
P. FS-series fiberoptic
sigmoidoscope
P. lithotripter
P. nasopharyngolaryngofiberscope
P. side-viewing endoscope
P. sigmoid fiberscope
P. Spotmatic camera
P. VSB-P-series pediatric
colonoscope
Pentax-Hitachi FG32UA endosonographic system
Penthrane analgizer
PEP
positive expiratory pressure
PEP mask
PEPS
peroral electronic pancreatoscope system
Perative enteral feeding container
Per-C-Cath catheter
Perc-DLE SpineWand
Perc-D SpineWand device
Perception scanner
Percival gastric balloon
Perclose
P. A-T vessel closure system
P. closure device
P. percutaneous vascular surgery
device
P. PVS device
P. suture device
P. vascular closure device
Percoll
P. bead
P. filter
Percor
P. dilator
P. dual-lumen intraaortic balloon
catheter
Percor-Stat-DL catheter
Percor-Stat intraaortic balloon
PercuCut cut-biopsy needle
Percufix catheter cuff kit
Percuflex
P. Amsterdam stent
P. biliary stent
P. endopyelotomy stent
P. flexible biliary stent
P. nephrostomy catheter
P. Plus ureteral stent
P. Tail Plus ureteral stent
PercuGuide needle

PercuPump disposable syringe and injector
percussion hammer
percussor
cup palm manual p.
English hospital reflex p.
Flimm Fighter p.
G5 Flimm-Fighter p.
G5 Neocussor p.
McGill neurological p.
mechanical p.
Neoguard p.
neurological p.
PalmCups p.
Percu-Stay catheter fastener
PercuSurge
P. GuardWire Plus temporary
occlusion and aspiration system
P. recovery system
percutaneous
p. access kit (PAK)
p. access needle
p. arterial closure device
p. brachial sheath
p. cardiopulmonary bypass support
p. central venous catheter
p. cutting needle
p. discoscope
p. dorsal column stimulator implant
p. drainage catheter
p. electrical nerve stimulation
p. endoscopic gastrostomy (PEG)
p. endoscopic jejunostomy
p. epidural electrode
p. epidural nerve stimulator
p. epidural neurostimulator
p. intraaortic balloon
counterpulsation catheter
p. introducer
p. mechanical thrombectomy system
p. needle
p. nephrostomy Malecot catheter
p. nephrostomy tube
p. pencil Doppler probe
p. pin
p. radiofrequency catheter
p. rotational thrombectomy catheter
p. spinal endoscope
p. stick
P. Stoller Afferent Nerve
Stimulation system
p. thecoperitoneal shunt

NOTES

P

percutaneous *(continued)*
   p. thrombolytic device (PTD)
   p. transhepatic biliary drainage (PTBD)
   p. transhepatic biliary drainage catheter
   p. transhepatic pigtail catheter
   p. transluminal angioplasty (PTA)
   p. transluminal angioplasty balloon
   p. transluminal coronary angioplasty (PTCA)
   p. transluminal coronary angioplasty catheter
   p. ultrasonic lithotripter
   p. ureteral stent
   p. vascular surgery
PercuTx percutaneous injection device
Percy
   P. amputating saw
   P. amputation retractor
   P. bone retractor
   P. clamp
   P. intestinal forceps
   P. plate
   P. tissue forceps
Percy-Wolfson
   P.-W. gallbladder forceps
   P.-W. gallbladder retractor
PerDUCER pericardial access device
Perdue
   P. hemostat
   P. tonsillar hemostat forceps
Pereyra
   P. ligature cannula
   P. ligature carrier
   P. needle
   P. needle driver
Pereyra-Raz ligature carrier
Perez-Castro forceps
Perfecta
   P. femoral stem
   P. hip prosthesis
   P. Interseal total hip system
Per-fit percutaneous tracheostomy kit
PerFixation
   P. screw
   P. system
PerFix Marlex mesh plug
Perflex biliary stent
perforating
   p. bur
   p. drill
   p. twist drill
perforation rasp
perforator
   Aesculap skull p.
   AmniHook amniotic membrane p.
   Anspach cranial p.
   antral p.

Baylor amniotic p.
Bishop antral p.
Boyd p.
Codman disposable p.
cranial p.
Cushing cranial p.
D'Errico p.
disposable p.
Dodd p.
p. drill
Heifitz skull p.
Hillis p.
Joseph antral p.
Kalinowski p.
Lasette laser finger p.
Lempert p.
membrane p.
Politzer ear p.
powered automatic skull p.
Royce tympanum p.
Smellie obstetrical p.
Smith p.
Stein membrane p.
Thornwald antral p.
tympanum p.
Wellaminski antral p.
Williams p.
Performa
   P. diagnostic ultrasound imaging system
   P. ultrasound
Performance
   P. knee prosthesis
   P. modular total knee system
performer ultralight knee brace
Perf-Plate cranial plate
perfusion
   p. balloon catheter
   p. cannula
   p. catheter
   p. monitor
   remote access p. (RAP)
perfusor
   Belsey p.
   P. compact S syringe pump
periapical curette
periaqueductal gray electrode
periareolar retractor
peribulbar needle
pericarbon bioprosthesis
pericardial
   p. patch
   p. prosthesis
   p. snare
pericardiocentesis needle
pericardiotomy scissors
Peri-Cold pack
Peri-Comfort seating cushion
pericortical clamp

Peries medicated hygienic wipe dressing
Periflow peripheral balloon angioplasty-
    infusion catheter
Periflux
    P. laser Doppler flowmeter
    P. PF 1 D blood-flow meter
Peri-Gel pack
Peri-Guard
    P.-G. vascular graft
    P.-G. vascular graft guard
perilimbal suction
perimeter
    Brombach p.
    Canon p.
    Cilco p.
    CooperVision imaging p.
    Digilab p.
    Ferree-Rand p.
    Goldmann p.
    Henson CFS 2000 p.
    Humphrey p.
    Interzeag bowl p.
    Medmont M600 p.
    Octopus 1-2-3 p.
    Ophthimus High-Pass Resolution p.
    Peritest p.
    Schweigger hand p.
Perimount
    P. mitral valve
    P. RSR pericardial bioprosthesis
perineal
    p. bandage
    p. prostatectomy retractor
    p. self-retaining retractor
    p. surgical apron
perineometer
    Gynos p.
    Kegel p.
    Peritron p.
Perio
    P. Pik irrigator
    P. Temp dental probe
periodontal
    p. probe
    p. prosthesis
PerioDontex bone graft substitute
PerioGlas
    P. bone graft particulate
    P. material
    P. synthetic bone graft
periosteal
    p. elevator

    p. raspatory
    p. spicule sweeper
periosteotome
    Alexander-Farabeuf costal p.
    Ballenger p.
    Brophy p.
    Brown p.
    costal p.
    Dean p.
    Doyen costal p.
    Ferris-Smith-Lyman p.
    Fomon p.
    Freer p.
    Jansen p.
    Joseph p.
    Moorehead p.
    Potts p.
    Speer p.
    Vaughan p.
    West-Beck p.
PerioTemp periodontal screening system
Periotest
    P. implant
    P. Implant Innovations gold screw
    P. system
PerioWise probe
peripheral
    p. blood vessel forceps
    p. indwelling intermediate infusion
        device
    p. interface adapter
    p. iridectomy forceps
    p. long-line catheter
    p. nerve glove
    p. quantitative computerized
        tomography scanner
    p. quantitative computer
        tomography (pQCT)
    p. vascular clamp
    p. vascular forceps
    p. vascular retractor
peripherally
    p. inserted central catheter (PICC)
    p. inserted central venous catheter
        (PICVC)
periscopic spectacles
peristaltic irrigation pump
Peri-Strips
    P.-S. Dry pericardial strip
    P.-S. Dry strip
Peritest perimeter

NOTES

P

peritoneal
- p. button
- p. clamp
- p. dialysis catheter
- p. forceps
- p. reflux control catheter

peritoneojugular shunt
peritoneoscope
- Menghini-Wildhirt p.

peritoneovenous shunt
Peritronics Medical Inc. fetal monitoring system
Peritron perineometer
periumbilical port
Peri-Warm pack
Perkin-Elmer model 5000 atomic absorption spectrophotometer
Perkins
- P. applanation tonometer
- P. elevator
- P. otologic retractor
- P. split-weight tractor
- P. traction

Per-Lee
- P.-L. equalizing tube
- P.-L. myringotomy tube
- P.-L. ventilation tube

Perlon suture
Perlstein
- P. brace
- P. joint
- P. orthosis

Permacol
- P. mesh
- P. permanent surgical implant

Perma-Cryl denture base material
Perma-Flow coronary bypass graft
Perma-Hand braided silk suture
Permalens lens
Permalock
- Weber P.

Permalume covering
PermaMesh
- P. hydroxyapatite woven sheet matrix
- P. material
- P. mesh

Perman cartilage forceps
PermaNeb nebulizer
permanent
- p. cardiac pacing lead
- p. myocardial pacemaker
- p. needle
- p. rate-responsive pacemaker
- p. transvenous demand pacemaker (PTDP)
- p. transvenous pacemaker
- p. ventricular pacemaker

Perman-Stille abdominal retractor

PermaRidge
- P. delivery syringe
- P. implant

Permark
- P. micropigmentation needle
- P. micropigmentation system

Perma-Seal dialysis access graft
PermaSoft reline material
Permathane
- P. lead
- P. Pacesetter lead pacemaker

Permatone denture material
PermCath dual-lumen hemodialysis catheter
permeable
- moisture vapor p. (MVP)

permeameter
- Corex digital probe p.

Perneczky aneurysm clip
Perone
- P. LASIK flap forceps
- P. LASIK marker

peroral
- p. electronic pancreatoscope system (PEPS)
- p. gastroscope

PerQ
- P. SANS
- P. SANS system

Per-Q-Cath CVP catheter
Perras mammary prosthesis
Perras-Papillon breast prosthesis
Perritt
- P. fixation forceps
- P. lens forceps

Perry
- P. forceps
- P. ileostomy bag
- P. latex Penrose drainage tubing
- P. Noz-Stop kit
- P. ostomy irrigator
- P. pediatric Foley latex catheter

PerryAnal/PerryVaginal EMG sensor
Perry-Foley catheter
PerryMeter EMG sensor
Perry/Pathway Anal EMG sensor
Perry/Pathway Vaginal EMG sensor
Persist skin prep swab
Personal
- P. Best peak flowmeter
- P. Catheter 100% silicone intermittent catheter

Persona monitoring kit
Personna
- P. Plus disposable Teflon scalpel
- P. surgical prep blade

Perspective
- P. chest imaging system
- P. dental imaging system

Perspex
> P. button
> P. CQ intraocular lens
> P. CQ-Shearing-Simcoe-Sinskey lens
> P. rod
> P. tube

Per-Stat-DL catheter
Perthes
> P. reamer
> P. sling

Pertrach percutaneous tracheostomy tube
pervenous catheter
PE-series implantable pronged unipolar electrode
pessary
> Albert-Smith p.
> Bioteque vaginal p.
> Biswas Silastic vaginal p.
> bladder neck support p.
> Blair modification of Gellhorn p.
> blue ring p.
> Chambers doughnut p.
> Chambers intrauterine p.
> cube p.
> cup p.
> diaphragm p.
> doughnut p.
> Dumontpallier p.
> Dutch p.
> Findley folding p.
> Gariel p.
> Gehrung p.
> Gellhorn p.
> Gold p.
> Gynefold prolapse p.
> Gynefold retrodisplacement p.
> Hodge p.
> intrauterine p.
> lever p.
> Maydl p.
> Mayer p.
> Menge p.
> Milex p.
> PelvX p.
> Plexiglas Gellhorn p.
> Prentif p.
> Prochownik p.
> prolapsus p.
> red p.
> retroversion p.
> ring p.

> safety p.
> Smith p.
> Smith-Hodge p.
> Smith retroversion p.
> stem p.
> tandem cube p.
> Thomas p.
> urethra cup p.
> Vimule p.
> White foam p.
> Wylie stem p.
> Zwanck radium p.

Pess lid everter
PET
> positron emission tomography
> PET balloon
> PET balloon Simpson atherectomy device
> PET scanner

Petanguy-McIndoe gouge
PET/CT scanner
Peter-Bishop forceps
Petersen rectal bag
Peterson
> P. cervical collar
> P. nail
> P. skeletal traction bow

Peters tissue forceps
Petit
> P. facial mask
> P. tourniquet

Petralit dental cement
Petri dish
petrolatum
> p. gauze
> p. gauze dressing

petroleum gauze
PET/SPECT camera
Pettigrove LASIK set
Peyman
> P. intraocular forceps
> P. vitrectomy unit
> P. vitrector
> P. vitreophage unit
> P. vitreous-grasping forceps
> P. vitreous scissors
> P. wide-field lens

Peyman-Green
> P.-G. vitrectomy lens
> P.-G. vitreous forceps

Peyman-Tennant-Green lens
Peyton brain spatula

NOTES

P

Pezzer
    P. drain
    P. mushroom-tipped catheter
    P. self-retaining urethral catheter
    P. suprapubic cystostomy catheter
PF
    PF Lee pediatric goniolens
    PF night splint
    PF Universal solder
Pfau
    P. atticus sphenoidal punch
    P. polyp forceps
PFC
    PFC component
    PFC offset tibial tray
    PFC Sigma total knee system
    PFC total hip replacement system
Pfeifer catheter
Pfeiffer-Grobety activator
Pfeiffer mechanical dosing pump
Pfister-Schwartz
    P.-S. basket forceps
    P.-S. sheath
    P.-S. stone basket
    P.-S. stone dislodger
    P.-S. stone retriever
Pfister stone basket
Pfizer scanner
PFM
    peak flow meter
    TruZone PFM
PFO-Star occluder
PGK stereotactic device
pH
    pH electrode
    pH meter
    pH probe
Phaco-4 diamond knife
phacoblade
    Myocure p.
Phaco Commander phacoemulsification system
phacodialysis spatula
phacoemulsifer-aspirator
phacoemulsification
    p. cautery
    p. handpiece
phacoemulsificator
phacoemulsifier
    Cavitron p.
    Kelman p.
    Legacy p.
    MVS p.
PhacoFlex
    P. II foldable intraocular lens implant
    P. II SI-30NB
Phacojack phaco system
Phakic 6 lens

phalangeal
    p. broach
    p. clamp
    p. forceps
Phaneuf
    P. arterial forceps
    P. clamp
    P. hysterectomy forceps
    P. peritoneal forceps
    P. uterine artery forceps
    P. uterine artery scissors
    P. vaginal forceps
phantom
    P. cardiac guidewire
    p. clamp
    Compass stereotactic p.
    3-dimensional SPECT p.
    p. frame
    p. interference screw
    p. nasal mask
    P. V Plus balloon dilatation catheter
Pharmacia
    P. corneal trephine
    P. Intermedics ophthalmics intraocular lens
    P. lancet
    P. Visco J-loop lens
Pharmaseal
    P. catheter
    P. closed drain
    P. disposable cervical dilator
    P. disposable uterine sound
    P. needle
PharmChek sweat patch drug detection system
Pharmex disposable catheter
pharyngeal
    p. airway
    p. retractor
pharyngometer
    EccoVision acoustic p.
pharyngoscope
    Hays p.
    Proud-Beck p.
pharyngotympanic tube
Phase-A-Caps alloy
Phaseafill dental composite
Phasealloy dental amalgam
phased-array
    p.-a. body coil MR imaging
    p.-a. coil
    p.-a. color-flow ultrasound system
    p.-a. extremity coil
    p.-a. probe
    p.-a. receiver coil
    p.-a. sector transducer
    p.-a. torso coil

p.-a. ultrasonographic device
p.-a. ultrasound-tipped catheter
phase-difference haloscope
3-phase generator
Phase II Multi-Podus foot orthosis
phase-sensitive detector
phase-shifted multielectrode catheter
Phazet lancet
PhD ergonomic pen and pencil
Pheifer-Young retractor
Phelan vein stripper
Phelps
P. brace
P. orthosis
P. splint
Phelps-Gocht osteoclast
PHEMA core-and-skirt keratoprosthesis
Phemister
P. biopsy trephine
P. brace
P. onlay bone graft
P. punch
P. raspatory
P. raspatory elevator
P. reamer
P. splint
Philadelphia
P. cervical collar
P. collar cervical traction
Philips
P. ACS-NT Gyroscan
P. CM-200 electron microscope
P. DVI 1 system
P. Easyguide navigation system
P. Gyroscan ACS-NT MR scanner
P. Gyroscan ACS scanner
P. Gyroscan NT-series scanner
P. Gyroscan S-series MR scanner
P. Gyroscan T5-NT MR scanner
P. linear accelerator
P. Orthoralix imaging
P. SensorTouch temple thermometer
P. small-bore system scanner
P. spiral CT scanner
P. toe force gauge
P. Tomoscan SR 6000 CT scanner
P. T-60 tomoscanner
P. ultrasound machine
Phillips
P. dilator
P. electronic stethoscope
P. fixation forceps

P. recessed-head screw
P. rectal clamp
P. screwdriver
P. swan neck forceps
P. urethral catheter
P. urethral whip bougie
P. urologic catheter
Philly bolt
Philos
P. DR pacemaker
P. DR-T pacemaker
phimosis forceps
Phinformer portable recorder
Phipps forceps
phlebograph
impedance p.
Phoenix
P. ancillary valve
P. Anti-Blok ventricular catheter
P. cruciform valve
P. fifth ventricle system
P. outrigger splint
P. 2 pacemaker
P. PX 115 Powerloft series II
alternating air flotation mattress
P. single-chamber pacemaker
P. total artificial heart
P. total hip prosthesis
phone
Picasso telemedicine p.
phonologic acquisition device
Phoresor II iontophoretic drug delivery
system
phorometer
phoro-optometer
Phoroptor
A-O minus cylinder P.
A-O plus cylinder P.
phosphate
potassium titanyl p. (KTP)
PhosphorImager system
photic-evoked response stimulator
photocathode
photocoagulator
American Optical p.
AO p.
argon laser p.
Coherent p.
Coherent argon laser p.
Ialo p.
infrared ray p.
Iolab I&A p.

NOTES

P

double-pronged p.
Farrior anterior footplate p.
Farrior oval-window p.
Farrior posterior footplate p.
fiberoptic p.
fixation p.
footplate p.
P. and Go monitor
Guilford-Wright stapes p.
Hayden footplate p.
Hoffmann scleral fixation p.
Hough stapedectomy footplate p.
House-Barbara p.
House obtuse p.
House oval-window p.
House strut p.
Kos p.
McGee footplate p.
Michel p.
Olk vitreoretinal p.
ophthalmic p.
Paparella footplate p.
posterior footplate p.
Rhein p.
Rice p.
Rosen p.
Saunders-Paparella p.
Scheer p.
Schuknecht p.
scleral p.
Shea p.
Sinskey p.
stapedectomy footplate p.
stapes p.
strut p.
Tabb knife p.
Trent p.
Wells scleral suture p.
Wilder p.
Wright-Guilford footplate p.
Wright-Guilford stapes p.
Picker
P. camera
P. Dyna Mo collimator
P. Edge MR scanner
P. Magnascanner
P. PQ helical CT scanner
P. Synerview 600 scanner
P. Vista HPQ MRI scanner
P. Vista MagnaScanner scanner

picket
P. Fence fiducial localization stereotactic system
p. fence guide
P. Fence leg positioner
Pickett scissors
Pickford-Nicholson
P.-N. analmoscope
P.-N. anomaloscope
Pickrell
P. hook
P. retractor
pickups
Adson p.
rat-tooth p.
Shoch foreign body p.
toothed p.
Pico-ST II low-profile balloon catheter
Picot
P. vaginal retractor
P. vaginal speculum
Pico-T II PTCA balloon catheter
Picotip
Endotak P.
Picture Archiving and Communications System (PACS)
picture-in-picture monitor
PICVC
peripherally inserted central venous catheter
Pidcock
P. nail
P. pin
PI disposable stapler
Pie
P. Medical CAAS II analysis system
P. Medical ultrasound
3-piece
3-p. acrylic intraocular lens
3-p. modified J-loop intraocular lens
3-p. silicone intraocular lens
Piedmont all-cotton elastic dressing
Pierce
P. antral trocar
P. antrum wash tube
P. attic cannula
P. cheek retractor
P. cryptotome
P. elevator
P. I&A vectis

NOTES

P

Pierce *(continued)*
    P. irrigating vectis
    P. nasal cup
    P. rongeur
    P. submucous dissector
Pierce-Donachy Thoratec ventricular assist device
Pierce-Kyle trocar
Pierse
    P. corneal forceps
    P. eye speculum
    P. fixation forceps
    P. tip forceps
Pierse-Colibri corneal forceps
Pierse-Hoskins forceps
piesimeter
piezoelectric
    p. accelerometer
    p. crystal
    p. shock wave lithotripter
    p. ultrasound transducer
piezoelectrical stimulator
Piezolith lithotripter
Piezo power microdissection
piezoresistive transducer
Piffard
    P. dermal curette
    P. placental curette
Pigg-O-Stat
    P.-O.-S. immobilization device
    P.-O.-S. x-ray chair
piggyback
    p. contact lens
    p. implant
    P. needle-knife papillotome
    Parker-Heath p.
    p. probe
Pigott forceps
pigskin graft
pigtail
    p. biliary stent
    p. catheter
    p. endoprosthesis
    p. nephrostomy drain
    p. nephrostomy tube
    p. probe
    p. rotation catheter
    p. tendon stripper
Pike jawed forceps
Pik Stick reacher
Pilcher
    P. catheter
    P. suprapubic hemostatic bag
pile clamp
pillar
    p. forceps
    p. retractor
pillar-and-post microsurgical retractor
pillar-grasping forceps

pill counter
Pillet hand prosthesis
Pilliar total hip replacement
Pilling
    P. bronchoscope
    P. collector
    P. dilator
    P. duralite tube
    P. Excalibur gauge
    P. fiberoptic illuminator
    P. forceps
    P. gouge
    P. laryngofissure shears
    P. microanastomosis clamp
    P. needle holder
    P. pediatric clamp
    P. retractor
    P. Weck Y-stent forceps
Pilling-Favaloro retractor
Pilling-Hartmann speculum
Pilling-Liston bone utility forceps
Pilling-Negus clamp-on aspirator
Pilling-Ruskin rongeur
Pilling-Wolvek sternal approximator
Pillo-Boot lower leg positioning device
Pillo-Pedic cervical traction pillow
Pillo Pro dressing
Pillo-Pump alternating pressure system
pillow
    abduction p.
    air p.
    Bedge p.
    Body buddy-body p.
    Capello slim-line abduction p.
    Carter p.
    cervical skull p.
    cervical sleep p.
    Core Sitback rest p.
    Core Slimrest lumbar p.
    Crescent memory p.
    Dream p.
    Flip-Flop p.
    foot p.
    FossFill Health p.
    Frejka hip p.
    Heart p.
    heel p.
    Hugg-L-O p.
    IMP-Capello slimline abduction p.
    Knee Pillo p.
    Max-Relax p.
    Mediflow waterbase p.
    Neckcare p.
    Neck-Hugger cervical support p.
    Nek-L-O hot & cold p.
    OrthoBone p.
    Orthosleep p.
    OsmoCyte p.
    Pillo-Pedic cervical traction p.

positioning p.
Pron p.
Richard p.
Rubens p.
Sand-Eze EGD p.
shoulder abduction p.
Softeze water p.
Tempur-Med p.
Tempur-Pedic pressure-relieving
  Swedish p.
T-Foam p.
Theracloud p.
Therapeutica sleeping p.
TherArc p.
Therasleep cervical p.
Tri-Core cervical support p.
vacuum p.
Wal-Pil-O neck p.
pillow-shaped balloon
Pil-O-Splint wrist splint
pilot
  P. audiometer
  p. bur
  p. drill
  p. needle
  P. point screw
  P. Spotlighter pen
Pilotip
  P. catheter
  P. catheter guide
pin
  Allofix cortical bone p.
  Apex p.
  Arthrex zebra p.
  ASIF screw p.
  Asnis p.
  Austin Moore p.
  Barr p.
  beaded hip p.
  Beath p.
  Belos compression p.
  bevel-point Rush p.
  Biofix system p.
  biphasic p.
  Böhler p.
  Böhler-Knowles hip p.
  Bohlman p.
  breakaway p.
  Breck p.
  calibrated p.
  Canakis beaded hip p.
  cancellous p.

Caspar distraction p.
Charnley p.
p. chuck
Co-Cr-Mo p.
Compere threaded p.
Conley p.
cortical p.
Craig p.
p. crimper
Crowe-tip p.
Crutchfield skull-tip p.
Davis p.
deluxe FIN p.
Denham p.
Deyerle p.
P. diode
distraction p.
distractor p.
duodenal p.
Ender p.
endodontic p.
femoral guide p.
Fisher half p.
fixation p.
Furness-Clute p.
Getz root canal p.
Gouffon hip p.
graft passing guide p.
p. guard
p. guide
Hagie p.
Hahnenkratt root canal p.
Hansen-Street p.
Hatcher p.
Haynes p.
p. headholder
p. headrest
Hegge p.
Hessel-Nystrom p.
Hewson breakaway p.
hexhead p.
Hoffmann apex fixation p.
Hoffmann transfixion p.
p. holder
p. implant
Intraflex intramedullary p.
intramedullary p.
Jones p.
Jurgan p.
Kirschner wire p.
Knowles hip p.
Kronendonk p.

NOTES

P

pin *(continued)*
    Kronfeld p.
    Küntscher femur guide p.
    lateral guide p.
    lead p.
    Link-Plus retention p.
    Lottes p.
    Marble bone p.
    Markley retention p.
    Mayfield skull clamp p.
    McBride p.
    mechanic's p.
    medullary p.
    metal p.
    Modny p.
    Moore fixation p.
    Moule screw p.
    Mt. Sinai skull clamp p.
    Neufeld p.
    Neurotips neurological
        examination p.
    Norman tibial p.
    Oris p.
    Ormco p.
    Orthofix p.
    orthopaedic p.
    OrthoSorb absorbable p.
    osseous p.
    Osteo-Pin p.
    osteotomy p.
    partially-threaded p.
    percutaneous p.
    Pidcock p.
    Pischel p.
    Pugh hip p.
    resorbable polydioxanone p.
    ReUnite orthopaedic p.
    Rhinelander p.
    Rica wire guide p.
    Riordan p.
    Rissler p.
    Rissler-Stille p.
    Roger Anderson p.
    Rush intramedullary fixation p.
    safety p.
    Safir p.
    Sage p.
    Scand p.
    Schanz p.
    Schneider self-broaching p.
    Schweitzer p.
    self-broaching p.
    self-tapering p.
    Shantz p.
    Shriners Hospital p.
    skeletal p.
    Slingshot cross p.
    Smillie p.
    Smith-Petersen fracture p.

SMo Moore p.
Snap fixation p.
spring p.
sprue p.
stabilizing guide p.
Stader p.
Steinmann calibrated p.
Street p.
strut-type p.
Surgin hemorrhage occluder p.
p. suture
Synthes guide p.
tapered p.
threaded guide p.
tibial guide p.
titanium half p.
torlone fixation p.
TransFix p.
trochanteric p.
tutoFix cortical p.
Venable-Stuck fracture p.
p. vise
von Saal medullary p.
Walker hollow quill p.
Watanabe p.
Watson-Jones guide p.
Webb p.
p. wheel
Zimfoam p.
Zimmer p.

Pinard
    P. fetal stethoscope
    P. horn fetoscope
pin-bending forceps
pince
    O'Shaughnessy p.
pincer
    overlapping p.
pinch
    p. forceps
    p. gauge
    P. Gauge and Jackson Strength
        evaluation system
    p. tree
pinchcock clamp
pinchometer
    Prestop p.
pin-deburring die
pineapple bur
Pineda LASIK Flap Iron
pinhole
    p. camera
    p. collimator
    p. occluder
pinion
    p. headholder
    p. headrest
Pinkerton balloon catheter
pink twisted cotton suture

Pinky ball
Pinnacle
    P. contact Nd:YAG fiber
    P. 3D radiotherapy planning system
    P. introducer sheath
    P. pacemaker
    P. reusable underpad
    P. R/O II introducer sheath
    P. R/O II radiopaque marker
Pinn-ACL guide system
2-pin passer
Pinpoint stereotactic arm
pin-seating forceps
pins and plaster
7-pin staple
Pinto
    P. dissector tip
    P. distractor
    P. superficial dissection cannula
pin-to-bar clamp
pinwheel
    CleanWheel disposable
     neurological p.
    Grafco p.
    Safe-T-Wheel p.
    Taylor p.
    Wartenberg p.
Pio root canal depth indicator
PIP/DIP strap
pipe
    endoscopic washing p.
    fiberoptic light p.
    light p.
    Mauch double-sheathed plastic
     wash p.
    p. tree
Pipelle
    P. catheter
    P. endometrial curette
    Unimar P.
Pipelle-deCornier endometrial curette
Piper
    P. lateral wall retractor
    P. obstetrical forceps
pipette
    Eppendorf Repeater Pro p.
    HandyStep electronic repeating p.
    Labpette FX p.
    light p.
    Pasteur p.
    SoftGrip p.

    Unopette capillary p.
    Wallace p.
Pipida scan
Piranha
    P. self-drilling screw
    P. uteroscopic biopsy forceps
Pirquet tongue depressor
Pisacano nucleus rotator
Pisces
    P. electrode
    P. implant
    P. spinal cord stimulation device
    P. spinal cord stimulation system
    P. Z Quad low-impedance lead
Pisces-Sigma lead
Pischel
    P. electrode
    P. micropin forceps
    P. needle
    P. pin
    P. scleral ruler
Pistofidis cervical biopsy forceps
pistol-grip hand drill
piston
    Austin p.
    Causse p.
    Guilford-Wright Teflon wire p.
    House p.
    McGee platinum/stainless steel p.
    MTS electrohydraulic p.
    p. stapes prosthesis
    Teflon p.
Pitanguy forceps
Pitha
    P. foreign body forceps
    P. urethral forceps
Pitie-Salpetriere saphenous vein hook
Pitkin
    P. dermatome
    P. spinal needle
    P. syringe
Pitot tube
Pitt
    P. talking tracheostomy
    P. talking tracheostomy tube
Pittman
    P. IMA retractor system
    P. needle holder
Pittsburgh triangular frame
pituitary
    p. curette
    p. forceps

NOTES

P

pituitary *(continued)*
    p. rongeur
    p. spoon
pivot
    p. aneurysm clip
    p. clip applier
    P. fixed-wire balloon catheter
    p. lock
    p. microanastomosis approximator
    P. Plate rehabilitation plate
pivoting
    p. surgical arm board
    p. table
Pixi bone densitometer
Pixie microlaparoscope
Pixsys
    P. FlashPoint camera
    P. FlashPoint digitizer
placement forceps
placental
    p. clamp
    p. curette
placenta previa forceps
Placer guidewire
Placido
    P. da Costa disc
    P. keratoscope
    P. 25-ring cone
placido ring
plagiocephaly
    p. headband
    p. helmet
plain
    p. catgut suture
    p. collagen suture
    p. ear hook
    p. ear spoon
    p. eye needle
    p. forceps
    p. gauze
    p. gut suture
    p. rib shears
    p. rotary scissors
    p. screwdriver
    p. wire speculum
plain-end grooved director
plain-line articulator
plain-pattern plate
Plak-Vac oral suction brush
planar
    p. blade
    p. circular coil
planer
    calcar p.
    Rubin cartilage p.
    Rubin nasal bone p.
Plange spud
planimeter

planimetry
    computerized p.
plano
    p. lens
    p. T-bandage
planoconcave lens
planoconvex
    p. disc
    p. eye implant
    p. lens
    p. nonridge lens
Planostretch stocking
plantar fasciitis night splint
plaque-cracker
    LeVeen p.-c.
plaque retriever
plasma
    p. clot diffusion chamber
    p. prothrombin conversion
     accelerator
    p. scalpel
    p. TFE vascular graft
PlasmaPlex bottle
plasma-sprayed
    low-pressure p.-s. (LPPS)
Plasorba BR plasma perfusion column
Plastalume
    P. bulb-ended splint
    P. straight splint
Plastazote
    P. arch support
    P. cervical collar
    P. foot bed
    P. orthotic
    P. orthotic device
    P. shoe
plaster
    p. bandage
    below-knee walking p.
    Hapset hydroxyapatite bone graft p.
    p. knife
    p. of Paris
    pins and p.
    p. saw
    p. shears
    p. spatula
    p. splint
    p. spreader
plaster-of-Paris
    p.-o.-P. bandage
    p.-o.-P. cast
    p.-o.-P. dressing
    p.-o.-P. jacket
    p.-o.-P. splint
Plastibell
    P. circumcision clamp
    P. circumcision device
    P. compression instrument

plastic
- p. bracket
- p. cannula
- p. collar
- p. connector
- p. corneal protector
- p. disposable irrigating vectis
- p. drape
- p. dressing
- p. endoprosthesis
- p. eye shield
- p. femoral plug
- p. forceps
- p. mouth guard
- p. orthosis
- p. prism
- p. scalp clip
- p. sewing ring
- p. sphere eye implant
- p. splint
- p. stent
- p. strip
- p. surgery scissors
- p. suture
- p. Tiemann catheter
- p. utility scissors

PlastiCast adjustable joint cast
plastic-cuffed tracheostomy tube
Plasticeph cephalometer
Plasticor prosthesis
Plasti-Pore ossicular replacement prosthesis
Plastizote collar
Plastodent
- P. dental impression adhesive
- P. wax

Plast-O-Fit thermoplastic bandage
plate
- absorbable p.
- acetabular reconstruction p.
- Alta channel bone p.
- Alta condylar buttress p.
- Alta distal fracture p.
- Alta femoral p.
- Alta supracondylar bone p.
- anchor p.
- AO blade p.
- AO compression p.
- AO condylar blade p.
- AO contoured T p.
- AO dynamic compression p.
- AO hook p.

- AO reconstruction p.
- AO semitubular p.
- AO small fragment p.
- AO spoon p.
- ASIF p.
- ASIF broad dynamic compression bone p.
- ASIF T p.
- Babcock p.
- Badgley p.
- Bagby compression p.
- Balser hook p.
- Batchelor p.
- Becton Colles fracture p.
- p. bender
- Berke-Jaeger lid p.
- Bimler elastic p.
- biodegradable p.
- Blackstone anterior cervical p.
- blade p.
- Blair talar body fusion blade p.
- Blair tibiotalar arthrodesis blade p.
- Blanchard traction device blade p.
- blood agar p.
- Blount blade p.
- bone flap fixation p.
- Bosworth spline p.
- breast p.
- Brophy p.
- buccal cortical p.
- butterfly-shaped monoblock vertebral p.
- buttress p.
- buttress-type p.
- Capener nail p.
- Caspar anterior cervical p.
- Caspar trapezoidal p.
- cervical p.
- cervical fusion p.
- CHS supracondylar bone p.
- coaptation p.
- cobra head p.
- Coffin p.
- CombiLock p.
- compression p.
- Concise side p.
- condylar lag screw p.
- connecting p.
- contoured anterior spinal p.
- cortical p.
- craniocervical p.
- craniomaxillofacial p.

NOTES

P

plate *(continued)*
Crockard midfacial osteotomy
  retractor p.
C-shaped p.
Dall-Miles p.
Danek cervical fusion p.
deck p.
depth p.
DePuy Peak anterior
  compression p.
Deyerle bone graft p.
double-angled blade p.
dynamic bridging p.
dynamic compression p.
eccentric dynamic compression p.
Eggers bone p.
Elliot knee p.
Elliott blade p.
Ellis buttress p.
fenestrated compression p.
finger p.
Foley p.
Fresnel zone p.
fusion p.
gait p.
Galveston p.
Gambro Liendia p.
Gambro Lundia p.
Gelfilm p.
Giebel blade p.
Haid cervical p.
Haid Universal bone p.
half-circle p.
Hansen-Street anchor p.
Hardy-Rand-Rittler p.
Harlow p.
Harm posterior cervical p.
Harris p.
Hawley bite p.
Hicks lugged p.
Hoen skull p.
2-hole p.
3-hole p.
7-hole p.
4-hole anteromedial Alta straight p.
6-hole mandibular p.
Hospidex microtiter p.
H-shaped p.
Hubbard p.
impactor p.
inner lip p.
interfragmentary p.
Ishihara pseudoisochromatic p.
Jaeger metal lid p.
Jewett double-angled osteotomy p.
Jewett slotted p.
Kessel osteotomy p.
keyed supracondylar p.
Kingsley orthodontic p.

Kleer base p.
lag screw p.
Laing osteotomy p.
Lane fracture p.
Lawson-Thornton p.
L buttress p.
lead p.
Leibinger 3-D bone p.
Leibinger Micro Plus p.
Leibinger mini Würzburg p.
Leibinger Würzburg p.
Letournel acetabular fracture
  bone p.
lid p.
limited-contact dynamic
  compression p.
lingual cortical p.
Liss locking distal femoral p.
locking reconstruction p.
Lorenz titanium screws and p.
low-contact dynamic compression p.
low-contact stress p.
L-plate p.
L-shaped p.
Luhr fixation p.
Luhr mandibular p.
Luhr MCS bone p.
Luhr microbone p.
Luhr microfixation cranial p.
Luhr minifixation bone p.
Luhr pan p.
Luhr Vitallium micromesh p.
Lundholm p.
Luque II p.
Lynch mucosa separator p.
mandibular bridging p.
mandibular staple bone p.
Massie II p.
May anatomical bone p.
McBride p.
McDonald bone p.
McLaughlin hip p.
Medoff sliding femoral fracture p.
metal reconstruction p.
Meurig Williams spinal fusion p.
Milch resection p.
Moberg bone p.
modified Grace p.
Moe intertrochanteric p.
Moore blade p.
Moore-Blount p.
Moore sliding nail p.
Morscher titanium anterior
  cervical p.
mucosal separator p.
Mueller-Hinton-supplemented agar p.
nail p.
narrow AO dynamic
  compression p.

Neufeld femoral nail p.
Newman toenail p.
Nicoll p.
Nord orthodontic p.
Ogden p.
Orion anterior cervical p.
Orozco p.
orthodontic base p.
orthopaedic p.
orthotic p.
Osborne osteotomy p.
palmar p.
Paulus chin p.
Paulus midfacial p.
pedicle p.
Percy p.
Perf-Plate cranial p.
Pivot Plate rehabilitation p.
plain-pattern p.
polydioxanone p.
PolyMedics p.
Profil-O-Plastic preshaped chin p.
Profil-O-Plastic preshaped
  midfacial p.
pseudoisochromatic p.
p. reader
reconstruction p.
resorbable p.
Rhinelander p.
Richards-Hirschhorn p.
Richards sideplate p.
Robin orthodontic p.
Rohadur gait p.
Roy-Camille p.
sacral p.
safety p.
Schwartz p.
Schweitzer spring p.
semitubular blade p.
Senn bone p.
Sensititre Streptococcus pneumoniae
  MIC p.
serpentine bone p.
Sherman bone p.
side p.
Silastic p.
Skirrow agar p.
skull p.
slotted bone p.
Smith-Petersen bone p.
Smith-Petersen intertrochanteric p.
SMo p.

snap-on inserter p.
Sofamor Danek anterior cervical p.
spring p.
Springlite p.
stabilization p.
Stahl calipers p.
staple bone p.
Steffee pedicle p.
Steffee screw p.
Steinhauser p.
Storz p.
superior border p.
supracondylar p.
Symmetrical thoracic vertebral p.
Synthes AO reconstruction p.
Synthes dorsal distal radius p.
Synthes maxillofacial locking
  reconstruction p.
Synthes maxillofacial titanium p.
Synthes stainless steel mini
  fragment p.
Synthes titanium mini fragment p.
Tacoma sacral p.
tantalum p.
T-buttress p.
Teflon p.
Temple University p.
tendon p.
Texas Scottish Rite Hospital
  crosslink p.
thoracolumbosacral p.
Thornton p.
THORP mandibular
  reconstruction p.
tibial p.
TiMesh orthognathic strap p.
titanium p.
titanium AO p.
titanium hollow osseointegrating
  reconstruction p.
titanium hollow screw
  osseointegrating reconstruction p.
titanium hollow screw
  reconstruction p. (THORP)
toe p.
tongue p.
Townsend-Gilfillan p.
tracheostomy p.
trochanteric p.
T-shaped AO p.
tubular p.
Tupman osteotomy p.

NOTES

plate *(continued)*
Universal bone p.
V-blade p.
Venable bone p.
Vitallium Elliott knee p.
Vitallium Hicks radius p.
Vitallium Wainwright blade p.
Vitallium Walldius mechanical
knee p.
V-type intertrochanteric p.
Wenger slotted p.
Whitman p.
Wilson spinal fusion p.
Wright knee p.
Würzburg p.
Y-bone p.
Z-plate p.
Zuelzer hook p.
plate-holding forceps
platelet
p. aggregometer
p. function analyzer
platelet-shaped knife
plate-spacer washer
platform
Aspen ultrasound p.
bariatric mat p.
Cemax PACS p.
p. forceps
Midline Hi-Lo Mat p.
operating p.
positioning p.
PSI-Tec aspiration p.
Servo ventilator p.
StealthStation treatment guidance p.
TomTec echo p.
Platina
P. clip lens
P. intraocular lens implant
plating
Caspar p.
dynamic compression p.
Gotfried percutaneous
compression p.
p. system
variable spinal p.
platinum
p. blade meatotomy electrode
p. embolization coil
p. eyelid implant
p. microcoil
p. oxygen electrode
P. Plus guidewire
p. probe
p. spatula
P. stationary table
p. wire

platinum-iridium
p.-i. electrode
p.-i. electrode wire
Platorit investment material
Platypus AV Fistula needle guard
platysma intrlocking suture sling
Playfair uterine caustic applicator
Pleatman
P. pouch
P. sac specimen container
pledget
cotton p.
cottonoid p.
Dacron p.
p. dressing
felt p.
Gelfoam p.
Meadox Teflon felt p.
neurosurgical p.
polypropylene p.
p. sponge
p. suture
Teflon p.
pledgeted
p. Ethibond suture
p. mattress suture
PlegiaGuard
P. pressure relief valve
P. safety device
Plenk-Matson raspatory
Plester retractor
plethysmograph
air p.
jerkin p.
Medgraphics body p.
mercury-in-rubber strain gauge p.
penile p.
respiratory inductance p. (RIP)
Respitrace inductive p.
RIP p.
venous occlusion p.
pleural
p. biopsy needle
p. biopsy needle shears
p. biopsy punch
p. dissector
p. peritoneal shunt
p. tube
**Pleura-Stay chest tube securement
device**
pleurectomy forceps
Pleur-evac
P.-e. autotransfusion system
P.-e. chest catheter
P.-e. device
P.-e. Sahara chest drainage system
P.-e. suction
P.-e. suction tube

Pleurx
- P. catheter drainage kit
- P. indwelling pleural catheter

Plexidure insole

Plexiglas
- P. eye implant
- P. Gellhorn pessary
- P. graft
- P. jig
- P. radiographic ruler
- P. spacer
- P. tissue equivalency block

PlexiPulse pneumatic sequential compression device

Pley extracapsular forceps

PLI-100 picoinjector pipette system

plication needle

pliers
- Allen root p.
- Beck p.
- Becker-Parkin p.
- bending p.
- Berbecker p.
- College p.
- crown-crimping p.
- debonding p.
- dental p.
- extraction p.
- Jacob-Swan goniotomy p.
- Jelenko p.
- KY p.
- ligature-locking p.
- Luhr microfixation system p.
- Mathieu p.
- needle-nose p.
- needle-nose vise-grip p.
- Ormco orthodontic p.
- orthopaedic surgical p.
- Power Grip p.
- Reill wire-cutting p.
- Risley p.
- root p.
- Schwarz arrow head clasp forming p.
- slip-joint p.
- SMIC p.
- Sontec p.
- square-end p.
- Stille flat p.
- threader rod holder p.
- vise-grip p.

Plondke uterine forceps

plug
- Air-Lon decannulation p.
- Alcock catheter p.
- Arthrex OATS bone p.
- Avina female urethral p.
- Berkeley Bioengineering brass scleral p.
- Bio-Plug canal p.
- bone femoral p.
- bone tunnel p.
- brass scleral p.
- Buck p.
- cannulated bone tunnel p.
- Catamaran swim p.
- catheter p.
- collagen p.
- Coloplast Conseal 1-piece, 2-piece p.
- Concept bone tunnel p.
- Counsellor p.
- Dittrich p.
- Dohlman p.
- dome hole p.
- EaglePlug tapered-shaft punctum p.
- EagleVision Freeman punctum p.
- ear putty ear p.
- Exeter intramedullary bone p.
- femoral p.
- Freeman punctum p.
- gastrostomy p.
- glass vaginal p.
- Herniamesh surgical p.
- Herrick lacrimal p.
- hydrogel p.
- intramedullary canal p.
- Isberg scleral p.
- Johnston gastrostomy p.
- Kirschner femoral canal p.
- Luer-Lok male adapter p.
- Mack ear p.
- Marlex PerFix p.
- methyl methacrylate cranioplasty p.
- Micro punctum p.
- Oasis collagen p.
- omental p.
- Osteonics acetabular dome hole p.
- PerFix Marlex mesh p.
- plastic femoral p.
- polypropylene p.
- punctum p.
- Reich-Nechtow p.
- R-Med p.

NOTES

P

plug *(continued)*
    scleral p.
    sealing window p.
    Seidel p.
    Shiley decannulation p.
    Sims vaginal p.
    tapered-shaft punctum p.
    TearSaver punctum p.
    Teflon p.
    Umbrella punctum p.
    Woodson p.
plug-finishing bur
plugged telescoping catheter
plugger
    amalgam p.
    Bredall amalgam p.
    endodontic p.
    Schilder p.
    serrated amalgam p.
    SMIC root canal p.
plugging instrument
plumbeous zirconate titanate tip
Plum-Blossom acupuncture needle
Plume-Away evacuator
PlumeSafe Whisper 602 smoke evacuation system
Plumicon camera tube
Plummer
    P. bag
    P. modified bougie
    P. water-filled pneumatic esophageal dilator
Plummer-Vinson
    P.-V. esophageal dilator
    P.-V. radium esophageal applicator
plunger
    dome p.
plunger-type femoral pressurizer
plus
    2010 P. Holter system
    4096 P. PET scanner
    p. power lens
    P. punctal occluder
Plyoback Rebounder medicine ball
Plyoball
    P. medicine ball
    P. system
PlyoSled exerciser
Plystan
    P. graft
    P. prosthesis
PMI implant
PMMA
    polymethyl methacrylate
    PMMA centering sleeve
    PMMA centralizer
    PMMA haptic
    PMMA hard contact lens
    PMMA implant
    PMMA intraocular lens
PMT
    PMT AccuSpan tissue expander
    PMT Cortac cortical electrode
    PMT Depthalon depth electrode
    PMT halo brace
    PMT Integra breast expander
    PMT InVac in-line suction control device
    PMT MacroVac suction-irrigator
    PMT MicroVac suction device
    PMT robotic fulcrumless tomographic system
PMV
    Passy-Muir valve
    PMV aqua, clear, purple, white ventilator connector
    PMV O_2 adapter
Pneu
    P. Care ICU dynamic low-air-loss bed
    P. Care Pedibed dynamic pediatric low-air-loss bed
    P. Knee brace
Pneu-Care Plus mattress
PneuGel postop knee brace
pneumatic
    p. ankle tourniquet
    p. antiembolic stocking
    p. bag
    p. balloon catheter
    p. balloon dilator
    p. 4-bar knee
    p. chair lift
    p. compression boot
    p. compression stocking
    p. cuff
    p. drill
    p. garment
    p. microscope
    p. otoscope
    p. tonometer
    p. tourniquet
    p. walker
pneumatonograph
pneumatonometer
    Micro One p.
    Modular One p.
pneumoballistic lithotripter
PneumoCheck spirometer
pneumodissector
    laparoscopic p.
pneumohydraulic capillary infusion system
Pneumo-Matic insufflation needle
Pneumomat laparoscopic insufflator
pneumoneedle
pneumoperitoneum needle

pneumoscope
pneumo sleeve
pneumostatic dilator
Pneumotach
pneumotach
    MicroTach p.
pneumotachograph
    Fleisch p.
    Gould p.
    Gould Godard p.
pneumotachometer
    Collins SurveyTach p.
    hot-wire p.
    MicroTach p.
    Rudolph linear p.
pneumothoracic
    p. apparatus
    p. injection needle
pneumotome
    Wappler p.
pneumotonometer
Pneumotron ventilator
pneumo-wrap ventilator
pneuPAC
    p. resuscitator
    p. ventilator
Pneu-Scale frameless air support
  therapy
Pneu-trac
    P.-t. cervical collar
    P.-t. cervical traction orthosis
PneuView
    P. single lung system
    P. ventilator testing and training
    system
PNS Unna boot
POC
  proximal occlusion catheter
    POC Bandit catheter
pocket
    P. pachymeter
    p. probe
    P. Starter device
Pocket-Dop
    P.-D. blood-flow detector
    P.-D. 3 fetal heart rate monitor
    P.-D. fetal stethoscope
Pocketpeak peak flowmeter
PocketView electrocardiograph
PodoSpray nail drill system
Pogon chair
Poh mouth mirror

point
    Crowe pilot p.
    Excell polishing p.
    p. forceps
    G-C diamond p.
    gutta-percha p.
    Mathews drill p.
    powered automatic stopping drill p.
    Raney-Crutchfield drill p.
    p. resolved spectroscopy
    self-stopping drill p.
    Universal drill p.
    William Dixon Cratex p.
3-point
    3-p. fixation intraocular lens
    3-p. head holder
    3-p. spreader bag
4-point
    4-p. cervical brace
    4-p. fixation intraocular lens
    4-p. spreader bag
2-point discriminator
pointed
    p. awl
    p. cone bur
pointed-tip electrode
pointer
    Baton laser p.
    P. 1-piece all-PMMA intraocular
    lens
6-point knee brace
point-of-care analysis
point-of-reduction clamp
point-search instrument
Polack
    P. corneal fixation forceps
    P. keratoscope
Polar
    P. Bair forced-air active cooling
    device
    P. Care 500 cryotherapy device
    P. coordinate system
    P. Pack
    P. Vantage XL heart rate monitor
    P. wrist monitor
polarimeter
  confocal scanning laser p.
  scanning laser p.
Polaris
    P. adjustable spinal cage implant
    P. cage
    P. CPAP

NOTES

P

Polaris *(continued)*
  P. electrode
  P. laparoscope
  P. LE catheter
  P. Mansfield/Webster deflectable tip
  P. 1.32 Nd:YAG laser
  P. reusable cutter
  P. reusable dissector
  P. reusable forceps
  P. reusable grasper
  P. steerable diagnostic catheter
Polaris-Dx steerable diagnostic catheter
polarizing ophthalmoscope
Polar-Mate
  P.-M. bipolar coagulator
  P.-M. bipolar microcoagulator
polarographic needle electrode
Polaroid
  P. CB-100 camera
  P. HealthCam system
  P. instant endocamera
  P. vectograph slide
Polaron sputter coater
Polarus
  P. humeral rod
  P. Plus humeral fixation system
  P. positional humeral fixation
  system
  P. Vantage XL heart rate monitor
Polatest vision tester
Polavision Land camera for endoscopy
Polcyn elevator
pole
  walking p.
20-pole
  20-p. deflectable halo catheter
  20-p. deflectable mapping catheter
Polhemus
  P. 3-D digitizer scanner
  P. Liberty 3D digitizer
Poliak eye retractor
poliglecaprone 25 suture
Polio laryngoscope
Polisar-Lyons
  P.-L. adapted tracheal tube
  P.-L. tracheal tube
polisher
  Anis ball reverse-curvature
  capsular p.
  Anis disc capsular p.
  Bechert capsular p.
  Buedding squeegee cortex extractor
  and p.
  capsule p.
  Deldent Jetsonic 2000 p.
  Drews posterior capsule p.
  Freeman posterior capsule p.
  Gill-Welsh capsular p.
  Holladay posterior capsular p.

Jensen capsular p.
  Knolle capsular p.
  Kraff capsular p.
  Kratz p.
  Kratz-Jensen p.
  Look capsular p.
  Tennessee capsular p.
  Terry silicone capsular p.
  Torchia capsular p.
  Yaghouti LASIK p.
polishing
  p. brush
  p. bur
  p. strip
Politzer
  P. air bag
  P. air-bag otoscope
  P. air syringe
  P. angular ear knife
  P. ear perforator
  P. ear speculum
  P. paracentesis knife
Politzer-Ralks knife
Polk
  P. finger goniometer
  P. placental forceps
  P. sponge forceps
Polle pod attachment for
  ophthalmoscope
Polley-Bickel trephine
Pollock
  P. catheter
  P. double corneal forceps
  P. punch
  P. sweetheart periosteal elevator
  P. wimp wire impactor
  P. zygoma elevator
Pollock-Dingman elevator
polly power grip
Polmedco endotracheal tube cuff
Polokoff rasp
Poloxamer 407 barrier material
Poly
  P. GIA stapler
  P. Surgiclip absorbable clip
polyamide
  p. mesh
  p. suture
polyanhydride biodegradable polymer
  wafer
polyaxial
  p. cervical screw
  p. spine system (PASS)
polybutester suture
polycarboxylate cement
Poly-Cath balloon catheter
polycationic histochemical probe
Polycel bone composite prosthesis
polycentric knee prosthesis

Polydek suture
Polyderm foam wound dressing
Poly-Dial insert
polydioxanone
    p. plate
    p. sheet
    p. suture (PDS)
Polydor Preforms orthotic
polyene thread
polyester fiber suture
polyether implant material
polyethylene
    ArCom compression-molded p.
    ArCom processed p.
    p. cannula
    carbon fiber-reinforced p.
    p. catheter
    p. collar button
    p. drain
    extruded bar p.
    p. foam
    p. glycol
    p. graft
    high density p.
    p. implant material
    p. liner
    porous p.
    p. retractor tape
    p. seat heart valve
    p. socket
    p. sphere implant
    p. stent
    p. strut
    p. suture
    p. talar prosthesis
    p. terephthalate balloon
    p. T-tube
    p. tube
    p. tubing
    ultra-high molecular weight p.
    (UHMWPe)
polyethylene-covered
    p.-c. Gianturco stent
    p.-c. Z-stent
polyethylene-faced
    p.-f. driver
    p.-f. mallet
polyfilament suture
PolyFlex
    P. implantable pacing lead
    pacemaker
    P. traction dressing

Polyfloat system II mattress
    replacement
PolyFlo peripherally inserted catheter
Polyflux
    P. hemodialyzer
    P. S dialyzer
Polyform splint
polygalactic acid suture
PolyGIA stapling device
polyglactin
    p. mesh
    p. 910 suture
polyglecaprone 25 suture
polyglycolate suture
polyglycolic
    p. acid mesh
    p. acid suture
polyglycolide implant
polyglyconate suture
polygoniometer
polygon mirror
polygraph
    Gould p.
    Mackenzie p.
    NightOwl pocket p.
polylactic acid arrow
polylactide
    p. absorbable screw
    p. implant
Polylite quilted underpad
poly-L-lysine-coated glass slide
Poly-Lock bonding
Polymed
    P. exam glove
    P. splint
PolyMedics plate
PolyMem adhesive surgical wound
    dressing
polymer
    Bioplastique p.
    HTR p.
    Hydrolene p.
    Hylamer orthopaedic bearing p.
    P.Q. viscoelastic p.
    p. stent
    p. tooth replica implant
polymer-coated, drug-eluting stent
PolymerFriction total knee
polymeric
    p. biomaterial
    p. endoluminal paving stent

NOTES

P

Poly-Mesam 7-channel ambulatory recording unit
polymethyl
- p. methacrylate (PMMA)
- p. methacrylate bone cement
- p. methacrylate ear splint
- p. methacrylate implant

polyolefin copolymer balloon
polypectomy snare
polyp forceps
polyphase generator
Poly-Plus Dacron vascular graft
Polyprep centrifuge
polypropylene
- p. button
- p. button suture
- p. catheter
- p. glycol ankle-foot orthosis
- p. glycol thoracolumbosacral orthosis
- p. hand brush
- p. intracardiac patch
- p. intraocular lens
- p. mesh
- p. needle
- p. pledget
- p. plug

polypus forceps
Polyrox fractal lead
Polysil-Foley catheter
Polyskin II dressing
polysomnograph
- Albert Grass Heritage p.
- Sleepscan p.

Polysorb
- P. absorbable staple
- P. heel cup
- P. liner
- P. 55 stapler
- P. suture

Polystan
- P. cardiotomy reservoir
- P. implant
- P. perfusion cannula
- P. venous return catheter

Polystim electrode
polysulfone
- p. dialyzer
- p. membrane

Polytec LaseAway Q-switched ruby laser
polytef
- p. paste
- p. soft tissue patch

polytef-sheathed needle
polytetrafluoroethylene (PTFE)
- expanded p. (ePTFE)
- p. implant
- p. mesh

- p. prosthesis
- p. sock
- p. stent
- p. stent graft

polytetrafluoroethylene-covered stent
polytome
- Massiot p.

PolyTome instrument
Polytrac Gomez retractor
PolyTrach dressing
Polytron PT 3000 homogenizer
polyurethane (PU)
- p. bandage
- p. catheter
- p. graft
- p. implant material
- p. nasoenteric catheter
- p. stent

polyurethane-coated silicone breast implant
polyvinyl
- p. alcohol foam
- p. alcohol splint
- p. alcohol sponge
- p. bougie
- p. chloride (PVC)
- p. chloride balloon
- p. chloride catheter
- p. chloride endotracheal tube
- p. dilator
- p. drain
- p. graft
- p. prosthesis
- p. sponge implant
- p. tubing

polyvinylsiloxane putty
Polyviolene polyester suture material
PolyWic
- P. dressing
- P. wound filling material

Pomard anthropomorphic measurement reference chart
Pomeranz
- P. aortic clamp
- P. hiatal hernia retractor

Pomeroy ear syringe
pommel cushion
poncho restraint
Ponseti splint
Ponsky
- P. Endo-Sock specimen retrieval bag
- P. PEG tube
- P. pull

Ponsky-Gauderer
- P.-G. PEG tube
- P.-G. type PEG

pontoon spica cast

pool

AquaMotion therapy p.
Endless Pool physical therapy p.
SwimEx p.

Poole

P. abdominal suction tube
P. trocar

Pool-Pfeiffer self-locking clip

Pope

P. halo dressing
P. Oto-Wick
P. rectal knife
P. wick

popliteal retractor

pop-off

p.-o. needle
p.-o. suture
p.-o. valve

**pop-on self-adhering male external
catheter**

Poppen

P. aortic clamp
P. electrosurgical coagulator
P. Gigli saw guide
P. intervertebral disc forceps
P. intervertebral disc rongeur
P. laminectomy rongeur
P. monopolar cautery cord
P. periosteal elevator
P. pituitary rongeur
P. Ridge Sensitometer
P. suction tube
P. sympathectomy scissors
P. ventricular needle

Poppen-Blalock carotid artery clamp
Poppen-Blalock-Salibi carotid clamp
**Poppen-Gelpi laminectomy self-retaining
retractor**
Poppers tonsillar guillotine
poppet

ball p.
barium-impregnated p.
prosthetic p.

pop rivet
Poracryl resin
porcine

p. bioprosthesis
p. graft
p. heart valve
p. prosthesis

Porex

P. drainage system

P. Medpor implant
P. nerve locator
P. paranasal implant
P. PHA implant

Porges

P. Neoflex dilator
P. stone dislodger

Pori and Rowe EEG receiver
Porites coral material
Porocoat

P. material
P. porous coating
Tri-Lock total hip prosthesis
with P.

Porocool prosthesis
Porolon sponge
Poron

P. cellular urethane
P. 400 insole

Poroplastic splint
porous

p. block hydroxyapatite
p. coating
Harris-Galante p. (HGP)
p. hydroxyapatite sphere
p. metallic stent
p. polyethylene
p. polyethylene implant

porous-coated

p.-c. anatomic (PCA)
p.-c. anatomic knee prosthesis

Porovin dental resin
PORP

partial ossicular reconstruction prosthesis
partial ossicular replacement prosthesis
prosthetic ossicular reconstruction
procedure
Richards hydroxyapatite PORP

port

A-Port implantable p.
BardPort implanted p.
Berkeley Bioengineering infusion
terminal p.
butterfly needle infusion p.
CathLink 20 implanted p.
Celsite brachial p.
Celsite pediatric p.
Cordis multipurpose access p.
Dialock access p.
endoscopic access p.
endoscopic threaded imaging p.
EndoTIP imaging p.

NOTES

P

725

port *(continued)*
    Gill-Welsh guillotine p.
    Hasson blunt p.
    implantable access p.
    implantable infusion p.
    Infuse-a-Port p.
    infusion p.
    Luer-Lok p.
    lumbar p.
    OmegaPort access p.
    periumbilical p.
    p. protector
    tangential p.
    Titanium VasPort p.
    treatment p.
    Universal catheter access p.
    Vasport access p.
    venous access p.
    Visiport p.
    Vortex Clear-Flow p.

portable
    p. blood gas analyzer
    p. blood irradiator
    p. cardiotachometer
    p. electronic goniometer
    p. insulin dosage-regulating
      apparatus
    p. insulin infusion pump
    p. monitoring device
    p. respirator
    p. sleep monitor
    p. suction aspirator
    p. volume ventilator

Port-A-Cath
    P.-A.-C. device
    P.-A.-C. implantable catheter

portacaval
    p. H graft
    p. shunt

Portadial kidney machine
PortaFlo urine collection system
portal
    AP p.
    p. cannula
    p. catheter
    fixed-beam p.
    integrated sideport access p.
    PA p.

portal-phased spiral CT scan
Portal Pro 3 treatment chair
Porta-Lung noninvasive extrathoracic
    ventilator
PortalVision radiation oncology system
Porta Pulse 3 portable defibrillator
Portaray dental x-ray unit
Porta-Resp monitor
Portazam portable exam chair
Porter duodenal forceps
Porterfield catheter

Porter-Kolpe biliary biopsy set
Porter-O-Surgical cutter
Portex
    P. bacterial filter
    P. Blue Line tracheostomy tube
    P. chorionic villus sampling
      catheter
    P. nasopharyngeal airway
    P. Neo-Vac meconium suction
      device
    P. nylon cannula
    P. Perfit tracheostomy tube
    P. preformed blue line tracheal
      tube
    P. Soft-Seal cuff system
    P. SS endotracheal tube cuff
    P. Thermovent heat and moisture
      exchanger
    P. XL endotracheal tube cuff

Portex-Gibbon catheter
Portmann
    P. drill
    P. retractor
    P. speculum holder

Portnoy
    P. DPV device
    P. multiflanged catheter
    P. ventricular cannula
    P. ventricular catheter

portogram
    SMA p.

portography
    arterial p.

Porto-Lift lift
portosystemic shunt
Porto-Vac
    P.-V. catheter
    P.-V. suction tube

PortSaver PercLoop device
Porvidx cancer screening technology
Porzett splint
Posada-Vasco orbital retractor
Posey
    P. bar
    P. bed cradle
    P. belt
    P. Cufflator
    P. drop seat
    P. grip
    P. Palm cone
    P. restraint
    P. SkinSleeves
    P. sling
    P. snare

Posicam HZ PET scanner
Posi-Grip umbilical cord clamp
Posilok instrument holder
Posi-Stop drill
Positex knee wedge

positional feedback stimulation trainer
positioner
- acetabular cup p.
- Allen hand p.
- Assistant Free Stulberg leg p.
- Bareskin knee p.
- beach chair p.
- body p.
- Body Wrap foam p.
- CAS-8000V angiography p.
- Cook stent p.
- cup p.
- eggcrate p.
- Foot Waffle p.
- Grasshopper p.
- Hold-and-Hold p.
- IMP Universal lateral p.
- Kirschenbaum foot p.
- knee p.
- lateral p.
- lateral hand p.
- leg p.
- p. Luer
- Mark II Stulberg hip p.
- Mark II Wixson hip p.
- McCaffrey p.
- McConnell shoulder p.
- McGuire pelvic p.
- Medline p.
- Miller bracket p.
- Montreal p.
- oblique hand p.
- Picket Fence leg p.
- Prep-Assist p.
- Profex arthroscopic leg p.
- ProForm p.
- Schlein shoulder p.
- shoulder abduction p.
- skull p.
- Starfish2 heart p.
- stent p.
- Stulberg hip p.
- Stulberg Mark II leg p.
- SurgAssist leg p.
- Ther-A-Shapes p.
- Thornton adjustable p.
- TMJ head p.
- Urchin heart p.
- Vac-Pac p.
- Waters p.
- Wixson hip p.

positioning
- p. needle
- p. pillow
- p. platform
Position Plus cushion
position-sensing catheter
positive
- p. end-expiratory pressure
- p. expiratory pressure (PEP)
- p. eyepiece
positive-intrinsic-negative diode
Positrap
- P. mini-retrieval basket
- P. retriever
Positrol
- P. II Bernstein catheter
- P. USCI catheter
positron
- p. emission tomography (PET)
- p. emission tomography balloon
- p. emission transaxial tomography scanner
- p. scintillation camera
Posner
- P. diagnostic lens
- P. diagnostic/surgical gonioprism
- P. slit lamp
Posner-Inglima applanator
Possis Perma-Seal dialysis access graft
post
- Brasseler Optipost root p.
- Caspar retraction p.
- Endowel p.
- Endowel dental p.
- Flexipost dental p.
- Hahnenkratt root canal p.
- PD crown p.
- PD root canal p.
- Prep-Tite p.
- Stalite root canal p.
- transosseous p.
postauricular
- p. ear dressing
- p. hearing aid
- p. retractor
4-poster frame
posterior
- p. capsule scrubber
- p. chamber intraocular lens
- p. chamber lens implant
- p. convex intraocular lens
- p. distraction instrumentation

NOTES

P

posterior *(continued)*
p. footplate pick
p. forceps
p. fossa retractor
p. hook-rod spinal instrumentation
p. leaf-spring ankle-foot orthosis
p. lumbar retractor
p. neck surface coil
p. reduction device
p. segment forceps
p. thigh bar
p. urethral retractor
postgadolinium scan
Post-Harrington erysiphake
postmortem
p. forceps
p. suture needle
postnasal
p. balloon
p. balloon tamponade
p. dressing
p. sponge forceps
postoperative
p. flexor tendon traction brace
p. mammary support
p. shoe
postpartum binder
postpyloric feeding tube
post-TUR irrigation clamp
Posture
P. Curve lumbar cushion
P. Pump Lordoticiser exerciser
P. S'port
P. Wedge seat cushion
post-urethroplasty review speculum
Pos-T-Vac vacuum erection device
Potain
P. aspirating trocar
P. aspirator
potassium
p. titanyl phosphate (KTP)
p. titanyl phosphate laser
potential acuity meter
potentiometer
linear p.
Potocky needle
Potta coarctation forceps
Potter
P. modified knife
P. needle
P. sickle knife
P. sponge forceps
P. tonsillar forceps
Potter-Bucky diaphragm
Potter-Elvehjem homogenizer
Potts
P. aortic clamp
P. bronchial forceps
P. bulldog forceps

P. cardiovascular clamp
P. coarctation clamp
P. coarctation forceps
P. dental elevator
P. dissector
P. divisional clamp
P. expansile dilator
P. expansile knife
P. expansile valvulotome
P. fixation forceps
P. infant rib shears
P. intestinal forceps
P. ligature
P. needle
P. patent ductus clamp
P. patent ductus forceps
P. periosteotome
P. pulmonic clamp
P. shunt
P. splint
P. tenaculum
P. tenotomy scissors
Potts-Cournand angiography needle
Potts-DeBakey clamp
Potts-DeMartel gall duct scissors
Potts-Nevins dressing forceps
Potts-Niedner aortic clamp
Potts-Riker
P.-R. dilator
P.-R. valvulotome
Potts-Satinsky clamp
Potts-Smith
P.-S. aortic clamp
P.-S. arterial scissors
P.-S. bipolar forceps
P.-S. dissecting scissors
P.-S. dressing forceps
P.-S. monopolar forceps
P.-S. needle holder
P.-S. pulmonic clamp
P.-S. reverse scissors
P.-S. thumb forceps
P.-S. tissue forceps
P.-S. vascular scissors
Potts-Yasargil scissors
pouch
Active Life urostomy p.
Assura EasiClose ostomy p.
Assura 1-piece postop drainable p.
Atlantic "O-Dor-Less" p.
Bard closed-end p.
Bard drainage adhesive p.
Bard security p.
bladder replacement urinary p.
Bongort Max-E-Pouch p.
Bongort urinary diversion p.
Coloplast 1-piece, 2-piece
drainable p.
Coloplast urostomy p.

ConvaTec ostomy p.
ConvaTec urostomy p.
Dansac Combi Colo F p.
Dansac Contour 1 p.
Denis Browne p.
DeRoyal Grab Bag specimen
  retrieval p.
Durahesive Wafer p.
female urinary p.
FirstChoice postoperative
  drainable p.
FirstChoice urostomy p.
Florida urinary p.
Grab Bag specimen retrieval p.
HolliGard seal closed stoma p.
Hollister First Choice p.
Hunt-Lawrence p.
Incise p.
Kataya seal closed stoma p.
Lap-Bag specimen retrieval p.
Le Bag urinary p.
Lo-Profile urostomy p.
Mainz p.
ManHood absorbent p.
Mansson urinary p.
Marsupial p.
Mentor absorbent p.
MicroSkin ostomy p.
Nu-Hope drainable urinary p.
Padua bladder urinary p.
Pagedas retrieval p.
Parks ileostomy p.
Parsonnet pulse generator p.
pediatric drainable p.
pediatric transfer p.
pediatric urostomy p.
Penn p.
Pleatman p.
Preemie p.
Premier drainable p.
Premier urostomy p.
Premium closed p.
Premium drainable p.
Reality vaginal p.
retracted penis p.
Rowland p.
Sheer Plus p.
Squibb urostomy p.
Studer p.
Sur-Fit flexible and drainable p.
Sur-Fit Natura p.
Sur-Fit urostomy p.

Tena p.
Tenador male p.
Torbot Plastic p.
Torbot Rubber p.
**Pouchkins pediatric ostomy belt
pouch-type sling
Pousson pigtail catheter
Poutasse**
  P. renal artery clamp
  P. renal artery forceps
powder
  p. blower
  p. board
**Powell wand
power**
  p. adapter
  p. amplifier
  P. Anthro shoe
  P. cannula
  p. drill
  P. Grip pliers
  p. injector
  p. peak filter
  P. Play knee brace
  P. Pogo stationary exerciser
  p. rasp
  p. router
  P. Trainer cycle
  P. Web hand exerciser
  p. wheelchair
PowerBath
  MacroSorb P.
**PowerBelt lower back and abdominal
  support belt
PowerCut drill blade
powered**
  p. automatic skull perforator
  p. automatic stopping drill point
Powerflex
  P. balloon catheter
  P. CMP exerciser
  P. Extreme PTA dilatation catheter
  P. PTA balloon
  P. tape
**Powerforma surgical drill
PowerGrip stent delivery system
PowerHeart AECD
Powerlink endoluminal graft
Powermatic table
PowerPen**
  MacroSorb P.
POWERPoint orthotic shoe insert

NOTES

P

PowerProxi Sonic toothbrush
PowerSculpt cosmetic surgery system
PowerStar bipolar scissors
PowerVision ultrasound
Pozzi
    P. tenaculum
    P. tenaculum forceps
PPG probe
PP knee air-brace
PPT
    PPT gel stirrup ankle brace
    PPT MXL soft molded insole
    PPT Plastazote insole
    PPT RX firm molded insole
    PPT sheet
pQCT
    peripheral quantitative computer
    tomography
    pQCT microscanner
    pQCT scanner
PQ premium heel cup
P.Q. viscoelastic polymer
PR-2 ventilator
Praeger iris hook
PRAFO
    pressure-relief ankle-foot orthosis
    PRAFO adjustable orthotic
    PRAFO KAFO attachment
Pram combination occluder
Pratt
    P. anoscope
    P. antral curette
    P. bivalve retractor
    P. bivalve speculum
    P. crypt hook
    P. cystic hook
    P. ethmoid curette
    P. hemostatic forceps
    P. nasal curette
    P. proctoscope
    P. rectal dilator
    P. rectal director
    P. rectal hook
    P. rectal probe
    P. rectal scissors
    P. rectal speculum
    P. tenaculum
    P. tissue forceps
    P. T-shaped hemostatic forceps
    P. urethral sound
    P. uterine dilator
    P. vulsellum forceps
Pratt-Smith hemostatic forceps
preamplifier
    Arzco p.
Preceder interventional guidewire
Precept DR pacemaker
prechopper
Precident stem

precipitation
    heparin-induced extracorporeal
    lipoprotein p. (HELP)
precise
    P. ACL guide system
    P. anastomotic coupler
    P. disposable skin stapler
    p. lesion measuring device
precision
    P. Cosmet lens
    P. hip system
    p. lancet cutting needle
    P. office transurethral needle
    ablation system
    P. Osteolock femoral prosthesis
    P. Osteolock stem
    P. Osteolock total hip
    P. QID glucose monitoring system
    P. refractor
    P. SpeedTac transvaginal anchor
    P. Strata hip system
    P. tack
    P. Twist transvaginal anchor
Precision-Cosmet intraocular lens
    implant
PrecisionGlide needle
Pre-Cision miniature and
    microminiature scalpel
Preci-Slot dental attachment
Precisor Direct Bite biopsy forceps
Preci-Vertix kit
PreClean soak system
Preclude
    P. Dura Substitute prosthesis
    P. IMA sleeve
    P. pericardial membrane
    P. peritoneal membrane
    P. spinal membrane
Precoat Plus femoral prosthesis
precollagenous filamentous material
precompression jig
precontoured unit rod
precordial
    p. lead
    p. stethoscope
precut papillotome
Predator balloon catheter
Preefer eye speculum
Preemie pouch
Preface braided guiding sheath
preformed
    p. clasp
    p. Cordis catheter
    p. polyvinyl chloride endotracheal
    tube
Premier
    P. cervical plate system
    P. drainable minipouch
    P. drainable pouch

P. I&A unit
P. pincore latex cushion
P. urostomy pouch
Premiere vitreous cutter
Premilene nonabsorbable suture
Premium
P. CEEA circular stapler
P. CEEA circular stapling device
P. closed pouch
P. drainable pouch
P. Plus CEEA disposable stapler
P. Poly CS-57 stapler
Premo guidewire
premounted stent
Prentif
P. cavity-rim cervical cap
P. pessary
Prentiss forceps
Prenyl jacket
Prep-Assist
P.-A. legholder
P.-A. positioner
preperitoneal distention balloon
Prep-IM kit
Preposition ColorCards
Preptic dressing
Prep-Tite post
prepuce forceps
presbyopia glasses
Presbyterian
P. Hospital forceps
P. Hospital occluding clamp
P. Hospital staphylorrhaphy elevator
P. Hospital T-clamp
P. Hospital ventricular needle
Prescriptor hearing aid
Presence bladder control pad
preshaped catheter
Preshaw clamp
presphenoethmoid suture
press
Cali-Press graft p.
CamStar power leg p.
fascial p.
House Gelfoam p.
Omni p.
Paparella tissue p.
p. plate needle holder
scleral shell p.
Sheehy fascial p.
tissue p.
press-button chuck

Press-Fit
P.-F. condylar total knee
P.-F. femoral component
P.-F. implant
P.-F. prosthesis
P.-F. stem
P.-F. total condylar knee system
Press-Mate model 8800T blood pressure monitor
Presso-Elastic dressing
pressometer
Jarcho p.
press-on prism
Pressoplast compression dressing
Pressore monitor
Presso-Superior dressing
PressPak dispenser
PresSsion pneumatic garment
pressure
Alladin Infant Flow nasal
continuous positive air p.
p. applied dressing (PAD)
p. bandage
biphasic positive airway p.
(BiPAP)
central venous p. (CVP)
continuous positive airway p.
(CPAP)
p. controller
p. cuff
p. earring
p. equalization tube
p. equalizing tube
p. forceps
p. gauge
p. glove
P. Guard guidewire
p. injector
intracranial p. (ICP)
p. length loop
p. mattress
p. patch dressing
positive end-expiratory p.
positive expiratory p. (PEP)
p. relief padding
p. relief shoe
p. ring
P. Sentinel reamer
sequential p.
p. shield
p. sling

NOTES

P

pressure *(continued)*
    p. sore status tool
    p. transducer
    p. transducer airflow sensor
    variable positive airway p. (VPAP)
    p. ventilator
pressure-activated safety valve
pressure-cycled ventilator
PressureEasy cuff inflation device
Pressurefuse automatic constant
    pressure device
PressureGuard
    P. IV alternating-pressure mattress
    P. Select patient adjustable pressure
      management system
pressure-point tension ring
pressure-preset ventilator
pressure-producing earring
pressure-relief
    p.-r. ankle-foot orthosis (PRAFO)
    p.-r. cushion
PressureSense monitor
PressureWire
    P. interface
    P. 3-300 sensor
pressurizer
    Oxyhood p.
    plunger-type femoral p.
Pressurometer blood pressure monitor
Presto cardiac device
Presto-Flash spirometer system
Preston
    P. ligamentum flavum forceps
    P. overhead pulley
    P. pinch gauge
    P. Traveler CPM exerciser
Preston-Hopkins ligator
Prestop pinchometer
pretapped Synthes lag screw
pretibial
    p. bearing (PTB)
    p. buttress (PTB)
Pre-Vent
    P.-V. boot style stirrup pad
    P.-V. elbow protector
    P.-V. heel protector
    P.-V. knee crutch pad
    P.-V. OR table pad
    P.-V. ulnar nerve protector
PreVENT Anti-Reflux filter
Prevent Plus training pant
preVent Pneumotach flowmeter
P.R. heat moldable insert
Pribram suction tube
Price
    P. corneal punch
    P. muscle clamp
Price-Thomas
    P.-T. bronchial clamp

    P.-T. bronchial forceps
    P.-T. rib stripper
Pricker needle
Pride Jazzy 1103 Mini electric
    wheelchair
Priessnitz
    P. bandage
    P. dressing
Priestley-Smith retinoscope
Priestly catheter
Priest wasp-waist laryngostat
Prima
    P. FX laser wire
    P. KTP/532 laser
    P. laser guidewire
    P. LEEP speculum
    P. pacemaker
    P. vaginal speculum
Primaderm foam dressing
Primallor alloy
Primapore
    P. absorptive wound dressing
    P. tape
primary
    p. clip
    p. trimming bur
Primbs-Circon indirect video
    ophthalmoscope system
Primbs suturing forceps
Prime
    P. balloon
    P. ECG electrocardiac mapping
      system
Primer
    P. compression dressing
    P. compression wrap
    P. flexible Unna boot
    P. modified Unna boot
PrimeTime
    P. disposable underpad
    P. Plus adult disposable brief
PrimoFocus hearing aid
primordial catheter tube
Primus
    P. flexible great toe implant
    P. prostate machine
Prince
    P. advancement forceps
    P. dissecting scissors
    P. eye cautery
    P. muscle clamp
    P. muscle forceps
    P. rongeur
    P. tonsillar scissors
    P. trachoma forceps
Prince-Potts scissors
PrinceStar electrophysiologic imaging
    study system
Pringle clamp

Printz aspirator
prism
bar p.
base-down p.
Becker gonioscopic p.
Berens p.
DermaGard p.
diopter p.
direct-vision p.
Drews inclined p.
Fresnel p.
Goldmann contact lens p.
gonioscopic p.
handheld rotary p.
Jacob-Swan gonioscopic p.
Keeler p.
p. loupe
Maddox p.
oblique p.
plastic p.
press-on p.
Risley rotary p.
scanning p.
square p.
P. 2000XP gamma camera
Prisma digital hearing aid
prismatic
p. contact lens
p. gonioscopic lens
p. spectacles
Prism-CL pacemaker
Pritchard
P. cannula
P. elevator
P. syringe
P. total elbow prosthesis
Pritikin scleral punch
Prizm
P. defibrillator
P. Electro-Mesh Sock electrode
P. Electro-Mesh Z-Stim-II
stimulator
Pro
P. Balance Master
P. infusion catheter
P. 50 KS 5 ACL brace
P. Peak decubitus pad
P. Pulse irrigator
P. Relief gel/foam wheelchair
cushion
P. traction table
Pro-8 ankle brace

ProAdvantage knee prosthesis
ProAire portable rotation system
Pro-Bal protected balloon-tipped
catheter
probe
AccuProbe 600 cryotherapy p.
Acolysis coronary p.
acoustic impedance p.
Actaeon p.
afterloading p.
Alcon vitrectomy p.
Aloka MP-PN ultrasound p.
Amoils p.
Amussat p.
Ando motor-driven p.
AnEber p.
Anel lacrimal p.
AngeLase combined mapping-
laser p.
angled p.
Arbuckle sinus p.
Arndorfer esophageal motility p.
arthroscopic p.
Aspir-Vac p.
back-stop laser p.
Bakes p.
p. balloon catheter
P. balloon-on-a-wire dilatation
system
Bard p.
Barr fistula p.
Barr rectal p.
4-beam laser Doppler p.
Becker p.
Beckman p.
Benger p.
Bermen-Werner p.
Beyer pigtail p.
BICAP bipolar hemostasis p.
BiLAP bipolar p.
biliary balloon p.
biometry p.
biopsy p.
Bipolar Circumactive P. (BICAP)
Bipolar EndoStasis p.
bipolar hemostasis p.
Birtcher electrocautery p.
blind endosonography p.
blood-flow p.
blunt p.
blunt-tip p.
Bodian lacrimal p.

NOTES

P

733

probe *(continued)*
Bodian minilacrimal p.
Bowman lacrimal p.
Brackett dental p.
brain p.
Brenner rectal p.
Bresgen frontal sinus p.
Brock p.
Brodie fistular p.
bronchoscopic p.
Bruel & Kjaer transvaginal
  ultrasound p.
Brunner p.
Brymill cryosurgical p.
Buck ear p.
Buie fistula p.
bullet p.
Bunnell dissecting p.
Bunnell forwarding p.
calibrated p.
Camino intracranial pressure p.
canaliculus p.
cardiac p.
Cardioscint nuclear p.
Castroviejo lacrimal sac p.
cataract p.
cDNA p.
Chandler transluminal V-pacing p.
Cherry brain p.
Circon ACMI electrohydraulic
  lithotriptor p.
Clinitex Charles
  endophotocoagulator p.
coagulation p.
Coakley nasal p.
Cody magnetic p.
CO$_2$ laser p.
common duct p.
conical p.
Contact Laser bullet p.
Contact Laser chisel p.
Contact Laser conical p.
Contact Laser flat p.
Contact Laser interstitial p.
Contact Laser round p.
continuously-perfused p.
convex p.
convex array ultrasound p.
Cook-Swartz Doppler flow p.
coronary artery p.
Corson needle electrosurgical p.
Crawford canaliculus p.
Criticare sensor p.
cross-sectional anal sphincter p.
cryogenic p.
CryoHit p.
cryopexy p.
cryotherapy p.
C-Trak handheld gamma p.

curved retinal p.
Dandy p.
Dekompressor percutaneous
  diskectomy p.
Desjardins gallstone p.
dilating p.
p. dilator
dilator p.
DioPexy p.
disposable p.
dissecting p.
dissection p.
Dix spud p.
Dobbhoff bipolar coagulation p.
Doppler 4-beam laser p.
Doppler flow echocardiographic p.
Doppler ultrasonic p.
dot-plotted p.
double-ended chrome p.
double-ended nickelene p.
double-ended silver p.
drum p.
Dymer excimer delivery p.
ear p.
Earle rectal p.
echo p.
echocardiographic p.
echo-tracking p.
electric p.
electrohydraulic lithotripsy p.
electromagnetic field p.
electromagnetic flow p.
electrosurgical monopolar spatula p.
Ellis foreign body spud p.
Emmet uterine p.
end-fire transrectal p.
endocavitary p.
Endocavity V33W p.
endocervical p.
endolaser p.
Endopath needle tip
  electrosurgery p.
Endo-P-Probe endorectal p.
endoscopic BICAP p.
endoscopic heat p.
endosonography p.
EndoSound ultrasound p.
EndoStasis p.
Endotrac ligament p.
Esmarch tin bullet p.
esophageal pH p.
esophageal temperature p.
eustachian p.
exocervical p.
extended sector ultrasonic p.
eye p.
Fenger gall duct p.
Fenger spiral gallstone p.
Ferguson esophageal p.

fiberoptic p.
filiform bougie p.
Fish antral p.
Fish sinus p.
fistula p.
flat p.
flexible endosonography p.
flow p.
Fluhrer bullet rectal p.
fluorescent p.
Fluoroptic thermometry p.
Fogarty biliary balloon p.
foreign body p.
fragmentation p.
Fränkel sinus p.
freehand p.
French lacrimal p.
Frigitronics freeze-thaw cryopexy p.
frontal sinus p.
Gabor p.
Gallagher bipolar mapping p.
gall duct p.
gallstone p.
galvanic p.
gamma p.
gamma detection p.
Gant rectal p.
gear shift pedicle p.
general p.
Gillquist-Oretorp-Stille p.
Gilmore p.
Girard Fragmatome p.
gold p.
Goldman-Fox p.
Gross p.
Hagar p.
handheld Doppler p.
handheld exploring electrode p.
handheld mapping p.
Harms trabeculotomy p.
Hayden p.
heater p.
Heller p.
Henning-Keinkel stomach p.
Hertzog pliable p.
Hewlett-Packard omniplane 5-MHz p.
high-frequency miniature p.
high-resolution p.
Hitachi convex-convex biplane p.
Hitachi convex ultrasound p.
Hitachi fingertip ultrasound p.

Hitachi linear ultrasound p.
Hitachi transrectal ultrasound p.
Hitachi transvaginal ultrasound p.
hockey-stick electrosurgical p.
Hoffrel transesophageal p.
Hotz ear p.
Huber p.
Hydromer coated bipolar
  coagulation p.
Ilg p.
Iliff lacrimal p.
illuminated p.
Injectate p.
injection gold p.
interstitial p.
intracavitary p.
IntraDop p.
intraductal ultrasound p.
intraluminal p.
intraoperative gamma p.
intraoperative ultrasonic p.
irrigating p.
Jacobson blood vessel p.
Jacobson vas deferens p.
Jacobson vessel p.
Jako laryngeal p.
Jannetta p.
Jansen-Newhart mastoid p.
Jobson-Horne p.
Josephberg p.
Jubileum 2.0 gastroesophageal
  pH p.
Kalk palpitation p.
Kartch pigtail p.
Keeler-Amoils curved cataract p.
Keeler-Amoils glaucoma p.
Keeler-Amoils long-shank retinal p.
Keeler-Amoils-Machemer retinal p.
Keeler-Amoils ophthalmic
  Machemer retinal p.
Keeler-Amoils ophthalmic
  vitreous p.
Kennerdell-Maroon p.
Killian p.
Kirschner guiding p.
Kistner p.
Kleinsasser p.
Knapp iris p.
Kocher p.
Koenig p.
Kron bile duct p.
KryMed 300 p.

NOTES

P

probe *(continued)*
KTP laser p.
lacrimal p.
lacrimal duct p.
lacrimal intubation p.
laparoscopic p.
laparoscopic Doppler p.
laparoscopic ultrasound p.
large-bore heat p.
Larry rectal p.
laryngeal p.
laser p.
laser-Doppler flowmetry p.
laser-Doppler Periflux PF-3 p.
Laserflow Doppler p.
Lente silver nitrate p.
L-hook electrosurgical p.
Liebreich p.
ligament chisel p.
light monitoring p.
Lilienthal p.
Lillie frontal sinus p.
Linde cryogenic p.
linear array ultrasound p.
lithotripter p.
localizing p.
Lockhart-Mummery p.
Lucae ear p.
magnetic eye p.
magnetometer p.
malleable p.
Mamtat p.
Manhattan Eye & Ear p.
Mannis suture p.
Martin uterine fistula p.
mastoid p.
Max-I-Probe irrigation p.
Mayo common duct p.
Mayo kidney stone p.
Mayo uterine p.
McKesson mouth p.
Meadox Surgimed Doppler p.
mechanical rotating p.
Medi-Tech bipolar p.
Medrad MRInnervu endorectal
    colon p.
Meerschaum p.
meniscectomy p.
Merit-B periodontal p.
microlaryngeal laser p.
MicroSmooth p.
Microvit p.
Microvit vitrectomy p.
miniature p.
miniaturized ultrasound catheter p.
Mixter common duct p.
Mixter Dilaprobe p.
Mixter dilating p.
Mixter gall duct p.

Mixter irrigating p.
Modulap p.
monitoring p.
Moynihan bile duct p.
Moynihan gallstone p.
Mui Scientific 6-channel esophageal
    pressure p.
multielectrode p.
multilumen p.
multiplane intracavitary p.
Myrtle leaf p.
Nabors p.
nasal p.
nasolacrimal duct p.
p. needle
needle p.
Nélaton bullet p.
NeoProbe gamma detection p.
Neo-Therm neonatal skin
    temperature p.
Nibbler laparoscopic p.
nuclear p.
Nucleotome Flex II cutting p.
Nucleotome Micro I p.
Ochsner-Fenger gallstone p.
Ochsner flexible spiral gallstone p.
Ochsner gall duct p.
Ochsner gallstone p.
Ochsner spiral p.
ocutome p.
O'Donoghue p.
Ohmeda p.
oligonucleotide p.
Olympus heat p.
Olympus MH-908 slim
    ultrasonic p.
Olympus ultrathin balloon-fitted
    ultrasound p.
Olympus UM-R-series miniature
    ultrasonic p.
Olympus UM-W-series
    endoscopic p.
Oratek thermal shrinking p.
Ossoff-Karlan microlaryngeal
    laser p.
over-the-wire p.
palpation p.
PA 120 Osypka radiofrequency p.
Paparella p.
Parker-Heath piggyback p.
Parsonnet coronary p.
Payr p.
Payr-Schmieden p.
pediatric biplane TEE p.
pencil Doppler p.
percutaneous pencil Doppler p.
periodontal p.
Perio Temp dental p.
PerioWise p.

pH p.
phased-array p.
piggyback p.
pigtail p.
platinum p.
pocket p.
p. point scissors
polycationic histochemical p.
PPG p.
Pratt rectal p.
Probex p.
pulpal microdialysis p.
quartz fiberoptic p.
QuickDop p.
Quickert-Dryden lacrimal p.
Quickert lacrimal p.
Radiometer p.
rectal p.
Reddick-Saye Lav-1 I&A p.
reflectance spectrophotometric p.
retinal p.
reverse-cutting meniscal p.
Rica ear p.
Richards p.
Ritleng p.
Robicsek vascular p.
Rockey dilating p.
Rohrschneider p.
Rolf lacrimal p.
Rollet lacrimal p.
Rosen ear p.
Rosen endaural p.
Rubinstein p.
salpingeal p.
Sandhill p.
Saphyre bipolar ablation p.
Sarns temperature p.
Schmieden p.
scintillation p.
sensor p.
p. sheath
Sheer p.
p. shield
Shirodkar p.
side-firing p.
side-hole cannulated p.
Siemens linear p.
Siemens vaginal p.
silver p.
Silverstein stimulator p.
Simpson sterling lacrimal p.
Sims uterine p.

simultaneous thermal diffusion blood flow and pressure p.
sinus p.
Skillern sinus p.
Skillern sphenoidal p.
SMIC periodontal abscess p.
SmokEvac electrosurgical p.
Softflo fiber optic p.
Somnus p.
Sonablate transrectal p.
Sonocath ultrasound p.
p. spatula
spatula p.
spatula electrosurgical p.
spear-ended chrome p.
spear-pointed nickelene p.
sphenoidal p.
Spiesman fistular p.
SpineStat side-directed diskectomy p.
spinning p.
spiral p.
Stacke p.
standard hook electrosurgical p.
Storz-Bowman lacrimal p.
Storz pigtail p.
straight retinal p.
suction p.
tactile p.
Teflon p.
temperature p.
Theobald sinus p.
thermistor p.
tin-bullet p.
trabeculotomy p.
transcranial Doppler p.
transesophageal echocardiography p.
Transonic flow p.
transrectal p.
TrueVision transvaginal p.
truncated NMR p.
Tufcote epilation p.
TULIP p.
tumor p.
ultrasound p.
ultrasound catheter p.
Universal vaginal p.
Urrets-Zavalia p.
USCI p.
uterine p.
vacuum intrauterine p.
Valliex uterine p.

NOTES

probe *(continued)*
Vasamedics PR-434 implantable prism laser p.
Versadopp Doppler p.
vertebrated p.
Vibrodilator p.
ViraType p.
vitrector p.
Vulcan ablator p.
V33W high-density endocavity p.
Vygantas-Wilder retinal drainage p.
Wasko common duct p.
water p.
Weaver sinus p.
Welch Allyn rectal p.
Werb right-angle p.
whalebone eustachian p.
whirlybird p.
Williams lacrimal p.
wire p.
Woodson p.
Worst double-ended pigtail p.
Xomed rectal p.
Yankauer salpingeal p.
Yellow Springs p.
Yeoman p.
YSI Foley p.
YSI neonatal temperature p.
Ziegler lacrimal p.
Ziegler needle p.
probe-ended grooved director
Probe-SV spectrometer
Probex probe
probing sheath exchange catheter
ProBloc insulated regional block needle
Probst Smiley[2] LASIK marker
Procath electrophysiology catheter
procedure
loop electrosurgical excision p. (LEEP)
prosthetic ossicular reconstruction p. (PORP)
total ossicular reconstruction p. (TORP)
Zaldivar anterior p. (ZAP)
Procel cast liner
Pro-Cell balloon catheter
Procera system
process
AuTolo cure p.
processed carbon implant
processor
array p.
Autotechnicon tissue p.
Clarion CII BTE sound p.
Clarion Platinum BTE sound p.
Cobe 2991 cell p.
Cordelle II sound p.
ESPrit ear level speech p.

Hope p.
Olympus EU-M-series endosonography image p.
output signal p.
Procomat small-tank semiautomatic p.
real-time video p.
ThinPrep 2000 p.
video p.
wearable speech p.
Prochownik pessary
Pro-Clude transparent wound dressing
Procol hydrocolloid wound dressing
Procomat small-tank semiautomatic processor
Pro-Comelastic abdominal belt
ProComp EMG
PRO/Covers ultrasound probe sheath
ProCross
P. Rely balloon
P. Rely over-the-wire balloon catheter
proctological
p. ball electrode
p. cotton carrier
p. grasping forceps
p. polyp forceps
Proctor
P. cheek retractor
P. laryngopharyngoscope
P. laryngostat
P. mucosal elevator
P. phrenectomy forceps
P. phrenicectomy forceps
P. suction tube
Proctor-Bruce mastoid searcher
Proctor-Hellens laryngostat
Proctor-Livingston endoprosthesis
proctoscope
ACMI p.
Bacon p.
Boehm p.
Fansler p.
Gabriel p.
Goldbacher p.
Hirschman p.
Hirschman-Martin p.
Kelly p.
Lieberman p.
Montague p.
Morgan p.
Morgan-Boehm p.
National p.
Newman p.
Pratt p.
Pruitt p.
Salvati p.
Sims p.
Tuttle p.

Welch Allyn p.
Yeoman p.
proctoscopic fulguration electrode
proctosigmoidoscope
ACMI fiberoptic p.
fiberoptic p.
ProCyte transparent film dressing
Proderm topical spray
Pro-Designed wrist guard
Prodigy
P. bone densitometer
P. lens inserter
Prodisc prosthetic lumbar disc
product
Innovative Medical P.'s (IMP)
ProDynamic monitor
Proetz
P. mouthgag
P. syringe
P. tongue depressor
Proetz-Jansen mouthgag
Profex
P. arthroscopic leg positioner
P. arthroscopic tourniquet
P. cast padding
P. finger cot
Profile
P. hip prosthesis
P. mammography system
P. pediatric polypectomy snare
P. Plus balloon dilatation catheter
P. total hip system
ProFile
P. file
P. orifice shaper
profilometer
Cottle p.
laryngoscope p.
Straith p.
Profil-O-Plastic
P.-O.-P. preshaped chin plate
P.-O.-P. preshaped midfacial plate
ProFinesse II ultrasonic handpiece
Profix
P. confirming tibial insert
P. metaphyseal tibial stem
P. nonporous tibial base
P. porous femoral component
P. total knee replacement system
proflavine wool dressing
Proflex dilatation catheter
ProFlex wrist support

Pro-Flo XT catheter
Profore
P. four-layer bandage
P. four-layer wound dressing
ProForm
P. maxim-VE pressure-reduction mattress
P. positioner
P. strata
ProForma
P. cannula
P. double-lumen papillotome
Progeny femoral stem
Progestasert intrauterine device
Pro-glide
P.-g. orthosis
P.-g. splint
Prograft Exluder bifurcated endograft
Programalith
P. AV pacemaker
P. II, III pacemaker
programmable
p. cardioverter-defibrillator (PCD)
p. pacemaker
p. pulse generator
p. pump
p. valve
p. VariGrip II prosthetic control system
programmer wand
progressive
P. ankle orthosis
p. dilators
P. palm guard
projection x-ray microscope
projector
acuity visual p.
fiberoptic light p.
Marco chart p.
NP-3S auto chart p.
Tagarno 35D cineangiography p.
Tagarno 35-series film p.
Topcon automatic chart p.
Project Research Ophthalmic specular microscope
Pro-Koester wide-field SCM microscope
Prokop intraocular lens
Prolapse coil
prolapser
Stone lens nucleus p.
prolapsus pessary

NOTES

Prolase
> P. fiber
> P. II lateral firing Nd:YAG laser

Prolene
> P. Hernia system patch
> P. mesh
> P. mesh sheet
> P. mesh silo
> P. polypropylene suture
> P. stitch
> P. suture

ProLine endoscopic instrument
Prolite fluorescent pulsed light
ProLite Plus runner's orthotic
Prolith pacemaker
Prolog pacemaker
PROloop instrument
Promag 2.2 biopsy gun
ProMax maxillofacial x-ray unit
Promex biopsy needle
Promise washable knit pant
Promoe enteral feeding container
Promogran matrix wound dressing
pronation spring control (PSC)
pronator drill
Proneb Ultra nebulizer
prone surgical saddle
Pronex
> P. cervical traction
> P. pneumatic device
> P. traction device

3-prong
> 3-p. fork
> 3-p. grasping forceps
> 3-p. rake blade retractor

4-prong
> 4-p. finger speculum
> 4-p. finger splint
> 4-p. retractor

3-pronged
> 3-p. grasper
> 3-p. polyp retriever
> 3-p. rake blade

pronged retractor
5-prong rake blade retractor
2-prong rake retractor
6-prong rake retractor
prongs
> curved nasal p.
> nasal p.
> Pro-Tech nasal p.

Pronova suture
Pron-Pillo head positioning device
Pron pillow
Pronto cement
Pro-Op frameless air support therapy
Pro-Ophtha
> P.-O. absorbent stick sponge
> P.-O. drape

> P.-O. dressing
> P.-O. eye pad
> P.-O. eye patch
> P.-O. stick
> P.-O. type-K, -S shield

ProOsteon
> P. implant 500 coralline hydroxyapatite bone void filler
> P. implant graft material
> P. synthetic bone implant

prop
> Moult mouth p.
> Oberto mouth p.

Propaq Encore vital signs monitor
Pro/Pel
> P./P. cannulated interference screw
> P./P. coating

Proplast
> P. graft
> P. HA
> P. I, II porous implant material
> P. preformed facial implant
> P. prosthesis
> P. TORP

Proplast-Teflon disc implant
Propoint multifunction knee brace
Pro-Post system
Propper
> P. binocular indirect ophthalmoscope
> P. Star retinoscope

Propper-Heine ophthalmoscope
Prop'r Toes hammer toe cushion
propylene dressing
ProROM walker
Proscan ultrasound imaging system
Proscope anoscope
Proshield collagen corneal shield
ProShifter ACL sports brace
Prosorba column
ProSound SSD-5500 ultrasound
Prospec disposable speculum
ProSpeed CT scanner
ProSport Cord
ProstaCoil self-expanding stent
ProstaJect ethanol injection system
Prostakath urethral stent
Prostalac total hip prosthesis
Prostalase laser
Prostaprobe catheter
Prostar-Plus percutaneous closure device
Prostar XL percutaneous closure device
ProstaScint scan
prostatectomy
> p. bag
> p. forceps
> transurethral ultrasound-guided laser-induced p. (TULIP)

**Prostathermer prostatic hyperthermia
system**
prostatic
- p. aluminum electrode
- p. biopsy needle
- p. bridge catheter
- p. dissector
- p. lobe forceps
- p. needle holder
- p. retractor
- p. stent
- p. tractor

**Prostatron transurethral thermotherapy
device**
prosthesis
- Abrams-Lucas mitral valve p.
- Accolade hip p.
- acrylic bar p.
- AcuMatch M Series modular
  femoral hip p.
- Advantage DP artificial leg p.
- Aequalis shoulder p.
- AGC knee p.
- Airlite monolithic p.
- Airprene hinged knee p.
- Allegretto unicompartmental knee p.
- Allen-Brown p.
- Allurion foot p.
- alumina cemented total hip p.
- Ambicor inflatable penile p.
- American Heyer-Schulte chin p.
- American Heyer-Schulte-Hinderer
  malar p.
- American Heyer-Schulte
  mammary p.
- American Heyer-Schulte-Radovan
  tissue expander p.
- American Heyer-Schulte
  rhinoplasty p.
- American Heyer-Schulte
  testicular p.
- AML total hip p.
- AMS Ambicor penile p.
- AMS 700CX-series penile p.
- AMS Hydroflex penile p.
- AMS malleable penile p.
- AMS M-series malleable penile p.
- AMS penile p.
- AMS Sphincter 800 urinary p.
- Amsterdam-type p.
- Amstutz cemented hip p.
- AMS Ultrex penile p.

- anatomic hip p.
- Anatomic Precoat hip p.
- Anderson acetabular p.
- Anderson columellar p.
- Angelchik antireflux p.
- antibiotic-loaded acrylic cement
  total joint p.
- antireflux p.
- aortofemoral p.
- Apollo hip p.
- Apollo knee p.
- Applebaum p.
- Arion rod eye p.
- arterial graft p.
- articulated chin p.
- artificial breast p.
- Ashley natural-Y breast p.
- Atkinson p.
- Atlas shoulder p.
- Attenborough total knee p.
- Aufranc-Turner hip p.
- auricular p.
- Austin Moore hip p.
- Balance hip p.
- ball-and-cage p.
- ball-and-socket p.
- ball valve p.
- Bankart shoulder p.
- Barnard mitral valve p.
- 4-bar polycentric knee p.
- Bateman finger p.
- Bateman UPF II shoulder p.
- Baxter mechanical valve p.
- Beall mitral valve p.
- Bechtol p.
- Becker breast p.
- Becker hand p.
- Becker tissue expander p.
- Beck-Steffee total ankle p.
- below-knee p.
- Bentall cardiovascular p.
- Bi-Angular shoulder p.
- BIAS p.
- Bicer-val mitral heart valve p.
- bicondylar knee p.
- bifurcation p.
- bileaflet p.
- Bi-Metric hip p.
- Bi-Metric Interlok femoral p.
- Bi-Metric porous primary
  femoral p.
- Bingham knee p.

NOTES

prosthesis *(continued)*
Bio-Chromatic hand p.
Bio-Clad acetabular p.
Bioglass p.
Bio-Groove acetabular p.
Bio-Groove Macrobond HA
  femoral p.
Biolox ball head p.
Biomet AGC knee p.
Biomet Discovery elbow p.
Biomet M2a-taper metal-on-metal
  hip system p.
Biometric p.
Biomet total toe p.
Bionic Ear p.
Bionit vascular p.
bisque-baked p.
Bivona-Colorado dummy p.
Bivona-Colorado voice p.
Bivona duckbill voice p.
Bivona Ultra Low voice p.
Björk-Shiley convexoconcave 60-
  degree valve p.
Björk-Shiley floating-disc p.
BK p.
bladder neck support p.
Blauth knee p.
Blom-Singer indwelling low-pressure
  voice p.
Blom-Singer tracheoesophageal p.
Bock knee p.
bovine collagen material p.
breast p.
Buchholz hip p.
Buechel-Pappas total ankle p.
Byars mandibular p.
Caffinière p.
caged-ball valve p.
Callender technique hip p.
Calnan-Nicolle synthetic digital
  joint p.
camouflage p.
Canadian hip disarticulation p.
Capetown aortic valve p.
CarboMedics cardiac valve p.
Carbon Copy HP foot p.
Carbon Copy II lightweight foot p.
Carbo-Seal Valsalva ascending
  aortic p.
Cardona keratoprosthesis p.
Carpentier annuloplasty ring p.
Carpentier-Edwards aortic valve p.
Carpentier-Edwards glutaraldehyde-
  preserved porcine xenograft p.
Carpentier-Rhone-Poulenc mitral
  ring p.
Carrion penile p.
Cartwright valve p.
Cathcart orthocentric hip p.

CDH Precoat Plus hip p.
Celestin endoesophageal p.
Centralign precoat hip p.
ceramic ossicular p.
Ceramion p.
Ceravital incus replacement p.
CFS hip p.
Charnley acetabular cup p.
Charnley cemented hip p.
Charnley-Hastings bipolar p.
Charnley hip p.
Charnley knee p.
Charnley-Mueller hip p.
Charnley total hip p.
chin p.
Chopart partial foot p.
Choyce MK II keratoprosthesis p.
Cintor knee p.
Cirrus foot p.
clamshell p.
cleft palate p.
C-Leg lower limb p.
Cloutier unconstrained knee p.
cobalt-chromium alloy p.
Co-Cr-W-Ni alloy p.
collar p.
College Park TruStep foot p.
combination gel/inflatable
  mammary p.
Conley mandibular p.
constrained rotating hinged knee p.
Cooley-Bloodwell mitral valve p.
Cooley Dacron p.
Coonrad-Morrey total elbow p.
C-2 OsteoCap hip p.
crimped Dacron p.
crimped-wire p.
Cronin Silastic mammary p.
Cross-Jones disc valve p.
Cross-Jones mitral valve p.
cruciate-retaining p.
cruciate-sacrificing p.
Crutchfield tongs p.
CSF p.
CUI artificial breast p.
CUI chin p.
CUI eye sphere p.
CUI gel-filled breast p.
CUI nasal p.
CUI saline mammary p.
CUI tendon p.
CUI testicular p.
Cutter-Smeloff aortic valve p.
Cutter-Smeloff cardiac valve p.
cylinder penile distensible p.
cylinder penile nondistensible p.
3D Accuscan facial p.
Dacron p.
Dacron arterial p.

Dacron bifurcation p.
Dallop-type fascial p.
Dana shoulder p.
Deane unconstrained knee p.
DeBakey ball-valve p.
DeBakey valve p.
Dee elbow p.
de la Caffiniére
  trapeziometacarpal p.
Delrin biomaterial joint
  replacement p.
Deon hip p.
DePalma hip p.
DePuy hip p.
Dilamezinsert penile p.
Dimension-C femoral stem p.
Dimension hip p.
Discovery elbow p.
distal radioulnar joint p.
double-pigtail p.
DRUJ p.
dual-lock total hip p.
duckbill voice p.
Duocondylar knee p.
Duo-Patellar knee p.
Duracon p.
Dura II positionable penile p.
DuraPhase inflatable penile p.
DuraPhase semirigid penile p.
Duromedics valve p.
dynamic penile p.
ear p.
ear pinna p.
ear piston p.
Eaton trapezium finger joint
  replacement p.
Edwards seamless p.
Edwards Teflon intracardiac
  patch p.
Ehmke ear p.
Eicher hip p.
Endoflex below-knee p.
Endo hinged knee p.
Endo rotating knee joint p.
Endo sled p.
Entegra p.
Epoca custom offset shoulder p.
ePTFE graft p.
Eriksson knee p.
ESKA-Jonas silicone-silver penile p.
EsophaCoil p.
esophageal p.

Esser p.
Ethicon Polytef paste p.
Ethrone p.
Evolution hip p.
Ewald elbow p.
expandable p.
fascia lata p.
femorofemoral crossover p.
Finn hinged knee replacement p.
First knee p.
fixed expansion p.
fixed femoral head p.
Flatow-Bigliani shoulder p.
Flatt finger p.
Flex-Foot p.
Flex H/A total ossicular p.
Flexi-Flate I, II penile p.
Flexi-Rod II penile p.
Flex-Walk foot p.
Fountain design p.
Fox p.
Free-Flow system p.
Freeman modular total hip p.
Freeman-Samuelson knee p.
Freeman-Swanson knee p.
fully constrained tricompartmental
  knee p.
Gaffney ankle p.
Galante hip p.
gel-filled breast p.
gel mammary p.
gel-saline Surgitek mammary p.
Gemini hip system p.
Geometric total knee p.
Georgiade breast p.
GFS Mark II inflatable penile p.
Gianturco p.
Gilbert p.
Giliberty acetabular p.
Gillette joint p.
Gillies p.
Girard keratoprosthesis p.
glass penile p.
glottic p.
Golaski vascular p.
Goodhill p.
Gore-Tex knee p.
Gott-Daggett heart valve p.
Gott low-profile p.
great toe p.
Greissinger foot p.
Gripper acetabular cup p.

NOTES

P

prosthesis *(continued)*

Groningen voice p.
Gruppe wire p.
GSB elbow p.
GSB knee p.
Guepar II hinged knee p.
Guilford-Wright p.
Gunston-Hult knee p.
Gunston polycentric knee p.
Gustilo knee p.
Haering esophageal p.
Hall-Kaster tilting-disc valve p.
Hamas upper limb p.
Hammersmith mitral valve p.
Hancock aortic valve p.
Hancock mitral valve p.
Hanger p.
Hanslik patellar p.
Harken p.
Harris cemented hip p.
Harris-Galante porous hip p.
Harris Micromini p.
Harrison interlocked mesh p.
Harris precoat p.
Hartley mammary p.
Haynes-Stellite implant metal p.
heart p.
Helanca seamless tube p.
Hemobahn endovascular p.
Henschke-Mauch SNS lower
   limb p.
Herbert knee p.
heterograft p.
Hexcel total condylar p.
Heyer-Schulte breast p.
HG Multilock hip p.
Hinderer malar p.
hinged constrained knee p.
hinged great toe replacement p.
hinged-leaflet vascular p.
hinged total knee p.
hingeless heart valve p.
hip disarticulation p.
Hittenberger p.
hollow sphere p.
homograft p.
Hosmer WALK p.
Hosmer weight-activated locking
   knee p.
House piston p.
House tantalum p.
House wire stapes p.
Howmedica Kinematic II knee p.
Howorth p.
Howse-Coventry hip p.
HPS II total hip p.
HSS total condylar knee p.
Hufnagel low-profile heart p.
Hunter tendon p.

hybrid p.
hydraulic knee unit p.
Hydroxial hip p.
hydroxyapatite ossicular p.
I-beam hemiarthroplasty hip p.
Icon foot p.
Identifit hip p.
Image custom external breast p.
immediate postoperative p. (IPOP)
Impact modular porous p.
implant-supported fixed p.
Impra collagen-impregnated
   Dacron p.
incus replacement p.
Indong Oh p.
Infinity modular hip p.
inflatable mammary p.
inflatable Mentor penile p.
inflatable penile p.
Inronail fingernail p.
Inronail toenail p.
Integral Interlok femoral p.
Intermedics Natural-Knee knee p.
internal ear p.
Introl bladder neck support p.
Ionescu-Shiley aortic valve p.
Iowa Precoat total hip p.
Iowa total hip p.
iridium p.
ischial weightbearing p.
isoelastic pelvic p.
Ivalon p.
Jenny mammary p.
Jewett p.
Jobst p.
Jonas penile p.
Jonathan Livingston Seagull
   patella p.
Joplin toe p.
Judet hip p.
KAFO p.
Kaster mitral valve p.
Kaufman III anti-incontinence p.
Kaufman male urinary
   incontinence p.
Kay-Shiley disc valve p.
Kay-Suzuki p.
K/B p.
KD chin p.
Keeler p.
Kessler p.
Kirschner Modular IIC shoulder p.
Kirschner total shoulder p.
KMC femoral stem p.
KMW/PC femoral p.
knee-bearing p.
knitted p.
knitted Teflon p.
knitted vascular p.

Koenig MPJ p.
Krause-Wolfe p.
Kudo elbow p.
Lacey p.
Lagrange-Letoumel hip p.
Lanceford p.
Landers-Foulks p.
Lattimer Silastic testicular p.
Leadbetter-Politano ureteral
 implant p.
Leake Dacron mandible p.
Leeds-Keio ligament p.
Leinbach head and neck total
 hip p.
Lewis expandable adjustable p.
 (LEAP)
Lezinski Flex-HA PORP ossicular
 chain p.
Lillehei-Cruz-Kaster valve p.
Link MP hip noncemented
 reconstruction p.
Lippman hip p.
Lippy modified p.
Liverpool knee p.
locking p.
Longevity V-Lign hip p.
Lord total hip p.
Lorenz SMO p.
lower limb p.
low-pressure voice p.
low-profile p.
Lubinus knee p.
lunate p.
MacIntosh tibial plateau p.
MacNab-English shoulder p.
Macrofit hip p.
madreporic hip p.
Magnuson valve p.
malleable p.
malleus-incus p.
Mallory-Head porous primary
 femoral p.
mammary p.
Mammatech breast p.
mandibular p.
Mangat curvilinear chin p.
Marlex mesh p.
Marlex methyl methacrylate p.
Marmor modular knee p.
Master step foot p.
M2a-taper metal-on-metal hip
 system p.

Matchett-Brown p.
Mathys p.
Matrol femoral head p.
maxillary p.
Mayo semiconstrained elbow p.
Mayo total ankle p.
McBride femoral p.
McBride-Moore p.
McCutchen SLT hip p.
McGee ear piston p.
McGehee elbow p.
McGhan breast p.
McKee-Farrar hip p.
McKee femoral p.
McKee totally constrained elbow p.
McKeever patellar cap p.
McNaught p.
MCP finger joint p.
Meadox-Cooley woven low-
 porosity p.
Meadox woven velour p.
mechanical p.
Mecring acetabluar p.
Medi-graft vascular p.
Medoc-Celestin endoprosthesis p.
Medtronic-Hall heart valve p.
Medtronic-Hall tilting-disc valve p.
Megasource penile p.
Meme breast p.
Mentor Alpha 1 inflatable
 penile p.
Mentor breast p.
Mentor GFS penile p.
Mentor IPP penile p.
Mentor malleable penile p.
Mentor Mark II penile p.
Mentor saline-filled testicular p.
Mentor Self-Cath penile p.
Mentor Spectrum mammary p.
mesh stent p.
metacarpophalangeal p.
metal bucket-handle p.
metal femoral head p.
metal-on-metal articulating
 intervertebral disc p.
Metasul hip p.
Meyerding p.
MGH knee p.
Microloc knee p.
Microvel p.
middle ear p.
Miller-Galante hip p.

NOTES

P

prosthesis *(continued)*
Milliknit arterial p.
Milliknit Dacron p.
Milliknit vascular graft p.
Minneapolis hip p.
Mittlemeir ceramic hip p.
modified Moore hip locking p.
modular Austin Moore hip p.
modular total hip p.
Monk hip p.
Monostrut cardiac valve p.
Moon-Robinson stapes p.
Moore femoral neck p.
Moretz p.
Moseley glenoid rim p.
Mueller-Charnley total hip p.
Mueller total hip p.
Mules p.
Mulligan Silastic p.
Murray knee p.
myoelectric p.
Naden-Rieth p.
nasal p.
natural-feel breast p.
Natural-Hip p.
Natural-Lok acetabular cup p.
NEB total hip p.
Neer I, II, III shoulder p.
neural p.
NeuroCybernetic p.
Neville tracheal reconstruction p.
Neville tracheobronchial p.
New Jersey hemiarthroplasty p.
New Jersey-LCS shoulder p.
New Jersey-LCS total knee p.
New Weavenit Dacron p.
Nexus hip p.
Nicoll tendon p.
Niebauer finger joint
  replacement p.
Niebauer trapezium replacement p.
Niehaber p.
Noiles posterior stabilized knee p.
Noiles rotating-hinge total knee p.
nonhinged knee p.
ocular p.
Odland ankle p.
offset modified p.
Oklahoma ankle p.
Omnicarbon heart valve p.
Omnifit knee p.
OmniPhase penile p.
Omniscience single-leaflet cardiac
  valve p.
orbital floor p.
Oregon p.
Orlon vascular p.
Orthofix p.
Ortron modular femoral p.

ossicular chain replacement p.
OsteoCap hip p.
Osteolock hip p.
Osteonics p.
Otto Bock electric hands p.
Otto Bock Greissinger Plus foot p.
Oxford p.
Padgett p.
palatal p.
Panje voice p.
partial ossicular reconstruction p.
  (PORP)
partial ossicular replacement p.
  (PORP)
patellar tendon-bearing below-
  knee p.
PC Performer knee p.
Pearman penile p.
pegged tibial p.
Perfecta hip p.
Performance knee p.
pericardial p.
periodontal p.
Perras mammary p.
Perras-Papillon breast p.
Phoenix total hip p.
Pillet hand p.
piston stapes p.
Plasticor p.
Plasti-Pore ossicular replacement p.
Plystan p.
Polycel bone composite p.
polycentric knee p.
polyethylene talar p.
polytetrafluoroethylene p.
polyvinyl p.
porcine p.
Porocool p.
porous-coated anatomic knee p.
Precision Osteolock femoral p.
Preclude Dura Substitute p.
Precoat Plus femoral p.
Press-Fit p.
Pritchard total elbow p.
ProAdvantage knee p.
Profile hip p.
Proplast p.
Prostalac total hip p.
Protasul femoral p.
Protek p.
Proud septal p.
Provox voice p.
PTB cast p.
PTS p.
Quantum foot p.
RAM knee p.
Ranawat-Burstein hip p.
Rashkind double-disc occluder p.
Rastelli p.

Reese p.
Reverdin p.
Revive system penile p.
R-HAB lighter weight ankle p.
Richards hydroxyapatite PORP p.
Richards hydroxyapatite TORP p.
Richards maximum contact cruciate-
  sparing p.
Richards Zirconia femoral head p.
Ring hip p.
Ring knee p.
Robinson incus replacement p.
Robinson middle ear p.
Robinson-Moon-Lippy stapes p.
Robinson-Moon stapes p.
Robinson piston p.
Robinson stapes p.
Rochester HKAFO p.
Rock-Mulligan p.
Rose L-type nose bridge p.
Rosenfeld hip p.
Rosen inflatable urinary
  incontinence p.
rotating-hinge knee p.
Rothman Institute femoral p.
Ruddy stapes p.
SACH p.
sacral segmental nerve stimulation
  implantable neural p.
saddle p.
Safian design p.
Safian rhinoplasty p.
Saint George knee p.
Saint Jude p.
saline mammary p.
Sampson p.
Sauerbruch p.
Sauvage fabric graft p.
Sauvage filamentous p.
Savastano Hemi-Knee p.
Sbarbaro p.
Scarborough p.
SCDT heart valve p.
Scheer Tef-wire p.
Schlein total elbow p.
Schlein trisurface ankle p.
Schuknecht Gelfoam wire p.
Schuknecht Teflon wire piston p.
Schurring ossicle cup p.
Scott AMS inflatable penile p.
Scurasil p.
seamless p.

Seattle Foot p.
Select ankle p.
Select shoulder p.
self-articulating femoral p.
self-centering Universal hip p.
semiconstrained knee p.
Sense-of-Feel p.
shaft p.
Shea polyethylene p.
Shea Teflon piston p.
Sheehan knee p.
Sheehy incus replacement p.
Shier knee p.
shoulder p.
Silastic ball spacer p.
Silastic chin p.
Silastic fimbrial p.
Silastic mammary p.
Silastic otoplasty p.
Silastic penile p.
Silastic sheeting keel p.
Silastic standard elastometer p.
Silastic testicular p.
Silflex intramedullary p.
silicone doughnut p.
silicone elastomer p.
silicone gel p.
silicone trapezium p.
silicone voice p.
Silima breast p.
Siloxane p.
Siltex Becker breast p.
Singer-Blom ossicular p.
Singh speech system voice
  rehabilitation p.
single-axis ankle p.
Sinterlock implant metal p.
Sivash hip p.
Small-Carrion penile p.
Smeloff-Cutter aortic ball valve p.
Smith-Petersen hip cup p.
Smith total ankle p.
SMo p.
Snyder breast p.
solid-ankle, cushioned-heel foot p.
solid silicone orbital p.
Sorin bicarbon bileaflet mitral
  valve p.
Souter-Strathclyde total elbow p.
Sparks mandrel p.
Spectron p.
spherocentric knee p.

NOTES

P

prosthesis *(continued)*

Springlite Advantage DP p.
Springlite lower limb p.
S-ROM femoral stem p.
stabilocondylar knee p.
Stanmore shoulder p.
stapedectomy p.
Starr ball heart p.
Starr-Edwards aortic valve p.
Starr-Edwards caged-ball valve p.
Starr-Edwards disc valve p.
STD+ titanium total hip p.
stemmed tibial p.
Stenzel rod p.
Stevens-Street elbow p.
St. George total elbow p.
St. Jude Medical mitral valve p.
Subrini penile p.
Sulzer p.
Supramid p.
Surgitek penile p.
Sutter double-stem silicone
  implant p.
Sutter MCP finger joint p.
Sutter-Smeloff heart valve p.
Swanson finger joint p.
Swanson flexible hallux valgus p.
Swanson great toe p.
Swanson metacarpal p.
Swanson metatarsal p.
Swanson Silastic elbow p.
Swanson wrist p.
Syme amputation p.
Syme foot p.
Synatomic total knee p.
Taperloc femoral p.
TARA total hip p.
TCCK unconstrained knee p.
Techmedica p.
Teflon tri-leaflet p.
Teflon woven p.
temporary p.
tendon p.
testicular p.
Tevdek p.
Thackray hip p.
Tharies hip replacement p.
Thiersch p.
T-28 hip p.
Thompson femoral head p.
Thompson femoral neck p.
Thompson hemiarthroplasty hip p.
threaded titanium acetabular p.
Thrust femoral p.
Ti-Bac II hip p.
tibial plateau p.
Ti/CoCr hip p.
Tilastin hip p.
tilting-disc aortic valve p.

titanium p.
tivanium hip p.
TMJ Fossa-Eminence p.
TMJ reconstruction p.
toe p.
Tornier radial head p.
TORP p.
torque-type p.
total alloplastic TMJ
  reconstruction p.
total ossicular p.
total ossicular replacement p.
Townley TARA p.
Townley total knee p.
trapeziometacarpal joint
  replacement p.
TR-28 hip p.
Triad p.
trial p.
triaxial semiconstrained elbow p.
Tricon-M cruciate-sparing p.
Tricon-M patellar p.
trileaflet p.
Trilicon external breast p.
Tronzo p.
trunnion-bearing hip p.
TruStep foot p.
Tygon endoesophageal p.
UCI p.
Ultima total hip p.
Ultra low-resistance voice p.
Ultrex Plus penile p.
umbrella-type p.
unconstrained p.
unicondylar p.
Uni-Flate 1000 penile p.
Universal p.
unsutured Dacron p.
upper extremity myoelectric p.
urinary incontinence p.
UroLume endourethral Wallstent p.
USCI bifurcated Vasculour II p.
USCI-DeBakey vascular p.
USCI Sauvage EXS side-limb p.
Usher Marlex mesh p.
Utah arm electronic p.
vaginal prolapse p.
Valls p.
valve p.
valved voice p.
Vanghetti limb p.
vascular graft p.
Vasculour-II vascular p.
Vascutek vascular p.
Vitallium cobalt-chrome alloy p.
Vitallium Moore self-locking p.
Vivosil p.
Voltz wrist joint p.
Wada hingeless heart valve p.

Wagner resurfaced p.
Walldius Vitallium mechanical
knee p.
Wallstent esophageal p.
Warsaw hip p.
Waugh p.
Wayfarer p.
Weaveknit vascular p.
Wehrs incus p.
Weller total hip joint p.
Wesolowski vascular p.
Wheeler p.
Whiteside p.
Wiles p.
Wilke boot p.
Wilson-Cook esophageal p.
wire-fat ear p.
wire stapes p.
Wolf p.
woven-tube vascular graft p.
Wright knee p.
Xenophor femoral p.
Zimaloy femoral head p.
Zimmer Centralign Precoat hip p.
Zimmer shoulder p.
Zimmer tibial p.
Ziramic femoral head p.
zirconia orthopaedic p.
Zweymuller-Alloclassic p.
Zweymuller hip p.

prosthetic
p. antibiotic-loaded acrylic cement
p. appliance
p. buttock contour
p. cup
p. foam
p. graft
p. heart valve
p. lens
p. ossicular reconstruction procedure
(PORP)
p. poppet
p. socket
p. valve holder
p. valve sewing ring
ProStretch exerciser
Prosurg RollerLoop electrode
ProSys
P. leg bag
P. Samec D, self-adhering,
nonlatex male external catheter,
short sheath

P. Samec NL, self-adhering
nonlatex male external catheter,
normal length sheath
P. silicone sterile 2-way, 3-way
Foley catheter
P. Urahesive system
Protasul femoral prosthesis
Pro-Tech nasal prongs
ProTect abutment
ProtectaCap
P. headgear
P. + Plus headgear
Protectaid contraceptive sponge
Protect-a-Pass suture passer
protected
p. bronchoscopic brush
p. knife handle
p. specimen brush
p. specimen microbiology brush
Protection Plus belted undergarment
protective
p. bandage
p. dressing
p. glasses
p. mattress cover
protector
Adson dural p.
Air-Limb amputation p.
alar p.
AquaShield bandage p.
AquaShield cast p.
Arroyo p.
Arruga p.
BIP breast implant p.
bite p.
Buratto flap p.
cast cutter p.
Cast Gard cast p.
CastGuard foot p.
Crouch corneal p.
dural p.
eggcrate p.
EpiFlex heel and elbow p.
eye p.
p. guide
hearing p.
Heelbo decubitus p.
Heeler inflatable heel p.
HP1035 gel heel p.
Isovis wound p.
Joseph saw p.
Jurgan pin p.

NOTES

P

protector *(continued)*
    KINS fitted mattress p.
    Kodel polyester elbow p.
    Lapwall wound p.
    Meds eye p.
    P. meniscus suturing system
    MF heel p.
    oculoplasty corneal p.
    Opti-Gard eye p.
    Patellar Band knee p.
    plastic corneal p.
    p. plus wire
    port p.
    Pre-Vent elbow p.
    Pre-Vent heel p.
    Pre-Vent ulnar nerve p.
    pulse ox p.
    Roho heel p.
    Seal-Tight cast p.
    ShowerSafe waterproof cast and
      bandage p.
    P. suturing device
    Terumo transducer p.
    The Heeler inflatable heel p.
    tissue p.
    Ultra-Care heel/elbow p.
    Vi-Drape wound p.
    Vinciguerra LASEK p.
    ViraGuard viral-blocking
      transducer p.
    X-Tend back p.
Protecto splint
Protect Point needle
Protégé
    P. Plus microscope
    P. self-expanding nitinol stent
    P. 3010 syringe infusion pump
Protege manual flexion distraction table
Protegen material
Protek
    P. joint implant
    P. prosthesis
Pro-Tex face shield
ProThotics orthotic
ProTime microcoagulation system
Protocult stool collection kit
protological biopsy forceps
proton-density axial MR scan
proton-density-weighted MRI
proton MR spectroscopy
ProTon tonometer
prototype cholangioscope
Protouch
    P. orthopaedic padding
    P. pad
ProTrac
    P. ACL tibial guide

    P. cruciate reconstruction
      measurement device
    P. cruciate reconstruction system
protractor
    cephalometric p.
    Dexterity p.
    Harrington p.
protrusio
    p. cage
    p. shell
Pro-Turn frameless air support therapy
Proud
    P. adenoidectomy forceps
    P. fascia crusher
    P. infant turbinate speculum
    P. septal prosthesis
Proud-Beck pharyngoscope
Proud-White uvula retractor
Pro-Vent
    P.-V. arterial blood sampling kit
    P.-V. Plus arterial blood sampling
      kit
Provide incontinence pad
Providence
    P. Hospital artery forceps
    P. Hospital clamp
    P. Hospital hemostat
    P. scoliosis system
Provider
    P. 6000 ambulatory dual-channel
      infusion pump
    P. 5500 patient-controlled analgesia
      device
Proview
    P. eye pressure monitor
    P. eye pressure tonometer
provisional liner
Pro-Vit cutter
Provit filling material
Provocative sensitivity balloon
Provox
    P. FreeHands heat/moisture
      exchanger
    P. tracheoesophageal speaking valve
    P. voice prosthesis
Prowler microcatheter
Proxiderm wound closure system
Proxi-Floss cleaning appliance
proximal
    p. cement spacer
    p. occlusion catheter (POC)
    p. over-shoulder strap
Proximate
    P. disposable skin stapler
    P. flexible linear stapler
    P. hemorrhoid circular stapler
    P. linear cutter
    P. Plus MD skin stapler
    P. PX skin stapler

P. RH skin stapler
P. TX linear stapler
Proximate-ILS curved intraluminal stapler
Proxi-Strip skin closure
ProYellow+ vascular treatment laser
Pruitt
P. anoscope
P. irrigation catheter
P. occlusion catheter
P. proctoscope
P. vascular shunt
Pruitt-Inahara
P.-I. balloon-tipped perfusion catheter
P.-I. carotid shunt
P.-I. vascular shunt
PRx implantable cardioverter-defibrillator
Pryor-Péan vaginal retractor
PS
PS Medical Flow Control valve
PS 153 stent
PS-2 needle
PSA thermoplastic orthosis
PSC
pronation spring control
PSC fertility monitor
pseudoisochromatic plate
PSI-Tec aspiration platform
psoas retractor
PSS
PSS Powered disposable skin stapler
PSS prostate seeding set
PTA
percutaneous transluminal angioplasty
PTA balloon catheter
PTB
patellar tendon bearing
pretibial bearing
pretibial buttress
PTB brace
PTB cast prosthesis
PTBD
percutaneous transhepatic biliary drainage
PTBD catheter
PTCA
percutaneous transluminal coronary angioplasty
PTCA catheter

Freeway PTCA
PTCA rapid exchange catheter
PTD
percutaneous thrombolytic device
Arrow-Trerotola PTD
PTDP
permanent transvenous demand pacemaker
pterygium
p. knife
p. scissors
pterygoid chisel
PTFE
polytetrafluoroethylene
PTFE Gore-Tex graft
PTFE mesh
PTFE shunt
PTFE-containing implant
PTFE-covered Palmaz stent
ptosis
p. clamp
p. forceps
p. knife
p. scissors
p. snare
PTS
PTS Panels test strip
PTS prosthesis
PU
polyurethane
PU catheter
Pucci
P. Air orthotic
P. inflatable knee orthosis
P. pediatrics hand orthosis
P. splint
Pucci-Seed
P.-S. hook
P.-S. spatula
Puck film changer
PuddleVac floor suction device
Puddu tibial aimer
pudendal
p. block anesthesia needle
p. needle guide
Pudenz
P. barium cardiac catheter
P. flushing valve
P. infant cardiac catheter
P. peritoneal catheter
P. reservoir
P. tube

NOTES

P

Pudenz *(continued)*
    P. valve-flushing shunt
    P. ventricular catheter
Pudenz-Heyer
    P.-H. clamp
    P.-H. vascular catheter
Pudenz-Schulte thecoperitoneal shunt
Puestow
    P. dilator
    P. guidewire
Puestow-Olander gastrointestinal tube
Pugh
    P. barrel component
    P. driver
    P. hip pin
    P. self-adjusting nail
Puig
    P. Massana annuloplasty ring
    P. Massana-Shiley annuloplasty ring
    P. Massana-Shiley annuloplasty
      valve
Puka chisel
Pulec needle
Pul-Ez
    P.-E. exerciser
    P.-E. shoulder pulley
pull
    p. knife
    Ponsky p.
pull-apart introducer
puller
pulley
    p. passer
    Preston overhead p.
    Pul-Ez shoulder p.
    Range-Master p.
    shoulder p.
pull-out button
pull-type gastrostomy tube
Pulmanex resuscitator
Pulmo-Aide
    P.-A. nebulizer
    P.-A. ventilator
PulmoMate nebulizer
Pulmo-Mist compressor
Pulmonair 40 bed
pulmonary
    p. arterial clamp
    p. arterial forceps
    p. arterial snare
    p. artery balloon pump
    p. artery catheter
    p. artery sling
    p. autograft valve
    p. balloon
    p. embolism clamp
    p. flotation catheter
    p. nodulectomy clamp

    p. retractor
    p. triple-lumen catheter
    p. vessel clamp
    p. vessel forceps
Pulmonex dynamic air therapy unit
pulmonic stenosis clamp
Pulmopak pump
PulmoSonic ultrasonic nebulizer
pulpal microdialysis probe
pulp canal file
Pulpdent
    P. cavity liner
    P. Ortho Band cement
pulped muscle dressing
Pulsair tonometer
Pulsar
    P. DDD pacemaker
    P. MAX II pacemaker
    P. Max II pacemaker system
    P. NI implantable pacemaker
    P. obstetrical 2-channel TENS unit
pulsatile jet lavage
pulsating low-air-loss bed
Pulsator
    P. anaerobic syringe
    P. dry heparin arterial blood gas
      kit
Pulsatron II handheld nerve stimulator
Pulsavac lavage
pulse
    p. amplifier
    p. lavage
    p. oximeter
    p. ox protector
    P. Pro heart rate monitor
    p. spray catheter
    p. wave Doppler
PulseCO hemodynamic monitor
pulsed
    p. angiolaser
    p. Doppler
    p. Doppler ultrasonic flowmeter
    p. Doppler ultrasound
    p. dye laser
    p. galvanic stimulator
    p. light
    p. metal vapor laser
    p. pump
    p. tunable dye laser
    p. ultrasonic velocity detector
    p. yellow dye laser
PulseDose oxygen conserver
pulsed-range gated Doppler
pulsed-wave Doppler transducer
pulse-height analyzer
PulseMaster laser
Pulse-Pak infusion kit
PulseSpray pulsed infusion system

Pulsolith
P. coumarin pulsed-dye laser
P. laser lithotripter
Pulsox-5
Pulsoxymeter P.-5
Pulsoxymeter Pulsox-5
pulverizer
Thermovac tissue p.
Pulvertaft suture
Pulvograft
Dembone demineralized cortical
powder P.
Osteomin Thermo-Ashed bone
powder P.
pumice stone
pump
Abbott infusion p.
ACAT 1 Plus intraaortic
balloon p.
AccurRx constant flow
implantable p.
ACMI Dolphin p.
Advanced Collection breast p.
Affinity blood p.
Alzet continuous-infusion
osmotic p.
ambulatory volumetric infusion p.
Ameda Egnell breast p.
aortic balloon p.
Arrow AutoCAT intraaortic
balloon p.
Arthrex AR-6400 Continuous Wave
II arthroscopy p.
Asahi blood plasma p.
Asid Bonz PP infusion p.
AutoCat intraaortic balloon p.
Autosyringe p.
Auto Syringe AS50 infusion p.
Avco intraaortic balloon p.
AV Impulse foot p.
Axiom double sump p.
balloon p.
Bard cardiopulmonary support p.
Bard Infus-OR syringe-type
infusion p.
Bard PCA p.
Bard TransAct intraaortic
balloon p.
Barron p.
Basis breast p.
battery-operated breast p.
Baxter ambulatory PCA p.

Baxter ambulatory volumetric
infusion p.
Baxter Flo-Gard 8200 volumetric
infusion p.
Betabed alternating pressure p.
bilateral breast p.
BioMedic microdelivery peel p.
Bio-Medicus centrifugal p.
Bio-Pump centrifugal blood p.
blood p.
Bluemle p.
breast p.
BVS p.
CADD-Plus intravenous infusion p.
CADD-TPN p.
cardiopulmonary bypass p.
Carones LASEK p.
Carrel-Lindbergh p.
centrifugal p.
Chicco breast p.
Chid breast p.
Clarus model 5169 peristaltic p.
Cobe Revolution centrifugal
blood p.
Colleague p.
Companion feeding p.
Compat enteral feeding p.
compression p.
computer-controlled infusion p.
Conjugate export p.
continuous subcutaneous insulin
infusion p.
Continuous Wave II arthroscopy p.
Cordis Hakim p.
Cordis implantable drug delivery p.
Cordis Secor implantable p.
Cormed ambulatory infusion p.
CPI #9100 insulin p.
CTI infusion p.
Curlin 2000 Plus p.
Datascope System 90 intraaortic
balloon p.
DeBakey VAD continuous-axial-
flow p.
Deltec-Pharmacia CADD p.
DeVilbiss suction p.
Disetronic infuser syringe p.
drug infusion p.
D-Tron insulin p.
DuraNeb portable nebulizer p.
ECMO p.
Egnell breast p.

P

pump *(continued)*
elastomeric p.
Elmed peristaltic irrigation p.
Entera-Flo enteral feeding p.
Enteroport feeding p.
external drug infusion p.
extracorporeal p.
extremity p.
EZ hand p.
Felig insulin p.
Fenwal hemapheresis p.
flexible p.
Flexiflo Companion enteral
  nutrition p.
Flexiflo feeding p.
Flocare 500 feeding p.
Flo-Gard p.
Frenta Mat feeding p.
Frenta System II feeding p.
Gemini PC1 IV p.
Gomco thoracic drainage p.
Grafco breast p.
Graseby anesthesia p.
Gynkotek p.
Hakim-Cordis p.
Hardy-Sella p.
Harvard 2 dual-syringe p.
heart p.
HeartMate portable p.
hepatic artery infusion p.
Hermes-Ready p.
Holter p.
H-TRON plus V100 insulin
  infusion p.
Imed Gemini PC-2 volumetric p.
Imed infusion p.
implantable osmotic p.
implanted infusion p.
Infumed p.
InfuO.R. drug delivery p.
Infusaid infusion p.
Infuse-a-Port p.
infusion p.
P. In Style breast pump
insulin infusion p.
Intelliject p.
intermittent extremity p.
intraaortic balloon p. (IABP)
ion p.
Isoflow p.
IsoMed implantable drug p.
IVAC volumetric infusion p.
Jobst athrombotic p.
Jobst extremity p.
KAAT II Plus intraaortic
  balloon p.
Kangaroo feeding p.
Kendall McGaw Intelligent p.
Keofeed II enteral feeding p.

Keofeed infusion p.
Klein p.
KM-1 breast p.
Lactina Select breast p.
Lamis Autofuse infusion p.
left ventricular bypass p.
Lifestream centrifugal p.
Lindbergh p.
Linvatec arthroscopic infusion p.
LVAS implantable p.
Lymphapress compression p.
MagMag breast p.
Mary Jane breast p.
MasterFlex p.
Master Flow Pumpette p.
McGaw volumetric p.
McKinley EpM p.
Medela Dominant vacuum
  delivery p.
Medela manual breast p.
Medex Protege 3010 syringe
  infusion p.
Medfusion 1001, 2001 syringe
  infusion p.
Medtronic MiniMed 508 insulin p.
Medtronic SynchroMed implantable
  infusion p.
MicroDelivery Peel p.
Microjet Quark portable p.
Miltex p.
MiniMed III infusion p.
Mityvac vacuum p.
Multipulse 1000 compression p.
Na-K exchange p.
Neuroperfusion p.
Nezhat-Dorsey hydrodissection p.
Norport p.
Nutromat Pad S feeding p.
Ohmeda 9000 computer-cotrolled
  infusion p.
On-Q p.
p. oxygenator
PainPump p.
Pancretec p.
Panomat infusion p.
Paradigm insulin infusion p.
Paragon ambulatory p.
patient-controlled analgesia p.
PCA p.
Perfusor compact S syringe p.
peristaltic irrigation p.
Pfeiffer mechanical dosing p.
portable insulin infusion p.
programmable p.
Protégé 3010 syringe infusion p.
Provider 6000 ambulatory dual-
  channel infusion p.
pulmonary artery balloon p.
Pulmopak p.

pulsed p.
Pump In Style breast p.
Quantum enteral p.
rapid infusion p.
roller p.
roller head perfusion p.
Sage Instruments syringe p.
Salem p.
Sarns 7000 MDX p.
Sarns Siok II blood p.
Sartorius breast p.
sequential extremity p.
Servo p.
Shiley Infusaid p.
Sigma 6000+ infusion p.
Space-Saver volumetric p.
S-Scort VX-2 suction p.
Stat 2 Pumpette disposable IV p.
Stryker PainPump p.
subcutaneous insulin infusion p.
subcutaneous morphine p.
sump p.
surgical suction p.
SurgiPeace analgesia p.
SynchroMed implantable
  programmable p.
syringe-type infusion p.
Talley p.
Thoratec p.
Tonkaflo p.
Travenol infusion p.
TurboStaltic p.
Unicare breast p.
Verifuse ambulatory infusion p.
Versaflow p.
volumetric infusion p.
pumped dye laser
Pumpette
  Master Flow P.
**Pump-It-Up pneumatic socket volume
  management system**
PumpPals insole
Pump-Vac Plus system
punch
  Abrams pleural biopsy p.
  Acufex rotary p.
  adenoid p.
  Adler attic ear p.
  Ainsworth p.
  Alexander antrostomy p.
  Anderson biopsy p.
  antral p.

aortic p.
arthroscopic p.
baby Tischler biopsy p.
backbiting bone p.
Bailey p.
Baker p.
Barron corneal p.
Baumgartner p.
Berens corneoscleral p.
biopsy p.
p. block
bone p.
bone hole p.
Brock infundibular p.
Brooks adenoidal p.
Bruening p.
Buerger p.
Carpel One-Step trabeculectomy p.
Caspari suture p.
Casteyer prostatic p.
Castroviejo corneoscleral p.
Cault p.
cervical p.
Charnley femoral prosthesis
  neck p.
Christensen ophthalmic p.
cigar handle basket p.
Citelli bone p.
Citelli laminectomy p.
Citelli-Meltzer atticus p.
CleanCut rotation aortic p.
Cloward bone p.
Cloward-Dowel p.
Cloward-English p.
Cloward-Harper cervical p.
Cloward intervertebral p.
Cloward square p.
Cone bone p.
cone skull p.
Cordes circular p.
Cordes ethmoidal p.
Cordes semicircular p.
Cordes sphenoidal p.
Cordes square p.
Corgill bone p.
corneal p.
corneoscleral p.
Cottingham p.
cruciate p.
cutaneous p.
Davol canal wall p.
Descemet membrane p.

NOTES

P

755

punch *(continued)*
Deyerle p.
disposable aortic rotating p.
Dorsey cervical foraminal p.
Dyonics suction p.
DyoVac suction p.
Ellison glenoid rim p.
Eppendorfer biopsy p.
ethmoid p.
Ferris-Smith-Kerrison bone p.
finned-stem p.
fluted-stem p.
p. forceps
Frangenheim hook p.
Frenckner-Stille p.
Gass cervical p.
Gass corneoscleral p.
Gass scleral p.
Gass sclerotomy p.
Gelfoam p.
Gellhorn uterine biopsy p.
Goldman cartilage p.
Goosen vascular p.
Gruenwald nasal p.
p. guide
Gusberg endocervical biopsy p.
hair transplant p.
Haitz canaliculus p.
Hajek-Koffler reversible p.
Hajek-Koffler sphenoidal p.
Hajek-Skillern sphenoidal p.
Hardy sellar p.
Harper cervical laminectomy p.
Hartmann biopsy p.
Hartmann-Citelli ear p.
Hartmann ear p.
Hartmann nasal p.
Hartmann tonsillar p.
Hirsch hypophyseal p.
Holth corneoscleral p.
Holth-Rubin p.
Holth scleral p.
Holth sclerectomy p.
Housepian sellar p.
I-beam cement p.
I-beam press-fit p.
infundibular p.
Ingraham skull p.
Jackson p.
Jacobson vessel p.
Jansen-Middleton septal p.
Johnson-Kerrison p.
Joseph p.
Karolinska-Stille p.
Karp aortic p.
Kelly p.
Kelly-Descemet membrane p.
Kerrison bone p.
Kerrison-Jacoby p.

Kerrison laminectomy p.
Kerrison-Rhoton sellar p.
Keyes cutaneous biopsy p.
Keyes dermatologic p.
Keyes skin p.
Keyes vulvar p.
keyhole p.
King adenoidal p.
Klause antral p.
Klause-Carmody antral p.
Klein p.
Knighton-Kerrison p.
Koffler-Hajek sphenoidal p.
Krause angular oval p.
Lange antral p.
Lebsche sternal p.
Leksell p.
Lempert malleus p.
Lermoyez nasal p.
Lewis-Resnik p.
linear scissor p.
Lineback adenoidal p.
Lund-Dodick p.
Luntz-Dodick p.
MacKenty sphenoidal p.
Mauermayer stone p.
McGoey Vitallium p.
Meltzer adenoid p.
Meltzer tonsillar p.
Mendez-Schubert aortic p.
Merz aortic p.
MGM glenoidal p.
Miltex disposable biopsy p.
Mixter brain biopsy p.
modified sclerectomy p.
Mulligan cervical biopsy p.
Murphy p.
Myerson biting p.
Myles nasal p.
nasal p.
Noyes chalazion p.
O'Connor hook p.
Orentreich p.
Osborne p.
ostrum antral p.
Pfau atticus sphenoidal p.
Phemister p.
pleural biopsy p.
Pollock p.
Price corneal p.
Pritikin scleral p.
Raney laminectomy p.
Rathke p.
Reaves p.
Rhoton sellar p.
Richter laminectomy p.
p. rongeur
Ronis adenoidal p.
Ronis tonsillar p.

Rothman-Gilbard corneal p.
Rowe glenoidal p.
Rubin-Holth sclerectomy p.
Sachs cervical p.
Scheicher laminectomy p.
Scheinmann biting p.
Schlesinger cervical p.
Schmeden tonsillar p.
Schnaudigel sclerotomy p.
Schubert-Van Doren uterine
  biopsy p.
scleral p.
sclerectomy p.
sclerotomy p.
Seiffert grasping p.
Seletz Universal Kerrison p.
sellar p.
side-biting ostrum p.
Skillern p.
skin p.
skull p.
Smeden tonsillar p.
Smillie nail p.
Smithuysen sphenoidal p.
Sparks atrioseptal p.
Spencer oval p.
sphenoidal bone p.
Spies ethmoidal p.
Spurling-Kerrison laminectomy p.
Stammberger antral p.
Stevenson capsular p.
Storz corneoscleral p.
Storz intranasal antral p.
Stough p.
Struyken p.
suction p.
suture p.
Swan corneoscleral p.
Sweet sternal p.
Takahashi ethmoidal p.
Takahashi nasal p.
Tanne corneal p.
Thompson p.
Tischler cervical biopsy p.
Tischler-Morgan biopsy p.
Tomey trabeculectomy p.
tonsillar p.
Townsend biopsy p.
p. trephine
Troutman p.
Turkel prostatic p.
uterine biopsy p.

Van Struyken nasal p.
Veenema-Gusberg prostatic p.
vessel p.
Wagner antral p.
Walser corneoscleral p.
Walton-Schubert p.
Watson-Williams ethmoidal p.
Weck endoscopic suture p.
Whitcomb-Kerrison laminectomy p.
Wilde ethmoidal p.
Wilde nasal p.
Williams-Watson ethmoidal p.
Wittner cervical biopsy p.
Woolley tibia p.
Yankauer antral p.
Yeoman biopsy p.
punched-out orchidometer
punctal
  p. dilator
  p. lens
punctum
  p. dilator
  p. plug
puncture
  p. needle
  p. transducer
puncture-tip needle
Punctur-Guard
  P.-G. needle
  P.-G. Revolution safety needle
  holder
Puno-Winter-Byrd (PWB)
  P.-W.-B. transpedicular spine
  fixation system
Puntenney
  P. forceps
  P. tying forceps
Puntowicz arterial forceps
pupil
  p. dilator
  p. spreader forceps
pupillary membrane scissors
pupillograph
pupillometer
  Colvard p.
  Pupilscan II p.
pupilloscope
Pupilscan II pupillometer
PuraPly wound dressing
Pura-Vario stent
**Purcell self-retaining abdominal
  retractor**

NOTES

P

purifier
- Air Supply air p.
- Bemis air p.

Purilon gel dressing

Puritan
- P. Bennett Aeris 590 concentrator
- P. Bennett 7250 metabolic monitor
- P. Bennett Simplicity spirometer
- P. Bennett ventilator
- P. Bennett volumetric spirometer
- P. Popule self-saturating swab

Purkinje image tracker

Purlon suture

Purstring disposable instrument

Pursuer CBD helical basket

Pursuit catheter

push
- p. cuff
- P. medical brace

Push-Ease
- P.-E. Quad cuff
- P.-E. wheelchair glove

pusher
- Aker lens p.
- Arrequi KPL laparoscopic knot p.
- p. catheter
- Charnley femoral prosthesis p.
- chorda tympani p.
- Clarke-Reich laparoscopic knot p.
- de la Vega lens p.
- Endo-Assist endoscopic knot p.
- Fresnel lens p.
- Gazayerli knot p.
- hemispherical p.
- hook p.
- Jacobson suture p.
- Jako knot p.
- knot p.
- Kuglen p.
- lens p.
- Mangum knot p.
- Martin Surefit lens p.
- Mershon band p.
- MetraTie knot p.
- Negus ligature p.
- Ranfac KPL laparoscopic knot p.
- Shuletz p.
- 6th Finger knot p.
- Visitec lens p.
- p. wire

push-pull catheter

push-up block

Puth abduction splint

Put-In driver

Putnam evacuator catheter

Putterman
- P. levator resection clamp
- P. ptosis clamp

Putterman-Chaflin ocular asymmetry device

Putti
- P. arthroplasty gouge
- P. bone file
- P. bone rasp
- P. frame
- P. splint

Putti-Platt/Bankart instrumentation

Putti-Platt director

putty
- AlloMatrix injectable p.
- Bishop p.
- Blue Brand therapy p.
- color-coded therapy p.
- DynaGraft p.
- Grafton moldable p.
- matrix Grafton p.
- Omnisil p.
- polyvinylsiloxane p.
- Thera-Plast p.
- Thera-Putty exercise p.

PVA eye spear

PVC
- polyvinyl chloride
  - PVC catheter
  - PVC drain
  - PVC tubing

P-wave-triggered ventricular pacemaker

PWB
- Puno-Winter-Byrd
  - PWB transpedicular spine fixation system

Pye cannula

pyeloureteral catheter

pylon
- P. intramedullary nail system
- Stratus impact reducing p.
- telescopic and torsional p.
- TT p.

pyloric stenosis dilator

pylorodilator

pylorus clamp

PyMaH
- P. nylon balanced bladder
- P. pre-gaged cuff
- P. Trimline sphygmomanometer system

Pynchol headband

Pynchon
- P. applicator
- P. cannula
- P. ear snare
- P. mouthgag
- P. nasal speculum
- P. suction tube
- P. tongue depressor

Pynchon-Lillie tongue depressor

pyoktanin catgut suture

Pyramesh cage
pyramid
    p. attachment
    p. cannula
    p. Toomey tip
pyramidal
    p. electrode
    p. eye implant

Pyrex
    P. eye sphere
    P. T-tube
pyroglycolic acid suture
Pyrolyte ball-cage heart valve
Pyrost bone replacement
PythonEC catheter
pyxigraphic sampling capsule

NOTES

P

QDR
quantitative digital radiography
QDR-series bone densitometer
Qiagen RNeasy Mini kit
QIAmp tissue kit
Q-LAS 0 YAG laser
Qlicksmart scalpel blade remover
Q-Maxx side-firing laser device
Q-Plex cardiopulmonary exercise system
Q-prep system
Q-Rad TOMO system tomography radiographic system
Q-Ray bracelet
QRS
Quantronic Resonance System
QSA dressing forceps
QS alexandrite laser
Q-Star
Q-S. IV pressure-relief mattress
Q-S. Voyager pressure-reduction mattress
Q-Stress treadmill
Q-switched
Q-s. alexandrite laser
Q-s. Er:YAG laser
Q-s. Nd:YAG laser
Q-s. neodymium:YAG laser
Q-s. neodymium:yttrium aluminum-garnet laser
Q-s. ruby laser
Q-Tee cleaning swab
QT interval sensing pacemaker
Q-Trak IAQ monitor
Quad
Q. cutting tip
Q. MRI scanner
Quadcat wire
Quad-Lumen catheter
QuadPediatric fundus lens
Quadpolar electrode
quad-ported LASIK irrigating cannula
Quadracut ACL shaver system
Quadra-Flo infusion catheter
QuadraLase advanced surgical fiber system
Quadrant shoulder brace
Quadra pipetting system
quadraplegic standing frame
quadrature
q. birdcage coil
q. body coil
Q. cervical spine coil
q. detector
q. head coil

q. phase detector
q. surface coil
quadriceps boot
quadricusp stentless mitral bioprosthetic valve
Quadrilite 6000 light source
quadripolar
q. cutting forceps
q. diagnostic catheter
q. electrode catheter
q. 6-French diagnostic electrophysiology catheter
q. pacing catheter
q. steerable electrode catheter
quadrisected minigraft dilator
Quadro dressing
Quadtro cushion
QualCare knee brace
QualCraft
Q. ankle support
Q. short elastic wrist support
Q. splint
Q. strap
Qualtex surgical drape
Quanam QP2 coronary stent
Quanta Lite ANA ELISA test kit
Quantec endodontic instrument
Quantico needle
Quanticor catheter
Quantimet 500 image analysis system
quantitative digital radiography (QDR)
Quantrex Sweep 650 ultrasonic cleansing system
Quantronic Resonance System (QRS)
Quantum
Q. biliary inflation device
Q. 400 chiropractic table
Q. enteral pump
Q. foot prosthesis
Q. hearing aid
Q. LP stent-graft
Q. Maverick catheter
Q. Monorail balloon catheter
Q. pacemaker
Q. PSV pressure support ventilator
Q. Ranger OTW balloon catheter
Q. 400 true intersegmental traction
Q. TTC biliary balloon dilator
quarantine drain
Quark PFT modular system
Quartet system
quartz
q. fiberoptic probe
q. lamp

quartz *(continued)*
  q. rod
  q. transducer
quartz-glass container
Quartzo device
Quattro mitral valve
Queen Anne dressing
Quervain
  Q. abdominal retractor
  Q. cranial forceps
  Q. elevator
  Q. rib spreader
  Q. rongeur
Quervain-Sauerbruch retractor
Quest
  Q. intersegmental roller traction
  table
  Q. MPS system
Questek laser tube
**Questus Leading Edge sheathed
  arthroscopy knife**
Quevedo
  Q. conjunctival forceps
  Q. suturing forceps
quick
  Q. Bend flex clamp
  q. connector
  Q. CT9800 scanner
  Q. Drain valve
  Q. Trak periosteal fixation system
QuickAnchor
  Mitek Micro Q.
  Mitek Mini Q.
  Resolve Q.
Quickbox container
QuickCast
  Q. splint
  Q. wrist immobilizer
Quick-Core biopsy needle
QuickDop probe
QuickDraw venous cannula
Quickert
  Q. lacrimal probe
  Q. suture
Quickert-Dryden lacrimal probe
Quicket tourniquet
QuickFlash arterial catheter
QuickFlow distal perfusion system
QuickFurl
  Q. double-lumen balloon
  Q. single-lumen balloon
Quickie
  Q. Carbon wheelchair
  Q. EX wheelchair
  Q. GPS wheelchair
  Q. GP Swing-Away wheelchair
  Q. GPV wheelchair
  Q. Kidz Pediatric wheelchair

  Q. Recliner wheelchair
  Q. Ti wheelchair
Quick-Lite lamp
Quicknet monitor interface
**QuickRinse automated instrument rinse
  system**
QuickSeal arterial closure device
Quick-Sil
  Q.-S. silicone system
  Q.-S. starter kit
QuickSilver hydrophilic-coated guidewire
QuickStick padding
**Quickswitch irrigation-aspiration
  ophthalmic device**
Quick-Tie ankle brace
QuickTrack coronary stent balloon
Quiet interference screw
**QuietTrak ambulatory blood pressure
  monitor**
Quiet-Vac vacuum
Quik
  Q. Connect fetal monitor
  Q. splint
Quikcoff device
QuikStrip adhesive bandage
Quik-Temp thermometer
quilt
  ThermaCare q.
Quimby
  Q. gum scissors
  Q. implant system
Quinaband dressing
Quinby curved scissors
Quincke
  Q. Babcock needle
  Q. spinal needle
  Q. tube
Quinn holder
**Quinones-Neubüser uterine-grasping
  forceps**
Quinones uterine-grasping forceps
Quinton
  Q. biopsy catheter
  Q. central venous catheter
  Q. dual-lumen catheter
  Q. peritoneal catheter
  Q. PermCath catheter
  Q. Q-Port catheter
  Q. Quik-Prep electrode
  Q. Scribner shunt
  Q. suction biopsy instrument
  Q. tube
**Quinton-Mahurkar dual-lumen peritoneal
  catheter**
Quinton-Scribner shunt
Quintron Microlyzer 12 chromatograph
Quire
  Q. foreign body forceps

Q. mechanical finger forceps
Q. mechanical finger snare
Quisling intranasal hammer
Quixil fibrin sealant

QUS-2 calcaneal ultrasonometer
Qwik-Clean dressing
Q-YAG 5 laser

Q

NOTES

R1 rapid exchange balloon dilatation catheter
RaAct NMES device
Raaf
R. Cath vascular catheter
R. dual-lumen catheter
R. flexible lighted spatula
R. forceps
Raaf-Oldberg
R.-O. intervertebral disc forceps
R.-O. rongeur
Rabbit mouthgag
Rabiner neurological hammer
Rabinov cannula
Racestyptine
R. cord
R. retraction ring
racetrack Microtron accelerator
rack
Hausmann weight r.
Jannetta sterilizing r.
Luneau retinoscopy r.
RackBeta scintillation counter
Racz catheter
Rad
R. airway laryngeal blade
R. 60 X-Treme curved blade
RAD40 sinus blade
Radcliff perineal retractor
RADenoid blade
radial
r. artery catheter
r. iridotomy scissors
R. Jaw bladder biopsy forceps
R. Jaw hot biopsy forceps
r. keratotomy (RK)
r. keratotomy knife
r. keratotomy marker
r. nerve glove
r. sector scanning echoendoscope
r. sponge
radiant heat warmer
radiation
r. beam monitor
r. detector
light activation by stimulated emission of r. (LASER)
r. seed
r. simulator
r. therapy system (RTS)
ultraviolet r. (UVR)
radiative hyperthermia device
Radical pulse oximeter
RadiMedical fiberoptic pressure-monitoring wire

Radin-Rosenthal implant
radioactive stent
radiocarpal implant
Radiofocus
R. Glidewire
R. Glidewire angiography catheter
R. guidewire
R. introducer B kit
radiofrequency (RF)
r. ablator
r. catheter
r. coil
r. generator
r. hot balloon
r. interstitial tissue ablation (RITA)
r. interstitial tissue ablation system
r. needle electrode system
r. pacemaker
r. thermal balloon catheter
r. tracer
radiofrequency-generated thermal balloon catheter
radio frequency generator
radiographic
r. grid
radiography
quantitative digital r. (QDR)
radioimmunoassay kit
radioimmunoguided surgery system
radioisotope
r. calibrator
r. camera
r. capsule
r. stent
radiologic portacaval shunt
radiolucent
r. cranial pin headholder
r. operating room table extension
r. plastic occluder
r. sound
r. spine frame
r. splint
RadioLucent wrist fixation system
Radiometer
R. ABL 500 blood gas analyzer
R. autotitrator
OSM3 R.
R. probe
scanning R.
Radionics
R. articulated arm system
R. bipolar coagulation unit
R. bipolar instrument
R. CRW stereotactic head frame
R. Optical Tracking System

R

Radionics *(continued)*
    R. OTS
    R. radiofrequency lesion generator
    R. stimulus generator
radionucleotide imaging
radionuclide
    r. camera
    r. carrier system
radiopaque
    r. calibrated catheter
    r. ERCP catheter
    r. gold marker
    r. nitinol stent
    r. silastic catheter
    r. tantalum stent
radioscope
    Lombart r.
radiosurgery
    CyberKnife SRS hypofractionated
      stereotactic r.
radiotranslucent rod
RadiStop radial compression system
radium needle
Radius
    R. enteral feeding tube
    R. self-expanding stent
Radix anchor
Radix-Raney jacket
RadNet radiology information system
Radnoid microdebrider
Radovan
    R. breast implant
    R. tissue expander
Radpour
    R. irrigator
    R. needle
Radpour-House
    R.-H. suction irrigator
    R.-H. suction tube
Radstat hemostasis device
RAE
    Ring-Adair-Elwyn
    RAE endotracheal tube
RAE-Flex tracheal tube
Ragnell
    R. double-ended retractor
    R. drain
    R. undermining scissors
Ragnell-Davis retractor
rail
    Ableware Bath+Safe deluxe tub
      safety r.
    Railguard bed r.
railway catheter
Raimondi
    R. hemostat
    R. low-pressure shunt
    R. peritoneal catheter

    R. scalp hemostatic forceps
    R. ventricular catheter
Rainbow
    R. 3D camera system
    R. drill
    R. envelope arm snare
    R. fracture frame
    R. vacuum
Raindrop medication nebulizer
Rainin
    R. iris hook
    R. lens hook
    R. lens spatula
Rainy Day playground bag
rake retractor
Ralks
    R. bone drill
    R. ear forceps
    R. ear retractor
    R. eye magnet
    R. fingernail drill
    R. mallet
    R. nasal gauze packer
    R. reversible knife
    R. sinus applicator
    R. splinter forceps
    R. thoracic clamp
    R. tuning fork
    R. wire-cutting forceps
Ralks-Davis mouthgag
Ramirez
    R. EndoFaceLift dissector
    R. EndoForehead suction coagulator
    R. periosteal elevator
    R. shunt
    R. Silastic cannula
    R. telescoping cannula
    R. winged catheter
Ramitec bite registration material
RAM knee prosthesis
Rampley sponge forceps
RAMS
    robot-assisted microsurgery
    RAMS workstation
Ramsbotham decapitating hook
Ramsden eyepiece
Ramses diaphragm
Ramsey County pyoktanin catgut suture
Ramstedt
    R. clamp
    R. pyloric stenosis dilator
ramus
    r. blade
    r. blade implant
    r. endosteal implant
    r. stripper
Ranawat-Burstein
    R.-B. hip prosthesis
    R.-B. porous stem

R

Rancho
- R. Los Amigos feeder
- R. Los Amigos orthosis
- R. Los Amigos splint

Rand
- R. bayonet ring curette
- R. forceps
- R. microballoon

Randall
- R. endometrial biopsy curette
- R. kidney stone forceps
- R. stone forceps
- R. uterine curette

Randelli modular shoulder system
Rand-House suction tube
Rand-Malcolm cranial x-ray frame
Randolph
- R. cyclodialysis cannula
- R. irrigator

random-zero sphygmomanometer
Randot circle
Rand-Radpour suction tube
Rand-Wells pallidothalmomectomy guide
Raney
- R. bone drill
- R. cranial drill
- R. dissector
- R. flexion jacket brace
- R. Gigli-saw guide
- R. jacket
- R. laminectomy punch
- R. laminectomy retractor
- R. laminectomy rongeur
- R. perforator drill
- R. periosteal elevator
- R. rongeur forceps
- R. scalp clip
- R. scalp clip applier
- R. scalp clip-applying forceps
- R. spinal fusion curette
- R. spring steel clip
- R. stirrup-loop curette
- R. straight coagulating forceps

Raney-Crutchfield
- R.-C. drill
- R.-C. drill point
- R.-C. skull tongs

Ranfac
- R. cholangiographic catheter
- R. KPL laparoscopic knot pusher
- R. soft-tissue needle
- R. stiffening cannula

range-gated transducer
Range-Master pulley
range-of-motion (ROM)
- r.-o.-m. brace
- cervical r.-o.-m. (CROM)

Ranger OTW balloon catheter
Ranieri clamp
Rankin
- R. anastomosis clamp
- R. arterial forceps
- R. hemostat
- R. hemostatic forceps
- R. intestinal clamp
- R. prostatic retractor
- R. prostatic tractor
- R. stomach clamp
- R. suture

Rankin-Crile forceps
Rankow forceps
Ransford loop
Ranzewski intestinal clamp
RAP
- remote access perfusion
- RAP cannula

rapid
- r. cuff inflator
- r. exchange balloon catheter
- r. exchange PTCA catheter
- r. infusion pump
- R. Loc device
- R. One Ecstasy dipstick
- R. One OXY dipstick

Rapide wound suture
RapidFire multiple band ligator
RapidFlap device
Rapidgraft
- R. arterial vessel substitute
- R. radial artery graft

Rapidlab 800 analyzer
RapidLoc meniscal repair system
Rapido dual-catheter system
RapidScreen RS-2000 computer-aided detection system
RapiSeal patch
Rappaport-Sprague stethoscope
Rappazzo
- R. foreign body scissors
- R. haptic scissors
- R. intraocular foreign body forceps
- R. intraocular lens
- R. intraocular manipulator

NOTES

Rappazzo *(continued)*
 R. iris hook
 R. speculum
Rapp forceps
Raptor
 R. over-the-wire delivery system
 R. PTCA balloon
 R. surgical grasper
rare earth magnet
Rascal II anesthetic monitor
Rashkind
 R. atrial septostomy balloon
  catheter
 R. balloon
 R. double-disc occluder prosthesis
 R. double-disc umbrella occluder
 R. double-umbrella device
 R. septostomy needle
 R. umbrella
Rasor blood pumping system
rasp *(See also* raspatory)
 acromioplasty r.
 Agris r.
 antral r.
 Arthrofile orthopaedic r.
 Aufricht diamond nasal r.
 Aufricht glabellar r.
 Aufricht-Lipsett nasal r.
 Austin Moore r.
 Bankart r.
 Bardeleben r.
 Barsky nasal r.
 Bartholdson-Stenstrom r.
 bell r.
 Berne nasal r.
 Bio-Modular humeral r.
 Bio-Moore r.
 Black r.
 bone r.
 Bowen r.
 Brawley sinus r.
 Bristow r.
 Brown r.
 Charnley r.
 Cohen sinus r.
 Concept arthroscopy r.
 Converse r.
 convex r.
 Cottle-MacKenty r.
 Cottle nasal r.
 Dean r.
 diamond r.
 Dolwick-Reich diamond r.
 Doyen rib r.
 ear r.
 Eicher r.
 Endotrac ligament r.
 Epstein bone r.
 facet r.

Farabeuf bone r.
Farabeuf-Collin r.
Farrior r.
FeatherTouch automated r.
femoral r.
Filtzer interbody r.
Fischer nasal r.
Fomon nasal r.
Friedman r.
frontal sinus r.
Gallagher antral r.
Gam-Mer r.
Georgiade r.
glabellar r.
Gleason r.
Good antral r.
Herczel rib r.
Hylin r.
interbody fusion r.
Israel nasal r.
Joseph nasal r.
Kalinowski r.
Kalinowski-Verner r.
Kessler podiatry r.
Key r.
Kleinert-Kutz r.
Koenig r.
Lamont nasal r.
Langenbeck periosteal r.
Leurs nasal r.
Lewis nasal r.
Lundsgaard r.
Lundsgaard-Burch corneal r.
Maliniac nasal r.
Mallory-Head Interlok r.
Maltz-Anderson nasal r.
Maltz-Lipsett nasal r.
Maltz nasal r.
Matchett-Brown stem r.
McCabe-Farrior r.
McCabe perforation r.
McCollough r.
McGee r.
McGee oval-window r.
McIndoe r.
Miller r.
Moore stem r.
nasal r.
Nicola r.
Ollier r.
orthopaedic r.
Parkes nasal r.
Peet nasal r.
perforation r.
Polokoff r.
power r.
Putti bone r.
Reidy r.
Ringenberg r.

Ritter r.
Robb-Roberts rotary r.
Rubin oblique r.
Saunders-Paparella window r.
Scheer oval window r.
side-cutting r.
snow plow r.
Southworth r.
Spratt nasofrontal r.
Stenstrom r.
Thompson frontal sinus r.
Thompson stem r.
Toriumi curved r.
triangular r.
ulnar r.
V. Mueller diamond r.
Watson-Williams sinus r.
Wiener antral nasal r.
Wiener-Pierce antral r.
Wiener Universal frontal sinus r.
window r.
Woodward antral r.
raspatory (*See also* rasp)
Alexander rib r.
Artmann r.
Babcock r.
Bacon periosteal r.
Ballenger r.
Barsky cleft palate r.
Bastow r.
Beck pericardial r.
Bennett r.
Berry rib r.
bronchocele sound r.
Brunner r.
cleft palate r.
Collin r.
Converse r.
Coryllos rib r.
Cushing r.
Davidson-Alexander rib r.
Doyen rib r.
Edwards r.
Farabeuf r.
Farabeuf-Lambotte r.
Farrior mushroom r.
fishtail spatula r.
French-pattern r.
Friedrich r.
Gam-Mer oblique r.
Hein r.
Hill nasal r.

Hoen periosteal r.
Hopkins Hospital periosteal r.
Howarth nasal r.
Jansen mastoid r.
Joseph nasal r.
Joseph periosteal r.
Joseph-Verner r.
Kirmisson periosteal r.
Kleesattel r.
Kocher r.
Kokowicz r.
Ladd r.
Lambert-Berry rib r.
Lambotte rib r.
Lane periosteal r.
Langenbeck-O'Brien r.
Lebsche r.
Mannerfelt r.
Mathieu r.
Matson r.
Matson-Alexander r.
Matson-Plenk r.
McIndoe r.
Moore r.
Mott r.
Nicola r.
Overholt rib r.
periosteal r.
Phemister r.
Plenk-Matson r.
rib r.
Sauerbruch-Frey r.
Scheuerlen r.
Schneider r.
Schneider-Sauerbruch r.
Semb r.
Sewall r.
Shuletz r.
Shuletz-Damian r.
skull r.
Stenstrom r.
Stille-Crafoord r.
Stille-Doyen r.
Stille-Edwards r.
Stillenberg r.
sympathetic r.
Trelat palate r.
Wiberg r.
Willauer r.
Williger r.
Yasargil r.

R

NOTES

raspatory *(continued)*
    Zenker r.
    Zoellner r.
Rastelli
    R. conduit
    R. graft
    R. implant
    R. prosthesis
Raster photogrammeter
ratchet
    r. clamp
    r. tourniquet
ratcheted grasper
ratchet-type brace
rate-modulated pacemaker
rate-responsive
    r.-r. pacemaker
    r.-r. pulse generator
Rathke punch
Rath mechanical treatment table
Ratliff-Blake gallstone forceps
Ratliff-Mayo gallstone forceps
rat-tail catheter
rat-tooth
    r.-t. forceps
    r.-t. pickups
    r.-t. rongeur
Rauchfuss
    R. sling splint
    R. snare
    R. suspension sling
Raulerson syringe
Raven Bacterial Spore strips
Ravich
    R. bougie
    R. clamp
    R. lithotriptoscope
    R. lithotrite
    R. needle holder
    R. ureteral dilator
Ray
    R. brain spatula
    R. brain spoon
    R. kidney stone forceps
    R. nasal speculum
    R. pituitary curette
    R. rhizotomy electrode
    R. RRE-TM thermistor electrode
    R. TFC device
    R. threaded fusion cage
Raylor
    R. bone impactor
    R. malleable retractor
Rayner-Choyce
    R.-C. eye implant
    R.-C. intraocular lens
Rayner lens
Raypaque resin

Ray-Parsons-Sunday staphylorrhaphy elevator
Rayport
    R. dural knife
    R. muscle clamp
Ray-Tec
    R.-T. band
    R.-T. dressing
    R.-T. x-ray detectable lap pad
    R.-T. x-ray detectable surgical
        sponge
Razi cannula introducer
razor
    American Safety R. (ASR)
    Bard-Parker r.
    r. blade
    r. blade holder
    r. blade knife
    r. blade trephine
    Castroviejo oscillating r.
    Emir r.
    r. scalpel
    Weck-Prep orderly r.
razor-tip needle
RazorVac ArthroWands
RB1 suture
R&B portable pneumothorax apparatus
RBS
    Rendell-Baker Soucek
    RBS face mask
RC1 catheter
RC-2 fundus camera
RCB
    Rotator Cuff Buttress
    RCB biopsy needle
reabsorbable suture
reach-and-pin forceps
reacher
    EZ r.
    Homecraft Folding EasiReach r.
    Pik Stick r.
ReAct NMES device
reactor
    breeder r.
    fast-breeder r.
Read
    R. chisel
    R. facial curette
    R. forceps
    R. gouge
    R. oral curette
    R. osteotome
    R. periosteal elevator
reader
    AutoPap r.
    Fisher microcapillary tube r.
    microplate r.
    microtitration plate r.

PapNet r.
plate r.
Real-EaSE neck and shoulder relaxer
Reality
    R. female condom
    R. vaginal pouch
Real scissors
real-time
    r.-t. B scanner
    r.-t. confocal scanning laser microscope
    r.-t. 2-dimensional Doppler flow-imaging system
    r.-t. format converter
    r.-t. position management tracking system
    r.-t. ultrasound
    r.-t. video processor
reamer
    acetabular r.
    acorn r.
    AMBI r.
    Anatomic/Intracone r.
    Arthrex coring r.
    Aufranc finishing ball r.
    Aufranc finishing cup r.
    Aufranc offset r.
    Austin Moore bone r.
    r. awl
    bone r.
    r. bushing
    calcar r.
    canal r.
    cannulated r.
    chamfer r.
    Charnley expanding r.
    Charnley taper r.
    Charnley trochanter r.
    r. clamp
    Con-Nex r.
    core r.
    Dentatus r.
    DePuy cannulated r.
    endodontic r.
    expanding r.
    femoral head bone removal r.
    femoral shaft r.
    flexible r.
    fluted r.
    Gray flexible intramedullary r.
    Green-Armytage r.
    Gruca hip r.

    Hall Versipower r.
    Harris brace-type r.
    Harris center-cutting acetabular r.
    Hewson-Richards r.
    humeral r.
    Indiana r.
    Intracone intramedullary r.
    intramedullary r.
    Jergensen r.
    Jergensen-Trinkle r.
    Jewett socket r.
    K r.
    Lorenz r.
    Lottes r.
    MacAusland finishing-ball r.
    MacAusland finishing-cup r.
    Mallory-Head Interlok r.
    Marin r.
    medullary canal r.
    Mira-Charnley r.
    Mira femoral head r.
    Moore bone r.
    Murphy ball r.
    Norton adjustable cup r.
    Norton ball r.
    orthopaedic r.
    Osteonics r.
    patellar shaft r.
    PD r.
    Pease r.
    Peeso r.
    Perthes r.
    Phemister r.
    Pressure Sentinel r.
    revision conical r.
    Rispi Micromega r.
    Rowe glenoidal r.
    Rush awl r.
    Schneider nail shaft r.
    shaft r.
    shelf r.
    Smith-Petersen hip r.
    Sovak r.
    spiral trochanteric r.
    Sturmdorf cervical r.
    Swanson r.
    taper r.
    tapered r.
    T-handle r.
    Tinel tapered r.
    Zimmer Orthair r.
reaming awl

NOTES

rear-entry ACL drill guide
rear-tip extender
Reaves punch
Rebar-18 microcatheter
Rebel knee orthosis
rebreathing
    r. bag
    r. mask
Récamier uterine curette
recanalization
    endovascular photoacoustic r.
    (EPAR)
receive-only circular surface coil
receiver
    Medtronic radiofrequency r.
    Pori and Rowe EEG r.
recessed balloon septostomy catheter
recession
    r. forceps
    r. ophthalmic muscle hook
reciprocal
    r. ohm meter
    r. planing instrument
reciprocating
    r. gait orthosis
    r. power handpiece
    r. saw
Recklinghausen tonometer
recliner
    Hydro Soothe r.
    Lumex Preferred Care r.
    Ortho-Biotic r.
reclining air chair
Recon reconstruction nail
reconstruction plate
recorder
    Accutracker ambulatory blood
      pressure r.
    Accutracker ambulatory BP r.
    Accutracker II ambulatory blood
      pressure r.
    ambulatory electrocardiographic r.
    blood pressure r.
    cardiac output r.
    circadian event r.
    Del Mar Avionics 3-channel r.
    Digitrapper III EGG r.
    Digitrapper Mark II pH r.
    DM-400 tape Holter r.
    Dopcord r.
    Eigon CardioLoop r.
    event r.
    Gould-Brush 481 8-channel r.
    Gould ES 1000 r.
    graphic level r.
    HeartCard cardiac event r.
    HeartWatch cardiac event r.
    Hellige electrocardiographic r.
    Honeywell r.

    24-hour ambulatory
      electrocardiographic r.
    intraocular tension r.
    iriscorder r.
    King of Hearts Express II cardiac
      event r.
    Leeds-Northrup Speedomax r.
    Medilog ambulatory ECG r.
    MicroDigitrapper apnea r.
    Narco Biosystems rectilinear r.
    Oxford Medilog frequency-
      modulated r.
    Phinformer portable r.
    Rectigraph-8K r.
    rectilinear r.
    Remmers sleep r.
    Reveal Plus insertable loop r.
    Sandhill-800 TDS chart r.
    Siesta physiologic data r.
    SNAP sleep r.
    Sphygmocorder r.
    video r.
recording
    r. electrode
    2120 r. spirometer
rectal
    r. balloon
    r. catheter
    r. clamp
    r. dilator
    r. forceps
    r. hook
    r. probe
    r. speculum
    r. trocar
    r. tube
rectangle
    Hartshill r.
    Luque r.
rectangular
    r. awl
    r. blade
    r. brain spatula
    r. tapper
    r. wire
rectifier
    full-wave r.
    silicon-controlled r.
    r. tube
Rectigraph-8K recorder
rectilinear
    r. recorder
    r. scanner
rectoromanoscope
rectoscope
    Storz r.
RectoSight disposable sigmoidoscope
rectosigmoidoscope
recumbent cycle

recurrent bandage
RED
    rigid external distraction
    RED system
red
    R. Cross adhesive dressing
    R. Cross graft
    r. laser
    r. lens occluder
    r. pessary
    R. Reflex Lens Systems lens
    r. Robinson catheter
    r. rubber catheter
    r. rubber endotracheal tube
    R. Witch bur
red-beam
    r.-b. laser
    r.-b. laser pen
Reddick cystic duct cholangiogram
catheter
Reddick-Saye
    R.-S. cannula
    R.-S. hydrosector
    R.-S. Lav-1 I&A probe
    R.-S. screw
    R.-S. screw catheter
    R.-S. trocar
ReDeuce pump tubing
Redfield IRC 2100 infrared coagulator
red-free filter
Redi-Around finger splint
Redi Bur
Rediform orthotic
RediFurl
    R. double-lumen balloon
    R. single-lumen balloon
    R. TaperSeal IAB catheter
RediGuard IAB catheter
Reditron refractometer
Redivac
    R. suction drain
    R. suction tube
Redmond retractor
Redo intestinal clamp
Redon drain
red-tip aspirator
reduced Snellen card
reducer
    cervical dislocation r.
    Endopath surgical trocar r.
    McCannel ocular pressure r.
    ocular pressure r.

reducing
    r. fracture frame
    r. stent
reduction
    r. instrument
    r. ring
Redy hemodialyzer
Reebok
    R. Slide system
    R. Step system
Reece
    R. orthopaedic shoe
    R. osteotomy guide
    R. PO shoe
Reed
    R. cast belt
    R. switch
Reeh stitch scissors
reel
    r. aspiration cannula
    suture tension adjustment r.
    (STAR)
Re-Entry Malecot catheter set
Reese
    R. advancement forceps
    R. dermatome
    R. dermatome blade
    R. muscle forceps
    R. prosthesis
    R. ptosis knife
    R. stimulator
Reese-Drum dermatome
reference
    r. catheter
    r. electrode
Refine fusion system
Refinity Coblation system
reflectance
    r. photometer
    r. spectrophotometer
    r. spectrophotometric probe
    r. TS-200 spectrum analyzer
Reflection acetabular cup
Reflec UV instant camera
reflex
    R. anterior cervical plate system
    R. articulating endoscopic cutter
    R. electrode
    R. gun
    r. hammer
    R. One skin stapler

R

NOTES

773

reflex *(continued)*
    R. pacemaker
    R. SuperSoft steerable guidewire
Re/Flex filter
ReFlexion implant system
ReFlex wand
Refobacin Palacos R cement
reformer
    Stott r.
reform eye implant
refractionometer
    Hartinger Coincidence r.
refractometer
    Abbe r.
    AMO r.
    Canon auto r.
    Hoya HDR objective r.
    Hoya MRM objective r.
    meridional r.
    Reditron r.
    Retinomax 2 Auto r.
    Speedy-1 Auto r.
    Zeiss vertex r.
refractor
    Amoils r.
    AR 1000 r.
    automated r.
    Barraquer-Krumeich-Swinger r.
    Berens r.
    Brawley r.
    Bronson-Turtz r.
    Campbell r.
    Canon r.
    Castallo r.
    Castroviejo r.
    Coburn r.
    CooperVision Diagnostic Imaging r.
    Elschnig r.
    Fink r.
    Goldstein r.
    Gradle r.
    Graether r.
    Green r.
    Groenholm r.
    Hartstein r.
    Hillis r.
    Humphrey automatic r.
    Kirby r.
    Knapp r.
    Kronfeld r.
    Kuglen r.
    Leland r.
    Marco ARK-2000 r.
    McGannon r.
    Mueller r.
    Nidek AR-2000 objective
     automatic r.
    Precision r.
    Reichert r.

    Remote Vision electronic r.
    Rizzuti r.
    Rollet r.
    Schepens r.
    SR-IV Programmed Subjective r.
    Stevenson r.
    Tomey auto r.
    Topcon RM-A2300 auto r.
    Ultramatic Rx Master Phoroptor r.
    Wilmer r.
Regain personal trainer EMG
Regal Acrylic Stretch prosthetic sock
Regan-Lancaster dial
Regan low-contrast acuity chart
Regaud radium colpostat
Regency
    R. pacemaker
    R. SR+ pulse generator
    R. XLC power wheelchair
Regentex GBR-200 membrane
Regugauge suction regulator
regulator
    aluminum oxygen r.
    Boehringer suction r.
    high-flow r.
    low-flow r.
    Medela membrane r.
    Ohmeda continuous-vacuum r.
    Ohmeda thoracic suction r.
    Optimed glaucoma pressure r.
    Regugauge suction r.
    Regu-Vac r.
    Vacutron suction r.
Regulus Navigator image-guided system
Regu-Vac regulator
Rehbein
    R. infant abdominal retractor
    R. internal steel strut
    R. rib spreader
Rehfuss
    R. duodenal tube
    R. stomach tube
Rehne
    R. abdominal retractor
    R. skin graft knife
Reich curette
Reichel-Mainster retina laser
Reichert
    R. antroscope
    R. binocular indirect
     ophthalmoscope
    R. camera
    R. flexible sigmoidoscope
    R. Ful-Vue binocular
     ophthalmoscope
    R. Ful-Vue spot retinoscope
    R. lensometer
    R. noncontact tonometer
    R. ophthalmodynamometer

R. radius gauge
R. refractor
R. slit lamp
R. stereotaxic brain apparatus
R. Ultramatic Rx Master Phoroptor refracting instrument
Reichert-Lenschek advanced logic lensometer
Reichert-Mundinger
R.-M. stereotactic head frame
R.-M. stereotactic system
Reichert-Mundinger-Fischer stereotactic frame
Reichling corneal scissors
Reich-Nechtow
R.-N. arterial clamp
R.-N. cervical biopsy curette
R.-N. dilator
R.-N. forceps
R.-N. hypogastric artery forceps
R.-N. plug
Reid
R. retinoscope
R. sleeve
Reidy rasp
Reif catheter
Reill
R. forceps
R. needle holder
R. wire-cutting pliers
reimplanted electrode
Reinecke-Carroll lacrimal tube
Reiner
R. curette
R. ear syringe
R. plaster knife
R. rongeur
Reiner-Alexander ear syringe
Reiner-Beck tonsillar snare
Reiner-Knight ethmoid-cutting forceps
Reinhart retractor
Reinhoff
R. arterial forceps
R. dissector
R. rib spreader
R. swan neck clamp
R. thoracic scissors
Reinhoff-Finochietto
R.-F. rib contractor
R.-F. rib spreader

Reipen
R. cannula
R. speculum
Reisinger lens-extracting forceps
Reitan CatheterPump
ReJuveness
R. pure silicone sheeting
R. scar therapy silicone sheet
Rekow system
relator
orthognathic occlusal r.
wide-tray bite r.
Relat vaginal speculum
Relax-a-Cizor exerciser
relaxer
Real-EaSE neck and shoulder r.
relaxograph
Datex r.
relaxometer
Bruker PC-10 r.
IBM field-cycling research r.
Relax SLH Deluxe massage chair
Relay
R. cardiac pacemaker
R. suture delivery system
release
R. nonadhering dressing
r. sleeve
Release-NF
R.-NF camera
R.-NF catheter
Reliance
R. CM femoral component
R. device
R. urinary control insert
R. urinary control insert catheter
R. urinary control stent
Relia-Vac drain
ReliefBand
R. nerve stimulation therapy
R. NST
R. RB-EL Explorer device
reliner
Brimms denture r.
Coe-Rect denture r.
Coe-Soft denture r.
Hydro-Cast r.
Simpa denture r.
Super-Soft denture r.
Reliquet lithotrite
Relton frame pad
Relton-Hall spinal frame

NOTES

Relume system
Remac system
Rema-Exakt investment material
Remak band
Remaloy wire
Remanium
 R. star alloy
 R. wire
Remedy
 R. colostomy appliance
 R. ileostomy appliance
 R. sleep therapy system
Remine mastectomy skin flap retractor
Remmers sleep recorder
remote
 r. access perfusion (RAP)
 r. access perfusion cannula
 r. afterloading system
 R. Vision electronic refractor
removable
 r. partial denture
 r. partial overdenture
Removatron epilator
Remove adhesive remover wipe
remover
 adhesive tape r.
 Atwood bridge/crown r.
 Bailey foreign body r.
 Bard adhesive and barrier film r.
 Biomet Ultra-Drive cement r.
 Braithwaite clip r.
 clip r.
 Crown-A-Matic crown and
  bridge r.
 Damon-Julian ring r.
 DMV contact lens r.
 Ferrolite crown r.
 foreign body r.
 frog cortex r.
 Macaluso stent r.
 Mead bridge/crown r.
 medical adhesive r.
 modular head r.
 Morrell crown r.
 Qlicksmart scalpel blade r.
 Richwil bridge/crown r.
 ring r.
 Schuknecht foreign body r.
 Universal clip r.
 Wart Stick wart r.
 Wölfe-Böhler cast r.
REM PolyHesive II patient return
 electrode
REMstar
 R. Plus CPAP system
 R. Pro CPAP system
Remy separator
Renaflo hollow fiber dialyzer

Renaissance
 R. crown system
 R. erbium laser
 R. II spirometry system
renal
 r. artery clamp
 r. artery forceps
 r. pedicle clamp
 r. sympathetic nerve activity
  recording electrode
 R. systems dialyzer
 R. Systems HF250 filter
Renalin dialyzer
Renata battery
Renatron II dialyzer
Rendell-Baker
 R.-B. Soucek (RBS)
 R.-B. Soucek face mask
Renegade microcatheter
RE-New laparoscopic instrument
Renolux convertible car seat
renovascular stent
Rentrop infusion catheter
Reo Macrodex suture
Rep Bands exercise bandage
Repela surgical glove
Repel-CV bioresorbable adhesion
 barrier film
reperfusion catheter
Repicci II unicompartment implant
Repiphysis pediatric bone replacement
 implant
replaceable blade
replacement
 Amstutz total hip r.
 Anatomical Vertebral Body R.
  (AVR)
 Biolox ceramic ball head for
  hip r.
 Biomet Liverpool radial head r.
 Bi-Wave plus mattress r.
 Calcitite bone r.
 r. collection bag
 Cosgrove mitral valve r.
 DressSkin skin r.
 hard tissue r. (HTR)
 Howmedica Centrax head r.
 KineMatch patellofemoral r.
 Kirschner Medical Dimension
  hip r.
 Liverpool radial head r.
 Manchester knee r.
 Mueller-type femoral head r.
 NexGen complete knee r.
 PCA E-Series hip r.
 Pilliar total hip r.
 Polyfloat system II mattress r.
 Pyrost bone r.
 SAF hip r.

self-articulating femoral hip r.
Silon-TSR temporary skin r.
temporary skin r.
replacer
Green iris r.
Smith-Fisher iris r.
Replace Select implant system
replant splint
RepliCare Thin hydrocolloid dressing
replicator
Steers r.
Replica total hip replacement system
Repliderm dressing
Repliform
R. dermal allograft
R. graft
Replogle
R. suction catheter
R. tube
Re-Ply TENS electrode
repositioner
Wilson-Cook prosthesis r.
repositor
iris r.
Knapp iris r.
Koman-Nair iris r.
Nettleship iris r.
reprocessor
automated endoscope r.
automatic r.
Bard automatic endoscope r.
Custom Ultrasonic automatic
endoscope r.
KeyMed automatic r.
Lutz automatic r.
MediVators DSD-91P endoscope r.
Orr automatic r.
Steris automatic r.
Reprodent acrylic tooth material
Repro head halter
Resano
R. sigmoid forceps
R. thoracic scissors
rescuing pacemaker
research
Alvarado Orthopedic R. (AOR)
R. Medical straight multiple-holed
aortic cannula
resection
r. clamp
r. intestinal forceps
r. ophthalmic double hook

resector
Dyonics full-radius r.
Friedrich-Petz machine r.
full-radius r.
Gator r.
Stryker r.
XPS Striaghtshot micro tissue r.
resectoscope
ACMI r.
Bard r.
Baumrucker r.
Boehm r.
continuous flow r.
r. curette
Elite System rotating r.
Ellik r.
foroblique microlens r.
Iglesias continuous-flow r.
Iglesias fiberoptic r.
Iglesias microlens r.
Kaplan r.
Mauermayer r.
McCarthy continuous-flow r.
McCarthy microlens r.
McCarthy miniature r.
McCarthy multiple r.
Nesbit r.
Olympus continuous-flow r.
Olympus OES 4000 r.
OPERA Star r.
Richard Wolf video r.
Scott rotating r.
r. sheath
Stern-McCarthy electrotome r.
Storz direct-view r.
Storz-Iglesias r.
Storz laser r.
Streak r.
Thompson direct full-vision r.
USA Elite System rotating
continuous-flow r.
Wolf r.
reservoir
Accu-Flo CSF r.
Braden flushing r.
Camey r.
Cardiometrics cardiotomy r.
cardiotomy r.
cerebral spinal fluid r.
Cobe cardiotomy r.
contiguous spinal fluid r.
CSF r.

R

NOTES

reservoir *(continued)*
    Denver r.
    double-dome r.
    r. face mask
    flat bottom r.
    flushing r.
    Foltz flushing r.
    Hakim r.
    Heyer-Schulte Jackson-Pratt wound-drainage r.
    Heyer-Schulte-Ommaya CSF r.
    Heyer-Schulte wedge-suction r.
    H-H Rickham cerebrospinal fluid r.
    Holter-Rickham ventriculostomy r.
    Holter-Salmon-Rickham ventriculostomy r.
    Holter-Selker ventriculostomy r.
    Holter ventriculostomy r.
    ICV r.
    Intersept cardiotomy r.
    inverted U-pouch ileal r.
    Jackson-Pratt large-volume suction r.
    Jostra cardiotomy r.
    J-Vac bulb suction r.
    Kock ileal r.
    LeBag r.
    Mainz pouch urinary r.
    Ommaya CSF r.
    Ommaya ventricular r.
    Parks ileoanal r.
    Polystan cardiotomy r.
    Pudenz r.
    Resipump pump r.
    retromastoid Ommaya r.
    Rickham r.
    Salmon-Rickham ventriculostomy r.
    Selker ventriculostomy r.
    Shiley cardiotomy r.
    sideport flat-bottomed Ommaya r.
    UNI r.
    William Harvey cardiotomy r.
    wound drainage r.

resin
    Aclec r.
    Astron r.
    Astron dental r.
    Bondeze r.
    Bowen r.
    Brilliant light-cured r.
    Celay Tech light curing r.
    r. cement
    Chelex ionic bead r.
    Coe orthodontic r.
    Concise r.
    Dentsply r.
    diacrylate r.
    Dynabond r.
    Effapoxy r.

    Endur r.
    Genie r.
    Ivocryl r.
    Lee orthodontic r.
    light-curing r.
    Myerson r.
    Nuvaseal r.
    Nuva-Tach r.
    orthodontic r.
    Orthomite r.
    Poracryl r.
    Porovin dental r.
    Raypaque r.
    Royale III denture r.
    Shur r.
    Solo-Tach r.
    r. sphere
    Technovit acrylic r.
    ultraviolet-light-polymerized r.
    unfilled r.
    Vynacron r.
    Vynagel dental r.

Resipump pump reservoir
Resist-A-Band exercise band
resistance wire heater
Resistex
    R. expiratory resistance exerciser
    R. PEP therapy device
resistive exerciser
ResMed CPAP Sullivan III device
Resnick
    R. button bipolar coagulator
    R. Tone Emitter I intraoral electrolarynx device
resolution
    low-energy ultra-high r. (LEUHR)
Resolve QuickAnchor
resonance
    magnetic r. (MR)
    nuclear magnetic r. (NMR)
resonance generator
resonator
    birdcage r.
    bridged loop-gap r.
    crossed-loop r.
    Faraday shielded r.
    flexible surface-coil-type r.
    multicoupled loop-gap r.
    Oudin r.
    transmission line r.
resorbable
    r. copolymer PGA/PLLA-Lactosorb miniplate fixation system
    r. plate
    r. plate and screw
    r. polydioxanone pin
ReSound
    R. CC4 hearing aid
    R. digital hearing aid

Respalert peak flowmeter
Respiradyne respiratory monitor
respiration bronchoscope
respirator
    Ambu r.
    Babybird II r.
    Bath r.
    Bear 5 r.
    Bennett r.
    Bird Mark 8 r.
    Bourns electronic adult r.
    Bourns infant r.
    Bragg-Paul r.
    Breeze r.
    cabinet r.
    Clevedan positive pressure r.
    cuirass r.
    Dann r.
    Drinker tank r.
    Emerson r.
    Engstrom r.
    Gill I r.
    Huxley r.
    MA-1 r.
    mechanical r.
    mechanically assisted r.
    Med-Neb r.
    Merck r.
    Monaghan r.
    Morch r.
    Morsch-Retec r.
    Moynihan r.
    particulate r.
    portable r.
    Sanders jet ventilation device r.
    volumetric diffusive r.
respiratory
    r. function monitor
    r. inductance plethysmograph (RIP)
respiratory-dependent pacemaker
Respirex incentive spirometer
Respirgard II nebulizer
respirometer
    Collins r.
    Dräger r.
    Fraser-Harlake r.
    Haloscale r.
    hot-wire r.
    Wright r.
Respironics
    R. BiPAP bilevel ventilator
    R. CPAP machine

    R. nasal mask
    R. Oasis humidifier
    R. pulse oximeter
Respitrace
    R. inductive plethysmograph
    R. machine
    R. monitor
    R. respiratory monitoring system
Respond wire
response
    automated brainstem auditory
      evoked r.
    R. cushion
    R. electrophysiology catheter
    R. R2930 4-Stack Multi-Station
      exercise system
Resposable Spacemaker surgical balloon
    dissector
Res-Q
    R.-Q ACD implantable cardioverter-
      defibrillator
    R.-Q arrhythmia control device
    R.-Q ICD generator
Res-Q-Vac emergency suction system
rest
    R. Assured oral appliance
    Cedar anesthesia face r.
    cervical r.
    Chan wrist r.
    ChiroFlow back r.
    Core Hibak R.
    Core Lobak R.
    face r.
    foot r.
    knee r.
    Krause arm r.
    Mayfield head r.
    Mouse Nest mouse r.
    Muirhead pelvic r.
    neck r.
    SutureMate needle r.
Restcue CC dynamic air therapy bed
resting
    r. foot sling
    r. orthosis
Reston
    R. hydrocolloid dressing
    R. padding
    R. polyurethane foam
    R. self-adhering foam
    R. sponge

NOTES

Restoration
    R. acetabular system
    R. GAP acetabular cup
    R. Secur-Fit X'tra acetabular shell
Restoration-HA hip system
Restore
    R. ACL guide system
    R. bone implant
    R. CalciCare dressing
    R. calcium alginate wound dressing
    R. Cx wound care dressing
    R. hydrocolloid dressing
    R. orthobiologic soft-tissue implant
    R. Plus wound care dressing
    R. X dental cement
restrainer
    Gulani globe stabilizer and flap r.
restraint
    r. calipers
    Circumstraint pediatric
      circumcision r.
    papoose board r.
    poncho r.
    Posey r.
    vacuum-operated viscous r.
    Velcro r.
restrictor
    BioStop G cement r.
    Buck femoral cement r.
    cement r.
    Charnley cement r.
    femoral canal r.
Resume electrode
Resurface laser resurfacing imaging
Resuscitaire neonatal resuscitation unit
resuscitation
    cardiopulmonary r. (CPR)
    r. cart
resuscitator
    ACD r.
    Ambu infant r.
    Ambu SPUR disposable r.
    BagEasy disposable manual r.
    bag-valve-mask r.
    Capno-Flo r.
    DMR2 disposable manual r.
    First Response manual r.
    Fisher-Paykel RD1000 r.
    heart-lung r.
    High Oxygen PRM r.
    Hope r.
    Hudson Lifesaver r.
    infant Ambu r.
    Laerdal infant r.
    Lifemask infant r.
    Lifesaver disposable r.
    NeoV0$_2$R volume control r.
    Ohio Hope r.
    Penlon infant r.

    pneuPAC r.
    Pulmanex r.
    Robertshaw bag r.
    Safe Response manual r.
    SureGrip manual r.
retainer
    r. arch bar
    r. closure
    continuous bar r.
    direct r.
    extracoronal r.
    Hahnenkratt r.
    Hawley r.
    r. insert
    intracoronal r.
    matrix r.
    McNealey-Glassman visceral r.
    Mectra tissue sample r.
    r. ring
    space r.
    SurgiFish visceral r.
    The Fish Glassman viscera r.
    Thermoskin heat r.
    Tofflemire r.
    viscera r.
Retcam 120 digital camera
retention
    r. bar
    r. catheter
    r. drill
    r. ring
    r. suture bolster
    r. suture bridge
rete peg
retinaculotome
    Paine r.
retinal
    r. detachment hook
    r. detachment pencil
    r. detachment syringe
    r. diathermy electrode
    r. Gelfilm implant
    r. laser ellipsometer
    r. probe
    r. thickness analyzer (RTA)
Retinomax
    R. 2 Auto refractometer
    R. cordless handheld autorefractor
    R. refractometry instrument
retinometer
    Heine Lambda 100 r.
Retinopan 45 camera
retinoscope
    Boilo r.
    Copeland 360 streak r.
    Ful-Vue spot r.
    Ful-Vue streak r.
    Keeler r.
    Macula r.

Priestley-Smith r.
Propper Star r.
Reichert Ful-Vue spot r.
Reid r.
spot r.
Welch Allyn standard r.
Welch Allyn streak r.
retracted penis pouch
retracting rod
retraction ring
retractor
Abadie self-retaining intestinal r.
abdominal vascular r.
Ablaza aortic wall r.
Ablaza-Blanco cardiac valve r.
Abramson r.
Adams r.
Adamson r.
Adson-Beckman r.
Adson brain r.
Adson cerebellar r.
Adson splanchnic r.
Agricola lacrimal sac r.
airgun r.
Airlift balloon r.
alar r.
Alden r.
Alexander r.
Alexander-Ballen orbital r.
Alexander-Matson r.
Alexian Hospital r.
Alfreck r.
Allen r.
Allis lung r.
Allison lung r.
Allport-Babcock r.
Allport-Gifford r.
Allport mastoid bayonet r.
Alm r.
Alm microsurgery r.
Alm self-retaining r.
Alter lip r.
aluminum cortex r.
Amenabar iris r.
American Heyer-Schulte brain r.
Amoils iris r.
amputation r.
anal r.
Anderson-Adson self-retaining r.
Anderson double-end r.
Andrews tracheal r.
Ankeney sternal r.

Ann Arbor phrenic r.
anterior prostatic r.
Anthony pillar r.
antral r.
AOR collateral ligament r.
Apfelbaum cerebellar r.
apicolysis r.
appendectomy r.
appendiceal r.
arch rake r.
Arem r.
Arem-Madden r.
arm r.
Army-Navy r.
Aronson esophageal r.
Aronson lateral sternomastoid r.
Arruga eye r.
Arruga globe r.
Ashley r.
Assistant Free r.
Aston nasal r.
Aston submental r.
Aufranc femoral neck r.
Aufranc hip r.
Aufranc psoas r.
Aufranc push r.
Aufricht nasal r.
Austin dental r.
automatic skin r.
Auvard weighted vaginal r.
Azar iris r.
Babcock r.
baby Adson brain r.
baby Balfour r.
baby Collin abdominal r.
baby Roux r.
baby Senn-Miller r.
baby Weitlaner r.
Backmann thyroid r.
Bacon cranial r.
Badgley laminectomy r.
Bahnson sternal r.
Bakelite r.
Balfour center-blade abdominal r.
Balfour pediatric abdominal r.
Balfour self-retaining abdominal r.
Ballantine hemilaminectomy r.
Ballen-Alexander orbital r.
ball-type r.
Bankart r.
Bankart shoulder r.
Barkan bident r.

NOTES

retractor *(continued)*
  Baron r.
  Barraquer-Krumeich-Swinger r.
  Barraquer lid r.
  Barrett-Adson cerebellum r.
  Barron r.
  Barr rectal r.
  Barr self-retaining rectal r.
  Barsky nasal r.
  Bauer r.
  Beardsley esophageal r.
  Beatty pillar r.
  beaver-tail r.
  Becker r.
  Beckman-Adson laminectomy r.
  Beckman-Eaton laminectomy r.
  Beckman goiter r.
  Beckman self-retaining r.
  Beckman thyroid r.
  Beckman-Weitlaner r.
  Bellfield wire r.
  Bellman r.
  Bellucci-Wullstein r.
  Benedict r.
  Beneventi self-retaining r.
  Bennett bone r.
  Bennett tibial r.
  Berens esophageal r.
  Berens lid r.
  Berens mastectomy skin flap r.
  Berens thyroid r.
  Bergen r.
  Bergman tracheal r.
  Bergman wound r.
  Berkeley r.
  Berkeley-Bonney self-retaining
    abdominal r.
  Berlind-Auvard r.
  Berna infant abdominal r.
  Bernay tracheal r.
  Bernstein nasal r.
  Bertin hip r.
  Bethune phrenic r.
  Bicek vaginal r.
  Biestek thyroid r.
  bifid gallbladder r.
  Biggs r.
  Billroth ovarian r.
  Billroth-Stille r.
  Bishop r.
  bivalved r.
  Black r.
  bladder r.
  blade r.
  r. blade
  Blair-Brown vacuum r.
  Blair 4-prong r.
  Blakesley uvular r.
  Blanco r.

  Bland perineal r.
  Blount double-prong r.
  Blount hip r.
  Blount knee r.
  Blount single-prong r.
  Bodnar knee r.
  Boley r.
  bone r.
  Bookwalter r.
  Bookwalter-Balfour r.
  Bookwalter-Goulet r.
  Bookwalter-Harrington r.
  Bookwalter-Hill-Ferguson rectal r.
  Bookwalter-Kelly r.
  Bookwalter-Magrina vaginal r.
  Bookwalter ring r.
  Bookwalter-St. Mark deep pelvic r.
  Bose r.
  Bosworth nerve root r.
  bowel r.
  Boyd r.
  Boyes-Goodfellow hook r.
  Braastad costal arch r.
  brain r.
  brain silicone-coated r.
  Brantley-Turner vaginal r.
  Brawley scleral wound r.
  Breen r.
  Breisky-Navratil straight r.
  Breisky vaginal r.
  Brewster r.
  Briggs r.
  Brinker hygienic tissue r.
  Bristow-Bankart humeral r.
  Bristow-Bankart soft tissue r.
  Britetrac r.
  Britetrac Taylor r.
  Brompton Hospital r.
  Bronson-Turtz iris r.
  Brophy r.
  Brown-Burr modified Gillies r.
  Brown uvular r.
  Bruch mastoid r.
  Bruening r.
  Brunner r.
  Brunschwig visceral r.
  Buck-Gramcko r.
  Bucy spinal cord r.
  Budde halo neurosurgical r.
  Buie r.
  Buie-Smith anal r.
  bulb r.
  Bulnes-Sanchez r.
  Burford rib r.
  Busenkell posterior hip r.
  Butler dental r.
  Butler pillar r.
  buttonhook nerve r.
  Bycroft-Brunswick thyroid r.

Byford r.
Cairns scalp r.
Callahan r.
Campbell lacrimal sac r.
Campbell nerve root r.
Campbell self-retaining r.
Campbell suprapubic r.
Canadian chest r.
Cardillo r.
Carlens-Stille tracheal r.
Carlens tracheotomy r.
Carmody-Brody r.
Caroline finger r.
Carroll-Bennett finger r.
Carroll offset hand r.
Carroll self-retaining spring r.
Carter r.
Caspar cervical r.
Castallo eyelid r.
Castaneda infant sternal r.
Castroviejo adjustable r.
Castroviejo lid r.
cat paw r.
Cave knee r.
cecostomy r.
cerebellar r.
cerebral r.
cervical r.
cervical disc r.
Cer-View lateral wall r.
chalazion r.
Chamberlain-Fries atraumatic r.
Chandler knee r.
Chandler laminectomy r.
channel r.
Charnley horizontal r.
Charnley pin r.
Charnley self-retaining r.
Charnley standard stem r.
Cheanvechai-Favaloro r.
cheek r.
Cherry laminectomy self-retaining r.
Cherry S-shaped brain r.
Cheyne r.
Children's Hospital pediatric r.
Chitten-Hill r.
Christie gallbladder r.
Cibis-Vaiser muscle r.
claw r.
Clayman lid r.
Clayman nucleus r.
Clevedent r.

Cleveland IMA r.
Cloward blade r.
Cloward cervical r.
Cloward-Cushing vein r.
Cloward dural r.
Cloward-Hoen laminectomy r.
Cloward laminectomy r.
Cloward nerve root r.
Cloward tissue r.
Cobb r.
cobra r.
Cocke large flap r.
Cohen r.
Cole duodenal r.
Coleman r.
collapsible tissue r.
collar button iris r.
Collin abdominal r.
Collin-Hartmann r.
Collins-Mayo mastoid r.
Collin sternal self-retaining r.
Collis anterior cervical r.
Collis posterior lumbar r.
Collis-Taylor r.
Colonial r.
Colver tonsillar r.
Colver tonsillar r.
Comyns-Berkeley r.
condylar neck r.
Cone laminectomy r.
Cone scalp r.
Cone self-retaining r.
Converse alar r.
Converse blade r.
Converse double-ended alar r.
Converse nasal r.
Converse nested r.
Conway lid r.
Cook rectal r.
Cooley r.
Cooley aortic r.
Cooley atrial r.
Cooley carotid r.
Cooley femoral r.
Cooley-Merz sternal r.
Cooley mitral valve r.
Cooley MPC cardiovascular r.
Cooley neonatal sternal r.
Cooley pediatric rib r.
Cooley rib r.
Cooley sternotomy r.
Cooley sternum r.

NOTES

retractor *(continued)*
Cope double-ended r.
corrugated forehead r.
cortex r.
Coryllos r.
Cosgrove mitral valve r.
costal arch r.
Costenbader r.
Coston-Trent iris r.
Cottle alar r.
Cottle hook r.
Cottle-Joseph r.
Cottle nasal r.
Cottle-Neivert nasal r.
Cottle pillar r.
Cottle 4-prong r.
Cottle pronged r.
Cottle sharp prong r.
Cottle single-blade r.
Cottle soft palate r.
Cottle upper lateral exposing r.
Cottle weighted r.
Crafoord r.
Craig-Sheehan r.
cranial r.
crank frame r.
Crawford aortic r.
Crawford-Beaver r.
Crego periosteal r.
Crile r.
Crile thyroid double-ended r.
Crockard r.
Crockard pharyngeal r.
Crotti goiter r.
Crotti thyroid r.
Crowe-Davis mouth r.
Cuda r.
Cushing aluminum r.
Cushing bivalve r.
Cushing brain r.
Cushing decompression r.
Cushing-Kocher r.
Cushing loop r.
Cushing nerve r.
Cushing nerve root r.
Cushing self-retaining r.
Cushing S-shaped r.
Cushing straight r.
Cushing subtemporal r.
Cushing vein r.
Czerny r.
dacryocystorhinostomy r.
Dallas r.
Danek self-retaining r.
Danis r.
Darling popliteal r.
Darrach r.
Dautrey r.
David-Baker lid r.

Davidoff trigeminal r.
Davidson erector spinae r.
Davidson scapular r.
Davis brain r.
Davis double-ended r.
Davis scalp r.
Deaver r.
DeBakey chest r.
DeBakey-Cooley Deaver-type r.
Decker r.
decompression r.
Dedo laser r.
deep abdominal r.
deep blunt rake r.
deep Deaver r.
de la Plaza transconjunctival r.
DeLee corner r.
DeLee Universal r.
DeLee vaginal r.
DeLee vesical r.
DeMartel self-retaining brain r.
Denis Browne abdominal r.
Denis Browne ring r.
dental r.
Denver-Wells atrial r.
Denver-Wells sternal r.
DePuy r.
D'Errico nerve root r.
Desmarres cardiovascular r.
Desmarres lid r.
Desmarres valve r.
Desmarres vein r.
Dingman flexible r.
Dingman Flexsteel r.
disposable iris r.
Dixon center-blade r.
Dockhorn r.
Dorsey nerve root r.
Dott r.
double-bent Hohmann acetabular r.
double-ended r.
Downing II laminectomy r.
Doyen abdominal r.
Doyen vaginal r.
Dozier radiolucent Bennett r.
Drews iris r.
Drews-Rosenbaum iris r.
dual nerve root suction r.
Duane r.
Dumont r.
duodenal r.
dural r.
Eastman vaginal r.
Eccentric Y finger r.
Edinburgh brain r.
Effenberger r.
Elite Farley r.
Elschnig lid r.
Emmet obstetrical r.

Emory EndoPlastic r.
endaural r.
Endoflex endoscopic r.
EndoRetract r.
Endotrac r.
epicardial r.
epiglottis r.
erector spinae r.
ESI long, narrow mammoplasty r.
esophageal r.
examination r.
eXpose r.
external r.
extraoral sigmoid notch r.
eyelid r.
facelift r.
Falk vaginal r.
fan elevator r.
fan liver r.
fan-shaped liver r.
Farabeuf double-ended r.
Farr self-retaining r.
Farr spring r.
Farr wire r.
Fasanella double-ended iris r.
fat pad r.
Favaloro atrial r.
Favaloro self-retaining sternal r.
Federspiel cheek r.
Feldman lid r.
Feldman lip r.
femoral r.
femoral neck r.
Ferguson r.
Ferguson-Moon rectal r.
Ferris-Smith orbital r.
Ferris-Smith-Sewall orbital r.
fiberoptic r.
finger rake r.
Fink lacrimal r.
Finochietto hand r.
Finochietto infant rib r.
Finochietto laminectomy r.
Finsen r.
Fisch dural r.
Fisher double-ended r.
Fisher fenestrated lid r.
Fisher lid r.
Fisher tonsil r.
fixed ring r.
flexible arm micro r.
flexible neck r.

flexible neck rake r.
flexible translimbal iris r.
FlexPosure endoscopic r.
Flexsteel ribbon r.
Foerster abdominal r.
Fomon double-hook r.
Fomon hook r.
Fomon nasal r.
force fulcrum r.
Ford-Deaver r.
Foss bifid gallbladder r.
Foss biliary r.
Fowler self-retaining r.
Franklin malleable r.
Franz abdominal r.
Frater intracardiac r.
Frazier cerebral r.
Frazier laminectomy r.
Frazier lighted r.
Freeman facelift r.
Freer dural r.
Freer skin r.
Freer submucous r.
Freiberg hip r.
Freiberg nerve root r.
French S-shaped brain r.
Friedman perineal r.
Friedman vaginal r.
Fritsch abdominal r.
Fujita snake r.
Fukuda humeral head r.
Fukushima r.
Fullerview flexible iris r.
Fulton r.
Gabarro r.
gallbladder r.
Gam-Mer medial esophageal r.
Gam-Mer occipital r.
Gant gallbladder r.
Garrett peripheral vascular r.
Garrigue vaginal r.
gastric resection r.
Gauthier r.
Gazayerli endoscopic r.
Geissendorfer rib r.
Gelpi-Lowrie r.
Gelpi perineal r.
Gelpi self-retaining abdominal r.
Gelpi vaginal r.
general r.
Gerbode sternal r.
Gifford mastoid r.

NOTES

retractor *(continued)*

Gifford scalp r.
Gillies single-hook skin r.
Gilvernet r.
Gil-Vernet lumbotomy r.
Glass abdominal r.
Glenner vaginal r.
Goelet double-ended r.
goiter r.
Goldstein lacrimal sac r.
Goligher modification of the Berkeley-Bonney r.
Goligher modified Berkeley-Bonney r.
Goligher sternal-lift r.
Gomez gastric r.
Gooch mastoid r.
Good r.
Goodhill r.
Goodyear tonsillar r.
Gosset abdominal r.
Gosset appendectomy r.
Gosset self-retaining r.
Gott malleable r.
Gradle eyelid r.
Graether r.
Grant gallbladder r.
Gray surgical r.
Greenberg Universal r.
Green goiter r.
Green thyroid r.
Greenwald r.
Grice r.
Grieshaber flexible iris r.
Grieshaber self-retaining r.
Grieshaber spring wire r.
Groenholm lid r.
Gross iris r.
Gross patent ductus r.
Gross-Pomeranz-Watkins atrial r.
Gruenwald r.
Guilford-Wright meatal r.
Guthrie r.
Guttmann obstetrical r.
Guttmann vaginal r.
Guzman-Blanco epiglottic r.
Haight-Finochietto rib r.
Haight pulmonary r.
Haight rib r.
Hajek antral r.
Hajek lip r.
half-moon r.
halo r.
Hamburger-Brennan-Mahorner thyroid r.
Hamby brain r.
Hamby-Hibbs r.
hand r.
handheld r.

hard palate r.
Hardy-Duddy vaginal r.
Hardy lip r.
Harken rib r.
Harrington bladder r.
Harrington Britetrac r.
Harrington-Deaver r.
Harrington-Pemberton sympathectomy r.
Harrington splanchnic r.
Harrington sympathectomy r.
Harrison chalazion r.
Hartstein irrigating iris r.
Hartzler rib r.
Haslinger palate r.
Haslinger soft palate r.
Haslinger uvular r.
Hasson r.
Haverfield hemilaminectomy r.
Haverfield-Scoville hemilaminectomy r.
Hawkins-Bell r.
Haynes r.
Hays finger r.
Hays hand r.
Heaney hysterectomy r.
Heaney-Simon hysterectomy r.
Heaney-Simon vaginal r.
Heaney vaginal r.
Hedblom rib r.
Heifitz r.
Heiss mastoid r.
Heiss soft tissue r.
Helfrick anal r.
Helveston "Great Big Barbie" r.
hemilaminectomy r.
Henderson self-retaining r.
Hendren self-retaining r.
Henley carotid r.
Henner T-model endaural r.
Henning meniscal r.
Henrotin r.
hernia r.
Hertzler baby rib r.
Hess nerve root r.
Heyer-Schulte brain r.
Hibbs self-retaining laminectomy r.
Hill-Ferguson rectal r.
Hillis eyelid r.
Hill rectal r.
Himmelstein sternal r.
Hind Site anal r.
Hirschman r.
Hoen hemilaminectomy r.
Hoen scalp r.
Hohmann r.
Holman lung r.
Holscher nerve r.
Holzbach abdominal r.

Holzheimer automatic skin r.
Holzheimer mastoid r.
r. hook
hook r.
Horgan r.
horizontal flexible bar r.
Hosel r.
House handheld double-end r.
House-Urban middle fossa r.
Howorth toothed r.
Huang Universal arm r.
Hubbard r.
Hudson bone r.
humeral r.
Hunt bladder r.
Hupp tracheal r.
Hurd pillar r.
Hurd tonsillar pillar r.
Hurson flexible r.
Hutchinson iris r.
hysterectomy r.
IMA r.
incision r.
infant abdominal r.
infant eyelid r.
infant rib r.
Inge laminectomy r.
intestinal occlusion r.
intracardiac r.
intradural r.
iris r.
Iron Intern r.
irrigating mushroom r.
Israel blunt rake r.
Jackson self-retaining goiter r.
Jackson tracheal r.
Jackson vaginal r.
Jacobson bladder r.
Jacobson goiter r.
Jaeger lid r.
Jaffe-Givner lid r.
Jaffe wire lid r.
Jako laser r.
Jannetta posterior fossa r.
Jansen-Gifford mastoid r.
Jansen mastoid r.
Jansen scalp r.
Jansen-Wagner mastoid r.
Jarit cross-action r.
Jarit-Deaver r.
Jarit P.E.E.R. r.
Jarit renal sinus r.

Jarit spring-wire r.
Jefferson self-retaining r.
Joe's hoe r.
Johns Hopkins gallbladder r.
Johnson cheek r.
Johnson hook r.
Johnson ventriculogram r.
Jones IMA epicardial r.
Jorgenson r.
Joseph skin hook r.
Joseph wound r.
Joystick r.
Judd-Allis intestinal r.
Judd-Mason bladder r.
Judd-Mason prostatic r.
Kalamarides dural r.
Kanavel-Senn r.
Kapp Surgical Instrument total
 knee r.
Karlin crank frame r.
Karmody vascular spring r.
Kartush insulated r.
Kasdan r.
Kaufer type II r.
Kaufman type II r.
Keeler-Fison tissue r.
Keeler-Rodger iris r.
Keizer-Lancaster lid r.
Keizer lid r.
Kelly abdominal r.
Kelly-Sims vaginal r.
Kelman iris r.
Kennerdell-Maroon orbital r.
Kennerdell medial orbital r.
Kerrison r.
kidney r.
Killey molar r.
Killian-King goiter r.
Kilner nasal r.
Kilner skin hook r.
Kilpatrick r.
King-Hurd r.
King self-retaining goiter r.
Kirby lid r.
Kirchner r.
Kirkland r.
Kirklin atrial r.
Kirschenbaum r.
Kirschner abdominal r.
Kirschner-Balfour abdominal r.
Kitner r.
Kleinert-Kutz hook r.

R

NOTES

retractor *(continued)*

Kleinert-Ragnell r.
Kleinsasser r.
Klemme appendectomy r.
Klemme gasserian ganglion r.
Klemme laminectomy r.
Kliners alar r.
Klippel r.
Knapp lacrimal sac r.
knee r.
Knighton hemilaminectomy self-
retaining r.
Kobayashi r.
Kocher bladder r.
Kocher blade r.
Kocher bone r.
Kocher-Crotti self-retaining goiter r.
Kocher gallbladder r.
Kocher-Langenbeck r.
Kocher self-retaining goiter r.
Kocher-Wagner r.
Koenig vein r.
Koerte r.
Koneg r.
Korte r.
Korte-Wagner r.
Kozlinski r.
Krasky r.
Kretschmer r.
Kristeller vaginal r.
Kronfeld eyelid r.
Krönlein-Berke r.
Kuglen lens r.
Kuyper-Murphy sternal r.
Kwapis subcondylar r.
Lack tongue r.
lacrimal sac r.
Lahey Clinic nerve root r.
Lahey goiter r.
Lahey thyroid r.
laminectomy self-retaining r.
Landau vaginal r.
Landon narrow-bladed r.
Lane r.
Lange bone r.
Lange-Hohmann bone r.
Langenbeck-Cushing vein r.
Langenbeck-Green r.
Langenbeck-Mannerfelt r.
Langenbeck periosteal r.
Laplace liver r.
Lapro-Flex laparoscopic r.
laryngeal r.
laryngofissure r.
lateral vaginal r.
lateral wall r.
Latrobe soft palate r.
Lawton-Balfour self-retaining r.
leaflet r.

Leasure tracheal r.
Leatherman trochanteric r.
Lee double-ended r.
Legen self-retaining r.
Legueu bladder r.
Legueu kidney r.
Lemmon self-retaining sternal r.
Lemole atrial valve self-retaining r.
Lemole mitral valve r.
Lempert r.
Lempert-Colver r.
Lempert endaural r.
LeVasseur-Merrill r.
Levinthal surgery r.
Levy articulating r.
Levy perineal r.
Lewis r.
Leyla self-retaining brain r.
Leyla-Yasargil self-retaining r.
lid r.
Liddicoat aortic valve r.
lighted r.
LightWare r.
Lilienthal-Sauerbruch r.
Lillehei r.
Lillie r.
LIMAvator chest wall r.
Linton splanchnic r.
lip r.
Little r.
liver r.
Lockhart-Mummery r.
Lofberg thyroid r.
Logan lacrimal sac self-retaining r.
London narrow-bladed r.
Lone Star r.
loop r.
Lorie cheek r.
Lothrop tonsillar r.
Lothrop uvular r.
Lovejoy r.
Love nasopharyngeal r.
Love nerve root r.
Love uvula r.
Lowman hand r.
Lowsley prostate r.
Luer r.
Luer double-ended tracheal r.
Luer S-shaped r.
Lukens double-ended tracheal r.
Lukens epiglottic r.
Lukens thymus r.
lumbar r.
lumbotomy r.
lung r.
Luongo hand r.
Luther-Peter lid r.
MacAusland-Kelly r.
MacAusland muscle r.

R

MacKay contour self-retaining r.
MacKool capsular r.
MacVicar double-end strabismus r.
Madlab conjunctival r.
Magrina-Bookwalter vaginal r.
Mahorner thyroid r.
Maison r.
Maliniac nasal r.
Malis cerebellar r.
Malis cerebral r.
malleable blade r.
malleable copper r.
malleable ribbon r.
malleable stainless steel r.
Maltz r.
mandibular body r.
Mannerfelt r.
Manning r.
Markham-Meyerding
  hemilaminectomy r.
Mark II Chandler total knee r.
Mark II lateral collateral
  ligament r.
Mark II modular weighted r.
Mark II Stubbs short-prong
  collateral ligament r.
Mark II wide PCL knee r.
Markley r.
Martin abdominal r.
Martin cheek r.
Martin lip r.
Martin nerve root r.
Martin palate r.
Martin rectal hook r.
Martin vaginal r.
Mason-Judd bladder r.
Mason-Judd self-retaining r.
mastectomy skin flap r.
mastoid self-retaining r.
Mathieu double-ended r.
Matson-Mead apicolysis r.
Mattison-Upshaw r.
Mayfield r.
Mayo abdominal r.
Mayo-Adams self-retaining
  appendectomy r.
Mayo-Collins appendectomy r.
Mayo-Collins double-ended r.
Mayo-Collins mastoid r.
Mayo-Lovelace abdominal r.
Mayo-Simpson r.
McBurney fenestrated r.

McBurney thyroid r.
McCabe antral r.
McCabe parotidectomy r.
McCabe posterior fossa r.
McCool capsule r.
McCullough externofrontal r.
McGannon iris r.
McGill r.
McIndoe r.
McNealey visceral r.
meat hook r.
Medicon rib r.
Mediflex r.
Mediflex Gazayerli r.
Meigs r.
Meller lacrimal sac r.
meniscal r.
Merrill-Levassier r.
metacarpal double-ended r.
Meyer biliary r.
Meyerding-Deaver r.
Meyerding finger r.
Meyerding laminectomy r.
Meyerding self-retaining
  laminectomy r.
microlumbar discectomy r.
microsurgical r.
microvascular modified Alm r.
Middledorpf r.
Middlesex-Pointe r.
Mikulicz abdominal r.
Mikulicz liver r.
Miles r.
Milex r.
Miller r.
Miller-Senn double-ended r.
Milligan self-retaining r.
Millin-Bacon bladder self-
  retaining r.
Millin-Bacon retropubic
  prostatectomy r.
Millin retropublic bladder r.
Millin self-retaining r.
Miltex Cottle r.
Minnesota r.
Miskimon cerebellar self-retaining r.
mitral valve r.
Moberg r.
Moberg-Stille r.
modified sternal r.
Mollison self-retaining r.
Moon rectal r.

NOTES

retractor *(continued)*

Moore bone r.
Moorehead cheek r.
Moorehead dental r.
Morrison-Hurd pillar r.
Morse modified Finochietto r.
Morse sternal r.
Morse valve r.
Mosher lifesaver r.
Mott double-ended r.
Mueller-Balfour self-retaining r.
Mueller lacrimal sac r.
Mufson-Cushing r.
Muldoon lid r.
Munro self-retaining r.
Murless head r.
Murphy-Balfour r.
Murphy gallbladder r.
Murphy rake r.
Murtagh self-retaining infant
    scalp r.
Muscle Jack orthopaedic r.
Naclerio diaphragm r.
nasal r.
Nathanson liver r.
Navratil r.
neck r.
Neivert double-ended r.
Nelson self-retaining rib r.
nerve r.
nerve root r.
Nevyas drape r.
newborn eyelid r.
Newell lid r.
Newton-Morgan r.
New tracheal r.
New York Hospital r.
Noblock r.
North-South r.
Nuttall r.
Nystroem r.
Nystroem-Stille r.
oardlike r.
Oberhill self-retaining r.
O'Brien phrenic r.
O'Brien rib r.
obstetrical r.
Obwegeser channel r.
Obwegeser periosteal r.
Ochsner-Favaloro self-retaining r.
Ochsner malleable r.
Ochsner ribbon r.
Ochsner vascular r.
O'Connor abdominal r.
O'Connor-O'Sullivan self-retaining
    vaginal r.
O'Connor vaginal r.
Octopus r.
Oertli wire lid r.

Oettingen abdominal self-
    retaining r.
offset hand r.
Oklahoma iris wire r.
Oldberg brain r.
Oldberg straight r.
Oliver scalp r.
Ollier rake r.
Omni r.
Omni-Tract vaginal r.
orbicular r.
orbital r.
O'Reilly esophageal r.
Orley r.
Osher iris r.
Osher lid r.
O'Sullivan-O'Connor self-retaining
    abdominal r.
O'Sullivan-O'Connor vaginal r.
O'Sullivan self-retaining
    abdominal r.
O'Sullivan vaginal r.
r. oval sprocket frame
Packiam r.
palate r.
Paparella self-retaining r.
Paparella-Weitlaner r.
Parker double-ended r.
Parker-Mott double-ended r.
Parker thumb r.
Parkes nasal r.
Parks anal r.
parotidectomy r.
Parsonnet epicardial r.
Paschall orthopaedic grasping r.
patent ductus r.
Paul lacrimal sac r.
Paulson knee r.
Payne r.
Payr abdominal r.
Peck rake r.
pectoralis r.
pediatric abdominal r.
pediatric self-retaining r.
Peet lighted splanchnic r.
Pemberton r.
Pemco r.
Penfield r.
Percy amputation r.
Percy bone r.
Percy-Wolfson gallbladder r.
periareolar r.
perineal prostatectomy r.
perineal self-retaining r.
peripheral vascular r.
Perkins otologic r.
Perman-Stille abdominal r.
pharyngeal r.
Pheifer-Young r.

phrenic r.
Pickrell r.
Picot vaginal r.
Pierce cheek r.
pillar r.
pillar-and-post microsurgical r.
Pilling r.
Pilling-Favaloro r.
Piper lateral wall r.
Plester r.
Poliak eye r.
Polytrac Gomez r.
Pomeranz hiatal hernia r.
popliteal r.
Poppen-Gelpi laminectomy self-
retaining r.
Portmann r.
Posada-Vasco orbital r.
postauricular r.
posterior fossa r.
posterior lumbar r.
posterior urethral r.
Pratt bivalve r.
Proctor cheek r.
4-prong r.
pronged r.
2-prong rake r.
6-prong rake r.
3-prong rake blade r.
5-prong rake blade r.
prostatic r.
Proud-White uvula r.
Pryor-Péan vaginal r.
psoas r.
pulmonary r.
Purcell self-retaining abdominal r.
Quervain abdominal r.
Quervain-Sauerbruch r.
Radcliff perineal r.
Ragnell-Davis r.
Ragnell double-ended r.
rake r.
Ralks ear r.
Raney laminectomy r.
Rankin prostatic r.
Raylor malleable r.
Redmond r.
Rehbein infant abdominal r.
Rehne abdominal r.
Reinhart r.
Remine mastectomy skin flap r.
retropubic prostatectomy r.

rib r.
ribbon malleable r.
Rica brain r.
Rica mastoid r.
Rica multipurpose r.
Rica posterior cranial fossa r.
Ricard abdominal r.
Rica scalp r.
Richards abdominal r.
Richardson abdominal r.
Richardson appendectomy r.
Richardson-Eastman double-ended r.
Richter vaginal r.
Rigby abdominal r.
Rigby appendectomy r.
Rigby bivalve rectal r.
Rigby vaginal r.
rigid neck rake r.
ring r.
ring abdominal r.
Rissler kidney r.
Rizzo r.
Rizzuti iris r.
Roberts thumb r.
Robin-Masse abdominal r.
Robinson lung r.
Rochester atrial septal r.
Rochester colonial r.
Rochester-Ferguson double-ended r.
Rochester rake r.
Rollet r.
Rollet eye r.
Rollet lake r.
Roos brachial plexus root r.
root and dural r.
Rose double-ended r.
Rosenbaum-Drews iris r.
Rosenbaum iris r.
Rosenberg full-radius blade
synovial r.
Rosenberg-Sampson r.
Rose tracheal r.
Ross aortic valve r.
Rotalok skin r.
Rothon r.
Roux double-ended r.
Rowe boathook r.
Rowe orbital floor r.
Rowe scapular neck r.
Rudolph trowel r.
Rultract internal mammary artery r.
Rumel r.

NOTES

retractor *(continued)*
Ryecroft r.
Ryerson bone r.
Sachs angled vein r.
Sachs-Cushing r.
Samb r.
Sanchez-Bulnes lacrimal sac self-
retaining r.
Sato lid r.
Sauerbruch r.
Sauerbruch-Zukschwerdt rib r.
Sawyer rectal r.
Sayre r.
scalp self-retaining r.
Scanlan pediatric r.
scapular r.
Schepens orbital r.
Schindler r.
Schink metatarsal r.
Schnitker scalp r.
Schoenborn r.
Scholten sternal r.
Schuknecht postauricular self-
retaining r.
Schuknecht-Wullstein r.
Schultz iris r.
Schwartz laminectomy self-
retaining r.
scleral wound r.
Scott ring penile r.
Scoville Britetrac r.
Scoville cervical disc self-
retaining r.
Scoville-Haverfield laminectomy r.
Scoville hemilaminectomy self-
retaining r.
Scoville laminectomy r.
Scoville nerve root r.
Scoville psoas muscle r.
Scoville-Richter self-retaining r.
Scoville self-retaining r.
Segond abdominal r.
Seldin flap r.
Seletz-Gelpi self-retaining r.
self-adhering lid r.
self-retaining abdominal r.
self-retaining bentback rotator
cuff r.
self-retaining brain r.
self-retaining laminectomy r.
self-retaining ring r.
self-retaining skin r.
self-retaining spring r.
Sellor rib r.
Semb lung r.
Semb self-retaining r.
Senn-Dingman double-ended r.
Senn double-ended r.
Senn-Green r.

Senn-Kanavel double-ended r.
Senn mastoid r.
Senn-Miller r.
Senn self-retaining r.
Senturia r.
serrated r.
serrefine r.
Sewall orbital r.
Shambaugh endaural self-
retaining r.
sharp-pronged r.
Shearer lip r.
Sheehan r.
Sheldon-Gosset self-retaining r.
Sheldon hemilaminectomy self-
retaining r.
Sherwin self-retaining r.
Sherwood r.
short Heaney r.
Shriners Hospital interlocking r.
Shuletz-Paul rib r.
Shurly tracheal r.
sigmoid notch r.
Silverstein lateral venous sinus r.
Simon vaginal r.
Sims double-ended r.
Sims-Kelly vaginal r.
Sims rectal r.
Sims vaginal r.
single-blade r.
single-hook r.
single-prong broad acetabular r.
Sisson-Love r.
Sisson spring r.
Sistrunk band r.
Sistrunk double-ended r.
skin flap r.
skin hook r.
skin self-retaining r.
Sloan goiter self-retaining r.
Sluder palate r.
Small rake r.
Small tissue r.
SMIC cheek r.
Smillie knee joint r.
Smith anal r.
Smith-Buie anal r.
Smith-Buie self-retaining rectal r.
Smith nerve root suction r.
Smith-Petersen capsular r.
Smith rectal self-retaining r.
Smith vaginal self-retaining r.
Smithwick nerve r.
Snitman endaural self-retaining r.
Sofamor Danek self-retaining r.
Sofield r.
soft palate r.
soft tissue blade r.
Spacekeeper r.

spike r.
spinal cord r.
Spivey iris r.
splanchnic r.
spoon r.
spring r.
spring-loaded self-retaining r.
spring-wire r.
Spurling r.
S-shaped r.
Stack r.
Stamey dorsal vein apical r.
stay suture r.
Steiner-Auvard vaginal r.
stereotactic r.
sternal r.
sternotomy r.
Stevens lacrimal r.
Stevens muscle hook r.
Stevenson lacrimal sac r.
Stille-Broback knee r.
Stille cheek r.
Stille heart r.
Stiwer r.
St. Luke's r.
St. Mark's Hospital r.
St. Mark's lipped r.
St. Mark's pelvis r.
Stookey r.
Storer thoracoabdominal r.
Storz r.
straight r.
Strandell r.
Strandell-Stille r.
Strully nerve root r.
Stuck self-retaining laminectomy r.
Suarez r.
submucous r.
suction r.
Sugita r.
suprapubic self-retaining r.
surgical r.
Sweeney posterior vaginal r.
Sweet amputation r.
sweetheart r.
Symmonds hysterectomy r.
sympathectomy r.
table-fixed r.
Tang r.
tapered brain r.
TARA retropubic r.
Taylor fiberoptic r.

Taylor spinal r.
T-bar r.
Tebbetts ribbon r.
Teflon iris r.
Temple-Fay laminectomy r.
Tepas r.
Terino facial implant r.
Tew cranial r.
Tew spinal r.
Theis self-retaining rib r.
Theis vein r.
Thomas r.
Thoma tissue r.
Thompson r.
Thompson-Farley spinal r.
Thorlakson deep abdominal r.
Thorlakson multipurpose r.
Thornton iris r.
thumb r.
Thurmond iris r.
thymus r.
thyroid r.
tibial r.
Tiko pliable iris r.
Tiko rake r.
Tillary double-ended r.
tissue r.
titanium wound r.
TLC r.
tongue r.
tonsillar pillar r.
toothed r.
Tower interchangeable r.
Tower rib r.
Tower spinal r.
tracheal r.
tracheotomy r.
transconjunctival r.
transoral r.
Trent eye r.
trigeminal self-retaining r.
Tubinger self-retaining r.
Tucker-Levine vocal cord r.
Tuffier abdominal r.
Tuffier-Raney laminectomy r.
Tuffier rib r.
Turner-Doyen r.
Turner-Warwick posterior urethral r.
Turner-Warwick prostate r.
Tyrer nerve root r.
Tyrrell hook r.
Ullrich-St. Gallen self-retaining r.

NOTES

retractor *(continued)*

Universal r.
Upper Hands self-retaining r.
upper-lateral exposing r.
Urban r.
U.S. Army double-ended r.
U-shaped r.
uvular r.
Vacher self-retaining r.
vacuum r.
vaginal r.
VagiTrac vaginal r.
vagotomy r.
Vail lid r.
Vaiser-Cibis muscle r.
Valin hemilaminectomy self-
  retaining r.
valve r.
Vasco-Posada orbital r.
vascular spring r.
Veenema retropubic self-retaining r.
vein r.
vein hook r.
ventriculogram r.
Verbrugge r.
vesical r.
Viboch iliac graft r.
Villalta r.
Vinke r.
Visitec iris r.
V. Mueller-Balfour abdominal r.
V. Mueller fiberoptic r.
Volkmann finger r.
Volkmann hand r.
Volkmann pocket r.
Volkmann rake r.
Wachtenfeldt-Stille r.
Walden-Aufricht nasal r.
Walker gallbladder r.
Walker lid r.
Walter-Deaver r.
Walter nasal r.
Wangensteen r.
W. D. Johnson epicardial r.
Weary nerve root r.
Webb r.
Webb-Balfour self-retaining
  abdominal r.
Webster abdominal r.
Weder r.
Weder-Solenberger pillar r.
Weder-Solenberger tonsillar r.
weighted posterior r.
Weinberg vagotomy r.
Weinstein horizontal r.
Weinstein intestinal r.
Weitlaner r.
Weitlaner brain r.
Weitlaner hinged r.

Weitlaner microsurgery r.
Weitlaner self-retaining r.
Wellington Hospital vaginal r.
Welsh iris r.
Wesson perineal self-retaining r.
Wesson vaginal r.
Wexler-Balfour r.
Wexler-Bantam r.
Wexler self-retaining abdominal r.
Wexler Universal joint
  abdominal r.
Wexler vaginal r.
Wexler X-P large abdominal r.
White-Lillie r.
White-Proud uvular r.
Wichman r.
Wieder dental r.
Wieder pillar r.
Wieder-Solenberger pillar r.
Wiet r.
Wigderson ribbon r.
Wilder scleral self-retaining r.
Wilkes self-retaining r.
Wilkinson ring-frame abdominal r.
Wilkinson self-retaining
  abdominal r.
Willauer-Deaver r.
Williams microlumbar r.
Williams rod self-retaining r.
Wills Eye lacrimal r.
Wilmer-Bagley r.
Wilmer iris r.
Wilson r.
Wiltse-Bankart r.
Wiltse-Gelpi self-retaining r.
Wiltse iliac r.
Winsburg-White r.
wiring r.
Wise orbital r.
Wolf meniscal r.
Wolfson gallbladder r.
Woodward r.
Worrall deep r.
Wort antral r.
Wullstein endaural r.
Wullstein self-retaining ear r.
Wullstein-Weitlaner self-retaining r.
Wylie renal vein r.
Wylie splanchnic r.
Yasargil-Leyla brain r.
Yasargil scalp flap r.
Young anterior prostatic r.
Young bifid r.
Young bladder r.
Young bulb r.
Young lateral prostatic r.
Young prostatic r.
Yu-Holtgrewe prostatic r.
Z r.

Zalkind-Balfour self-retaining r.
Zalkind lung r.
Zenker r.
Zimberg esophageal hiatal r.
Zylik-Michaels r.

Retract-O-Tape surgical vessel loop

retrieval
r. balloon
r. forceps
r. loop

retriever
basket r.
Brimfield magnetic r.
Carroll tendon r.
Concentric foreign body r.
Curry intravascular r.
Entract stone r.
foreign body r.
Golden R.
Kleinert-Kutz tendon r.
magnetic r.
Penetrator suture r.
Pfister-Schwartz stone r.
plaque r.
Positrap r.
3-pronged polyp r.
snail-headed catheter r.
Soehendra stent r.
stone r.
ureteral stone r.
Utrata foldable lens r.
Vantec loop r.
Warren-Wilder r.
Wilson-Cook mini stent r.

retrobulbar needle
retroflexed cystoscopy sheath
retrograde
r. bougie
r. compression nail
r. curette
r. electrode
r. femoral catheter
r. knife
r. meniscal blade
r. occlusion balloon catheter
r. valvulotome

retrograde-cutting hook-shaped knife
retromastoid Ommaya reservoir
Retromax endopyelotomy stent
retroperfusion catheter
retropubic prostatectomy retractor
retroreflective marker

retroscopic lens
retrospective bronchoscopic telescope
retroversion pessary
Retrox Fractal active fixation lead
RetroX hearing system
Retter aneurysm needle
return-flow
r.-f. cannula
r.-f. hemostatic catheter
r.-f. retention catheter

Retzius system
Reul
R. aortic clamp
R. coronary artery scissors
R. coronary forceps

ReUnite
R. hammertoe implant
R. hand fixation
R. orthopaedic pin
R. orthopaedic screw
R. resorbable orthopaedic fixation system
R. VersaTile fixation

Reuse Expanda-graft dermatome
Reuss table
Reuter
R. bobbin collar button
R. bobbin implant
R. bobbin ventilation tube

Reveal
R. MLR+ camera
R. Plus insertable loop recorder
R. single lens reflex camera

Revelation
R. handpiece
R. hip system
R. Tx microcatheter

Reverdin
R. abdominal spatula
R. graft
R. holder
R. implant
R. prosthesis
R. suture needle

reverse
r. adenotome
r. cystotome
r. head scissors
r. intraocular lens
r. Kingsley splint
r. knuckle-bender splint

reverse-action hypophysectomy forceps

NOTES

reverse-angle skid curette
reverse-bevel laryngoscope
reverse-curve
  r.-c. adenoid curette
  r.-c. clamp
reverse-cutting
  r.-c. meniscal probe
  r.-c. needle
  r.-c. scissors
reverse-shape implant
reverse-threaded screw
reversible lid speculum
reversion pacemaker
revised
ReVision
  R. hip stem
  R. nail
revision
  anatomic porous r. (APR)
  r. conical reamer
RevitaLase erbium cosmetic laser
Revivac catheter
Reviva Microbrade Duo system
Revive system penile prosthesis
Revo
  R. retrievable cancellous screw
  R. suture anchor
Revolution lens
Revots vulsellum tenaculum
Rew-Wyly
  R.-W. blade
  R.-W. mouthgag
Rexton hearing aid
Reynolds
  R. dissecting clamp
  R. dissecting scissors
  R. infusion catheter
  R. Pathfinder 3 analyzer
  R. resection clamp
  R. skull traction tongs
  R. vascular clamp
Reynolds-Jameson vessel scissors
Reynold-Southwick H-graft portacaval
  shunt
Rezaian interbody external fixation
  device
Rezek forceps
Rezifilm dressing
Reziplast spray-on dressing
RF
  radiofrequency
  RF ablation system
  RF Ablatr ablation catheter
  RF balloon catheter
  RF coil
  RF Mariner catheter
  RF Performer catheter
RF2000 radiofrequency generator
RFb respiratory biofeedback system

RFG-3C Plus lesion generator
R-HAB lighter weight ankle prosthesis
rHead radial implant
Rhein
  R. Advantage diamond knife
  R. capsulorrhexis cystotome forceps
  R. clear-cornea diamond knife
  R. 3-D trapezoid diamond blade
  R. pick
Rheinberg microscope
Rheinstaedter
  R. flushing curette
  R. uterine curette
rheolytic thrombectomy catheter
rheometer
Rhinelander
  R. clamp
  R. guide
  R. pin
  R. plate
Rhino
  R. Cruiser Pavlik harness
  R. Kicker Pavlik harness
  R. Rocket dressing
  R. Rocket epistaxis sponge
  R. Rocket nasal pack
  R. Triangle hip abduction brace
RhinoBur rhinoplasty bur
rhinolaryngoscope
  Olympus ENF-P2 r.
rhinolaryngostroboscopy system
rhinolarynx stroboscope
Rhinoline endoscopic sinus surgery
  system
rhinomanometer
  Storz r.
rhinometer
  Hood Laboratories Eccovision
    acoustic r.
  2-microphone acoustical r.
rhinoplasty
  r. diamond bur
  r. implant
rhinoscope
  Wolf-Post r.
  Wylie-Post r.
rhinoscopic mirror
Rhinotec
  R. blade
  R. shaver blade
Rhinotherm controlled temperature
  system
rhodamine laser
Rhode Island Secto dissector
rhodium
  r. anode
  r. filter
Rhoton
  R. ball dissector

R. bayonet needle holder
R. bayonet scissors
R. bipolar forceps
R. blunt-ring curette
R. cup forceps
R. dural forceps
R. elevator
R. enucleator
R. grasping forceps
R. horizontal-ring curette
R. loop curette
R. microcup forceps
R. microcurette
R. microdissecting forceps
R. microdissector
R. microforceps
R. microneedle holder
R. microscissors
R. microsurgical scissors
R. microtying forceps
R. microvascular forceps
R. nerve hook
R. osteotome
R. pituitary curette
R. 3-prong fork
R. ring tumor forceps
R. round dissector
R. sellar punch
R. spatula dissector
R. spoon curette
R. straight point needle
R. tissue forceps
R. transsphenoidal bipolar forceps
R. tying forceps
R. vertical ring curette

Rhoton-Adson
R.-A. dressing forceps
R.-A. tissue forceps

Rhoton-Cushing tissue forceps

Rhoton-Merz
R.-M. rotatable coupling head
R.-M. suction tube

Rhoton-Tew bipolar forceps

Rhyder diagnostic catheter

RhythmScan monitor

rhytidectomy scissors

Riahl coronary compressor

rib
r. approximator
r. brad awl
r. contractor
r. cutter

r. edge stripper
r. elevator
r. raspatory
r. retractor
r. shears
r. spreader

Riba
R. electrical ureteral meatotome
R. electrourethrotome electrode
R. urethrotome

Riba-Valeira forceps

Ribble
R. bandage
R. dressing

ribbon
r. arch appliance
r. blade
r. gauze dressing
r. gut needle
r. gut suture
r. malleable retractor

RiboPrinter microbial characterization system

Rica
R. anesthetic laryngoscope
R. aneurysm needle
R. anterior commissure laryngoscope
R. arterial clamp
R. bone drill
R. bone hammer
R. bone mallet
R. bone rongeur
R. brain retractor
R. brain spatula
R. cerebral angiography puncture needle
R. cerumen hook
R. clip-applying forceps
R. cotton carrier
R. cranial rongeur
R. cranioclast
R. cross-action towel clip
R. dermatome
R. ear curette
R. ear polypus scissors
R. ear probe
R. ear speculum
R. esophagoscopy set
R. eustachian catheter
R. forceps holder
R. hemostatic forceps

NOTES

Rica *(continued)*
R. infant laryngoscope
R. laminectomy rongeur
R. lipoma curette
R. malleus head nipper
R. mastoid chisel
R. mastoid curette
R. mastoid gouge
R. mastoid retractor
R. mastoid rongeur
R. mastoid suction tube
R. microarterial clamp
R. multipurpose retractor
R. myringotome
R. nasal septal speculum
R. nylon
R. pelvimeter
R. pneumatic otoscope
R. posterior cranial fossa retractor
R. powder blower
R. scalp retractor
R. silver clip
R. skull perforator set
R. spinal rongeur
R. stem clamp
R. surgical catgut
R. suture clip
R. suturing needle
R. tracheostomy cannula
R. trigeminal knife
R. tuning fork
R. Universal trocar
R. uterine curette
R. uterine sound
R. vaginal speculum
R. vessel clamp
R. wire guide pin
R. wire saw
Rica-Adson forceps
Ricard abdominal retractor
Rice pick
Richard
R. Gruber speculum
R. pillow
R. Wolf arthroscope
R. Wolf laparoscopic trocar
R. Wolf Medical Instruments diagnostic/operating laparoscope
R. Wolf nasal epistaxis system
R. Wolf video resectoscope
Richard-Allan surgical ruler
Richards
R. abdominal retractor
R. bone clamp
R. bone curette
R. bone hook
R. bone tap
R. chisel
R. classic compression hip screw

R. Colles fracture frame
R. combination mallet
R. drape
R. drill guide
R. ethmoid curette
R. fixation staple
R. forceps
R. headrest
R. hydroxyapatite PORP
R. hydroxyapatite PORP prosthesis
R. hydroxyapatite TORP prosthesis
R. lag screw compression device
R. locking rod
R. mastoid curette
R. maximum contact cruciate-sparing prosthesis
R. ministaple
R. modular hip system
R. Phillips screwdriver
R. pistol-grip drill
R. probe
R. sideplate plate
R. tamp
R. tonsillar forceps
R. wire twister
R. Zirconia femoral head prosthesis
Richards-Andrews forceps
Richards-Cobb
R.-C. spinal elevator
R.-C. spinal gouge
Richards-Hibbs
R.-H. chisel
R.-H. gouge
R.-H. osteotome
Richards-Hirschhorn plate
Richards-Lovejoy bone drill
Richards-Moeller pneumatic air-filled dilator
Richardson
R. abdominal retractor
R. appendectomy retractor
R. periosteal elevator
R. polyethylene tube introducer
R. rod
R. shaver
Richardson-Eastman double-ended retractor
Riches
R. bladder syringe
R. diathermy artery forceps
R. diathermy forceps
Richet
R. bandage
R. dressing
Rich forceps
Richie brace
Rich-Mar 510 external ultrasound
Richmond
R. bolt

R. forceps
R. subarachnoid screw
R. subarachnoid twist drill
R. subarachnoid wrench
Richnau-Holmgren ear speculum
Richter
R. bone drill
R. forceps
R. laminectomy punch
R. screwdriver
R. surgical scissors
R. vaginal retractor
Richter-Heath clip-removing forceps
Richwil bridge/crown remover
Rickett facebow
Rickham
R. cup
R. reservoir
R. reservoir shunt
Rickshaw Rehab exerciser
Riddle coagulator
Rider-Moeller
R.-M. dilator
R.-M. needle
ridge forceps
ridge-form mesh
Ridley
R. anterior chamber lens implant
R. forceps
R. Mark II lens implant
Ridlon
R. plaster knife
R. spreader
Ridpath ethmoid curette
Riechert-Mundinger apparatus
Riecker-Kleinsasser laryngoscope
Riecker respiration bronchoscope
Riedel corneal needle
Riepe-Bard gastric balloon
Riester otoscope
Rife machine
Rigby
R. abdominal retractor
R. appendectomy retractor
R. bivalve rectal retractor
R. vaginal retractor
Rigg cannula
right
R. 3200 Advantage ultrasound
scanner
r. angle ArthroWands
R. Clip applier

r. coronary catheter
r. heart catheter
r. internal jugular (RIJ)
r. Judkins catheter
r. ventricular assist device
r. ventricular coil
rigid
r. biopsy forceps
r. external distraction (RED)
r. external distraction system
r. gas-permeable contact lens
r. holding rod
r. internal fixation device
r. intranasal endoscope
r. intraocular lens
r. neck rake retractor
r. pedicle screw
r. sigmoidoscope
r. ventilation bronchoscope
r. ventriculoscope
rigidometer
digital inflection r.
Rigiflator handheld inflation/deflation device
Rigiflex
R. ABD balloon dilatation catheter
R. achalasia balloon
R. achalasia balloon dilator
R. biliary balloon dilatation
catheter
R. esophageal TTS
R. OTW balloon dilatation catheter
R. TTS balloon dilatation catheter
RigiScan
R. device
R. penile tumescence and rigidity
monitor
R. Plus rigidity assessment system
RIJ
right internal jugular
RIJ catheter
Rik
Rik Defender prevention mattress
Rik fluid overlay
Rik FootHugger fluid heel boot
Riley arterial needle
ring
r. abdominal retractor
Ace-Colles half r.
AnnuloFlex flexible annuloplasty r.
AnnuloFlo annuloplasty r.
r. applicator

R

NOTES

ring (continued)

atrioventricular valve r.
Bac-Stat drainage r.
Bickel r.
biofragmentable anastomotic r.
 (BAR)
blepharostat r.
Bloomberg lens ophthalmic r.
Bloomberg SuperNumb anesthetic r.
Bonaccolto-Flieringa scleral r.
Bonaccolto scleral r.
Bookwalter retractor r.
Bookwalter segmented r.
Bookwalter vaginal retractor r.
Bores twist fixation r.
Brown-Roberts-Wells base r.
Budde halo r.
Burr corneal r.
Buzard-Thornton fixation r.
Carpentier r.
Carpentier-Edwards Physio
 annuloplasty r.
cataract mask r.
CBI stereotactic r.
centering r.
Charnley centering r.
circumaortic venous r.
r. clamp
r. clip
Confidence r.
constriction r.
Cook continence r.
corenal suture r.
corneal r.
corneal suture r.
corneal transplant centering r.
Crawford suture r.
CRW MRI stereotactic r.
r. cushion
Dell ophthalmic fixation r.
R. drainage catheter needle
Duran annuloplasty r.
r. electrode
Estring estradiol vaginal r.
Estring silicone vaginal r.
Falope r.
Falope tubal sterilization r.
Fine crescent fixation r.
Fine-Thornton scleral fixation r.
fixation r.
Fleischer-Kayser fixation r.
Flieringa fixation r.
Flieringa scleral r.
foam r.
r. forceps
Gimbel stabilization r.
Gimbel stabilizing r.
Girard scleral r.
gold r.

half r.
head r.
R. hip prosthesis
Ilizarov r.
incontinence r.
Intacs intrastromal corneal r.
intrastromal corneal r. (ICR)
intravaginal r.
invalid r.
Japanese erection r.
Johnston fixation r.
Katena r.
Kayser-Fleischer r.
KeraVision Intacs intracorneal r.
R. knee prosthesis
knitted sewing r.
Kraff hyperopic fixation r.
Landers irrigating vitrectomy r.
Landolt C r.
laparotomy sponge r.
r. lens expressor
Lyon r.
Martinez corneal transplant
 centering r.
Martinez scleral centering r.
McKinney fixation r.
McNeill-Goldmann blepharostat r.
McNeill-Goldmann corneal
 transplant r.
McNeill-Goldmann scleral r.
Mertz keratoscopy r.
metal sewing r.
Moran-Karaya r.
Moretsky LASIK hinge protector
 fixation r.
Mose concentric r.
Muller acetabular roof
 reinforcement r.
Nakayama r.
Nichamin fixation r.
Nuvaring contraceptive vaginal r.
Ochsner r.
olive r.
Osbon pressure-point tension r.
pediatric perineal retractor r.
r. pessary
placido r.
plastic sewing r.
pressure r.
pressure-point tension r.
prosthetic valve sewing r.
Puig Massana annuloplasty r.
Puig Massana-Shiley annuloplasty r.
Racestyptine retraction r.
reduction r.
r. remover
retainer r.
retention r.
retraction r.

r. retractor
r. retractor blade
roof-reinforcement r.
r. rotation forceps
r. scanner
Schatzki r.
Sculptor flexible annuloplasty r.
Seguin annuloplasty r.
sewing r.
Silastic r.
silicone elastomer r.
SIM-Seguin annuloplasty r.
sizing r.
SJM Sequin annuloplasty r.
SJM Tailor annuloplasty r.
sponge r.
stereotactic r.
St. Jude annuloplasty r.
r. stripper
Suarez continence r.
suction r.
suture r.
symblepharon r.
Tano r.
Thornton-Fine r.
Thornton fixation r.
r. tongue blade
Tru-Arc blood vessel r.
Turner-Warwick pediatric perineal
  retractor r.
vacuum fixation r.
Valtrac absorbable biofragmentable
  anastomosis r.
V1 halo r.
Villasenor-Navarro fixation r.
Waldeyer r.
Walsh pressure r.
Whitten fixation r.
Wolf-Yoon r.
Yoon tubal sterilization r.
zipper r.
Ring-Adair-Elwyn (RAE)
ring-curette
  Fukushima r.-c.
ring-cutting saw
Ring-Derlan TM biliary endoprosthesis
ringed formed forceps
Ringenberg
  R. electrode
  R. rasp
  R. stapedectomy forceps
ring-handled bulldog clamp

ring-jawed holding clamp
Ringlite fiberoptic light
RingLoc instrument
RingMASTER guide wire
Ring-McLean
  R.-M. catheter
  R.-M. sump drainage set
  R.-M. sump tube
ring-tip forceps
ring-type
  r.-t. imaging system
  r.-t. rigidity measuring device
Rinn
  R. XCP film holder
  R. XCP radiographic paralleling
    device
Rinoflow nasal wash and sinus system
Rionet hearing aid
Riordan
  R. flexible silver cannula
  R. pin
RIP
  respiratory inductance plethysmograph
  RIP plethysmograph
rip-cord suture
Ripstein
  R. arterial forceps
  R. tissue forceps
RI Rapid Exchange balloon catheter
Rish
  R. cartilage knife
  R. chisel
  R. osteotome
Risley
  R. pliers
  R. rotary prism
Rispi Micromega reamer
Risser
  R. cast table
  R. frame
  R. localizer
  R. localizer scoliosis cast
  R. turnbuckle cast
  R. wedging jacket
Risser-Cotrel body cast
Rissler
  R. kidney retractor
  R. mallet
  R. periosteal elevator
  R. pin
  R. vein sound
Rissler-Stille pin

NOTES

Ristow osteotome
RITA
    radiofrequency interstitial tissue ablation
    RITA ablation system
Ritch
    R. contact lens
    R. nylon suture laser lens
    R. trabeculoplasty laser lens
Ritch-Krupin-Denver eye valve insertion
forceps
RiteBite biopsy forceps
Ritleng probe
Ritter
    R. Bovie cautery
    R. coagulator
    R. forceps
    R. meatal dilator
    R. rasp
    R. sound
    R. suprapubic suction drain
    R. suprapubic suction tube
Ritter-Bantam Bovie coagulator
Rival coronary stent system
Riva-Rocci sphygmomanometer
Rivas vascular catheter
rivet
    r. gun
    pop r.
Rivetti-Levinson intraluminal shunt
Riwomat respirator jet
Riza-Ribe needle
Rizzo
    R. dorsal implant
    R. retractor
Rizzoli osteoclast
Rizzuti
    R. double-prong forceps
    R. fixation forceps
    R. graft carrier spatula
    R. graft carrier spoon
    R. iris expressor
    R. iris retractor
    R. keratoplasty scissors
    R. lens expressor
    R. refractor
    R. scleral forceps
    R. superior rectus forceps
Rizzuti-Bonaccolto instrument
Rizzuti-Fleischer instrument
Rizzuti-Furness cornea-holding forceps
Rizzuti-Kayser-Fleischer instrument
Rizzuti-Lowe instrument
Rizzuti-Maxwell instrument
Rizzuti-McGuire corneal section scissors
Rizzuti-Soemmering instrument
Rizzuti-Spizziri cannula knife
Rizzuti-Verhoeff forceps

RK
    radial keratotomy
    RK marker
r\LS red blood cell filtration system
RLS videostroboscopy system
R-Med
    R-M. miniretractor
    R-M. plug
RM stereotaxic system
RNeasy Mini kit
Roach
    R. ball precision attachment
    R. clasp
Roadrunner
    R. PC guidewire
    R. wire
ROAM
    roaming optical access multiscope
roaming optical access multiscope
(ROAM)
Roane bullet tip
Robb
    R. antral cannula
    R. needle
    R. tonsillar forceps
    R. tonsillar knife
Robbins
    R. Acrotorque hand engine
    R. automatic tourniquet
Robb-Roberts rotary rasp
Robert
    R. Jones bandage
    R. Jones bulky soft compressive
      dressing
    R. Jones splint
    R. nasal snare
Robertazzi nasopharyngeal airway
Roberts
    R. abdominal trocar
    R. applicator
    R. artery forceps
    R. bronchial forceps
    R. dental implant
    R. episiotomy scissors
    R. esophageal speculum
    R. folding esophagoscope
    R. headrest
    R. hemostatic forceps
    R. hip dissecting chisel
    R. needle
    R. oval esophagoscope
    R. oval speculum
    R. self-retaining laryngoscope
    R. thumb retractor
Roberts-Gill periosteal elevator
Robertshaw
    R. bag resuscitator
    R. pediatric laryngoscope blade
    R. tube

Roberts-Jesberg esophagoscope
Roberts-Nelson
    R.-N. lobectomy tourniquet
    R.-N. rib stripper
Robertson
    R. corneal trephine
    R. suprapubic drain
    R. tonsillar forceps
    R. tonsillar knife
Roberts-Singley
    R.-S. dressing forceps
    R.-S. thumb forceps
Robicsek vascular probe
Robin
    R. chalazion clamp
    R. orthodontic plate
Robinject needle injector
Robin-Masse abdominal retractor
Robinson
    R. artificial pneumothorax apparatus
    R. bag
    R. equalizing tube
    R. flap knife
    R. incus replacement prosthesis
    R. lung retractor
    R. middle ear prosthesis
    R. piston prosthesis
    R. pocket arthrometer
    R. stapes prosthesis
    R. stone basket
    R. stone dislodger
    R. strut
    R. urethral catheter
Robinson-Moon
    R.-M. prosthesis inserter
    R.-M. stapes prosthesis
Robinson-Moon-Lippy stapes prosthesis
Robinson-Smith
    R.-S. needle
    R.-S. tamp
Robles cutting point cannula
Robodoc robot
Roboprep G device
robot
    Aesop 2000, 3000 endoscopic
      stabilizer r.
    da Vinci r.
    Long Beach stereotactic r.
    Minerva r.
    Minerva neurosurgical r.
    NanoWalker r.
    NeuroMate stereotactic r.

    Robodoc r.
    R. Starr II camera
robot-assisted
    robot-assisted microsurgery (RAMS)
    robot-assisted microsurgery
      workstation
robotic-automated assist device
robotics-controlled stereotactic frame
Robotrac passive retraction system
Robson intestinal forceps
Roc
    R. EZ anchor
    R. suture fastener
    R. XS bone anchor
    R. XS suture anchor
    R. XS suture fastener
Rocabado posture gauge
Rochester
    R. aortic vent needle
    R. atrial septal retractor
    R. awl
    R. bone trephine
    R. bone trephine device
    R. colonial retractor
    R. dressing
    R. gallstone forceps
    R. harvest bone cutter
    R. hip-knee-ankle-foot orthosis
    R. HKAFO prosthesis
    R. hook clamp
    R. lamina elevator
    R. laminar dissector
    R. Medical self-adhering male
      external catheter
    R. mitral stenosis knife
    R. needle holder
    R. oral tissue forceps
    R. rake retractor
    R. recipient bone cutter
    R. Russian tissue forceps
    R. scissors
    R. sigmoid clamp
    R. spinal elevator
    R. suction tube
    R. syringe
    R. tissue forceps
    R. tracheal tube
Rochester-Carmalt
    R.-C. hemostatic arterial forceps
    R.-C. hysterectomy forceps
Rochester-Davis forceps
Rochester-Ewald tissue forceps

R

NOTES

Rochester-Ferguson
 R.-F. double-ended retractor
 R.-F. scissors
Rochester-Harrington forceps
Rochester-Kocher clamp
Rochester-Meeker needle
Rochester-Mixter
 R.-M. arterial forceps
 R.-M. gall duct forceps
Rochester-Mueller forceps
Rochester-Ochsner
 R.-O. forceps
 R.-O. hemostat
 R.-O. scissors
Rochester-Péan
 R.-P. clamp
 R.-P. forceps
 R.-P. hemostat
 R.-P. hysterectomy forceps
Rochester-Rankin arterial forceps
Rochette bridge
Rock
 R. endometrial suction curette
 R. & Roller exercise board
rocker
 r. board
 r. boot
 Carolina r.
 hematology r.
 r. knife
 Uniplane r.
 Wooden Uniplane r.
rocker-bottom
 r.-b. cast boot
 r.-b. cast shoe
Rockert dilator
Rocket coronary dilatation catheter
Rockey
 R. dilating probe
 R. endoscope
 R. forceps
 R. mediastinal cannula
 R. tracheal cannula
 R. vascular clamp
Rockey-Thompson catheter
Rock-Mulligan prosthesis
Rockwood shoulder screw
rod
 Alta CFX reconstruction r.
 Alta femoral intramedullary r.
 Alta tibial-humeral r.
 Amset R-F r.
 r. bender
 Bickel intramedullary r.
 Biofix biodegradable fixation r.
 cold rolled r.
 colostomy r.
 compression r.
 condylar r.

Cotrel-Dubousset pediatric r.
Danek r.
degradable polyglycolide r.
Delrin push r.
Delta r.
DePuy Summit r.
distraction r.
double-L spinal r.
dual square-ended Harrington r.
Edwards-Levine r.
Edwards Universal r.
r. electrode
enamel r.
Ender r.
Fixateur Interne r.
flared spinal r.
glass retracting r.
Green-Armytage polythene r.
Hamby r.
Harrington r.
Harrington dual square-ended r.
Harris condylocephalic r.
Hopkins r.
House measuring r.
Hunter tendon r.
impactor r.
impingement r.
intramedullary alignment r.
intramedullary Rush r.
Jackson r.
Jacobs distraction r.
Jacobs locking hook spinal r.
Kaneda r.
Knodt distraction r.
Kostuik r.
laser r.
Lincoff sponge r.
Luque r.
Maddox r.
McLaughlin laser vaginal
 measuring r.
McLaughlin quartz r.
measuring r.
Meckel r.
medullary r.
Mira silicone r.
modified Harrington r.
Moe modified Harrington r.
Moe subcutaneous r.
Moss r.
Mouradian humeral r.
Olerud PSF r.
orthopaedic r.
Perspex r.
Polarus humeral r.
precontoured unit r.
quartz r.
radiotranslucent r.
retracting r.

Richards locking r.
Richardson r.
rigid holding r.
Rogozinski r.
round extension r.
Rush r.
Russell-Taylor Delta r.
Schneider r.
scleral sponge r.
screw alignment r.
Shaw-Sgarlato hammertoe implant
  prosthesis r.
Shaw-SHIP r.
SHIP-Shaw r.
silicone flexor r.
SinuScope rigid r.
slotted intramedullary r.
spinal r.
square-ended distraction r.
Stader connecting r.
Stenzel fracture r.
sterile transverse r.
Sur-Fit loop ostomy r.
R. TAG suture anchor system
telescoping r.
r. template
threaded r.
vaginal laser measuring r.
Veirs canaliculus r.
Williams r.
Wiltse system spinal r.
Wissinger r.
Zickel II subtrochanteric r.
Zickel supracondylar r.
Zielke r.
Rodenstock
  R. Modular Focusing system
  R. panfundoscope
  R. panfundus lens
  R. scanning laser ophthalmoscope
  R. slit lamp
rod-hook construct
Rodin orbital implant
rod-lens system
Rodriguez-Alvarez catheter
Rodriguez catheter
Roe aortic tourniquet clamp
Roeder
  R. towel clamp
  R. towel forceps
Roeltsch forceps

roentgen
  R. knife
  R. knife stereotaxic radiosurgical
    device
  R. meter
  r. tube
roentgenographic opaque marker
Rogan teleradiology system
Roger
  R. Anderson apparatus
  R. Anderson external skeletal
    fixation device
  R. Anderson pin
  R. Anderson pin fixation appliance
  R. Anderson well-leg splint
  R. septal elevator
  R. septal knife
  R. submucous dissector
  R. system
  R. vascular-toothed hysterectomy
    forceps
  R. wire-cutting scissors
Rogers
  R. mammotome
  R. needle holder
  R. sphygmomanometer
  R. wire cutter
Rogozinski
  R. hook
  R. rod
  R. spinal fixation system
Rohadur gait plate
Rohadur-Polydor orthotic
Rohadur-Schaefer orthotic
Rohadur-Whitman orthotic
**Rohm and Haas PMMA intraocular
lens**
Roho
  R. bed
  R. Dry Flotation wheelchair pad
  R. enhancer cushion
  R. heel pad
  R. heel protector
  R. high-profile cushion
  R. mattress
  R. Pack-It cushion
  R. pediatric seating system
  R. quadtro cushion
  R. solid seat insert
Rohrschneider
  R. cannula
  R. probe

R

NOTES

Roland dilator
rolandometer
Rolf
    R. jeweler's forceps
    R. lacrimal probe
    R. lance
    R. lance needle
    R. muscle hook
    R. punctum dilator
    R. utility forceps
Rolf-Jackson cannula
roll
    ACCO cotton r.
    Akton positioning r.
    Celluron dental r.
    cervical r.
    r. control bolster
    Dutchman's r.
    Fluftex gauze r.
    intrascapular r.
    Kerlix bandage r.
    Kling fluff r.
    Krinkle gauze r.
    Lakeside cotton r.
    lumbar r.
    McKenzie cervical r.
    McKenzie lumbar r.
    McKenzie night r.
    Medline r.
    3M Reston self-adhering foam r.
    neck r.
    octagon r.
    Original McKenzie CPM r.
    silver mylar r.
    Skillbuilder half r.
    Stretch gauze r.
    Tensor elastic bandage r.
    Tumble Forms r.
    Veratex cotton r.
Roll-A-Bout mobility device
Rollator Nova walker
rolled Instat stent
roller
    r. bandage
    Devonshire r.
    r. dressing
    r. electrode
    r. forceps
    r. head perfusion pump
    r. knife
    Lindstrom LASIK flap r.
    r. pump
    Spence cranioplastic r.
    Toledo r.
    tubing hand r.
RollerBack self-massage device
rollerball electrode
roller-bar electrode
roller-barrel electrode

Rollerbottom Xtra Depth shoe
RollerLoop electrode
Roller pump suction tube
Rollet
    R. anterior chamber irrigator
    R. chisel
    R. eye retractor
    R. I&A unit
    R. lacrimal probe
    R. lacrimal sac hook
    R. lake retractor
    R. refractor
    R. retractor
    R. rugine
    R. strabismus hook
Rolnel catheter
Rolo-dermatome
    Stryker R.-d.
Rolodermatome dermatome
Rolon spatula
Rolyan
    R. arm elevator
    R. Firm D-Ring wrist brace
    R. foot support
    R. Gel Shell splint
    R. Reach-N-Range pulley system
    R. tibial fracture brace
ROM
    range-of-motion
    ROM knee brace
Roman laryngostat
Romano curved surgical drill
romanoscope
Romhilt-Estes point scoring system
Rommel
    R. cautery
    R. electrocautery
Rommel-Hildreth
    R.-H. cautery
    R.-H. electrocautery
Rondic sponge dressing
Rondo inhaler
rongeur
    Adson bone r.
    Adson cranial r.
    Andrews-Hartmann r.
    Bacon bone r.
    Baer bone r.
    Bailey aortic valve r.
    Bane r.
    Bane-Hartmann bone r.
    Bane mastoid r.
    Belz lacrimal r.
    Beyer bone r.
    Beyer endaural r.
    Beyer laminectomy r.
    Beyer-Lempert r.
    Beyer-Stille bone r.
    biting r.

Blakesley laminectomy r.
Blumenthal bone r.
Bogle r.
Böhler r.
Boise-Lombard mastoid r.
bone r.
bone-biting r.
bone-cutting r.
bone punch r.
Bruening-Citelli r.
Bucy laminectomy r.
Cairns r.
Callahan lacrimal r.
Campbell laminectomy r.
Campbell nerve r.
Carroll r.
Caspar r.
cervical r.
Cherry-Kerrison laminectomy r.
Cicherelli bone r.
Citelli sphenoid r.
Cleveland bone r.
Cloward-English r.
Cloward-Harper laminectomy r.
Cloward intervertebral disc r.
Cloward laminectomy r.
Codman cervical r.
Codman-Kerrison laminectomy r.
Codman laminectomy r.
Codman-Leksell laminectomy r.
Codman-Schlesinger cervical
  laminectomy r.
Cohen r.
Colclough laminectomy r.
Colclough-Love-Kerrison
  laminectomy r.
Converse-Lange r.
Converse nasal root r.
Corbett bone r.
Costen-Kerrison r.
Cottle-Jansen r.
Cottle-Kazanjian r.
cranial r.
cranial bone r.
Cushing bone r.
Cushing disc r.
Cushing laminectomy r.
Cushing pituitary r.
Dahlgren r.
Dale first rib r.
Dale thoracic r.
Dawson-Yuhl-Kerrison r.

Dawson-Yuhl-Leksell r.
Dean bone r.
Decker microsurgical r.
Defourmental bone r.
Defourmental nasal r.
delicate intervertebral disc r.
Dench r.
dental r.
DePuy pituitary r.
DeVilbiss cranial r.
disc r.
double-action r.
duckbill r.
Echlin bone r.
Echlin duckbill r.
Echlin laminectomy r.
Ferris-Smith-Gruenwald r.
Ferris-Smith intervertebral disc r.
Ferris-Smith-Kerrison
  laminectomy r.
Ferris-Smith pituitary cup jaw r.
Ferris-Smith-Spurling disc r.
Ferris-Smith-Takahashi r.
FlexTip intervertebral r.
r. forceps
Friedman bone r.
Frykholm bone r.
Fukushima r.
Fulton laminectomy r.
Gam-Mer r.
Glover r.
Goldman-Kazanjian r.
gooseneck r.
Gruenwald-Love intervertebral
  disc r.
Gruenwald pituitary r.
Guleke bone r.
Hajek antral r.
Hajek-Claus r.
Hajek downbiting r.
Hajek-Koffler laminectomy r.
Hajek-Koffler sphenoidal r.
Hajek upbiting r.
Hakansson bone r.
Hakansson-Olivecrona r.
Hardy r.
Hartmann bone r.
Hartmann ear r.
Hartmann-Herzfeld ear r.
Hartmann mastoid r.
Hein r.
Henny laminectomy r.

NOTES

rongeur *(continued)*

Hoen intervertebral disc r.
Hoen laminectomy r.
Hoen pituitary r.
Hoffmann ear r.
Horsley cranial bone r.
Houghton r.
Husk mastoid r.
Innomed Ortho r.
intervertebral disc r.
Ivy mastoid r.
Jackson intervertebral disc r.
Jansen bayonet r.
Jansen bone r.
Jansen-Cottle r.
Jansen ear r.
Jansen-Middleton r.
Jansen-Zaufel r.
Jarit-Kerrison r.
Jarit-Ruskin r.
jaw r.
Juers-Lempert endaural r.
Kazanjian-Goldman r.
Kerrison cervical r.
Kerrison-Costen r.
Kerrison-Ferris Smith r.
Kerrison lumbar r.
Kerrison mastoid r.
Kerrison-Morgenstein r.
Kerrison-Schwartz r.
Kerrison-Spurling r.
Killearn r.
Kleinert-Kutz bone r.
Kleinert-Kutz synovectomy r.
Koffler-Hajek laminectomy r.
lacrimal sac r.
laminectomy r.
Lange-Converse nasal root r.
Lebsche r.
Leksell bone r.
Leksell cardiovascular r.
Leksell laminectomy r.
Leksell-Stille thoracic r.
Lempert bone r.
Lempert endaural r.
Lempert-Juers r.
Lillie r.
Liston-Littauer r.
Liston-Luer-Whiting r.
Littauer r.
Littauer-West r.
Lombard r.
Lombard-Beyer r.
Lombard-Boise mastoid r.
Love-Gruenwald cranial r.
Love-Gruenwald intervertebral
 disc r.
Love-Gruenwald laminectomy r.
Love-Gruenwald pituitary r.

Love-Kerrison r.
Love pituitary r.
Lowman r.
Luer bone r.
Luer-Friedman bone r.
Luer-Hartmann r.
Luer-Liston-Wheeling r.
Luer-Stille r.
Luer thoracic r.
Luer-Whiting r.
Markwalder bone r.
Markwalder rib r.
Marquardt bone r.
mastoid r.
Mead bone r.
Mead dental r.
micropituitary r.
Middleton r.
Mollison mastoid r.
Montenovesi cranial r.
Morgenstein-Kerrison r.
needle-nose r.
Nichols infundibulectomy r.
Nicola pituitary r.
Noyes r.
O'Brien r.
Oldberg intervertebral disc r.
Oldberg laminectomy r.
Oldberg pituitary r.
Olivecrona endaural r.
Ortho r.
orthopaedic r.
peapod intervertebral disc r.
Peiper-Beyer bone r.
Pennybacker r.
Pierce r.
Pilling-Ruskin r.
pituitary r.
Poppen intervertebral disc r.
Poppen laminectomy r.
Poppen pituitary r.
Prince r.
punch r.
Quervain r.
Raaf-Oldberg r.
Raney laminectomy r.
rat-tooth r.
Reiner r.
Rica bone r.
Rica cranial r.
Rica laminectomy r.
Rica mastoid r.
Rica spinal r.
Ronjair air-powered r.
Röttgen-Ruskin bone r.
Rowland nasal r.
Ruskin bone r.
Ruskin duckbill r.
Ruskin-Jay r.

Ruskin mastoid r.
Ruskin multiple-action r.
Ruskin-Storz r.
Sauerbruch r.
Sauerbruch-Coryllos rib r.
Sauerbruch-Lebsche r.
Scaglietti r.
Schlesinger cervical r.
Schlesinger intervertebral disc r.
Schlesinger laminectomy r.
Schwartz-Kerrison r.
Selverstone intervertebral disc r.
Selverstone laminectomy r.
Semb r.
Semb-Sauerbruch r.
Shearer bone r.
side-cutting r.
single-action r.
SMIC bone r.
SMIC cranial r.
SMIC laminectomy r.
SMIC mastoid r.
Smith-Petersen laminectomy r.
Smolik curved r.
Smolinski endaural r.
Spurling intervertebral disc r.
Spurling-Kerrison r.
Spurling laminectomy r.
Spurling-Love-Gruenwald-Cushing r.
Spurling pituitary r.
Stellbrink synovectomy r.
Stille-Beyer r.
Stille bone r.
Stille-Horsley r.
Stille-Leksell r.
Stille-Liston r.
Stille-Luer angular duckbill r.
Stille-Luer bone r.
Stille-Luer-Echlin r.
Stille-Ruskin r.
Stille-Zaufal-Jansen r.
St. Luke's double-action r.
Stookey r.
Storz duckbill r.
Struempel r.
Strully-Kerrison r.
Super Cut laminectomy r.
synovectomy r.
Takahashi r.
Tobey ear r.
Universal Kerrison r.
Urschel r.

Urschel-Leksell r.
von Seemen r.
Voris intervertebral disc r.
Wagner r.
Walton r.
Walton-Ruskin r.
Watson-Williams intervertebral
   disc r.
Weil-Blakesley pituitary r.
Weingartner r.
Whitcomb-Kerrison r.
Whiting mastoid r.
Young cystoscopic r.
Zaufal bone r.
Zaufel-Jansen bone r.
Ronis
   R. adenoidal punch
   R. cutting forceps
   R. tonsillar punch
Ronjair air-powered rongeur
roof-reinforcement ring
roof wedge
Rooke perioperative boot
room humidifier
Roos
   R. brachial plexus root retractor
   R. first rib shears
Roosen clamp
Roosevelt
   R. gastroenterostomy clamp
   R. gastrointestinal clamp
root
   r. canal broach
   r. canal drill
   r. canal file
   r. canal spreader
   r. and dural retractor
   r. needle
   r. pliers
   r. rubber dam clamp
   R. ZX apex locator
root-form dental implant
rope
   Bard AlgiDerm r.
   Kaltostat r.
   The R. stretch/traction device
Roper alpha-chymotrypsin cannula
Roper-Hall
   R.-H. foreign body locator
   R.-H. localizer
Roper-Rumel tourniquet
Rosa-Berens orbital implant

NOTES

rosary bougie
Rosato fascial splitter
Rosch catheter
Roschke dropper sponge
Rosch-Thurmond fallopian tube catheter
Rösch-Uchida
   R.-U. needle
   R.-U. transjugular liver access set
Rose
   R. bed dressing
   R. disimpaction forceps
   R. double-ended retractor
   R. L-type nose bridge prosthesis
   R. tracheal retractor
Rosebud dissector
rosehead bur
Rosen
   R. angular elevator
   R. bayonet separator
   R. bur
   R. cartilage knife
   R. dissector
   R. ear incision knife
   R. ear probe
   R. endaural probe
   R. fenestrator
   R. fenestrometer
   R. incontinence device
   R. inflatable urinary incontinence
     prosthesis
   R. J-guide guidewire
   R. knife curette
   R. middle ear instrument
   R. nucleus paddle
   R. phaco splitter
   R. pick
   R. splint
   R. suction
   R. suction tube
Rosenbaum
   R. iris retractor
   R. pocket vision screener
Rosenbaum-Drews
   R.-D. iris retractor
Rosenberg
   R. dissecting cannula
   R. dissector tip
   R. full-radius blade synovial
     retractor
   R. gynecomastia dissection
     instrument
   R. meniscal repair kit
Rosenberg-Sampson retractor
Rosenblatt scissors
Rosenblum rotating adapter
Rosenfeld hip prosthesis
Rosenkranz pedatric retractor system
Rosenmüller curette

Rosenthal
   R. aspiration needle
   R. urethral speculum
Rosenthal-French nebulization dosimeter
Roser
   R. mouthgag
   R. needle
Roser-Koenig mouthgag
Rosner tonometer
Ross
   R. aortic valve retractor
   R. catheter
   R. needle
   R. pulmonary porcine valve
Rosser crypt hook
Rossmax automatic wristwatch blood
   pressure monitor
Rotablator
   R. atherectomy device
   R. catheter
   Heart Technology R.
   R. RotaLink system
   R. rotating bur
   R. wire
Rotacamera camera
Rotacs
   R. guidewire
   R. motorized catheter
   R. rotational atherectomy device
Rotaflex exerciser
Rotafloppy wire
Rotaglide total knee system
Rotahaler inhaler
RotaLink Plus rotational atherectomy
   device
Rotalok
   R. acetabular cup
   R. skin retractor
   R. wrist strap
rotary
   r. basket
   r. bur
   r. cutting instrument
   r. dissector
   r. scaler
rotatable
   r. pigtail catheter
   r. polypectomy snare
rotating
   r. adapter
   r. anode x-ray tube
   r. arm impactor
   r. cutter catheter
   r. disc electrode
   r. endoprobe
   r. forceps
   r. gamma camera
   r. hemostatic valve

r. morcellator
r. speculum anoscope
rotating-hinge knee prosthesis
rotational
r. ablation laser
r. atherectomy device
r. dynamic air therapy bed
rotation-stop washer
rotator
Bechert-Hoffer nucleus r.
Bechert-Kratz nucleus r.
Bechert nucleus r.
R. Cuff Buttress (RCB)
Hosmer above-knee r.
Howmedica monotube external r.
Jaffe-Bechert nucleus r.
Jarit r.
Maloney nucleus r.
nucleus r.
Osher globe r.
Pisacano nucleus r.
R. polypectomy snare
Tennant nuclear ball r.
rotatory-variable-differential transducer
RotaWire floppy gold guidewire
Rotex II biopsy needle
Roth
R. arch form
R. dental cement
R. Grip-Tip suture guide
R. Net retrieval device
R. polyp retrieval net
Rothene catheter
Rothman
R. Institute femoral prosthesis
R. Institute porous femoral component
Rothman-Gilbard corneal punch
Rothon retractor
Roticulator
Cabot Optima laparoscopic R.
R. stapler
Roto
R. Kinetic bed
R. Rest delta kinetic therapy treatment table
RotoClix tubing fixation system
rotoextractor
Douvas r.
Rotograph Plus dental radiography machine
roto-osteotome

rotor
Beckman J5.0 elutriation r.
Beckman JE10X elutriation r.
Kontron TFT 45.6 r.
Ti r.
Roto-Rest bed
Rotorod sampler
Rotosnare device
rotosteotome rotary handpiece
Röttgen-Ruskin bone rongeur
Rotunda perineum needle
Roubaix forceps
Roubin-Gianturco flexible coil stent
Roubin LuMax flexible guiding catheter
Roughton-Scholander
R.-S. apparatus
R.-S. syringe
round
r. body needle
r. chuck-end Kirschner wire
r. cutting bur
r. diamond bur
r. dissector
r. extension rod
r. Gigli saw
r. optical zone marker
r. punch forceps
r. ruby knife
r. speculum
Rousek extender
Roush tonometer
Roussel-Fankhauser contact lens
router
power r.
trochanteric r.
Vortex r.
Roux
R. double-ended retractor
R. spatula
Roveda lid everter
Rovenstine catheter-introducing forceps
Rovers Viba-Brush
Rowden uterine manipulator injector
Rowe
R. blanket
R. boathook retractor
R. bone-drilling forceps
R. bone elevator
R. disimpaction forceps
R. glenoidal punch
R. glenoidal reamer
R. maxillary disimpaction forceps

R

NOTES

Rowe *(continued)*
    R. modified-Harrison forceps
    R. orbital floor retractor
    R. scapular neck retractor
    R. zygomatic elevator
Rowe-Harrison bone-holding forceps
Rowe-Killey forceps
Rowen
    R. spatula
    R. spinal fusion gouge
Rowland
    R. double-action forceps
    R. hump forceps
    R. keratome
    R. nasal rongeur
    R. osteotome
    R. pouch
Rowland-Hughes osteotomy spline
Rowsey fixation cannula
Royal
    R. crown
    R. disposable skin stapler
    R. Flush angiographic flush catheter
    R. Hospital dilator
    R. spoon
Royale III denture resin
Royalite body jacket
Roy-Camille plate
Royce
    R. bayonet ear knife
    R. forceps
    R. tympanum perforator
Roylan
    R. ergonomic hand exerciser
    R. Gel Shell spica splint
Royl-Derm wound hydrogel nonadherent dressing
RPM tracking system
RS4 pacemaker
R-synchronous VVT pacemaker
RT
    RT 3200 Advantage ultrasound
    RT nail
RTA
    retinal thickness analyzer
RTS
    radiation therapy system
    MammoSite RTS
RT/SC 2000 frameless air support therapy
RTV total artificial heart
rubber
    r. acorn tip
    r. airway
    r. band ligator
    r. bite liner
    r. catheter
    r. dam clamp

    r. dam drain
    r. finger cot
    r. Scan spray dressing
    r. spa bowl
    r. spacer
    r. sponge
    r. suture
    r. walking heel
rubber-reinforced bandage
rubber-shod
    r.-s. clamp
    r.-s. forceps
Rubbs aortic dilator
Rubens pillow
Rubicon embolic filter
Rubin
    R. blade
    R. bronchial clamp
    R. cartilage planer
    R. fallopian tube cannula
    R. gouge
    R. nasal bone planer
    R. nasal chisel
    R. needle
    R. oblique rasp
    R. osteotome
    R. septal morcellizer
Rubin-Arnold needle
Rubin-Holth sclerectomy punch
Rubin-Lewis periosteal elevator
Rubinstein
    R. cryoextractor
    R. cryophake
    R. cryoprobe
    R. probe
Rubin-Wright forceps guard
Rubio
    R. needle holder
    R. scissors
    R. wire-holding clamp
Rubovits clamp
ruby
    R. II DDD pacemaker
    r. diamond knife
    r. knife scalpel
    r. laser
RubyStar tattoo removal laser
Rudd
    R. Clinic hemorrhoidal forceps
    R. ligator
Rudderman Frelevator fragment elevator
Ruddock laparoscope
Ruddy
    R. dissector
    R. stapes calipers
    R. stapes prosthesis
Rudolf-Buck suturing device

Rudolph
- R. breathing system
- R. calibrated super syringe
- R. linear pneumotachometer
- R. mask
- R. trowel retractor
- R. 1-way respiratory valve

Ruedemann
- R. eye implant
- R. lacrimal dilator
- R. tonometer

Ruedemann-Todd tendon tucker
Ruese bone graft
Rugby deep-surgery forceps
Rugelski arterial forceps
Ruggles
- R. microcurette
- R. neurosurgical instrument

rugine
- Farabeuf r.
- Rollet r.

Ruiz
- R. adjustable marker
- R. fundal contact lens
- R. fundal laser lens
- R. microkeratome
- R. plano fundal lens
- R. plano fundal lens implant

Ruiz-Cohen round expander
Ruiz-Shepard marker
rulangemeter
ruler
- Berndt hip r.
- Bio-Pen biometric r.
- bronchoscopic r.
- r. calipers
- centimeter subtraction r.
- Charnow notched r.
- Helveston scleral marking r.
- Hyde astigmatism r.
- Hyde-Osher keratometric r.
- Joseph measuring r.
- Krinsky-Prince accommodation r.
- metal r.
- Pischel scleral r.
- Plexiglas radiographic r.
- Richard-Allan surgical r.
- stainless steel flexible r.
- steel r.
- Tabb r.
- Thornton corneal press-on r.
- Thornton double corneal r.

- V. Mueller r.
- Walker scleral r.
- Webster r.
- Weck astigmatism r.

Rultract internal mammary artery retractor
Rumel
- R. aluminum bridge splint
- R. catheter
- R. dissecting forceps
- R. lobectomy forceps
- R. myocardial clamp
- R. ratchet tourniquet
- R. ratchet tourniquet eyed stylet
- R. retractor
- R. rubber clamp
- R. thoracic clamp
- R. thoracic forceps
- R. tourniquet
- R. tourniquet-eyed obturator

Rumel-Belmont tourniquet
Rumex titanium instrument
RUMI
- RUMI system
- RUMI uterine manipulator

Rumison side port fixation occluder
running nylon penetrating keratoplasty suture
ruptured disc curette
Rusch
- R. bougie
- R. bronchial catheter
- R. cleaning brush
- R. coudé catheter
- R. endotracheal tube cuffed
- R. esophageal stethoscope
- R. external catheter
- R. filiform
- R. follower
- R. head strap
- R. laryngectomy reinforced tracheostomy tube
- R. laryngoscope
- R. laryngoscope blade
- R. laryngoscope handle
- R. laryngoscope lamp
- R. leg bag
- R. mucous trap
- R. perineal drape
- R. red rubber rectal tube
- R. retrievable esophageal stent

R

NOTES

Ruschelit
- R. catheter
- R. endotracheal tube
- R. urethral bougie

Rusch-Foley catheter

Rush
- R. awl reamer
- R. bone clamp
- R. driver
- R. extractor
- R. intramedullary fixation pin
- R. intramedullary nail
- R. mallet
- R. pin reamer awl
- R. rod

Rushkin balloon

Ruskin
- R. antral trocar
- R. antral trocar needle
- R. bone-cutting forceps
- R. bone rongeur
- R. duckbill rongeur
- R. mastoid rongeur
- R. multiple-action rongeur
- R. rongeur forceps
- R. sphenopalatine ganglion needle

Ruskin-Jay rongeur

Ruskin-Liston bone-cutting forceps

Ruskin-Rowland bone-cutting forceps

Ruskin-Storz rongeur

Russ
- R. tumor forceps
- R. vascular forceps

Russell
- R. forceps
- R. frame
- R. gastrostomy kit
- R. gastrostomy tray
- R. hydrostatic dilator
- R. hysterectomy forceps
- R. peel-away sheath dilator
- R. percutaneous endoscopic gastrostomy
- R. skeletal traction
- R. splint
- R. suction tube
- R. traction device

Russell-Beck extension tractor

Russell-Davis forceps

Russell-Taylor
- R.-T. Delta rod
- R.-T. Delta tibial nail
- R.-T. femoral interlocking nail system
- R.-T. interlocking medullary nail
- R.-T. screw

Russian
- R. four-pronged fixation hook
- R. Péan forceps
- R. thumb forceps
- R. tissue forceps

Rust amputation saw

Ruth-Hedwig
- R.-H. pneumothorax apparatus
- R.-H. splitter

Rutkow sutureless plug and patch

Rutner
- R. balloon dilation stone extractor
- R. biopsy needle
- R. nephrostomy balloon catheter
- R. stone basket
- R. Universal wedge ureteral catheter

Rutzen ileostomy bag

Ruuska meniscotome

RX
- RX Comet VP coronary dilatation catheter
- RX CrossSail coronary dilatation catheter
- RX Herculink Plus biliary stent
- RX Multi-Link stent
- RX Rocket coronary dilatation catheter
- RX Solaris coronary dilatation catheter
- RX Streak balloon catheter
- RX Viatrac 14 peripheral dilatation catheter

Rx Rocker wheelchair

Rychener-Weve electrode

Rycroft
- R. cannula
- R. lamp
- R. needle
- R. tying forceps

Rydell nail

Rydel-Seiffert tuning fork

Ryder
- R. needle holder
- R. scissors

Ryecroft retractor

Ryerson
- R. bone retractor
- R. bone skid
- R. tenotome
- R. tenotome knife

Ryle duodenal tube

RZ mandibular matrix system

S

S root canal file
S stylet

Saalfeld comedo extractor
Sabbatsberg septum elevator
Sabel cast walker
Saber

S. ArthroWands
S. Bisector ArthroWands
S. BT blunt-tip surgical trocar

saber-back scissors
Sabina lift
sable

S. balloon catheter
s. brush
S. PTCA balloon catheter

Sableflex anterior chamber intraocular lens
Sabra OMS 45 handpiece
Sabre all-in-1 deluxe otoscope
Sabreloc

S. spatula needle
S. suture

Sac

Lap S.

SACH

solid ankle-cushion heel
SACH foot
SACH orthopaedic appliance
SACH prosthesis

Sachs

S. angled vein retractor
S. brain-exploring cannula
S. cervical punch
S. dural hook
S. dural separator
S. needle
S. nerve separator
S. skull bur
S. spatula
S. suction tube
S. tissue forceps
S. urethrotome

Sachs-Cushing retractor
Sachs-Freer dissector
sack

entrapment s.
LapSac collection s.

Sacker trephine
Sacks

S. biliary drain
S. QuickStick catheter
S. Single-Step catheter

Sacks-Vine

S.-V. gastrostomy kit
S.-V. PEG tube

sacral

s. alar screw
s. Dish pressure relief back cushion
s. fixation device
s. pedicle screw
s. plate
s. screw
s. segmental nerve stimulation implantable neural prosthesis
s. spine modular instrumentation
s. spine Universal instrumentation
s. support

sacroiliac cinch belt
saddle

cervical s.
Cloward surgical s.
s. coil
s. locator
prone surgical s.
s. prosthesis
surgical s.

saddlebag

Seidel s.

Sadler

S. bone hook
S. cartilage scissors

Sadowsky hook wire
SAE cast
Saeed Six-Shooter multiband ligator
Saenger

S. ovum forceps
S. placental forceps
S. suture

Safar-S airway
Safar ventilation bronchoscope
Safco

S. alloy
S. diamond instrument
S. polycarbonate crown

Safe

S. & Dry undergarment
S. Response manual resuscitator
S. spine thoracic-lumbar-sacral support

SafeClean instrument cleaning brush
SafeCrit microhematocrit tube
Safe-Cuff blood pressure cuff
Safe-Dwel Plus catheter
Safeset blood sampling system
SafeSheath

S. CSG introducer

S

SafeSheath *(continued)*
    S. introducer sheath
    S. Long introducer
SafeSorb fluid solidifier
Safe-Steer
    S.-S. to Crossing coronary
        guidewire system
    S.-S. guidewire
Safestretch incontinence system
SafeTap tapered spinal needle
**Safe-T-Coat heparin-coated
    thermodilution catheter**
SafeTrak
    S. epidural catheter adapter
    S. ESP system
Safe-T-Tube
    Montgomery S.-T.-T.
SafeTway mouthpiece
Safe-T-Wheel pinwheel
safety
    S. AV fistula needle
    s. belt
    S. Clear Plus endotracheal tube
    s. glasses
    s. guidewire
    s. handle
    s. J-wire
    s. pessary
    s. pin
    s. pin splint
    s. plate
    S. syringe
safety-bolt suture
SafetySURE transfer gurney
Safe-Wrap gauze
**Saf-Gel hydrating dermal wound
    dressing**
SAF hip replacement
SAFHS
    sonic accelerated fracture healing system
    SAFHS 2000 ultrasound fracture
        healing system
Safian
    S. design prosthesis
    S. nasal splint
    S. rhinoplasty prosthesis
**Safil synthetic absorbable surgical
    suture**
Safir pin
Safsite
    S. IV therapy system
    S. valve
Saf-T
    S.-T EZ set
    S.-T J guidewire
    S.-T shield
Saf-T-Coil intrauterine device
Saf-T-Fit amalgamator capsule
Saf-T-Flo T-tube connector

**Saf-T-Intima integrated IV catheter
    safety system**
SafTouch catheter
Saf-T-Pass retractable scalpel
Saf-T-Sound uterine sound
Safyre synthetic sling
Sage
    S. driver-extractor
    S. Instruments syringe pump
    S. pin
    S. tonsillar snare
    S. wire
sagittal oscillating saw
Sahara
    S. clinical bone sonometer
    S. portable bone densitometer
    S. super absorbent reusable
        underpad
    S. ultrasound system
Sahli needle
Saint
    S. George knee prosthesis
    S. Jude prosthesis
    S. Mark dilator
Sajou laryngeal forceps
Sakler erysiphake
SAL
    self-aligning
Salah sternal puncture needle
Salem
    S. pump
    S. sump drain
    S. sump nasogastric tube
Salenius meniscal knife
Salera HKAFO orthosis
SalEst preterm labor test system
Salibi carotid artery clamp
SaliCept
    S. dressing
    S. oral patch
saline
    s. dressing
    s. mammary prosthesis
saline-filled
    s.-f. anatomical breast implant
    s.-f. expander
saline-saturated wool dressing
Saling amnioscope
Salinger reduction instrument
salivary bypass tube
Salman FES stent
**Salmon-Rickham ventriculostomy
    reservoir**
salpingeal
    s. curette
    s. probe
salpingograph
    Schultze s.
Salvage catheter

Salvati proctoscope
Salvatore-Maloney tracheotome
Salvatore umbilical cord ligator
Salzburg
    S. biconcave washer
    S. screw
Salz nucleus splitter
SAM
    subcutaneous augmentation material
    SAM facial implant
    SAM module
    SAM system
Sam
    S. Roberts bronchial biopsy forceps
    S. Roberts esophagoscope
    S. splint
Samadhi cushion
Samb retractor
Samco tube
Sammons biplane goniometer
SampleMaster biopsy needle
sampler
    Cervex-Brush cervical cell s.
    chorionic villus s.
    Cordguard umbilical cord s.
    Cytobrush Plus endocervical cell s.
    Endocell disposable endometrial
      cell s.
    Endopap endometrial s.
    Gynoscann cell s.
    inertial suction s.
    Isaacs endometrial cell s.
    Johnson swab s.
    Mucat cervical s.
    Rotorod s.
    Sartorius air s.
    SelectCells Mini endometrial s.
    Wallach Endocell endometrial
      cell s.
sampling
    chorionic villus s. (CVS)
Sampson
    S. fluted nail
    S. prosthesis
Samson-Davis infant suction tube
Samuels
    S. Hemoclip-applying forceps
    S. valvulotome
    S. vein stripper
Samuels-Weck Hemoclip clip
Samway tourniquet
Sana-Lok syringe

Sanarus Visica treatment system
Sanborn metabolator
Sanchez-Bulnes lacrimal sac self-
    retaining retractor
Sanchez-Perez automatic film cassette
    changer
sandal
    Dr. Scholl exercise s.
    exercise s.
Sandalthotics orthotic
sandbag
    pediatric s.
Sanders
    S. intubation laryngoscope
    S. jet ventilation device respirator
    S. oscillating bed
    S. valve
    S. vasectomy forceps
    S. ventilation adapter
    S. Venturi injector system
Sanders-Brown needle
Sanders-Brown-Shaw aneurysm needle
Sanders-Castroviejo suturing forceps
Sand-Eze EGD pillow
Sandhill
    S. esophageal motility system
    S. probe
Sandhill-800 TDS chart recorder
Sandia Decon foam
Sandman system
Sandoz
    S. balloon replacement tube
    S. Caluso PEG gastrostomy tube
    S. feeding/suction tube
    S. nasogastric feeding tube
    S. suction tube
sandpaper dermabrader
Sandt
    S. suture forceps
    S. utility forceps
sandwich
    Marlex methyl methacrylate s.
sandwich-type splint
Sanford ligator
Sani-Cloth
    S.-C. HB disposable wipe
    S.-C. Plus germicidal disposable
      wipe
Sani-Garm waterproof pant
Sani-Grinder grinder
Sani-Spec vaginal speculum

S

NOTES

sanitizer
    HandClens instant hand s.
Sani Vac
Sano clip applier
SANS
    Stoller afferent nerve stimulation system
    PerQ SANS
Santa Casa wrench
Santulli clamp
saphenous vein cannula
SaphFinder surgical balloon dissector
SaphLite
    S. II retractor system
    S. saphenous vein system
SAPHtrak balloon dissector
Saphyre bipolar ablation probe
sapphire
    s. crystal infrared photocoagulator
    s. knife
    s. lens
    S. premium closed wound drainage system
    S. View arthroscope
Sapporo shunt tube
Saqalain dressing forceps
Saratoga
    S. cycle
    S. sump catheter
Sargis uterine tenaculum
Sargon implant
Sarmiento
    S. brace
    S. cast
Sarnoff aortic clamp
Sarns
    S. aortic arch cannula
    S. intracardiac suction tube
    S. 7000 MDX pump
    S. membrane oxygenator
    S. Siok II blood pump
    S. soft-flow aortic cannula
    S. 2-stage cannula
    S. sternal saw
    S. temperature probe
    S. venous drainage cannula
    S. ventricular assist device
    S. wire-reinforced catheter
Sarot
    S. arterial clamp
    S. arterial forceps
    S. bronchus clamp
    S. intrathoracic forceps
    S. knife
    S. needle
    S. needle holder
    S. pleurectomy forceps
    S. thoracoscope
Sarot-Vital needle holder
Sarstedt system

Sartorius
    S. air sampler
    S. breast pump
SAS
    static adjustable stretch
    SAS II brace
    SAS shoe
Sat-A-Lite contoured wedge seat cushion
Satellight needle holder forceps
Satellite
    S. ear endoscope
    S. Plus pulse oximeter
    S. spirometer
Saticon pickup tube
SatinCrescent implant knife
Satin Plus glove
SatinShortCut implant knife
Satinsky
    S. anastomosis clamp
    S. aortic clamp
    S. forceps
    S. pediatric clamp
    S. vascular clamp
    S. vena cava clamp
    S. vena caval scissors
SatinSlit
    S. implant knife
    S. keratome
Sato
    S. cataract needle
    S. corneal knife
    S. lid retractor
    S. speculum
Satterlee
    S. advancement forceps
    S. amputating saw
    S. aseptic saw
    S. bone saw
    S. bone saw blade
    S. muscle forceps
saturated calomel electrode
SaturEyes contact lens
Saturn splint
Satvioni cryptoscope
Sauer
    S. corneal debrider
    S. eye speculum
    S. hemostatic tonsillectome
    S. infant eye speculum
    S. outer ring forceps
    S. suture forceps
    S. tonometer
Sauerbruch
    S. implant
    S. pickup forceps
    S. prosthesis
    S. retractor
    S. rib elevator

S. rib forceps
S. rib guillotine
S. rib shears
S. rongeur
Sauerbruch-Britsch rib shears
Sauerbruch-Coryllos
S.-C. rib rongeur
S.-C. rib shears
Sauerbruch-Frey
S.-F. raspatory
S.-F. rib elevator
S.-F. rib shears
Sauerbruch-Lebsche
S.-L. rib shears
S.-L. rongeur
Sauerbruch-Lillienthal rib spreader
Sauerbruch-Zukschwerdt rib retractor
Sauer-Sluder tonsillectome
Sauer-Storz
S.-S. tonometer
S.-S. tonsillectome
Sauflon PW hydrophilic contact lens
Saunders
S. cataract needle
S. cervical HomeTrac traction
S. eye speculum
S. mobilization wedge
Saunders-Paparella
S.-P. marker
S.-P. needle
S.-P. pick
S.-P. stapes hook
S.-P. window rasp
Saurex spreader
Sauvage
S. Bionit graft
S. Dacron graft
S. fabric graft prosthesis
S. filamentous prosthesis
S. filamentous velour graft
Savage decompressor
Savant imaging system
Savariaud-Reverdin needle
Savary
S. bronchoscope
S. esophageal dilator
S. tapered thermoplastic dilator
Savary-Gilliard
S.-G. esophageal dilator
S.-G. metal olive-tipped dilator
S.-G. over-the-wire dilator
S.-G. Silastic flexible bougie

S.-G. wire guide
S.-G. wire-guided bougie
Savastano Hemi-Knee prosthesis
Save-A-Tooth emergency tooth preserving system
Saver
Haemonetics Cell S.
Shin S.
Saverburger I&A tip
Savlon splint
Savvi synchronous pacemaker
Savvy PTA dilatation catheter
saw
Accutome low-speed diamond s.
Adams s.
Adson Gigli s.
air s.
air-driven s.
Albee bone s.
amputation s.
aseptic s.
Bailey wire s.
Becker-Joseph s.
Bergman plaster s.
Bier amputation s.
Bishop oscillatory bone s.
Bodenham s.
bone s.
Bosworth s.
Bosworth-Joseph nasal s.
Brown s.
Brown-Joseph s.
Butcher s.
chain s.
Charnley s.
Charriére amputation s.
Charriére aseptic metacarpal s.
Charriére bone s.
Codman sternal s.
Converse nasal s.
Cottle-Joseph s.
Cottle Universal nasal s.
Crego-Gigli s.
crown s.
crurotomy s.
Delrin-handle bone s.
DeMartel conductor s.
DeMartel T-wire s.
diamond wafering s.
Engel plaster s.
Farabeuf s.
finger ring s.

S

NOTES

saw *(continued)*
Gigli s.
Gigli solid-handle s.
Gigli-Strully s.
Gigli wire s.
gold s.
Goldman s.
Gottschalk transverse s.
Hall sagittal s.
Hall Versipower oscillating s.
Hall Versipower reciprocating s.
s. handle
helical tube s.
Hetherington circular s.
Hey skull s.
Hill-Bosworth s.
Hough crurotomy s.
Hub s.
humeral s.
Isomet low-speed s.
Isomet Plus precision s.
Joseph bayonet s.
Joseph-Farrior s.
Joseph-Maltz angular nasal s.
Joseph nasal s.
Joseph-Stille s.
Joseph-Verner s.
Lamont nasal s.
Langenbeck metacarpal
  amputation s.
laryngeal s.
Lebsche wire s.
Lell laryngofissure s.
Luck-Bishop s.
Luck bone s.
Luxation patellar s.
Macewen s.
Magnuson circular twin s.
Magnuson double counter-rotating s.
Magnuson single circular s.
Maltz bayonet s.
McCabe crurotomy s.
metacarpal s.
Micro-Aire oscillating bone s.
microreciprocating s.
microsagittal s.
Miltex bone s.
Mueller s.
Myerson laryngectomy s.
nasal s.
Ogura nasal s.
Olivecrona-Gigli wire s.
Olivecrona wire s.
Orthair oscillating s.
Osada s.
oscillating s.
patellar bone s.
Percy amputating s.
plaster s.

reciprocating s.
Rica wire s.
ring-cutting s.
round Gigli s.
Rust amputation s.
sagittal oscillating s.
Sarns sternal s.
Satterlee amputating s.
Satterlee aseptic s.
Satterlee bone s.
Schwartz antral trocar s.
Seltzer s.
Shrady s.
single-sided bone s.
Skil s.
Sklar bone s.
Slaughter nasal s.
spinal s.
Stedman s.
sternal s.
Stille-Gigli wire s.
Stryker autopsy s.
surgical s.
Tuke bone s.
Tyler-Gigli s.
Tyler spiral Gigli s.
Universal nasal s.
V. Mueller amputating s.
V. Mueller-Gigli s.
Wigmore plaster s.
wire s.
Woakes nasal s.
Zimmer s.

sawblade
Stablecut s.

sawdust bed

Sawtell
S. arterial forceps
S. gallbladder forceps
S. hemostat
S. laryngeal applicator
S. tonsillar forceps

Sawtell-Davis
S.-D. forceps
S.-D. hemostat

saw-toothed curette

Sawyer
S. rectal retractor
S. rectal speculum

SAXX renal stent

Sayre
S. bandage
S. double-end periosteal elevator
S. dressing
S. head snare
S. jacket
S. retractor
S. sling
S. splint

S. suspension apparatus
S. suspension traction
Sbarbaro prosthesis
SB Charite III intervertebral dynamic disc spacer
SBE cast
SBQC cane
SC
　suprapubic catheter
Scabbard needle holder
SCA-Ex ShortCutter catheter
scaffold
　biodegradable polymer s.
　collagen s.
　3-dimensional biocompatible s.
Scaglietti rongeur
scalar lead
scale
　balance beam s.
　bedside s.
　Braden s.
　Digitron dialysis chair s.
　Epworth Sleepiness s.
　Esterman s.
　Gosnell s.
　Kenna knee s.
　Scotty the Scale stand-on s.
　Symptom Rating s.
scaler
　Amdent ultrasonic s.
　Brahler ultrasonic dental s.
　Buffalo ultrasonic s.
　Cavitron SPS ultrasonic s.
　Columbia s.
　Deldent Delsonic 2000 s.
　Densco ultrasonic s.
　dental s.
　Eilman rotary s.
　loop s.
　Nordent s.
　rotary s.
　Sonatron ultrasonic s.
　Steele s.
　Tamsco periodontic s.
　Titan s.
　ultrasonic s.
　Vivant ultrasonic s.
scaling device
scalp
　s. clip-applying forceps
　s. electrode
　s. flap forceps

s. forceps
s. hemostasis clip
s. hemostat
s. self-retaining retractor
s. vein needle
scalpel
ASR s.
Bard-Parker s.
Bergman s.
blade s.
s. blade handle
bone s.
Bowen double-bladed s.
carbon dioxide laser s.
Cavitron s.
Contact Laser s.
Dieffenbach s.
disposable s.
Downing cartilage s.
s. electrode
electrosurgical s.
Endo-Assist retractable s.
Endotron-Lipectron ultrasonic s.
Epitome s.
feather s.
Green pendulum s.
s. guard
Guyton-Lundsgaard s.
Hamer s.
Jackson tracheal s.
John Green pendulum s.
laser s.
LaserSonics Nd:YAG LaserBlade s.
lid s.
Lipectron ultrasonic s.
long s.
Myocure blade s.
Otocap myringotomy s.
pendulum s.
Personna Plus disposable Teflon s.
plasma s.
Pre-Cision miniature and microminiature s.
razor s.
ruby knife s.
Saf-T-Pass retractable s.
sculpturing s.
Shaw I, II s.
Smart s.
tracheal s.
UltraCision harmonic s.
ultrasonically activated s.

S

NOTES

scalpel *(continued)*
    ultrasonic harmonic s.
    water s.
ScalpelTec keratome slit blade
scalpene needle
scan
    bladder s.
    Cardiac Protect s.
    CardioTec s.
    computed tomography s.
    CT s.
    DentaScan s.
    DEXA s.
    duplex s.
    fluorodopa positron emission
     tomographic s.
    gadolinium s.
    magnetic resonance imaging s.
    MRI s.
    s. pattern generator
    Pipida s.
    portal-phased spiral CT s.
    postgadolinium s.
    ProstaScint s.
    proton-density axial MR s.
    sestamibi s.
    SPECT s.
    s. spray dressing
    tagged s.
    T2-weighted s.
    ZeroRad body s.
Scanditronix PET scanner
Scand pin
scanhead
    Entos vascular and abdominal
     intraoperative s.
Scanlan
    S. aneurysm clip
    S. bipolar coagulator
    S. laparoscopic forceps
    S. ligator
    S. ligature guide
    S. microforceps
    S. microneedle holder
    S. micronerve hook
    S. microrasp
    S. microscissors
    S. microvessel hook
    S. pediatric retractor
    S. plaster shears
    S. rib shears
    S. scissors
    S. vascular tunneler
    S. vessel dilator
Scanlan-Crafoord contractor
ScanLite
    S. Computer Pattern Generator
    laser accessory
    S. scanner

ScanMaker 9600XL scanner
Scanmaster D, DX x-ray film digitizer
scanned-slot detector system
scanner
    AccuScan CO_2 laser s.
    Acoma s.
    Acuson model 128XP ultrasound s.
    Acuson ultrasound s.
    Acuson XP10 s.
    Advanced NMR Systems s.
    Agfa s.
    All-Tronics s.
    Aloka SSD-720 real-time s.
    Aloka ultrasound linear s.
    Aloka ultrasound sector s.
    American Shared CuraCare s.
    Analogic Anatom 2000 mobile
     CT s.
    Aquilion CT s.
    Artoscan MRI s.
    A-scan s.
    ATL duplex s.
    ATL Mark 600 real-time sector s.
    ATL Neurosector real-time s.
    ATL ultrasound s.
    Aurora MR breast imaging s.
    Bergmann Optical laser s.
    Biosound wide-angle monoplane
     ultrasound s.
    BladderManager portable
     ultrasound s.
    BladderScan s.
    Bruker s.
    Canon s.
    CardioData MK-3 Holter s.
    Cemax/Icon s.
    Cencit facial s.
    Cencit surface s.
    charge-coupled device s.
    cine CT s.
    computed tomographic s.
    computerized axial tomography s.
    Corometrics Doppler s.
    C-PET s.
    CT body s.
    CTI 933/04 ECAT PET s.
    CTI positron emission
     tomography s.
    CT Max 640 s.
    dedicated head s.
    dedicated PET s.
    Del Mar Avionics s.
    DermaScan laser s.
    Diasonics Cardiovue SectOR s.
    digital slide s.
    Dine digital s.
    DMetrix digital slide s.
    Dornier s.
    3D surface digitizer s.

DuPont s.
dynamic spatial reconstructor s.
Eastman Kodak s.
EBT s.
ECAT Reveal PET/CT s.
electrical sector s.
electron beam tomography s.
electron beam x-ray CT s.
Elscint Excel 905 CT s.
Elscint MR s.
Elscint Twin CT s.
Emed s.
EMI 7070 s.
EMI brain s.
EMI CT s.
Evolution s.
Evolution EBCT s.
Evolution XP s.
Fonar Quad MRI s.
Fonar Stand-Up MRI s.
Footfax-SL portable foot s.
full-ring s.
Galen Scan s.
gamma ray s.
Gammex RMI s.
GE Advance PET s.
GE CT Advantage s.
GE CT Max s.
GE CT Pace s.
GE CT/T s.
GE Genesis CT s.
GE 9800 high-resolution CT s.
GE HiSpeed Advantage helical
 CT s.
GE MR Max s.
GE MR Signa s.
GE MR Vectra s.
GE Omega 500-MHz s.
GE single-axis SR-230
 echoplanar s.
GE Spiral CT s.
GF-UM3 s.
Gyroscan ACS NT MRI s.
Gyroscan NT-series MR s.
Gyroscan S-series s.
Gyroscan T5-NT MR s.
Heidelberg laser tomographic s.
high-field open MRI s.
high-resolution real-time s.
Hilight Advantage System CT s.
HiSpeed Advantage CT s.
HiSpeed Advantage helical s.

Hitachi CT s.
Hitachi EUB-405 ultrasound s.
Hitachi MR s.
Hitachi PCT-3600W PET s.
Hologic QDR 1000W dual-energy
 x-ray absorptiometry s.
Horizon LX s.
Howtek Scanmaster DX s.
Imatron C-150XL ultrafast CT s.
Imatron electron beam
 tomography s.
Imatron Fastrac C-100 cine x-ray
 CT s.
Indomitable s.
infrared liver s.
Innervision MR s.
InstaScan s.
intensified radiographic imaging
 system s.
Interad whole body CT s.
iris s.
JustVision 400 diagnostic
 ultrasound s.
Konica KFDR-S laser film s.
Kretz Combison 330 ultrasound s.
large-bore imaging system s.
s. laser ophthalmoscope
LightSpeed multidetector CT s.
LightSpeed QX/i CT s.
LightSpeed Ultra CT s.
linear convex array s.
Lintro-Scan s.
low-field MR s.
Lumiscan s.
Lumisys s.
Lunar DPX total-body s.
3M s.
Magna-SL s.
Magnes 2500 whole-blood s.
Magnetom Symphony whole-
 body s.
Magnex MR s.
Mallinckrodt s.
Max Plus MR s.
MedImage s.
Medison s.
MedX s.
megavoltage CT s.
Microtek ScanMaker 9600XL s.
MKII automated s.
mobile spiral computed
 tomography s.

S

NOTES

scanner *(continued)*

mPower PET s.
multidetector CT s.
multiplane s.
multisensory structured light range digitizer s.
multislice CT s.
NeuroFocus scanned focal point s.
Neurolite SPECT perfusion s.
neurSector s.
NewTom s.
Nishimoto Sangyo s.
Norland pQCT XCT2000 s.
nuclear s.
OctreoScan s.
Ohio Nuclear Delta s.
Olympus endoscopic ultrasound s.
OmniMedia XRS s.
Opthascan Mini-A s.
Optiscan 2000 s.
Oxford 2-T large-bore imaging system s.
Pace Plus System s.
Park Medical Systems s.
Perception s.
peripheral quantitative computerized tomography s.
PET s.
PET/CT s.
Pfizer s.
Philips Gyroscan ACS s.
Philips Gyroscan ACS-NT MR s.
Philips Gyroscan NT-series s.
Philips Gyroscan S-series MR s.
Philips Gyroscan T5-NT MR s.
Philips small-bore system s.
Philips spiral CT s.
Philips Tomoscan SR 6000 CT s.
Picker Edge MR s.
Picker PQ helical CT s.
Picker Synerview 600 s.
Picker Vista HPQ MRI s.
Picker Vista MagnaScanner s.
4096 Plus PET s.
Polhemus 3-D digitizer s.
Posicam HZ PET s.
positron emission transaxial tomography s.
pQCT s.
ProSpeed CT s.
Quad MRI s.
Quick CT9800 s.
real-time B s.
rectilinear s.
Right 3200 Advantage ultrasound s.
ring s.
Scanditronix PET s.
ScanLite s.

ScanMaker 9600XL s.
scintillation s.
SCU-series digital color ultrasound s.
sector s.
Shimadzu 5000 CT s.
Siemens DRH CT s.
Siemens ECAT 951/31R PET s.
Siemens Evolution EBCT s.
Siemens Magnetom GBS II s.
Siemens Magnetom Vision s.
Siemens Somatom DR2, DR3 whole-body s.
Siemens 1.5 Tesla s.
Signa I.S.T. MRI s.
Signa whole-body MRI s.
SilkTouch CO_2 laser s.
single-detector helical s.
single-detector row s.
Sinvision ultrasound s.
Skinscan s.
small-bore s.
SmartPrep s.
Softscan laser s.
Somatom DR CT s.
Somatom Plus S whole-body CT s.
spiral computed tomography s.
spiral CT s.
spiral XCT s.
SwiftLase s.
Swissray s.
Symphony whole-body s.
Technicare Delta 2020 s.
Tecmag Libra-S16 system s.
thermographic s.
tomographic s.
Tomomatic brain s.
Tomoscan M CT s.
Tomoscan SR 7000 s.
Toshiba brain s.
Toshiba helical CT s.
Toshiba MR s.
Toshiba TCT-900S helical CT s.
Toshiba Xpress SX helical CT s.
Toshiba Xvision s.
Trionix s.
Twin Flash s.
Ultrafast CT s.
Ultra-Image A-scan s.
Varian CT s.
Vidar s.
Vision MRI s.
Vision Ten V-scan s.
Vista Tesla MRI s.
whole-body digital s.
Xpress/SW helical CT s.
Xpress/SX helical CT s.

scanning
- s. arm
- s. beam digital system
- s. echoendoscope
- s. electron microscope
- s. excimer laser
- s. fluorometer
- s. laser acoustic microscope
- s. laser ophthalmoscope
- s. laser polarimeter
- s. prism
- s. Radiometer
- s. retinal thickness analyzer
- s. slit confocal microscope
- s. transmission electron microscope
- s. tunneling microscope

S-cannula
- Clagett S-c.

Scanpor
- S. acrylate adhesive
- S. surgical tape

Scanzoni forceps
Scaphoid-Microstaple system
scaphoid screw guide
scapular retractor
Scarborough prosthesis
scarf bandage
Scar Fx lightweight silicone sheeting
scarifier
- Berkeley s.
- Desmarres s.
- Graefe s.
- s. knife
- Kuhnt corneal s.

scarifying curette
scarlet red gauze dressing
scattering
- s. foil
- s. foil compensator
- s. system

scavenging tube
SCD
- sequential compression device
- SCD MaleFactor Pak
- SCD stocking

SCDT heart valve prosthesis
Sceratti goniometer
Schaaf foreign body forceps
Schachar
- S. blepharostat
- S. lens

Schachne-Desmarres lid everter

Schacht colostomy appliance
Schaedel
- S. clip
- S. cross-action towel clamp

Schaefer
- S. ethmoid curette
- S. fixation forceps
- S. mastoid curette
- S. sponge holder

Schaldach electrode pacemaker
Schall laryngectomy tube
Schaltenbrand-Wahren stereotactic atlas
Schamberg comedo extractor
Schanz
- S. blade
- S. cannula
- S. cautery
- S. collar
- S. collar brace
- S. electrocautery
- S. knife
- S. needle
- S. pin
- S. screw
- S. trephine

Schanzioni craniotomy forceps
Scharff
- S. bipolar forceps
- S. lens

Schatzki ring
Schatz-Palmaz tubular mesh stent
Schatz utility forceps
Schecter-Bryant aortic vent needle
Schede bone curette
Scheer
- S. crimper forceps
- S. elevator knife
- S. hook
- S. knife elevator
- S. middle ear instrument
- S. needle
- S. oval window rasp
- S. pick
- S. Tef-wire prosthesis

Scheer-Wullstein cutting bur
Scheicher laminectomy punch
Scheie
- S. anterior chamber cannula
- S. blade
- S. cataract-aspirating cannula
- S. cataract-aspirating needle
- S. electrocautery

S

NOTES

Scheie *(continued)*
S. goniopuncture knife
S. goniotomy knife
S. ophthalmic cautery
S. trephine
Scheie-Graefe fixation forceps
Scheie-Westcott corneal scissors
Scheimpflug camera
Scheinmann
S. biting punch
S. biting tip
S. esophagoscopy forceps
S. laryngeal forceps
Schein syringe
Schepens
S. binocular indirect camera
S. boat silicone
S. eye cautery
S. forceps
S. grooved rubber silicone
S. hollow hemisphere implant
S. ophthalmoscope
S. orbital retractor
S. pad silicone
S. refractor
S. scleral depressor
S. spoon
S. surface electrode
S. tantalum clip
Schepens-Pomerantzeff ophthalmoscope
Scherback-Porges vaginal speculum
Scheuerlen raspatory
Schick forceps
Schiek back support
Schilder plugger
Schillinger suture support
Schimelbusch inhaler
Schindler
S. gastroscope
S. optical esophagoscope
S. peritoneal forceps
S. retractor
Schink
S. dermatome
S. metatarsal retractor
Schiötz tonometer
Schirmer tear test strip
Schlein
S. clamp
S. shoulder holder
S. shoulder positioner
S. total elbow prosthesis
S. trisurface ankle prosthesis
Schlesinger
S. cervical punch
S. cervical punch forceps
S. cervical rongeur
S. clamp

S. Gigli-saw guide
S. intervertebral disc forceps
S. intervertebral disc rongeur
S. laminectomy rongeur
S. meniscus-grasping forceps
S. rongeur forceps
Schmeden tonsillar punch
Schmidt optics system
Schmid vascular spatula
Schmieden
S. needle
S. probe
Schmieden-Dick needle
Schmieden-Taylor
S.-T. dissector
S.-T. dural scissors
Schmiedt tube
Schmitt fan
Schmuth modification activator
Schnaudigel sclerotomy punch
Schneider
S. catheter
S. driver-extractor
S. esophageal Wallstent
S. extractor
S. intramedullary nail
S. Magic Wallstent
S. nail driver
S. nail shaft reamer
S. pelvimeter
S. PTCA instrument
S. raspatory
S. rod
S. self-broaching pin
S. stent
S. trefoil balloon catheter
S. Wallstent biliary endoprosthesis
Schneider-Meier magnum system
Schneider-Sauerbruch raspatory
Schneider-Shiley
S.-S. balloon
S.-S. dilatation catheter
Schnidt
S. clamp
S. gall duct forceps
S. hemostat
S. thoracic forceps
S. tonsillar forceps
Schnidt-Rumpler forceps
Schnitker scalp retractor
Schnitman skin hook
Schocket
S. scleral depressor
S. tube implant
Schoemaker
S. intestinal clamp
S. scissors
Schoemaker-Loth scissors

Schoenberg
    S. intestinal forceps
    S. uterine forceps
Schoenborn retractor
Schoenrock laser instrument set
Scholander apparatus
Scholar II vital sign monitor
Scholda style sponge
Scholl
    S. meniscal knife
    S. pad
Scholten
    S. endomyocardial biopsy forceps
    S. endomyocardial bioptome
    S. sternal retractor
Schonander film changer
SchonCath long-term catheter
Schon hemodialysis catheter
SchonXL temporary catheter
Schoonmaker femoral catheter
Schroeder
    S. episiotomy scissors
    S. interlocking uterine sound
    S. operating scissors
    S. tenaculum
    S. tissue forceps
    S. uterine curette
    S. uterine scoop
    S. uterine vulsellum forceps
    S. vulsellum forceps
Schroeder-Braun
    S.-B. uterine forceps
    S.-B. uterine tenaculum
Schroeder-Van Doren tenaculum forceps
Schrotter catheter
Schubert
    S. cervical biopsy forceps
    S. uterine biopsy forceps
Schubert-Van Doren uterine biopsy punch
Schuco 2000 nebulizer
Schuknecht
    S. chisel
    S. cutter
    S. elevator
    S. foreign body remover
    S. Gelfoam wire prosthesis
    S. gouge
    S. middle ear instrument
    S. needle
    S. pick

    S. postauricular self-retaining retractor
    S. roller knife
    S. sickle knife
    S. spatula
    S. stapes hook
    S. suction tip
    S. suction tube
    S. Teflon wire piston prosthesis
    S. temporal trephine
    S. whirlybird excavator
    S. wire crimper
    S. wire-cutting scissors
Schuknecht-Paparella wire-bending die
Schuknecht-Wullstein retractor
Schulec silver clip
Schuler aspiration/irrigation tube
Schuletz
    S. antral curette
    S. pacemaker
Schuletz-Simmons ethmoidal curette
Schultz-Crock binocular ophthalmoscope
Schultze
    S. embryotomy knife
    S. salpingograph
Schultz iris retractor
Schumacher
    S. aortic clamp
    S. biopsy forceps
    S. sternum shears
    S. umbilical cord scissors
Schumann giant eye magnet
Schumann-Schreus dermabrader
Schurring ossicle cup prosthesis
Schutte shovel-nose basket
Schutt needle
Schutz
    S. clamp
    S. clip
    S. forceps
Schwaber otologic implant
Schwarten
    S. balloon dilatation catheter
    S. LP balloon catheter
    S. LP guidewire
    S. Microglide LP balloon
Schwartz
    S. antral trocar saw
    S. arterial aneurysm clamp
    S. bulldog clamp
    S. cervical tenaculum hook
    S. clip

S

NOTES

Schwartz *(continued)*
    S. clip applier
    S. clip-applying forceps
    S. cordotomy knife
    S. endocervical curette
    S. intracranial clamp
    S. laminectomy self-retaining
      retractor
    S. multipurpose forceps
    S. obstetrical forceps
    S. plate
    S. temporary vessel clamp-applying
      forceps
    S. trocar
    S. vascular clamp
Schwartz-Blajwas-Marcinko irrigation
  system
Schwartze chisel
Schwartz-Kerrison rongeur
Schwarz
    S. arrow head clasp forming pliers
    S. bow activator
    S. finger extension bow
    S. traction bow
Schwasser
    S. brain clip
    S. microclip clip
Schwed Flexicut file
Schweigger
    S. capsular forceps
    S. extracapsular forceps
    S. hand perimeter
Schweitzer
    S. pin
    S. spring plate
Schweizer
    S. cervix-holding forceps
    S. speculum
    S. uterine forceps
Schwinn
    S. Air-Dyne bicycle
    S. light commercial treadmill
Scialom dental implant material
Science-Med balloon catheter
Scientech calorimeter
Scientronics magnet
Scimed
    S. angioplasty catheter
    S. Express Monorail coronary stent
    S. guiding catheter
    S. rTRA-GC guiding catheter
    S. SSC Skinny catheter
Scimed-Choice floppy wire
scimitar blade
Scinticore multicrystal scintillation
  camera
scintigraphic balloon
scintillation
    s. camera

    s. counter
    s. detector
    s. probe
    s. scanner
    s. spectrometer
scintillator
    aqueous s.
    benzene s.
    cyclohexane s.
    organic liquid s.
scintimammography prone breast
  cushion
scintiscanner
Scintron IV computer
scissors
    abdominal s.
    Ada s.
    Adson ganglion s.
    Aebli corneal s.
    Aebli-Manson s.
    Aebli tenotomy s.
    Alio MICS s.
    alligator s.
    alligator MacCarty s.
    American umbilical s.
    Anderson converse iris s.
    angled s.
    angular s.
    anterior chamber synechia s.
    arteriotomy s.
    ArthroForce hook s.
    arthroscopic s.
    Aslan endoscopic s.
    Aston facelift s.
    Atkinson corneal s.
    Atkinson-Walker s.
    AtrauGrip Weck s.
    Aufricht facelift s.
    Azar corneal s.
    baby Metzenbaum s.
    Bahama suture s.
    Bakst cardiac s.
    Baltimore nasal s.
    bandage s.
    Bantam wire-cutting s.
    Barkan s.
    Barnes perineorrhaphy s.
    Barnes vessel s.
    Barraquer corneal section s.
    Barraquer-DeWecker iris s.
    Barraquer iris s.
    Barraquer-Karakashian s.
    Barraquer vitreous strand s.
    Barsky nasal s.
    Baruch circumcision s.
    bayonet s.
    Beall circumflex artery s.
    Becker corneal section spatulated s.
    Becker septum s.

Becker spatulated corneal section s.
Beckman nasal s.
Beebe wire-cutting s.
Bellucci alligator s.
Bellucci middle ear s.
Berens corneal transplant s.
Berens iridocapsulotomy s.
Bergman plaster s.
Berkeley Bioengineering
  mechanized s.
bipolar s.
Birks Mark II trabeculectomy s.
Blanco s.
Blum arterial s.
blunt-nose s.
Boettcher tonsil s.
Bonn iris s.
Bowman iris s.
Bowman strabismus s.
Boyd dissecting s.
Boyd-Stille tonsillar s.
Boyd tonsillar s.
Bozeman s.
Braun episiotomy s.
Braun-Stadler episiotomy s.
Brooks gallbladder s.
Brophy s.
Brown dissecting s.
Brun plaster s.
Buerger-McCarthy s.
Buie rectal s.
bulldog s.
Bunge s.
Burnham bandage s.
Busch umbilical cord s.
calcified tissue s.
canalicular s.
cannula s.
Caplan angular s.
Caplan dorsal s.
Caplan nasal s.
Caplan septal s.
capsulotomy s.
Carb-Edge s.
cardiovascular s.
cartilage s.
Castanares facelift s.
Castroviejo anterior synechia s.
Castroviejo corneal s.
Castroviejo corneal transplant s.
Castroviejo iridocapsulotomy s.
Castroviejo iris s.

Castroviejo keratoplasty s.
Castroviejo-McPherson
  keratectomy s.
Castroviejo microcorneal s.
Castroviejo tenotomy s.
Castroviejo-Troutman s.
Castroviejo Universal corneal s.
Castroviejo-Vannas capsulotomy s.
cataract s.
cautery s.
Caylor s.
Chadwick s.
Charnley cup-trimming s.
Cherry S-shape s.
Chevalier Jackson s.
Church pediatric s.
Cinelli-Fomon s.
circumflex artery s.
Classon s.
Clayman-Troutman corneal s.
Clayman-Vannas s.
Clayman-Westcott s.
clip-removing s.
Codman s.
Cohan-Vannas iris s.
Cohan-Westcott s.
Cohney s.
cold s.
conjunctival s.
Converse s.
Converse nasal tip s.
Converse-Wilmer conjunctival s.
Cooley arteriotomy s.
Cooley cardiovascular s.
Cooley neonatal s.
Cooley probe-point s.
Cooley reverse-cut s.
corneal s.
corneal section-enlarging s.
corneal section spatulated s.
corneal spatulated s.
corneal transplant s.
corneoscleral s.
coronary artery s.
Costa wire suture s.
Cottle s.
Cottle bulldog s.
Cottle dorsal s.
Cottle dressing s.
Cottle heavy septal s.
Cottle spring s.
Crafoord lobectomy s.

S

NOTES

scissors *(continued)*

Crafoord lung s.
Crafoord thoracic s.
Craig s.
craniotomy s.
crown s.
curved iris s.
curved-on-flat s.
curved operating s.
curved tenotomy s.
cuticle s.
Dahlgren iris s.
Dandy trigeminal s.
Davis rhytidectomy s.
Dean dissecting s.
Dean iris s.
Dean tonsillar s.
Deaver operating s.
DeBakey endarterectomy s.
DeBakey-Metzenbaum s.
DeBakey-Potts s.
DeBakey stitch s.
DeBakey valve s.
DeBakey vascular s.
Decker microsurgical s.
DeMartel neurosurgical s.
DeMartel vascular s.
Derf s.
DeWecker iridectomy s.
diamond-edge s.
diathermy s.
Diethrich circumflex artery s.
Diethrich coronary artery s.
Diethrich-Hegemann s.
Diethrich-Potts s.
Diethrich valve s.
disposable s.
dissecting s.
dissection s.
Dixon collar s.
dorsal s.
Douglas nasal s.
Doyen abdominal s.
Doyen uterine s.
dressing s.
Dubois decapitation s.
Duffield cardiovascular s.
Dumont thoracic s.
dural s.
Durotip s.
ear s.
East-Grinstead s.
Eiselsberg ligature s.
Electroscope disposable s.
electrosurgical s.
Emmet uterine s.
endoscopic s.
enterotomy s.
enucleation s.

episiotomy s.
E-series s.
Esmarch bandage s.
esophageal s.
Essrig dissecting s.
Evershears bipolar laparoscopic s.
Evershears LP bipolar s.
eye s.
eye stitch s.
eye suture s.
facelift s.
facial plastic surgery s.
Favaloro coronary s.
Federspiel s.
Ferguson abdominal s.
Ferguson-Metzenbaum s.
Fine suture s.
Finochietto lobectomy s.
Finochietto thoracic s.
Fisch microcrurotomy s.
Fiskars s.
fistula s.
Fomon angular s.
Fomon facelift s.
Fomon lower lateral s.
Fomon saber-back s.
Fomon upper lateral s.
s. forceps
Foster s.
Frahur s.
Frazier dural s.
Freeman rhytidectomy s.
Frost s.
Fukushima-Giannotta s.
Fulton pediatric s.
gallbladder s.
ganglion s.
gauze s.
Gene s.
general utility s.
Giertz-Stille s.
Gill s.
Gill-Hess s.
Gillies suture s.
Gill-Welsh s.
Gill-Welsh-Vannas capsulotomy s.
Girard corneoscleral s.
Glasscock s.
Glassman thin-point s.
goiter s.
Goldman-Fox gum s.
Goldman septal s.
Good tonsillar s.
Gorney facelift s.
Gorney rhytidectomy s.
Gradle stitch s.
Graham pediatric s.
Grieshaber vertical cutting s.
Grieshaber vitreous s.

Guggenheim s.
Guilford s.
Guilford-Wright s.
guillotine s.
Guist enucleation s.
Guyton s.
Haenig irrigating s.
Haglund plaster s.
Haimovici arteriotomy s.
Halsey nail s.
Halsted strabismus s.
harmonic s.
Harrington deep surgical s.
Harrington-Mayo s.
Harrison suture-removing s.
Harvey wire-cutting s.
Haynes s.
Heath clip-removing s.
Heath suture s.
Heath suture-cutting s.
Heath wire-cutting s.
heavy septal s.
Hegemann s.
Heymann nasal s.
Heyman-Paparella angular s.
Hipp & Sohn dental s.
Hoen laminectomy s.
Holinger curved s.
Holmes s.
hook rotary s.
Hooper pediatric s.
Hoskins-Castroviejo corneal s.
Hoskins-Westcott tenotomy s.
Hough s.
House alligator s.
House-Bellucci alligator s.
House-Bellucci-Shambaugh
  alligator s.
Huey s.
Huger diamond-back nasal s.
Hunt chalazion s.
IMA s.
insulated curved s.
insulated straight s.
iridectomy s.
iridocapsulotomy s.
iridotomy s.
iris s.
Irvine corneal s.
Irvine probe-pointed s.
Jabaley s.
Jabaley-Stille s.

Jackson esophageal s.
Jackson laryngeal s.
Jackson turbinate s.
Jacobson bayonet-shaped s.
Jacobson spring-handled s.
Jako microlaryngeal s.
Jameson facelift s.
Jameson-Metzenbaum s.
Jameson-Werber s.
Jannetta bayonet s.
Jannetta bayonet-shaped s.
Jannetta-Kurze dissecting s.
Jansen-Middleton s.
Jarit dissecting s.
Jarit endarterectomy s.
Jarit flat-tip s.
Jarit lower lateral s.
Jarit microstitch s.
Jarit microsurgery s.
Jarit peripheral vascular s.
Jarit stitch s.
Jesco s.
Jones dissecting s.
Jones IMA s.
Jorgenson dissecting s.
Jorgenson gallbladder s.
Jorgenson thoracic s.
Joseph-Maltz s.
Joseph nasal s.
Joseph serrated s.
Kahn s.
Karakashian-Barraquer s.
Karmody venous s.
Katzeff cartilage s.
Katzin corneal transplant s.
Katzin-Troutman s.
Kaye blepharoplasty s.
Kaye facelift s.
Kaye fine dissecting s.
Kazanjian s.
Keeler intravitreal s.
Kelly fistular s.
Kelly uterine s.
keratectomy s.
keratoplasty s.
Kirby s.
Kitner dissecting s.
Kleinsasser microlaryngeal s.
Klinkenbergh-Loth s.
Knapp iris s.
Knapp strabismus s.
Knight nasal s.

NOTES

S

scissors *(continued)*
 Knowles bandage s.
 Koenig nail-splitting s.
 Koenig-Stille s.
 Koros EndoMax s.
 Kramp s.
 Kreiger-Spitznas vibrating s.
 Kreuscher semilunar cartilage s.
 Kurze dissecting s.
 Lagrange eye s.
 Lagrange sclerectomy s.
 Lahey Carb-Edge s.
 Lahey delicate s.
 Lahey dissecting s.
 Lahey operating s.
 Lahey thyroid s.
 Lakeside nasal s.
 Lambert-Heiman s.
 Landolt enucleation s.
 laparoscopic s.
 laryngeal s.
 Laschal suture s.
 Lawrie modified circumflex s.
 Lawton corneal s.
 Leather-Karmody in situ valve s.
 left-handed cornea s.
 Lexer Durotip dissecting s.
 ligature s.
 Lillie tonsillar s.
 Lincoln-Metzenbaum s.
 Lincoln pediatric s.
 Lindley s.
 Lipshultz epididymovasostomy
  microdissection s.
 Lister bandage s.
 Liston plaster-of-Paris s.
 Littauer dissecting s.
 Littauer suture s.
 Littler dissecting s.
 Littler suture-carrying s.
 Litwak mitral valve s.
 Litwin s.
 Lloyd-Davies rectal s.
 lobectomy s.
 loop s.
 Lorenz PC/TC s.
 lung dissecting s.
 Lynch s.
 MacKenty s.
 Maclay tonsillar s.
 Maki s.
 Malis neurosurgical s.
 Mancusi-Ungaro s.
 Manson-Aebli corneal section s.
 Marbach episiotomy s.
 marking s.
 Martin ballpoint s.
 Martin cartilage s.
 Martin throat s.

 Mattis corneal s.
 Mattox-Potts s.
 Maunoir iris s.
 Max Fine s.
 Mayo curved s.
 Mayo-Harrington dissecting s.
 Mayo-Lexer s.
 Mayo long dissecting s.
 Mayo-New s.
 Mayo-Noble dissecting s.
 Mayo operating s.
 Mayo-Potts dissecting s.
 Mayo round blade s.
 Mayo-Sims dissecting s.
 Mayo-Stille operating s.
 Mayo straight s.
 Mayo uterine s.
 McAllister s.
 McClure iris s.
 McGuire corneal s.
 McIndoe s.
 McLean capsulotomy s.
 McPherson-Castroviejo corneal
  section s.
 McPherson-Castroviejo
  microcorneal s.
 McPherson corneal section s.
 McPherson microconjunctival s.
 McPherson microtenotomy s.
 McPherson-Vannas iris s.
 McPherson-Westcott conjunctival s.
 McPherson-Westcott stitch s.
 McReynolds pterygium s.
 meatotomy s.
 mechanized s.
 meniscal hook s.
 meniscectomy s.
 Metzbaum curved operating s.
 Metzbaum operating s.
 Metzenbaum delicate s.
 Metzenbaum dissecting s.
 Metzenbaum-Lipsett s.
 Metzenbaum operating s.
 microlaryngeal s.
 MicroPoint suture s.
 microscopic s.
 microsurgical s.
 Microtek s.
 microvascular s.
 Microvit s.
 Microwec s.
 Miller dissecting s.
 Miller operating s.
 Miller rectal s.
 Millesi s.
 Mills circumflex s.
 Milteck s.
 Mixter operating s.
 Mohr endoscopic s.

Moore-Troutman corneal s.
Morse backward-cutting aortic s.
MPC automated intravitreal s.
Munro brain s.
Murphy s.
Nadler superior radial s.
nail s.
nasal s.
Nelson lobectomy s.
Nelson lung-dissecting s.
Nelson-Metzenbaum s.
Nelson-Vital dissecting s.
Neumann s.
neurosurgical s.
neurovascular s.
New suture s.
Noble s.
Northbent suture s.
Noyes iridectomy s.
Noyes iris s.
Noyes-Shambaugh s.
Nugent-Gradle stitch s.
Nu-Tip laparoscopic s.
O'Brien-Mayo s.
O'Brien stitch s.
O'Brien suture s.
Ochsner s.
Ochsner ball-tipped s.
Ochsner diamond-edged s.
Olivecrona angular s.
Olivecrona dural s.
Olivecrona guillotine s.
O'Neill cardiac surgical s.
Ong capsulotomy s.
operating s.
Ormco band s.
orthopaedic s.
Osher corneal s.
otologic s.
Panzer gallbladder s.
Paparella wire-cutting s.
Par s.
pattern umbilical s.
Péan s.
Peck-Joseph s.
pericardiotomy s.
Peyman vitreous s.
Phaneuf uterine artery s.
Pickett s.
plain rotary s.
plastic surgery s.
plastic utility s.

Poppen sympathectomy s.
Potts-DeMartel gall duct s.
Potts-Smith arterial s.
Potts-Smith dissecting s.
Potts-Smith reverse s.
Potts-Smith vascular s.
Potts tenotomy s.
Potts-Yasargil s.
PowerStar bipolar s.
Pratt rectal s.
Prince dissecting s.
Prince-Potts s.
Prince tonsillar s.
probe point s.
pterygium s.
ptosis s.
pupillary membrane s.
Quimby gum s.
Quimby curved s.
radial iridotomy s.
Ragnell undermining s.
Rappazzo foreign body s.
Rappazzo haptic s.
Real s.
Reeh stitch s.
Reichling corneal s.
Reinhoff thoracic s.
Resano thoracic s.
Reul coronary artery s.
reverse-cutting s.
reverse head s.
Reynolds dissecting s.
Reynolds-Jameson vessel s.
Rhoton bayonet s.
Rhoton microsurgical s.
rhytidectomy s.
Rica ear polypus s.
Richter surgical s.
Rizzuti keratoplasty s.
Rizzuti-McGuire corneal section s.
Roberts episiotomy s.
Rochester s.
Rochester-Ferguson s.
Rochester-Ochsner s.
Roger wire-cutting s.
Rosenblatt s.
Rubio s.
Ryder s.
saber-back s.
Sadler cartilage s.
Satinsky vena caval s.
Scanlan s.

S

NOTES

scissors *(continued)*

Scheie-Westcott corneal s.
Schmieden-Taylor dural s.
Schoemaker s.
Schoemaker-Loth s.
Schroeder episiotomy s.
Schroeder operating s.
Schuknecht wire-cutting s.
Schumacher umbilical cord s.
Scott dissecting s.
Scott right-angle s.
Scoville s.
Sealy dissecting s.
Seiler turbinate s.
Semb dissecting s.
serrated iris s.
Serratex s.
Seutin s.
Shapshay-Healy laryngeal s.
Shea-Bellucci s.
Shea vein graft s.
Shepard-Westcott s.
Shield iridotomy s.
Shortbent suture s.
Shutt s.
sickle s.
Siebold uterine s.
Sims-Siebold uterine s.
Sims uterine s.
Sistron s.
Sistrunk dissecting s.
in situ valve s.
in situ venous valve s.
Slip-N-Snip s.
Smellie obstetrical s.
SMIC collar s.
SMIC ear polypus s.
Smith bandage s.
Smith suture wire s.
Snowden-Pencer Super-Cut s.
Southbent s.
Spencer eye suture s.
Spencer stitch s.
Spetzler s.
spring-handled s.
Spring iris s.
Stalzner rectal s.
StaySharp face lift Super-Cut s.
Stevens eye s.
Stevenson alligator s.
Stevens stitch s.
Stevens tenotomy s.
Stille dissecting s.
Stille-Mayo dissecting s.
Stille Super Cut s.
stitch s.
Stiwer s.
Storz intraocular s.
Storz iris s.

Storz stitch s.
Storz-Westcott conjunctival s.
Storz wire-cutting s.
strabismus s.
straight tenotomy s.
Strully cardiovascular s.
Strully dissecting s.
Strully dural s.
Strully hook s.
Strully neurosurgical s.
Sullival gum s.
Supercut s.
Sutherland s.
Sutherland-Grieshaber s.
suture wire-cutting s.
Sweet delicate pituitary s.
Sweet esophageal s.
Switch-Blade s.
Take-apart s.
Tamsco wire-cutting s.
Taylor dural s.
tenotomy s.
thin-shaft nasal s.
Thomas s.
Thomson-Walker s.
thoracic s.
Thorek-Feldman gallbladder s.
Thorek gallbladder s.
Thorek thoracic s.
Thorpe-Castroviejo cataract s.
Thorpe pupillary membrane s.
Thorpe-Westcott cataract s.
Tindall s.
tissue s.
Toennis-Adson dissecting s.
Toennis dissecting s.
tonsillar s.
Torchia conjunctival s.
Torchia microcorneal s.
Torchia-Vannas micro-iris s.
trigeminal s.
Troutman-Castroviejo conjunctival s.
Troutman-Castroviejo corneal
  section s.
Troutman-Katzin corneal
  transplant s.
Troutman microsurgical s.
Troutman suture s.
Trusler-Dean s.
tubal s.
turbinate s.
turbinectomy s.
Turner-Warwick diathermy s.
Twisk s.
umbilical s.
Universal wire s.
upper lateral s.
U.S. Army gauze s.
U.S. Army umbilical s.

uterine s.
utility bandage s.
valve s.
valve leaflet excision s.
Vannas capsulotomy s.
Vannas corneal s.
Vannas iridocapsulotomy s.
vascular s.
Verhoeff dissecting s.
Verner-Joseph s.
Vernon wire-cutting s.
Vezien abdominal s.
vibrating s.
Vital-Cooley operating s.
Vital-Cooley wire-cutting s.
Vital-Cottle dorsal angled s.
Vital-Fomon angular s.
Vital-Knapp iris s.
Vital-Knapp strabismus s.
Vital-Mayo dissecting s.
Vital-Metzenbaum dissecting s.
Vital-Nelson dissecting s.
Vital operating s.
Vital wire-cutting s.
vitreous s.
V. Mueller curved operating s.
V. Mueller laser tubal s.
V. Mueller operating s.
V. Mueller-Vital laser Mayo
  dissecting s.
Wadsworth s.
Walker-Apple s.
Walker-Atkinson s.
walker corneal s.
Walton s.
Weber tissue s.
Weck iris s.
Weck-Spencer suture s.
Weck suture s.
Weck suture-removal s.
Weck wire-cutting s.
Weller cartilage s.
Werb s.
Wertheim deep surgery s.
Westcott conjunctival s.
Westcott curved tenotomy s.
Westcott double-end s.
Westcott micro s.
Westcott-Scheie s.
Westcott spring-action s.
Westcott stitch s.
Westcott tenotomy s.

Westcott utility s.
Wester meniscectomy s.
White s.
Wiechel s.
Wiechel-Stille bile duct s.
Wiet otologic s.
Wilde-Blakesley s.
Willauer s.
Williamson-Noble s.
Wilmer conjunctival s.
Wilmer-Converse conjunctival s.
Wilmer iris s.
Wilson intraocular s.
Wincor enucleation s.
wire s.
wire-cutting suture s.
Wong-Staal s.
Wullstein ear s.
Wutzler s.
Yankauer s.
Yasargil Aesculap s.
Yasargil bayonet s.
Yasargil microvascular bayonet s.
Zaldivar iridectomy s.
Zoellner s.
Z-Scissors hysterectomy s.
Zylik-Michaels s.

scleral
s. blade
s. buckle eye implant
s. buckling catheter
s. depressor
s. exoplant
s. hook
s. implant
s. marker
s. pick
s. plug
s. punch
s. resection knife
s. shell press
s. shield
s. shortening clip
s. spatula needle
s. sponge rod
s. trephine
s. twist fixation hook
s. twist-grip forceps
s. wound retractor

sclerectomy
s. punch
s. punch forceps

NOTES

S

ScleroLaser laser
ScleroPLUS
> S. HP laser system
> S. LongPulse dye laser

sclerostomy needle
sclerotherapy needle
sclerotome
> Alvis-Lancaster s.
> Atkinson s.
> s. blade
> Castroviejo s.
> Curdy s.
> Guyton-Lundsgaard s.
> Lancaster s.
> Lundsgaard s.
> Lundsgaard-Burch s.
> s. pain chart
> Walker-Lee s.

sclerotomy punch
Scobee-Allis forceps
Scobee oblique muscle hook
Scoi brace
scoliometer
scoliosis brace
scoop
> Abbott s.
> abdominal s.
> abortion s.
> Arlt fenestrated lens s.
> Asch uterine secretion s.
> Beck abdominal s.
> Beck gastrostomy s.
> Berens common duct s.
> Berens lens s.
> Boyd bone s.
> Bruus s.
> common duct stone s.
> cystic duct s.
> Daviel lens s.
> Desjardins gall duct s.
> Desjardins gallstone s.
> s. dish
> duct s.
> Elschnig lens s.
> enucleation s.
> Ferguson gallstone s.
> Ferris common duct s.
> French s.
> gallbladder s.
> gall duct s.
> gallstone s.
> Green lens s.
> Hess lens s.
> Hibbs s.
> Klebanoff gallstone s.
> Knapp lens s.
> Lang eye s.
> lens enucleation s.
> Lewis lens s.

> Luer s.
> Luer-Koerte gallstone s.
> Mayo common duct s.
> Mayo cystic duct s.
> Mayo gallbladder s.
> Mayo gall duct s.
> Mayo gallstone s.
> Mayo-Robson gallstone s.
> Moore gall duct s.
> Moore gallstone s.
> Moynihan gallstone s.
> Mules s.
> Pagenstecher lens s.
> Schroeder uterine s.
> Simon uterine s.
> Snellen lens s.
> Syrrat s.
> S. transtracheal catheter
> uterine s.
> Volkmann s.
> Wallich abortion s.
> Wallich placental s.
> Weber lens s.
> Wells enucleation s.
> Wilder lens s.
> Yasargil s.
> Zarski gallstone s.

Scooter
> K9 S.

Scoot-Gard mat
scope
> Augustine s.
> baby s.
> Electro-Acuscope s.
> ENT s.
> fixed-focus s.
> Gamboscope s.
> KeraCorneoScope s.
> KeyMed fiberoptic s.
> Olympus fiberoptic s.
> variable-focus s.
> Welch Allyn pocket s.

3Dscope laparoscope
Scopemaster contact hysteroscope
ScopeTrac support device
Scorpio total knee system
Scotch boot
Scotchcast
> S. 2 casting tape
> S. custom length splint system

scotometer
> Bjerrum s.

Scott
> S. AMS inflatable penile prosthesis
> S. attic cannula
> S. chronic wound care system
> S. dissecting scissors
> S. ear speculum
> S. humeral splint

S. lens-insertion forceps
S. nasal suction tube
S. right-angle scissors
S. ring penile retractor
S. rotating resectoscope
S. rubber ventricular cannula
Scott-Craig orthosis
Scott-Harden tube
Scottish
S. Rite brace
S. Rite hip orthosis
S. Rite splint
Scott-McCracken periosteal elevator
Scott-RCE osteotomy guide
Scotty
S. the Scale stand-on scale
S. stainless ankle joint
Scoville
S. blunt hook
S. brain forceps
S. Britetrac retractor
S. cervical disc self-retaining retractor
S. clip
S. clip applier
S. clip-applying forceps
S. curved nerve hook
S. dural hook
S. flat brain spatula
S. hemilaminectomy self-retaining retractor
S. laminectomy retractor
S. nerve root retractor
S. psoas muscle retractor
S. retractor blade
S. retractor hook
S. ruptured disc curette
S. scissors
S. self-retaining retractor
S. skull trephine
S. ventricular needle
Scoville-Drew clip applier
Scoville-Greenwood bipolar forceps
Scoville-Haverfield laminectomy retractor
Scoville-Hurteau forceps
Scoville-Lewis
S.-L. aneurysm clip
S.-L. clamp
Scoville-Richter self-retaining retractor
Scram emergency escape breathing device

scraper
amalgam s.
Bradley femoral canal preparation s.
capsular s.
Charnley acetabular s.
drum s.
epithelial s.
Hough drum s.
Knolle capsular s.
Kratz capsular s.
Lewicky capsular s.
Simcoe capsular s.
Tano membrane s.
scraping brush
scratcher
Jensen capsular s.
Knolle capsular s.
Kratz capsular s.
Kratz-Jensen capsular s.
screen
Bernell tangent s.
Bjerrum s.
ether s.
Hess diplopia s.
Hess-Lee s.
homogeneous s.
intensifying s.
Lancaster red-green s.
Lanex medium s.
split s.
tangent s.
screener
Algo newborn hearing s.
AutoPap 300 QC automatic Pap s.
Noise Stik II pediatric hearing s.
Rosenbaum pocket vision s.
SmartScreener infant hearing s.
SureSight vision s.
screw
Absolute absorbable s.
Acutrak s.
Acutrak Mini s.
Acutrak Plus s.
alar s.
s. alignment bar
s. alignment rod
Alta cancellous s.
Alta cortical s.
Alta cross-locking s.
Alta lag s.
Alta supracondylar s.

NOTES

screw *(continued)*

Alta transverse s.
amputation s.
Amset R-F s.
anchor s.
AO cancellous s.
AO cortex s.
AO lag s.
AO spongiosa s.
Arthrex sheathed interference s.
Asnis guided s.
Asnis 2 guided s.
Asnis III cannulated s.
Aten olecranon s.
Barouk cannulated bone s.
Basile hip s.
bicortical s.
bicortical superior border s.
bioabsorbable interference s.
BioCuff s.
biodegradable s.
Biofix absorbable s.
biointerference s.
Biologically Quiet interference s.
Biologically Quiet reconstruction s.
Bionx BioCuff s.
BioRCI s.
BioScrew bio-absorbable
  interference s.
BioSorb endoscopic browlift s.
Bio-Tenodesis s.
bone s.
Bone Mulch s.
Bosworth coracoclavicular s.
Calcitek retaining s.
Camino subdural s.
cancellous bone s.
cannulated cancellous lag s.
carpal scaphoid s.
Carrel-Girard s.
Caspar cervical s.
CeraOne abutment/implant s.
Clearfix meniscal s.
Cohort bone s.
Collison s.
compression hip s.
s. compressor
Concise compression hip s.
CorIS interference s.
cortex s.
cortical s.
cortical pin s.
Cotrel pedicle s.
cover s.
craniomaxillofacial s.
Crites laryngeal cotton s.
crown drill s.
cruciate head bone s.
cruciform head bone s.

Cubbins s.
dental implant cover s.
Dentatus s.
s. depth calibrator
s. depth gauge
DePuy interference s.
Deyerle s.
distal locking s.
distraction s.
Doyen myoma s.
Dwyer spinal s.
dynamic condylar s. (DCS)
dynamic hip s.
EBI Omega21 expandable s.
Edwards sacral s.
Eggers s.
encased s.
endobrow push s.
EndoFix absorbable interference s.
expansion s.
Fixateur Interne s.
fixation s.
foreign body s.
Gentle Threads interference s.
glenoid fixation s.
s. grip
Guardsman femoral interference s.
Hahn s.
Hall-Morris biphase s.
Hall spinal s.
healing s.
Heck s.
Helio cortical lag s.
Herbert bone s.
Herbert scaphoid s.
Herbert-Whipple bone s.
Hiploc compression hip s.
Howmedica Universal
  compression s.
iliac s.
iliosacral s.
Ilizarov s.
ImplaMed gold s.
implant cover s.
Implant Innovations titanium s.
Implant Support Systems
  titanium s.
Instrument Makar biodegradable
  interference s.
interference s.
interfragmentary lag s.
intracranial pressure monitor s.
Isola vertebral s.
Jeter lag s.
Jeter position s.
Jewett pickup s.
Johannson lag s.
Johannson-Stille lag s.
KLS Centre-Drive s.

KLS-Martin Centre-Drive s.
Kostuik s.
Kristiansen eyelet lag s.
Kurosaka interference-fit s.
lag s.
Lane bone s.
lateral s.
Leibinger Micro Plus s.
Leibinger Mini Würzburg s.
Leibinger Würzburg s.
Leinbach olecranon s.
Leone expansion s.
Lewis tonsillar s.
Lindorf lag s.
Lindorf position s.
Linvatec bioabsorbable
  interference s.
Linvatec cannulated interference s.
locking s.
Lorenz s.
Luhr implant s.
Luhr Vitallium s.
lumbar pedicle s.
Lundholm s.
Luque II s.
MacroSorb StarBurst surgical s.
Marion s.
maxillofacial bone s.
McLaughlin carpal scaphoid s.
medial bicortical s.
medial unicortical s.
metallic s.
Micro Plus s.
Mille Pattes s.
mini lag s.
monocortical s.
Morris biphase s.
Moss Miami polyaxial s.
multiaxial s.
navicular s.
Neufeld s.
Nobelpharma gold prosthetic
  retaining s.
No-Lok compression s.
s. occlusive clamp
Olerud PSF s.
Omega compression hip s.
Omega21 expandable s.
Orion plate and s.
Orthex cannulated titanium bone s.
Orthofix s.
orthopaedic s.

OsteoMed s.
OsteoTite bone s.
Palex expansion s.
pedicle s.
PerFixation s.
Periotest Implant Innovations
  gold s.
Phantom interference s.
Phillips recessed-head s.
Pilot point s.
Piranha self-drilling s.
polyaxial cervical s.
polylactide absorbable s.
pretapped Synthes lag s.
Pro/Pel cannulated interference s.
Quiet interference s.
Reddick-Saye s.
resorbable plate and s.
ReUnite orthopaedic s.
reverse-threaded s.
Revo retrievable cancellous s.
Richards classic compression hip s.
Richmond subarachnoid s.
rigid pedicle s.
Rockwood shoulder s.
Russell-Taylor s.
sacral s.
sacral alar s.
sacral pedicle s.
Salzburg s.
Schanz s.
Scuderi s.
self-tapping bone s.
self-tapping Leibinger lag s.
set s.
Sharpey s.
Sherlock self-tapping s.
Sherman bone s.
silk s.
Simmons double-hole spinal s.
Simmons-Martin s.
SmartScrew s.
Smith & Nephew s.
Spiessel lag s.
Spin s.
stainless steel s.
Steinhauser lag s.
Steinhauser position s.
step s.
Stryker lag s.
subarachnoid s.
syndesmotic s.

S

NOTES

screw (*continued*)
Synthes compression hip s.
s. tap
Thatcher s.
thoracic pedicle s.
thoracolumbar pedicle s.
ThreadLoc retaining s.
Ti alloy s.
TiMesh s.
titanium s.
Townley bone graft s.
Townsend-Gilfillan s.
TPS-coated s.
transarticular s.
transfixing s.
transfixion s.
transpedicular s.
Triad facet s.
triangulated pedicle s.
tulip-headed pedicle s.
tumor s.
Universal fixation s.
Venable s.
Vilex cannulated s.
Virgin hip s.
Vitallium s.
Weise jack s.
Wisorb malleolar s.
Wood s.
Woodruff s.
Yuan s.
Zielke s.
Zimmer tibial locking s.
screwdriver
Allen-headed s.
automatic s.
Becker s.
Bosworth s.
Children's Hospital s.
Collison s.
cross-slot s.
cruciform s.
Cubbins s.
DePuy s.
Dorsey s.
Hall s.
heavy cross-slot s.
hexhead s.
Johnson s.
Ken s.
KLS Centre-Drive s.
Lane s.
light cross-slot s.
Lok-it s.
Lok-screw double-slot s.
MacroSorb surgical s.
Massie s.
Master s.
Moore-Blount s.

Phillips s.
plain s.
Richards Phillips s.
Richter s.
Shallcross s.
Sherman s.
Sherman-Pierce s.
skull plate s.
Stab-and-Grab s.
straight hex s.
Stryker s.
Trinkle s.
Universal s.
Universal hex s.
V. Mueller s.
White s.
Williams s.
Woodruff s.
Zimmer s.
screw-holding forceps
screw-in
s.-i. epicardial electrode
s.-i. pacemaker lead
s.-i. sutureless myocardial electrode
screw-on lead
screw-tipped intraosseous needle
screw-to-screw compression construct
screw-type implant
Screw-Vent
S.-V. implant
S.-V. implant system
Scribner shunt
Script Stat, Inc. dispensing system
scrotal
s. dressing
s. truss
scrub
s. brush
s. file
scrubber
capsular s.
posterior capsule s.
Simcoe anterior chamber capsule s.
Simcoe posterior capsule s.
Scudder
S. intestinal clamp
S. intestinal forceps
S. skid
S. stomach clamp
Scuderi
S. bipolar coagulating forceps
S. screw
Scuderi-Callahan flange
Scully Hip S'port functional hip support
sculp knife
sculps
Concise cementing s.
Sculptor flexible annuloplasty ring

sculpturing scalpel
Scultetus
> S. bandage
> S. binder

scultetus binder band
Scurasil prosthesis
SCU-series digital color ultrasound scanner
Scutan temporary splint material
SD
> SD Sorb E-Z TAC suture anchor
> SD sorb meniscal stapler

SDS
> slow deflate system

SDU-400 EchoView ultrasound machine
SE-100 smoke aspiration tip
SeaBands acupressure wristband
seal
> AccuPort s.
> a-fiX cannula s.
> Asherman chest s.
> Bennett s.
> iLEX stomal s.
> No-React Pneumo-Pledgets staple-line s.

sealant
> BioGlue surgical s.
> CoSeal resorbable synthetic s.
> CoSeal surgical s.
> FloSeal matrix hemostatic s.
> FocalSeal liquid s.
> FocalSeal-L lung s.
> FocalSeal-S surgical s.
> Helioseal dental s.
> Hemaseel APR fibrin s.
> Quixil fibrin s.
> Tisseel VH fibrin s.

SealEasy resuscitation mask
Sealed Ice
sealer
> TissueLink BPS5.0 bipolar s.
> TissueLink DS3.0 dissecting s.

sealing window plug
Seal-On spray
Seal-Tight cast protector
Seal-Tite adhesive gasket
Sealy dissecting scissors
SeamGuard staple line reinforcement material
seamless
> s. graft
> s. prosthesis

seam-sealer gun
searcher
> Allport-Babcock mastoid s.
> Allport mastoid s.
> mastoid s.
> Proctor-Bruce mastoid s.
> Shuletz s.

Searcy
> S. capsular forceps
> S. chalazion trephine
> S. fixation anchor
> S. fixation hook
> S. oval cup erysiphake
> S. tonsillectome

Searle volume ventilator
Sears Wee Alert
SeaSorb alginate wound dressing
seat
> Carrie car s.
> Dream Ride car s.
> Flofit ComfortFluid s.
> Heffington lumbar s.
> Ingram bicycle s.
> Maddacare child bath s.
> orthopaedic positioning s.
> Posey drop s.
> Renolux convertible car s.
> Snug s.
> Spelcast car s.
> Tall-ette toilet s.
> Tubsider kneeling s.
> Versa bath s.

seated hamstring curl exercise chair
Seattle
> S. Foot prosthesis
> S. orthosis
> S. splint

Sebbin ultrasound-assisted lipoplasty machine
Sebileau periosteal elevator
Sebra arm tourniquet
Sechrist
> S. Millenium infant/pediatric ventilator
> S. monoplace hyperbaric chamber

second
> s. generation lithotripter
> S. Look computer-aided detection system
> s. skin knee pad

Secor system

S

NOTES

Secto
 S. dissector
 S. tonsillar sponge
sector
 s. scanner
 s. scanning echoendoscope
 s. transducer
Secu clip
Securat suction tube
SeCure
 S. therapeutic mattress
Secure
 S. closed pressure monitoring and
  blood sampling system
 S. Yet Gentle surgical dressing
  system
SecureEasy endotracheal harness
**Secureline operating room camera
 drape**
SecureStrand
 S. cable
 S. cervical fusion system
Secur-Fit HA hip system
Secur-Its silicon cushion mat
security
 S. blade
 s. clip
Security+ Self-Sealing Urisheath
Sedan goniometer
Sedan-Nashold
 S.-N. biopsy cannula
 S.-N. needle
Seddon nerve graft
Sédillot periosteal elevator
Seeburger implant
Seecor pacemaker
seed
 BrachySeed brachytherapy s.
 s. implant
 I-Plant brachytherapy s.
 Isostar iodine-125 brachytherapy s.
 radiation s.
seeker
 ball-tipped s.
 Kuhn-Bolger s.
 ostium s.
Seeker guidewire
Seeman-Seiffert mouthgag
Seep-Pruf ileostomy appliance
SeeQuence disposable contact lens
Seer cardiac monitor
segmental
 s. compression construct
 s. spinal instrumentation
segmented ring tripolar lead
Segond
 S. abdominal retractor
 S. hysterectomy forceps
 S. myomatome

 S. tumor forceps
 S. vaginal spatula
Segond-Landau hysterectomy forceps
Seguin
 S. annuloplasty ring
 S. formboard
Segura
 S. CBD basket
 S. Hemisphere stone retrieval
  basket
 S. stone basket
Segura-Dretler stone basket
Segway hydrophilic guidewire
Sehrt
 S. clamp
 S. compressor
Seibel
 S. LASIK flap irrigator and
  squeegee cannula
 S. LASIK flap lifter
 S. nucleus chopper
 S. ophthalmic paracentesis valve
  adjuster
 S. vertical safety quick chopper
Seidel
 S. bone-holding clamp
 S. catheter
 S. humeral locking nail
 S. intramedullary fixation
 S. plug
 S. saddlebag
Seiffert
 S. esophagoscopy forceps
 S. grasping punch
 S. laryngeal forceps
 S. tonsillectome
Seiff frontalis suspension set
Seiler
 S. MC-M900 surgical microscope
 S. tonsillar knife
 S. turbinate scissors
Seirin
 S. acupuncture needle
 S. LaserPen device
 S. ProPoint acupuncture point-
  search pen
Seitzinger tripolar cutting forceps
seizing forceps
Selby II hook
Seldin
 S. elevator
 S. flap retractor
 S. periosteal elevator
Seldinger
 S. apparatus
 S. arterial needle
 S. cardiac catheter
 S. gastrostomy needle
 S. retrograde wire

Selecon coronary angiography catheter
Select
> S. ankle prosthesis
> S. GT blood glucose testing
> system
> S. joint orthosis
> S. shoulder prosthesis

Selecta 7000 glaucoma laser
SelectCells Mini endometrial sampler
Selective-HI catheter
selector
> Leksell s.
> sleeve s.

Selector ultrasonic aspirator
Selectron system
Selenia full-field digital mammography system
Seletz
> S. catheter
> S. foramen-plugging forceps
> S. Universal Kerrison punch
> S. ventricular cannula

Seletz-Gelpi self-retaining retractor
self-adhering lid retractor
self-aligning (SAL)
> s.-a. knee

self-articulating
> s.-a. femoral hip replacement
> s.-a. femoral prosthesis

self-aspirating cut-biopsy needle
Selfast dental cement
self-broaching pin
Self-Cath coudé tipped catheter
self-catheter
> Mentor female s.-c.

self-centering
> s.-c. micromanipulator
> s.-c. Universal hip prosthesis

self-contained underwater breathing apparatus
self-expandable stainless steel braided endoprosthesis
self-expanding
> s.-e. coil stent
> s.-e. Easy Wallstent
> s.-e. metallic endoprosthesis
> s.-e. stainless steel stent
> s.-e. tulip sheath
> s.-e. Wallstent endoprosthesis

self-fixating sideport diamond knife
self-guiding catheter

self-inflating
> s.-i. bulb
> s.-i. tissue expander

self-opening
> s.-o. forceps
> s.-o. rigid snare

self-propelling wheelchair
self-retaining
> s.-r. abdominal retractor
> s.-r. bentback rotator cuff retractor
> s.-r. bone holding forceps
> s.-r. brain retractor
> s.-r. brain retractor frame
> s.-r. catheter
> s.-r. chamber maintainer
> s.-r. coil stent
> s.-r. infusion cannula
> s.-r. irrigating cannula
> s.-r. laminectomy retractor
> s.-r. laryngoscope
> s.-r. retractor blade
> s.-r. ring retractor
> s.-r. skin retractor
> s.-r. spring retractor

self-sealing
> s.-s. cannula
> s.-s. latex balloon

Self Snag strap
self-stabilizing vitrectomy lens
self-stopping drill point
self-tapering pin
self-tapping
> s.-t. bone screw
> s.-t. Leibinger lag screw
> s.-t. screw-type implant

Selker ventriculostomy reservoir
sellar punch
Sellheim
> S. elevating spoon
> S. obstetrical lever
> S. uterine catheter

Sellor
> S. clamp
> S. mitral valve knife
> S. rib contractor
> S. rib retractor
> S. valvulotome

Sellotape
> S. dressing
> S. tie-over dressing

Selman
> S. clamp

S

NOTES

Selman *(continued)*
S. clip
S. lung tissue forceps
S. nonslip tissue forceps
S. peripheral blood vessel forceps
S. vessel forceps
Selofix dressing
Selopor dressing
Seloris balloon
Selrodo
S. bulb
S. nebulizer
Selsi sport telescope
Seltzer saw
Selverstone
S. carotid artery clamp
S. cordotomy hook
S. embolus forceps
S. intervertebral disc forceps
S. intervertebral disc rongeur
S. laminectomy rongeur
S. rongeur forceps
Semb
S. bone-cutting forceps
S. bone-holding clamp
S. bone-holding forceps
S. bronchus clamp
S. dissecting forceps
S. dissecting scissors
S. ligature-carrying forceps
S. ligature forceps
S. lung retractor
S. raspatory
S. rib-holding forceps
S. rib shears
S. rongeur
S. rongeur forceps
S. self-retaining retractor
S. vaginal speculum
Semb-Ghazi dissecting forceps
Semb-Sauerbruch rongeur
semiadjustable articulator
semicircular gouge
semicompressive dressing
semiconstrained knee prosthesis
semiflat tip electrode
semiflexible
s. endoscope
s. intraocular lens
semilunar cartilage knife
semilunar-tip blade
semiocclusive moisture-retentive dressing
semipermeable membrane dressing
semipressure dressing
semirigid
s. catheter
s. endoscope
s. fiberglass cast

s. intraocular lens
s. polypropylene ankle-foot orthosis
semishell eye implant
semitubular blade plate
Semken
S. bipolar forceps
S. dressing forceps
S. infant forceps
S. microbipolar neurosurgical
forceps
S. thumb forceps
S. tissue forceps
Semm
S. endocoagulator
S. morcellator
S. Pelvi-Pneu insufflator
S. pneumoperitoneum apparatus
S. uterine vacuum cannula
S. uterine vacuum catheter
Semmes
S. curette
S. dural forceps
Semmes-Weinstein
S.-W. monofilament instrument
S.-W. nylon monofilament
S.-W. pressure aesthesiometer
filament
S.-W. pressure anesthesiometer
Sendax MDI system
**SenDx 100 blood gas/electrolyte analysis
system**
Seneliners
Senepads underpad
Sengstaken
S. balloon
S. nasogastric tube
Sengstaken-Blakemore
S.-B. esophageal balloon
S.-B. esophagogastric tamponade
tube
Senn
S. bone plate
S. double-ended retractor
S. mastoid retractor
S. self-retaining retractor
Senn-Dingman double-ended retractor
Senn-Green retractor
Senning
S. cardiovascular forceps
S. featherweight bulldog clamp
S. intraatrial baffle
Senning-Stille clamp
Senn-Kanavel double-ended retractor
Senn-Miller retractor
Senographe
S. 2000D digital mammography
system
S. 2000D mammography machine
S. DMR+ mammography system

Senoran aspirator
**SenoScan full-field digital
 mammography system**
Sensar
> S. acrylic intraocular lens
> S. foldable acrylic posterior
> chamber intraocular lens
> S. OptiEdge acrylic intraocular lens

**Sens-A-Ray digital dental imaging
 system**
Sensatec
> S. endoscope
> S. fall prevention system

Sensation
> S. intraaortic balloon catheter
> S. Short Throw snare
> S. vacuum assist device

Sens dissector
Sense-of-Feel prosthesis
**SensiCare synthetic powder-free surgical
 glove**
SensiCath
> S. blood gas monitoring system
> S. optical sensor

Sensimatic electrosurgical unit
sensing
> s. catheter
> s. coil

**Sensititre Streptococcus pneumoniae
 MIC plate**
Sensitometer
> Poppen Ridge S.

**Sensi-Touch regional anesthesia delivery
 system**
Sensiv endotracheal tube
Senso
> S. listening device

Sensolog II, III pacemaker
Sensonic plaque removal instrument
sensor
> Albin-Bunegin pressure s.
> BreastAlert differential
> temperature s.
> capacitive s.
> Capnostat Mainstream CO_2 s.
> CardioSearch s.
> ClipTip reusable s.
> Cross Top replacement oxygen s.
> Datex-Ohmeda infrared s.
> DC Squid s.
> DermaTemp infrared
> thermographic s.

Diasensor 1000 s.
differential temperature s.
3-dimensional magnetic s.
disposable Doppler-constant
 thermocouple s.
Dymedix pediatric airflow s.
Dymedix sleep s.
electromyogram s.
Endex apex s.
fiberoptic PCO_2 s.
FilterWatch s.
finger clip s.
Infinity s.
S. Kelvin pacemaker
Ladd intracranial pressure s.
manometric s.
Masimo Set oximeter s.
MEG s.
MicroMirror gold s.
multiparameter s.
MyoScan s.
Nellcor FS-series oximeter s.
Novametrix combination $0_2/CO_2$ s.
oximetry s.
OxyTip s.
s. pad
Paratrend 7+ s.
Paratrend 7 fiberoptic PCO_2 s.
pediatric finger clip s.
PerryAnal/PerryVaginal EMG s.
PerryMeter EMG s.
Perry/Pathway Anal EMG s.
Perry/Pathway Vaginal EMG s.
pressure transducer airflow s.
PressureWire 3-300 s.
s. probe
S. PTFE-nitinol guidewire with
 hydrophilic tip
SensiCath optical s.
Servo Pro force s.
SET oximeter s.
Shell s.
SpiroSense flow s.
S. surgical guidewire
telemetric intracranial pressure s.
ultrasonic tactile s.

sensor-based single-chamber pacemaker
SensorHand device
sensory
> Dymedix airflow/snore s.
> s. stimulation kit

SensoScan mammography system

NOTES

Sentalloy digital calipers
SentiLite neurological monitor
Sentinel-4 neurological monitor
Sentinel implantable cardioverter-
  defibrillator
Sentron
  S. pigtail angiographic
    micromanometer catheter
  S. transducer
Senturia
  S. forceps
  S. pharyngeal speculum
  S. retractor
separator
  Allen stereo s.
  Amicus blood collection s.
  Asahi Plasmaflo plasma s.
  bayonet s.
  Benson baby pyloric s.
  blood cell s.
  Cascadeflo plasma component s.
  cone finger s.
  Davis nerve s.
  Dorsey dural s.
  dural s.
  Fenwal CS3000 Plus cell s.
  Ferrier s.
  finger s.
  Frazier dural s.
  Grant dural s.
  Harris s.
  head spoon s.
  Hoen dural s.
  Horsley dural s.
  House ear s.
  Hunter s.
  iliac graft s.
  Kirby curved zonular s.
  Kirby cylindrical zonular s.
  Kirby double-ball s.
  Kirby flat zonular s.
  Lig-A-Ring s.
  Luys s.
  mechanical s.
  noninterfering s.
  Remy s.
  Rosen bayonet s.
  Sachs dural s.
  Sachs nerve s.
  Sep-A-Ring s.
  Silverstein nerve s.
  stem spoon s.
  synovial s.
  s. tube
  Woodson dural s.
  zonule s.
Sep-A-Ring separator
Sephadex bead

Seprafilm
  S. adhesion barrier
  S. bioresorbable membrane
  S. sheet
Sepramesh biosurgical composite
septal
  s. bone forceps
  s. chisel
  s. clamp
  s. compression forceps
  s. dissector
  s. elevator
  s. knife
  s. needle
  s. occluder system
  s. ridge forceps
  s. straightener
Septer closed wound drainage system
Septi-Chek blood culture system
Septisol soap dressing
Septobal bead
Septoject needle
Septopack periodontal dressing
Septopal implant
Septosil impression material
septostomy balloon catheter
septum-cutting forceps
septum-straightening forceps
Sep-T-Vac suction cannister
Sequel compression system
sequencer
  automated laser fluorescence s.
sequencing
  s. bead patterns set
sequential
  s. circulator
  s. compression device (SCD)
  s. compression stocking
  s. demand pacemaker
  s. extremity pump
  S. Multiple Analyzer Computer
    (SMAC)
  s. pressure
  s. video converter
Sequestra 1000 autotransfusion system
sequestrum forceps
Sequicor II, III pacemaker
Sequoia
  S. Acuson system
  S. echocardiography system
Seraflo AV fistular needle
Seraphim clip
Seraton dialysis control system
Serature spur clip
Serdarevic
  S. speculum
  S. suture adjuster
Ser Form silicone orthotic
Series-II humeral head

Serola sacroiliac belt
Seroma-Cath wound drainage catheter
Serono SR1 FSH analyzer
serpentine bone plate
serrated
- s. amalgam plugger
- s. blade
- s. catheter
- s. conjunctival forceps
- s. curette
- s. fine-cutting knife
- s. iris scissors
- s. retractor
- s. suture
- s. T-spatula

Serratex scissors
serrefine
- Blair s.
- Brunswick s.
- s. clamp
- Dieffenbach s.
- s. forceps
- Hess s.
- s. implant
- Lemoine s.
- Mack s.
- s. retractor

Serter
- C-wire S.

server
- AquariusNET streaming 2D/3D medical imaging s.

Servo
- S. Pro force sensor
- S. pump
- S. ventilator platform

servomechanism sphincter
Servo-series ventilator
Servox
- S. amplifier
- S. device
- S. electronic speech aid
- S. Inton speech aid

sesamoidectomy dissector
sestamibi scan
set
- Ackrad Tampa catheter s.
- Acland-Banis arteriotomy s.
- Alken s.
- Amicon arteriovenous blood tubing s.
- Amplatz dilator s.

Arnold-Bruening intracordal injection s.
Baker amniocentesis needle s.
Bankart shoulder repair s.
Bantam irrigation s.
Bio-Medicus percutaneous cannula s.
Biostil blood transfusion s.
Bloomberg trabeculotome s.
Borst-Tuohy side-arm introducer s.
Brodmerkel colon decompression s.
Brown-Mueller T-fastener s.
Bruening-Arnold intracordal injection s.
Bruening intracordal injection s.
Bruening otoscope s.
Buretrol solution s.
Catalano lacrimal intubation s.
Ciaglia Blue Rhino percutaneous tracheostomy introducer s.
Cliniset infusion s.
Colapinto transjugular cholangiography/liver biopsy s.
Collis Universal laminectomy s.
Coloplast economy irrigation s.
colostomy irrigation s.
Cone-Bucy suction cannula s.
Cook drainage pouch s.
Cope gastrointestinal suture anchor s.
Corpak enteral Y extension s.
Cotton-Leung biliary stent s.
Craig vertebral body biopsy instrument s.
Crampton-Tsang percutaneous endoscopic biliary stent s.
Crawford lacrimal s.
Criticare HN-Isocal tube feeding s.
Dansac colostomy irrigation s.
DePuy small-joint arthroscopy instrument s.
Dotter intravascular retriever s.
DSP Micro Diamond-Point microsurgery s.
Dynacor vaginal irrigator s.
Echosight Jansen-Anderson intrauterine catheter s.
Echosight Patton coaxial catheter s.
Echotip Baker amniocentesis needle s.
Echotip Dominion needle s.

NOTES

set *(continued)*

Echotip Kato-Asch coaxial needle s.
Elliptosphere cardiac catheter s.
Entrex small-joint arthroscopy instrument s.
Fine bimanual ophthalmic handpiece s.
Freiburg biopsy s.
Garcia endometrial biopsy s.
Guibor canaliculus intubation s.
Henning instrument s.
Heyer-Schulte Small-Carrion sizing s.
Hobbs stent s.
Hulbert endo-electrode s.
Impex/Lerner foldable lens removing s.
Inpersol peritoneal dialysis s.
Insuflon infusion s.
Jackson lacrimal intubation s.
Jackson magnification ruler s.
Janacek reimplantation s.
Jeffrey introducer s.
Kawasumi infusion s.
Leung endoscopic nasal biliary drainage s.
Level One normothermic IV fluid s.
Loversan infusion s.
Maciol suture needle s.
Malis irrigation tubing s.
Marcon colon decompression s.
McIntyre infusion s.
MegaFlo infusion s.
Mentanium vitreoretinal instrument s.
Messerklinger sinus endoscopy s.
Mills coronary endarterectomy s.
Mi-Mark endocervical curette s.
Moore nail s.
Mullan percutaneous trigeminal ganglion microcompression s.
Mullan trigeminal ganglion microcompression s.
Myelo-Nate lumbar puncture s.
Neff percutaneous access s.
Novack special extraction s.
Ochsner total enarterectomy s.
Palex colostomy irrigation starter s.
Parker-Glassman intestinal clamp s.
parquetry s.
Patton coaxial catheter s.
Pettigrove LASIK s.
Porter-Kolpe biliary biopsy s.
PSS prostate seeding s.
Re-Entry Malecot catheter s.
Rica esophagoscopy s.
Rica skull perforator s.

Ring-McLean sump drainage s.
Rösch-Uchida transjugular liver access s.
Saf-T EZ s.
Schoenrock laser instrument s.
s. screw
Seiff frontalis suspension s.
sequencing bead patterns s.
Simcoe lens-positioning s.
Sobel-Kaplitt-Sawyer gas endarterectomy s.
Soehendra lithotripsy s.
Soluset IV s.
Steinert laser-assisted intrastromal keratomileusis s.
Surewing winged infusion s.
Surflo winged infusion s.
Tebbetts rhinoplasty s.
Tender subcutaneous infusion s.
Toomey surgical stainless steel instrument s.
Turkel bone biopsy trephine s.
U-Mid-O_2 Jet s.
Uri-Cath s.
Veirs dacryocystorhinostomy s.
Vennes pancreatic dilation s.
Visi-Flow irrigation starter s.
VPI-Jacobellis microhematuria catheter s.
Wiegerinck culdocentesis puncture s.
Wissinger s.
Wylie endarterectomy s.
Zimmon endoscopic biliary stent s.
Zimmon endoscopic pancreatic stent s.
Zimmon esophagogastric balloon tamponade s.

Setacure denture repair acrylic
Setma hydrotherapy system
seton

s. drain
s. hip brace
Molteno s.
s. needle
s. suture

Set-Op myringotomy kit
Setopress

S. dressing
S. high-compression bandage

SET oximeter sensor
SetPoint coronary catheter
setter

Eby band s.
Klauber band s.
Ormco band s.
orthodontic band s.

Seutin

S. bandage

S. plaster shears
S. scissors
Seven-Star Plum Blossom acupuncture needle
severance transurethral bag
Severin
S. implant
S. multiple closed-loop intraocular lens
Severinghaus electrode
Sewall
S. antral cannula
S. antral trocar
S. brain clip-applying forceps
S. ethmoidal chisel
S. ethmoidal elevator
S. mucoperiosteal elevator
S. orbital retractor
S. raspatory
Sewell system
sewing ring
sewn-in waterproof drape
sew-on electrode
Sexton ear knife
Seyand vulsellum
Seyfert
S. forceps
S. vaginal speculum
SFB-I right-angled bronchoscope
SFS
small fragment system
SG
Swan-Ganz
SG catheter
Sgarlato hammertoe implant
SGIA 50 disposable stapler
Shaaf
S. eye forceps
S. foreign body forceps
Shack-Hartmann aberrometer
shadow
S. balloon
S. over-the-wire balloon catheter
s. shield
shadow-free laryngoscope
Shadow-Line ACF spine retractor system
Shadow-Stripe catheter
Shaeffer rigid orthosis
Shaffer modification of Barkan knife
Shaffner orthopaedic inserter

shaft
Adante Monorail catheter s.
Cloward drill s.
cup pusher s.
Marlow Primus s.
s. prosthesis
s. reamer
Shah
S. aural dressing
S. grommet
S. myringotomy tube
S. nasal splint
S. permanent ventilation tube
Shahan thermopore
Shahinian lacrimal cannula
Shah-Shah intraocular lens
shaker
Gyrotwister laboratory s.
Shaldach pacemaker
Shaldon catheter
Shallcross
S. cystic duct forceps
S. gallbladder forceps
S. hemostat
S. nasal forceps
S. screwdriver
Shallcross-Dean gall duct forceps
Shambaugh
S. adenoidal curette
S. endaural hook
S. endaural self-retaining retractor
S. fistula hook
S. irrigator
S. knife
S. microscopic hook
S. narrow elevator
S. palpating needle
S. reverse adenotome
Shambaugh-Derlacki
S.-D. chisel
S.-D. duckbill elevator
S.-D. microhook
Shambaugh-Lempert knife
Shampaine
S. headholder
S. orthopaedic table
Shamp AK casting brief
Shandon
S. Candenza immunostainer
S. cytospin chamber
shank
Crowley s.

S

NOTES

shank *(continued)*
Hudson s.
taper with Zimmer s.
Zimmer-Hudson s.
Shank electrode
Shannon bur
Shantz
S. dressing
S. pin
shape
S. Maker system
Trimensional augmentation 3-D s.
shape-memory
s.-m. alloy (SMA)
s.-m. alloy recoverable technology
(SMART)
s.-m. alloy recoverable technology
stent
shaper
automated corneal s.
Chiron automated corneal s.
interspace s.
ProFile orifice s.
Shapleigh
S. curette
S. ear wax curette
Shapshay-Healy
S.-H. laryngeal alligator forceps
S.-H. laryngeal scissors
S.-H. operating laryngoscope
S.-H. phonatory laryngoscope
Shapshay laser bronchoscope
Sharbaro driver
shark
S. disposable biopsy forceps
s. fin papillotome
s. fin sphincterotome
The S. disposable biopsy forceps
shark-mouth cannula
shark-tooth forceps
Sharman curette
sharp
s. dermal curette
s. hook
s. loop curette
S. point-tip cystotome
s. trocar
Sharpey screw
Sharplan
S. argon laser
S. CO₂ laser
S. Erbium SilkLaser
S. FeatherTouch SilkLaser
S. Laser 710 Acuspot
S. Medilas Nd:YAG surgical laser
S. sight system
S. SilkTouch flashscan surgical
laser
S. Ultra ultrasonic aspirator

SharpLase Nd:YAG laser
Sharplav laparoscope
Sharpley hook
Sharpoint
S. knife
S. microsuture
S. ophthalmic microsurgical suture
S. spoon blade
S. Ultra-Guide ophthalmic needle
V-lance S.
S. V-lance blade
sharp-pointed forceps
sharp-pronged retractor
SharpShooter meniscal repair system
Sharptome
S. crescent blade
S. microblade
Shar-Tek foot positioning grid
Sharvelle side port splitter
Shasta alloy
shattering needle
shaver
Aggressor meniscal s.
arthroscopic s.
s. catheter
Concept s.
Cuda s.
DORC vitreous s.
Gator s.
Grierson meniscal s.
Microsect s.
motorized meniscal s.
Richardson s.
Skimmer RRP laryngeal s.
Stryker s.
sucker s.
Xomed Skimmer s.
Shaw
S. carotid artery clot stripper
S. catheter
S. I, II scalpel
**Shaw-Sgarlato hammertoe implant
prosthesis rod**
Shaw-SHIP rod
Shea
S. bur
S. curette
S. ear drill
S. elevator
S. fenestration hook
S. fistular hook
S. forceps
S. headrest
S. incision knife
S. irrigator
S. microdrill
S. middle ear instrument
S. oblique hook
S. pick

S. polyethylene prosthesis
S. speculum
S. speculum holder
S. stapes hook
S. Teflon piston prosthesis
S. vein graft scissors

Shea-Anthony
S.-A. bag
S.-A. balloon

Shea-Bellucci scissors
Shealy facet rhizotomy electrode
ShearBan orthotic material
Shearer
S. bone rongeur
S. chicken-bill forceps
S. lip retractor

ShearGuard low-friction interface
Shearing
S. J-Loop intraocular lens
S. posterior chamber intraocular lens
S. S-style anterior chamber intraocular lens

shears
ADC Medicut s.
Bacon s.
Baer rib s.
bandage s.
Bethune-Coryllos rib s.
Bethune rib s.
Bortone s.
Braun-Stadler sternal s.
Brunner rib s.
Brun plaster s.
Clayton laminectomy s.
Collin rib s.
Cooley first-rib s.
Cooley-Pontius sternal s.
Cooley rib s.
Coryllos-Bethune rib s.
Coryllos-Moure rib s.
Coryllos rib s.
Eccentric locked rib s.
Esmarch plaster s.
felt s.
first rib s.
Frey-Sauerbruch rib s.
Giertz rib s.
Giertz-Shoemaker rib s.
Giertz-Stille rib s.
Gluck rib s.
Harmonic Scalpel II curved s.

Hercules plaster s.
Horgan-Coryllos-Moure rib s.
Horgan-Wells rib s.
infant rib s.
Jackson esophageal s.
Jackson-Moore s.
Jarit plaster s.
Jarit utility s.
LaparoSonic coagulating s.
Lebsche sternal s.
Lefferts rib s.
Liston s.
Liston-Key-Horsley rib s.
Liston-Ruskin s.
Moure-Coryllos rib s.
Nelson-Bethune s.
Pilling laryngofissure s.
plain rib s.
plaster s.
pleural biopsy needle s.
Potts infant rib s.
rib s.
Roos first rib s.
Sauerbruch-Britsch rib s.
Sauerbruch-Coryllos rib s.
Sauerbruch-Frey rib s.
Sauerbruch-Lebsche rib s.
Sauerbruch rib s.
Scanlan plaster s.
Scanlan rib s.
Schumacher sternum s.
Semb rib s.
Seutin plaster s.
Shoemaker rib s.
Shuletz rib s.
sternal s.
Stille-Aesculap plaster s.
Stille-Ericksson rib s.
Stille-Giertz s.
Stille-Horsley s.
Stille plaster s.
Stille rib s.
Stille-Stiwer plaster s.
Thompson rib s.
Thomsen rib s.
Tudor-Edwards rib s.
utility s.
Walton rib s.
Weck s.

sheath
Amplatz s.
Angetear tear-away introducer s.

NOTES

S

sheath *(continued)*
    angioplasty s.
    Appel-Bercie s.
    Arrow-Flex s.
    arthroscopic s.
    Bakelite cystoscopy s.
    Bakelite rectoscope s.
    beaked s.
    catheter s.
    Check-Flo introducer s.
    Colapinto s.
    convex s.
    Cordis s.
    Cordis Bioptone s.
    Desilets-Hoffman s.
    s. and dilator system
    Disposashielf s.
    double-channel operating s.
    Electroshield reusable s.
    ERA resectoscope s.
    excimer s.
    femoral introducer s.
    fiberoptic s.
    French s.
    Futura resectoscope s.
    Hemaflex s.
    Hemaquet PTCA s.
    hysteroscope s.
    incandescent s.
    Insul-Sheath vaginal speculum s.
    Intradyn tear-away introducer s.
    introducer s.
    irrigating s.
    IVT percutaneous catheter
     introducer s.
    Klein transseptal introducer s.
    Lee-Ahn sinus injection needle s.
    Mapper hemostasis EP mapping s.
    Medi-Tech s.
    MicroSpan s.
    Mullins transseptal catheterization s.
    s. and obturator
    O'Connor s.
    Passager introducing s.
    Peel-Away s.
    percutaneous brachial s.
    Pfister-Schwartz s.
    Pinnacle introducer s.
    Pinnacle R/O II introducer s.
    Preface braided guiding s.
    probe s.
    PRO/Covers ultrasound probe s.
    ProSys Samec D, self-adhering,
     nonlatex male external catheter,
     short s.
    ProSys Samec NL, self-adhering
     nonlatex male external catheter,
     normal length s.
    resectoscope s.

    retroflexed cystoscopy s.
    SafeSheath introducer s.
    self-expanding tulip s.
    short monorail polyethylene
     imaging s.
    Silipos Distal Dip prosthetic s.
    single-channel operating s.
    Spectranetics laser s.
    Storz s.
    Storz continuous-flow
     resectoscope s.
    Super Arrow-Flex catheterization s.
    tear-away introducer s.
    Teflon s.
    Terumo s.
    TorFlex transseptal guiding s.
    transseptal s.
    TULIP s.
    UMI Cath-Seal s.
    Universal s.
    vascular s.
    Warne penile s.
    water-filled balloon s.

sheathed flexible sigmoidoscope
Sheathes ultrasound probe cover
Shea-type parasol myringotomy tube
Sheehan
    S. gouge
    S. knee prosthesis
    S. nasal chisel
    S. osteotome
    S. retractor
Sheehan-Gillies needle holder
Sheehy
    S. canal knife
    S. collar button
    S. collar-button ventilating tube
    S. fascial press
    S. incus replacement prosthesis
    S. myringotomy knife
    S. ossicle-holding clamp
    S. ossicle-holding forceps
    S. Pate collector
    S. round knife
    S. Tytan ventilation tube
Sheehy-House
    S.-H. chisel
    S.-H. curette
    S.-H. knife
Sheehy-Urban sliding lens adapter
Sheen tip graft
sheepskin
    s. boot
    s. dressing
Sheer
    S. Plus pouch
    S. probe
    S. wire crimper

sheet
 Abanda drape s.
 Barrier lower extremity s.
 Biobrane s.
 casting wax s.
 Causse stapes s.
 craniomaxillofacial s.
 Derma-Gel hydrogel s.
 Diab-A-Sheet ThermoThotic s.
 Elasto-Gel hydrogel s.
 Flexderm hydrogel s.
 foil s.
 Grafton flexible s.
 HK s.
 s. holder
 hydrogel s.
 impervious U-sheet s.
 Ioban 2 iodophor cesarean s.
 iodoform-impregnated plastic s.
 KINS draw s.
 Korex cork s.
 MacroSorb PS macroporous
  protective s.
 mandibular s.
 Moran-Karaya s.
 polydioxanone s.
 PPT s.
 Prolene mesh s.
 ReJuveness scar therapy silicone s.
 Seprafilm s.
 Silastic s.
 Silk Skin s.
 sterile s.
 Subortholen s.
 Supramid s.
 Teflon s.
 Tegagel hydrogel s.
 Teknamed drape s.
 U-sheet s.

sheeting
 Carboplast II s.
 Dimisil gel s.
 Epi-Derm silicone gel s.
 gel s.
 Kelocote s.
 micromesh s.
 New Beginnings GelShapes silicone
  gel s.
 NovaGel silicone gel s.
 Oleeva fabric s.
 Oleeva scar s.
 ReJuveness pure silicone s.

 Scar Fx lightweight silicone s.
 silicone gel s.
 Silon silicone elastomer s.
Sheets
 S. closed-loop posterior chamber
  intraocular lens
 S. intraocular glide
 S. iris hook
 S. irrigating vectis
 S. irrigating vectis cannula
 S. lens cutter
 S. lens forceps
 S. lens glide
 S. lens spatula
Sheets-Hirsch spatula
Sheets-McPherson
 S.-M. angled forceps
 S.-M. tying forceps
sheet-wadding dressing
Sheffield
 S. gamma unit
 S. pedobarograph
 S. splint
Sheinmann laryngeal forceps
Sheldon
 S. clamp
 S. hemilaminectomy self-retaining
  retractor
 S. spreader
Sheldon-Gosset self-retaining retractor
Sheldon-Pudenz dissector
Sheldon-Spatz vertebral arteriogram
  needle
Sheldon-Swann needle
shelf reamer
shelf-type implant
Shelhigh
 S. No React VascuPatch
 S. pulmonic valve conduit
 S. suture organizer
shell
 elastomer s.
 s. eye implant
 Hansen ophthalmic s.
 Harris protrusio s.
 s. impactor
 implant elastomer s.
 s. implant material
 Integrity s.
 Inter-Op acetabular s.
 KM-series s.
 Ossoinig ophthalmic s.

S

NOTES

shell *(continued)*
    protrusio s.
    Restoration Secur-Fit X'tra
      acetabular s.
    S. sensor
    Terino malar s.
shellac-covered catheter
Shenstone tourniquet
Shepard
    S. bipolar forceps
    S. calipers block
    S. curved intraocular lens forceps
    S. drain tube
    S. flexible anterior chamber
      intraocular lens
    S. grommet
    S. grommet ventilation tube
    S. incision depth gauge
    S. incision irrigating cannula
    S. intraocular lens implant
    S. lens forceps
    S. optical center marker
    S. radial keratotomy irrigating
      cannula
    S. reversed iris hook
    S. tying forceps
    S. Universal intraocular lens
Shepard-Kramer calipers block
Shepard-Reinstein intraocular lens
  forceps
Shepard-Westcott scissors
shepherd's hook catheter
Shepherd Tomahawk chopper
Sherform silicone insole
Sheridan
    S. endotracheal tube
    S. endotracheal tube cuff
Sherlock
    S. self-tapping screw
    S. soft tissue fixation system
    S. threaded suture anchor
Sherman
    S. bone plate
    S. bone screw
    S. knife
    S. remote podiatric vacuum system
    S. screwdriver
    S. suction tube
Sherman-Pierce screwdriver
Sherman-Stille drill
Sherpa guiding catheter
Sherwin self-retaining retractor
Sherwood
    S. intrascopic suction/irrigation
      system
    S. retractor
ShiatsuBACK support
shield
    aluminum eye s.

AME PinSite s.
American Medical Electronics
  PinSite s.
Atkins-Tucker surgical s.
Barraquer eye s.
binocular s.
Buller eye s.
bunion s.
Carapace face s.
collagen s.
ComPly panty s.
corneal light s.
Cox III LaserSecure s.
Cox II ocular laser s.
Dacron s.
Dalkon s.
dental s.
Durette dental s.
Durette external ocular laser s.
Electroshield cylindrical
  conductive s.
Expo Bubble eye s.
eye s.
face s.
Face-It protective s.
Faraday s.
Fox aluminum eye s.
Fuller perianal s.
Garter s.
gastric s.
Goffman blue eye garter s.
gonad s.
Grafco eye s.
Green eye s.
Hessburg corneal s.
Hessburg eye s.
high-humidity tracheostomy s.
S. iridotomy scissors
Jardon eye s.
Jet s.
Katena scleral s.
lead eye s.
Lea's vaginal s.
metal Fox s.
metal scleral s.
Mueller eye s.
Nolan system collimator mounted
  contact s.
Paton eye s.
plastic eye s.
pressure s.
probe s.
Pro-Ophtha type-K, -S s.
Proshield collagen corneal s.
Pro-Tex face s.
Saf-T s.
scleral s.
shadow s.
Simmons eye s.

SlimStem metal scleral s.
Sof-Gel palm s.
Soft Shield collagen corneal s.
Sportelli system collimator mounted
  contact s.
Storz Easy s.
Surety s.
Surgical Patient Arm s.
Sutcliffe laser s.
Trelles metal scleral s.
tungsten eye s.
Tungsten syringe s.
universal eye s.
Visitec corneal s.
Weck eye s.
Zerowet Splashfield s.
shielded
  s. gradient coil
  s. open-end cone
shielding block
Shields forceps
Shier knee prosthesis
Shiffrin bone wire tightener
shifter
  all-optical frequency s.
  frequency s.
shifting pacemaker
Shikani middle meatal antrostomy stent
Shiley
  S. cardioplegia system
  S. cardiotomy reservoir
  S. catheter distention system
  S. convexoconcave heart valve
  S. cuffless fenestrated tracheostomy
    tube
  S. decannulation plug
  S. disposable cannula low-pressure
    cuffed tracheostomy tube
  S. distention kit
  S. fenestrated low-pressure cuffed
    tracheostomy tube
  S. French sump tube
  S. guiding catheter
  S. Infusaid pump
  S. irrigation catheter
  S. laryngectomy tube
  S. monostrut heart valve
  S. MultiPro catheter
  S. neonatal tracheostomy tube
  S. oxygenator
  S. pediatric tracheostomy tube
  S. Phonate speaking valve

  S. pressure-relief adapter
  S. single-cannula cuffed
    tracheostomy tube
  S. soft-tip guiding catheter
  S. Tetraflex vascular graft
  S. TracheoSoft XLT tracheostomy
    tube
  S. tracheostomy tube
Shiley-Ionescu catheter
shim
  s. coil
  s. magnet
Shimadzu
  S. cardiac ultrasound
  S. 5000 CT scanner
  S. DAR-2400 coronary
    arteriographic analyzer
  S. IIQ ultrasound
  S. RF-5301 PC spectrometer
  S. SDU-400 ultrasound
  S. ultrasound system
Shimano stainless steel cutting forceps
shimmed magnet
Shimstock occlusion foil
shin
  S. Ice sleeve
  S. Saver
  s. splint compression sleeve
SHIP hammertoe implant
SHIP-Shaw rod
Shirakabe nasal implant
Shirlee spline
Shirley wound drain
Shirodkar
  S. aneurysm needle
  S. cervical needle
  S. probe
  S. suture
SHO
  shoulder holster orthosis
  Lerman SHO
Shoch
  S. foreign body pickups
  S. suture
shock
  s. block
  s. suit
  s. wave lithotripter
shocker
  Take-Me-Along Personal Shocker
  pocket s.

NOTES

ShockMaster heel cushion
Shockwave Therapy Systems (STS)
shoe
>Ambulator H1200 healing s.
Anywear s.
Balmoral s.
beach bum rocker-bottom cast sandal s.
Blucher low-quarter s.
cast s.
Castaway surgical s.
Comed postoperative s.
S. Curl no-tie shoe lace
Darby surgical s.
Darco MedSurg s.
Darco OrthoWedge healing s.
decubitus boot s.
diabetic pressure relief s.
Dynaslipper night s.
extra-depth s.
GentleStep s.
Goldenberg footplate s.
healing s.
HeelWedge healing s.
Hi-Top s.
ipos heel relief s.
Kunzli orthopaedic sports s.
s. lift
low-quarter Blucher s.
Mala-paedic s.
Markell Mobility S.'s
Markell open-toe s.
Markell tarso medius straight s.
Markell tarso pronator outflare s.
OrthoWedge healing s.
Pedors orthopaedic s.
Plastazote s.
postoperative s.
Power Anthro s.
pressure relief s.
Reece orthopaedic s.
Reece PO s.
rocker-bottom cast s.
Rollerbottom Xtra Depth s.
SAS s.
Softie s.
s. stretcher
Thera-Medic s.
Tru-Fit custom-molded s.
Tru-Mold s.
Vibram rockerbottom s.
WACH s.
wedge adjustable cushioned heel s.

shoehorn speculum
Shoemaker
>S. intraocular lens forceps
S. rib shears

Shoethotic orthotic
Shofu dental cement

Shone catheter
4,6,10 Shooter Saeed multiband ligator
short
>s. above-elbow cast
s. arm cylinder cast
s. arm navicular cast
s. arm plaster splint
s. arm posterior molded splint
s. below-elbow cast
S. bridge
s. C-loop intraocular lens
s. Heaney retractor
s. leg caliper brace
s. leg cylinder cast
s. leg nonwalking cast
s. leg nonweightbearing cast
s. leg plaster cast
s. leg splint
s. leg walker
s. leg walking cast
s. monorail polyethylene imaging sheath
s. needle
S. Speedy balloon
s. stent
s. taper
s. tooth forceps

short-arm Grollman catheter
Shortbent suture scissors
short-bore magnet
ShortCut A-OK small-incision knife
ShortCutter catheter
shorthand vertical mattress stitch
Shorti limbal relaxing inciusion diamond knife
short-stretch bandage
short-term
>flow-assisted s.-t. (FAST)

short-tip hemostatic bag
ShotBlocker pain reduction device
shot compressor
shotted suture
shoulder
>s. abduction immobilizer
s. abduction pillow
s. abduction positioner
s. blade
s. brace
s. controller
s. cuff
S. Ease abduction support
s. holster orthosis (SHO)
s. ladder
s. orthosis
s. prosthesis
s. pulley
s. ROM arc
s. saddle sling
s. subluxation inhibitor brace

s. surface coil
s. traction and rotation sleeve
s. wheel
shoulder-elbow-wrist-hand orthosis
Shoulder-Float adjustable axillary support
shoulderRAP wrap
shower
s. chair
Hydrokinetic Vichy s.
ShowerSafe
S. protector material
S. waterproof cast and bandage cover
S. waterproof cast and bandage protector
Show'rbag cast and dressing cover
SH pop-off suture
Shrader fitting
Shrady saw
Shriners
S. Hospital interlocking retractor
S. Hospital pin
shrinker
Juzo s.
Shuco-Myst nebulizer
Shug male contraceptive device
Shulec adenotome
Shuletz
S. pusher
S. raspatory
S. rib shears
S. searcher
S. spring
Shuletz-Damian raspatory
Shuletz-Paul rib retractor
Shulitz catheter
shunt
Accura hydrocephalus s.
Allen-Brown vascular access s.
Ames ventriculoperitoneal s.
Anastaflo intravascular s.
angiographic portacaval s.
aortopulmonary s.
aqueous tube s.
Austin endolymph dispersement s.
Baerveldt s.
balloon s.
bidirectional s.
bidirectional cavopulmonary s.
Blalock s.
Blalock-Taussig s.

Brenner carotid bypass s.
Brescia-Cimino s.
Brisman-Nova carotid endarterectomy s.
Buselmeier s.
cavernospongiosum s.
cerebrospinal fluid s.
Cimino s.
Cimino-Brescia arteriovenous s.
Cimino dialysis s.
s. clamp
ClearView intracoronary s.
Codman Accu-Flow s.
Cordis-Hakim s.
coronary anastomotic s.
CSF T-tube s.
CUI s.
Denver s.
Denver ascites s.
Denver hydrocephalus s.
Denver peritoneovenous s.
Denver pleural effusion s.
Denver pleuroperitoneal s.
Denver valve s.
dialysis s.
Diamond Valve flow-regulating s.
endolymphatic-subarachnoid s.
extracardiac right-to-left s.
extrahepatic s.
s. filter
Flo-Thru intraluminal s.
flow-regulating s.
Gibson inner ear s.
Glenn s.
Gore-Tex s.
Gott s.
Hakim s.
Hallin carotid endarterectomy s.
Hashmat s.
Hashmat-Waterhouse s.
hepatofugal porto-systemic venous s.
Heyer-Schulte hydrocephalus s.
Heyer-Schulte-Spetzler lumbar peritoneal s.
H-H neonatal s.
Holter s.
House endolymphatic s.
House and Pulec otic-periotic s.
hydrocephalus s.
indwelling nonvascular s.
intracardiac s.

S

NOTES

shunt *(continued)*
  Javid carotid s.
  jejunoileal s.
  Kasai peritoneal venous s.
  s. kit
  LaRivetti-Levinson intraluminal s.
  LeVeen ascites s.
  LeVeen dialysis s.
  LeVeen peritoneal s.
  LeVeen peritoneovenous s.
  loop s.
  mesocaval s.
  mesocaval H-graft s.
  Mischler s.
  Mischler-Pudenz s.
  Ommaya s.
  Orbis-Sigma s.
  parietal s.
  PC s.
  percutaneous thecoperitoneal s.
  peritoneojugular s.
  peritoneovenous s.
  pleural peritoneal s.
  portacaval s.
  portosystemic s.
  Potts s.
  Pruitt-Inahara carotid s.
  Pruitt-Inahara vascular s.
  Pruitt vascular s.
  PTFE s.
  Pudenz-Schulte thecoperitoneal s.
  Pudenz valve-flushing s.
  Quinton-Scribner s.
  Quinton Scribner s.
  radiologic portacaval s.
  Raimondi low-pressure s.
  Ramirez s.
  Reynold-Southwick H-graft
    portacaval s.
  Rickham reservoir s.
  Rivetti-Levinson intraluminal s.
  Scribner s.
  side-to-side portacaval s.
  Silastic Ames s.
  Silastic ventriculoperitoneal s.
  Simeone-Erlik side-to-end
    portorenal s.
  Sof-Flo coronary s.
  Spetzler lumbar-peritoneal s.
  splenorenal bypass s.
  subduroperitoneal s.
  Sundt carotid endarterectomy s.
  Sundt hemodynamic s.
  syrinx s.
  TDMAC-heparin s.
  Thomas s.
  Thomas femoral s.
  Thomas vascular access s.
  TIPS s.

  TIPSS s.
  Torkildsen s.
  tracheoesophageal s.
  tracheopharyngeal s.
  transhepatic portacaval s.
  transjugular intrahepatic
    portosystemic s. (TIPS, TIPSS)
  T-shaped Edwards-Barbaro syringo-
    peritoneal s.
  T-tube s.
  s. tube
  s. tubing
  Uni-Shunt hydrocephalus s.
  UreSil Vascu-Flo carotid s.
  USCI s.
  VA s.
  valve s.
  Vascushunt carotid balloon s.
  ventriculoatrial s.
  ventriculoperitoneal s.
  vesicoamniotic s.
  Vitagraft arteriovenous s.
  VP s.
  VS s.
  Warren splenorenal s.
  Waterston s.
  Waterston-Cooley s.
  White glaucoma pump s.
Shuppe biting forceps
Shur-Band self-closure elastic bandage
Shurly tracheal retractor
Shur resin
Shur-Strip wound closure tape
Shuster
  S. suture forceps
  S. tonsillar forceps
shutoff clamp
Shutt
  S. Aggressor forceps
  S. alligator forceps
  S. basket forceps
  S. B-scoop forceps
  S. grasping forceps
  S. Mantis retrograde forceps
  S. microscissors
  S. Mini-Aggressor forceps
  S. minibasket
  S. retrograde forceps
  S. scissors
  S. shovel-nosed forceps
  S. suction forceps
  S. suture punch system
shuttle
  S. Balance balance trainer
  Caspari s.
Shuttle-Relay suture passer
sialendoscope
  Marchal interventional s.
sialography needle

Siamese twin bracket
Sibel-Home-300 sleep diagnostic system
Sichel
    S. iris knife
    S. movable orbital implant
Sichi implant
sickle
    s. blade
    s. knife
    s. scissors
Sickle-Chex control
sickle-shaped Beaver blade
Sicor cardiac catheterization recording system
side
    s. blade
    s. mouthgag
    s. plate
    S. Rester cushion
side-arm
    s.-a. adapter
    s.-a. nebulizer
side-biting
    s.-b. clamp
    s.-b. ostrum punch
    s.-b. spatula
    s.-b. Stammberger punch forceps
side-curved forceps
side-cutter
    heavy-duty pliers with s.-c.
side-cutting
    s.-c. basket forceps
    s.-c. blade
    s.-c. cannula
    s.-c. irrigating cystotome
    s.-c. rasp
    s.-c. rongeur
    s.-c. spatula
    s.-c. spatulated needle
    s.-c. Swanson bur
4-sided cutting needle
SideFire laser
Side-Fire reflecting dish
side-firing probe
side-flattened needle
side-grasping forceps
side-hole
    s.-h. cannulated probe
    s.-h. catheter
    s.-h. pigtail catheter
Sidekick foot support
side-lip forceps

side-opening laminar hook
sideport
    s. cannula
    s. flat-bottomed Ommaya reservoir
Sideris adjustable buttoned device
SideStream nebulizer
sidestream spirometer
side-to-side portacaval shunt
side-viewing
    s.-v. duodenoscope
    s.-v. endoscope
    s.-v. fiberscope
sidewall
    s. holed needle
    s. infusion cannula
sidewinder
    s. aortic clamp
    s. percutaneous intraaortic balloon catheter
Sidney Stephenson corneal trephine
Siebold uterine scissors
Siegel-Cohen dilating catheter
Siegel stent
Sieger insufflator
Siegle
    S. antique pneumatic otoscope
    S. ear speculum
Siegler biopsy forceps
Siegler-Hellman clamp
Sielaff gastroscope
Siemens
    S. BICOR cardioscope
    S. custom tinnitus control instrument
    S. DRH CT scanner
    S. ECAT 951/31R PET scanner
    S. Endo-P endorectal transducer
    S. Evolution EBCT scanner
    S. Hicor angiography machine
    S. Hicor cardioscope
    S. linear probe
    S. Magnetom GBS II scanner
    S. Magnetom Vision scanner
    S. Mevatron 74 linear accelerator
    S. Mingograph
    S. MRI unit
    S. open-heart table
    S. Orbiter gamma camera
    S. PTCA open-heart suture
    S. Quantum 2000 Color Doppler
    S. Satellite CT evaluation console
    S. Servo-series ventilator

NOTES

S

Siemens *(continued)*
    S. Siecure implantable cardioverter-defibrillator
    S. SI 400 ultrasound
    S. Somatom DR2, DR3 whole-body scanner
    S. Somatom DRH CT analyzer unit
    S. Somatom Plus 4 CT system
    S. Sonoline Elegra ultrasound
    S. Sonoline Prima ultrasound
    S. Sonoline SI-400 ultrasound system
    S. Sonoline SL-2 echocardiograph
    S. 1.5 Tesla scanner
    S. vaginal probe
    S. Vision MRI
Siemens-Albis bicycle ergometer
Siemens-Elema
    S.-E. AG bicycle ergometer
    S.-E. multiprogrammable pacemaker
    S.-E. Servo-series 900C ventilator
Siemens-Pacesetter pacemaker
Sienna ultrasound system
Siepser intraocular lens
Sierra alloy
Sierra-Sheldon tracheotome
SieScape
    S. imaging
    S. ultrasound
Siesta physiologic data recorder
sieve
    s. graft
    Mobin-Uddin s.
    molecular s.
Sievers model 280 nitric oxide analyzer
Sifoam padding
Sigma
    S. II Dualplace hyperbaric system
    S. 6000+ infusion pump
    S. 34 Monoplace hyperbaric system
sigmoid
    s. anastomosis clamp
    s. notch retractor
sigmoidoscope
    ACMI flexible s.
    adult s.
    Boehm s.
    Buie s.
    disposable sheathed flexible s.
    Eder s.
    ESI s.
    fiberoptic s.
    flexible s.
    Frankfeldt s.
    Fujinon ES-series s.
    Fujinon flexible s.
    Fujinon FS-series s.
    Gorsch s.

    Heinkel s.
    Hopkins s.
    Kelly s.
    KleenSpec fiberoptic disposable s.
    Lieberman s.
    s. light carrier
    Lloyd-Davies s.
    Montague s.
    Olympus CF-L-series flexible s.
    Olympus CF-OSF-series flexible s.
    Olympus CF-series flexible s.
    Olympus fiberoptic s.
    Olympus OSF flexible s.
    Pentax flexible s.
    Pentax FS-series fiberoptic s.
    RectoSight disposable s.
    Reichert flexible s.
    s. replacement lamp
    rigid s.
    sheathed flexible s.
    Solow s.
    Strauss s.
    Turrell s.
    Tuttle s.
    Vernon David s.
    Visiline disposable s.
    VSI 2000 s.
    Welch Allyn fiberoptic s.
    Welch Allyn flexible s.
    Welch Allyn KleenSpec fiberoptic disposable s.
    Yeoman s.
Signa
    S. Advantage system
    S. Horizon LX MRI system
    S. imager
    S. Infinity MRI system
    S. I.S.T. MRI scanner
    S. pad
    S. 1.5 Tesla unit
    S. whole-body MRI scanner
SignaDress hydrocolloid dressing
signal
    optical intrinsic s. (OIS)
signal-averaged electrocardiograph
Signature Edition infusion system
Signet
    S. disposable skin stapler
    S. Optical lens
Signorini tourniquet
Sigvaris
    S. compression stocking
    S. medical stocking
Siker mirror laryngoscope
silanated slide
Silastic
    S. Ames shunt
    S. ball
    S. ball spacer prosthesis

S. band
S. catheter
S. chin implant
S. chin prosthesis
S. corneal eye implant
S. coronary artery cannula
S. Cronin implant
S. cup extractor
S. elastomer infusion catheter
S. eustachian tube
S. eye implant
S. fimbrial prosthesis
S. finger implant
S. foam dressing
S. gel dressing
S. Gel-filled testicular implant
S. graft
S. grommet
S. ileal reservoir catheter
S. indwelling ureteral stent
S. intestinal tube
S. mammary prosthesis
S. medical adhesive
S. midfacial malar implant
S. mold
S. mushroom catheter
S. obstetrical vacuum cup
S. otoplasty prosthesis
S. penile implant
S. penile prosthesis
S. plate
S. rhinoplasty implant
S. ring
S. scleral buckle implant
S. scleral buckler eye implant
S. sheet
S. sheeting keel prosthesis
S. silicone rubber implant
S. sling
S. sphere
S. sponge
S. spring-loaded silo
S. standard elastometer prosthesis
S. strain gauge
S. strap
S. subdermal implant
S. sucker suction tube
S. suture button
S. tape
S. tape
S. testicular prosthesis
S. thoracic drain

S. thyroid drain
S. toe implant
S. tracheostomy tube
S. tubing
S. ventriculoperitoneal shunt
S. wick
Silber
S. microneedle holder
S. microvascular clamp
S. vasovasostomy clamp
Silberg E.U.A. system
Silcath subclavian catheter
Silc extractor
Silcock dissection forceps
Silent
S. Nite alarm
S. Nite snore prevention device
S. Speaker communication system
Silesian bandage
Silflex intramedullary prosthesis
Silhouette
S. endoscopic laser
S. massager
S. spinal fixation system
S. therapeutic massage system
S. therapeutic mattress
silica contact lens
silicate cement
Silicon
S. Graphics Indigo 2 computer
S. Graphics Reality Engine system
silicon-controlled
s.-c. rectifier
s.-c. switch
silicone
s. adhesive
s. ball heart valve
Biocell textured s.
s. block
s. buckling implant
s. button
s. button eye implant
s. cannula
s. conformer
s. diode dosimeter
s. disc heart valve
s. doughnut prosthesis
s. dressing
s. elastomer
s. elastomer band
s. elastomer infusion catheter
s. elastomer lens

S

NOTES

silicone *(continued)*
- s. elastomer prosthesis
- s. elastomer ring
- s. elastomer rubber ball implant
- s. epistaxis catheter
- s. exoplant
- s. eye sphere
- s. flexor rod
- s. gel prosthesis
- s. gel sheeting
- s. hubless flat drain
- s. insole
- s. introducer
- s. lead
- s. membrane
- s. meshed motility implant
- s. microimplant
- s. mold
- s. MP implant
- s. nasal strut implant
- s. oil removal cannula
- s. pad eye implant
- s. Robinson catheter
- s. rod implant
- s. rod and sleeve forceps
- s. round drain
- s. rubber Dacron-cuffed catheter
- Schepens boat s.
- Schepens grooved rubber s.
- Schepens pad s.
- s. sizer
- s. sleeve eye implant
- s. sponge
- s. sponge forceps
- s. sponge implant
- s. stent
- s. strip
- s. strip eye implant
- s. sump drain
- s. textured mammary implant
- s. thoracic drain
- s. tire
- s. tire eye implant
- tire-grooved s.
- s. trapezium prosthesis
- s. T-tube
- s. tube
- s. voice prosthesis

silicone-coated, metallic self-expanding stent
silicone-filled
- s.-f. anatomical breast implant
- s.-f. mammary implant
- s.-f. round breast implant

silicone-gel breast implant
silicone-lubricated endotracheal tube
silicone-spiked mat
silicone-treated surgical silk suture

Silicore catheter
Si(Li) detector
Sili-Gel impression material
Silikon 1000 retinal tamponade
Silima breast prosthesis
Silipos
- S. digital pad
- S. Distal Dip prosthetic sheath
- S. mesh cap
- S. mesh tubing
- S. silicone wonder cup
- S. suspension sleeve

Silitek
- S. catheter
- S. Uropass stent

silk
- s. braided suture
- s. guidewire
- S. Laser
- s. Mersilene suture
- s. nonabsorbable suture
- Owens s.
- s. pop-off suture
- s. screw
- S. Skin sheet
- s. stay suture
- s. suture
- s. traction suture

silk-and-wax catheter
SilkLaser
- erbium S.
- FeatherTouch S.
- S. laser
- S. laser system
- Sharplan Erbium S.
- Sharplan FeatherTouch S.

Sil-K OB barrier
SilkTouch CO_2 laser scanner
silkworm gut suture
Silky Polydek suture
Sil-Med
- S.-M. catheter
- S.-M. instrument paws

silo
- Prolene mesh s.
- Silastic spring-loaded s.

SI-LOC sacroiliac belt
SiloLiner interface material
Silon
- S. Dual-Dress wound dressing
- S. silicone elastomer sheeting
- S. silicone thermoplastic splinting material
- S. tent
- S. wound dressing

Silon-LTS low temperature splinting
Silon-TEX silicone-bonded textile
Silon-TSR temporary skin replacement

Silopad
  S. body sleeve
  S. toe sleeve
Silosheath
  S. gel liner
  S. sock
Siloskin dressing
SiloSplint thumb splint
Silovi saphenous vein graft
Siloxane
  S. graft
  S. implant
  S. prosthesis
Silsoft extended wear contact lens
Siltex
  S. Becker breast prosthesis
  S. mammary implant
Silva-Packer
silver
  s. bead electrode
  S. Bullet blade
  s. catheter
  S. chisel
  s. clip
  S. endaural forceps
  S. knife
  s. mylar roll
  S. nasal osteotome
  s. needle
  s. probe
  s. suture
  S. trachea cannula
silver-coated
  s.-c. catheter
  s.-c. stent
silvered contact lens
silverized catgut suture
Silverlon wound packing strip
Silverman biopsy needle
Silverman-Boeker
  S.-B. cannula
  S.-B. needle
silver-silver chloride electrode
SilverSpeed hydrophilic guidewire
Silverstein
  S. arachnoid dissector
  S. auditory canal dissector
  S. dressing
  S. dural elevator
  S. facial nerve monitor
  S. lateral venous sinus retractor
  S. micromirror

  S. nerve separator
  S. permanent aeration tube
  S. round knife
  S. sickle knife
  S. stimulator probe
Silver-Thera stocking
Simal cervical stabilization system
Simcoe
  S. anterior chamber capsule
    scrubber
  S. anterior chamber receiving
    needle
  S. anterior chamber retaining wire
  S. cannula tip
  S. capsular scraper
  S. C-loop intraocular lens
  S. connecting tubing
  S. corneal marker
  S. cortex cannula
  S. cortex extractor
  S. double-barreled cannula
  S. double-end lens loop
  S. eye speculum
  S. I&A system
  S. II PC aspirating needle
  S. II PC double cannula
  S. II posterior chamber nucleus
    delivery loop
  S. implantation forceps
  S. interchangeable tip
  S. intraocular lens implant
  S. irrigating needle
  S. lens-inserting forceps
  S. lens-positioning set
  S. microhook
  S. notched irrigating spatula
  S. nucleus delivery cannula
  S. nucleus erysiphake
  S. nucleus forceps
  S. nucleus lens loop
  S. nucleus spatula
  S. posterior capsule scrubber
  S. posterior chamber forceps
  S. reverse-aperture cannula
  S. reverse I&A cannula
  S. superior rectus forceps
  S. suture needle
  S. wire speculum
Simcoe-AMO eye implant
Simcoe-Barraquer eye speculum
**Simeone-Erlik side-to-end portorenal
  shunt**

S

NOTES

863

Simmonds
- S. cricothyrotomy needle
- S. vaginal speculum

Simmons
- S. catheter
- S. chisel
- S. double-hole spinal screw
- S. eye shield
- S. plating system
- S. sidewinder catheter

Simmons-Kimbrough glaucoma spatula
Simmons-Martin screw
Simon
- S. bone curette
- S. cup uterine curette
- S. dermatome
- S. expansion arch
- S. fistula hook
- S. fistula knife
- S. nitinol inferior vena caval filter
- S. spinal curette
- S. uterine scoop
- S. vaginal retractor

Simonart
- S. band
- S. bar

Simons
- S. cleft palate knife
- S. stone-removing forceps

Simpa denture reliner
Simplastic catheter
Simple-Ject
- S.-J. auto-injector
- S.-J. auto-injector system

Simplex
- S. cement adhesive
- S. P bone cement

Simplicity contoured pant
SimpliCT interventional guidance system
Simplus PE/t dilatation catheter
Simply Wet table
Simpson
- S. antral curette
- S. atherectomy catheter
- S. coronary AtheroCath
- S. coronary AtheroCath catheter
- S. directional coronary atherectomy device
- S. endoscope
- S. epistaxis balloon
- S. forceps
- S. lacrimal dilator
- S. obstetrical forceps
- S. peripheral AtheroCath
- S. PET balloon atherectomy device
- S. sterling lacrimal probe
- S. suction catheter
- S. sugar-tong splint

- S. Ultra Lo-Profile II balloon catheter
- S. uterine dilator
- S. uterine sound

Simpson-Braun obstetrical forceps
Simpson-Luikart obstetrical forceps
Simpson-Robert
- S.-R. ACS dilatation catheter
- S.-R. vascular dilation system

Simpulse
- S. irrigation system
- S. pulsing lavage

Simrock speculum
Sims
- S. abdominal needle
- S. anoscope
- S. cannula
- S. double-ended retractor
- S. double-ended vaginal speculum
- S. irrigating uterine curette
- S. knife
- S. Per-fit percutaneous tracheostomy kit
- S. proctoscope
- S. rectal retractor
- S. rectal speculum
- S. sponge holder
- S. suction tip
- S. suture
- S. uterine depressor
- S. uterine dilator
- S. uterine probe
- S. uterine scissors
- S. uterine sound
- S. vaginal decompressor
- S. vaginal plug
- S. vaginal retractor
- S. vaginal speculum

SIM-Seguin annuloplasty ring
Sims-Kelly vaginal retractor
Sims-Maier
- S.-M. clamp
- S.-M. dressing forceps

Sims-Siebold uterine scissors
simulator
- AcQSIM CT s.
- Boston Dynamics surgical s.
- BTE Work s.
- Ergos work s.
- flexible bronchoscopy s.
- Lido WorkSet work s.
- Maxwell 3D field s.
- MR s.
- Nucletron s.
- radiation s.
- spinal physiotherapy s.
- surgical s.
- virtual reality s.
- Ximatron s.

simultaneous thermal diffusion blood flow and pressure probe
Sinai system
SI-30NB
    PhacoFlex II SI-30NB
Sinclair spatula
Sine-U-View nasal endoscope
Sinexon dilator
Singer
    S. needle
    S. portable pneumothorax apparatus
Singer-Blom
    S.-B. ossicular prosthesis
    S.-B. tube
    S.-B. valve
Singh speech system voice rehabilitation prosthesis
single-action rongeur
single-armed suture
single-axis
    s.-a. ankle prosthesis
    s.-a. friction knee
    s.-a. locking knee
    s.-a. Syme DYCOR foot
single-base cane
single-beveled cutting instrument
single-blade retractor
single-chamber
    s.-c. pacemaker
    s.-c. pulse generator
single-channel
    s.-c. analyzer
    s.-c. cochlear implant
    s.-c. electromyograph oscilloscope
    s.-c. fiberoptic bronchoscope
    s.-c. nonfade oscilloscope
    s.-c. operating sheath
    s.-c. in vivo light dosimeter
    s.-c. wire-guided sphincterotome
single-crystal gamma camera
Single-Day Baxter infuser
single-detector
    s.-d. helical scanner
    s.-d. row scanner
single-energy x-ray absorptiometer
single-fiber EMG electrode
single-head
    s.-h. rotating gamma camera
    s.-h. SPECT camera
single-hole collimator
single-hook retractor
single-J urinary diversion stent

single-lead VDD pacemaker
single-loop tourniquet
single-lumen
    s.-l. balloon stone extractor catheter
    s.-l. cannula
    s.-l. infusion catheter
single-mirror goniolens
single-needle device
single-pass
    s.-p. lead
    s.-p. pacemaker
single-photon
    s.-p. densitometer
    s.-p. electrospinal orthosis
    s.-p. emission computed tomography (SPECT)
single-plane instrument
single-prong broad acetabular retractor
single-reference-point instrument
single-rod construct
single-running suture
single-sided bone saw
single-stage
    s.-s. catheter
    s.-s. screw implant
single-stemmed silicone hemiprosthesis
SingleStitch PhacoFlex lens
Singleton empyema trocar
single-tooth
    s.-t. forceps
    s.-t. retractor blade
    s.-t. subperiosteal implant
    s.-t. tenaculum
single-use
    s.-u. dermatome
    s.-u. electrode
single-wall needle
single-wire electrode
Singley
    S. intestinal clamp
    S. intestinal forceps
    S. tissue forceps
Singley-Tuttle
    S.-T. dressing forceps
    S.-T. intestinal forceps
    S.-T. tissue forceps
Singular oval polypectomy snare
Siniscal eyelid clamp
Siniscal-Smith lid everter
sinoscopy
    s. cannula
    s. trocar

S

NOTES

Sinskey
    S. intraocular lens forceps
    S. iris hook
    S. J-loop intraocular lens
    S. lens implant
    S. lens-manipulating hook
    S. lens manipulator
    S. microlens hook
    S. microtying forceps
    S. needle holder
    S. nucleus spatula
    S. pick
    S. tying forceps
Sinskey-McPherson forceps
Sinskey-Wilson foreign body forceps
sintered titanium mesh
Sinterlock
    S. implant
    S. implant metal prosthesis
SinuNEB system
sinus
    s. antral cannula
    s. balloon
    s. bur
    s. chisel
    s. curette
    s. dilator
    s. irrigating cannula
    s. irrigator
    s. lift osteotome
    s. mask
    s. node pacemaker
    s. probe
    s. stent
    s. trephine
    s. tympani excavator
SinuScope
    S. rigid rod
    S. rigid rod lens optics
SinuSeal resorbable nasal packing
SinuSpacer turbinate stent
Sinvision ultrasound scanner
siphon
    Moniz carotid s.
    Nichols nasal s.
    s. suction tube
Sippy
    S. esophageal dilator
    S. esophageal dilator pusher wire
Sirecust 404N neonatal monitoring system
Siremobil Iso-C-arm
Sirognathograph analyzing system
Sirus intramedullary nail
Sisco spectrometer
Sisler
    S. lacrimal trephine
    S. punctum dilator

Sisson
    S. forceps
    S. fracture-reducing elevator
    S. spring hook
    S. spring retractor
Sisson-Cottle speculum
Sisson-Love retractor
Sisson-Vienna speculum
Sister Helen Mustard ENT table
sister-hook forceps
Sistron scissors
Sistrunk
    S. band retractor
    S. dissecting scissors
    S. double-ended retractor
Site
    S. argon laser
    S. guillotine cutting tip
    S. I&A needle
    S. TXR phacoemulsification system
SiteGuard
    S. MVP
    S. MVP transparent dressing
Site-Rite II ultrasound system
SiteSelect percutaneous incisional breast biopsy system
SITEtrac spinal surgery system
sit/stand chair
Sit Straight coccyx relief wheelchair cushion
Sitzmarks radiopaque marker
Sivash hip prosthesis
sizer
    Björk-Shiley heart valve s.
    Brannock device shoe s.
    Meadox graft s.
    silicone s.
    voice prosthesis s.
sizing
    s. balloon
    s. ring
SJM
    St. Jude Medical
    SJM Masters series valve
    SJM pericardial patch
    SJM Quattro mitral valve
    SJM Regent valve
    SJM Sequin annuloplasty ring
    SJM Tailor annuloplasty ring
    SJM X-Cell cardiac bioprosthesis
SkareKare silicon gel-filled cushion
Skatron apparatus
Skeele
    S. chalazion curette
    S. corneal curette
    S. eye curette
Skeeter otologic drill
skeletal pin
Skeleton fine forceps

Skene
- S. catheter
- S. tenaculum forceps
- S. uterine forceps
- S. uterine spoon
- S. uterine tenaculum
- S. vulsellum
- S. vulsellum forceps

skiameter
skiascope
skiascopy bar
skid
- acetabular s.
- Austin Moore-Murphy bone s.
- bone s.
- s. curette
- Davis bone s.
- hip s.
- MacAusland hip s.
- Meyerding bone s.
- Meyerding hip s.
- Meyerding hip bone s.
- Meyerding shoulder s.
- Murphy bone s.
- Murphy-Lane bone s.
- Ryerson bone s.
- Scudder s.
- Yund acetabular s.

SkiFlex Plus orthotic
Skil-Care
- S.-C. Alarm cushion
- S.-C. cushion grip
- S.-C. reclining wheelchair

Skillbuilder half roll
Skillern
- S. phimosis forceps
- S. punch
- S. sinus probe
- S. sphenoidal probe
- S. sphenoid cannula

Skillman
- S. arterial forceps
- S. mosquito forceps
- S. prepuce forceps

Skil saw
Skimmer
- S. blade
- S. laryngeal blade tip
- S. RRP laryngeal shaver

skin
- s. clip
- composite cultured s.

- s. elevator
- s. flap retractor
- s. graft expander
- s. graft expander mesh
- s. graft mesher
- s. grinder
- s. gun
- s. hook
- s. hook retractor
- Integra artificial s.
- s. marker
- s. marking pen
- s. punch
- s. self-retaining retractor
- S. Skribe marker
- S. Skribe pen
- s. splint
- s. staple

Skin-Bond skin cement
ski needle
skinfold calipers
SkinLaser system
Skinlight
- S. erbium yttrium-aluminum-garnet laser
- S. Er:YAG laser

SkinMaster
- S. MD7 microdermabrader
- S. MD7 skin rejuvenation system

Skinny
- S. Chiba needle
- S. over-the-wire balloon catheter

Skin-Prep protective dressing
Skinscan scanner
Skinsense glove
SkinSleeves
- Posey S.

SkinTech medical tattooing device
SkinTegrity hydrogel dressing
SkinTemp biosynthetic skin dressing
Skirrow agar plate
skiving knife
Sklar
- S. anoscope
- S. bone drill
- S. bone saw
- S. brush
- S. evacuator
- S. ligature needle
- S. medical breast stamp
- S. pin cutter

S

NOTES

Sklar *(continued)*
    S. tonometer
    S. wire tightener
Sklar-Junior Tompkins aspirator
Sklar-Schitz jewel tonometer
SklarScribe skin marker
Skoog nasal chisel
skull
    s. block
    s. bur
    s. clamp
    s. elevator
    s. plate
    s. plate screwdriver
    s. positioner
    s. punch
    s. raspatory
    s. traction drill
    s. traction tongs
    s. trephine
Sky-Boot stirrup system
Sky epidural pain control system
Skylark
    S. surface electrode
    S. TENS unit
Skylight
    S. gantry-free nuclear medicine
        gamma camera
    S. system
Skytron
    S. air-fluidized bed
    S. surgical table
slab
    2-dimensional MRA s.
    3-dimensional MRA s.
Slade cannula
Slalom balloon
Slam'r wheelchair
Slant
    S. haptic
    S. haptic intraocular lens
slant-hole collimator
slaphammer
    BIAS s.
Slatis frame
slatted plinth table
Slattery-McGrouther dynamic flexion
  splint
Slaughter nasal saw
Sled implant
Sleds
    Penco Walker S.
Sleek catheter
sleep
    s. apnea monitor
    S. Right device
    S. Right nasal strip

Sleepscan
    S. airflow pressure transducer
    S. polysomnograph
sleeve
    s. adapter
    s. bag
    Bard irrigation s.
    Biocompression pneumatic s.
    Charles anterior segment s.
    Charles infusion s.
    Charles vitrector with s.
    Coloplast disposable irrigation s.
    Coloplast transparent irrigation s.
    Cunningham-Cotton s.
    delivery assistance s.
    Dexterity Surgical Pneumo S.
    drug infusion s.
    Dunlop s.
    Easy s.
    Edwards-Levine s.
    elbow s.
    Electro-Mesh s.
    forefoot compression s.
    gel suspension s.
    heel s.
    Iceflex Endurance suction
      suspension s.
    Iceross s.
    s. implant
    implant s.
    infusion s.
    Jobst s.
    Ken drive s.
    Knit-Rite suspension s.
    Labtician oval s.
    laparoscopic s.
    LocalMed catheter infusion s.
    malleolar gel s.
    Mediven lymphedema s.
    Mica 3x s.
    neoprene elbow s.
    OrthoGuard AB bone pin s.
    PMMA centering s.
    pneumo s.
    Preclude IMA s.
    Reid s.
    release s.
    s. selector
    Shin Ice s.
    shin splint compression s.
    shoulder traction and rotation s.
    Silipos suspension s.
    Silopad body s.
    Silopad toe s.
    STaR s.
    Steri-Sleeve tube s.
    Stevens-Charles s.
    supine driver nail drill s.
    SupraSLEEVES nylon s.

Sur-Fit colostomy irrigation s.
Ultra Duet colostomy irrigating s.
Watzke silicone s.
sleeved nut
sleeve-spreading forceps
Sleuth
ETO S.
Slick stylette endotracheal tube guide
slide
CytoRich cervical cytology s.
Fisher-plus s.
gelatin-subbed s.
s. hammer
Hemoccult Sensa s.
Polaroid vectograph s.
poly-L-lysine-coated glass s.
silanated s.
Tanner s.
Testsimplets prestained s.
Slide-On EndoSheath
SlidePro 15 compact slide heater
Slider
S. balloon
S. catheter
Slidewire extension guide
sliding
s. barrel hook
s. capsular forceps
s. hammer
s. laryngoscope
s. lock
sliding-rail catheter
Slik-Pak nonstick nasal pack
Slim
S. Fit flex clamp
S. Option shoe orthosis
S. and Trim brief
slimcut blade
Slimfit lens
SlimLine
S. cast boot
S. disposable brief
SlimSIGHT ultraslim GI videoscope
SlimStem metal scleral shield
Slimthetics orthotic
sling
Aldridge rectus fascia s.
Ampoxen s.
Arjo s.
arm elevator s.
Barton s.
Biosling urethral s.

Böhler-Braun leg s.
cardiac s.
clip-reinforced cotton s.
Colles s.
Core envelope arm s.
cradle arm s.
CVA s.
Dacron mesh s.
DLP cardiac s.
s. dressing
envelope arm s.
finger s.
Fits-All s.
FortaPerm surgical s.
s. frame
hanging cast s.
Harris Hemi Arm s.
Harris splint s.
head s.
Hemi s.
Kodel s.
leg s.
Mersilene mesh s.
Murphy s.
Nada-Chair Back-Up portable
  back s.
Perthes s.
platysma intrlocking suture s.
Posey s.
pouch-type s.
pressure s.
pulmonary artery s.
Rauchfuss suspension s.
resting foot s.
Safyre synthetic s.
Sayre s.
shoulder saddle s.
Silastic s.
slinger-style envelope s.
sling and swathe s.
Stratasis urethral s.
suburethral s.
SurgiSis s.
Suspend s.
s. and swathe
Thomas Kodel s.
triangular arm s.
UltraSling glenohumeral joint s.
Uni-Versatil s.
Uretex pubourethral s.
Velpeau s.

S

NOTES

sling *(continued)*
 Weil pelvic s.
 Westfield-style envelope s.
sling-and-swathe bandage
slinger-style envelope sling
Slingshot
 S. ACL fixation system
 S. cross pin
Slinky
 S. balloon
 S. balloon catheter
 S. PTCA catheter
Slip-Coat tip
slip-ins
 Gulden red and green s.-i.
slip-joint pliers
Slip-N-Snip scissors
slipper-tipped guidewire
Slippery Slider transport board
slip-ring camera
Slip-Sheen catheter
slit
 s. blade
 s. blade knife
 s. illuminator
 s. lamp
slit-lamp
 s.-l. cup
 s.-l. fluorophotometer
 Gullstrand s.-l.
 s.-l. microscope
SLM-8000 fluorescence spectrophotometer
Sloan
 S. goiter flap dissector
 S. goiter self-retaining retractor
Sloane LASEK micro hoe
Slocum meniscal clamp
Slocum-Smith-Petersen nail
Slo-Mo ball
slot
 S. distraction device
 s. table
slot-scanning detector
slotted
 s. anoscope
 s. bone plate
 s. instrument
 s. intramedullary rod
 s. laryngoscope
 s. mallet
 s. nail
 s. needle
 s. nerve clamp
 s. tendon stripper
 s. tube articulated stent
 s. whisker
 s. wrench
slotting bur

slotting-bur osteotome
slow
 s. deflate system (SDS)
 s. palatal expander
SL-Plus stem
SLS Chromos long pulse ruby laser system
SLT
 Surgical Laser Technologies
 SLT CL MD/Dual Contact laser
 SLT Contact MTRL laser
 SLT FiberTact/Contact laser fiber
Sluder
 S. adenotome
 S. cautery electrode
 S. headband
 S. knife
 S. needle
 S. palate retractor
 S. sphenoidal hook
 S. sphenoidal speculum
 S. tonometer
 S. tonsillar guillotine
 S. tonsillar tonsillectome
Sluder-Ballenger
 S.-B. tonsillar punch forceps
 S.-B. tonsillectome
Sluder-Demarest
 S.-D. tonometer
 S.-D. tonsillectome
Sluder-Ferguson mouthgag
Sluder-Jansen mouthgag
Sluder-Mehta electrode
Sluder-Sauer
 S.-S. tonsillar guillotine
 S.-S. tonsillectome
Sluijter-Mehta SMK-C10 cannula
SMA
 shape-memory alloy
 SMA portogram
SMAC
 Sequential Multiple Analyzer Computer
small
 s. aperture Steri-Drape drape
 s. fragment system (SFS)
 s. nail spicule bur
 S. rake retractor
 S. tissue retractor
small-based quad cane
small-bore
 s.-b. cannula
 s.-b. needle
 s.-b. scanner
small-caliber needle
Small-Carrion
 S.-C. penile implant material
 S.-C. penile prosthesis
 S.-C. Silastic rod for penile implant

small-diameter endosonographic
   instrument
small-loop electrode
small-particle aerosol generator
small-volume nebulizer
SMART
   shape-memory alloy recoverable
      technology
      SMART nitinol self-expandable
         stent
      SMART stent
smart
   S. Balance Master
   S. scalpel
   S. splint
   S. Trigger Bear 1000 ventilator
SmartAnchor-D suture anchor
SmartAnchor-L suture anchor
SmartBrace brace
Smartdop Doppler
SmartDose infusion system
SmartEpil laser
SmartFlow Multiple Lesion device
Smartglove orthopaedic wrist glove
SmartKard digital Holter system
SmartKnit seamless sock
SmartLine low vision aid
SmartMist asthma management system
SmartNeedle
   S. inserter
   S. vascular access device
SmartPins fastener
SmartPrep scanner
SmarTracking
SmartScreener infant hearing screener
SmartScrew
   S. bioabsorbable implant
   S. screw
SmartSite needleless system
SmartSpot high-resolution digital
   imaging system
SmartTack absorbable bone anchor
SmartWrap elbow brace
Smedberg
   S. brace
   S. dilator
Smeden tonsillar punch
Smedley dynamometer
SMEI ultrasound-assisted lipoplasty
   machine
Smellie
   S. obstetrical forceps

S. obstetrical hook
S. obstetrical perforator
S. obstetrical scissors
Smeloff-Cutter
   S.-C. aortic ball valve prosthesis
   S.-C. ball-cage prosthetic valve
Smeloff heart valve
SMIC
   SMIC abdominal spatula
   SMIC anterior commisure
      laryngoscope
   SMIC auricular tourniquet
   SMIC bone chisel
   SMIC bone file
   SMIC bone hammer
   SMIC bone rongeur
   SMIC brain spatula
   SMIC burnisher
   SMIC carver
   SMIC cerumen hook
   SMIC cheek retractor
   SMIC collar scissors
   SMIC cranial rongeur
   SMIC dermatome
   SMIC ear curette
   SMIC ear polypus scissors
   SMIC ear speculum
   SMIC eustachian catheter
   SMIC excavator
   SMIC explorer
   SMIC intestinal clamp
   SMIC laminectomy rongeur
   SMIC malleus head nipper
   SMIC mastoid chisel
   SMIC mastoid curette
   SMIC mastoid gouge
   SMIC mastoid rongeur
   SMIC mastoid suction tube
   SMIC mouth mirror
   SMIC myringotome
   SMIC nasal septal speculum
   SMIC nylon thread
   SMIC periodontal abscess probe
   SMIC periodontal file
   SMIC periosteal elevator
   SMIC pituitary curette
   SMIC pliers
   SMIC pneumatic otoscope
   SMIC powder blower
   SMIC root canal plugger
   SMIC sternal chisel
   SMIC sternal drill

NOTES

S

SMIC *(continued)*
    SMIC sternal knife
    SMIC surgical catgut
    SMIC surgical mallet
    SMIC suture needle
    SMIC tonsillar guillotine
    SMIC tuning fork
Smiley-Williams arteriography needle
SmiLine abutment system
Smillie
    S. cartilage chisel
    S. knee joint retractor
    S. meniscal cartilage knife
    S. meniscectomy chisel
    S. meniscotome
    S. nail
    S. nail punch
    S. pin
Smirmaul
    S. eyelid speculum
    S. nucleus extractor
Smith
    S. anal retractor
    S. anal speculum
    S. aneurysm clip
    S. anoscope
    S. bandage scissors
    S. bone clamp
    S. cartilage knife
    S. cataract knife
    S. cordotomy clamp
    S. cordotomy knife
    S. drill
    S. endoscopic electrode
    S. expressor hook
    S. eye speculum
    S. grasping forceps
    S. intraocular capsular amputator
    S. intraocular implant lens
    S. lens expressor
    S. lid expressor
    S. lid-retracting hook
    S. lion-jaw forceps
    S. marginal clamp
    S. & Nephew barbed staple
    S. & Nephew ENT
      nasopharyngoscope
    S. & Nephew Reflection Interfit
      acetabular cup implant component
    S. & Nephew Richards bipolar
      forceps
    S. & Nephew screw
    S. nerve root suction retractor
    S. obstetrical forceps
    S. orbital floor implant
    S. perforator
    S. pessary
    S. posterior cartilage stripper
    S. rectal self-retaining retractor

    S. retroversion pessary
    S. suture wire scissors
    S. tonsillar dissector
    S. total ankle prosthesis
    S. tube
    S. vaginal self-retaining retractor
Smith-Buie
    S.-B. anal retractor
    S.-B. rectal spreader
    S.-B. self-retaining rectal retractor
Smith-Fisher
    S.-F. cataract knife
    S.-F. cataract spatula
    S.-F. iris replacer
    S.-F. iris spatula
Smith-Green
    S.-G. cataract knife
    S.-G. double-ended spatula
Smith-Hodge pessary
Smith-Leiske
    S.-L. cross-action intraocular lens
      forceps
    S.-L. lens manipulator
**Smith-Miller-Patch cryosurgical
  instrument**
Smith-Petersen
    S.-P. bone gouge
    S.-P. bone plate
    S.-P. cannulated nail
    S.-P. capsular retractor
    S.-P. chisel
    S.-P. cup
    S.-P. curette
    S.-P. curved gouge
    S.-P. curved osteotome
    S.-P. elevator
    S.-P. extractor
    S.-P. femoral neck nail
    S.-P. forceps
    S.-P. fracture pin
    S.-P. hammer
    S.-P. hip cup prosthesis
    S.-P. hip reamer
    S.-P. impactor
    S.-P. intertrochanteric plate
    S.-P. laminectomy rongeur
    S.-P. mallet
    S.-P. spatula
    S.-P. straight osteotome
    S.-P. transarticular nail
    S.-P. tucker
Smith-Richards instrumentation
Smithuysen sphenoidal punch
Smithwick
    S. anastomotic clamp
    S. buttonhook
    S. buttonhook button
    S. clip-applying forceps
    S. ganglion hook

S. hook
S. nerve dissector
S. nerve hook
S. nerve retractor
S. silver clip
S. sympathectomy hook
Smithwick-Hartmann forceps
SMo
S. Moore pin
S. plate
S. prosthesis
smoke
s. Controller device
s. Control Porta-Pack aversive stimulator
s. evacuator
s. evacuator suction tube
s. evacuator tubing
s. removal tube
Smokeeter tube
SmokEvac
S. electrosurgical probe
S. smoke evacuator
S. trumpet valve
Smolik curved rongeur
Smolinski endaural rongeur
S-Monovette blood collection system
Smoothbeam dermatologic laser
Smoothie Junior bur
smooth-tipped jeweler's forceps
smooth-tooth forceps
Smuckler tucker
SMZ-1 microscope
SMZ zoom stereo microscope
snail-headed catheter retriever
Snap
S. EEG device
S. fixation pin
Snap-Gauge impotence screening device
snap-lock brace
snap-on inserter plate
Snap-Pak anchor
SNAP sleep recorder
snare
AcuSnare s.
Alfred s.
Amplatz gooseneck s.
Amplatz retinal s.
ASSureBite hot polypectomy s.
Beck-Schenck tonsil s.
Beck-Storz tonsillar s.
BiSNARE bipolar polypectomy s.

Boettcher-Farlow s.
Bosworth nasal s.
Brown tonsillar s.
Bruening ear s.
Bruening nasal s.
Buerger s.
Captiflex polypectomy s.
Captivator polypectomy s.
Castroviejo enucleation s.
s. catheter
cautery s.
coaxial s.
Colles s.
Cox polypectomy s.
Crapeau nasal s.
crescent s.
diathermic s.
diathermy s.
Douglas nasal s.
Douglas tonsillar s.
ear polyp s.
electrosurgery s.
enucleation wire s.
s. enucleator
EUE tonsillar s.
Eves tonsillar s.
Farlow tonsillar s.
fascial s.
Foerster enucleation s.
Förster enucleation s.
Frankfeldt diathermy s.
Frankfeldt rectal s.
Glegg nasal polyp s.
gooseneck s.
hand cock-up s.
Harris s.
hexagon s.
Hobbs polypectomy s.
Hoyer s.
Jarvis s.
Krause ear polyp s.
Krause laryngeal s.
Krause nasal polyp s.
laryngeal s.
lasso s.
levator s.
Lewis tonsillar s.
Marlex mesh s.
Martin s.
Mason-Allen s.
Meek s.
Microvena Amplatz Goose Neck s.

S

NOTES

snare *(continued)*
    Milwaukee s.
    Myles tonsillectome s.
    nasal s.
    Neivert-Eves tonsillar s.
    Nesbit tonsillar s.
    Newhart-Casselberry s.
    nitinol s.
    Norwood rectal s.
    Olympus SD-5L semicircular s.
    oval s.
    pelvic s.
    pericardial s.
    polypectomy s.
    Posey s.
    Profile pediatric polypectomy s.
    ptosis s.
    pulmonary arterial s.
    Pynchon ear s.
    Quire mechanical finger s.
    Rainbow envelope arm s.
    Rauchfuss s.
    Reiner-Beck tonsillar s.
    Robert nasal s.
    rotatable polypectomy s.
    Rotator polypectomy s.
    Sage tonsillar s.
    Sayre head s.
    self-opening rigid s.
    Sensation Short Throw s.
    Singular oval polypectomy s.
    standard endoscopy polypectomy s.
    Stewart lenticular nuclear s.
    Stiegler unipolar nasal s.
    Storz-Beck tonsillar s.
    Stutsman nasal s.
    Supramid s.
    surgical s.
    Teare s.
    tonsillar s.
    transvenous s.
    Tydings automatic ratchet s.
    Tydings tonsil s.
    UroSnare cystoscopic tumor s.
    Veeder tip s.
    Velpeau s.
    Wappler polypectomy s.
    Weil pelvic s.
    Weston rectal s.
    Wilde-Bruening ear s.
    Wilde-Bruening nasal s.
    Wilde ear polyp s.
    Wilde nasal s.
    Wilson-Cook polypectomy s.
    wire s.
    Wright nasal s.
    Wright tonsillar s.
    Zimmer s.
Snarecoil bone marrow biopsy needle

Snellen
    S. chart
    S. conventional reform eye implant
    S. entropion forceps
    S. lens loop
    S. lens scoop
    S. reform implant
    S. soft contact lens
    S. suture
    S. vectis
Sniper Elite hydrophilic guidewire
Snitman endaural self-retaining retractor
SnorNoMor device
Snowden-Pencer
    S.-P. insufflator
    S.-P. internal heater
    S.-P. laparoscopic cholecystectomy instrument
    S.-P. Super-Cut scissors
Snowflake laparotomy sponge
snow plow rasp
Snug
    S. denture cushion
    S. seat
Snugfit eye patch
Snuggle Warm convective warming system
Snugs
    S. dressing
    S. tapeless wound care system
Snyder
    S. breast prosthesis
    S. corneal spring forceps
    S. Hemovac evacuator
    S. Hemovac silicone sump drain
    S. Hemovac suction tube
    S. suction device
    S. Surgivac drainage
    S. Surgivac suction tube
    S. Urevac suction tube
    S. Urevac trocar
Soaker catheter
Sobel-Kaplitt-Sawyer gas endarterectomy set
Soccer Sporthotic
sock
    AFO brace s.
    s. aid
    Bauerfeind Champion Powersox s.
    Bio-Wick s.
    Carolon AFO s.
    Comfort S.'s
    Comfort Ag prosthetic s.
    Creative diabetic s.'s
    Dero hole-in-one prosthetic s.
    diabetic s.
    edema s.
    electrode s.

Electro-Mesh electrode s.
gel stump s.
molding s.
NouveauDerm s.'s
polytetrafluoroethylene s.
Regal Acrylic Stretch prosthetic s.
Silosheath s.
SmartKnit seamless s.
Soft Walk gel s.
STS molding s.

socket
APOPPS transtibial prosthetic s.
flexible s.
Flo-Tech prosthetic s.
hard s.
Icex s.
ischial containment s.
metal-backed s.
polyethylene s.
prosthetic s.
SuperClearPro suction s.
supracondylar s.
suspension-type s.
s. wrench

Socon spinal system
Socrates
S. Robotic telecollaboration system
S. telementoring system
Sodem high-speed system
Soderstrom-Corson electrode
sodium
s. alginate wool mold
s. chloride-impregnated gauze
s. hyaluronate-based bioresorbable membrane
s. hyaluronate viscoelastic
s. iodide detector
Soehendra
S. BII papillotome/sphincterotome
S. catheter system
S. endoscopic biliary stent system
S. lithotripsy set
S. Precut papillotome/sphincterotome
S. rotary dilator
S. stent extractor
S. stent retrieval device
S. stent retriever
S. Universal dilating catheter
Sofamor
S. Danek anterior cervical plate
S. Danek self-retaining retractor
S. spinal instrument

Sof-Band bulky bandage
Sof-Care
S.-C. chair cushion
S.-C. mattress
S.-C. Plus cushion
Sofflex mattress
Sof-Flo coronary shunt
Sof-Foam dressing
Sof-Form conforming gauze
Sof Gel HeelCup orthosis
Sof-Gel palm shield
Sofield
S. retractor
S. retractor blade
S. retractor clip
Sof-Kling conforming bandage
Soflens contact lens
SoFlex lens
Sof-Matt pressure reducing mattress
Sofnit
S. Birdseye reusable underpad
S. 300 fitted brief
SofPulse electrotherapy device
Sof-Rol
S.-R. cast padding
S.-R. dressing
SofSeat pressure relief pad
Sofsilk
S. coated and braided suture
S. nonabsorbable silk suture
SofSorb absorptive dressing
SofStep wheelchair footplate cover
Sof-T
S.-T guidewire
S.-T guiding catheter
soft
s. cataract aspirator
s. contact lens
S. Guard XL fecal incontinence bag
s. intraocular lens
S. N Dry Merocel sponge
s. palate retractor
s. rubber curette
s. scrub brush
S. Seal cervical catheter
S. & Secure pouch system
S. Shield collagen corneal shield
S. & Silent diaper pant
s. silicone sphere implant
s. silicone sponge
S. Super Sport orthotic

NOTES

S

soft *(continued)*
S. Support Preforms orthotic
S. Thoracoport
s. tissue blade retractor
s. tissue graft clamp
s. tissue shaving cannula
S. Torque uterine catheter
S. Touch cup
S. Touch hand exerciser
S. Touch lancet device
S. Walk gel sock
s. wire loop
s. x-ray film
Soft-Cell permanent dual-lumen catheter
SoftCloth absorptive dressing
SofTec
S. genu knee brace
S. Lens Delivery system
S. Lumbo orthosis
Softech endotracheal tube
Softepil tweezer epilation device
Softexe non-adherent sub-bandage padding
Softeze
S. self-adhering foam pad
S. water pillow
Soft-EZ reusable electrode
SoftFit ultra nasal CPAP mask
Softflo fiber optic probe
SoftForm
S. facial implant
S. tube
SoftGrip pipette
Softgut surgical chromic catgut suture
Softie shoe
Softip
S. arteriography catheter
S. diagnostic catheter
SofTip monofilament
Softjaw
S. clamp
S. insert
SoftLight
S. laser
S. laser hair removal system
soft-lined denture
Softopac intraoral film
Softouch
S. angiography catheter
S. Cobra 1, 2 catheter
S. cold/hot pack
S. Headhunter 1 catheter
S. Multipurpose B2 catheter
S. Simmons 1, 2 catheter
S. UHF cardiac pigtail catheter
SofTouch vacuum erection device
Softrace gel electrode
Softrac-PTA catheter
Softscan laser scanner

SoftSITE high add aspheric multifocal contact lens
Softsplint foot splint
soft-tip catheter
soft-tipped cannula
soft-tissue Super Sport orthotic
Soft-Touch A-Probe
Soft-Vu
S.-V. angiographic catheter
S.-V. Omni flush catheter
Soft-Wand atraumatic tissue manipulator balloon
Sof-Wick
S.-W. drain
S.-W. drain sponge
S.-W. dressing
S.-W. lap pad
Sohes pacemaker
Soileau Tytan ventilation tube
Sokolec elevator
Sola
S. Optical USA Spectralite high-index lens
S. VIP lens
SolAiris III oxygen concentrator
Solar
S. Beam medical examination light
S. pacemaker
SolarEar hearing aid
Solaris
S. coronary dilatation catheter
S. MR injection system
SolaTone artificial larynx
Solcotrans
S. autotransfusion system
S. Plus drainage-reinfusion system
Solcovac
S. closed wound drainage system
S. suction evacuator
solder
PF Universal s.
tissue s.
soldering tweezers
sole
D-Soles foot s.
S. Primeur 33D analyzer
solenoid surface coil
Solera thrombectomy catheter
SOLEutions custom orthosis
Solfy ZX ultrasonic unit
solid
s. ankle-cushion heel (SACH)
S. Creation System
s. silicone buttock implant
s. silicone exoplant implant material
s. silicone orbital prosthesis
s. silicone with Supramid mesh implant

solid-ankle, cushioned-heel foot prosthesis
solid-core guidewire
solidifier
SafeSorb fluid s.
solid-phase
s.-p. extraction chromatograph
s.-p. extraction tube
solid-rod rigid telescope
solid-state
s.-s. esophageal manometry catheter
s.-s. instrument
s.-s. nuclear track detector
solid-tip catheter
SoLight breast form
Solis pacemaker
Solitaire needle
Solitens
S. TENS unit
S. transcutaneous electrical nerve stimulation unit
Soll suture and incision marker
SoloCath catheter
SoloPass Percuflex biliary stent
Solos endoscopy diagnostic laparoscope
SoloSite hydrogel dressing
Solo-Tach resin
Solow sigmoidoscope
Soluset
intravenous S.
S. IV set
Solus pacemaker
Solvang graft
Soma
S. Gonio system
S. pulley system
S. sacroiliac stabilization belt
Somanetics Invos 3100 cerebral oximeter
SomaSensor
S. cerebral oximeter monitoring system
S. device
S. pad
Somatics
S. monitoring electrode
S. mouth guard
Somatom
S. DR CT scanner
S. Plus S whole-body CT scanner
S. Volume Zoom

Somers
S. uterine clamp
S. uterine forceps
Somerset bur
SOMI
sternal occipital mandibular immobilizer
SOMI brace
SOMI Jr. brace
SOMI orthosis
Somjee-Crabtree temporal bone support clamp
SOMNOlab sleep diagnostic system
SOMNOmask sleep apnea mask
Somnoplasty system
SomnoStar apnea testing device
SOMNOvent S sleep apnea therapy device
Somnus
S. probe
S. Somnoplasty system
Sonablate
S. ablation device
S. 200 system
S. transrectal probe
Sonata imager
Sonatron ultrasonic scaler
Sonde enteroscope
Sones
S. Cardio-Marker catheter
S. coronary catheter
S. guidewire
S. hemostatic bag
S. Hi-Flow catheter
S. Positrol catheter
S. vent catheter
S. woven Dacron catheter
Songbird disposable hearing aid
Song covered duodenal stent
Songer
S. cable
S. spinal cable system
S. tonsillar forceps
sonic
s. accelerated fracture healing system (SAFHS)
S. Air handpiece
S. Boom alarm clock
S. Hedgehog signaling molecule
Sonicaid
S. Axis monitor

S

NOTES

Sonicaid *(continued)*
    S. Team system 8000 fetal monitor
    S. Vasoflow Doppler system
Sonicare Plus toothbrush
Sonicath
    S. endoluminal ultrasound catheter
    S. intravascular ultrasound catheter
Sonicator
    S. Plus 930 therapy unit
    S. portable ultrasound
    S. therapeutic ultrasound
SonicWave phacoemulsification system
Sonifer sonicating system
Sonix 2000 ultrasonic nebulizer
Sonnenschein nasal speculum
SonoAce 6000 II ultrasound system
Sonocath ultrasound probe
Sonoclot coagulation analyzer
Sonocur Basic system
Sonocut ultrasonic aspirator
Sonogage ultrasound pachymeter
sonogram
    Acuson transvaginal s.
sonography
    Acuson computed s.
    Toshiba SSA-340A Doppler s.
    s. unit
SonoHeart ELITE personal hand-carried echocardiography system
Sonolayer SSA-270A-30 ultrasound
Sonoline
    S. Elegra ultrasound system
    S. Prima ultrasound
    S. Sienna ultrasound system
Sonolith Praktis lithotripter
Sonomed A/B-Scan system
sonometer
    Omnisense 7000S bone s.
    Sahara clinical bone s.
    SoundScan Compact bone s.
    UBIS 5000 ultrasound bone s.
Sonometric Ocuscan
Sonoprobe
    Fujinon S.
Sonopsy ultrasound-guided breast biopsy system
Sonop ultrasonic aspirator
Sonoran dehumidifier
SonoSite
    S. digital ultrasound
    S. imaging device
    S. 180 ultrasound system
Sonos-series imaging system
Sonos 2000-series, 5000-series ultrasound imager
Sono-Stat Plus sound device
Sonotrode lithotripter

Sonotron
    S. electronic therapeutic device
    S. Vingmed CFM 800 imaging system
SonoVu US aspiration needle
Sontec pliers
Sony CCD/RGB DXC-151 color video camera
Soonawalla
    S. uterine elevator
    S. vasectomy forceps
Sopha Medical gamma camera
Sopher ovum forceps
Sophie mammography unit
Sophy programmable valve
Soprano
    S. cryoablation system
    S. cryotherapy unit
SorbaView
    S. composite wound dressing
    S. window dressing
Sorbex hydrocolloid wound dressing
Sorbiclear dialyzer
Sorbie-Questor total elbow system
Sorb-It II dressing
Sorbothane orthotic device
Sorbsan
    S. calcium alginate dressing
    S. gel block topical wound dressing
Sorbuthane II heel cup
Sorensen
    S. reusable cannister
    S. uterine aspirator
Sorenson thermodilution catheter
Soresi cannula
Sorin
    S. bicarbon bileaflet mitral valve prosthesis
    S. pacemaker
Sorrells Mark II hip arthroplasty retractor system
sorter
    FACSVantage cell s.
    fluorescence-activated cell s.
    magnetically activated cell s.
Sorvall Discovery SE ultracentrifuge
SOS Omni catheter
Soto USCI balloon
Soucek
    Rendell-Baker S. (RBS)
Soules intrauterine insemination catheter
sound
    Allport mastoid s.
    Bellocq s.
    Béniqué s.
    bladder s.
    bronchocele s.
    Campbell-French s.

Campbell miniature urethral s.
Davis interlocking s.
Dittel urethral s.
Dittel uterine s.
Ellik s.
female s.
flexible s.
Fowler urethral s.
French steel s.
Gouley tunneled urethral s.
Greenwald s.
Guyon-Bénlqué urethral s.
Guyon dilating s.
Guyon urethral s.
Hishida pine-needle s.
Hunt metal s.
interlocking s.
Jewett urethral s.
Jewett uterine s.
Klebanoff common duct s.
Kocher bronchocele s.
Korotkoff s.
lacrimal s.
LeFort urethral s.
LeFort uterine s.
s. level meter
Martin uterine s.
McCrea infant s.
meatal s.
Mercier s.
Otis urethral s.
Pharmaseal disposable uterine s.
Pratt urethral s.
radiolucent s.
Rica uterine s.
Rissler vein s.
Ritter s.
Saf-T-Sound uterine s.
Schroeder interlocking uterine s.
Simpson uterine s.
Sims uterine s.
urethral s.
uterine s.
Van Buren canvas roll s.
Van Buren dilating s.
Van Buren urethral s.
Walther urethral s.
Winternitz s.
Woodward s.

sounder

mini-echo s.
pedicle s.

SoundScan Compact bone sonometer
Soundtec hearing aid
source

Arclite light s.
dummy s.
Dyonics DyoBrite light s.
ESI fiberoptic light s.
fiberoptic light s.
halogen dual light s.
Heyman-Simon s.
Maxenon Xi 300 xenon light s.
Maxillume 250 watt quartz halogen
  light s.
Medicam light s.
Minimax 200 watt light s.
MX2-300 xenon quality light s.
Quadrilite 6000 light s.
xenon light s.
Zeiss Super Lux 40 light s.

Sourdille forceps
Souter-Strathclyde total elbow prosthesis
Southbent scissors
Southey

S. anasarca trocar
S. cannula
S. capillary drainage tube

Southey-Leech trocar
Southwick

S. clamp
S. screw extractor

Southworth rasp
Souttar

S. cautery
S. esophageal conductor
S. tube

Sovak reamer
Sovally suprapubic suction cup drain
Sovereign

S. bifocal lens
S. Shield system

Soviet mechanical bronchial stapler
SP-10 spirometer
Spa

S. Ready-To-Wear gradient pressure
  therapy hosiery
S. SoftBasics gradient pressure
  therapy hosiery
S. UltraSilk Sheers gradient
  pressure therapy hosiery

space-age wire
Spacekeeper retractor
SpaceLabs Holter monitor

S

NOTES

space-maintaining barrier
Spacemaker
    S. breast balloon dissector
    S. hernia balloon dissector
    S. II balloon
spacer
    Accu-Space plain gut seeding s.
    AeroChamber s.
    Barouk s.
    Barouk button s.
    Bio-Moore II provisional neck s.
    button s.
    ceramic vertebral s.
    dummy s.
    Ellipse compact s.
    eyelid s.
    Kinemax s.
    methyl methacrylate s.
    Plexiglas s.
    proximal cement s.
    rubber s.
    SB Charite III intervertebral
      dynamic disc s.
    suture s.
    Synthes vertebral s.
    telescopic plate s.
    vertebral s.
space retainer
Space-Saver volumetric pump
SpaceSEAL balloon tip cannula
spade-shaped valvotome
spaghetti drain
Spaleck forceps
Span-American wheelchair cushion
Spandage
    S. bandage
    S. elastic
Spand-Gel primary hydrogel dressing
Span+Guard mattress overlay
Spanish blue virgin silk suture
spanner
    Codman s.
    s. gauge
    s. wrench
spanning external fixator
SPARC sling system
spark-gap
    s.-g. instrument
    s.-g. shock wave generator
Spark handheld dynamometer
Sparks
    S. atrioseptal punch
    S. mandrel prosthesis
Spartan jaw wire cutter
SpaTouch PhotoEpilation system
spatula
    Ayers s.
    Aylesbury s.
    Aylesbury cervical s.

Ayre s.
Ayre cervical s.
Bakelite s.
Banaji LASIK flap s.
Bangerter s.
Barraquer cyclodialysis s.
Barraquer iris s.
Barraquer irrigator s.
Bechert s.
Berens s.
Birks Mark II micro push/pull s.
brain s.
s. cannula
s. cannula tip
Carones LASEK s.
Castroviejo cyclodialysis s.
Castroviejo double-end s.
Castroviejo synechia s.
Cave scaphoid s.
cement s.
Children's Hospital brain s.
Clayman s.
Cleasby iris s.
corneal fascia lata s.
corneal graft s.
coronary endarterectomy s.
Crile s.
Culler iris s.
Cushing brain s.
Cushing S-shaped brain s.
cyclodialysis s.
Cytobrush s.
Davis brain s.
DeBakey S-shaped brain s.
D'Errico brain s.
DeWecker iris s.
s. dissector
Dixey s.
Dorsey s.
double-vector brain s.
Doyen s.
Drews-Sato capsular fragment s.
Drews-Sato suture-pickup s.
electrosurgical s.
s. electrosurgical probe
Elschnig cyclodialysis s.
endarterectomy s.
Fisher-Smith s.
fishtail s.
flat s.
s. forceps
Fox LASIK s.
Freer nasal s.
French hook s.
French lacrimal s.
French-pattern s.
Fukushima malleable brain s.
Galin lens s.
Gill-Welsh s.

Girard synechia s.
Green double s.
Green lens s.
Green replacer s.
Gross brain s.
Guimaraes ophthalmic flap s.
Haberer s.
Halle vascular s.
Heifitz s.
Hersh LASIK retreatment s.
Hertzog lens s.
Hirschman iris s.
Hirschman lens s.
s. hook
hook s.
Hough s.
Interstate s.
iridodialysis s.
iris s.
irrigating notched s.
Jacobson endarterectomy s.
Jaffe intraocular s.
Jaffe lens s.
Johnson s.
Kader intestinal s.
Kallmorgen vaginal s.
Katena iris s.
Katena spoon and s.
Kellman-Elschnig s.
Kennerdell s.
Killian laryngeal s.
Kimura platinum s.
Kirby angulated iris s.
Knapp cyclodialysis s.
Knapp iris s.
Knolle lens cortex s.
Knolle lens nucleus s.
Kocher bladder s.
Korte abdominal s.
Krause-Davis s.
Kummel intestinal s.
Kwitko lens s.
Laird s.
Legueu s.
lens s.
Leriche s.
Lewicky IOL s.
Lieppman s.
Lindner cyclodialysis s.
lingual s.
Lynch s.
Maddox LASIK s.

malleable s.
Manhattan Eye & Ear s.
Masket phaco s.
Maumenee-Barraquer vitreous
  sweep s.
Maumenee vitreous sweep s.
Mayfield malleable brain s.
McIntyre irrigating s.
McPherson iris s.
McReynolds eye s.
Medscand cervical s.
Meller cyclodialysis s.
Mikulicz s.
Milex s.
Millin bladder s.
Mills coronary endarterectomy s.
Morgenstein s.
needle s.
nerve separator s.
nucleus s.
O'Brien s.
Obstbaum lens s.
Obstbaum synechia s.
Olivecrona brain s.
Olk retinal s.
Olk vitreoretinal s.
Ousley insertion s.
Pallin lens s.
Paton double s.
Paton single s.
Paton transplant s.
Peyton brain s.
phacodialysis s.
plaster s.
platinum s.
probe s.
s. probe
Pucci-Seed s.
Raaf flexible lighted s.
Rainin lens s.
Ray brain s.
rectangular brain s.
Reverdin abdominal s.
Rica brain s.
Rizzuti graft carrier s.
Rolon s.
Roux s.
Rowen s.
Sachs s.
Schmid vascular s.
Schuknecht s.
Scoville flat brain s.

S

NOTES

spatula *(continued)*
    Segond vaginal s.
    Sheets-Hirsch s.
    Sheets lens s.
    side-biting s.
    side-cutting s.
    Simcoe notched irrigating s.
    Simcoe nucleus s.
    Simmons-Kimbrough glaucoma s.
    Sinclair s.
    Sinskey nucleus s.
    SMIC abdominal s.
    SMIC brain s.
    Smith-Fisher cataract s.
    Smith-Fisher iris s.
    Smith-Green double-ended s.
    Smith-Petersen s.
    s. split needle
    spoon s.
    s. spoon
    Sterling iris s.
    Suker cyclodialysis s.
    surgical s.
    suture s.
    synechia s.
    Tan s.
    Tennant s.
    Thomas s.
    Thornton malleable s.
    Tooke s.
    Troutman-Barraquer iris s.
    Troutman lens s.
    Tuffier abdominal s.
    University of Kansas s.
    vaginal s.
    Vinciguerra-Carones LASEK s.
    Vinciguerra PRK/LASEK s.
    vitreous sweep s.
    wax-removing s.
    Weary brain s.
    Wheeler cyclodialysis s.
    Wheeler iris s.
    Wills spoon with s.
    Woodson s.
    Wullstein transplant s.
    Wurmuth s.
    Wylie s.

spatulated
    s. half-circle needle
    s. needle

speaking
    s. tube
    s. valve

spear
    Bac-Stat LASIK s.
    s. blade
    eye s.
    K-Sponge s.
    LASIK s.

    Merocel surgical s.
    ML eye s.
    PVA eye s.
    Weck-Cell surgical s.

Speare dural hook
spear-ended chrome probe
spear-pointed nickelene probe
Spears USCI laser balloon
special Colles splint
specimen
    s. brush
    s. forceps

SPECT
    single-photon emission computed
      tomography
      SPECT camera
      SPECT high-resolution brain system
      SPECT scan

spectacles
    compound s.
    decentered s.
    Franklin s.
    Fresnel nystagmus s.
    Masselon s.
    mica s.
    periscopic s.
    prismatic s.
    tinted s.

Spect-Align laser system
Spectra
    S. 400 extended surveillance and
      alert system
    S. quilted underpad

Spectra-Cath STP catheter
Spectra-Diasonics ultrasound
Spectraflex pacemaker
spectral Doppler
Spectralite Transitions lens
Spectramed
    S. L2000 color therapy system
    S. transducer

Spectranetics
    S. CVX-300 excimer laser
    S. excimer laser system
    S. Extreme peripheral catheter
    S. laser sheath
    S. support catheter

Spectra-Physics
    S.-P. argon laser
    S.-P. microsurgical laser

SpectraScience optical biopsy system
Spectra-System implant
Spectrax
    S. bipolar pacemaker
    S. programmable Medtronic
      pacemaker
    S. SX, SX-HT, SXT, VL, VM,
      VS pacemaker

Spectris
  S. power injector
  S. Solaris MR injection system
spectrocolorimeter
spectrometer
  Amis 2000 respiratory mass s.
  Bruker AMX 300 NMR s.
  Bruker Avance s.
  Centronic 200 MGA respiratory
    mass s.
  Compton suppression s.
  continuous-wave laser s.
  Digilab FTS 40A s.
  EDXRF s.
  gamma ray s.
  gas isotope ratio mass s.
  GE NMR s.
  hard x-ray imaging s.
  IBM NMR s.
  InSpectra tissue s.
  IntraSpectra tissue s.
  liquid scintillation s.
  mass s.
  Mossbauer s.
  Nicolet NMR s.
  NMR s.
  nuclear magnetic resonance s.
  Probe-SV s.
  scintillation s.
  Shimadzu RF-5301 PC s.
  Sisco s.
  Varian NMR s.
  x-ray s.
Spectron
  S. EF total hip system
  S. prosthesis
Spectronic 20 spectrophotometer
spectrophotofluorometer
spectrophotometer
  absorption s.
  atomic absorption s.
  Beckman UV s.
  digital imaging s.
  F-series fluorescence s.
  Hitachi U-series s.
  liquid scintillation s.
  mass s.
  Perkin-Elmer model 5000 atomic
    absorption s.
  reflectance s.
  SLM-8000 fluorescence s.
  Spectronic 20 s.

  U-1100 UV-Vis s.
  Varian Cary-118C s.
spectroscope
  Auger electron s.
  direct vision s.
  near-infrared s.
  Ohmeda Rascal II Raman s.
  2-wavelength near-infrared s.
spectroscopy
  Fourier transform infrared s.
  gas chromatography/mass s.
  H-1 MR s.
  laser-Doppler s.
  magnetic resonance s.
  MR proton s.
  point resolved s.
  proton MR s.
  in vivo image-guided H-magnetic
    resonance s.
  in vivo optical s. (INVOS)
spectroscopy-directed laser
spectrum
  S. antibiotic-impregnated central
    venous catheter
  S. breast implant
  DermaGard s.
  S. Designs facial implant
  S. K1 laser
  S. Lensographer lens analysis
    system
  S. Q-switched ruby laser
  S. stethoscope
  S. tissue repair system
SPECTurn chair
Specular
  S. reflectance attachment
  S. reflex slit lamp
speculoscopy
  Pap Plus s.
speculum
  adolescent vaginal s.
  Adson s.
  Agricola eye s.
  Alfonso eyelid s.
  Allen-Heffernan nasal s.
  Allingham rectal s.
  Amko vaginal s.
  anal s.
  s. anoscope
  Arruga eye s.
  Arruga globe s.
  Artisan wide-angle vaginal s.

NOTES

speculum *(continued)*
Aufricht septal s.
aural s.
Auvard Britetrac s.
Auvard-Remine vaginal s.
Azar lid s.
Bárány s.
Barr anal s.
Barraquer s.
Barraquer-Colibri eye s.
Barraquer-Douvas eye s.
Barraquer eye s.
Barraquer-Floyd s.
Barraquer wire s.
Barr rectal s.
Barr-Shuford s.
Beard eye s.
Becker-Park s.
Beckman-Colver nasal s.
Beckman nasal s.
Bedrossian eye s.
Bercovici wire lid s.
Berens eye s.
Berlind-Auvard weighted vaginal s.
Bionix nasal s.
bivalved anal s.
blackened s.
Bodenheimer rectal s.
Bosworth nasal wire s.
Boucheron ear s.
Bovin-Stille vaginal s.
Bovin vaginal s.
Bowman s.
Bowman eye s.
Bozeman s.
Braun s.
Breisky-Navratil vaginal s.
Breisky-Stille s.
Breisky vaginal s.
Brewer vaginal s.
Brinkerhoff rectal s.
Britetrac s.
Bronson s.
Bronson-Park s.
Bronson-Turtz s.
Brown ear s.
Bruening s.
Bruner vaginal s.
Buie-Smith rectal s.
Burnett Sani-Spec disposable s.
Callahan modification s.
Carpel s.
Carter septal s.
Caspar s.
Castallo eye s.
Castroviejo eye s.
Chelsea-Eaton anal s.
Chevalier Jackson laryngeal s.
Clarke eye s.
Coakley nasal s.
Collin vaginal s.
Conway lid s.
Cook eye s.
Cook rectal s.
Cottle s.
Cottle nasal s.
Cottle septum s.
Critchett eye s.
Culler iris s.
Cusco vaginal s.
Cushing-Landolt transsphenoidal s.
Czerny rectal s.
DeLee s.
Desmarres eye s.
DeVilbiss vaginal s.
disposable nasal s.
Douglas mucosal s.
Downes nasal s.
Doyen vaginal s.
duckbill s.
Duplay nasal s.
Dynacor vaginal s.
ear s.
Eastman vaginal s.
Eaton nasal s.
Econo Vienna nasal s.
Eisenhammer s.
endaural s.
ENT s.
Erhardt ear s.
eye s.
eyelid s.
Fansler-Ives rectal s.
Fansler rectal s.
Farrior ear s.
Farrior oval s.
Fergusson tubular vaginal s.
fiberoptic vaginal s.
fine-wire s.
flat-bladed nasal s.
Flint glass s.
Floyd-Barraquer wire s.
Forbes esophageal s.
s. forceps
Foster-Ballenger nasal s.
Fox eye s.
Fränkel s.
Garrigue weighted vaginal s.
Gerzog nasal s.
Ginsberg eye s.
Gleason s.
Global Healthcare disposable vaginal s.
Goldbacher anoscope s.
Goldstein septal s.
Goligher s.
Graefe eye s.
Grandon-Barraquer eye s.

Graves bivalve s.
Graves Britetrac vaginal s.
Graves Coldlite s.
Graves open-side vaginal s.
Gruber ear s.
Guilford-Wright bivalve s.
Guist s.
Guist-Black eye s.
Guist-Bloch s.
Gutter s.
Guttmann vaginal s.
Guyton-Maumenee s.
Guyton-Park eye s.
Gyn-A-Lite vaginal s.
Haglund-Stille vaginal s.
Haglund vaginal s.
Halle infant nasal s.
Halle-Tieck nasal s.
1-hand s.
Hansa ophthalmic s.
Hardy bivalve s.
Hardy-Duddy s.
Hardy nasal bivalve s.
Hartmann dewaxer s.
Hartmann ear s.
Hartmann nasal s.
Hayes vaginal s.
Heffernan nasal s.
Helmholtz s.
Helmont s.
Henrotin weighted vaginal s.
Hertel nephrostomy s.
Higbee vaginal s.
Hinkle-James rectal s.
Hirschman anoscope rectal s.
s. holder
Holinger infant esophageal s.
Hood-Graves vaginal s.
Hough-Boucheron ear s.
House stapes s.
Huffman-Graves adolescent
  vaginal s.
Huffman infant vaginal s.
Iliff-Park s.
illuminated vaginal s.
Ingals nasal s.
iris s.
Ives rectal s.
Jackson vaginal s.
Jaffe eyelid s.
Jarit-Graves vaginal s.
Jarit-Pederson vaginal s.

Jonas-Graves vaginal s.
Kahn-Graves vaginal s.
Kaiser s.
Kalinowski ear s.
Kalinowski-Verner ear s.
Kammann ophthalmic s.
Katena s.
Keeler-Pierse eye s.
Keizer-Lancaster eye s.
Kelly rectal s.
Kershner reversible eyelid s.
Killian-Halle nasal s.
Killian nasal s.
Killian rectal s.
Killian septal s.
Klaff septal s.
KleenSpec disposable vaginal s.
Knapp-Culler s.
Knapp eye s.
Knolle lens s.
Kogan endocervical s.
Kogan urethra s.
Kramer ear s.
Kratz aspirating s.
Kratz-Barraquer wire s.
Kristeller vaginal s.
Kyle nasal s.
Lancaster eye s.
Lancaster lid s.
Lancaster-O'Connor s.
Landau s.
Landolt pituitary s.
Lang eye s.
Lawford s.
LeeSpec s.
LeFort s.
Lempert-Beckman-Colver endaural s.
Lempert-Colver endaural s.
Lempert endaural s.
Lester-Burch eye s.
lid s.
LidFix s.
Lieberman aspirating s.
Lieberman K-Wire s.
lighted s.
Lillie nasal s.
Lindstrom-Chu aspirating s.
Lister-Burch eye s.
Lofberg vaginal s.
Lucae ear s.
Luer eye s.

S

NOTES

speculum *(continued)*
Machat adjustable aspirating
  wire s.
Macon Hospital s.
Mahoney intranasal antral s.
Manche LASIK s.
Martin rectal s.
Martin vaginal s.
Mason-Auvard weighted vaginal s.
Mathews rectal s.
Matzenauer vaginal s.
Maumenee-Park eye s.
Mayer s.
McBratney aspirating s.
McHugh oval s.
McKee s.
McKinney eye s.
McLaughlin s.
McPherson eye s.
Mellinger-Axenfeld eye s.
Mellinger eye s.
Mellinger fenestrated blades s.
Merz-Vienna nasal s.
Metcher eye s.
Miller vaginal s.
Milligan s.
Montgomery-Bernstine s.
Montgomery vaginal s.
Moria s.
Mosher nasal s.
Mosher urethral s.
Moynihan s.
Mueller eye s.
Muir rectal s.
Murdock eye s.
Murdock-Wiener eye s.
Murdoon eye s.
Myles nasal s.
Myles-Ray s.
nasal bivalve s.
Nasa-Spec nasal s.
nasopharyngeal s.
National ear s.
National Graves vaginal s.
Nott-Gutmann vaginal s.
Nott vaginal s.
Noyes s.
Omni-Park s.
O'Sullivan-O'Connor vaginal s.
oval s.
Pannu-Kratz-Barraquer s.
Park eye s.
Park-Guyton-Callahan eye s.
Park-Guyton eye s.
Park-Guyton-Maumenee s.
Park-Maumenee s.
Parks anal s.
Patton septal s.
Patton vaginal s.

Pearce eye s.
Pederson vaginal s.
pediatric s.
pediatric lid s.
Pennington rectal s.
Picot vaginal s.
Pierse eye s.
Pilling-Hartmann s.
plain wire s.
Politzer ear s.
post-urethroplasty review s.
Pratt bivalve s.
Pratt rectal s.
Preefer eye s.
Prima LEEP s.
Prima vaginal s.
4-prong finger s.
Prospec disposable s.
Proud infant turbinate s.
Pynchon nasal s.
Rappazzo s.
Ray nasal s.
rectal s.
Reipen s.
Relat vaginal s.
reversible lid s.
Rica ear s.
Rica nasal septal s.
Rica vaginal s.
Richard Gruber s.
Richnau-Holmgren ear s.
Roberts esophageal s.
Roberts oval s.
Rosenthal urethral s.
round s.
Sani-Spec vaginal s.
Sato s.
Sauer eye s.
Sauer infant eye s.
Saunders eye s.
Sawyer rectal s.
Scherback-Porges vaginal s.
Schweizer s.
Scott ear s.
Semb vaginal s.
Senturia pharyngeal s.
Serdarevic s.
Seyfert vaginal s.
Shea s.
shoehorn s.
Siegle ear s.
Simcoe-Barraquer eye s.
Simcoe eye s.
Simcoe wire s.
Simmonds vaginal s.
Simrock s.
Sims double-ended vaginal s.
Sims rectal s.
Sims vaginal s.

Sisson-Cottle s.
Sisson-Vienna s.
Sluder sphenoidal s.
SMIC ear s.
SMIC nasal septal s.
Smirmaul eyelid s.
Smith anal s.
Smith eye s.
Sonnenschein nasal s.
stapes s.
Stearnes s.
Steiner-Auvard weighted s.
Stop eye s.
Storz nasal s.
Storz septal s.
Storz-Vienna nasal s.
Sutherland-Grieshaber s.
Sweeney posterior vaginal s.
Swiss-pattern s.
Swolin self-retaining vaginal s.
Tauber s.
Taylor vaginal s.
Terson s.
Thornton open-wire lid s.
Thudichum nasal s.
Thudichum self-retaining ear s.
Tieck-Halle infant nasal s.
Tieck nasal s.
Torchia eye s.
Toynbee ear s.
transsphenoidal s.
Trelat vaginal s.
Troeltsch ear s.
Turner-Warwick post-urethroplasty
  review s.
Ullrich vaginal s.
Universal s.
vaginal s.
Vaginard metal s.
Vauban s.
Verner s.
Verner-Kalinowski s.
Vienna Britetrac nasal s.
Vienna nasal s.
Voltolini nasal s.
Vu-Max vaginal s.
Watson s.
Weeks eye s.
weighted vaginal s.
Weiner s.
Weisman-Graves open-sided
  vaginal s.

Weiss s.
Weissbarth vaginal s.
Welch Allyn illuminated s.
Welch Allyn KleenSpec vaginal s.
Wellington Hospital vaginal s.
Wiener eye s.
Williams eye s.
Wilson-Kirbe s.
wire bivalve vaginal s.
wire lid s.
Worcester City Hospital s.
Yankauer nasopharyngeal s.
Ziegler eye s.
Zower s.
Zylik-Michaels s.
Speed
  S. brace
  S. hand splint
  S. Lok soft stent
  S. osteotomy graft
Speedband
  S. ligature
  S. multiple-band ligator
SpeedBlocks head immobilizer
Speed-E-Rim denture bite block
Speedi-Pak sinus pack
SpeedLink transverse connector
SpeedReducer instrument
Speed-Sprague knife
Speedy-1 Auto refractometer
Speedy balloon catheter
Speer
  S. periosteotome
  S. suture hook
Spelcast car seat
Spembly cryoprobe
Spence
  S. cranioplastic roller
  S. rongeur forceps
Spence-Adson forceps
Spencer
  S. biopsy forceps
  S. cannula
  S. chalazion forceps
  S. eye suture scissors
  S. oval punch
  S. oval tip
  S. probe depth electrode
  S. stitch scissors
Spencer-Wells
  S.-W. arterial forceps
  S.-W. chalazion forceps

NOTES

Spenco
  S. boot
  S. external breast form
  S. insole
  S. Orthotic arch support
  S. orthotic device
  S. top-cover
Sperma-Tex preshaped mesh
Sperm Select sperm recovery system
Spero meibomian forceps
Spetzler
  S. dissector
  S. forceps
  S. lumbar-peritoneal shunt
  S. scissors
  S. subarachnoid catheter
  S. titanium aneurysm clip
SpF spinal fusion stimulator
sphenoidal
  s. bone punch
  s. bur
  s. cannula
  s. probe
  s. punch forceps
sphenoid cannula
sphenopalatine ganglion needle
sphere
  AccuPoint targeting s.
  American Heyer-Schulte s.
  Carter s.
  Doherty s.
  s. introducer
  Mules vitreous s.
  porous hydroxyapatite s.
  Pyrex eye s.
  resin s.
  Silastic s.
  silicone eye s.
spherical
  s. bur
  s. eye implant
spherocentric knee prosthesis
spherocylinder
spherocylindrical lens
Sphero Flex implant
sphincter
  AMS 800 artificial urethral s.
  artificial s.
  AS-800 artificial s.
  s. dilator
  double-cuff urinary s.
  Hydroflex s.
  servomechanism s.
sphincteroscope
  Kelly s.
sphincterotome
  bipolar s.
  Bitome bipolar s.

  Cotton s.
  Cremer-Ikeda s.
  Doubilet s.
  double-channel s.
  ERCP s.
  Frimberger-Karpiel 12 o'clock s.
  Howell rotatable BII s.
  Huibregtse-Katon s.
  Koch-Julian s.
  needle-tipped s.
  shark fin s.
  single-channel wire-guided s.
  Tapertome s.
  Tri-Tome s.
  Ultratome XL triple-lumen s.
  Wilson-Cook double-channel s.
  Wilson-Cook wire-guided s.
  wire-guided s.
  Zimmon s.
sphincterotomy basket
Sphygmocorder recorder
SphygmoCor noninvasive aortic blood pressure system
sphygmomanometer
  Baumanometer s.
  cuff s.
  s. cuff
  Erlanger s.
  Faught s.
  Hader aneroid s.
  Hawksley random zero mercury s.
  Janeway s.
  Mosso s.
  Physio-Control Lifestat 200 s.
  random-zero s.
  Riva-Rocci s.
  Rogers s.
sphygmometer
  Honan s.
sphygmoscope
  Bishop s.
SPI-Argent II peritoneal dialysis catheter
spica
  s. bandage
  s. cast
  s. dressing
  s. splint
  s. table
spicule forceps
Spiegel-Wycis
  S.-W. stereoencephalotome
  S.-W. stereotactic apparatus
Spielberg
  S. dilator
  S. sinus cannula
Spies ethmoidal punch
Spiesman fistular probe

Spiessel
S. internal screw fixation
S. lag screw
Spigelman baseball finger splint
spike
Gissane s.
s. retractor
s. staple
sterile vent s.
spiked washer
SPI-Lite sleep position indicator
spinal
s. adjusting instrument
s. arthroscope
s. catheter
s. cord retractor
s. cord stimulator
s. frame
s. fusion chisel
s. fusion curette
s. fusion gouge
s. needle
s. physiotherapy simulator
s. retractor blade
s. rod
s. rod cross-bracing
s. saw
s. slip wrench
S. Technology bivalve TLSO brace
s. turning frame
SpinaLase Nd:YAG surgical laser system
Spinalator table
SpinaLogic 1000 bone growth stimulator
SpinalPak fusion stimulator
spinal-perforating forceps
SpineCATH
S. IDET therapy
S. intradiscal catheter
SpineLink anterior cervical spinal system
Spinelli biopsy needle
Spine Power pelvic stabilizer belt
SpineStat side-directed diskectomy probe
SpineWand
Perc-DLE S.
Spinhaler Turbo-Inhaler inhaler
spinner
DiffSpin slide s.

spinning
s. disc nebulizer
s. probe
Spinoscope noninasive imaging system
spinous
s. process spreader
s. process wire
Spin screw
spiral
s. coil stent
s. computed tomography scanner
s. CT
s. CT scanner
s. drill
s. electrode
s. endosteal implant
s. filler
s. fluted tungsten carbide bur
s. forceps
S. Mark V portable ultrasonic drug inhaler
s. multidetector CT
s. probe
s. reverse bandage
s. stone dislodger
s. trochanteric reamer
s. vein stripper
s. XCT scanner
SpiralGold oxygenator
spiral-tipped
s.-t. bougie
s.-t. catheter
spiral-wound endotracheal tube
SpiraStent stent
Spirea adjustable foldable wheelchair
Spirec drill
SpiroFlo bioabsorbable prostate stent
Spir-O-Flow peak flowmeter
Spirolyte 201 bedside spirometer
spirometer
AT-10 s.
Barnes s.
bedside s.
Benedict-Roth s.
Bennett monitoring s.
Buhl s.
Calculair s.
Capnomac Ultima sidestream s.
Cardiovit s.
CDX Spiro 850 portable s.
closed-circuit s.
Coach incentive s.

S

NOTES

spirometer *(continued)*
    Collins Dry s.
    Collins survey s.
    Collis s.
    Compact s.
    Compact II s.
    Datex Ultima s.
    Discovery handheld s.
    Douglas bag s.
    dry s.
    Eagle II survey s.
    Flash portable s.
    flow-sensing s.
    incentive s.
    Inspirx incentive s.
    KoKo Mate s.
    KoKo Trek s.
    Krogh apparatus s.
    low-resistance rolling seal s.
    MedicAIR s.
    MicroLoop II s.
    MicroLoop ML3535 s.
    Micro Plus s.
    PneumoCheck s.
    Puritan Bennett Simplicity s.
    Puritan Bennett volumetric s.
    2120 recording s.
    Respirex incentive s.
    Satellite s.
    sidestream s.
    SP-10 s.
    Spirolyte 201 bedside s.
    SpiroVision-3 s.
    Spirovit SP-1, SP-2 portable s.
    Timeter pocket s.
    Tissot s.
    Tri-flow incentive s.
    Venturi s.
    Vitalograph Escort s.
    volume displacement s.
    Volurex incentive s.
    water-sealed s.
    wedge s.
    Welch Allyn PneumoCheck s.
    Welch Allyn Schiller SP-series s.
    Wright s.
SpiroSense
    S. flow sensor
    S. system
Spiros inhalation delivery system
SpiroVision-3 spirometer
Spirovit SP-1, SP-2 portable spirometer
Spitz-Holter
    S.-H. flushing device
    S.-H. valve
    S.-H. valve implant material
Spivack valve
Spivey iris retractor
Spizziri cannula knife

Spizziri-Simcoe cannula
splanchnic retractor
splenorenal bypass shunt
splice
    breakaway s.
spline
    Bosworth osteotomy s.
    Calcitek s.
    S. dental implant system
    Keys-Briston type s.
    Rowland-Hughes osteotomy s.
    Shirlee s.
    S. Twist microtextured titanium
      implant
splint
    abduction s.
    abduction finger s.
    Accuform nasal s.
    acrylic s.
    acrylic cap s.
    acrylic wafer TMJ s.
    Adam and Eve rib belt s.
    Adjusta-Wrist s.
    aeroplane s.
    A-Force dorsal night s.
    Agnew s.
    Ainslie acrylic s.
    air s.
    AirFlex carpal tunnel s.
    airfoam s.
    airplane s.
    AliMed diabetic night s.
    AliMed Freedom thumb spica s.
    AliMed PF night s.
    Allen s.
    Alumafoam nasal s.
    aluminum fence s.
    aluminum/foam cot s.
    anchor s.
    Anderson s.
    angle s.
    ankle-foot orthotic s.
    Aquaplast s.
    Asch nasal s.
    Ashhurst leg s.
    A-splint dental s.
    Atkins nasal s.
    Balkan femoral s.
    ball-peen s.
    banana split s.
    banjo s.
    baseball finger s.
    Basswood s.
    Bavarian s.
    Baylor adjustable cross s.
    Baylor metatarsal s.
    Bend-A-Boot foot s.
    Bilson fixable-removable cross arch
      bar s.

birdcage s.
bivalve s.
bivalve nasal s.
Blount s.
board s.
Body prop positioning s.
Böhler-Braun s.
Böhler wire s.
Bond arm s.
boutonniere s.
Bowlby arm s.
bracketed s.
Brady balanced suspension s.
Brant aluminum s.
bridge s.
Bridgemaster nasal s.
Brooke Army Hospital s.
Brown nasal s.
Buck extension s.
Buck traction s.
Budin hammertoe s.
Budin toe s.
Bunnell active hand s.
Bunnell finger extension s.
Bunnell gutter s.
Bunnell knuckle-bender s.
Bunnell outrigger s.
Bunnell reverse knuckle bender s.
Bunnell safety-pin s.
Bunny Boot foot s.
Burget nasal s.
Cabot leg s.
calibrated clubfoot s.
Camo disposable dental s.
Campbell airplane s.
Campbell traction s.
Cannon Bio-Flek nasal s.
cap s.
Capener coil s.
Capener finger s.
carpal lock cockup wrist s.
carpal lock wrist s.
Carter intranasal s.
cast lingual s.
Cawood nasal s.
Chandler felt collar s.
Chatfield-Girdlestone s.
clubfoot s.
coaptation s.
cock-up s.
cock-up ankle s.
cock-up wrist s.

Colles s.
Comfort Cool D-ring wrist s.
Comfy s.
Comprifix ankle s.
cone s.
Converse s.
copper band-acrylic s.
Cordon Colles fracture s.
counterrotation s.
Craig abduction s.
Cramer wire s.
crib s.
CTS Gripfit s.
Culley ulna s.
Curry walking s.
Darco toe alignment s.
Davis metacarpal s.
Denis Browne clubfoot s.
Denis Browne hip s.
Denis Browne talipes hobble s.
Denver s.
Denver nasal s.
DePuy aeroplane s.
DePuy any-angle s.
DePuy open-thimble s.
DePuy rocking leg s.
DePuy rolled Colles s.
DeRoyal/LMB finger s.
digit s.
Digit Aid s.
DonJoy knee s.
dorsal wrist s.
Dorsiwedge night s.
Doyle bi-valved airway s.
Doyle Combo nasal airway s.
Doyle intranasal airway s.
Doyle Shark nasal s.
Doyle spacer s.
drop foot s.
Dupuytren s.
dynamic s.
Easy Access foot s.
Eclipse gel wrist s.
Eggers contact s.
elbow extension s.
elbow flexion s.
EnduraSplint s.
Engen palmar wrist s.
Erich maxillary s.
Erich nasal s.
Extend-It finger s.
Ezeform s.

NOTES

splint *(continued)*
EZ-Splint PM TMJ s.
Fasplint s.
fence s.
Ferciot tip-toe s.
Fillauer night s.
finger s.
finger cot s.
finger extension clockspring s.
finger flexion s.
Finger-Hugger s.
Flexi-Guard s.
fold-over finger s.
foot s.
foot drop night s.
Forrester head s.
Fox clavicular s.
FracSure s.
Fractomed s.
fracture s.
Framer s.
Freedom Neutral Position s.
Freedom Omni progressive s.
Freedom Progressive resting s.
Freedom Sportsfit s.
Freedom Ultimate Grip s.
Frejka pillow s.
Friedman s.
frog s.
full-occlusal s.
functional resting position s.
Futuro s.
gait lock s.
Gallows s.
Galveston s.
Ganley s.
Gibson s.
Gilmer dental s.
Gilmer tooth s.
Goldsmith inflatable airway s.
Gooch s.
Goode Magne-Splint magnetic
    nasal s.
Gordon s.
Granberry s.
Guastella/Mantovani internal
    nasal s.
Gunning jaw s.
Hammond orthodontic s.
hand cock-up s.
Hare compact traction s.
Hart extension finger s.
Haynes-Griffin mandibular s.
HealWell night s.
Heel Free s.
Hexcelite sheet s.
hinged Thomas s.
HIPciser abduction s.
Hirschtick utility shoulder s.

Hodgen hip s.
Hodgen leg s.
HV NightSplint s.
HV SoftSplint s.
Hydro-Splint II s.
Ilfeld s.
indexed s.
infant abduction s.
inflatable elbow s.
Innoboot night s.
Inro surgical nail s.
interdental s.
intermediate s.
intranasal bivalve s.
Isoprene plastic s.
Jacoby heel s.
Jelenko s.
Jet-Air s.
Joint-Jack finger s.
Jonell countertraction finger s.
Jonell thumb s.
Jones arm s.
Jones forearm s.
Jones metacarpal s.
Jones nasal s.
Jones traction s.
Joseph nasal s.
Joseph septal s.
Kanavel cock-up s.
Kazanjian nasal s.
Keller-Blake leg s.
Kenny-Howard s.
Kerr abduction s.
Keystone s.
kidney internal s.
Kingsley s.
Kirschner wire s.
Kleinert s.
Klenzak double-upright s.
knee brace s.
knee immobilizer s.
knuckle-bender s.
Lambrinudi s.
leaf s.
Levis arm s.
Lewin baseball finger s.
Lewin-Stern finger s.
Lewin-Stern thumb s.
Liberty One s.
s. liner
Link stack split s.
Link toe s.
Liston s.
long arm s.
long leg s.
long leg posterior molded s.
Love nasal s.
Lynch septal s.
Lytle metacarpal s.

MacKay nasal s.
magnet s.
Magnuson abduction humeral s.
malleable metal finger s.
Mason s.
Mason-Allen hand s.
maxillary s.
Mayer nasal s.
McGee s.
McIntire s.
McLeod padded clavicular s.
memory s.
metacarpal s.
metal s.
Middledorpf s.
MindSet toe s.
modified Oppenheimer s.
Mohr finger s.
Morris s.
Murphy ring finger s.
Murray-Jones arm s.
Murray-Thomas arm s.
nasal s.
Neiman nasal s.
Neubeiser adjustable forearm s.
neutral position s.
New Mind Set toe s.
N'ice Stretch night s.
nose guard s.
OCL volar s.
O'Donoghue knee s.
O'Donoghue stirrup s.
O'Malley jaw fracture s.
Oppenheimer knuckle-bender s.
Oppenheim spring wire s.
opponens s.
Orfit s.
Ortho-last s.
Orthomedics Stretch and Heel s.
Ortho-Mold s.
orthopaedic strap clavicle s.
Orthoplast isoprene s.
outrigger s.
padded aluminum s.
padded board s.
padded plywood s.
s. padding
palmar wrist s.
Pavlik harness s.
Peabody s.
PF night s.
Phelps s.

Phemister s.
Phoenix outrigger s.
Pil-O-Splint wrist s.
plantar fasciitis night s.
Plastalume bulb-ended s.
Plastalume straight s.
plaster s.
plaster-of-Paris s.
plastic s.
Polyform s.
Polymed s.
polymethyl methacrylate ear s.
polyvinyl alcohol s.
Ponseti s.
Poroplastic s.
Porzett s.
Potts s.
Pro-glide s.
4-prong finger s.
Protecto s.
Pucci s.
Puth abduction s.
Putti s.
QualCraft s.
QuickCast s.
Quik s.
radiolucent s.
Rancho Los Amigos s.
Rauchfuss sling s.
Redi-Around finger s.
replant s.
reverse Kingsley s.
reverse knuckle-bender s.
Robert Jones s.
Roger Anderson well-leg s.
Rolyan Gel Shell s.
Rosen s.
Roylan Gel Shell spica s.
Rumel aluminum bridge s.
Russell s.
safety pin s.
Safian nasal s.
Sam s.
sandwich-type s.
Saturn s.
Savlon s.
Sayre s.
Scott humeral s.
Scottish Rite s.
Seattle s.
Shah nasal s.
Sheffield s.

NOTES

splint *(continued)*
short arm plaster s.
short arm posterior molded s.
short leg s.
SiloSplint thumb s.
Simpson sugar-tong s.
skin s.
Slattery-McGrouther dynamic
  flexion s.
Smart s.
Softsplint foot s.
special Colles s.
Speed hand s.
spica s.
Spigelman baseball finger s.
spreading hand s.
spring cock-up s.
spring wire safety pin s.
Stack s.
Stader s.
Stax fingertip s.
Stock finger s.
Strampelli eye s.
Stretch and Heel Night s.
Stromeyer s.
Stuart Gordon hand s.
Stulberg HIPciser abduction s.
sugar-tong s.
Supramead nose s.
swan-neck s.
Swanson dynamic toe s.
Swanson hand s.
synergistic wrist motion s.
Synergy s.
SynthoSplint fiberglass s.
talipes hobble s.
Taylor s.
Teare arm s.
tennis elbow s.
T-finger s.
therapeutic s.
thermoplastic s.
Thomas full-ring s.
Thomas knee s.
Thomas leg s.
Thomas posterior s.
Thomas suspension s.
Thompson modification of Denis
  Browne s.
Thumbfit s.
thumb spica s.
ThumZ'Up functional thumb s.
Ticonium s.
Titus forearm s.
Titus wrist s.
TMJ acrylic s.
Toad finger s.
Tobruk s.

toe alignment s.
Toronto s.
torsion bar s.
turnbuckle elbow s.
turnbuckle functional position s.
Universal support s.
Urias pressure s.
U-splint s.
Valentine s.
Velcro extenders s.
Volkmann s.
von Rosen s.
Wertheim s.
Wheaton bunion s.
Winter s.
wire s.
Xomed Doyle nasal airway s.
Xomed Silastic s.
Yucca wood s.
Zimfoam finger s.
Zimmer airplane s.
Zimmer clavicular cross s.
Zim-Trac traction s.
Zim-Zip rib belt s.
Zollinger s.
Zucker s.
splinter forceps
splinting
Silon-LTS low temperature s.
Splintline acrylic
Splintrex instrument
SplintsRite stabilization device
split
s. drape
s. overtube
s. Russell skeletal traction
s. screen
split-finger hook
split-sheath
s.-s. catheter
s.-s. introducer
splitter
beam s.
Brierley nucleus s.
Gillum nucleus s.
Goldberg side port s.
Koch-Salz nucleus s.
Kraff nucleus s.
Lindstrom Trident ophthalmic s.
Rosato fascial s.
Rosen phaco s.
Ruth-Hedwig s.
Salz nucleus s.
Sharvelle side port s.
Tooke angled s.
Troutman corneal s.
Zeiss small beam s.
split-thickness implant

splitting
  s. chisel
  s. forceps
Spondex sponge ball
spondylitic bar
sponge
  absorbable gelatin s.
  Accu-Sorb gauze s.
  Actifoam collagen s.
  Alcon s.
  Avitene Ultrafoam collagen s.
  Bernay s.
  Bicol collagen s.
  Bohm dropper s.
  Boston gauze s.
  bronchoscopic s.
  Bulkee super fluff s.
  s. carrier
  cellulose surgical s.
  cherry s.
  s. clamp
  Codman Bicol s.
  collagen s.
  Collatamp G hemostatic s.
  Collostat s.
  cotton ball s.
  C-sponge s.
  Curity cover s.
  Curity disposable laparotomy s.
  Curity gauze s.
  cylindrical s.
  DeRoyal laparotomy s.
  s. dissector
  s. dressing
  s. ear curette
  EndoZime s.
  Excilon dressing s.
  Expandacell s.
  s. forceps
  Fuller silicone s.
  gauze s.
  gauze dissector s.
  gauze rosebud s.
  gelatin s.
  Gelfoam s.
  s. graft
  Graham Clark silicone s.
  grooved silicone s.
  Helistat absorbable collagen
    hemostatic s.
  Helitene absorbable collagen
    hemostatic s.

  Heros chiropody s.
  Hibbs s.
  s. implant
  implant s.
  Incert bioabsorbable implantable s.
  InstruWipes surgical s.
  Ivalon s.
  Ivalon embolic s.
  Johnson gauze s.
  Johnson & Johnson gauze s.
  K dissector s.
  Kenwood laparotomy s.
  Kerlix disposable laparotomy s.
  Kerlix packing s.
  Kerlix super s.
  Kling s.
  Krukenberg s.
  K-Sponge hydrocellulose s.
  laminectomy wedge s.
  laparotomy s.
  Lapwall laparotomy s.
  Lincoff lens s.
  lint-free s.
  Lisco ss.
  Masciuli silicone s.
  Mediskin hemostatic s.
  Medline gauze s.
  Merocel s.
  Microsponge Teardrop s.
  Mikulicz s.
  Mirasorb s.
  nasal tampon s.
  Naso-Tamp nasal packing s.
  NeuroCol neurosurgical s.
  nonwoven s.
  Nu-Brede packing and
    debridement s.
  Nu Gauze s.
  ophthalmic s.
  Optipore wound-cleaning s.
  Packer tunnel silicone s.
  peanut dissector s.
  Pedic s.
  pledget s.
  polyvinyl alcohol s.
  Porolon s.
  Pro-Ophtha absorbent stick s.
  Protectaid contraceptive s.
  radial s.
  Ray-Tec x-ray detectable
    surgical s.
  Reston s.

S

NOTES

sponge *(continued)*
>Rhino Rocket epistaxis s.
>s. ring
>Roschke dropper s.
>rubber s.
>Scholda style s.
>Secto tonsillar s.
>Silastic s.
>silicone s.
>s. silicone implant material
>Snowflake laparotomy s.
>Soft N Dry Merocel s.
>soft silicone s.
>Sof-Wick drain s.
>s. stick
>2×2 strung s.
>Surgidine s.
>Surgifoam absorbable gelatin s.
>Taka microneurosurgical s.
>tonsil s.
>Topper dressing s.
>tracheotomy s.
>Vaiser s.
>Venture s.
>Versalon all purpose s.
>VersaTool eye s.
>Visi-Spear eye s.
>Vistec x-ray detectable s.
>vitrectomy s.
>Weck s.
>Weck-Cel s.
>Wextran s.
>x-ray detectable laparotomy s.

sponge-holding forceps
spongiosa bone graft
spoon
>s. anastomosis clamp
>Ballance mastoid s.
>Bunge evisceration s.
>Bunge exenteration s.
>Castroviejo lens s.
>cataract s.
>Coyne s.
>Culler lens s.
>s. curette
>Cushing pituitary s.
>Cushing spatula s.
>Cutler lens s.
>Daviel cataract s.
>Daviel lens s.
>ear s.
>Elschnig cataract s.
>Elschnig eye s.
>Elschnig lens s.
>evisceration s.
>exenteration s.
>Falk appendectomy s.
>Fisher eye s.
>s. forceps

>gallbladder s.
>Graefe cataract s.
>Gross ear s.
>Hardy pituitary s.
>Hatt s.
>Hess lens s.
>Hiebert esophageal suture s.
>Hoke s.
>Hoke-Roberts s.
>Kalt eye s.
>Kirby intracapsular lens s.
>Knapp cataract s.
>Knapp lens s.
>Kocher brain s.
>laser-assisted intrastromal keratomileusis aspiration s.
>LASIK aspiration s.
>lens s.
>Lindner cyclodialysis s.
>MacNamara cataract s.
>maroon s.
>meniscal s.
>Moore gallbladder s.
>s. needle
>needle s.
>obstetrical s.
>Olivecrona brain s.
>pituitary s.
>plain ear s.
>Ray brain s.
>s. retractor
>Rizzuti graft carrier s.
>Royal s.
>Schepens s.
>Sellheim elevating s.
>Skene uterine s.
>spatula s.
>s. spatula
>Turner-Warwick malleable s.
>Volkmann s.
>Wells enucleation s.
>Woodson obstetrical s.

spoon-shaped forceps
S'port
>S. Max back support
>Posture S.

Sport
>S. Cord
>S. Preforms orthotic

Sportape tape
Sportelli system collimator mounted contact shield
Sporthotic
>Soccer S.

Sportorno cementless hip arthroplasty system
Sports
>S. Breather lung power optimizer
>S. Plus II back belt

Sports-Caster I, II knee brace
SportsFit thumb orthosis
SportsRAC arm care system
SportsTape tape
SportStim muscle stimulation electrode
Sport-Stirrup orthosis
SporTX
    S. pulsed direct current stimulator
    S. stimulation device
spot
    s. compression paddle
    s. retinoscope
SpotCheck+ handheld pulse oximeter
spotlight
    KDC-Healthdyne nonfluorescent s.
Sprague ear curette
Spratt
    S. ear curette
    S. mastoid curette
    S. nasofrontal rasp
spray
    s. bandage
    S. Band dressing
    Proderm topical s.
    Seal-On s.
    Stopain analgesic s.
SprayGel adhesion barrier system
spreader
    Assistant Free calibrated femoral-
      tibial s.
    Assistant Free coated femoral-
      tibial s.
    Athens suture s.
    baby Inge bone s.
    baby Inge laminar s.
    Bailey rib s.
    s. bar
    Beeson cast s.
    Benson pylorus s.
    Blanco valve s.
    Blount bone s.
    Blount laminar s.
    Bobechko s.
    Bores incision s.
    Burford-Finochietto infant rib s.
    Burford rib s.
    calcaneal s.
    Caspar disc space s.
    Caspar vertebral body s.
    cast s.
    Cloward s.
    Cloward vertebral s.

    conjunctival s.
    Costenbader incision s.
    Cox metatarsal s.
    Davis modified Finochietto rib s.
    Davis rib s.
    DeBakey infant rib s.
    Doyen rib s.
    Endotec s.
    Finochietto-Burford rib s.
    Finochietto infant rib s.
    Frederick sleeve s.
    Gerbode modified Burford rib s.
    Gerbode rib s.
    Gill incision s.
    s. graft
    Gross ductus s.
    Haglund plaster s.
    Haglund-Stille plaster s.
    Haight baby rib s.
    Haight-Finochietto rib s.
    Haight pediatric rib s.
    Haight rib s.
    Harken rib s.
    Harrington s.
    Henning cast s.
    Hertzler rib s.
    incision s.
    Inge lamina s.
    intervertebral s.
    Jarit 3-prong cast s.
    jaw s.
    Kimpton vein s.
    Kirschner wire s.
    Kwitko conjunctival s.
    lamina s.
    Landolt s.
    Lefferts rib s.
    Leksell sternal s.
    Lemmon sternal s.
    Lilienthal rib s.
    Lilienthal-Sauerbruch rib s.
    McGuire rib s.
    Medicon rib s.
    Millin-Bacon bladder neck s.
    Millin bladder neck s.
    Miltex rib s.
    Mity s.
    Morris mitral valve s.
    Morse sternal s.
    M-Pact cast s.
    Nelson rib s.
    Nissen rib s.

S

NOTES

spreader *(continued)*
 Overholt-Finochietto rib s.
 Overholt rib s.
 Park rectal s.
 plaster s.
 Quervain rib s.
 Rehbein rib s.
 Reinhoff-Finochietto rib s.
 Reinhoff rib s.
 rib s.
 Ridlon s.
 root canal s.
 Sauerbruch-Lillienthal rib s.
 Saurex s.
 Sheldon s.
 Smith-Buie rectal s.
 spinous process s.
 sternal s.
 Stille plaster s.
 Stille-Quervain s.
 Struck s.
 Suarez s.
 Sweet-Burford rib s.
 Sweet rib s.
 Tessier s.
 Texas Scottish Rite Hospital eyebolt s.
 Theis infant rib s.
 Tudor-Edwards rib s.
 Tuffier rib s.
 Turek spinous process s.
 Turner-Warwick bladder neck s.
 USA plaster s.
 Ventura s.
 vertebral s.
 Weinberg rib s.
 Wilder band s.
 Wilson rib s.
 Wiltberger spinous process s.
 Wölfe-Böhler plaster cast s.
 wound s.
spreading
 s. forceps
 s. hand splint
spring
 s. ball valve
 S. catheter
 s. clip
 s. cock-up splint
 coiled s.
 compression s.
 Gruca s.
 Gruca-Weiss s.
 s. hook
 INSTRA-mate instrument-holding s.
 internal fixation s.
 S. iris scissors
 Kesling tooth-spacing s.
 s. loaded biopsy instrument

 s. needle holder
 s. pin
 s. plate
 s. retractor
 Shuletz s.
 Weiss s.
 s. wire loop
 s. wire safety pin splint
spring-assisted syringe
spring-eye needle
spring-handled
 s.-h. forceps
 s.-h. needle holder
 s.-h. scissors
spring-hook wire needle
Springlite
 S. Advantage DP prosthesis
 S. G foot component
 S. II foot component
 S. Lo Rider prosthetic foot
 S. lower limb prosthesis
 S. plate
spring-loaded
 s.-l. biopsy gun
 s.-l. biopsy needle
 s.-l. nail
 s.-l. self-retaining retractor
 s.-l. vascular stent
spring-lock
 Sumpter clasp s.-l.
spring-mounted electromagnet
spring-tipped guidewire
spring-wire retractor
Sprint
 S. catheter
 S. Climber
 S. crosstrainer
Spri Xercise board
Sprotte
 S. epidural needle
 S. spinal needle
SPR.Plus II mattress
sprue pin
SPTL vascular lesion laser
SPTU Soviet stapler
spud
 Alvis foreign body s.
 Bahn s.
 Bennett foreign body s.
 Bishop-Harman s.
 Corbett foreign body s.
 corneal s.
 curved needle s.
 Davis foreign body s.
 s. dissector
 Dix eye s.
 Dix foreign body s.
 Ellis foreign body s.
 Fisher s.

flat needle s.
foreign body s.
foreign body needle s.
Francis s.
Francis knife s.
Goldstein golf club s.
golf-club s.
gouge s.
s. gouge
Gross ear s.
Hosford foreign body s.
knife s.
LaForce golf-club knife s.
Levine curetting s.
Levine foreign body s.
needle s.
s. needle
Nicati foreign body s.
O'Brien foreign body s.
Plange s.
s. tool
Walter corneal s.
Walton round gauge s.
Whittle s.

spur-crushing clamp
Spurling
S. intervertebral disc forceps
S. intervertebral disc rongeur
S. laminectomy rongeur
S. periosteal elevator
S. pituitary rongeur
S. retractor
S. tissue forceps

Spurling-Kerrison
S.-K. laminectomy punch
S.-K. rongeur
S.-K. rongeur forceps

Spurling-Love-Gruenwald-Cushing
rongeur
Sputnik Russian razor blade
Spyglass angiography catheter
Spyrogel hydrogel wound dressing
spyrolace shoe lace
SQS-20 subcuticular skin stapler
square
s. module seating system
s. prism
s. specimen forceps
s. wire

square-ended
s.-e. distraction rod
s.-e. hook

square-end pliers
square-hole broach
square-tipped arterial dissector
squeeze ball
squeeze-handle forceps
Squeeze-Mark surgical marker
Squibb
S. catheter
S. urostomy pouch

squint hook
Squire catheter
Squirt wound irrigation system
SR
Microny K SR

Sr-90 eye applicator
SRI automated immunoassay analyzer
SR-Isosit dental restorative material
SR-Ivocap denture material
SR-Ivolen impression material
SR-Ivoseal impression material
SR-IV Programmed Subjective refractor
S-ROM
S-ROM acetabular cup
S-ROM femoral stem prosthesis
S-ROM hip replacement system
S-ROM modular total knee system
S-ROM Poly-Dial insert
S-ROM proximally modular total
hip system

SRR-5 digital-analogue converter
SS
SS bobbin drain tube
SS bobbin myringotomy tube
SS suture
SS White clamp

S-Scort
S-S. new-Duet suction unit
S-S. VX-2 suction pump

S-series sleep system
S-shaped retractor
S-Soles insole
S.S.T. orthopaedic nail
St.
S. Bartholomew barium catheter
S. Clair forceps
S. Clair-Thompson adenoidal curette
S. Clair-Thompson adenoidal
forceps
S. Clair-Thompson adenotome
S. Clair-Thompson peritonsillar
abscess forceps
S. George total elbow prosthesis

S

NOTES

St. *(continued)*
S. Jude annuloplasty ring
S. Jude cardiac device
S. Jude composite valve graft
S. Jude Medical (SJM)
S. Jude Medical aortic connector system
S. Jude Medical bileaflet tilting-disc aortic valve
S. Jude Medical Biocor valve
S. Jude Medical BioImplant valve
S. Jude Medical Masters series valve
S. Jude Medical mitral valve prosthesis
S. Jude Medical pericardial patch
S. Jude Medical Quattro mitral valve
S. Jude Medical Regent valve
S. Luke's double-action rongeur
S. Luke's retractor
S. Mark clamp
S. Mark pudendal electrode
S. Mark's Hospital retractor
S. Mark's lipped retractor
S. Mark's pelvis retractor
S. Martin eye forceps
S. Martin-Franceschetti cataract hook
S. Martin suturing forceps
S. Vincent tube clamp
S. Vincent tube-occluding forceps
ST3 stethoscope
Staar
S. foldable intraocular lens
S. glaucoma wick
S. implantable contact lens
S. low-diopter IOL
S. toric IOL
S. toric lens
stab
s. electrode
s. needle
Stab-and-Grab screwdriver
Stabident system
Stability total hip system
stabilization
Oscillating Techniques for Isometric S.
s. plate
stabilizer
Access MV coronary s.
Axius Vacuum 2 s.
Cadlow shoulder s.
Claussen fragment s.
Cohn Cardiac s.
dynamic foot s.
EndoOctopus s.
foot s.

Freedom Thumb s.
Goldstein Grasp atraumatic cervical s.
Heel Hugger therapeutic heel s.
Insall-Burstein posterior s.
Kwik Board IV and arterial line s.
Medline lateral s.
Medtronic Octopus 2 tissue s.
Palumbo ankle s.
Stamler corneal transplant s.
subpectoral s.
stabilizing
s. bar
s. guide pin
stabilocondylar knee prosthesis
Stabilor alloy
stab-in epicardial electrode
stable access cannula
Stablecut sawblade
Stableflex lens
Stableloc
S. Colles fracture external fixator
S. II external wrist fixation system
Stable-Lok nut
stab-wound drain
Stack
S. autoperfusion balloon
S. perfusion coronary dilatation catheter
S. retractor
S. splint
Stacke
S. gouge
S. probe
stacking cone
STA Compact hemostasis system
Stader
S. connecting rod
S. extraoral apparatus
S. pin
S. pin guide
S. splint
S. wrench
Stadie-Riggs microtome
stadiometer
digital s.
Harpenden s.
Heightronic s.
Hite-Rite s.
Photonic s.
Sta-Fix tape
2-stage
2-s. cannula
2-s. Sarns cannula
Stage-1 single-stage dental implant system
Stagnara gouge

Stahl
- S. calipers block
- S. calipers plate
- S. lens gauge
- S. nucleus expressor
- S. ophthalmic calipers

stainless
- s. steel balloon expandable stent
- s. steel blade
- s. steel clamp
- s. steel crown
- s. steel cup
- s. steel flexible ruler
- s. steel guidewire
- s. steel implant
- s. steel jaw forceps
- s. steel mesh
- s. steel mesh stent
- s. steel screw
- s. steel wire
- s. steel wire suture

StairClimber assist device
StairMaster exercise system
Stalite root canal post
Stallard
- S. blunt dissector
- S. head clamp
- S. scleral hook
- S. stricturotome

Stallard-Liegard suture
stall bar
Stallerpointe needle
Stalzner rectal scissors
Stamey
- S. dorsal vein apical retractor
- S. needle
- S. open-tip ureteral catheter

Stamler
- S. corneal transplant stabilizer
- S. sideport fixation hook

Stamm
- S. bone-cutting forceps
- S. gastrostomy tube

Stammberger
- S. antral punch
- S. side-biting punch forceps

stamp
- Sklar medical breast s.

StanceGuard internal support
stand
- Brown-Roberts-Wells floor s.
- Cherf cast s.

- Contraves s.
- Grand stand support s.
- IMP turnstile casting s.
- Keeler lightsource s.
- Mayo s.
- turnstile casting s. (TCS)
- Wilson-Mayo s.

standard
- s. above-elbow cast
- s. arterial forceps
- S. Care sterile urethral catheter
- s. duodenoscope
- s. endoscopy polypectomy snare
- s. full-lumen esophagoscope
- s. head halter
- s. hook electrosurgical probe
- s. Jackson laryngoscope
- s. needle
- s. pattern mallet
- s. wire gauge

standby pacemaker
standing
- s. frame orthosis
- S. Ovation MRI system

Stanford
- S. bioptome
- S. end-hole pigtail catheter
- S. and Wheatstone stereoscope

Stanford-Caves bioptome
Stangel
- S. fallopian tube cannula
- S. fallopian tube miniclip

Stange laryngoscope
Stanicor
- S. Gamma pacemaker
- S. Lambda demand pacemaker

Stankiewicz iris clip intraocular lens
Stanmore
- S. modular hip system
- S. shoulder arthroplasty
- S. shoulder prosthesis
- S. total knee

Stanton cautery clamp
Stanzel needle holder
Staodyne EMS+2 neurostimulator
Staodyn Insight point locator
stapedectomy
- s. footplate pick
- s. forceps
- s. knife
- s. prosthesis

STA-Pen Writer

NOTES

stapes
    s. chisel
    s. curette
    s. dilator
    s. elevator
    s. excavator
    s. forceps
    s. hoe
    s. hook
    s. needle
    s. pick
    s. speculum
Staph-Chek pad
staphylorrhaphy
    s. elevator
    s. needle
staple
    arcuate skin s.
    Arthrotek meniscus s.
    barbed Richards s.
    bioabsorbable s.
    Biologically Quiet s.
    Blount epiphyseal s.
    Blount fracture s.
    s. bone plate
    Bostick s.
    DePalma s.
    duToit shoulder s.
    Ellison fixation s.
    s. forceps
    GIA s.
    Hernandez-Ros bone s.
    Krackow HTO blade s.
    Lactomer absorbable subcuticular
      skin s.
    meniscal s.
    metallic s.
    Nakayama s.
    orthopaedic s.
    7-pin s.
    Polysorb absorbable s.
    Richards fixation s.
    skin s.
    Smith & Nephew barbed s.
    spike s.
    stone s.
    TA metallic s.
    TA Premium-series s.
    titanium s.
    titanium mandibular s.
    Wiberg fracture s.
    Zimaloy epiphyseal s.
stapler
    American vascular s.
    Appose skin s.
    Auto Suture Multifire Endo GIA
      30 s.
    Auto Suture Premium CEEA s.
    CDH s.

circular s.
circular intraluminal s.
Cobe gun s.
Concorde disposable skin s.
copolymer s.
Coventry s.
Cricket disposable skin s.
curved intraluminal s.
Day s.
disposable skin s.
Downing s.
duToit s.
Dwyer spinal mechanical s.
EEA s.
end-end s.
Endo Babcock s.
Endo GIA 30 suture s.
endohernia s.
Endopath EMS hernia s.
Endopath endoscopic articulating s.
Endopath ES endoscopic s.
Endopath Stealth s.
endostapler s.
Ethicon Endo-Surgery circular s.
gastroplasty s.
Graftac-S skin s.
Hall double-hole spinal s.
hernia s.
ILA s.
Imagyn surgical s.
Inokucki vascular s.
intraluminal s.
Lactomer copolymer absorbable s.
ligating and dividing s.
linear s.
mechanical s.
Multifire GIA-series s.
Multifire TA-series s.
Multifire VersaTack s.
Nakayama microvascular s.
Ni-Ti Shape Memory alloy
  compression s.
One-Time disposable skin s.
Oswestry-O'Brien spinal s.
PCEEA s.
PC EEA s.
PI disposable s.
Poly GIA s.
Polysorb 55 s.
Precise disposable skin s.
Premium CEEA circular s.
Premium Plus CEEA disposable s.
Premium Poly CS-57 s.
Proximate disposable skin s.
Proximate flexible linear s.
Proximate hemorrhoid circular s.
Proximate-ILS curved
  intraluminal s.
Proximate Plus MD skin s.

Proximate PX skin s.
Proximate RH skin s.
Proximate TX linear s.
PSS Powered disposable skin s.
Reflex One skin s.
Roticulator s.
Royal disposable skin s.
SD sorb meniscal s.
SGIA 50 disposable s.
Signet disposable skin s.
Soviet mechanical bronchial s.
SPTU Soviet s.
SQS-20 subcuticular skin s.
STI-1 needle-shaped tissue s.
SureLine skin s.
Surgeons Choice surgical s.
SurgiMate skin s.
Surgiport s.
thoracoabdominal s.
United States Surgical circular s.
UPO-16 s.
VersaTack s.
Vista disposable skin s.
Vital skin s.
Vogelfanger-Beattie s.
Vogelfanger blood vessel s.
Wiberg fracture s.
Yamagishi s.

Staples osteotomy nail
STAR
suture tension adjustment reel
STAR system
Star
S. Optica hearing aid
S. S3 ActiveTrak Excimer laser
S. S2 SmoothScan excimer laser system
S. ventilator
S. X carbon dioxide laser
StarCam camera
starch bandage
starch-based copolymer dressing
Starck dilator
Starfish2 heart positioner
StarFlex occluder
Stargate falloposcopy catheter
STA-R hemostasis system
Starion thermal cautery hook
Starkey
S. hearing aid
S. stethoscope
Stark vulsellum forceps

Starlinger uterine dilator
Starlite Omni-AT bur
Star-Lock Press-Fit cylinder implant
Starr
S. ball heart prosthesis
S. fixation forceps
Starr-Edwards
S.-E. aortic valve prosthesis
S.-E. caged-ball valve prosthesis
S.-E. cloth-covered metallic ball heart valve
S.-E. disc valve prosthesis
S.-E. hermetically-sealed pacemaker
S.-E. pacemaker
S.-E. prosthetic aortic valve
S.-E. prosthetic mitral valve
S.-E. Silastic valve
S.-E. silicone rubber ball valve
STARRT falloposcopy system
STaR sleeve
STart-4 clot detection system
Startanius blade implant
starter
s. awl
s. broach
Star/Vent 1-stage dental screw implant
Stat
S. aspirator
S. Profile pHOx blood gas/critical care analyzer
S. 2 Pumpette disposable IV pump
S. Scrub handwasher machine
Statak
S. anchor system
S. soft tissue attachment device
S. suture anchor
Statham
S. cautery
S. electromagnetic flowmeter
S. external transducer
static
s. adjustable stretch (SAS)
s. air mattress
stationary
s. angle guide
s. ankle flexible endoskeleton
Sta-Tite
S.-T. gauze dressing
S.-T. 2ply elastic roll gauze
STATLase-SDL diode laser
StatLock-Foley catheter
StatLock hemodyalysis catheter

NOTES

STAT-Site M Hgb test system
StatSpin Express centrifuge
Stat-Temp
    S.-T. II liquid crystal temperature
       monitor
    S.-T. II temperature device
Stat-Trace electrode
Status Cup Plus testing system
Status-X machine
Staude
    S. tenaculum forceps
    S. uterine tenaculum
Staude-Jackson uterine tenaculum
Staude-Moore
    S.-M. uterine tenaculum
    S.-M. uterine tenaculum forceps
Staurenghi 230 scanning laser
Stavis fixation forceps
Stax fingertip splint
Stayce adjustable clamp
Stay-Erec system
Stayoden 9000F TENS unit
Stay-Rite clamp
StaySharp face lift Super-Cut scissors
stay suture retractor
STC 900-series travel chair
STD+ titanium total hip prosthesis
Steady Step walker
Stealth
    S. angioplasty balloon catheter
    S. catheter balloon
    S. DBO diamond blade
    S. DBO free-hand diamond knife
    S. frame
    S. occlusion system
    S. surgical clip
StealthStation
    S. image-guided system
    S. treatment guidance platform
steam
    s. box
    s. tent
steam-shaping mandrel
Stearnes speculum
Stecher
    S. arachnoid knife
    S. microruler
Stedman
    S. awl
    S. continuous suction tube
    S. saw
    S. suction pump aspirator
steel
    s. embolization coil
    s. mesh suture
    s. ruler
Steele
    S. articulator
    S. bronchial dilator

S. fiberoptic system
S. filling instrument
S. periosteal elevator
S. scaler
steel-slotted plastic bracket
steel-winged butterfly needle
Steeper Powered Gripper
steerable
    s. angioplastic guidewire
    s. catheter
    s. DecaPolar electrode catheter
    s. electrode catheter
    s. guidewire catheter
steering catheter
Steerocath-A, -T ablation catheter
Steerocath-Dx valve mapping catheter
Steers replicator
Steffee
    S. pedicle plate
    S. pedicle screw-plate system
    S. screw plate
    S. spinal instrumentation
Steffensmeier board
Steigmann-Goff endoscopic ligature
    overtube
Steinbach mallet
Steiner
    S. bracket
    S. electromechanical morcellator
Steiner-Auvard
    S.-A. vaginal retractor
    S.-A. weighted speculum
Steinert
    S. double-ended claw chopper
    S. II irrigating claw chopper
    S. laser-assisted intrastromal
       keratomileusis set
Steinert-Deacon incision gauge
Steinhauser
    S. bone clamp
    S. electromucotome
    S. internal screw fixation
    S. lag screw
    S. orotome
    S. plate
    S. position screw
Steinhauser-Castroviejo electromucotome
Steinmann
    S. calibrated pin
    S. extension bow
    S. extension nail
    S. holder
    S. intestinal forceps
    S. pin chuck
    S. tendon forceps
    S. traction
    S. traction tractor
Stein membrane perforator
Steis bone marrow transplant needle

Stela electrode lead
Steldent alloy
Stellbrink
    S. fixation device
    S. synovectomy rongeur
Stellite
    S. ball-cage heart valve
    S. ring material
    S. ring material of prosthetic valve
stem
    APR I femoral s.
    Austin Moore standard s.
    autologous s.
    Bio-Groove s.
    calcar s.
    s. cell concentrator
    Cementless Sportorno hip
      arthroplasty s.
    collarless s.
    Corin Hi-Nek total hip s.
    Deon s.
    Extend s.
    s. extractor
    femoral s.
    fenestrated Moore-type femoral s.
    F2L Multineck femoral s.
    HA-coated s.
    Howmedica hip fracture s.
    hydroxyapatite-coated s.
    Iowa s.
    KMP fenestrated femoral s.
    Linear hip s.
    Link microporous hip s.
    Lubinus SP II hip s.
    modular calcar replacement s.
    Morse taper s.
    Natural-Hip titanium hip s.
    nonfenestrated Moore-type
      femoral s.
    Omnifit HA hip s.
    Opteon femoral s.
    Osteonics Omnifit-HA hip s.
    PCA total hip s.
    Perfecta femoral s.
    s. pessary
    Precident s.
    Precision Osteolock s.
    Press-Fit s.
    Profix metaphyseal tibial s.
    Progeny femoral s.
    Ranawat-Burstein porous s.
    ReVision hip s.

    SL-Plus s.
    s. spoon separator
    Strata hip s.
    Taperloc femoral s.
    TC femoral s.
    VS femoral s.
stemmed tibial prosthesis
Stemp clamp
stencil
    Etch-Master electronic s.
stenopaic goggles
Stenosimeter
stenosis clamp
Stenstrom
    S. nerve holder
    S. rasp
    S. raspatory
stent
    absorbable s.
    Acculink self-expanding s.
    ACMI ureteral s.
    ACS Multi-Link Duet coronary s.
    ACS Multi-Link OTW Duet s.
    ACS Multi-Link RX Duet s.
    ACS Multi-Link RX Ultra
      coronary s.
    ACS Multi-Link Tristar coronary s.
    ACS Multi-Link Ultra coronary s.
    ACS RSX Multi-Link s.
    ACT-one coronary s.
    adjustable vaginal s.
    American Heyer-Schulte s.
    Amplatz ureteral s.
    Amsterdam biliary s.
    AMS urethral s.
    Anastaflo s.
    AngioStent balloon-expandable
      coronary s.
    antegrade internal s.
    antegrade ureteral s.
    antibiotic-coated s.
    Atkinson tube s.
    AVE bridge biliary s.
    AVE GFX coronary s.
    AVE Microstent II coronary s.
    AVE S-series coronary s.
    bailout s.
    balloon-expandable flexible coil s.
    balloon-expandable intravascular s.
    Bard coil s.
    Bardex s.
    Bard Memotherm colorectal s.

S

NOTES

stent *(continued)*
    Bard soft double-pigtail ureteral s.
    Bard XT coronary s.
    bare-metal s.
    Beamer s.
    Benestent I, II s.
    BeStent balloon-expandable s.
    BeStent 2 coronary s.
    BeStent Rival s.
    bifurcated s.
    biliary s.
    bioabsorbable s.
    bioabsorbable double-spiral s.
    biocompatible s.
    biodegradable s.
    BioDiamond bare s.
    BioDiamond coronary s.
    BioDiamond F s.
    BioDiamond Micro F12 s.
    BiodivYsio AS s.
    BiodivYsio OC s.
    BiodivYsio PC coated coronary s.
    BiodivYsio SV s.
    BioSorb resorbable urology s.
    Biostent s.
    Black Beauty ureteral s.
    Black spanner s.
    Braun s.
    Bx IsoStent s.
    Bx Sonic coronary s.
    Bx Velocity coronary artery s.
    Carbostent coronary s.
    Carcon s.
    CardioCoil coronary s.
    Carey-Coons soft s.
    carotid s.
    CarotidCoil s.
    Carpentier s.
    Carson-Bush internal/external
        endopyelotomy s.
    Carson internal/external
        endopyelotomy s.
    cell-seeded s.
    C-Flex Amsterdam s.
    C-Flex ureteral s.
    Champion drug eluding s.
    cobalt alloy s.
    coil s.
    compliance matching s.
    Conley tracheal s.
    Contour closed-end s.
    Contour VL Percuflex s.
    Cook Amplatz ureteral s.
    Cook FlexStent s.
    Cook intracoronary s.
    Cook Urosoft s.
    Cook-Z s.
    Cordis coronary s.
    Cordis Crossflex s.
    Cordis radiopaque tantalum s.
    Cordis SMART s.
    Corinthian transhepatic biliary s.
    coronary s.
    Corvita s.
    Cotton-Huibregtse double-biliary
        pigtail s.
    Cotton-Leung biliary s.
    Cragg EndoPro nitinol s.
    Cragg Endopro System I s.
    CrossFlex LC coronary s.
    Crown s.
    Cypher sirolimus-eluting coronary s.
    Dart coronary s.
    Devon-Pura s.
    DISA S-Flex coronary s.
    diversion s.
    Dobbhoff biliary s.
    double-J s.
    double-J dangle s.
    double-J indwelling catheter s.
    double-J silicone internal ureteral
        catheter s.
    double-J ureteral s.
    double-pigtail ureteral s.
    Doyle II silicone s.
    s. dressing
    Driver coronary s.
    drug-coated s.
    Dua s.
    Duet coronary s.
    Dumon silicone s.
    Dumon tracheobronchial s.
    Dynalink 0.035 biliary self-
        expanding s.
    dynamic Y s.
    Easy Wallstent s.
    Elastalloy esophageal s.
    Eliminator biliary s.
    eluting s.
    endobiliary s.
    Endocare Horizon prostatic s.
    EndoCoil-T biliary s.
    endoluminal s.
    Endo-Sof double pigtail s.
    Entract s.
    EsophaCoil self-expanding
        esophageal s.
    esophageal s.
    esophageal Strecker s.
    Esophageal Z-Stent s.
    expandable esophageal s.
    expandable intrahepatic portacaval
        shunt s.
    expandable metallic s.
    expanded polytetrafluoroethylene-
        covered s.
    Fanelli laparoscopic endobiliary s.
    fibrin-film s.

Flamingo s.
flat wire coil s.
flexible s.
flexible coil s.
Flexima biliary s.
FlexStent flexible esophageal s.
FlexStent memory s.
foam rubber vaginal s.
FocalSeal-R neurosurgical s.
Focustent coronary s.
Freedom coronary s.
Freeman frontal sinus s.
freestanding s.
Freitag s.
French s.
Geenan pancreatic s.
Gelfilm s.
GFX coronary s.
Gianturco expandable metallic
  biliary s.
Gianturco metal urethral s.
Gianturco-Rosch metallic s.
Gianturco-Rosch self-expandable
  biliary Z s.
Gianturco-Roubin flexible coil s.
Gianturco-Roubin FlexStent
  coronary s.
Gianturco-Roubin II s.
Gianturco zigzag s.
Gibbon indwelling ureteral s.
Global Therapeutics Freedom s.
Global Therapeutics V-Flex s.
GRII coronary s.
Guidant s.
hand-crimped s.
hand-mounted s.
Harrell Y s.
heat-activated recoverable
  temporary s.
heat-expandable s.
helical coil s.
helical-ridged ureteral s.
Hepamed-coated Wiktor s.
heparin-coated Palmaz-Schatz s.
Hood stoma s.
Hood-Westaby T-Y s.
Horizon prostatic s.
Huibregtse biliary s.
Hydromer coated polyurethane s.
HydroPlus s.
Igaki-Tamai s.
iliac artery s.

indwelling s.
indwelling ureteral s.
inflow coronary s.
InStent CardioCoil s.
InStent CarotidCoil s.
interdigitating coil s.
internal biliary s.
internal ureteral s.
IntraCoil self-expanding
  peripheral s.
intracoronary s.
intraoral s.
Intra-Prostatic s.
intravascular s.
s. introducer
INX stainless steel s.
IRIS coronary s.
J s.
s. jail
Jasin Frontal Ostent s.
J-Maxx s.
Johnson & Johnson biliary s.
Johnson & Johnson coronary s.
Jomed s.
Jostent bifurcation s.
Jostent coronary s.
Jostent Flex s.
Jostent peripheral s.
Jostent Plus s.
Jostent SelfX endoscopic s.
Jostent side branch s.
Kaminsky s.
keel s.
kidney internal s.
kissing s.
lacrimal s.
laryngeal s.
Liberte coronary s.
lighted s.
Lubri-Flex ureteral s.
luminal s.
Luminexx biliary s.
Mac-Loc Ultrathane Cope
  nephroureterectomy s.
Magic-Wall s.
Magic Wallstent s.
magnetic internal ureteral s.
main pancreatic duct s.
Mardis-Dangler ureteral s.
Mardis soft s.
Medinol NIR s.
Medinol NIRside slotted s.

NOTES

stent *(continued)*

Medivent self-expanding coronary s.
Medivent vascular s.
Medtronic AVE S660 coronary s.
Medtronic Bestent s.
Medtronic interventional vascular s.
Medtronic S-series small vessel s.
MegaLink biliary s.
Memotherm colorectal s.
Memotherm endoscopic biliary s.
Memotherm Flexx biliary s.
Memotherm nitinol self-
  expandable s.
Mentor biliary s.
MeroGel s.
mesh s.
metal-augmented polymer s.
metal-coated s.
metallic s.
Metal Z s.
methyl methacrylate ear s.
Microstent II coronary s.
Microvasive s.
Miller s.
Mini Crown s.
Montgomery laryngeal s.
MPD s.
MSM-BMS coronary s.
multicellular s.
Multi-Link OTW Ultra coronary s.
Multi-Link RX Ultra coronary s.
Multi-Link Tetra coronary s.
Multi-Link Tristar coronary s.
Navius s.
nephroureteral s.
Neville s.
NexStent carotid s.
Nexus coronary s.
NIR s.
NIRflex coronary s.
NIR ON Ranger premounted s.
Niroyal Advance balloon
  expandable s.
NIR Primo balloon expandable s.
NIR with SOX over-the-wire
  coronary s.
nitinol mesh s.
nitinol self-expanding coil s.
nitinol Strecker s.
nitinol subglottic stenosis s.
nitinol thermal memory s.
Novastent s.
nuclear s.
Omniflex PTCA s.
OmniLink biliary s.
OmniStent s.
Orbus coronary R s.
Orbus R stent SVS s.
Orlowski s.

Ossoff-Sisson surgical s.
osteomeatal s.
paclitaxel-coated coronary s.
Palmaz arterial s.
Palmaz balloon-expandable iliac s.
Palmaz biliary s.
Palmaz Corinthian transhepatic
  biliary s.
Palmaz Genesis transhepatic
  biliary s.
Palmaz-Schatz balloon-expandable s.
Palmaz-Schatz biliary s.
Palmaz-Schatz coronary s.
Palmaz-Schatz Crown balloon-
  expandable s.
Palmaz vascular s.
pancreatic duct s.
Paragon Champion s.
Paragon coronary s.
Paragon nitinol s.
Passager s.
patent s.
Percuflex Amsterdam s.
Percuflex biliary s.
Percuflex endopyelotomy s.
Percuflex flexible biliary s.
Percuflex Plus ureteral s.
Percuflex Tail Plus ureteral s.
percutaneous ureteral s.
Perflex biliary s.
piano-style guidewire s.
pigtail biliary s.
plastic s.
polyethylene s.
polyethylene-covered Gianturco s.
polymer s.
polymer-coated, drug-eluting s.
polymeric endoluminal paving s.
polytetrafluoroethylene s.
polytetrafluoroethylene-covered s.
polyurethane s.
porous metallic s.
s. positioner
premounted s.
ProstaCoil self-expanding s.
Prostakath urethral s.
prostatic s.
Protégé self-expanding nitinol s.
PS 153 s.
PTFE-covered Palmaz s.
Pura-Vario s.
Quanam QP2 coronary s.
radioactive s.
radioisotope s.
radiopaque nitinol s.
radiopaque tantalum s.
Radius self-expanding s.
reducing s.
Reliance urinary control s.

renovascular s.
Retromax endopyelotomy s.
rolled Instat s.
Roubin-Gianturco flexible coil s.
Rusch retrievable esophageal s.
RX Herculink Plus biliary s.
RX Multi-Link s.
Salman FES s.
SAXX renal s.
Schatz-Palmaz tubular mesh s.
Schneider s.
Scimed Express Monorail
  coronary s.
self-expanding coil s.
self-expanding stainless steel s.
self-retaining coil s.
shape-memory alloy recoverable
  technology s.
Shikani middle meatal
  antrostomy s.
short s.
Siegel s.
Silastic indwelling ureteral s.
silicone s.
silicone-coated, metallic self-
  expanding s.
Silitek Uropass s.
silver-coated s.
single-J urinary diversion s.
sinus s.
SinuSpacer turbinate s.
slotted tube articulated s.
SMART s.
SMART nitinol self-expandable s.
SoloPass Percuflex biliary s.
Song covered duodenal s.
Speed Lok soft s.
spiral coil s.
SpiraStent s.
SpiroFlo bioabsorbable prostate s.
spring-loaded vascular s.
stainless steel balloon
  expandable s.
stainless steel mesh s.
straight s.
Strecker balloon-expandable
  esophageal s.
Strecker coronary s.
Strecker tantalum s.
s. strut
Stryker s.
Supramid occluding s.

Surgitek Double-J II closed-tip
  ureteral s.
Surgitek Quadra-Coil ureteral s.
Surgitek UroPass II ureteral s.
Symbiot s.
Symbiot vascular s.
Symphony nitinol biliary s.
synthetic s.
tandem s.
Tannenbaum s.
tantalum balloon-expandable s.
tantalum coil s.
Tenax coronary s.
Tensum coronary s.
Terumo s.
thermal memory s.
ThermaStent prostatic s.
thermoexpandable s.
thermoplastic s.
Titan s.
titanium urethral s.
Tower s.
tracheal s.
transhepatic biliary s.
transpapillary pancreatic s.
Trimble suture s.
T-tube s.
tubular s.
tubular slotted s.
TY s.
Ultraflex Microvasive s.
Ultraflex nitinol expandable
  esophageal s.
Ultraflex self-expanding s.
Ultrathane Amplatz ureteral s.
uncoated mesh s.
Universal s.
ureteral s.
UroCoil self-expanding s.
Uro-Guide s.
UroLume urethral s.
Urosoft s.
Urospiral urethral s.
U-tube s.
vaginal s.
Vantec urinary s.
VascuCoil peripheral vascular s.
vascular s.
vein graft s.
Velocity s.
s. and vent system
V-Flex Plus PTX s.

NOTES

S

stent *(continued)*
    Wallstent self-expanding s.
    Wallstent spring-loaded s.
    Westaby s.
    whistle s.
    Wilson-Cook s.
    wire mesh s.
    wire mesh self-expandable s.
    XT radiopaque coronary s.
    Y s.
    Z s.
    Za-Stent biliary s.
    Zeta coronary s.
    zigzag s.
    Zilver biliary s.
    Zimmon biliary s.
stented bioprosthetic valve
stent-graft
    Ancure s.-g.
    AneuRx aortic aneurysm s.-g.
    Dacron-covered s.-g.
    endovascular s.-g.
    Excluder endovascular s.-g.
    FreeFlo s.-g.
    Gore Excluder endovascular s.-g.
    Quantum LP s.-g.
    Talent LPS endoluminal s.-g.
    Wallgraft endoprosthesis s.-g.
stenting catheter
stentless porcine aortic valve
stent-mounted
    s.-m. allograft valve
    s.-m. heterograft valve
Stenzel
    S. fracture rod
    S. rod prosthesis
step
    s. drill
    S. laparoscopic trocar
    s. screw
1-step
    1-s. button gastrostomy device
    1-s. limbar relaxing incision
      diamond knife
step-down
    s.-d. cannula
    s.-d. drill
    s.-d. transformer
Stephen-Slater valve
Stephenson needle holder
Stephens soft IOL-inserting forceps
Stepita meatal clamp
Step-Knife diamond blade knife
stepped-down cautery
stepper
    NuStep total body recumbent s.
Stepty P hemostasis device
step-up transformer
stereo campimeter

Stereocrepe crepe bandage
stereoencephalotome
    Spiegel-Wycis s.
stereofly
    Titmus s.
StereoGuide
    S. breast biopsy equipment
    S. collimator
    S. needle
    S. stereotactic breast biopsy system
stereolithography cage
stereoscope
    Krumeich s.
    Stanford and Wheatstone s.
stereoscopic microscope
stereotactic *(See also* stereotaxic)
    s. apparatus
    s. atlas
    s. breast biopsy needle
    s. breast biopsy system
    s. coordinate frame
    s. head frame
    s. localization frame
    s. retractor
    s. ring
stereotactic-assisted radiation therapy kit
stereotaxic *(See also* stereotactic)
    s. instrument
    s. laser
Stereotaxis magnetic surgery system
Steri-Band bandage
SteriCam Endoscopic camera
Stericare
    S. copolymer absorbent dressing
    S. glycerin hydrogel
    S. hydrogel gauze dressing
Steri-Cath catheter
Steri-Cuff disposable tourniquet cuff
Steri-Dent dry heat sterilizer
Steri-Drape 2 incise drape
Steriflex-Braun bacterial filter
Steriking sterilization system
sterile
    s. drape
    s. electrodermatome blade
    s. field barrier
    s. forceps holder
    s. isolation bag
    s. sheet
    s. specimen trap
    s. stockinette
    s. transverse rod
    s. vent spike
sterilizer
    Anprolene s.
    autoclave s.
    Bard s.
    s. box
    Cox s.

dry heat s.
Esquire dental s.
s. forceps
glass bead s.
Harvey vapor s.
hot salt s.
Steri-Dent dry heat s.
Stermatic s.
Wallach Bio-Tool s.
sterilizing
    s. basket
    s. forceps
Steri-Oss
    S.-O. dental implant device
    S.-O. endosteal dental implant
Steri-Pad
    S.-P. dressing
    S.-P. gauze pad
Steri-Probe explorer
Steris automatic reprocessor
Steriseal disposable cannula
Steri-Sleeve tube sleeve
Steri-Strip skin closure
Steritapes closure
Steritek ICP mini monitor
Steri-Vac drain
Sterling
    S. arthroscopy blade
    S. iris spatula
Sterling-Spring orthodontic wire
Sterling-Sylva irrigator
Stermatic sterilizer
Sterna-Band self-locking suture
sternal
    s. approximator
    s. blade
    s. knife
    s. needle holder
    s. notch stethoscope
    s. occipital mandibular immobilizer
    (SOMI)
    s. punch forceps
    s. puncture needle
    s. retractor
    s. retractor blade
    s. saw
    s. shears
    s. spreader
    s. wire suture
Stern-Castroviejo
    S.-C. locking forceps
    S.-C. suturing forceps

Stern dental attachment
Stern-McCarthry panendoscope
Stern-McCarthy
    S.-M. electrode
    S.-M. electrotome
    S.-M. electrotome resectoscope
sterno-occipital-mandibular
    s.-o.-m. immobilization orthosis
    s.-o.-m. immobilizer brace
sternooccipitomanubrial immobilizer
sternotome
sternotomy retractor
steroid-eluting electrode
Sterrad sterilization system
Stertzer brachial guiding catheter
Stertzer-Myler extension wire
stethoscope
    Acoustascope esophageal s.
    Allen fetal s.
    Andries s.
    Argyle esophageal s.
    bell s.
    Boston s.
    Cammann s.
    Cardiocare s.
    Cardiology II s.
    CareTone I, II telephonic s.
    Classic II s.
    DeLee s.
    DeLee-Hillis fetal s.
    Doppler fetal s.
    Doppler ultrasound s.
    Doptone fetal s.
    electronic-amplified s.
    E-Scope electronic s.
    esophageal s.
    EST40 electronic s.
    fetal s.
    First Beat ultrasound s.
    Harvey Elite s.
    Hillis fetal s.
    Labtron s.
    Leff s.
    pacing esophageal s.
    Phillips electronic s.
    Pinard fetal s.
    Pocket-Dop fetal s.
    precordial s.
    Rappaport-Sprague s.
    Rusch esophageal s.
    Spectrum s.
    ST3 s.

S

NOTES

stethoscope *(continued)*
    Starkey s.
    sternal notch s.
    Tapscope esophageal pacing s.
    Tria handheld Doppler
      ultrasound s.
    ultrasound s.
Stetten
    S. intestinal clamp
    S. spur crusher
Stevens
    S. eye scissors
    S. fixation forceps
    S. iris forceps
    S. lacrimal retractor
    S. muscle hook
    S. muscle hook retractor
    S. needle holder
    S. stitch scissors
    S. tenotomy hook
    S. tenotomy scissors
Stevens-Charles sleeve
Stevenson
    S. alligator forceps
    S. alligator scissors
    S. capsular punch
    S. clamp
    S. cupped-jaw forceps
    S. grasping forceps
    S. lacrimal sac retractor
    S. microsurgical forceps
    S. needle holder
    S. refractor
Stevenson-LaForce adenotome
Stevens-Street elbow prosthesis
Stewart
    S. cartilage knife
    S. cruciate ligament guide
    S. crypt hook
    S. lenticular nuclear snare
    S. rectal hook
STI-1 needle-shaped tissue stapler
Stichs wound clip
stick
    bite s.
    dextrose s.
    dressing s.
    FMS Intracell s.
    Grafco seizure s.
    Intracell Sprinter s.
    lollipop s.
    percutaneous s.
    Pro-Ophtha s.
    sponge s.
    switching s.
"stick-and-carrot" appliance
stick-on electrode
Stiegler unipolar nasal snare
Stieglitz splinter forceps

Stiegmann-Goff Clearvue endoscopic ligator
Stierlen lens loop
Stifcore transbronchial aspiration needle
stiff
    s. guidewire
    s. shaft Glidewire
stiffening wire
Stik-Temp thermometer
stiletto
    Berkeley Bioengineering s.
    Blair s.
    s. knife
    s. ureteroscope
Stilith implantable cardiac pulse generator
Stille
    S. bone chisel
    S. bone drill
    S. bone gouge
    S. bone rongeur
    S. brace
    S. bur
    S. cast cutter
    S. cheek retractor
    S. coarctation hook
    S. conchotome
    S. cranial drill
    S. dissecting scissors
    S. flat pliers
    S. gallstone forceps
    S. Gigli-saw guide
    S. hand drill
    S. heart retractor
    S. insufflator
    S. kidney clamp
    S. kidney forceps
    S. laryngeal applicator
    S. mallet
    S. osteotome
    S. periosteal elevator
    S. plaster shears
    S. plaster spreader
    S. rib shears
    S. rongeur forceps
    S. Super Cut scissors
    S. tissue forceps
    S. trephine
    S. uterine dilator
    S. vessel clamp
    S. wrench
Stille-Adson forceps
Stille-Aesculap plaster shears
Stille-Babcock forceps
Stille-Bailey-Senning rib contractor
Stille-Barraya
    S.-B. intestinal forceps
    S.-B. vascular forceps
Stille-Beyer rongeur

Stille-Björk forceps
Stille-Broback knee retractor
Stille-Crafoord
    S.-C. forceps
    S.-C. raspatory
Stille-Crawford coarctation clamp
Stille-Crile forceps
Stille-Doyen raspatory
Stille-Edwards raspatory
Stille-Ericksson rib shears
Stille-French cardiovascular needle
  holder
Stille-Giertz shears
Stille-Gigli wire saw
Stille-Halsted forceps
Stille-Horsley
    S.-H. bone-cutting forceps
    S.-H. rib forceps
    S.-H. rongeur
    S.-H. shears
Stille-Langenbeck elevator
Stille-Leksell rongeur
Stille-Liston
    S.-L. bone forceps
    S.-L. rib-cutting forceps
    S.-L. rongeur
Stille-Luer
    S.-L. angular duckbill rongeur
    S.-L. bone rongeur
    S.-L. rongeur forceps
Stille-Luer-Echlin rongeur
Stille-Mayo dissecting scissors
Stille-Mayo-Hegar needle
Stillenberg raspatory
Stille-Quervain spreader
Stille-Ruskin rongeur
Stille-Russian forceps
Stille-Seldinger needle
Stille-Sherman bone drill
Stille-Stiwer
    S.-S. gouge
    S.-S. osteotome
    S.-S. plaster shears
Stille-Waugh forceps
Stille-Zaufal-Jansen rongeur
Stimitrode electrode
Stimoceiver implant
Stim Plus handheld microcurrent
  stimulator
Stimprene
    S. electrotherapy brace
    S. wrap

Stimson
    S. dressing
    S. pedicle clamp
StimuCath nerve block catheter
stimulating
    s. catheter
    s. electrode
stimulation
    electrical muscle s. (EMS)
    percutaneous electrical nerve s.
    transcutaneous electrical nerve s.
    (TENS)
stimulator
    Acuscope microcurrent s.
    AME bone growth s.
    Anustim electronic neuromuscular s.
    Arzco transesophageal cardiac s.
    Atrostim phrenic nerve s.
    Axostim nerve s.
    Axxess spinal cord s.
    Baltimore Therapeutic Equipment
      work s.
    Bionicare s.
    Biopulse s.
    BioStim digital NMS muscle s.
    Bloom programmable s.
    bone growth s.
    Butler s.
    CAM s.
    Concept nerve s.
    constant current s.
    Digitimer pattern reversal s.
    direct-current bone growth s.
    direct electrical nerve s.
    Dormed cranial electrotherapy s.
    dorsal column s.
    DTU-series cardiac digital s.
    EBI SPF-2 implantable bone s.
    electrical brain s.
    electrical nerve s.
    electronic muscle s.
    EMG s.
    EMHI galvanic electrode s.
    EMS 2000 neuromuscular s.
    Endo Multi-Mode s.
    external functional neuromuscular s.
    facial nerve s.
    fastSTART EMS neuromuscular s.
    fastSTART HVPC pulsed s.
    Freedom Micro Pro s.
    galvanic electrode s.
    Ganzfeld s.

S

NOTES

stimulator *(continued)*
    G5 Porta-Plus muscle s.
    Grass Model S9 s.
    Grass S88 muscle s.
    Hilger facial nerve s.
    implantable neural s.
    Innova pelvic floor s.
    InSync cardiac s.
    Intelect Legend Combo s.
    Intelect 600MP microcurrent s.
    interferential s.
    JACE-Stim electrical s.
    Liberty electrical s.
    magnetic s.
    Magnum s.
    Magstim 200 s.
    Master-Stim interferential s.
    Maxima II transcutaneous electrical
      nerve s.
    Medi-Stim s.
    metabolic heat load s.
    Micro-Z neuromuscular s.
    Myogyn II s.
    Myopulse muscle s.
    Myosynchron muscle s.
    Myotest train-of-four nerve s.
    nerve s.
    neuromuscular electronic s. (NMES)
    neuromuscular III s.
    Neuro Stim 2000 Mk$_1$ s.
    Nicolet SM-300 s.
    oculogyric s.
    optokinetic s.
    Ortho Dx electromedical s.
    Orthofix Cervical-Stim s.
    Orthofuse implantable growth s.
    OrthoGen bone growth s.
    OrthoLogic bone growth s.
    OrthoPak II bone growth s.
    OsteoGen-D bone s.
    OsteoGen implantable s.
    OsteoStim implantable bone
      grown s.
    percutaneous epidural nerve s.
    photic-evoked response s.
    Physio-Stim Lite bone growth s.
    piezoelectrical s.
    Prizm Electro-Mesh Z-Stim-II s.
    Pulsatron II handheld nerve s.
    pulsed galvanic s.
    Reese s.
    smoke Control Porta-Pack
      aversive s.
    SpF spinal fusion s.
    spinal cord s.
    SpinaLogic 1000 bone growth s.
    SpinalPak fusion s.
    SporTX pulsed direct current s.
    Stim Plus handheld microcurrent s.

    Stimuplex HNS 11 nerve s.
    Stimuplex-S nerve s.
    Super Stimm MF s.
    surgical nerve s.
    Synchrosonic s.
    SysStim muscle s.
    Theramini 1, 2 electrotherapy s.
    Theratouch 4.7 s.
    ThermaStim muscle s.
    transcutaneous cranial electrical s.
    transcutaneous electrical nerve s.
    transcutaneous electrical
      neuromuscular s.
    transmural electrical s.
    URYS 800 nerve s.
    Vari-Stim III handheld nerve s.
    Waters muscle s.
    Whistle-Stop wireless aversive s.
Stimulite
    S. honeycomb mattress overlay
    S. honeycomb seating pad
Stimuplex
    S. block needle
    S. HNS 11 nerve stimulator
Stimuplex-S nerve stimulator
Stinger M, S ablation catheter
sting mat
stirrup
    Allen laparoscopic s.'s
    s. brace
    candy cane s.'s
    Comfort Cast s.
    Finochietto s.
    Infinity s.
    Lloyd-Davies s.'s
    Navratil s.
    Swivel-Strap ankle s.
stirrup-loop curette
stitch
    Allgower s.
    Endo S.
    Frost s.
    Kessler s.
    Mersilene Kessler s.
    Prolene s.
    s. scissors
    shorthand vertical mattress s.
    tracheal safety s.
stitch-removing knife
Stitt catheter
Stiwer
    S. biopsy forceps
    S. bone-holding forceps
    S. curette
    S. dressing forceps
    S. furuncle knife
    S. grooved director
    S. hand drill
    S. laryngeal mirror

S. retractor
S. scalpel handle
S. scissors
S. sponge forceps
S. tendon dissector
S. tissue forceps
S. towel clamp
S. trocar
STKS hematology analyzer
S&T Lalonde hook forceps
Stock
S. eye trephine
S. finger splint
Stocker cyclodiathermy puncture needle
Stockert cardiac pacing electrode
Stockfisch appliance
stockinette
s. amputation bandage
bias s.
s. dressing
impervious s.
orthopaedic s.
sterile s.
Velpeau s.
stocking
adjustable thigh antiembolism s.
antiembolic s.
antiembolism s.
A-T antiembolism s.
Atkins-Tucker antiembolism s.
Bellavar support s.
Camp-Sigvaris s.
Carolon antiembolism s.
CircAid elastic s.
compression s.
Compriform support s.
Comtesse medical support s.
elastic s.
Fast-Fit compression s.
Florex medical compression s.
graduated compression s.
Jobst-Stride support s.
Jobst-Stridette support s.
Jobst Vairox support s.
Jobst VPGS s.
Juzo s.
Juzo-Hostess compression s.
Juzo-Hostess two-way stretch
compression s.
Kendall compression s.
Linton elastic s.
Medi Plus compression s.

Medi-Strumpf s.
Medi vascular s.
Orthawear antiembolism s.
Planostretch s.
pneumatic antiembolic s.
pneumatic compression s.
SCD s.
sequential compression s.
Sigvaris compression s.
Sigvaris medical s.
Silver-Thera s.
Stride support s.
TED antiembolism s.
TheraPress Duo compression s.
TheraPress Duo Lite
compression s.
thigh-high antiembolic s.
thromboembolic disease s.
True Form support s.
Twee alternating cut-off
compressor s.
Vairox high-compression vascular s.
Vairox support s.
Venofit medical compression s.
Venoflex medical compression s.
venous pressure gradient support s.
Zimmer antiembolism s.
Zipzoc medicated s.
Stockman
S. meatal clamp
S. penile clamp
Stoesser stripper
Stokes lens
**Stoller afferent nerve stimulation
system (SANS)**
Stolte
S. capsulorrhexis forceps
S. tonsillar dissector
Stolte-Stille elevator
Stoltz laparoscope
stoma
Bard regular one-piece s.
s. button
s. cone
s. irrigator drain
stoma-centering guide
stomach
s. brush
s. clamp
s. tube
Stomahesive sterile wafer
stomal bag

NOTES

stoma-measuring device
Stomate
    S. decompression tube
    S. extension tube
    S. low-profile gastrostomy kit
stone
    s. basket
    S. clamp-applying forceps
    S. clamp-locking device
    S. Cone nitinol retrieval device
    s. dislodger
    S. eye implant
    s. forceps
    S. intestinal clamp
    S. intestinal forceps
    S. lens nucleus prolapser
    pumice s.
    s. retriever
    s. staple
    S. stomach clamp
    S. tissue forceps
stone-crushing forceps
stone-extraction forceps
stone-grasping forceps
Stone-Holcombe
    S.-H. anastomosis clamp
    S.-H. intestinal clamp
stone-holding basket
Stoneman forceps
stone-retrieval
    s.-r. balloon
    s.-r. basket
stone-tissue
    s.-t. detection system
    s.-t. recognition system
Stonetome stone removal device
Stony splenorenal shunt clamp
Stookey
    S. retractor
    S. rongeur
stool
    s. collector
    Fuchs surgical s.
STOO Series Ten Thousand ocutome
stop
    Bowman needle s.
    s. cock
    s. collar telescope
    Devonshire-Mack s.
    Endo s.
    S. eye speculum
    foot drop s.
    Krueger instrument s.
    s. needle
Stopain analgesic spray
stopcock
    Accel s.
    Burron s.

    Discofix s.
    Luer-Lok s.
4-stopcock manifold
Stop-Leak
    S.-L. gel flotation cushion
    S.-L. gel flotation mattress
Storer thoracoabdominal retractor
Storey
    S. clamp
    S. gall duct forceps
    S. thoracic forceps
Storey-Hillar dissecting forceps
Stormby brush
Stormer balloon catheter
Storm Von Leeuwen chamber
Storq guidewire
Story orbital elevator
Storz
    S. adjustable headrest
    S. anterior commissure
      laryngoscope
    S. arthroscope
    S. aspiration biopsy needle
    S. biopsy forceps
    S. bronchial catheter
    S. bronchoscope
    S. bronchoscopic forceps
    S. bronchoscopic telescope
    S. calipers
    S. camera
    S. cannula
    S. capsular forceps
    S. chalazion trephine
    S. cholangiograsper
    S. ciliary forceps
    S. cleaning brush
    S. continuous-flow resectoscope
      sheath
    S. corneal bur
    S. corneal forceps
    S. corneal trephine
    S. corneoscleral punch
    S. cotton carrier
    S. curved forceps
    S. cystoscope
    S. cystoscopic electrode
    S. cystoscopic forceps
    S. diagnostic/operating laparoscope
    S. direct-view resectoscope
    S. duckbill rongeur
    S. Easy shield
    S. endoscope
    S. esophagoscopic forceps
    S. flexible injection needle
    S. folding-handle ear knife
    S. grasping biopsy forceps
    S. hair transplant trephine
    S. hysteroscope
    S. infant bronchoscope

S. inserter
S. intranasal antral punch
S. intraocular scissors
S. iris hook
S. iris scissors
S. keratome
S. keratometer
S. kidney stone forceps
S. Laparocam
S. Laparoflator insufflator
S. laser
S. laser resectoscope
S. meatal clamp
S. microcalipers
S. microscope
S. MicroSeal
S. microserrefine
S. Millennium microsurgical system
S. miniature forceps
S. Monolith lithotripter
S. nasal speculum
S. nasopharyngeal biopsy forceps
S. needle holder
S. nephroscope
S. operating esophagoscope
S. optical biopsy forceps
S. optical esophagoscope
S. panendoscope
S. pediatric esophagoscope
S. pigtail probe
S. plate
S. Premiere Microvit vitrector
S. radial incision marker
S. rectoscope
S. resectoscope curette
S. retractor
S. rhinomanometer
S. scleral buckling balloon catheter
S. septal speculum
S. sheath
S. sheath-handle ear knife
S. Sine-U-View endoscope
S. sinus biopsy forceps
S. 27022 SK ureteroscope
S. stitch scissors
S. stone-crushing forceps
S. stone dislodger
S. stone-extraction forceps
S. thoracoscope
S. tonometer
S. tracheoscope
S. trocar

S. Universal lens loop
S. urethrotome
S. wire-cutting scissors
Storz-Atlas eye magnet
Storz-Beck tonsillar snare
Storz-Bell erysiphake
Storz-Bonn suturing forceps
Storz-Bowman lacrimal probe
Storz-Bruening
  S.-B. anastigmatic aural magnifier
  S.-B. diagnostic head
Storz-DeKock 2-way bronchial catheter
Storz-Duredge
  S.-D. keratome
  S.-D. steel cataract knife
Storz-Hopkins
  S.-H. bronchoscope
  S.-H. telescope
Storz-Iglesias resectoscope
Storz-Kirkheim urethrotome
Storz-LaForce adenotome
Storz-LaForce-Stevenson adenotome
Storz-Lieberman DiaPhine trephine
Storz-Moltz tonsillectome
Storz-Riecker laryngoscope
Storz-Schitz tonometer
Storz-Shapshay tracheoscope
Storz-Utrata forceps
Storz-Vienna nasal speculum
Storz-Walker retinal detachment unit
Storz-Westcott conjunctival scissors
Stott reformer
Stough punch
stout-neck curette
strabismus
  s. forceps
  s. hook
  s. needle
  s. scissors
straight
  s. bipolar pencil
  s. bistoury
  s. burnisher
  s. catheter guide
  s. chest tube
  s. coagulating forceps
  s. connector
  s. Connor irrigating wand
  s. fissure crosscut bur
  s. flush percutaneous catheter
  s. guidewire
  s. hex screwdriver

S

NOTES

straight *(continued)*
  s. inclined plane elevator
  s. knot-tying forceps
  s. lacrimal cannula
  s. laryngeal mirror
  s. line bayonet forceps
  s. magnifying mirror
  s. Maryland forceps
  s. microbipolar forceps
  s. micromonopolar forceps
  s. microscissors
  s. monopolar electrosurgical dissector
  s. mosquito clamp
  s. mosquito hemostat
  s. nerve hook
  s. osteotome
  s. periosteal elevator
  s. retinal probe
  s. retractor
  s. ring curette
  s. shank bur
  s. single tenaculum forceps
  s. spring-handled microscissors
  s. stent
  s. suturing needle
  s. tenaculum
  s. tenotomy scissors
  s. tying forceps
  s. tympanoplasty knife
  s. walker brace
straight-blade
  s.-b. electrode
  s.-b. laryngoscope
straight-end cup forceps
straightener
  Asch septal s.
  Cottle-Walsham septal s.
  septal s.
  Walsham septal s.
straightening cannula
straight-fibered Guglielmi detachable coil
Straight-In
  S.-I. male sling system
  S.-I. surgical system
straight-needle electrode
StraightShot
  S. arterial cannula
  S. Magnum handpiece
straight-tip
  s.-t. bipolar forceps
  s.-t. electrode
straight-tipped catheter
straight-wire electrode
Straith
  S. chin implant
  S. nasal implant

  S. nasal splint kit
  S. profilometer
Strampelli
  S. eye splint
  S. implant
  S. lens
Strandell retractor
Strandell-Stille
  S.-S. retractor
  S.-S. tendon hook
strands
  AcryDerm s.
  FlexiGel s.
strap
  API Universal foam chin s.
  Band-It tennis elbow s.
  Bard catheter s.
  Bard wide leg bag s.
  Beta Pile II, III splint s.
  buddy s.
  catheter leg s.
  Cho-Pat Achilles tendon s.
  Cho-Pat dual-action knee s.
  Cho-Pat elbow s.
  Cho-Pat knee s.
  Circumpress chin s.
  Conveen leg bag s.
  deluxe leg bag s.
  Dermicel Montgomery s.
  distal over-shoulder s.
  D-ring s.
  DynaWraps s.
  Eclipse gel elbow s.
  EpiLock tennis elbow s.
  extremity mobilization s.
  figure-of-8 clavicle s.
  Fitz-all fabric leg s.
  forearm flexion control s.
  front support s.
  latex rubber tourniquet s.
  leg bag s.
  LEMA s.
  S. Lok ankle brace
  lower extremity mobility aid s.
  Meek-style clavicular s.
  Mentor deluxe leg bag s.
  Montgomery s.
  neoprene wrist s.
  Nylatex s.
  over-shoulder s.
  PIP/DIP s.
  proximal over-shoulder s.
  QualCraft s.
  Rotalok wrist s.
  Rusch head s.
  Self Snag s.
  Silastic s.
  stretch-out s.
  tourniquet s.

Strap-Pad
Daw S.-P.
strapping
loop & hook s.
LowDye s.
Strasbourg-Fairfax in vitro fertilization needle
Strassburger tissue forceps
Strassmann uterine forceps
Strata
S. hip stem
S. hip system
strata
ProForm s.
Stratasis urethral sling
StrataSorb composite dressing
Strategy coronary wire guide
Stratis II MRI system
Stratos orthotic
Stratte
S. forceps
S. kidney clamp
S. needle holder
Stratus impact reducing pylon
Straus curved retrobulbar needle
Strauss
S. cannula
S. meatal clamp
S. penile clamp
S. sigmoidoscope
Strauss-Valentine penile clamp
Strayer meniscal knife
Streak resectoscope
2-stream irrigating forceps
Streamline peripheral catheter
Strecker
S. balloon-expandable esophageal stent
S. coronary stent
S. tantalum stent
Street pin
Streli forceps
Strelinger
S. catheter-introducing forceps
S. colon clamp
Strempel dermatome
stress
s. echo bed
low-contact s. (LCS)
StressCath catheter
Stress-Ray varus-valgus device

stretch
S. balloon
S. cardiac device
S. gauze roll
S. and Heel Night splint
S. Net wound dressing
static adjustable s. (SAS)
stretcher
Brandy front closure scalp s.
Kuttner wound s.
Lumex shower s.
shoe s.
stretch-out strap
Stretta catheter
Stretzer bent-tip USCI catheter
striascope
Stribs strut
Strichman SME-810 camera
stricturotome
Stallard s.
Werb angled s.
Stride
S. analyzer
S. cardiac pacemaker
S. support stocking
string drawing board
Stringer
S. catheter-introducing forceps
S. newborn throat forceps
S. tracheal catheter
stringing peg
strip
blood glucose reagent s.
bovine pericardium s.
boxing s.
Breathe Right nasal s.
CarraGauze packing s.
Codman surgical s.
Color Bar Schirmer s.
ColorpHast pH indicator s.
Cover-Strip wound closure s.
demineralized flexible laminar bone s.
DermAssist hydrogel packing s.
DisIntek reagent s.
Excel GE blood glucose monitoring test s.
EyeClose adhesive s.
flexible laminar bone s.
Fluor-i-Strip ophthalmic s.
G-C polishing s.
GHM polishing s.

NOTES

S

strip *(continued)*
    Gore-Tex s.
    LC s.
    leucocyte detection s.
    Medline packing s.
    Microflo test s.
    Mosher s.
    Multistix Pro urinalysis test s.
    Neuray neurosurgical s.
    Nu-Hope skin barrier s.
    Pacific Coast flexible laminar
      bone s.
    packing s.
    PD polishing s.
    Peri-Strips Dry s.
    Peri-Strips Dry pericardial s.
    plastic s.
    polishing s.
    PTS Panels test s.
    Raven Bacterial Spore s.'s
    Schirmer tear test s.
    silicone s.
    Silverlon wound packing s.
    Sleep Right nasal s.
    Suture S.
    Suture Strip Plus wound closure s.
    tear s.
    Telfa s.
    Thera-Band s.
    UC s.
    Urihesive moldable adhesive s.
    Urofoam-1, -2 adhesive foam s.
    Visidex II blood glucose testing s.

stripper
    Babcock jointed vein s.
    Bartlett fascial s.
    Brand tendon s.
    Bunnell tendon s.
    Bunt tendon s.
    Carroll forearm tendon s.
    chest tube s.
    Codman vein s.
    Cole polyethylene vein s.
    Crawford fascial s.
    Crile vagotomy s.
    DeBakey intraluminal s.
    Doyen rib s.
    Doyle vein s.
    Dunlop thrombus s.
    Emerson vein s.
    Endostat fiber s.
    external vein s.
    fascial s.
    fascia lata s.
    Fischer tendon s.
    Friedman olive-tip vein s.
    Grierson tendon s.
    Hall-Chevalier s.
    hydraulic vein s.

    IM tendon s.
    interchangeable vein s.
    intraluminal s.
    Joplin tendon s.
    Keeley vein s.
    Kurtin vein s.
    LaVeen helical s.
    Lempka vein s.
    Levy-Okun s.
    Linton vein s.
    Martin endarterectomy s.
    Masson fascial s.
    Matson-Alexander rib s.
    Matson-Mead periosteum s.
    Matson rib s.
    Mayo external vein s.
    Mayo-Myers external vein s.
    Meyer olive-tipped vein s.
    Meyer spiral vein s.
    Nabatoff vein s.
    Nelson rib s.
    Nelson-Roberts s.
    New Orleans endarterectomy s.
    Oesch s.
    orthopaedic surgical s.
    Phelan vein s.
    pigtail tendon s.
    Price-Thomas rib s.
    ramus s.
    rib edge s.
    ring s.
    Roberts-Nelson rib s.
    Samuels vein s.
    Shaw carotid artery clot s.
    slotted tendon s.
    Smith posterior cartilage s.
    spiral vein s.
    Stoesser s.
    Stukey s.
    surgical s.
    tendon s.
    thrombus s.
    Trace hydraulic vein s.
    vagotomy s.
    vein s.
    Verner s.
    Webb interchangable vein s.
    Wilson vein s.
    Wurth vein s.
    Wylie endarterectomy s.
    Zollinger-Gilmore vein s.
    zonule s.

Stripseal catheter
Strobex Mark II electrosurgical unit
stroboscope
    Kay rhinolaryngeal s.
    rhinolarynx s.
Stromeyer splint
Stromgren ankle brace

Stronghands hand exerciser
strontium-90 ophthalmic beta ray
    applicator
Stropko irrigator
Stroud-Baron ear suction tube
Strow corneal forceps
Strubel lid everter
Struck spreader
structured coil electromagnet
Struempel
    S. ear alligator forceps
    S. ear punch forceps
    S. rongeur
Struempel-Voss
    S.-V. ethmoidal forceps
    S.-V. nasal forceps
Strully
    S. cardiovascular scissors
    S. dissecting scissors
    S. dressing forceps
    S. dural scissors
    S. dural twist hook
    S. Gigli-saw handle
    S. hook scissors
    S. nerve root retractor
    S. neurosurgical scissors
    S. ruptured-disc curette
    S. tissue forceps
Strully-Kerrison rongeur
2 × 2 strung sponge
strut
    Adkins s.
    Anderson nasal s.
    s. bar
    s. bar hook
    s. calipers
    s. forceps
    s. graft
    Harrington s.
    House calipers s.
    Judet s.
    Magnuson s.
    s. measuring instrument
    miniplate s.
    Nalebuff-Goldman s.
    s. pick
    polyethylene s.
    Rehbein internal steel s.
    Robinson s.
    stent s.
    Stribs s.
    Teflon s.

TORP s.
    tricuspid valve s.
    valve outflow s.
    wire-loop s.
strut-type pin
Struyken
    S. angular punch tip
    S. conchotome
    S. ear forceps
    S. nasal-cutting forceps
    S. nasal forceps
    S. punch
    S. turbinate forceps
Stryker
    S. arthrometer
    S. arthroscope
    S. autopsy saw
    S. blade
    S. bur
    S. cartilage knife
    S. cast cutter
    S. chip camera
    S. chondrotome
    S. CircOlectric bed
    S. CircOlectric fracture frame
    S. CPM exerciser
    S. drain
    S. drill
    S. fracture table
    S. lag screw
    S. leg exerciser
    S. PainPump pump
    S. power instrumentation
    S. resector
    S. Rolo-dermatome
    S. screwdriver
    S. SE3 arthroscopy system
    S. shaver
    S. stent
    S. suction irrigator
    S. turning fracture frame
    S. wedge suture anchor
Stryker-School meniscal knife
STS
    Shockwave Therapy Systems
    STS lithotripsy system
    STS molding sock
Stuart
    S. articulator
    S. Gordon hand splint
Stubbs adenoidal curette

NOTES

Stuckrad magnifying laryngopharyngoscope
Stuck self-retaining laminectomy retractor
Studer pouch
study
    IsoStents for Restenosis Intervention S. (IRIS)
Stuhler-Heise fixator
Stukey stripper
Stulberg
    S. HIPciser abduction splint
    S. hip positioner
    S. Mark II leg positioner
Stumer perforating bur
Sturmdorf
    S. cervical needle
    S. cervical reamer
    S. pedicle needle
    S. suture
Stutsman nasal snare
STx Saunders lumbar disc device
Stycar graded ball
Styles forceps
stylet
    Bard malleable tip catheter s.
    Bing s.
    Bruening forceps s.
    cardiovascular s.
    Cook locking s.
    Cooper endotracheal s.
    endotracheal s.
    Frazier s.
    Frigitronics disposable cryosurgical s.
    illuminating s.
    Inrad HiLiter ultrasound-enhanced s.
    S. internal esophageal MRI coil
    Jelco intravenous s.
    jet s.
    K s.
    Liberator Universal locking s.
    lighted s.
    locking s.
    Malis irrigating forceps s.
    malleable s.
    MAPcath s.
    Rumel ratchet tourniquet eyed s.
    S s.
    surgical s.
    The Hockey Stick articulating s.
    tourniquet-eyed ratchet s.
    Trachlight lighted intubating s.
    transmyocardial pacing s.
    transthoracic pacing s.
    Tubestat lighted s.
    ureteral s.
    wire s.

stylus
    S. cardiovascular suture
    IM/EM tibial resection s.
    S. suture needle
    tibial s.
S-type dental implant
Styrofoam dressing
Suarez
    S. continence ring
    S. retractor
    S. spreader
subannular mattress suture
subarachnoid screw
subclavian
    s. apheresis catheter
    s. cannula
    s. dialysis catheter
    s. hemodialysis catheter
    s. vein access catheter
Subco needle
subconjunctival needle
subcostal trocar
subcutaneous
    s. augmentation material (SAM)
    s. insulin infusion pump
    s. morphine pump
    s. patch electrode
    s. polytef patch
subcuticular suture
subdermal implant
subdural
    s. grid electrode
    s. strip electrode
subduroperitoneal shunt
subgaleal drain
subglottic forceps
subglottiscope
    Healy-Jako pediatric s.
sublaminar wire
Sub-Lite-Wall tubing
submammary dissector
submicroinfusion catheter
submucosal implant
submucous
    s. chisel
    s. curette
    s. dissector
    s. retractor
Subortholen sheet
subpectoral stabilizer
subperiosteal
    s. implant
    s. tissue expander
Sub-Q-Set subcutaneous continuous infusion device
Subramanian sidewinder aortic clamp
subretinal fluid cannula
Subrini penile prosthesis

substitute
> AlloMatrix injectable putty bone
>   graft s.
> Biobrane/HF experimental skin s.
> Biobrane skin s.
> Calcigen-S calcium sulfate bone s.
> Centurion gel moisturizer saliva s.
> Dermagraft skin s.
> Dermagraft-TC temporary skin s.
> dural s.
> Durashield dural s.
> HemAssist blood s.
> OrthoDyn bone s.
> OsteoDONTEX bone graft s.
> OsteoSet bone graft s.
> PerioDontex bone graft s.
> Rapidgraft arterial vessel s.
> Thoralon biomaterial TransCyte
>   skin s.
> TransCyte temporary skin s.
> U-channel stripping dural s.

sub-tenon anesthesia cannula
subtraction
> intraarterial digital s. (IDIS)

suburethral sling
Sub-Vent implant system
sucker
> Churchill s.
> intercardiac s.
> intracardiac s.
> Kam Super S.
> malleable s.
> s. shaver
> s. tip

suction
> s. adapter
> s. apparatus
> s. aspirator
> Barton s.
> s. biopsy curette
> s. biopsy needle
> s. biter
> Bowen s.
> S. Buster catheter
> s. cannula
> s. catheter
> s. cautery
> s. connector
> s. cup
> s. cylinder
> s. dissector
> s. drain

> ear forceps with s.
> s. elevator
> Ferguson s.
> s. forceps
> Frazier s.
> s. irrigator
> s. magnet
> Ortholav s.
> perilimbal s.
> Pleur-evac s.
> s. probe
> s. punch
> s. retractor
> s. ring
> Rosen s.
> SureTran s.
> s. tip
> s. tip curette
> Tis-U-Trap endometrial s.
> s. tube
> s. tube holder
> Wangensteen s.

suction-coagulation tube
suction-coagulator
suction/irrigation tube
suction-irrigator
> Brackmann s.-i.
> FlowGun s.-i.
> Jako s.-i.
> Kurze s.-i.
> Nezhat-Dorsey s.-i.
> PMT MacroVac s.-i.
> William-House s.-i.

Sudan needle
Sudarsky cryoprobe
Sudbury system
Suetens-Gybels-Vandermeulen
** angiographic localizer**
Sugar aneurysm clip
Sugarbaker retrocolic clamp
Sugar-Chex II glucose control
sugar-tong
> s.-t. cast
> s.-t. splint

Suggs catheter
Sugita
> S. aneurysm clip
> S. catheter
> S. cross-legged clip
> S. head clamp
> S. head holder
> S. jaws clip applier

S

NOTES

Sugita (*continued*)
    S. microsurgical table
    S. multipurpose head frame
    S. retractor
    S. side-curved bayonet clip
    S. temporary straight clip
Sugita-Ikakogyo clip
Suh ventilation tube
suit
    anti-G s.
    antigravity s.
    antishock s.
    Life S.
    MAST s.
    shock s.
    total-body compression s.
Suker
    S. cyclodialysis spatula
    S. iris forceps
    S. spatula knife
Sukhtian-Hughes fixation device
Sulcabrush brush
Sulfix-6 cement
Sullival gum scissors
Sullivan
    S. bubble cushion
    S. HumidAire heated humidifier
    S. III CPAP
    S. variable stiffness cable
Sully shoulder stabilizer brace
SULP II balloon catheter
Sulze diamond-point needle
Sulzer prosthesis
Summar alloy
SummaSketch III digitizing board
Summit
    S. alloy
    S. channel plate fixation system
    S. Excimed UV 200 laser
    S. Krumeich-Barraquer
      microkeratome
    S. Omnimed excimer laser
    S. rod fixation system
    S. SVS Apex Plus excimer laser
Sumner clamp
sump
    Argyle silicone Salem s.
    Cooley ventricular s.
    DLP pericardial s.
    s. drain
    s. drainage catheter
    Grice laparoscopic s.
    s. pump
    s. tube
    ventricular s.
Sumpter clasp spring-lock
SunBox light therapy box
sunburst mechanism
Sunday staphylorrhaphy elevator

Sundt
    S. AVM clip system
    S. booster clip
    S. carotid endarterectomy shunt
    S. cross-legged clip
    S. encircling clip
    S. hemodynamic shunt
    S. straddling clip
    S. suction system
Sundt-Kees
    S.-K. aneurysm clip
    S.-K. booster clip
    S.-K. encircling patch clip
    S.-K. Slimline clip
Sung reverse nucleus chopper
Sunrise LTK system
Sun SPARCstation system
SunVideo frame grabber
Super
    S. Arrow-Flex catheterization sheath
    S. Arrow-Flex transseptal sheath
      introducer
    S. Constructa foam
    S. Cut laminectomy rongeur
    S. Eidersoft bed pad
    S. Field NC slit lamp lens
    S. M vacuum extractor cup
    S. Pak posterior nasal pack
    S. Pinky ball
    S. Pinky pressure device
    S. Revo suture anchor
    S. Stimm MF stimulator
    S. Torque Plus catheter
Super-4 catheter ablation system
Super-9 guiding catheter
super-absorptive polymer dressing
Superblade
    Bishop-Harman S.
SuperCat self-tapping implant
SuperClearPro suction socket
superconducting
    s. magnet
    s. quantum interference device
superconductive
    s. magnetic system
Supercut
    S. blade
    S. diamond bur
    S. scissors
Super-Dent orthodontic cement
SuperEBA cement
superficial implant
superfine
    s. fiberscope
    S. Microbrush brush
Superflex elastic dressing
Superflow guiding catheter
Superform Contours orthotic
Superglue adhesive

superior
    s. border plate
    s. rectus forceps
    S. suction catheter
Super-Plus Trimshield pad
SuperQuad assistive device
Superscript preamplification system
Superselector Y-K guidewire
Superset exercise system
SuperSkin thin film dressing
Super-Soft denture reliner
Superstabilizer
    S. cemented stem extender
    S. press-fit stem extender
super-stiff guidewire
SuperStitch vascular closure device
Supertorque MB 5F marker band flush catheter
Super-Trac adhesive traction dressing
supervoltage generator
super wrap
supine
    S. C-Trax cervical traction system
    s. driver nail drill sleeve
Supolene suture
supply
    Air S.
    Japanese Medical S. (JMS)
    Kinder Incontinence S.'s (KINS)
support
    Achillotrain active Achilles tendon s.
    Act joint s.
    Airprene hinged knee s.
    AliMed Freedom arthritis s.
    AliMed QualCraft neoprene thigh s.
    AliMed QualCraft wrist s.
    arch s.
    BabyHugger prenatal back and abdominal s.
    Back-Huggar lumbar s.
    BackThing lumbar s.
    BIOflex magnet lumbar back s.
    BioSkin s.
    BioWrap s.
    Birkenstock blue footbed arch s.
    Birkenstock high-flange arch s.
    Body Gard neoprene s.
    Carabelt lower back s.
    Carabelt lumbar s.
    Castech extremity s.

    chin s.
    ChiroFlow adjustable back s.
    Cho-Pat ankle s.
    cock-up wrist s.
    Comfort Cool neoprene s.
    Comprifix ankle s.
    Conve back s.
    Corfit System 7000 Series lumbosacral s.
    Dale oxygen cannula s.
    Dale ventilator tubing s.
    DayTimer carpal tunnel s.
    DePuy s.
    Desk-Rest arm s.
    Dr. Gibaud thermal health s.
    Dr. Kho's CMC S.
    EpiLock tennis elbow s.
    Epitrain active elastic elbow s.
    Ergo Cush back s.
    Ezy Wrap lumbosacral s.
    Firm D-Ring wrist s.
    flat brain spatula s.
    FlexLite hinged knee s.
    Foot Hugger foot s.
    Freedom arthritis s.
    Freedom back s.
    Freedom Elastic Long Wrist S.
    Futuro wrist s.
    Genutrain P3 active knee s.
    geriatric chair trunk s.
    Grotena abdominal s.
    Hand-Aid arterial wrist s.
    IMP-Capello arm s.
    Kallassy ankle s.
    lateral lumbar s.
    Lo Bak spinal s.
    Malleo-med soft ankle s.
    MalleoTrain ankle s.
    ManuTrain wrist s.
    McKenzie AirBack s.
    MKG knee s.
    Mold-In-Place back s.
    Momma-Too Maternity S.
    Monitor Master monitor s.
    Morton toe s.
    Mother-To-Be abdominal s.
    MouseMitt Keyboarders wrist s.
    neck s.
    Nek-L-O orthopaedic s.
    neoprene ankle s.
    neoprene back s.
    Nightimer carpal tunnel s.

S

NOTES

support *(continued)*
 Norco ulnar deviation s.
 Obus back s.
 Olympia Vacpac s.
 OmoTrain shoulder s.
 Orion lumbar s.
 OrthoKnit joint s.
 Ortho-Pal body s.
 OSI Well Leg S.
 oxygen cannula s.
 Parham s.
 Patellamed knee s.
 PattStrap knee s.
 percutaneous cardiopulmonary
  bypass s.
 Plastazote arch s.
 postoperative mammary s.
 ProFlex wrist s.
 QualCraft ankle s.
 QualCraft short elastic wrist s.
 Rolyan foot s.
 sacral s.
 Safe spine thoracic-lumbar-sacral s.
 Schiek back s.
 Schillinger suture s.
 Scully Hip S'port functional hip s.
 ShiatsuBACK s.
 Shoulder Ease abduction s.
 Shoulder-Float adjustable axillary s.
 Sidekick foot s.
 Spenco Orthotic arch s.
 S'port Max back s.
 StanceGuard internal s.
 Surgi-Bra breast s.
 Taylor clavicle s.
 Tecnol back s.
 Tecnol hand-aid wrist s.
 Tecnol Rebound neoprene elbow s.
 Tecnol Rebound neoprene knee s.
 Thermo comforter hand s.
 Thermo comforter knee s.
 Thompson chin s.
 Three-D worker's back s.
 Warm 'n Form lumbosacral
  back s.
 wedge-shaped s.
 well-leg s.
 Whitman arch s.
 Wristaleve s.
supracondylar
 s. knee-ankle-foot orthosis
 s. nail
 s. plate
 s. socket
SupraFoley
 S. suprapubic catheter
 S. suprapubic introducer
suprahepatic caval clamp

Supralen
 S. cradle orthotic
 S. Schaefer orthotic
supramalleolar orthosis
Supramead nose splint
Supramid
 S. collagen suture
 S. Extra suture
 S. graft
 S. implant
 S. lens
 S. occluding stent
 S. polyamide mesh
 S. prosthesis
 S. sheet
 S. snare
 S. suture
Supramid-Allen implant
suprapubic
 s. cannula
 s. catheter (SC)
 s. hemostatic bag
 s. self-retaining retractor
 s. trocar
suprarenal Greenfield filter
SupraSLEEVES nylon sleeve
Supreme
 S. electrophysiology catheter
 S. II blood glucose meter
Suraci
 S. elevator hook
 S. zygoma hook elevator
Surbaugh legholder
Surcan
 S. knee holder
 S. leg holder
Sur-Catch paired-wire basket
Sur-Cut guillotine knife
Sure
 S. Seal Golden Drain catheter
 S. Sport pad
 S. Step ankle support system
 S. Step brace
SureBite biopsy forceps
Surecan safety Huber needle
SureCare/Medical disposable underpad
SureCath port access catheter
Sure-Closure
 S.-C. closure
 S.-C. skin stretching system
 S.-C. wound closure tape
SureCuff tissue ingrowth cuff
Sure-Cut biopsy needle
Surefit intraocular lens
Sure-Flex III prosthetic foot
SureFlex nickel-titanium file
Sure-Gait folding walker

SureGrip
S. manual resuscitator
S. resuscitation bag
SureLine skin stapler
Surelite blood lancet
SurePress
S. absorbent padding
S. compression dressing
S. compression wrap
S. high compression bandage
SureScan
S. scanning handpiece
S. system
Sureseal
S. cellulose sponge bandage
S. pressure bandage
Suresharp
S. blood collecting needle
S. dental needle
SureSight vision screener
SureSite transparent adhesive film dressing
Sure-Snare tourniquet
SureStart
S. contrast tracking system
S. imaging system
SureStep
S. glucose meter
S. glucose monitor
SureStepPro professional blood glucose management system
Suretac fixation device
SureTemp4 oral thermometer
SureTemp electronic thermometer
SureTrans autotransfusion system
SureTran suction
Surety shield
Surevue contact lens
Surewing winged infusion set
surface
Advance Zoneaire sleep s.
Alpha Active pressure-relieving support s.
Carmeda BioActive s.
s. coil
DeCube therapeutic s.
DermaGard II seating s.
DermaGard Triad seating s.
s. electrode
Isch-Dish CFT pressure-relieving seat s.
NewLife therapeutic s.

surface-coil MRI
Surfasoft dressing
Sur-Fast needle
Sur-Fit
S.-F. colostomy bag
S.-F. colostomy irrigation sleeve
S.-F. disposable convex insert
S.-F. flange cap
S.-F. flexible and drainable pouch
S.-F. irrigation adapter faceplate
S.-F. irrigation sleeve tail closure
S.-F. loop ostomy rod
S.-F. minipouch
S.-F. Natura pouch
S.-F. night drainage container tubing
S.-F. urinary drainage bag
S.-F. urostomy pouch
S.-F. wafer
Sur-Fit/Active Life tail closure
Surfit adhesive
Surflo
S. IV catheter
S. winged infusion set
Surgairtome air drill
Surgaloy metallic suture
Surgamid polyamide suture material
SurgAssist
S. leg positioner
S. surgical leg holder
Surgenomic endoscope
Surgeons Choice surgical stapler
surgery
Bosker TMI s.
computer-assisted stereotactic s. (CASS)
Elite Farley retractor for spinal s.
fracture computer-aided s. (FRACAS)
InstaTrak System image-guided s.
microincision cataract s. (MICS)
percutaneous vascular s.
Surg-E-Trol
S.-E.-T. I/A/R system
S.-E.-T. I/A system
SurgiBlade laser
Surgibone
Unilab S.
Surgi-Bra breast support
Surgica K6 laser
surgical
s. appliance

S

NOTES

surgical *(continued)*
s. aspirator
s. binder
s. bur
s. cannula
s. chromic suture
s. clip
s. clip applier
s. compression garment
s. drape
s. dressing
s. electrode
s. exhaust apparatus
s. file
s. gouge
s. gut suture
s. hammer
s. handle
s. hood
s. instrument guide
s. keratometer
s. laser
S. Laser Technologies (SLT)
s. loupe
s. mallet
s. marking pen
s. mask
s. mesh
s. microscope
s. nerve stimulator
S. Nu-Knit collagen hemostatic material
s. orthopaedic drill
s. otoscope
S. Patient Arm shield
s. pedestal
s. retractor
s. saddle
s. saw
s. saw blade
s. silk suture
S. Simplex P radiopaque adhesive
S. Simplex P radiopaque bone cement
s. simulator
s. snare
s. spatula
s. stapling gun
s. steel suture
s. stripper
s. stylet
s. suction pump
s. telescope
Surgicel
S. collagen hemostatic material
S. fibrillar absorbable hemostat
S. gauze
S. gauze dressing

S. implant
S. Nu-Knit
S. Nu-Knit absorbable hemostat
S. Nu-Knit absorbable hemostatic material
S. Nu-Knit dressing
Surgicenter 40 CO_2 laser
Surgiclip
S. clip applier
McDermott S.
McFadden S.
Surgicraft
S. pacemaker electrode
S. suture
S. suture needle
Surgicraft-Copeland fetal scalp electrode
Surgicutt incision device
Surgidac suture
Surgidev
S. iris clip
S. Leiske anterior chamber intraocular lens
S. suture
Surgidine sponge
Surgi-Fine reusable cannula tip
SurgiFish visceral retainer
Surgifix dressing
Surgiflex
S. bandage
S. dressing
S. WAVE XP suction-irrigation system
Surgi-Flo leg bag
Surgifoam absorbable gelatin sponge
Surgigut suture
Surgikit Velcro tourniquet
Surgikos disposable drape
Surgilar suture
Surgilase
S. CO_2 laser
S. 150 high-powered CO_2 laser
S. Nd:YAG laser
Surgilast tubular elastic dressing
SurgiLav Plus irrigator
Surgilene monofilament suture
SurgiLight OptiVision YAG laser
Surgiloid suture
Surgilon
S. braided nylon suture
S. monofilament polypropylene suture
Surg-I-Loop silicone loop
Surgilope suture
SurgiMate skin stapler
SurgiMed
S. clamp
S. suture
S. umbiliclamp

Surgimedics
> S. cholangiography catheter
> S. TMP air aspirator needle

Surgin
> S. hemorrhage occluder pin
> S. insufflation tubing

Surgineedle pneumoperitoneum needle
Surgi-Pad combined dressing
SurgiPeace analgesia pump
Surgi-PEG replacement gastrostomy feeding system
Surgiport
> S. disposable trocar
> S. stapler

Surgi-Prep sponge brush
Surgi-Press pressure infuser
Surgipro
> S. mesh
> S. monofilament polypropylene suture
> S. prolene mesh
> S. suture

Surgipulse XJ 150 CO$_2$ laser
SurgiScope navigational device
Surgiscribe surgical marking pen
Surgiset suture
SurgiSis
> S. Gold hernia repair graft
> S. mesh
> S. sling

Surgi-Site Incise drape
Surgi-Spec telescope
Surgistar
> S. corneal trephine
> S. ophthalmic blade

Surgi Stim postsurgical therapy system
SurgiStitch
> Auto Suture S.

Surgitable hand surgery table
Surgitek
> S. button
> S. Double-J II closed-tip ureteral stent
> S. Double-J ureteral catheter
> S. Flexi-Flate II penile implant
> S. graduated cystoscope
> S. handpiece
> S. mammary implant
> S. OM-5 urodynamic system
> S. One Step percutaneous endoscopic gastrostomy
> S. penile prosthesis

> S. Quadra-Coil ureteral stent
> S. UroPass II ureteral stent

Surgitite ligating loop
Surgitome bur
Surgitron
> S. portable radiosurgical unit
> S. radiofrequency unit
> S. ultrasound-assisted lipoplasty machine
> S. 3000 ultrasound device

Surgi-Tron thoracoscopic instrument
Surgitube
> S. dressing
> S. tubular gauze

Surgivac drain
Surgiview multi-use laparoscope
Surgi-Vision
> S.-V. Intercept urethral coil
> S.-V. internal MR coil

Surgiwand suction/irrigation device
Surgiwip suture ligature
Surgtech glove
Surpass
> S. catheter
> S. guidewire

Surusil braided silk suture
Surveyor monitor
SURx transvaginal system
Suspend
> S. sling
> S. Tutoplast processed fascia lata

suspended operating illuminator
suspension
> s. apparatus
> s. laryngoscope

suspension-type socket
suspensor
> elastic s.

suspensory
> s. bandage
> s. dressing

Sussman 4-mirror gonioscope
Sustagen nasogastric tube
Sustain
> S. dental implant system
> S. HA-coated threaded implant
> S. hydroxyapatite biointegrated dental implant

sustainer
> Akahoshi nucleus s.

Sutcliffe laser shield

S

NOTES

Sutherland
- S. lens
- S. rotatable intraocular forceps
- S. scissors
- S. vitreous forceps

Sutherland-Grieshaber
- S.-G. forceps
- S.-G. scissors
- S.-G. speculum

Sutralon suture

SutraSilk suture

Sutter
- S. double-stem silicone implant prosthesis
- S. hinged great toe implant
- S. MCP finger joint prosthesis

Sutter-CPM knee device

Sutter-Smeloff heart valve prosthesis

Sutton biopsy needle

Sutupak suture

Suturamid suture

Sutura Superstitch vascular closure device

suture
- absorbable s.
- Acier stainless steel s.
- Acufex bioabsorbable Suretac s.
- Acutrol s.
- alar cinch s.
- Alcon nylon s.
- aluminum-bronze wire s.
- American silk s.
- Ancap braided silk s.
- s. anchor
- s. applicator
- Arthrex Bio-Corkscrew s.
- Arthrex FiberWire s.
- S. Assistant
- S. Assistant system
- atraumatic braided silk s.
- atraumatic chromic s.
- Aureomycin s.
- Barraquer silk s.
- bastard s.
- basting s.
- Biosyn s.
- black braided nylon s.
- black braided silk s.
- black twisted s.
- Blalock s.
- blanket s.
- blue-black monofilament s.
- blue twisted cotton s.
- bolster s.
- Bondek absorbable s.
- bone wax s.
- Bozeman s.
- braided Ethibond s.
- braided Mersilene s.
- braided Nurolon s.
- braided nylon s.
- braided polyamide s.
- braided polyester s.
- braided silk s.
- braided Vicryl s.
- braided wire s.
- Bralon s.
- bridle s.
- bronze wire s.
- Brown-Sharp gauge s.
- Bunnell wire pull-out s.
- s. button
- cable wire s.
- capitonnage s.
- Caprolactam s.
- Caprosyn s.
- cardinal s.
- Cardioflon s.
- Cardionyl s.
- cardiovascular Prolene s.
- cardiovascular silk s.
- Carrel s.
- s. carrier
- catgut s.
- celluloid linen s.
- Chinese fingertrap s.
- Chinese twisted silk s.
- chloramine catgut s.
- chromated catgut s.
- chromic blue dyed gut s.
- chromic catgut s.
- chromic collagen s.
- chromic gut s.
- chromicized catgut s.
- circular s.
- s. clip forceps
- coated polyester s.
- coated Vicryl Rapide s.
- cocoon thread s.
- collagen s.
- compound s.
- Connell s.
- coronal s.
- cotton Deknatel s.
- cotton nonabsorbable s.
- cottony Dacron tape s.
- cranial s.
- s. cushion
- Czerny s.
- Czerny-Lembert s.
- Dacron bolstered s.
- Dacron traction s.
- Dafilon s.
- Dagrofil s.
- Davis-Geck s.
- deep dermal s.
- Deklene II polypropylene s.
- Deknatel silk s.

DermaGlide cosmetic surgery s.
dermal s.
Dermalon cuticular s.
Dexon absorbable s.
Dexon II s.
Dexon Plus s.
DG Softgut s.
Docktor s.
double-armed s.
double-running penetrating
  keratoplasty s.
Dupuytren s.
Edinburgh s.
EEA Auto S.
elastic s.
Endoknot s.
Endoloop s.
ePTFE vascular s.
Ethibond polybutilate-coated
  polyester s.
Ethibond polyester s.
Ethicon Micropoint s.
Ethicon Sabreloc s.
Ethicon silk s.
Ethilon nylon s.
Ethi-pack s.
expanded polytetrafluoroethylene s.
FiberWire s.
figure-of-8 s.
filament s.
fine chromic s.
fine silk s.
fingertrap s.
Flaxedil s.
Flexon steel s.
Foster s.
Frater s.
Frost s.
Gaillard-Arlt s.
Gambee s.
gastrointestinal s.
gastrointestinal surgical gut s.
gastrointestinal surgical linen s.
gastrointestinal surgical silk s.
Gély s.
general closure s.
Gillies horizontal dermal s.
GI pop-off silk s.
glue-in s.
Gore-Tex s.
Gould s.
Grams nylon nonabsorbable s.

Gramsorb s.
Grams polypropylene
  nonabsorbable s.
Grams silk nonabsorbable s.
green braided s.
green Mersilene s.
green monofilament
  polyglyconate s.
groove s.
s. guide
Gussenbauer s.
gut s.
Guyton-Friedenwald s.
Halsted mattress s.
Heaney s.
heavy monofilament s.
heavy retention s.
heavy silk retention s.
heavy wire s.
helical s.
hemostatic s.
Herculon s.
s. holder
s. hole drill
s. hook
Horsley s.
Hu-Friedy PermaSharp s.
IKI catgut s.
India rubber s.
interrupted pledgeted s.
intraluminal s.
Investa s.
iodine catgut s.
iodized surgical gut s.
iodochromic catgut s.
Ivalon s.
Jobert de Lamballe s.
Kal-Dermic s.
kangaroo tendon s.
Kessler-Kleinert s.
Kirschner s.
Krackow s.
Küstner s.
lacidem s.
lambdoidal s.
s. lancet
lancet s.
Lang s.
lateral trap s.
lead s.
lead-shot tie s.
LeFort s.

NOTES

S

suture *(continued)*
    Lembert s.
    Ligapak s.
    Linatrix s.
    Lindner corneoscleral s.
    linen s.
    Linvatec meniscal BioStinger
      anchor s.
    S. Lok device
    Look s.
    Lukens catgut s.
    malar periosteum-SMAS flap
      fixation s.
    Mannis s.
    Marlex s.
    Maxam s.
    Maxon absorbable s.
    Maxon polyglyconate
      monofilament s.
    Mayo linen s.
    McCannel s.
    McLean s.
    Measuroll s.
    Medrafil wire s.
    Meigs s.
    Mersilene braided nonabsorbable s.
    Mersilk s.
    metallic s.
    Micrins microsurgical s.
    Micro-Glide corneal s.
    MicroMite anchor s.
    Millipore s.
    Miralene s.
    Monocryl poliglecaprone s.
    monofilament absorbable s.
    monofilament clear s.
    monofilament green s.
    monofilament nylon s.
    monofilament polypropylene s.
    monofilament skin s.
    monofilament steel s.
    monofilament wire s.
    Monograms s.
    Monosof s.
    Monosyn s.
    multifilament steel s.
    multistrand s.
    nasofrontal s.
    natural s.
    s. needle
    neurosurgical s.
    Nissen s.
    nonabsorbable s.
    nonabsorbable surgical s.
    Novafil s.
    Nurolon s.
    nylon 66 s.
    nylon monofilament s.
    nylon retention s.

oiled silk s.
Ophthalon s.
Oyloidin s.
Pagedas self-locking s.
Pagenstecher linen thread s.
Palfyn s.
Panacryl absorbable s.
Panalok absorbable s.
Pancoast s.
Paré s.
Parker-Kerr basting s.
s. passer
PDS II Endoloop s.
PDS Vicryl s.
Pearsall Chinese twisted s.
Pearsall silk s.
Perlon s.
Perma-Hand braided silk s.
pin s.
pink twisted cotton s.
plain catgut s.
plain collagen s.
plain gut s.
plastic s.
pledget s.
pledgeted Ethibond s.
pledgeted mattress s.
poliglecaprone 25 s.
polyamide s.
polybutester s.
Polydek s.
polydioxanone s. (PDS)
polyester fiber s.
polyethylene s.
polyfilament s.
polygalactic acid s.
polyglactin 910 s.
polyglecaprone 25 s.
polyglycolate s.
polyglycolic acid s.
polyglyconate s.
polypropylene button s.
Polysorb s.
pop-off s.
Premilene nonabsorbable s.
presphenoethmoid s.
Prolene s.
Prolene polypropylene s.
Pronova s.
Pulvertaft s.
s. punch
Purlon s.
pyoktanin catgut s.
pyroglycolic acid s.
Quickert s.
Ramsey County pyoktanin catgut s.
Rankin s.
Rapide wound s.
RB1 s.

reabsorbable s
Reo Macrode
ribbon gut s.
s. ring
rip-cord s.
rubber s.
running nylon penetrating
  keratoplasty s.
Sabreloc s.
Saenger s.
safety-bolt s.
Safil synthetic absorbable
  surgical s.
serrated s.
seton s.
Sharpoint ophthalmic
  microsurgical s.
Shirodkar s.
Shoch s.
shotted s.
SH pop-off s.
Siemens PTCA open-heart s.
silicone-treated surgical silk s.
silk s.
silk braided s.
silk Mersilene s.
silk nonabsorbable s.
silk pop-off s.
silk stay s.
silk traction s.
silkworm gut s.
Silky Polydek s.
silver s.
silverized catgut s.
Sims s.
single-armed s.
single-running s.
Snellen s.
Sofsilk coated and braided s.
Sofsilk nonabsorbable silk s.
Softgut surgical chromic catgut s.
s. spacer
Spanish blue virgin silk s.
s. spatula
SS s.
stainless steel wire s.
Stallard-Liegard s.
steel mesh s.
Sterna-Band self-locking s.
sternal wire s.
S. Strip
S. Strip Plus wound closure strip

rmdorf s.
lus cardiovascular s.
annular mattress s.
cuticular s.
polene s.
supramid s.
Supramid collagen s.
Supramid Extra s.
Surgaloy metallic s.
surgical chromic s.
surgical gut s.
surgical silk s.
surgical steel s.
Surgicraft s.
Surgidac s.
Surgidev s.
Surgigut s.
Surgilar s.
Surgilene monofilament s.
Surgiloid s.
Surgilon braided nylon s.
Surgilon monofilament
  polypropylene s.
Surgilope s.
SurgiMed s.
Surgipro s.
Surgipro monofilament
  polypropylene s.
Surgiset s.
Surusil braided silk s.
Sutralon s.
SutraSilk s.
Sutupak s.
Suturamid s.
Sutureloop colposuspension
  needle s.
swaged s.
swaged-on s.
Swedgeon s.
Swiss blue virgin silk s.
synthetic absorbable s.
Synthofil s.
s. tag forceps
tantalum wire monofilament s.
Tapercut s.
Teflon-coated Dacron s.
Teflon-pledgeted s.
s. tension adjustment reel (STAR)
s. tension adjustment reel system
tension-requiring s.
tentalum wire tension s.
Tevdek pledgeted s.

S

NOTES

suture *(continued)*
- Thermo-Flex s.
- Thiersch s.
- thread s.
- through-and-through reabsorbable s.
- Ti-Cron s.
- tiger gut s.
- Tinel s.
- traction s.
- transfixion s.
- transosseous s.
- transscleral s.
- twisted cotton s.
- twisted dermal s.
- twisted linen s.
- twisted silk s.
- twisted virgin silk s.
- Tycron s.
- tympanomastoid s.
- Tyrrell-Gray s.
- U s.
- UltraFix MicroMite anchor s.
- unabsorbable s.
- undyed s.
- Vascufil s.
- vascular silk s.
- Verhoeff s.
- Vicryl pop-off s.
- Vicryl Rapide s.
- Vicryl SH s.
- Vienna wire s.
- virgin silk s.
- Viro-Tec s.
- white braided silk s.
- white nylon s.
- white twisted s.
- s. wing
- s. wire
- s. wire-cutting scissors
- wire Zytor s.

sutured plaque electrode
SutureGroove gold eyelid weight
SutureLasso orthopaedic instrument
sutureless pacemaker electrode
Sutureloop colposuspension needle suture
SutureMate
- S. needle rest
- S. suture assist device

suture-tying platform forceps
suturing
- s. forceps
- s. needle

Sven
- S. Johansson driver
- S. Johansson extender
- S. Johansson femoral neck nail

SVS Apex Plus excimer laser

swab
- calcium alginate s.
- Calgiswab calcium alginate s.
- chamois s.
- Janet bladder s.
- KBM gauze s.
- Koenig tonsillar s.
- Merthiolate s.
- Persist skin prep s.
- Puritan Popule self-saturating s.
- Q-Tee cleaning s.

swaged
- s. needle
- s. suture

swaged-on
- s.-o. needle
- s.-o. suture

Swan
- S. aortic clamp
- S. corneoscleral punch
- S. discission knife
- S. eye needle holder
- S. lancet
- S. needle
- S. spade-type needle knife

Swan-Brown arterial forceps
Swan-Ganz (SG)
- S.-G. balloon flotation catheter
- S.-G. bipolar pacing catheter
- S.-G. flow-directed catheter
- S.-G. pacing TD catheter
- S.-G. pulmonary artery catheter
- S.-G. thermodilution catheter

Swank high-flow arterial blood filter
swan-neck
- s.-n. clamp
- s.-n. gouge
- s.-n. Missouri catheter
- s.-n. pediatric Coil-Cath catheter
- s.-n. splint

Swann-Morton surgical blade
Swanson
- S. carpal lunate implant
- S. dynamic toe splint
- S. elevator
- S. finger joint implant
- S. finger joint prosthesis
- S. flexible hallux valgus prosthesis
- S. great toe implant
- S. great toe prosthesis
- S. Grip-X isometric exerciser
- S. hand splint
- S. intramedullary broach
- S. mallet
- S. metacarpal prosthesis
- S. metacarpophalangeal implant
- S. metatarsal broach
- S. metatarsal prosthesis
- S. osteotome

S. radial head implant
S. radiocarpal implant
S. reamer
S. scaphoid awl
S. Silastic elbow prosthesis
S. Silastic implant
S. small joint implant
S. titanium carpal scaphoid implant
S. trapezium implant
S. ulnar head implant
S. wrist joint implant
S. wrist prosthesis
Swartz SL Series Fast-Cath introducer
swathe
    sling and s.
Sweaper curette
Sweat-Chek analyzer
Swede-O
    S.-O. ankle brace
    S.-O. Arch Lok brace
    S.-O. Inner Lok 8 ankle brace
Swede-O-Universal
    S.-O.-U. brace
    S.-O.-U. orthosis
Swede-Vent TL self-tapping external
  hex implant
Swedgeon
    S. already-threaded needle
    S. suture
Swedish
    S. Helparm device
    S. knee cage
Swedish-pattern chisel
Sween-A-Peel wound dressing
Sweeney
    S. posterior vaginal retractor
    S. posterior vaginal speculum
sweep
    Barraquer s.
sweeper
    Cottle spicule s.
    Fossa ureteral stone s.
    periosteal spicule s.
    Tiko zonule s.
Sweet
    S. amputation retractor
    S. antral trocar
    S. clip-applying forceps
    S. delicate pituitary scissors
    S. dissecting forceps
    S. esophageal scissors
    S. eye magnet

S. ligature forceps
S. locator
S. original magnet
S. rib spreader
S. sternal punch
S. Tip bipolar lead
S. two-point discriminator
Sweet-Burford rib spreader
sweetheart retractor
Swenko
    S. bag
    S. gastric-cooling apparatus
Swenson
    S. cholangiography tube
    S. papillomatome
    S. papillotome
    S. ring-jawed holding clamp
Swets
    S. goniotomy cannula
    S. goniotomy knife
Swiderski nasal chisel
swift-cut phaco incision knife
SwiftLase scanner
SwimEx
    S. hydrotherapy system
    S. pool
swimmer's goggles
Swing
    S. DR1 DDDR pacemaker
    S. exerciser machine
SwingAlong walker caddie
Swinger car bed
Swiss
    S. Balance orthotic
    S. ball
    S. blade
    S. bladebreaker
    S. blade holder
    S. blue virgin silk suture
    S. bulldog clamp
    S. Kiss intrastent balloon inflation
      device
    S. LithoClast lithotripter
    S. MP joint implant
    S. Precision cannula system
    S. Therapy eye mask
Swissedent wax
Swiss-pattern speculum
Swissray scanner
switch
    s. box
    internal Reed s.

S

NOTES

switch *(continued)*
    Reed s.
    silicon-controlled s.
    Trigger S.
Switch-Blade scissors
switching stick
Switzerland dilatation catheter
swivel
    s. adapter
    Erich s.
    s. joint suture holder
    s. knife
    Universal s.
swivel-arm system
Swivel-Strap
    S.-S. ankle brace
    S.-S. ankle stirrup
Swive-Strap
    Aircast S.-S.
Swolin self-retaining vaginal speculum
sword knife
Swyrls swim mold
Syark vulsellum forceps
Sydenham mouthgag
Syed
    S. template
    S. template implant
Syed-Neblett
    S.-N. gynecological template
    S.-N. implant
Syed-Puthawala-Hedger esophageal applicator
Sylva
    S. anterior chamber irrigator
    S. I&A unit
    S. irrigating cannula
Sylver-Wax dental wax
Symbion
    S. biventricular assist device
    S. Jarvik-7 artificial heart
Symbion/CardioWest 100 mL total artificial heart
Symbios pacemaker
Symbiot
    S. stent
    S. vascular stent
symblepharon ring
Syme
    S. amputation prosthesis
    S. Dycor prosthetic foot
    S. foot prosthesis
Symmetrical thoracic vertebral plate
Symmetry endobipolar generator
Symmonds
    S. hysterectomy retractor
    S. needle
sympathectomy
    s. hook
    s. retractor

sympathetic raspatory
Symphonix Vibrant Soundbridge implant
Symphony
    S. graft delivery system
    S. monitoring system
    S. MRI system
    S. nitinol biliary stent
    S. whole-body scanner
Symptom Rating scale
Syms
    S. traction
    S. tractor
Synaptic 2000 pain management system
Synatomic total knee prosthesis
SynchroMed
    S. drug administration device
    S. implantable programmable pump
    S. infusion system
Synchron
    S. CX-series automated analyzer
    S. LX20 Pro chemical analyzer
synchronizer
    CardioSync cardiac s.
synchronous
    s. burst pacemaker
    s. mode pacemaker
    s. pacemaker
Synchrony I, II pacemaker
Synchrosonic stimulator
Syncrus low-energy internal cardioversion system
syndesmotic screw
syndrome
    carpal tunnel s. (CTS)
synechia spatula
Synectics-Dantec Flo-Lab II uroflowmeter
Synectics 6000 digital pH meter
synergistic wrist motion splint
Synergist vacuum erection device
SynerGraft heart valve
Synergy
    S. frameless air support therapy
    S. neurostimulation system
    S. posterior titanium spinal system
    S. Pulse frameless air support therapy
    S. splint
    S. ultrasound system
Synergyst
    S. DDD pacemaker
    S. II pacemaker
Synevac vacuum curettage system
SynMesh mesh
Syn-optics camera
synoptoscope
Synovator arthroscopic blade

synovectomy
  s. blade
  s. rongeur
synovector
  arthroscopic s.
synovial
  s. dissector
  s. separator
synovium biopsy forceps
Syntel
  S. embolectomy catheter
  S. graft cleaning catheter
  S. latex-free embolectomy catheter
Synthaderm occlusive wound dressing
Synthes
  S. AO reconstruction plate
  S. CerviFix system
  S. compression hip screw
  S. dorsal distal radius plate
  S. drill
  S. facial curette
  S. genioplate
  S. guide pin
  S. ligament washer
  S. maxillofacial locking
    reconstruction plate
  S. maxillofacial titanium plate
  S. mini-depth gauge
  S. mini L-plate
  S. Schuhli implant system
  S. stainless steel mini fragment
    plate
  S. titanium elastic nail
  S. titanium mini fragment plate
  S. transbuccal trocar
  S. Universal spinal system
  S. vertebral spacer
Syntheses critical care analyzer
synthetic
  s. absorbable suture
  S.'s dual-channel, solid-state
    Digitrapper
  s. hygroscopic cervical dilator
  s. mesh
  s. sapphire tip
  s. stent
SynthoCast hgh-performance casting
  tape
Synthofil suture
SynthoSplint fiberglass splint
Syracuse anterior I-plate
Syrex syringe

Syrijet Mark II needleless injector
syringe
  Accuguide s.
  Alcock bladder s.
  Alexander-Reiner ear s.
  Anel s.
  Arnold-Bruening s.
  Arrow Raulerson spring-wire
    introduction s.
  Asepto bulb irrigation s.
  aspirating s.
  Autoblock safety s.
  BD Luer s.
  Boehm drop s.
  Bruening pressure s.
  bulb s.
  bulbous-tip ear s.
  s. cap
  Cardizem Lyo-Ject s.
  Carti-Loid s.
  Centrix s.
  Cilacalcin double-chambered s.
  Concord line draw s.
  C-R resin s.
  Cuchica s.
  Davidson s.
  DeVilbiss aerosol s.
  DigiTrace sleep/EEG monitoring s.
  Dynacor ear s.
  Dynacor ulcer s.
  ear s.
  electric s.
  Ensi s.
  Epiquick s.
  Exel Zero Dead Space s.
  EZ s.
  Fluorescite s.
  FNA-21 s.
  Fortuna s.
  Fragmatome flute s.
  Fuchs retinal detachment s.
  Fuchs 2-way eye s.
  Gabriel s.
  Gas-Lyte ABG s.
  Gas-Lyte arterial blood gas s.
  G-C s.
  Gemini s.
  glycerine s.
  Goldstein anterior chamber s.
  Goldstein lacrimal s.
  Green-Armytage s.
  Higginson irrigation s.

S

NOTES

syringe *(continued)*

Ilopan disposable s.
Imbibe bone marrow aspiration s.
impression material s.
Infuset GP s.
intraligamentary s.
Ipas s.
Irrigo s.
Irrivac s.
Isosal s.
laryngeal s.
LeVeen inflation s.
Lewy Teflon glycerine-mixture s.
Ligmajet s.
Luer s.
Luer-Lok B-D s.
Max-I-Probe endodontic irrigation s.
MPL aspirating s.
Multi-Fit Luer-Lok control
  tonsillar s.
Namic angiographic s.
Neisser s.
Nourse bladder s.
Osciflator balloon inflation s.
OutBound s.
Pallin spring-assisted s.
Parker-Heath anterior chamber s.
PDL intraligamentary s.
PermaRidge delivery s.
Pitkin s.
Politzer air s.
Pomeroy ear s.
Pritchard s.
Proetz s.
Pulsator anaerobic s.
Raulerson s.
Reiner-Alexander ear s.
Reiner ear s.
retinal detachment s.
Riches bladder s.
Rochester s.
Roughton-Scholander s.
Rudolph calibrated super s.
Safety s.
Sana-Lok s.
Schein s.
spring-assisted s.
Syrex s.
tapered-tip ear s.
Teflon glycerine-mixture s.
Terumo insulin s.
Tobald s.
tonsillar s.
Toomey s.
tuberculin s.
Tubex metal s.
Ultraject contrast media s.
Ultraject prefilled s.
VanishPoint s.

Visitec s.
Yale Luer-Lok s.
syringe-type infusion pump
syrinx shunt
Syrrat scoop
Sysmex

S. NE-8000 CBC analyzer
S. R-1000 reticulocyte counter

SysStim muscle stimulator
System-1
system

ABaer newborn hearing
  screening s.
ABBI breast biopsy s.
Abbott LifeCare PCA Plus II
  infusion s.
Abbott Lifeshield needleless s.
Abbott Plum infusion s.
ABG cement-free hip s.
Abiomed biventricular support s.
Abiomed BVS 5000 biventricular
  support s.
ABI Vest airway clearance s.
Ablatherm HIFU s.
Ablatherm high-intensity focused
  ultrasound s.
ABL520 blood gas measurement s.
AbMap electrophysiologic
  imaging s.
AbMap imaging s.
above-knee suction enhancement s.
Accents micropigmentation s.
Access immunoassay s.
Access MV stabilizer s.
AccuBrush dental s.
accuDEXA bone mineral density
  assessment s.
AccuLength arthroplasty
  measuring s.
AccuMeter cholesterol test s.
Accunet embolic protection s.
AccuProbe 450 cryosurgical s.
Accur hemofiltration s.
Accurus vitrectomy s.
AccuStick II introducer s.
AccuSway balance measurement s.
AccuTrack eye-tracking s.
Ace intramedullary femoral nail s.
Achieve off-pump s.
ACIST injection s.
Acolysis ultrasound thrombolysis s.
ACP plating s.
Acra-clip s.
Acragun s.
Acryl-X-II bone cement removal s.
Acryl-X orthopaedic cement
  removal s.
ACS Concorde over-the-wire
  catheter s.

Actalyke activated clotting time test s.
Action traction s.
Activa Parkinson control s.
Activa tremor control s.
Active Can defibrillator lead s.
Active Can-RV defibrillator lead s.
ACT MicroCoil delivery s.
AcuBlade robotic laser microsurgery s.
Acucair continuous airflow s.
Acufex MosaicPlasty comprehensive s.
AcuFix anterior cervical plate s.
Acumed bone graft s.
Acuson cardiovascular ultrasound s.
AcuSyst-Xcell cell culturing s.
Acutrak bone fixation s.
Acutrak bone replacement s.
Acutrak fusion s.
Adapteur power s.
AddOn-Bucky image acquisition s.
Adeza TLi s.
Adjustaback wheelchair backrest s.
Adjustable Postoperative Protective and Preparatory S.'s (APOPPS)
Adolph Gasser camera s.
Advanced Breast Biopsy Instrumentation s.
Advanced Cardiovascular S. (ACS)
Advanced Medical Systems fetal monitoring s.
Advancit guidewire s.
Advantage ultrasound s.
Advantim revision knee s.
Advantx-E Legacy s.
Advantx LC+ cardiovascular imaging s.
Aegis ICD s.
Aegis implantable cardioverter-defibrillator s.
Aegis sonography management s.
AEM current flow monitoring s.
AER+ automated endoscope reprocessing s.
AeroNOx nitric oxide delivery and analysis s.
AeroView optical intubation s.
AERx diabetes management s.
AERx pain management s.
AERx pulmonary drug delivery s.
Aesculap ScalpFix scalp clip s.

Aesculap Unitrac retraction and retention s.
Aesculap Vascu Cut punch s.
Aesculap Verio wound hook s.
Affirm VP microbial identification s.
Affymetrix GeneChip s.
AFx DR AutoCapture pacing s.
Agee carpal tunnel release s.
Agee WristJack fracture reduction s.
Agfa CR s.
Agfa PACS s.
Aim titanium femoral nail s.
AirBack spinal s.
Aircast knee s.
AirFlo alternating pressure s.
Airis II MRI s.
Air-Limb edema control s.
Aladdin II nasal CPAP s.
Aladdin infant flow s.
Aladdin nasal CPAP s.
Alara DenOptix filmless dental imaging s.
Alara MetriScan bone density s.
AlaStat allergy immunoassay s.
Albert Grass Heritage digital EEG s.
Albert Grass Heritage PSG s.
Alcon closure s.
Alexa 1000 breast diagnostic s.
Alice 4 sleep diagnostic s.
All Access laser s.
Allen traction s.
Allen Universal stirrup s.
Alliance integrated inflation s.
Alliance rehabilitation s.
Alloclassic hip s.
Allofit acetabular cup s.
allogeneic cellular immune therapy s.
AlloMune s.
Allon thermoregulation s.
Allo-Pro hip s.
Aloka SD, SSD ultrasound s.
Aloka SSD-500 ultrasound s.
Alphatec large cannulated screw s.
Alphatec small fragment s.
Altaire open MRI s.
Alta modular trauma s.
Alterns therapeutic seating s.
AMBI compression hip screw s.

S

NOTES

system *(continued)*

A-Med A-Syst right heart support s.
American Medical S.'s (AMS)
AMK total knee s.
AML total hip s.
AMO Diplomax phacoemulsification s.
AMO Prestige advanced cataract extraction s.
Amplatz anchor s.
Amplatz TractMaster s.
Amplicor automated PCR s.
Amset anterior locking plate s.
Amset R-F reduction fixation s.
AMS SPARC sling s.
Anatomic hip s.
Anatomic Medullary Locking total hip s.
Anchor IIa osseointegrated titanium implant s.
AnchorLok s.
Ancor imaging s.
Ancure balloon catheterization s.
Ancure bifurcated s.
Ancure endograft s.
AneuRx AAA stent graft s.
AneuRx bifurcated stent graft s.
AneuRx DTA stent graft s.
AneuRx endograft s.
AneuRx stent graft s.
AngeCool RF catheter ablation s.
AngePass lead s.
Anger gamma camera s.
AngioJet rapid thrombectomy s.
AngioJet Rheolytic thrombectomy s.
Angiomat 6000 contrast delivery s.
Angiomat Illumena injector s.
AngioRad radiation s.
Angio-Seal hemostasis s.
AngioSurf scan s.
AngioVista angiographic s.
Angstrom II ICD s.
Angstrom II implantable cardioverter-defibrillator s.
AnkleTough ankle rehabilitation s.
AnnuloFlex annuloplasty s.
AnnuloFlo annuloplasty ring s.
Anspach 65K instrument s.
anterior cervical plate s.
anterior cervical plate fixation s. (ACFS)
anterior locking plate s. (ALPS)
anterior plate s.
Antlantis ACP plating s.
AOA/Chick ambulatory halo s.
AO/ASIF titanium craniofacial s.
AO mandibular s.
aortic connector s.

Apex irrigation s.
ApexPro telemetry s.
Apogee CX-series echocardiography s.
Apogee RX-series diagnostic ultrasound s.
Apollo DXA bone densitometry s.
Apollo 95E tooth-whitening and curing s.
Apollo hip s.
Apollo knee s.
Apollo Light S.'s
APR total hip s.
Aqua-Cel Aqua-Relief heating pad s.
Aqualase cataract removal s.
Aquanex hydrodynamic measurement s.
Aqua-Seal s.
AquaSens FMS 1000 fluid monitoring s.
Aqua Spray debridement s.
arcitumomab diagnostic imaging s.
arc-quadrant stereotactic s.
Argyle Turkel safety thoracentesis s.
Argyle-Turkel safety thoracentesis s.
Aria LX CPAP s.
Arndorfer infusion s.
Arndorfer pneumohydraulic capillary infusion s.
Arnett-TMP s.
arrhythmia mapping s.
Arrow LionHeart left ventricular assist s.
Arrow UserGard injection cap s.
arterial port catheter s.
ArthroCare arthroscopic s.
ArthroCare Coblation-based cosmetic surgery s.
Arthro-Flo powered irrigation s.
Arthro-Lok s.
Arthroscan imaging s.
ArthroSew suturing s.
Artoscan MRI s.
Artus power s.
ASAP automated biopsy s.
ASAP Stacker automated multisample biopsy s.
Ascent total knee s.
ASDOS double umbrella s.
Aspen CTO s.
Aspen digital ultrasound s.
Aspen echocardiography s.
Aspen ultrasound s.
AspenVAC smoke evacuation s.
Aspire continuous imaging s.
Assistant Free self-retaining hip surgery retractor s.

Assure blood glucose monitoring s.
Asteion computed tomography s.
Aston cartilage reduction s.
Astra Tech dental implant s.
Astro-Med Albert Grass Heritage digital EEG s.
Atakr RF ablation s.
Atavi atraumatic spine fusion s.
Atavi MDS s.
Atavi TiTLE top-loading rod fixation s.
AT-1 3-channel resting ECG s.
Athena high frequency mammography s.
Atlantis anterior cervical plating s.
Atlas 2.0 diagnostic ultrasound s.
AtLast blood glucose s.
ATL HDI-series cardiovascular ultrasound s.
ATL high definition imaging s.'s
A-Trac atraumatic clamping s.
Atrauclip ligating clip s.
atrial septal defect occlusion s. (ASDOS)
Atridox drug s.
Atrigel drug delivery s.
Atrium blood recovery s.
ATS 500/1500 tourniquet s.
AuRA cemented total hip s.
Aura laser s.
Aurora dedicated breast MRI s.
Aurora diode-based dental laser s.
AutoCapture Pacing S. (APS)
AutoCyte image analysis s.
autoLog autotransfusion s.
automated cellular imaging s.
AutoPap Pap smear s.
Autoread centrifuge hematology s.
AutoSet portable riveting s.
AutoSet T titration s.
Auto Suture ABBI s.
autotransfusion s.
Autovac autotransfusion s.
Autovac LF autotransfusion s.
Avera breast imaging s.
AVE stent s.
Avi lens s.
Aviva mammography s.
AVR spinal reconstruction s.
Axcis percutaneous myocardial revascularization laser s.
Axiom modular knee s.

Axya bone anchor s.
AxyaWeld bone anchor s.
AxyaWeld J-tip suture welding s.
AxyaWeld laparoscopic sonic J s.
Babe OB ultrasound reporting s.
Babyflex heated ventilation s.
BacFix s.
BacT/Alert automated blood culture s.
Bactec automated blood culture s.
Bacti-Swab II collection and transport s.
Bacti-Swab NPG collection and transport s.
Badal stimulus s.
Bagby and Kuslich interbody fusion s.
Bair Hugger patient warming s.
BAK/C interbody fusion s.
BAK interbody fusion s.
BAK/T interbody fusion s.
Balance Master training and assessment s.
Bambi cell analysis s.
Bard cardiopulmonary support s.
Bard CPS s.
Bard EndoCinch suturing s.
Bard endoscopic suture s.
Bard rotary atherectomy s.
Bard urinary sterile collection s.
Bard Urolase fiber laser s.
BariKare advanced power s.
Bateman UPF II bipolar knee s.
Baxter InterLink needle s.
Baylor rapid autologous transfusion s.
BCell-HDM filtering s.
BDProbeTec ET s.
BD Vacutainer s.
beachchair shoulder positioning s.
Beamer injection stent s.
Beaver clear cornea incision s.
Becker orthopaedic spinal s. (BOSS)
Becker-Rojas Sub-Sonic surgical s.
Becker thermoformable ankle s.
Becker vibrating cannula s.
Beckman ICS Nephelometer s.
Beekley skin marking s.
Bennett contour mammography s.
Benzaquen-Chajchir extraction/reinjection s.

S

NOTES

system *(continued)*

Berkeley Vacurette curettage s.
BeStent Rival coronary stent s.
Beta-Cath delivery s.
Betaseron needle-free delivery s.
Better Than Another Pair of
Hands retractor s.
Bevalac s.
Biacore s.
Biad SPECT imaging s.
BIAS total hip s.
bilateral variable screw
placement s.
BiliBlanket Plus high-output
phototherapy s.
BiliLight phototherapy s.
Bi-Metric hip s.
Biocell breast implant s.
Biodex balance s.
Biodex Unweighing s.
BioDimensional breast
reconstruction s.
Biodynamic molding s.
Bio-Esthetic abutment s.
Bio-Fit total hip s.
Bio Flote air flotation s.
Biogel Reveal puncture
indication s.
Bio-Groove HA hip s.
BioGun automated biopsy s.
Biojector 2000 needle-free injection
management s.
BioLab modular motility s.
BioLogic-DT s.
BioLogic-HT s.
Biologic Ingrowth Anatomic S.
(BIAS)
BioMedx portable air flotation s.
Biomet AGC knee s.
Biomet Ascent total knee s.
Biomet Finn salvage/oncology knee
reconstruction s.
Biomet MARS acetabular
reconstructive s.
Biomet Maxim revision knee s.
Biomet tripolar acetabular s.
Biomet Ultra-Drive ultrasonic
revision s.
Bio-Modular total shoulder s.
Bionicare stimulator s.
Bio-Optics Bambi image analysis s.
Bioplate rigid fixation s.
Bioport collection and transport s.
Biopsys Mammotome vacuum
biopsy s.
bioptic amorphic lens s.
BioRad 5000 titanium s.
bioresorbable drug delivery s.

Biorigid Nail unreamed tibial
nailing s.
Biosearch anorectal biofeedback s.
Biosense DMR s.
Biosense intracardiac mapping s.
Biosense NOGA catheter-based
endocardial mapping s.
BioSorb FX tack s.
Biosound AU-series
echocardiography s.
Biosound Phase 2 ultrasound s.
BioSpec MR imaging s.
BioSpec MRI/MRS s.
BioStinger meniscal repair s.
biotelemetry s.
BioTwist soft tissue anchor s.
BioZtect sensor s.
BiPAP Duet LX s.
BiPAP Pro s.
BiPAP S/T-D ventilatory support s.
BiPAP Vision s.
biphasic s.
Bi-Rads breast imaging and
reporting s.
BIRO s.
Bitome bipolar s.
Blackstone spinal fixation s.
Blade-Vent implant s.
Blajwas-Schwartz-Marcinko
irrigation/drainage s.
Blue multi-vector external
distraction s.
BMC radiofrequency perforation s.
BodPod body composition s.
Body Logic rehabilitation s.
Body Masters MD 510 hi-lo
pulley s.
Body Response s.
Boehringer Autovac
autotransfusion s.
Bolin x-ray filter s.
Bonchek-Shiley vein distention s.
Bone-Lok bone fixation s.
bone tack s.
Bosker TMI Reconstruction s.
Bosker transmandibular
reconstructive surgical s.
BosPac cardiopulmonary bypass s.
Boston elbow s.
Bottoms-Up posture s.
Bracco s.
BrachyVision brachytherapy
planning s.
Brackmann II EMG s.
BrainLab VectorVision
neuronavigational s.
BrainSCAN Linac radiosurgery s.
BrainSCAN stereotactic s.
Brånemark implant s.

Brava breast enhancement and shaping s.
Bremer halo Crown s.
Bridge hip s.
Bridge X3 renal stent s.
BriteSmile laser tooth whitening s.
Broselow/Hinkle pediatric resuscitation s.
Browlift Bone Bridge s.
Brown-Roberts-Wells computerized tomography stereotaxic guidance s.
Bruker BioSpec s.
Bruker CSI MR s.
Bruker/GE CSI Omega MR s.
BRW stereotactic s.
BTA S-2000 biofeedback s.
Burette multiple patient delivery s.
Buzard-Barraquer Diamond Microkeratome s.
BVS-5000 biventricular support s.
BWM spine s.
cable s.
CADD-Prizm pain control s.
CADD-TPN ambulatory infusion s.
Cadence tiered therapy defibrillator s.
CADx SecondLook computer-aided detection s.
CAFET speech therapy s.
Calasept delivery s.
Calcitek implant s.
Calvitron hair replacement s.
canal finder s.
Candela videoimaging s.
Cannulated Plus screw s.
cannulated screw s.
Can-Opt dual-lumen ERCP s.
Canyons wound irrigation s.
Capasee diagnostic ultrasound s.
Capintec VEST s.
Capiox-E bypass oxygenator s.
Capiox SX gas and heat exchange oxygenation s.
CAPIS bone plate s.
CarboJet lavage s.
Cardioblate surgical ablation s.
CardioCamera imaging s.
CardioCard s.
CardioCOOL myocardial cooling s.
Cardio3DScope imaging s.
Cardiofreezer cryosurgical s.

CardioGenesis PMR s.
CardioLab 7000 electrophysiology monitoring s.
Cardiovascular Angiography Analysis S. (CAAS)
Cardiovascular Imaging S.'s (CVIS)
Cardiovit AT-series ECG s.
Cardiovit CS-series ECG s.
cartesian reference coordinate s.
Carto electrophysiology navigation s.
Carto EP navigation s.
Cascade Up and About s.
CASE computerized exercise EKG s.
CASE Marquette 16-exercise s.
CASS whole-brain mapping s.
CastAlert cast pressure sensing s.
Castle Daystar surgical television s.
Catalyst microsurgical s.
Catarex cataract removal s.
Cath-Finder catheter tracking s.
CathTrack catheter locator s.
CatsEye digital camera s.
Cavi-Endo ultrasonic s.
Cavitron I&A s.
Cavitron-Kelman I&A s.
C-AVR spinal reconstruction s.
CC Rider closed-chain rehabilitation s.
CD Horizon Eclipse spinal s.
CD Horizon Sextant spinal s.
CDRPan digital x-ray s.
Ceegraph 128 EEG s.
cell analysis s.
CellFIT acquisition s.
cell recovery s.
Cell Saver Haemolite autotransfusion s.
Cell Saver Haemonetics autotransfusion s.
Cencit imaging s.
CenterPointLock 2-piece ostomy s.
Centrax bipolar s.
Centrica rotational core biopsy s.
CeraOne implant s.
CerviFix s.
Cervi-Lok cervical fixation s.
CFC BioScanner s.
CFix cable fixation s.
CGR biplane angiographic s.
Chair-Mate s.

S

NOTES

system *(continued)*

ChamberLift 2000 patient lift s.
Champy miniplate rigid fixation s.
Charnley Howorth ExFlow s.
Chattanooga balance s.
Checkmate intravascular
  brachytherapy s.
ChemoBloc vial venting s.
Chemo-Port implantable vascular
  access s.
Chemo-Port perivena catheter s.
Chirotech x-ray s.
Chocstruct chondral repair s.
Cholestech LDX office lab s.
Chromos imager s.
ChromoVision video s.
Cineloop image review
  ultrasound s.
CineView Plus Freeland s.
CircAid compression s.
CircPlus bandage/wrap s.
Circulaire aerosolized drug
  delivery s.
Circul'Air shoe s.
CIS-2 s.
CKS knee s.
Clarion CII Bionic Ear s.
Claris spinal clip s.
Clarity newborn hearing s.
Clave needleless IV s.
ClearESS irrigation and suction s.
Clearglide endoscopic vessel
  harvesting s.
Clensicair incontinence
  management s.
Clinac 600SR stereotactic radiation
  treatment s.
Clini-Float flotation therapy bed s.
Closure vein reflux s.
CMI vacuum delivery s.
CMS AccuProbe 450
  cryosurgical s.
CMSI warming s.
CoaguChek s.
Cobe Spectra apheresis s.
Cobe Trima automated blood
  component collection s.
Coburn I&A s.
Codman external drainage s.
Codman Ti-Frame posterior
  fixation s.
COER-24 delivery s.
Cofield 2 total shoulder s.
COGNIShunt CNS fluid shunt s.
Cohort anterior plate s.
CO$_2$ject s.
Coleman microinfiltration s.
Colin Electronics BP-508
  tonometry s.

CollectFirst s.
Coltene direct inlay s.
Combi Multi-Traction s.
Command hip instrumentation s.
Companion 300-series nasal
  CPAP s.
Compass CT stereotaxic
  adaptation s.
Compass Cygnus portable frameless
  stereotactic s.
Compliant pre-stress s.
ComPreSs compliant pre-stress bone
  implant s.
Compton suppression s.
CompuMed computer-controlled
  local anesthetic delivery s.
Computed Anatomy corneal
  modeling s.
Computer-Aided Patient
  Information S. (CAPIS)
computer-assisted neurosurgical
  navigational s.
computer-controlled infusion
  pump s.
computer-controlled neurological
  stimulation s.
computerized bedside transfusion
  identification s.
computerized morphometric s.
computerized radiographic image
  analysis s.
Concentrix dual-aspiration pump s.
Concept beachchair shoulder
  positioning s.
Concept Precise ACL guide s.
Concept rotator cuff repair s.
Concept self-compressing cannulated
  screw s.
Concept Sterling arthroscopy
  blade s.
Conceptus fallopian tube
  catheterization s.
Concept video imaging s.
Concept zone-specific cannula s.
condom catheter collecting s.
Conforma 3000 proton beam
  treatment s.
ConstaVac autoreinfusion s.
Contact lightweight telemedicine s.
contact-tip laser s.
continuous insulin delivery s.
continuous-wave high-frequency
  Doppler ultrasound s.
Continuum knee s.
Continuum MR-compatible
  infusion s.
Contour Genesis ultrasonic-assisted
  liposuction s.
Contour II ICD s.

Contour mammography s.
Contrajet ERCP contrast delivery s.
Convertible trocar s.
Cook stereotactic s.
CoolGlide aesthetic laser s.
CoolTouch II facial laser s.
Coombs bone biopsy s.
CooperSurgical LEEP s.
Coordinate complete revision
 knee s.
Corail total hip replacement s.
cord blood collection s. (CBCS)
Cordguard II cord blood
 collection s.
Cordis Checkmate s.
Cordis endovascular s.
Core Dynamics cannula s.
Corin taper-fit total hip s.
corneal topography s.
CorneaSparing LTK s.
Corometrics Medical Systems Inc.
 fetal monitoring s.
coronary angiography analysis s.
Coroscop C cardiac imaging s.
Corvita graft s.
Cosgrove-Edwards annuloplasty s.
Cosman ICP Tele-Sensor s.
Cotrel-Dubousset distraction s.
Cotrel-Dubousset screw-rod s.
Counter Rotational S. (CRS)
cranial osteosynthesis s.
cranial plating s.
craniomaxillofacial plating s.
CritiCore monitoring s.
CritSpin hematocrit s.
Crockard retractor s.
Crown mattress s.
Crown recliner s.
CRS tibial torsion s.
CRW stereotactic s.
CRYOcare cryoablation s.
CryoCor s.
CryoCor cardiac cryoablation s.
CryoGuide ultrasound guidance s.
CryoHit cryotherapy s.
Cryomedics electrosurgery s.
CryoPen cryosurgical s.
cryotherapy s.
Cryo-Vac-Away cryostat vacuum s.
Cryovial s.
CrystalEyes endoscopic video s.
CSZ Electri-Cool cold therapy s.

CTDx electrostimulation s.
C-Tek anterior cervical plate s.
CTI Cyclotron s.
CT-MRI-compatible stereotactic
 head frame s.
C-Trak surgical guidance s.
Cuidant s.
CurvTek bone tunneling s.
CUSA CEM s.
Cusp-Lok cuspid traction s.
CustomCornea wavefront
 measurement s.
C-Vest radiation detection s.
CVIS information s.
CVIS/InterTherapy intravascular
 ultrasound s.
CyberKnife stereotactic
 radiosurgery s.
Cybex Norm testing and
 rehabilitation s.
Cygnet Laboratories fetal
 monitoring s.
Cygnus PFS image-guided s.
Cytomax brush cytology s.
CytoRich cervical cytology
 monolayer preparation s.
Dall-Miles cable s.
Danniflex CPM s.
Dansac irrigation s.
Dantec 12-channel Urocolor
 video s.
Dantec Etude s.
DAR breathing s.
DataHand s.
da Vinci surgical s.
Davol irrigation s.
DawSkin flexible protective skin s.
DCI-S automated coronary
 analysis s.
DCS condylar screw s.
DCS dynamic hip s.
DebioClip single-dose delivery s.
Deknatel autotransfusion s.
Delphia II massage and
 microdermabrasion s.
Delta 32 digital stereotactic s.
Deltaloc anterior cervical plate s.
DELTAmanager MedImage s.
Delta 32 TACT 3-dimensional
 breast imaging s.
Deltoid-Aid arm counterbalance s.
DentiCAD s.

S

NOTES

system *(continued)*

DentiPatch lidocaine transoral delivery s.
Dent manometry s.
Dentsply implant s.
Dent-X dental imaging s.
DePuy Bremer AirFlo halo vest s.
DePuy Kaneda s.
DePuy M-2 Anterior Plate s.
DePuy Profile s.
DePuy Songer cable s.
DePuy TiMX comprehensive low back s.
DePuy total hip s.
DePuy University Plate s.
DePuy VSP plate and screw s.
Dermablate hair transplantation s.
Derma-K laser s.
DermaLase laser s.
Dermapulse wound management s.
DermMaster macrodermabrasion s.
DFS 2 mattress replacement s.
Diab-A-Foot protection s.
DIAGNOdent caries detection s.
Dialys-Aids s.
Diapact CRRT s.
Diapulse wound treatment s.
Diasonics Sonotron Vingmed CFM 800 imaging s.
dichroic filter s.
Difco ESP testing s.
Digi-Flex exercise s.
Digital B s.
digital holography s.
digital selenium-based chest imaging s.
Digital Traumex s.
Digitron digital subtraction imaging s.
dilator-sheath s.
3-dimensional Viewnix software s.
Dimension hip s.
Dingman oral retraction s.
Dioptimum s.
Director Guidewire s.
DirectView CR 900 imaging s.
Discovery PET/CT imaging s.
Dispos-a-ject microinjection s.
distal perfusion s.
Disten-U-Flo fluid s.
Dobbhoff G/J s.
DOBI breast cancer diagnostic s.
Dodick laser Photolysis s.
Dolphin II fluid management s.
Doppler Quantum color flow s.
DORC diathermy s.
DORC fast freeze cryosurgical s.
Dormia extracorporeal shockwave lithotripsy s.

Drake-Willock automatic delivery s.
DryView laser imaging s.
DSX ELISA s.
DTR-one UltraSure imaging ultrasound s.
Dualer Plus s.
Dual Quattrode spinal cord stimulation s.
Dual Range Limiter s.
Dumbach mandibular reconstruction s.
Dumon-Gilliard endoprosthesis s.
Dunlap cold compression wrap s.
Duoloid impression s.
Duovisc viscoelastic s.
Dupel iontophoretic drug delivery s.
DuPont rare earth imaging s.
Duracon PS total knee s.
Duraloc acetabular cup s.
Dur-A-Sil silicone impression s.
Durasul large diameter head s.
DX-PC spirometry s.
Dymer excimer excimer laser delivery s.
Dyna-Care pressure pad s.
DynaFix external fixation s.
Dynaflex multilayer compression s.
DynaGuard LAL low-air-loss pressure management s.
Dynalink biliary self-expanding stent s.
Dyna-Lok plating s.
dynamic optical breast imaging s.
Dynamite mattress s.
DynaRad portable x-ray s.
Dynasplint shoulder s.
Dynasty delivery s.
Dyonics Dyosite office arthroscopy s.
Dyonics IntelliJet fluid management s.
Easy Analysis s.
EasyGuide Neuro image-guided surgery s.
Easy Introduction s.
EBI bone healing s.
EBI gravity cold therapy s.
EBI SpineLink anterior cervical spinal s.
EBI XFix DynaFix s.
E.CAM dual-head emission imaging s.
Eccocee CX ltrasound s.
EccoVision acoustic rhinometry s.
EchoEye imaging s.
EchoFlow blood velocity meter s.
Echovar Doppler s.
Eclipse Axcis PTMR s.

S

Eclipse Highfield MRI s.
Eclipse infusion s.
Eclipse magnetic resonance s.
ECTRA s.
Edentrace sleep s.
EDG s.
Eductor fluid management s.
Edwards modular spinal s.
Eklund breast positioning s.
Elan-E electronic motor s.
ElastaTrac home lumbar traction s.
Electri-Cool cold therapy s.
Electro-Acuscope myopulse
  therapy s.
Electroshield monitoring s.
Elite hip s.
Ellman press-form s.
Elscint tomography s.
Embletta portable diagnostic s.
Embol-X arterial cannula and
  filter s.
Emerald implantation s.
Emergence Profile implant s.
EnAbl thermal ablation s.
Enac ultrasonic endodontic s.
Encore ceramic hip joint
  replacement s.
Encore ceramic knee joint
  replacement s.
Encore Poly-Axial Spine S.
Endermologie adipose destruction s.
Endius Atavi spine surgery s.
Endius EndoFusion s.
Endius endoscopic access s.
Endius TiTLE implant and
  instrument s.
Endius WAVE polyaxial plate s.
Endobag laparoscopic specimen
  retrieval s.
Endocam video camera s.
endocavitary applicator s.
EndoCinch suturing s.
endocoagulator laser s.
Endodermologie LPG s.
Endoflex endoscopic instrument s.
EndoMed LSS laparoscopy s.
Endopath Optiview s.
Endopore dental implant s.
Endo-Ring surgical retraction s.
EndoSaph vein harvest s.
endoscopic carpal tunnel release s.
EndoSheath endoscopy s.

Endotak lead s.
Endotek urodynamics s.
Endo Tip port s.
Endotrac blade s.
Endotrac endoscopic carpal tunnel
  release s.
Endovasix endovascular
  photoacoustic recanalization s.
Endovasix EPAR s.
EnGuard double-lead ICD s.
EnGuard pacing and defibrillation
  lead s.
EnSite 3000 cardiac mapping s.
ENTec Coblator Plasma Surgery s.
Entre II trocar and cannula s.
ENTrak electromagnetic surgical
  navigation s.
Entree II laparoscopic trocar s.
Entree II trocar and cannula s.
Entree Plus trocar and cannula s.
EntriStar skin level gastrostomy s.
EntSol nasal wash s.
Envision targeted dose drug
  delivery s.
Envision TD implantable drug
  delivery s.
Envoy middle ear implantable s.
EPAR laser s.
Epic ophthalmic 3-in-1 laser s.
EpiLaser laser-based hair
  removal s.
EpiLight hair removal s.
EpiTouch ruby SilkLaser hair
  removal s.
EPT-1000 XP cardiac ablation s.
Equinox EEG neuromonitoring s.
ErecAid Esteem external vacuum
  therapy s.
Ergo irrigation s.
ErgoTec vitreoretinal instrument s.
Ero-Scan otoacoustic emissions
  test s.
E-series hip s.
ESI Lav gastric lavage s.
Esprit microdermabrasion s.
ESSential shaver s.
Essure sterilization s.
Estilux ultraviolet s.
EuroPeel s.
ExAblate 2000 MR
  scanner/ultrasound delivery s.
Exact-Fit ATH hip replacement s.

NOTES

system *(continued)*

Exakt cutting/grinding s.
Exogen 2000+ ultrasound fracture healing s.
Exonix Ultrasonic Surgical s.
Explorer common bile duct exploration s.
Explorer X 70 intraoral radiography s.
Express 2 coronary stent s.
Extend total hip s.
extracorporeal membrane oxygenation s.
extracorporeal shockwave lithotripsy s.
eyeFix speculum s.
EyeMap EH-290 corneal tomography s.
EyeSys 2000 corneal topographic mapping s.
EZE-Fit IOL s.
E-Z-EM BioGun automated biopsy s.
EZ Flap titanium miniplate s.
EZ-On traction belt s.
EZ Tac s.
facet screw s.
F.A.S.T.1 adult intraosseous infusion s.
FastPack s.
FastTake blood glucose monitoring s.
FeatherTouch SilkLaser s.
femtosecond laser s.
Fenlin total shoulder s.
Ferno AquaCiser II underwater treadmill s.
Ferno Recline-a-Bath bathing s.
FiberLase beam delivery s.
fiberoptic catheter delivery s.
fiberTome s.
Fillauer endoskeletal alignment s.
Filtresse surgical smoke filtration s.
Finesse dilating trocar s.
Finger Phantom pulse oximeter testing s.
Fischer modular stereotaxic s.
Fitnet joint testing s.
Fixateur Interne fixation s.
Fixion IL nailing s.
Fixion PF nailing s.
Fletcher-Suit-Delclos s.
Flexiflo gastrostomy tube enteral delivery s.
Flexi-Therm liquid crystal s.
FlexStent flexible esophageal stent s.
Flipper detachable embolization coil delivery s.

Flo-Stat fluid management s.
FloVAC Hi-Flo laparoscopic suction-irrigation s.
FlowPlus therapeutic pneumatic compression s.
Flowtron Excel DVT prophylaxis s.
FluoroNav virtual fluoroscopy s.
Fluoroptic thermometry s.
FluoroTrak 3500 navigation s.
flying spot excimer laser s.
F-Mat screening s.
Foamart foot impression s.
Fonar Standing Ovation MRI s.
Fonix 6500-CX hearing aid test s.
Foot-Station 3-D foot imaging s.
Force GSU argon-enhanced electrosurgery s.
Foundation 4-part fracture s.
Foundation total hip s.
Foundation total knee s.
Foundation total shoulder s.
FracSure total hip s.
frameless stereotaxy s.
Frank EKG lead placement s.
Freedom leg bag collection s.
Freehand neuroprosthetic s.
FreeStyle Tracker diabetes management s.
French Pharmacovigilance s.
Fresenius volumetric dialysate balancing s.
Frialit-2 system dental implant s.
Frostline linear cryoablation s.
F-Scan foot force and gait analysis s.
Fuji AC2 storage phosphor computed radiology s.
Fuji FCR9000 computed radiology s.
Fujinon SP-501 sonoprobe s.
full-field digital mammography s.
Galaxy IVUS s.
Galen teleradiology s.
Galileo III intravascular radiotherapy s.
Gambro hemofiltration s.
Gamma locking nail s.
GastrograpH ambulatory pH monitoring s.
Gastroscan motility s.
GDLH posterior spinal s.
GD Regainer s.
GE CT Hi-Speed Advantage s.
Gel-U-Sleep series III floatation mattress s.
Gemini combined PET/CT s.
Gem PCL Plus coagulation s.
Gem SensiCath blood gas mesaurement s.

General Electric Advantx s.
generator s.
GenESA closed-loop delivery s.
Genesis II foot/ankle s.
Genesis II total knee s.
GenesisXP neurostimulation s.
Genotropin s.
GentleLASE laser s.
GentleLASE Plus laser s.
GentlePeel skin exfoliation s.
Gentle Touch colostomy/ileostomy
postoperative s.
Gentle Touch loop ostomy s.
Genucom ACL laxity analysis s.
Genucom knee flexion analysis s.
Genzyme Hind Site 20/20 s.
GE Senographe 2000D
mammography s.
GFX2 coronary stent s.
Gillette double-flexure ankle
joint s.
Given diagnostic imaging s.
Global Advantage total shoulder s.
Global Fx shoulder fracture s.
Glucometer II home glucose
monitoring s.
GlyMed Camouflage s.
gNomos stereotactic s.
Goldenberg implant s.
golf exercise s.
GoodKnight nasal auto-PAP s.
GoodKnight nasal CPAP s.
Graf stabilization s.
Granberg cervical traction s.
Grasping Stitcher s.
Grass Neurodata s.
gravity cold therapy s.
Gravity Lumbar Traction s.
Greenberg retracting s.
Grieshaber power injector s.
Guardian limb salvage s.
Guardian 2-piece ostomy s.
GuardWire Plus s.
Guidant Heart Rhythm
Technologies Linear Ablation s.
Guidant Multi-Link Tetra coronary
stent s.
Guidant Triad 3-electrode energy
defibrillation s.
Guldmann Overhead Trac s.
Gx-99 vibratory endermatherapie s.

Gynecare tension-free vaginal
tape s.
Gynecare Thermachoice uterine
balloon therapy s.
Gynecare Verascope hysteroscopy s.
Gyroscan HP Philips 15S whole-
body s.
Gyrus endourology s.
HA-biointegrated dental implant s.
Haemolite autologous blood
recovery s.
Hakim valve s.
Hall mandibular implant s.
Hall modular acetabular reamer s.
Hall Osteon drill s.
halo cervical traction s.
Halo CO_2 laser s.
Hammer mini-tubular external
fixation s.
HandiCare adult disposable pant
and pad s.
HandMaster s.
Hands Free knee retractor s.
Hanger ComfortFlex socket s.
Hariri-Heifetz microsurgical s.
Harrington rod and hook s.
Hausmann Work-Well work
hardening s.
HCMI chiropractic s.
HDI cardiovascular ultrasound s.
heads-up imaging s.
Healthy Back s.
Heartflow automated anastomosis s.
Heartport Precision-OP s.
HEARTrac I cardiac monitoring s.
HeatProbe water irrigation/lavage s.
Helios diagnostic imaging s.
Helix multihead nuclear imaging s.
HELP s.
Hematome s.
HemoCue B-hemoglobin s.
Hem-o-lok polymer ligation clip s.
Hemo-Nate blood filtration s.
Hemopump cardiac assist s.
Hemopure oxygen-based
therapeutic s.
Hemostatix thermal scalpel s.
HepatAssist bioartificial liver s.
HEPAtech Air Purification s.
Herculite XRV lab s.
Heritage hip s.

S

NOTES

system *(continued)*

Hermes Evolution tricompartmental knee s.
Hermetic II drainage management s.
Hessburg subpalpebral lavage s.
Hewlett-Packard 5 MHz phased-array TEE s.
Hewlett-Packard Sonos 1000, 1500 ultrasound s.
Hex-Fix s.
Hexon illumination s.
Hi-Care pulmonary hygiene s.
high-field MRI s.
high-resolution brain SPECT s.
hipGRIP pelvic positioning s.
Hipokrat bimodular shoulder s.
hipRAP pelvic positioning s.
Hi-Star midfield MRI s.
Histofreezer cryosurgical s.
Hitachi Altaire open MRI s.
Hitachi EUB-405 ultrasound s.
Hitachi open MRI s.
Hitachi UB 420 digital ultrasound s.
Hix-Fix fracture fixation s.
Hoek-Bowen cement removal s.
Hoffman II Compact external fixation s.
Hologic EP 2000 electrophysiology imaging s.
Holter external drainage s.
Holter hydrocephalus shunt s.
Homepump infusion s.
HomMed monitoring s.
homonuclear spin s.
Horizon AutoAdjust CPAP s.
Horizon LT nasal CPAP s.
Horizon phacoemulsification s.
Housecall transtelephonic ICD monitoring s.
House grading s.
Howmedica HNR s.
Howmedica pediatric osteotomy s.
Howmedica total ankle s.
Howmedica Unitrax hip fracture s.
HP Sonos ultrasound imaging s.
Humphrey Atlas Eclipse corneal topography s.
Humphrey Mastervue corneal topography s.
Hunsaker Mon-Jet tube anesthesia s.
Hunstad tumescent anesthesia s.
hybrid capture s.
HybridFit total hip s.
HybridFit total knee s.
HydraClearTM endoscopic cleansing s.

Hydradjust urology s.
hydraulic capillary infusion s.
Hydra Vision ES urology s.
Hydra Vision IV urology imaging s.
Hydra Vision Plus DR urological imaging s.
Hydra Vision Plus HP urological imaging s.
hydrodynamic thrombectomy s.
HydroFlex irrigation s.
HydroThermAblator endometrial ablation s.
HygieniKit breast milk collection s.
HyperPACS s.
Hypobaric transfemoral s.
Hypobaric transtibial s.
Hysteroser contact hysteroscopy s.
Hy-Tec Plus Automated EIA s.
I&A s.
IDIS angiography s.
Igloo Heatshield s.
IL 1640 blood/gas electrolyte s.
Ilizarov limb-lengthening s.
Illumena injector s.
ImageChecker CT LN-1000 s.
ImageNet image digitizing s.
Image-View s.
Imatron s.
Imcor No-Touch implant placement s.
Imexlab vascular diagnostic s.
Immediate Implant Impression s.
Impact drug and alcohol testing s.
Impact modular total hip s.
Impax PACS s.
ImplaMed implant s.
Implatome dental tomography s.
IMx PSA s.
INCA infant CPAP s.
Incardia valve s.
InCare pelvic floor therapy office s.
In Charge diabetes control s.
Indiana tome carpal tunnel release s.
Indigo LaserOptic treatment s.
Infant Flow nasal CPAP s.
In-Fast bone screw s.
In-Fast female sling s.
Infiniti vision s.
InFix interbody fusion s.
InfraGuide delivery s.
Infuse-a-Port vascular access s.
Inhale deep lung delivery s.
InjecAid s.
Injex needle-free injector s.
Innomed arthroplasty measuring s.

Innova feminine incontinence treatment s.
Innovator Holter s.
INOvent delivery s.
InPath cervical cancer screening s.
Insall-Burstein II modular knee s.
Insight knee positioning and alignment s.
InSight manometry s.
InstaTrak s.
InsulScan insulation testing s.
InSync ICD s.
In-Tac bone anchoring s.
Integral hip s.
Integrity AFx DR AutoCapture pacing s.
IntelliJet arthroscopic fluid management s.
Intensified Radiographic Imaging S. (IRIS)
Inteq small joint suturing s.
Interax total knee s.
Intermedics natural hip s.
International 10-20 s.
International Biomedical Mode 745-100 microcapillary infusion s.
International compression s.
Interpore IMZ implant s.
IntraArc 9963 arthroscopic power s.
Intrabeam intraoperative radiotherapy s.
intraluminal Safe-Steer guidewire s.
Intra-Op autotransfusion s.
Intrel 3 spinal cord stimulation s.
Invacare Venture II HomeFill complete home oxygen s.
InVance male sling s.
Inverter vitrectomy s.
Ionalyzer ion measurement s.
iON intraoperative navigation s.
Iontopatch transdermal drug delivery s.
Iontophor drug delivery s.
ipos arch support s.
Iriscorder portable infrared video pupillography s.
IRMA SL blood analysis s.
IRMA SL blood gas analysis s.
Irri-Cath suction s.
Irrijet DS irrigation s.

Irvine viable organ-tissue transport s.
IS1000 gel documentation imaging s.
ISKD internal limb lengthening s.
Isobar TTL posterior spinal s.
Isocam SPECT imaging s.
Isoflex portable pressure relief s.
Isola spinal instrumentation s.
Isolator blood culture s.
Isolex 300i magnetic stem cell selection s.
IsoMed constant-flow infusion s.
Isosleeve needle delivery s.
Isotechnologies B-200 back testing and rehabilitation s.
ITI dental implant s.
Itrel II, III spinal cord stimulation s.
IVAC needleless IV s.
Jace continuous passive motion ankle s.
Jackson staging s.
Jay Care wheelchair seating s.
Jewel AF implantable cardioverter defibrillator s.
Jimmy John colonic irrigation s.
Jinotti closed suctioning s.
Jobst athrombic pump s.
Johnson & Johnson PFC Sigma s.
joint activated s. (JAS)
Jostent Flex Supreme s.
Joyce-Loebl Magiscan image analysis s.
JS Quick-fill s.
J-Vac closed wound drainage s.
Kaneda anterior scoliosis s.
Karl Storz pediatric bronchoscopy s.
Katena Quick Switch I/A s.
KaVo oral surgery s.
K-Centrum anterior spinous fixation s.
Keeler loupe mounting s.
Kellan capsular sparing s.
Kelley-Goerss Compass stereotactic s.
Kelly stereotactic s.
Kendall A-V impulse s.
Kendall Ventex wound dressing s.
Keratom excimer laser s.
Khouri phacofragmentation s.

S

NOTES

system *(continued)*

Kinamed Exact-Fit ATH s.
Kin-Con isokinetic exercise s.
Kinematic II rotating-hinge total knee s.
Kinemax Plus total knee s.
Kinemetric guide s.
Kinetec ECT s.
Kinetik great toe implant s.
King double-umbrella closure s.
Kirschner hip replacement s.
Kirschner II-C shoulder s.
Kirschner integrated shoulder s.
Kleen-Needle s.
KLS-Martin modular osteosynthesis s.
Knee Signature s.
KnightStar 335 respiratory support s.
Koehler illumination s.
Koenig MPJ implant and arthroplasty s.
Koh colpotomizer s.
Komet XK-95 surgical drill s.
Kostuik-Harrington anterior distraction s.
Kostuik internal spine fixation s.
Kowa fluorescein s.
KTP/Nd:YAG XP surgical laser s.
KTP/532 surgical laser s.
Kulzer inlay s.
laboratory automation s.
Lact-Aid STARTrainer nursing s.
LactoSorb anterior cruciate ligament crosspin s.
Ladd fiberoptic s.
LAGB s.
Laitinen CT guidance s.
Lambotte exhaust s.
laminar flow s.
Lamis infusion s.
Laparolift s.
Laparomed cholangiogram vacuum s.
laparoscopic manipulator s.
laparoscopic retraction s.
Laparo Vac I&A s.
LaseAway ruby laser s.
Laser Advanced Interventional S.'s (LAIS)
laser CHRP rigid fiberscope s.
Laser I bubble s.
Laseroptic treatment s.
LaserScan LSX excimer laser s.
LaTIS intravascular laser s.
LCS mobile bearing knee s.
LCS total knee s.
LEAP s.
Lectromed urinary investigation s.

LEEP s.
left ventricular assist s. (LVAS)
Leibinger locking s.
Leibinger miniplate s.
Leibinger plating s.
Leibinger Profyle hand s.
Leibinger titanium mini Würzburg implant s.
Leibinger titanium Würzburg mandibular reconstruction s.
Leitz image analysis s.
Leksell stereotactic s.
Lenbach hip s.
Lens Comfort ultrasound cleaning and disinfecting s.
Leukotrap red cell storage s.
Level Anchorage s.
Level I normothermic irrigating s.
Lewis expandable adjustable prosthesis s.
Liberty spinal s.
Licox brain tissue oxygen monitoring s.
Lido Active Multijoint s.
Lidoback isokinetic dynamometry s.
Lido Passive Multijoint s.
Liebel-Flarsheim CT 9000 contrast delivery s.
Life-Air 1000 hypothermic therapy s.
Lifecore Restore wide diameter implant s.
LIFE-Lung fluorescence endoscopy s.
LifeNest portable seating s.
Lifepath AAA endovascular graft s.
LifeScan blood glucose monitoring s.
LifeShirt s.
LifeSite hemodialysis access s.
LiftStation lifting assessment s.
LigaSure vessel sealing s.
LightSheer laser hair removal s.
Liko Golvo lift s.
LIMA-Lift spreading s.
LimaLoop shoe s.
LINAC-based radiosurgical s.
linear accelerator s.
Linear total hip s.
Link Lubinus AP hip s.
Link Lubinus SP II total hip replacement s.
Link Saddle Prosthesis Endo-Model hip replacement s.
LionHeart ventricular assist s.
Lipoprint cholesterol subfraction test s.
Liquid Embolic s.
LiteNest portable seating s.

Lithovac Master suction and aspiration s.
Lixiscope pocket-size x-ray imaging s.
Localisa cardiac navigation s.
LogiCal pressure transducer s.
Lorad M-IV mammography s.
Lorad Selenia full-field digital mammography s.
Lordex lumbar spine s.
Lorenz Micro-Power dense bone drilling and cutting s.
Lorenz osteosynthesis s.
Lorenz plating s.
Lubinus AP hip s.
Lubinus SP II hip s.
Luhr maxillofacial fixation s.
Luhr microfixation s.
Luhr MRS s.
Luhr pan fixation s.
Luma cervical imaging s.
lumbar external drainage s.
Luxtec fiberoptic s.
LX 20 laser s.
LymphoScan nuclear imaging s.
Lynco biomechanical orthotic s.
LySonix TTD cannula s.
Macroduct s.
MacroPore OS reconstruction s.
MadaJet XL jet-injection anesthesia s.
Maestro MRI s.
Magerl hook-plate s.
Magerl plate-screw s.
Magna-Site locating s.
Magnes biomagnetometer s.
Magnetic Surgery s.
Magnetom Open MRI s.
Magnetron MRI s.
Magnex Alpha MR s.
Magnum-Meier s.
Malcolm-Lynn radiolucent spinal retraction s.
Malcolm-Rand radiolucent headrest and retraction s.
Malis bipolar coagulating/cutting s.
Malis CMC-III electrosurgical s.
malleable retractor s.
Mallinckrodt Hi-Care pulmonary hygiene s.
Mallinckrodt sensor s.
Mallory-Head modular calcar s.

Mammex TR computer-aided mammography diagnosis s.
Mammo-Lume imaging s.
Mammomat C3 mammography s.
MammoReader computer-aided detection s.
Mammoscan digital imaging s.
MammoSite radiation therapy s.
MammoSite radiation therapy s.
Mammotest Plus breast biopsy s.
Mammotest Select breast biopsy s.
Mammotome ultrasound biopsy s.
Manchester LDR implant s.
manometry s.
Maramed Miami fracture brace s.
Marex MRI s.
Marion oxygen resuscitation s.
Mark III halo s.
Mark II Sorrells hip arthroplasty retractor s.
Marlen UltraLite one-piece convex disposable s.
Marquette Case-12 electrocardiographic s.
MARS acetabular reconstructive s.
Marx bridging plate s.
Mason-Likar 12-lead EKG s.
Mastel compass-guided arcuate keratotomy s.
MatScan s.
Mattrix spinal cord stimulation s.
Maturna bra s.
Mauch GaitMaster s.
Max FiberScan laser s.
Maxilift Combi patient lifting s.
Maxim modular knee s.
Maxim revision knee s.
Maxi-Myst nebulizer s.
Mayfield surgical headrest s.
McCain TMJ arthroscopic s.
McGinnis balloon s.
McGuire I&A s.
McIntyre coaxial I&A s.
Mectra I&A s.
Meddars cardiac catheterization analysis s.
Medelec-Van Gogh electroencephalographic recording s.
Medex Secure s.
medical implant s. (MIS)
Medical Management S. (MMS)

S

NOTES

system *(continued)*

MediClenze therapy s.
Medi-Duct ocular fluid management s.
Mediflex MD-7 endoscopic video s.
Medi-Ject needle-free insulin injection s.
Medisorb drug delivery s.
Medi-Tech catheter s.
Mednext bone dissecting s.
Medos mechanical circulatory support s.
MedSelect-R X s.
Medspec MR imaging s.
Medstone IRIS s.
Medstone STS lithotripsy s.
Medtronic AVE stent s.
Medtronic Bridge X3 renal stent s.
Medtronic GFX 2 coronary stent s.
Medtronic GuardWire Plus s.
Medtronic Hemopump s.
Medtronic Interactive Tachycardia Terminating s.
Medtronic Interstim sacral nerve stimulation s.
Medtronic Pulsor Intrasound s.
Medtronic spinal cord stimulation s.
Medtronics Sequestra 1000 autotransfusion s.
Medwatch telemetry s.
Med-Wick medication delivery s.
Mega Peel resurfacing s.
MEG head-based coordinate s.
Meier magnum s.
Meniscus Mender II s.
Mentor cinch bladder neck suspension anchor s.
Mentor Contour Genesis s.
Mentor Contour Genesis ultrasonic lipoplasty s.
MetaFluor s.
Metalift crown and bridge removal s.
Metasul metal-on-metal hip prosthesis s.
Metrix atrial defibrillation s.
METRx s.
MG II total hip s.
MG II total knee s.
MHS modular hip screw s.
MIBB breast biopsy s.
MicroAire carpal tunnel release s.
Micro-Aire pulse lavage s.
MicroChoice electric powered surgical s.
microdebrider s. (MDS)

Micro Delta s.
microdilution s.
MicroGuide microelectrode recording s.
MicroHartzler ACS balloon catheter s.
MicroLap Gold microlaparoscopy s.
Microloc knee s.
MicroLux video camera s.
micromanometer catheter s.
MicroMax drill s.
Micro-Mill knee instrument s.
MicroPeel Plus s.
MicroPhor iontophoretic drug delivery s.
MicroPlex coil s.
Micro Plus plating s.
MicroShape keratome s.
Micros infusion s.
MicroSpan microhysteroscopy s.
MicroSpan minihysteroscopy s.
Microsponge delivery s.
Microstar dialysis s.
microvascular anastomotic coupler s.
Microvasive biliary stent s.
Microvasive Ultraflex esophageal stent s.
MicroVein vascular s.
microvitrectomy s. (MVS)
MicroWrist robotic surgical s.
Midas Rex instrumentation s.
Millennium CX microsurgical s.
Millennium LX microsurgical s.
Miller-Galante I condylar total knee s.
Miller-Galante revision knee s.
Miller-Galante total knee s.
Milli-Q water purification s.
Mimix bone replacement s.
MiniMed continuous glucose monitoring s.
Mirage nasal ventilation mask s.
Mirage spinal s.
Mirage top-tightening spinal s.
Mitek GII suture anchor s.
Mitek Vapr tissue removal s.
Mityvac vacuum delivery s.
MKM AutoPilot stereotactic s.
MLS small cannulated cancellous screw s.
MMG/O'Neil sterile-field urinary catheter s.
Mobetron intraoperative radiation therapy treatment s.
modular acetabular reconstruction s. (MARS)
Modular Acetabular Revision S. (MARS)

modular clip application s. (MCAS)
modular S-ROM total hip s.
Modulus CD anesthesia s.
Mojave cataract extraction s.
Monarch II IOL delivery s.
MonitorMate ergonomic monitor positioning control s.
MoniTorr ICP CSF drainage and monitoring s.
Monogram total knee instrument s.
Monotube external fixator s.
Montgomery thyroplasty implant s.
Monticelli-Spinelli circular external fixation s.
Moonwalker weightbearing s.
Morganstern aspiration/injection s.
Moss fixation s.
MotoVate rehabilitation s.
Mot-R-Pak vitrectomy s.
Mouradian humeral fixation s.
MPM I multi-parameter monitoring s.
Mport foldable lens placement s.
M4 rigid fixation s.
MR imaging s.
MSM-CIS s.
M-TEC 2000 surgical s.
Mui Scientific pressurized capillary infusion s.
Mulholland growth guidance s.
Mullins sheath s.
multidetector s.
MultiDop XS s.
MultiLight s.
Multi-Link Pixel coronary stent s.
Multi Podus foot s.
multiport illumination s. (MIS)
Multipulse laser s.
MultiSPIRO s.
Myocardial Protection s.
MyoSight dedicated nuclear cardiology camera s.
MYOtherm XP cardioplegia delivery s.
Nanoduct neonatal sweat analysis s.
nasal CPAP s.
Natchez Mobil-Trac s.
Natural-Knee II s.
Natural Profile abutment s.
Navigus cranial electrode s.

NaviPro Image-Free navigation s.
Navitrack computer-assisted navigation s.
NC-stat nerve conduction s.
NeedleBuster transdermal drug delivery s.
needle trephination s.
Neer II total knee s.
Neff femorotibial nail s.
Nellcor N-series fetal oxygen saturation monitoring s.
Nellcor OxiFirst fetal oxygen saturation monitoring s.
Nellcor Puritan Bennett 840 ventilator s.
Nellcor-Puritan Bennett 840 ventilator s.
NeoControl pelvic floor therapy s.
Neotrend s.
Neuroform microdelivery stent s.
Neurogard TCD s.
NeuroLink II EEG data acquisition s.
Neuropak 8 s.
NeuroPlan CRW stereotactic s.
Neuroprobe 500 pain management s.
NeuroPro rigid fixation s.
NeuroSector ultrasound s.
NeuroShield filter s.
NeuroStation frameless s.
Neurostat Mark II cryoanalgesia s.
Neurotrac II neurological monitoring s.
Neurotrend continuous multiparameter s.
Neuroview integrated visualization s.
NeuroVision s.
NeuroVision intraoperative nerve guidance s.
New Vision magnification s.
Nexerciser Plus exercise s.
NexFlex total hip s.
NexFlex total knee s.
Nexus wheelchair seating s.
Niamtu video imaging s.
Nicolet Biomedical UltraSom NT polysomnography s.
Nicolet Viking II electrophysiologic s.
Nidek MK-2000 keratome s.

NOTES

system (*continued*)

NIR Primo Monorail stent s.
NLite laser collagen
  replenishment s.
Nobelpharma implant s.
Nomos stereotactic s.
NonSpil drug delivery s.
nonthoracotomy defibrillation
  lead s.
NordiCare Back Therapy s.
Norwegian s.
No-Touch delivery s.
Novacor left ventricular assist s.
NovaLine excimer laser s.
Nova Microsonics Image Vue s.
NovaPulse laser s.
NovaSure endometrial ablation s.
Novoste Beta-Cath s.
NS2000 bipolar generator s.
Nucleus 24 Contour cochlear
  implant s.
Nu-Trake Weiss emergency
  airway s.
Nuvolase 660 laser s.
Oasis sheet introducer s.
Obtura II gutta percha s.
OCL PolyLite synthetic splinting s.
OCL Splint Roll Contour
  splinting s.
Octopus 2, 2+, 3 tissue
  stabilization s.
OctreoScan s.
Oculex drug delivery s.
Ocutech Vision Enhancing s.
Ocutome II fragmentation s.
Odyssey phacoemulsification s.
OEC-Diasonics 9400 fluoroscopy
  C-arm s.
OEC Mini 6600 imaging s.
OEC-series FluoroTrak navigation s.
Ogden tissue reattachment mini s.
OIS image digitizing s.
Olerud PSF fixation s.
OligoDetect s.
Olson calibrated cornea trephine s.
Olympus CLV-series fiberoptic s.
Olympus MAJ363 FNA needle s.
Olympus OSP fluorescence
  measuring s.
Olympus video urology
  procedure s.
Omega CSI MR s.
Omega Plus compression hip s.
Ommaya intraventricular reservoir s.
Omnifit HA hip s.
Omnifit Plus hip s.
Omni-Flow 4000 Plus medication
  management s.
Omni-LapoTract support s.

Omni-Tract retractor s.
One Action Stent Introduction S.
One Touch II hospital blood
  glucose monitoring s.
OnLine ABG monitoring s.
On-Q pain management s.
Opart MRI imaging s.
Opdima digital mammography s.
OpenGene automated DNA
  sequencing s.
open-loop insulin delivery s.
open MRI s.
OPERA s.
Operating Arm s.
Opmilas 144 Plus laser s.
Opsis DistalCam video s.
Optetrak comprehensive knee s.
Optetrak total knee s.
Optical Biopsy s.
optical multichannel analyzer s.
Optical Tracking S. (OTS)
Opti-Fix total hip s.
OptiHaler drug delivery s.
Optimaze surgical ablation s.
Option hip s.
Opti-Pure s.
Opti-Qvue CCO pulmonary artery
  catheter s.
Optistar MR contrast delivery s.
OptiVu HDVD s.
OptoTrak motion-analysis s.
Orbasone s.
Orbscan corneal topography s.
Orfizip casting s.
Orion cardiovascular information
  management s.
Orion continence s.
Orlando tibial plateau fracture
  bracing s.
OrlandoTPFx bracing s.
Orth-evac autotransfusion s.
Orthodoc presurgical planning s.
Ortho-evac postoperative
  autotransfusion s.
Orthofix ISKD s.
Ortholoc Advantim revision knee s.
Orthomet Axiom total knee s.
Orthomet Perfecta total hip s.
OrthoPak bone growth stimulator s.
Orthotec pressurized fluid
  irrigation s.
OrthPAT autotransfusion s.
Oscar ultrasonic bone cement
  removal s.
OscilloMate 930 blood pressure
  measurement s.
OSI modular table s.
OssaTron extracoporeal
  shockwave s.

OsseoFix implant s.
Osseous Coagulum Trap
collecting s.
Osteobond vacuum mixing s.
Osteochondral Autograft Transfer S.
(OATS)
Osteo-Clage cable s.
OsteoMed bioresorbable fixation s.
Osteonics Omnifit-C long stem s.
Osteonics Scorpio posterior cruciate
retaining total knee s.
Osteonics spinal s.
Osteonics total shoulder s.
Osteopatch test s.
OsteoView desktop hand x-ray s.
Ostreg spinal marker s.
OtoScan ear aeration s.
Oulu neuronavigator s.
Outpatient Endometrial Resection
and Ablation S.
Ovation falloposcopy s.
oxalate s.
oxalate dentin bonding s.
OxiFirst fetal monitoring s.
OxiMax pulse oximetry s.
Oxycure topical oxygen s.
Oxydome oxygen therapy s.
Oxylator-EM 100 resuscitation s.
OxyLite oxygen conserving s.
Oxy-Ultra-Lite ambulatory
oxygen s.
Paceart complete pacemaker
testing s.
Pacefinder lead placement s.
Packard radioimmunoassay s.
PadKit sample collection s.
PainBuster infusion delivery s.
PainDoc computerized support s.
Panasol II home phototherapy s.
PanoView arthroscopic s.
Papnet computer-assisted Pap smear
testing s.
Pap-Perfect supply s.
Parabath paraffin s.
ParaFlow right heart support s.
Paragon single-stage dental
implant s.
ParaMax cruciate guide s.
Parastep I s.
Paratrend 7 intravenous blood gas
monitoring s.

Parisian Peel Prestige medical
microdermabrasion s.
Paris ultrasound s.
Park-O-Tron drill s.
Parr closed-irrigation s.
Pathfinder microcatheter s.
PathSpeed picture archiving
communication s.
Patil stereotactic s.
Paulus trocar s.
PCA modular total knee s.
Peak anterior compression plate s.
Pedar in-shoe pressure
measurement s.
pediatric circle s.
Pediatric Nutrition Surveillance S.
Pegasus Airwave pressure relief s.
Pelorus surgical s.
pelvic floor therapy s.
Pelvic Organ Prolapse-Quantified s.
PenRad mammography
information s.
Pentax endoPRO s.
Pentax-Hitachi FG32UA
endosonographic s.
Perclose A-T vessel closure s.
PercuSurge GuardWire Plus
temporary occlusion and
aspiration s.
PercuSurge recovery s.
percutaneous mechanical
thrombectomy s.
Percutaneous Stoller Afferent Nerve
Stimulation s.
Perfecta Interseal total hip s.
PerFixation s.
Performa diagnostic ultrasound
imaging s.
Performance modular total knee s.
PerioTemp periodontal screening s.
Periotest s.
Peritronics Medical Inc. fetal
monitoring s.
Permark micropigmentation s.
peroral electronic pancreatoscope s.
(PEPS)
PerQ SANS s.
Perspective chest imaging s.
Perspective dental imaging s.
PFC Sigma total knee s.
PFC total hip replacement s.

NOTES

system *(continued)*
  Phaco Commander
    phacoemulsification s.
  Phacojack phaco s.
  PharmChek sweat patch drug
    detection s.
  phased-array color-flow
    ultrasound s.
  Philips DVI 1 s.
  Philips Easyguide navigation s.
  Phoenix fifth ventricle s.
  Phoresor II iontophoretic drug
    delivery s.
  PhosphorImager s.
  PhotoDerm bright light delivery s.
  PhotoDerm MultiLight s.
  PhotoGenica T laser s.
  photon-activated drug delivery s.
  Photon cataract removal s.
  Photon laser s.
  Photon Ocular Surgery s.
  Photon Radiosurgery s.
  Phototome s.
  pH-Response reflux diagnostic s.
  Physios CTM 01 s.
  Picket Fence fiducial localization
    stereotactic s.
  Picture Archiving and
    Communications S. (PACS)
  Pie Medical CAAS II analysis s.
  Pillo-Pump alternating pressure s.
  Pinch Gauge and Jackson Strength
    evaluation s.
  Pinnacle 3D radiotherapy
    planning s.
  Pinn-ACL guide s.
  Pisces spinal cord stimulation s.
  Pittman IMA retractor s.
  plating s.
  Pleur-evac autotransfusion s.
  Pleur-evac Sahara chest drainage s.
  PLI-100 picoinjector pipette s.
  PlumeSafe Whisper 602 smoke
    evacuation s.
  2010 Plus Holter s.
  Plyoball s.
  PMT robotic fulcrumless
    tomographic s.
  pneumohydraulic capillary
    infusion s.
  PneuView single lung s.
  PneuView ventilator testing and
    training s.
  PodoSpray nail drill s.
  Polar coordinate s.
  Polaroid HealthCam s.
  Polarus Plus humeral fixation s.
  Polarus positional humeral
    fixation s.

  polyaxial spine s. (PASS)
  Porex drainage s.
  PortaFlo urine collection s.
  PortalVision radiation oncology s.
  Portex Soft-Seal cuff s.
  PowerGrip stent delivery s.
  PowerSculpt cosmetic surgery s.
  Precise ACL guide s.
  Precision hip s.
  Precision office transurethral needle
    ablation s.
  Precision QID glucose
    monitoring s.
  Precision Strata hip s.
  PreClean soak s.
  Premier cervical plate s.
  Press-Fit total condylar knee s.
  PressureGuard Select patient
    adjustable pressure management s.
  Presto-Flash spirometer s.
  Primbs-Circon indirect video
    ophthalmoscope s.
  Prime ECG electrocardiac
    mapping s.
  PrinceStar electrophysiologic
    imaging study s.
  ProAire portable rotation s.
  Probe balloon-on-a-wire dilatation s.
  Procera s.
  Profile mammography s.
  Profile total hip s.
  Profix total knee replacement s.
  programmable VariGrip II
    prosthetic control s.
  Pro-Post s.
  Proscan ultrasound imaging s.
  ProstaJect ethanol injection s.
  Prostathermer prostatic
    hyperthermia s.
  ProSys Urahesive s.
  Protector meniscus suturing s.
  ProTime microcoagulation s.
  ProTrac cruciate reconstruction s.
  Providence scoliosis s.
  Proxiderm wound closure s.
  Pulsar Max II pacemaker s.
  PulseSpray pulsed infusion s.
  Pump-It-Up pneumatic socket
    volume management s.
  Pump-Vac Plus s.
  Puno-Winter-Byrd transpedicular
    spine fixation s.
  PWB transpedicular spine
    fixation s.
  Pylon intramedullary nail s.
  PyMaH Trimline
    sphygmomanometer s.
  Q-Plex cardiopulmonary exercise s.
  Q-prep s.

Q-Rad TOMO system tomography radiographic s.
Quadracut ACL shaver s.
QuadraLase advanced surgical fiber s.
Quadra pipetting s.
Quantimet 500 image analysis s.
Quantrex Sweep 650 ultrasonic cleansing s.
Quantronic Resonance S. (QRS)
Quark PFT modular s.
Quartet s.
Quest MPS s.
QuickFlow distal perfusion s.
QuickRinse automated instrument rinse s.
Quick-Sil silicone s.
Quick Trak periosteal fixation s.
Quimby implant s.
radiation therapy s. (RTS)
radiofrequency interstitial tissue ablation s.
radiofrequency needle electrode s.
radioimmunoguided surgery s.
RadioLucent wrist fixation s.
Radionics articulated arm s.
Radionics Optical Tracking S.
radionuclide carrier s.
RadiStop radial compression s.
RadNet radiology information s.
Rainbow 3D camera s.
Randelli modular shoulder s.
RapidLoc meniscal repair s.
Rapido dual-catheter s.
RapidScreen RS-2000 computer-aided detection s.
Raptor over-the-wire delivery s.
Rasor blood pumping s.
real-time 2-dimensional Doppler flow-imaging s.
real-time position management tracking s.
RED s.
Reebok Slide s.
Reebok Step s.
Refine fusion s.
Refinity Coblation s.
Reflex anterior cervical plate s.
ReFlexion implant s.
Regulus Navigator image-guided s.
Reichert-Mundinger stereotactic s.
Rekow s.

Relay suture delivery s.
Relume s.
Remac s.
Remedy sleep therapy s.
remote afterloading s.
REMstar Plus CPAP s.
REMstar Pro CPAP s.
Renaissance crown s.
Renaissance II spirometry s.
Replace Select implant s.
Replica total hip replacement s.
resorbable copolymer PGA/PLLA-Lactosorb miniplate fixation s.
Respitrace respiratory monitoring s.
Response R2930 4-Stack Multi-Station exercise s.
Res-Q-Vac emergency suction s.
Restoration acetabular s.
Restoration-HA hip s.
Restore ACL guide s.
RetroX hearing s.
Retzius s.
ReUnite resorbable orthopaedic fixation s.
Revelation hip s.
Reviva Microbrade Duo s.
RF ablation s.
RFb respiratory biofeedback s.
rhinolaryngostroboscopy s.
Rhinoline endoscopic sinus surgery s.
Rhinotherm controlled temperature s.
RiboPrinter microbial characterization s.
Richards modular hip s.
Richard Wolf nasal epistaxis s.
rigid external distraction s.
RigiScan Plus rigidity assessment s.
ring-type imaging s.
Rinoflow nasal wash and sinus s.
RITA ablation s.
Rival coronary stent s.
r\LS red blood cell filtration s.
RLS videostroboscopy s.
RM stereotaxic s.
Robotrac passive retraction s.
Rodenstock Modular Focusing s.
rod-lens s.
Rod TAG suture anchor s.
Rogan teleradiology s.

S

NOTES

system *(continued)*

Roger s.
Rogozinski spinal fixation s.
Roho pediatric seating s.
Rolyan Reach-N-Range pulley s.
Romhilt-Estes point scoring s.
Rosenkranz pedatric retractor s.
Rotablator RotaLink s.
Rotaglide total knee s.
RotoClix tubing fixation s.
RPM tracking s.
Rudolph breathing s.
RUMI s.
Russell-Taylor femoral interlocking nail s.
RZ mandibular matrix s.
Safeset blood sampling s.
Safe-Steer to Crossing coronary guidewire s.
Safestretch incontinence s.
SafeTrak ESP s.
SAFHS 2000 ultrasound fracture healing s.
Safsite IV therapy s.
Saf-T-Intima integrated IV catheter safety s.
Sahara ultrasound s.
SalEst preterm labor test s.
SAM s.
Sanarus Visica treatment s.
Sanders Venturi injector s.
Sandhill esophageal motility s.
Sandman s.
SaphLite II retractor s.
SaphLite saphenous vein s.
Sapphire premium closed wound drainage s.
Sarstedt s.
Savant imaging s.
Save-A-Tooth emergency tooth preserving s.
scanned-slot detector s.
scanning beam digital s.
Scaphoid-Microstaple s.
scattering s.
Schmidt optics s.
Schneider-Meier magnum s.
Schwartz-Blajwas-Marcinko irrigation s.
ScleroPLUS HP laser s.
Scorpio total knee s.
Scotchcast custom length splint s.
Scott chronic wound care s.
Screw-Vent implant s.
Script Stat, Inc. dispensing s.
Second Look computer-aided detection s.
Secor s.

Secure closed pressure monitoring and blood sampling s.
SecureStrand cervical fusion s.
Secure Yet Gentle surgical dressing s.
Secur-Fit HA hip s.
Select GT blood glucose testing s.
Selectron s.
Selenia full-field digital mammography s.
Sendax MDI s.
SenDx 100 blood gas/electrolyte analysis s.
Senographe 2000D digital mammography s.
Senographe DMR+ mammography s.
SenoScan full-field digital mammography s.
Sens-A-Ray digital dental imaging s.
Sensatec fall prevention s.
SensiCath blood gas monitoring s.
Sensi-Touch regional anesthesia delivery s.
SensoScan mammography s.
septal occluder s.
Septer closed wound drainage s.
Septi-Chek blood culture s.
Sequel compression s.
Sequestra 1000 autotransfusion s.
Sequoia Acuson s.
Sequoia echocardiography s.
Seraton dialysis control s.
Setma hydrotherapy s.
Sewell s.
Shadow-Line ACF spine retractor s.
Shape Maker s.
Sharplan sight s.
SharpShooter meniscal repair s.
sheath and dilator s.
Sherlock soft tissue fixation s.
Sherman remote podiatric vacuum s.
Sherwood intrascopic suction/irrigation s.
Shiley cardioplegia s.
Shiley catheter distention s.
Shimadzu ultrasound s.
Shockwave Therapy S.'s (STS)
Shutt suture punch s.
Sibel-Home-300 sleep diagnostic s.
Sicor cardiac catheterization recording s.
Siemens Somatom Plus 4 CT s.
Siemens Sonoline SI-400 ultrasound s.
Sienna ultrasound s.

Sigma II Dualplace hyperbaric s.
Sigma 34 Monoplace hyperbaric s.
Signa Advantage s.
Signa Horizon LX MRI s.
Signa Infinity MRI s.
Signature Edition infusion s.
Silberg E.U.A. s.
Silent Speaker communication s.
Silhouette spinal fixation s.
Silhouette therapeutic massage s.
Silicon Graphics Reality Engine s.
SilkLaser laser s.
Simal cervical stabilization s.
Simcoe I&A s.
Simmons plating s.
Simple-Ject auto-injector s.
SimpliCT interventional guidance s.
Simpson-Robert vascular dilation s.
Simpulse irrigation s.
Sinai s.
SinuNEB s.
Sirecust 404N neonatal
  monitoring s.
Sirognathograph analyzing s.
Site-Rite II ultrasound s.
SiteSelect percutaneous incisional
  breast biopsy s.
SITEtrac spinal surgery s.
Site TXR phacoemulsification s.
SkinLaser s.
SkinMaster MD7 skin
  rejuvenation s.
Sky-Boot stirrup s.
Sky epidural pain control s.
Skylight s.
Slingshot ACL fixation s.
slow deflate s. (SDS)
SLS Chromos long pulse ruby
  laser s.
small fragment s. (SFS)
SmartDose infusion s.
SmartKard digital Holter s.
SmartMist asthma management s.
SmartSite needleless s.
SmartSpot high-resolution digital
  imaging s.
SmiLine abutment s.
S-Monovette blood collection s.
Snuggle Warm convective
  warming s.
Snugs tapeless wound care s.
Socon spinal s.

Socrates Robotic telecollaboration s.
Socrates telementoring s.
Sodem high-speed s.
Soehendra catheter s.
Soehendra endoscopic biliary
  stent s.
SofTec Lens Delivery s.
SoftLight laser hair removal s.
Soft & Secure pouch s.
Solaris MR injection s.
Solcotrans autotransfusion s.
Solcotrans Plus drainage-
  reinfusion s.
Solcovac closed wound drainage s.
Solid Creation s.
Soma Gonio s.
Soma pulley s.
SomaSensor cerebral oximeter
  monitoring s.
SOMNOlab sleep diagnostic s.
Somnoplasty s.
Somnus Somnoplasty s.
Sonablate 200 s.
Songer spinal cable s.
sonic accelerated fracture healing s.
  (SAFHS)
Sonicaid Vasoflow Doppler s.
SonicWave phacoemulsification s.
Sonifer sonicating s.
SonoAce 6000 II ultrasound s.
Sonocur Basic s.
SonoHeart Elite personal hand-
  carried echocardiography s.
Sonoline Elegra ultrasound s.
Sonoline Sienna ultrasound s.
Sonomed A/B-Scan s.
Sonopsy ultrasound-guided breast
  biopsy s.
SonoSite 180 ultrasound s.
Sonos-series imaging s.
Sonotron Vingmed CFM 800
  imaging s.
Soprano cryoablation s.
Sorbie-Questor total elbow s.
Sorrells Mark II hip arthroplasty
  retractor s.
Sovereign Shield s.
SPARC sling s.
SpaTouch PhotoEpilation s.
Spect-Align laser s.
SPECT high-resolution brain s.

S

NOTES

system *(continued)*

Spectra 400 extended surveillance and alert s.
Spectramed L2000 color therapy s.
Spectranetics excimer laser s.
SpectraScience optical biopsy s.
Spectris Solaris MR injection s.
Spectron EF total hip s.
Spectrum Lensographer lens analysis s.
Spectrum tissue repair s.
Sperm Select sperm recovery s.
SphygmoCor noninvasive aortic blood pressure s.
SpinaLase Nd:YAG surgical laser s.
SpineLink anterior cervical spinal s.
Spinoscope noninasive imaging s.
SpiroSense s.
Spiros inhalation delivery s.
Spline dental implant s.
Sportorno cementless hip arthroplasty s.
SportsRAC arm care s.
SprayGel adhesion barrier s.
square module seating s.
Squirt wound irrigation s.
S-ROM hip replacement s.
S-ROM modular total knee s.
S-ROM proximally modular total hip s.
S-series sleep s.
Stabident s.
Stability total hip s.
Stableloc II external wrist fixation s.
STA Compact hemostasis s.
Stage-1 single-stage dental implant s.
StairMaster exercise s.
Standing Ovation MRI s.
Stanmore modular hip s.
STAR s.
STA-R hemostasis s.
STARRT falloposcopy s.
Star S2 SmoothScan excimer laser s.
STart-4, -8 clot detection s.
Statak anchor s.
STAT-Site M Hgb test s.
Status Cup Plus testing s.
Stay-Erec s.
Stealth occlusion s.
StealthStation image-guided s.
Steele fiberoptic s.
Steffee pedicle screw-plate s.
stent and vent s.

StereoGuide stereotactic breast biopsy s.
stereotactic breast biopsy s.
Stereotaxis magnetic surgery s.
Steriking sterilization s.
Sterrad sterilization s.
St. Jude Medical aortic connector s.
Stoller afferent nerve stimulation s. (SANS)
stone-tissue detection s.
stone-tissue recognition s.
Storz Millennium microsurgical s.
Straight-In male sling s.
Straight-In surgical s.
Strata hip s.
Stratis II MRI s.
Stryker SE3 arthroscopy s.
STS lithotripsy s.
Sub-Vent implant s.
Sudbury s.
Summit channel plate fixation s.
Summit rod fixation s.
Sundt AVM clip s.
Sundt suction s.
Sunrise LTK s.
Sun SPARCstation s.
Super-4 catheter ablation s.
superconductive magnetic s.
Superscript preamplification s.
Superset exercise s.
Supine C-Trax cervical traction s.
Sure-Closure skin stretching s.
SureScan s.
SureStart contrast tracking s.
SureStart imaging s.
Sure Step ankle support s.
SureStepPro professional blood glucose management s.
SureTrans autotransfusion s.
Surg-E-Trol I/A s.
Surg-E-Trol I/A/R s.
Surgiflex WAVE XP suction-irrigation s.
Surgi-PEG replacement gastrostomy feeding s.
Surgi Stim postsurgical therapy s.
Surgitek OM-5 urodynamic s.
SURx transvaginal s.
Sustain dental implant s.
Suture Assistant s.
suture tension adjustment reel s.
SwimEx hydrotherapy s.
Swiss Precision cannula s.
swivel-arm s.
Symphony graft delivery s.
Symphony monitoring s.
Symphony MRI s.
Synaptic 2000 pain management s.

SynchroMed infusion s.
Syncrus low-energy internal
  cardioversion s.
Synergy neurostimulation s.
Synergy posterior titanium spinal s.
Synergy ultrasound s.
Synevac vacuum curettage s.
Synthes CerviFix s.
Synthes Schuhli implant s.
Synthes Universal spinal s.
TAG open instrument s.
Talairach bicommissural reference s.
Talairach-Tournoux s.
Talent LPS endoluminal stent-
  graft s.
Talos laser delivery s.
Taperloc hip s.
TargetCath steerable catheter s.
Targis s.
Tarsys tilt and recline s.
Taylor Wharton Model 27K
  cryostorage s.
TBird ventilatory s.
TCI Heartmate mechanical
  circulatory support s.
TD glucose monitoring s.
Tebbetts EndoPlastic instrument s.
TEC atherectomy s.
Tech-Attach connection s.
Technolas 217 excimer laser s.
Technos ultrasound s.
Techstar XL percutaneous vascular
  surgical s.
TEC interface s.
TEGwire ST s.
Telefactor beehive s.
telemanipulator s.
TelePACS remote diagnostic s.
Terumo Steri-Cell s.
Tesla MRI s.
Testoderm testosterone
  transdermal s.
Tetra coronary stent s.
Tetrax interactive balance s.
Texas Scottish Rite Hospital
  pedical screw and rod s.
ThAIRapy vest airway clearance s.
The Bodyguard emboli
  containment s.
Therabite jaw motion
  rehabilitation s.
Thera Cool cold therapy s.

TheraPEP positive expiratory
  pressure therapy s.
Thera-turn rotational s.
ThermaChoice uterine balloon
  therapy s.
ThermaCool TC s.
ThermoChem-HT s.
Thermo-Flo irrigation s.
ThermoPulse pain relief therapy s.
Thermo-STAT rewarming s.
Thompson-Farley spinal retractor s.
Thompson hip endoprosthesis s.
thoracic drainage s.
thoracolumbosacroiliac implant s.
Thora-Drain III chest drainage s.
Thora-Klex chest drainage s.
Thoraseal chest tube drainage s.
Thoratec mechanical circulatory
  support s.
Thoravision s.
thrombectomy s.
Thrombex PMT clot removal s.
Thumper CPR s.
tibial torsion s.
Ti-Fit total hip s.
Ti-Frame posterior fixation s.
time-of-flight PET imaging s.
TiMesh cranial plating s.
TiMesh craniofacial s.
TiMesh craniomaxillofacial
  plating s.
TiMesh rigid fixation bone
  plating s.
TiMesh titanium bone plating s.
TiMX comprehensive low-back s.
tissue anchor guide s.
Titan intramedullary nail s.
titanium hollow screw-plate s.
TMJ Concepts patient-fitted TMJ
  prosthesis s.
TMS 3-dimensional radiation
  therapy treatment planning s.
Tomey topographic modeling s.
Tomolex tomographic s.
TomTec imaging s.
Topcon IMAGEnet digital
  imaging s.
Top Notch automated biopsy s.
topographic scanning s.
TopSS topographic scanning s.
Tosic external fixation s.
Total O₂/Oxylite oxygen s.

NOTES

system *(continued)*

Total Recall digital imaging s.
Total Synchrony s.
TPL-6 hip s.
Trac knee s.
Tranquility Auto CPAP s.
Tranquility bilevel s.
Tranquility Quest CPAP s.
transesophageal pacing s.
TransFix ACL s.
TransFx external fixation s.
transluminal lysing s.
TransScan 200 breast imaging s.
TransScan TS2000 electrical
   impedance breast scanning s.
transtelephonic ambulatory
   monitoring s.
transurethral needle ablation s.
TraumaJet wound debridement s.
Traveler portable oxygen s.
Treon ENT image guidance s.
Trex digital mammography s.
Triad defibrillator s.
Triad SPECT imaging s.
TriaDyne II therapy s.
Triage cardiac s.
tricomponent coaxial s.
TriFix spinal instrumentation s.
Trima automated blood
   collection s.
Tri-Motion knee s.
Trinica s.
Trinica anterior cervical plate s.
triple-lumen perfused catheter s.
Triton power surgical instrument s.
Tri-Wedge total hip s.
trocar-cannula s.
TroGARD Finesse dilating trocar s.
Trubyte Alma gauge s.
Tru-Close wound drainage s.
True/Fit femoral intramedullary
   rod s.
True/Flex intramedullary rod s.
TrueMax 2400 metabolic s.
Trufill n-BCA liquid embolic s.
TruPulse CO_2 laser s.
TruTrak data sampling s.
TS2000 breast imaging s.
T-TAC s.
T2 thermoablation s.
TULIP syringe s.
Tumble Forms Tortoise Shell
   therapy s.
TurnAide therapeutic s.
Turning Board exercise s.
Turnsoft automatic turning s.
TwinMic hearing s.
Tylok high-tension cerclage
   cabling s.

UlcerJet s.
Ulson fixator s.
Ultima hip replacement s.
UltiMA mammography s.
Ultima OPCAB s.
Ultimax distal femoral
   intramedullary rod s.
Ultimax Haig II nail s.
UltraBag s.
Ultra-Drive bone cement
   removal s.
UltraFix rotator cuff suture
   anchor s.
Ultraflex dynamic splint s.
Ultraflex esophageal stent s.
Ultraflex stent delivery s.
Ultra-Guard hip orthosis s.
UltraLite one-piece convex
   disposable s.
UltraPACS diagnostic imaging s.
UltraPak enteral closed feeding s.
UltraPower drill s.
Ultrascan digital B s.
Ultraseed ultrasound-guided
   brachytherapy s.
UltraShaper Automate durable
   keratome s.
UltraSom NT polysomnography s.
Ultra Twin bag s.
Ultra-X external fixation s.
Ultra Y-set s.
underwater seal drainage s.
Unfolder intraocular lens
   implantation s.
Unica CO_2 laser s.
Uniflex nailing s.
Uni-frame patient immobilization s.
Uni-Lead ECG electrode s.
Unilink hand surgery s.
UniPlast Imaging and Archiving s.
UniPort Plus vein harvesting s.
Unison bone plate s.
UniSpacer knee s.
Unistep delivery s.
United Sonics J shock phaco
   fragmentor s.
Unitek II convoluted innerspring
   mattress s.
Unitrax unipolar s.
Uni-Vent Eagle portable
   ventilation s.
Universal F breathing s.
Universal Plus instrument s.
Uni-Yeast-Tek s.
Unopette s.
Up and About s.
uPACS picture archiving s.
UPS 2020 ambulatory
   manometry s.

Uro-Cup female vaginal urinary collection s.
Urocyte diagnostic cytometry s.
UroVive s.
Urowave microwave thermotherapy s.
USCI Probe balloon-on-a-wire dilatation s.
UT bag s.
Vac-Lok patient immobilization s.
V.A.C. Therapy wound healing s.
Vacupac portable vacuum s.
Vacutainer specimen tube s.
Vakutage suction s.
Valleylab CUSA CEM s.
Valleylab REM s.
Valley Vac smoke evacuation s.
Vapr arthroscopic s.
Var-A-Pulse wound debridement s.
Variable Anesthesia Monitoring S. (VAMOS)
variable screw placement s.
Varian brachytherapy s.
Varian MLC s.
VariCare s.
Varigrip spine fixation s.
Varis radiation oncology s.
VasoExtor lead extraction s.
Vasotrac blood pressure monitoring s.
VasoView balloon dissection s.
VasoView Uniport Plus endoscopic vein harvesting s.
Vector low back analysis s.
VectorVision neuronavigation s.
VenaFlow compression s.
Venodyne venous compression s.
venous arterial blood management protection s. (VAMP)
VentAire bottle s.
VentNet remote monitoring s.
Ventritex TVL s.
Ventrix tunnelable ventricular intracranial pressure monitoring s.
VentTrak monitoring s.
Venture II HomeFill complete home oxygen s.
Venturi-Flo valve s.
Verruca-Freeze clinical freezing s.
Versaback Safe Station back s.
VersaDoc Model 5000 imaging s.
Versa-Fracture femoral fixation s.

Versalok low-back fixation s.
VersaPoint s.
Versaport trocar s.
Versatrac lumbar retractor s.
VerSys hip s.
VertAlign spinal support s.
Vertetrac ambulatory traction s.
Vertex reconstruction s.
Vertis PNT s.
vesicular transport s.
vessel occlusion s.
VestaBlate balloon s.
Vest airway clearance s.
Vet-Co vacuum s.
Viatronix V3D virtual colonoscopy s.
VidaMed TUNA s.
Vidas automated immunoassay s.
Viewing Wand s.
Vigilance monitoring s.
virtual biopsy s.
Virtuoso LX Smart CPAP s.
Virtuoso portable three-dimensional imaging s.
Visica cryoablation s.
Visica treatment s.
Visio-Gem color s.
Vision Magnetom 1.5-tesla s.
Vision Sciences bronchoscope EndoSheath s.
Vision Sciences VSI 2000 flexible sigmoidoscope s.
Visitec surgical vitrectomy s.
Visulab s.
Visx Star S2 excimer laser s.
Visx Twenty/Twenty s.
Visx Wavefront s.
Visx WaveScan wavefront s.
Vitrea 3D s.
Vnus Closure vein reflux s.
Vocare bladder s.
Voluson ultrasound s.
Vortex stabilization s.
Voxel s.
VoxelView s.
Voxgram digital holography s.
VPAP II ST-A ventilatory assistance s.
VPI nonadhesive colostomy s.
VPI nonadhesive ileostomy s.
VPI nonadhesive urostomy s.
VueCath spinal endoscopic s.

S

NOTES

system *(continued)*
VueLock anterior cervical plate s.
Vulcan EAS ElectroThermal
 Arthorscopy s.
Waffle mattress replacement s.
Wagner revision hip s.
Wallaby II phototherapy s.
Wallach LL100 cryosurgical s.
WarmTouch patient warming s.
Warm-Up active wound therapy s.
WaveMap intracoronary pressure s.
WaveScan wavefront s.
WaveWire guidewireXact graft-
 fixation s.
Wedge TAG suture anchor s.
Wheeler cyclodialysis s.
whole-body MR imaging s.
Wiktor GX Hepamed coated
 coronary artery stent s.
Wiltse cross-bracing spinal
 fixation s.
Wiltse pedicle screw fixation s.
Window cervical plate s.
Winquest tibial/femoral extraction s.
Wisorb spinal fusion s.
Wit portable TENS s.
Wolf aspiration/injection s.
Wolf delivery s.
Wrightlock spinal fusion s.
Würzburg maxillofacial plating s.
WuScope s.
Xact graft-fixation s.
XFix DynaFix s.
Xia spinal s.
Xillix LIFE-GI fluorescence
 endoscopy s.
Xillix LIFE-Lung s.
XKnife stereotactic radiosurgery s.
Xplorer 1000 digital imaging s.
X-Press vascular closure s.
XPS Sculpture s.
XPS Straightshot micro tissue
 resector s.

Xsensor Pressure Mapping s.
Xtrac laser s.
X-Trel spinal cord stimulation s.
YagLazr s.
ZAAG dental implant s.
ZA-Stent endoscopic biliary stent s.
Zeiss OPMI CS-NC2 surgical
 microscope s.
Zephir anterior cervical plate s.
Zest Anchor Advanced Generation
 implant s.
Zeus computer-controlled robotic s.
Zeus surgical s.
Zeus voice-controlled robotic s.
Zimmer anatomic hip prosthesis s.
Zimmer CPT hip s.
Zimmer-Hall drive s.
Zimmer Pulsavac wound
 debridement s.
ZMR hip s.
ZMS intramedullary fixation s.
Zone Specific II meniscal repair s.
Zplate-ATL anterior spinal
 fixation s.
Zuni exercise s.
systemic arterial catheter
System-S soft skeletal implant
Syticon 5950 bipolar demand
 pacemaker
Szabo-Berci
 S.-B. needle
 S.-B. needle driver
Sztehlo umbilical clamp
Szulc
 S. bone cutter
 S. grommet
 S. orbital implant
 S. vascular dilator
Szuler
 S. eustachian bougie
 S. vascular forceps
Szultz corneal forceps

T

T bandage
T bar
T clamp
T Philips ACS-II Gyroscan
T rotating joint
T self-retaining drainage tube
T tube

T-28 hip prosthesis
T2 thermoablation system
T2-weighted scan
TA

thoracoabdominal
TA II loading unit
TA metallic staple
TA Premium-series staple

Tabb

T. crural nipper
T. double-ended flap knife
T. ear curette
T. ear elevator
T. ear knife
T. knife pick
T. myringoplasty knife
T. ruler

table

ActiveTrac traction treatment t.
Adapta massage t.
Advocate electric flexion
  distraction t.
Air-Drop chiropractic t.
Air-Flex chiropractic t.
Akron tilt t.
Albee orthopaedic fracture t.
Allen arm surgery t.
Alliance cable system t.
AlphaStar operating room t.
American Sterilizer operating t.
Anatomotor traction/massage t.
Andrews spinal surgery t.
Aqua Thermassage t.
Back Specialist t.
t. band
Betaclassic surgical t.
Biodex XYZ imaging t.
Chandler t.
chemonucleolysis t.
Chick CLT operating t.
Chick-Langren t.
Chick surgical t.
circumductor t.
crank t.
Crystal adjusting exam lift t.
cutout t.
Diamond biomechanical t.

Dornier Urotract cysto t.
Ergo style flexion t.
Eurotech Diamond t.
Eurotech Emerald t.
Eurotech Platinum t.
Eurotech Sapphire t.
EZ Lift t.
floating t.
fracture t.
friction-reduced segmented t.
Galaxy 900HS adjusting t.
Galaxy McManis hylo t.
Hadlock t.
harmonic attenuation t.
Hawley t.
Heidelberg-R t.
Hercules t.
Hercules drop-adjusting t.
Hill Air-Drop HA90C t.
Hill Air-Flex t.
HiLo MultiPro t.
HiLo PowerTilt t.
HiLo PowerTilt massage t.
Hixon-Oldfather prediction t.
Hydradjust IV t.
hydromassage t.
IMSI-Metripond operating room t.
intersegmental t.
Jackson imaging t.
Jackson spinal surgery t.
Kanavel t.
Leander chiropractic t.
Leander motorized flexion t.
lithotripsy t.
Lloyd chiropractic t.
Lloyd flexion/distraction t.
Magnum 101 Plus t.
Maquet operating t.
Massage Time Pro hydromassage t.
Mayo instrument t.
McKee t.
Med-Fit cranial-sacral t.
Meridian intersegmental t.
Midland tilt t.
Multilok hand operating t.
MultiPro t.
Orthostar surgical t.
over-bed t.
Paris manual therapy t.
pedestal massage t.
pivoting t.
Platinum stationary t.
Powermatic t.
Protege manual flexion
  distraction t.

T

table *(continued)*
    Pro traction t.
    Quantum 400 chiropractic t.
    Quest intersegmental roller traction t.
    Rath mechanical treatment t.
    Reuss t.
    Risser cast t.
    Roto Rest delta kinetic therapy treatment t.
    Shampaine orthopaedic t.
    Siemens open-heart t.
    Simply Wet t.
    Sister Helen Mustard ENT t.
    Skytron surgical t.
    slatted plinth t.
    slot t.
    spica t.
    Spinalator t.
    Stryker fracture t.
    Sugita microsurgical t.
    Surgitable hand surgery t.
    Telos fracture t.
    tilt t.
    Titan Apollo electric flexion distraction t.
    Topaz flexion t.
    traction t.
    treatment t.
    VAX-D therapy t.
table-fixed retractor
Tab-Strap knee immobilizer
TAC2 atrial caval cannula
TAC atherectomy catheter
Tach-EZ dental attachment
tachycardia-terminating pacemaker
Tachylog pacemaker
Tacit
    T. craniofacial instrumentation
    T. threaded anchor
tack
    Ace bone screw t.
    biodegradable surgical t.
    Cody sacculotomy t.
    Effler t.
    Graftac absorbable skin t.
    membrane t.
    Precision t.
    titanium retinal t.
tack-and-pin forceps
tacker
    Origin t.
Tacoma sacral plate
Tactaid
    T. hearing aid
    T. VII vibrotactile aid
Tacticon
    T. peripheral neuropathy kit

    T. peripheral neuropathy screening device
Tactilaze
    T. angioplasty laser
    T. angioplasty laser catheter
tactile probe
Tactyl 1 glove
Tactylon synthetic surgical glove
T-adapter
    Universal T.-a.
TAD tapered steerable guidewire
TAF175 dialyzer
TAG
    TAG open instrument system
    TAG Rod II suture anchor
Tagarno
    T. 35D cineangiography projector
    T. 35-series film projector
tagged scan
Taheri-Leonhardt catheter
Tahoe Surgical Instruments ligature
4-tailed
    4-t. bandage
    4-t. dressing
Takagi arthroscope
Takahashi
    T. cutting forceps
    T. ethmoidal forceps
    T. ethmoidal punch
    T. iris retractor forceps
    T. nasal forceps
    T. nasal punch
    T. neurosurgical forceps
    T. rongeur
Taka microneurosurgical sponge
Takaro clip
Takata laser
Take-apart
    T.-a. grasping forceps
    T.-a. scissors
Take-Me-Along Personal Shocker pocket shocker
Take-Out extractor
Takumi PTCA catheter
Talairach
    T. bicommissural reference system
    T. stereotactic frame
Talairach-Tournoux system
Talent
    T. bifurcated endograft
    T. LPS endoluminal stent-graft
    T. LPS endoluminal stent-graft system
    T. stent graft
talipes hobble splint
Talker
    Light T.
Tallerman apparatus
Tall-ette toilet seat

Talley pump
Talon
    T. balloon dilatation catheter
    T. curved needle driver
Talos laser delivery system
Tamai clamp approximator
Tamarack flexure joint
tamp
    inflatable bone t.
    interbody graft t.
    Kiene bone t.
    KyphX inflatable bone t.
    Richards t.
    Robinson-Smith t.
    tension band wire t.
tamper
    McIntyre suture t.
tampon
    t. forceps
    Merocel t.
    nasal t.
    Trendelenburg t.
tamponade
    balloon t.
    Cook liver balloon t.
    esophageal balloon t.
    nasal t.
    postnasal balloon t.
    Silikon 1000 retinal t.
Tamsco
    T. curette
    T. forceps
    T. periodontic scaler
    T. wire-cutting scissors
tandem
    t. applicator
    t. connector
    t. cube pessary
    Fleming afterloading t.
    Fletcher-Suit afterloading t.
    Fletcher-Suit-Delclos t.
    t. and ovoid applicator
    t. scanning confocal microscope
    t. stent
    T. thin-shaft transureteroscopic
      balloon dilatation catheter
    T. XL triple-lumen ERCP cannula
TandemHeart ventricular assist device
tangential
    t. forceps
    t. occlusion clamp
    t. occlusion forceps

    t. pediatric clamp
    t. port
tangent screen
Tang retractor
Tanita Professional body composition
  analyzer
tank
    Hubbard hydrotherapy t.
    Imhoff t.
    oxygen t.
Tanne
    T. corneal cutting block
    T. corneal patch
    T. corneal punch
Tannenbaum stent
Tanner
    T. mesher
    T. mesh graft dermacarrier
    T. slide
Tanner-Vandeput mesh dermatome
Tano
    T. double-mirror peripheral
      vitrectomy lens
    T. eraser
    T. membrane scraper
    T. ring
Tan spatula
tantalum
    t. balloon-expandable stent
    t. balloon-expandable stent with
      helical coil
    t. coil stent
    t. gauze
    t. hemostasis clip
    t. mesh
    t. mesh eye implant
    t. plate
    t. wire
    t. wire monofilament suture
tantalum-178 generator
tantalum-ball marker
Tant cystic duct catheter
tap
    AO t.
    t. drill
    Richards bone t.
    screw t.
    t. water wet dressing
Tapcath esophageal electrode
tape
    Blenderm t.
    Blenderm surgical t.

T

NOTES

tape *(continued)*
t. board
Broselow t.
Catheter-Secure t.
Cath-Secure t.
CollaTape t.
ColorZone t.
Cosmolon hook and loop t.
Dacron t.
Deknatel wound closure t.
Delta-Lite casting t.
Dermicare hypoallergenic paper t.
Dermicel hypoallergenic cloth t.
Dermiclear t.
Dermiform hypoallergenic knitted t.
Dermiview hypoallergenic
 transparent t.
Durapore t.
Elastikon elastic t.
EnduraFix t.
EnduraSports t.
EnduraTape t.
foam t.
Glow 'N Tell t.
Hypafix retention t.
Hy-Tape latex-free surgical t.
Hy-Tape waterproof adhesive t.
instrument coding t.
Johnson & Johnson waterproof t.
Kinesio Tex t.
lap t.
Leukopore t.
Leukotape P sports t.
t. marker
MaxCast fiberglass casting t.
Medipore H soft cloth surgical t.
Meditape t.
Mefix adhesive t.
Megazinc Pink adhesive t.
Mersilene t.
Microfoam conformable foam
 elastic t.
Microfoam surgical t.
Micropore surgical t.
3M matrix t.
3M Micropore surgical t.
Omnifix t.
polyethylene retractor t.
Powerflex t.
Primapore t.
Scanpor surgical t.
Scotchcast 2 casting t.
Shur-Strip wound closure t.
Silastic t.
silastic t.
Sportape t.
SportsTape t.
Sta-Fix t.
Sure-Closure wound closure t.

SynthoCast hgh-performance
 casting t.
Transpore clear t.
TSH-01 transdermal t.
umbilical t.
Vascor sterile retraction t.
vascular t.
Zonas porous t.

taper
collarless polished t.
funnelform t.
T. guidewire
t. hand file
laser t.
Morse t.
t. needle
t. reamer
short t.
t. with Zimmer shank

Tapercut
T. needle
T. suture

tapered
t. blade
t. brain retractor
t. catheter
t. fissure bur
t. Micro-Vent implant
t. needle
t. pin
t. reamer
t. torque guidewire

tapered-shaft punctum plug
tapered-spring needle holder
tapered-tip
t.-t. ear syringe
t.-t. hydrophilic-coated guiding
 catheter

Taperloc
T. femoral component
T. femoral prosthesis
T. femoral stem
T. hip system

Taper-Lock external hex implant
taper-point suture needle
TaperSeal hemostatic device
Tapertome sphincterotome
taping
LowDye t.

tapper
rectangular t.

tapping hammer
Tapscope esophageal pacing stethoscope
Tapsul pill electrode
Taq extender
TARA
total articular replacement arthroplasty
TARA retropubic retractor
TARA total hip prosthesis

Tardy
    T. Microbur instrument
    T. osteotome
Targa+ image capture board
TargetCath steerable catheter system
targeted
    t. cryoablation device
    t. dose (TD)
targeter
    bone screw t.
    IMP bone screw t.
targeting drill guide
Targis
    T. BPH microwave technology
    T. system
Tarlov nerve elevator
Tarnier
    T. axis-traction forceps
    T. basiotribe
    T. cephalotribe
    T. cranioclast
    T. obstetrical forceps
tarsal bar
tarsoconjunctival composite graft
Tarsys tilt and recline system
Tascon prosthetic valve
Tasserit shoulder attachment
Tassett vaginal cup bag
tattooing needle
Tatum
    T. meatal clamp
    T. Tee intrauterine device
    T. ureteral transilluminator
Tauber
    T. ligature carrier
    T. ligature hook
    T. male urethrographic catheter
    T. needle
    T. speculum
Taufic cholangiography clamp
Taut
    T. capillary drain
    T. cholangiographic catheter
    T. cystic duct catheter
    T. M-series catheter
    T. percutaneous introducer
    T. Safety Klip clip
Taveras injector
tax double needle
Taylor
    T. aspirator

    T. catheter holder
    T. clavicle support
    T. curette
    T. dissecting forceps
    T. dural scissors
    T. fiberoptic retractor
    T. gastric balloon
    T. gastroscope
    T. halter device
    T. knife
    T. laminectomy blade
    T. lateral mandibular angle implant
    T. pinwheel
    T. pulmonary dilator
    T. reflex percussion hammer
    T. spinal blade
    T. spinal frame
    T. spinal retractor
    T. spinal support apparatus
    T. spine brace
    T. splint
    T. thoracolumbosacral orthosis
    T. tissue forceps
    T. vaginal speculum
    T. Wharton Model 27K cryostorage system
Taylor-Cushing dressing forceps
Taylor-Knight brace
T-bandage
    T-b. dressing
    plano T-b.
T-bar
    T-b. retractor
T-binder pressure dressing
TBird
    T. ventilator
    T. ventilatory system
T-buttress plate
TC
    TC CO_2 monitor
    TC femoral stem
    TC needle holder
    TC pin cutter
TC-7 adhesion barrier
TCCK unconstrained knee prosthesis
TCI Heartmate mechanical circulatory support system
T-clamp
    Presbyterian Hospital T-c.
TCS
    turnstile casting stand

NOTES

T

TD
targeted dose
TD glucose monitoring system
TDMAC-heparin shunt
T-drain
Teale
T. gorget
T. gorget lithotrite
T. tenaculum
T. tenaculum forceps
T. vulsellum
T. vulsellum uterine forceps
tear
t. duct tube
t. strip
tear-away introducer sheath
teardrop
t. dissector
T. microsponge
Teare
T. arm splint
T. snare
TearSaver punctum plug
Tearscope
Keeler T.
Tear-Trough implant
Tebbetts
T. EndoPlastic instrument system
T. rhinoplasty set
T. ribbon retractor
TEC
transluminal extraction catheter
TEC atherectomy device
TEC atherectomy system
TEC catheter
TEC interface system
TEC liner
TEC 2100 positioning laser
Tech-Attach connection system
Techmedica
T. implant
T. prosthesis
Technicare
T. camera
T. Delta 2020 scanner
T. Omega 500 gamma camera
technique
TechnoGel insole
Technolas 217 excimer laser system
technology
Advanced Coronary T. (ACT)
Aesthetic and Reconstructive T.'s
(AART)
Angiographic Contrast Injection
System T. (ACIST)
Arrow Cardiac Assist T. (ACAT)
ARTMA virtual patient t.
CardioFix pericardium with
PhotoFix t.

Cochlea Dynamics sound
processing t.
Concentrix Fluidics t.
Fox Hollow T.'s (FHT)
PEARL t.
Porvidx cancer screening t.
shape-memory alloy recoverable t.
(SMART)
Surgical Laser T.'s (SLT)
Targis BPH microwave t.
WhiteStar power modulation t.
TechnoMed C-Scan videokeratoscope
Technos ultrasound system
Technovit
T. acrylic resin
T. 7210 VLC adhesive
Techstar
T. percutaneous closure device
T. XL percutaneous vascular
surgical system
Tecmag Libra-S16 system scanner
Tecnol
T. ankle wrap
T. back support
T. hand-aid wrist support
T. Rebound neoprene elbow
support
T. Rebound neoprene knee support
Tectonic magnet
TED
thromboembolic disease
TED antiembolism stocking
TED hose
Tedlar bag
Tefcat intrauterine insemination catheter
Tefcor core wire guide
**TefGen-FD guided tissue regeneration
membrane**
Teflo-Kapton freezing bag
Teflon
T. clip
T. coating
T. collar button
T. cutting block
T. ERCP cannula
T. ERCP catheter
T. felt
T. glycerine-mixture injection
needle
T. glycerine-mixture syringe
T. graft
T. guiding catheter
T. injection catheter
T. injector
T. intracardiac patch
T. iris retractor
T. liner
T. mesh
T. mesh implant

T. mold
T. nasobiliary drain
T. orbital floor implant
T. piston
T. plate
T. pledget
T. pledget suture buttress
T. plug
T. probe
T. sheath
T. sheet
T. Silastic loop
T. strut
T. tri-leaflet prosthesis
T. tubing
T. woven prosthesis
Teflon-coated
T.-c. Dacron suture
T.-c. guidewire
T.-c. hollow-bore needle
T.-c. stimulation needle
Teflon-covered needle
Teflon-pledgeted suture
Teflon-tipped catheter
Tegaderm semipermeable occlusive dressing
Tegagel
T. hydrogel dressing
T. hydrogel sheet
Tegagen HG, HI alginate wound dressing
Tegam microprocessor thermometer
Tegapore contact-layer wound dressing
Tegasorb occlusive dressing
Tegtmeier hand board
TEGwire
T. balloon
T. balloon dilatation catheter
T. guide
T. ST system
Tehl clamp
Tei-Shin spring modulator
Tekna mechanical heart valve
Teknamed drape sheet
Tekno
T. coagulator
T. forceps
Tek-Pro needle
Tekscan in-shoe monitoring device
Tektronix
T. digital oscilloscope
T. digital photometer

Tel-A-Fever forehead thermometer
telebinocular
TeleCaption decoder
telecentric fundus camera
Telectronics
T. Accufix pacing lead
T. Guardian ATP II ICD
T. Guardian ATP implantable cardioverter-defibrillator
T. pacemaker
Telefactor beehive system
telemanipulator system
telemeter
Bio-sentry t.
telemetric intracranial pressure sensor
TelePACS remote diagnostic system
telescope
ACMI microlens foroblique t.
Atkins esophagoscopic t.
Best direct forward-vision t.
biopsy t.
bioptic t.
Bridge t.
Broyles t.
Burns bridge t.
direct forward-vision t.
direct-vision t.
double-catheterizing t.
endoscopic t.
Eschenbach monocular t.
examining t.
fiberoptic right-angle t.
foroblique bronchoscopic t.
forward-vision t.
High-Vision surgical t.
Holinger bronchoscopic t.
Hopkins direct-vision t.
Hopkins forward-oblique t.
Hopkins lateral t.
Hopkins nasal endoscopy t.
Hopkins pediatric t.
Hopkins retrospective t.
Hopkins rod lens t.
infant t.
Keeler panoramic surgical t.
Kramer direct-vision t.
lateral microlens t.
Lumina operating t.
Lumina-SL t.
Luxtec illuminated surgical t.
Luxtec surgical t.
McCarthy foroblique operating t.

T

NOTES

telescope *(continued)*
McCarthy miniature t.
Microlens direct-vision t.
Microlens foroblique t.
Mueller t.
Negus t.
pediatric t.
retrospective bronchoscopic t.
Selsi sport t.
solid-rod rigid t.
stop collar t.
Storz bronchoscopic t.
Storz-Hopkins t.
surgical t.
Surgi-Spec t.
transilluminating t.
Tucker direct-vision t.
Vest direct forward-vision t.
Walden t.
Zeiss binocular prism t.
telescopic
t. distractor
t. plate spacer
t. and torsional (TT)
t. and torsional pylon
t. view guide
telescoping
t. brace
t. guide
t. plugged catheter
t. rod
Telestill photo adapter
telethermometer
YSI t.
Teletrast gauze
Telfa
T. adhesive pad
T. bolster
T. Clear nonadherent wound dressing
T. gauze
T. gauze pad
T. island dressing
T. Plus barrier island dressing
T. strip
T. 4 x 4 bandage
T. Xtra absorbent island dressing
Telfamax ultra absorbent dressing
TeliCam intraoral camera
Teller acuity card
Telos
T. fracture table
T. stress device
Temco hoist
Temens curette
Temno
T. biopsy needle
T. II cutting needle
TE MOO mode beam laser

Tempa-DOT
T.-DOT axillary thermometer
Tempa-Dot B thermometer
Tempbond dental cement
Temper
T. Foam cube
T. Foam cushion
temperature probe
temperature-sensing pacemaker
Temperlite saw blade
Temp-Kuff blood pressure cuff
template
Bivona-Colorado t.
breast keyhole t.
Charnley t.
dermal regeneration t.
Integra dermal regeneration t.
interimplant papillary t.
Jacobsen t.
Kuske breast t.
Mallory-Head modular acetabular t.
Marchac forehead t.
Martinez Universal interstitial t.
McKissock keyhole areolar t.
Mick prostate t.
Moore t.
rod t.
Syed t.
Syed-Neblett gynecological t.
thermoplastic t.
tissue expander t.
Temple
T. University nail
T. University plate
Temple-Fay laminectomy retractor
Tempo denture liner
temporal
t. bone holder
t. electrode
temporary
t. AV sequential pacemaker
t. crown
t. pacing catheter
t. percutaneous SCS electrode
t. pervenous lead
t. prosthesis
t. skin replacement
t. transvenous pacemaker
t. vascular clip
t. vessel clip
temporomandibular
t. joint (TMJ)
t. joint implant
TempTrac temperature monitor
Tempur-Med
T.-M. hospital mattress
T.-M. hospital overlay
T.-M. lumbar pad
T.-M. O.R. table pad

T.-M. pillow
T.-M. stretch pad
T.-M. wheelchair cushion
Tempur PC seat wedge
Tempur-Pedic
T.-P. pressure-relieving Swedish
mattress
T.-P. pressure-relieving Swedish
pillow
Tempur-Plus mattress
Temrex dental cement
tenaculum
Abel-Aesculap-Pratt t.
Aesculap-Pratt t.
Braun-Schroeder single-tooth t.
Braun uterine t.
breast t.
Brophy t.
cervical t.
Coakley t.
Collen-Pozzi t.
Corey t.
Cottle t.
double-tooth t.
Duplay uterine t.
Emmet cervical t.
t. forceps
Gynex Emmett t.
t. holder
t. hook
t. hook loop
Hulka uterine t.
Jackson tracheal t.
Jacobs uterine t.
Jarcho uterine t.
Kahn traction t.
Kelly uterine t.
Kennett t.
Küstner t.
Lahey goiter t.
lion jaw t.
Martin t.
Museux t.
nasal t.
New t.
Newman t.
Potts t.
Pozzi t.
Pratt t.
Revots vulsellum t.
Sargis uterine t.
Schroeder t.

Schroeder-Braun uterine t.
single-tooth t.
Skene uterine t.
Staude-Jackson uterine t.
Staude-Moore uterine t.
Staude uterine t.
straight t.
Teale t.
Thoms t.
thyroid t.
toothed t.
tracheal t.
uterine t.
Watts t.
Weisman t.
White t.
Wylie uterine t.
tenaculum-reducing forceps
Tenador male pouch
Tena pouch
Tenax coronary stent
Tenckhoff
T. 2-cuff catheter
T. peritoneal dialysis catheter
Tender
T. subcutaneous infusion set
T. Touch extractor
T. Touch Ultra vacuum cup
TenderCloud pressure pad
**TenderCups postoperative breast
dressing**
Tenderfoot incision-making device
Tenderlett device
Tendersorb ABD pad
Tenderwrap Unna boot
tendon
t. forceps
t. gouge
t. hook
t. implant
t. knife
t. needle
t. passer
t. plate
t. prosthesis
t. stripper
t. tucker
Tutoplast anterior tibialis t.
tendon-holding forceps
tendon-passing forceps
tendon-pulling forceps
tendon-retrieving forceps

NOTES

tendon-seizing forceps
Tendril
    T. DX implantable pacing lead
    T. lead
    T. SDX active-fixation lead
Tennant
    T. Anchorflex anterior chamber
       intraocular lens
    T. Anchorflex lens implant
    T. anchor lens-insertion hook
    T. intraocular lens forceps
    T. iris hook
    T. lens forceps
    T. needle holder
    T. nuclear ball rotator
    T. spatula
    T. titanium suturing forceps
    T. tying forceps
Tennant-Colibri corneal forceps
Tennant-Maumenee forceps
Tennant-Troutman superior rectus
forceps
Tenner lacrimal cannula
Tennessee capsular polisher
tennis
    t. elbow splint
    T. Racquet angiographic catheter
Ten-O-Matic TENS unit
Tenoplast elastic adhesive dressing
tenotome
    Dieffenbach t.
    Ryerson t.
tenotomy
    t. hook
    t. scissors
TENS
    transcutaneous electrical nerve
       stimulation
    TENS machine
    Nuwave TENS
    TENS pad
    TENS unit
Tensilon implant
tension
    t. band wire tamp
    t. clamp
    t. Isometer
tensioner
tension-requiring suture
Tensmax TENS unit
Tensor
    T. elastic bandage roll
    T. elastic dressing
Tensum coronary stent
Ten system balloon catheter
tent
    Cam t.
    croup t.
    croupette t.

    hydrophilic t.
    Hypan t.
    KTK laminaria t.
    laminaria cervical t.
    mist t.
    Mizutani laminaria t.
    oxygen t.
    Silon t.
    steam t.
tentalum wire tension suture
Tenzel
    T. bipolar forceps
    T. calipers
    T. double-end periosteal elevator
Tepas retractor
Tepperwedge wedge
Teq-Trode electrode
teres knife
Terino
    T. anatomical chin implant
    T. facial implant retractor
    T. malar shell
terminal
    t. electrode
    t. electrode adapter
    t. extensor mechanism
Ternamian EndoTIP access cannula
Ter-Pogossian cervical radium
applicator
Terry
    T. astigmatome
    T. keratometer
    T. nail
    T. silicone capsular polisher
    T. trephine
Terry-Mayo needle
Terson
    T. capsular forceps
    T. extracapsular forceps
    T. speculum
Terumo
    T. AV fistula needle
    T. dental needle
    T. dialyzer
    T. Doppler fetal heart rate monitor
    T. Glidewire
    T. guidewire
    T. hydrophilic guidewire
    T. hypodermic needle
    T. insulin syringe
    T. Radiofocus introducer
    T. sheath
    T. SP coaxial catheter
    T. SP hydrophilic-coated
       microcatheter
    T. stent
    T. Steri-Cell system
    T. Surflo intravenous catheter
    T. transducer protector

Terumo-Clirans dialyzer
Terumo/Meditech guidewire
Tesa S.A. handheld electronic digital calipers
Tesberg esophagoscope
Tesio catheter
Tesla
- T. magnet
- T. MRI system
- T. Signa magnetic resonance imager
- T. superconductive magnet unit

Tessier
- T. craniofacial instrument
- T. dislodger
- T. elevator
- T. osteomicrotome
- T. osteotome
- T. rib bender
- T. spreader

Tes Tape dressing
tester
- Accu-Measure personal body fat t.
- Polatest vision t.

testicular
- t. implant
- t. prosthesis

testing drum knife
Testoderm
- T. patch
- T. testosterone transdermal system

Testsimplets prestained slide
Test-Size orchidometer
Tetra coronary stent system
tetrapolar esophageal catheter
Tetrax interactive balance system
Teufel cervical brace
Teurlings wrist brace
Tevdek
- T. implant
- T. pledgeted suture
- T. prosthesis

Tew
- T. cranial retractor
- T. needle
- T. spinal retractor

Texal-Muller chest binder
Texas
- T. cannula
- T. condom catheter
- T. Goodstein sharp tip
- T. Heart Institute (THI)

- T. Scottish Rite Hospital (TSRH)
- T. Scottish Rite Hospital crosslink plate
- T. Scottish Rite Hospital eyebolt spreader
- T. Scottish Rite Hospital pedical screw and rod system

textile
- Silon-TEX silicone-bonded t.

Textor vasectomy clamp
TFE-coated wireguide
T-finger splint
T-Foam
- T-F. cushion
- T-F. flotation pad
- T-F. pillow

T-Gel cushion
TG Osseotite single-stage procedure implant
T-grommet ventilation tube
Thackray
- T. dental forceps
- T. hip prosthesis
- T. mouthgag

Thackston retropubic bag
ThAIRapy
- T. vest
- T. vest airway clearance system

Thal-Mantel obturator
Thal-Quick chest tube
T-handle
- T-h. bone awl
- T-h. cup curette
- T-h. elevator
- T-h. Jacob chuck
- T-h. nut wrench
- T-h. reamer
- T-h. wrench
- T-h. Zimmer chuck

Tharies
- T. femoral resurfacing component
- T. hip component
- T. hip replacement prosthesis

Thatcher
- T. nail
- T. screw

THC:YAG laser
Theden bandage
The Hockey Stick articulating stylet
Theis
- T. infant rib spreader

NOTES

Theis *(continued)*
- T. self-retaining rib retractor
- T. vein retractor

Theobald
- T. lacrimal dilator
- T. sinus probe

Thera
- T. Cane massager wand
- T. Cane shoulder exerciser
- T. Cool cold therapy system
- T. DR pacemaker

Thera-Band
- T.-B. Assist
- T.-B. exercise ball
- T.-B. exercise band
- T.-B. FlexBar bar
- T.-B. handle
- T.-B. Max band
- T.-B. Slow Deflate System exercise ball
- T.-B. strip
- T.-B. tubing

Therabath paraffin therapy bath
TheraBeads microwaveable moist heat pack
Therabite
- T. jaw exerciser
- T. jaw motion rehabilitation system
- T. mobilizer

Thera-Boot compression bandage
Theracloud pillow
Thera-Fit exerciser
Theraflex wrist exerciser
Theraform Selectives orthotic
Theragym ball
Ther-A-Hoop exerciser
TheraKair air pulsation mattress
Thera-Loop exerciser
Thera-Med cold pack
Thera-Medic shoe
Theramini 1, 2 electrotherapy stimulator
Thera-P bar
TheraPEP positive expiratory pressure therapy system
therapeutic
- t. side-viewing duodenoscope
- t. splint

Therapeutica sleeping pillow
Thera-Plast putty
Therap-Loop
- T.-L. door anchor
- T.-L. door handle

Thera-Pos
- T.-P. elbow orthosis
- T.-P. knee orthosis

TheraPress
- T. Duo compression stocking
- T. Duo Lite compression stocking

TheraPulse pulsating air suspension bed
Thera-Putty exercise putty
therapy
- aerosol respiratory t.
- 600 Asta air support t.
- t. ball
- Burke Plus frameless air support t.
- circulator boot t.
- Cool-Aid continuous controlled cold t.
- Electri-Cool continuous controlled cold t.
- electroconvulsive t. (ECT)
- Enterra t.
- Epos Ultra orthopaedic shock wave t.
- Facial-Flex t.
- First Option uterine cryoblation t.
- frameless air support t.
- GeriMend skin tear t.
- gold probe hemostasis t.
- high-output extended aerosol respiratory t.
- InFerno moist heat t.
- InSync cardiac resynchronization t.
- integrated massage t. (IMT)
- interferential t.
- InterStim t.
- Kelsey unloading exercise t.
- magnet t.
- Medtronic Activa tremor-control t.
- Moxa heat t.
- nerve stimulation t. (NST)
- Pedi Asta frameless air support t.
- Pneu-Scale frameless air support t.
- Pro-Op frameless air support t.
- Pro-Turn frameless air support t.
- ReliefBand nerve stimulation t.
- RT/SC 2000 frameless air support t.
- SpineCATH IDET t.
- Synergy frameless air support t.
- Synergy Pulse frameless air support t.
- VersaLight photodynamic t.
- XKnife software for stereotactic radiation t.

TherArc pillow
TheraRest mattress
TheraSeed therapeutic implant
Ther-A-Shapes positioner
TheraSkin wound dressing
Therasleep cervical pillow
TheraSnore oral appliance
Thera-Soft hand/wrist orthosis
Therasonics lithotripter
Therasound transducer
Thera-SR pacemaker
Therastream microcatheter

Theratotic
  T. firm foot orthosis
  T. soft foot orthosis
Theratouch 4.7 stimulator
Thera-turn rotational system
ThermaCare
  T. HeatWrap
  T. quilt
ThermaChoice
  T. catheter
  T. thermal balloon ablation
  T. uterine balloon
  T. uterine balloon therapy system
ThermaCool TC system
Thermaderm epilator
Thermafil
  T. plastic carrier
  T. Plus obturator
Therma Jaw hot urologic forceps
thermal
  t. conductivity detector
  t. energy analyzer
  t. knife
  t. memory stent
  t. plastic wrap
  T. responsive nitrile surgical glove
  t. space blanket
Thermalator heating unit
ThermalSoft hot & cold pack
Thermapad cryotherapy cooler
Thermasonic gel warmer
ThermaSplint heating bath
ThermaStent prostatic stent
ThermaStim muscle stimulator
Thermedics HeartMate 10001P left anterior assist device
Thermex-II transurethral prostate heating device
thermistor
  t. catheter
  t. needle
  t. probe
  t. rectal thermometer
  t. thermodilution catheter
  t. thermometer
Thermo
  T. Cardiosystems left ventricular assist device
  T. comforter hand support
  T. comforter knee support
  T. HK/Rohadur orthotic
  T. HK/Tepefom orthotic

ThermoChem-HT system
thermocoagulator
  Olympus CD-Z-series heat probe t.
thermocouple
  Chromel-Alumel t.
  low impedance t.
  needle t.
thermocycler
thermodeltameter
thermodilution
  t. balloon catheter
  t. cardiac output computer
  t. pacing catheter
  t. Swan-Ganz catheter
thermoexpandable stent
ThermoFlex
  T. liner
  T. thermotherapy unit
Thermo-Flex suture
Thermo-Flo irrigation system
ThermoFX mesh
thermographic scanner
Thermograph temperature monitor
thermography
  laser-induced t. (LITT)
  Varicoscreen contact t.
thermoluminescent dosimeter
thermometer
  AccuProbe t.
  basal body t.
  Core-Check tympanic t.
  Coretemp deep tissue t.
  Diatek 9000 Insta-Temp t.
  EZ Temp t.
  Fahrenheit flat bath t.
  First Temp Genius 3000A tympanic t.
  FirstTemp Genius tympanic t.
  infrared t.
  instant fever tester t.
  Iso-Thermex 16-channel electronic t.
  IVAC Temp Plus II t.
  LighTouch Neonate t.
  Mon-a-Therm 6510 two-channel t.
  NexTemp Precision Phase Change t.
  Ototemp 3000 tympanic t.
  Philips SensorTouch temple t.
  Quik-Temp t.
  Stik-Temp t.
  SureTemp electronic t.

T

NOTES

thermometer *(continued)*
    SureTemp4 oral t.
    Tegam microprocessor t.
    Tel-A-Fever forehead t.
    Tempa-DOT axillary t.
    Tempa-Dot B t.
    thermistor t.
    thermistor rectal t.
    Thermoscan Pro-1 instant t.
    Thermoscan tympanic instant t.
    TraxIt continuous-reading precision
      phase-change t.
    tympanic membrane t.
Thermophore
    T. hot pack
    T. moist heat pad
thermoplastic
    t. elastomer (TPE)
    t. splint
    t. stent
    t. template
thermopore
    Shahan t.
Thermoprep heating oven
ThermoPulse pain relief therapy system
Thermoscan
    T. Pro-1 instant thermometer
    T. tympanic instant thermometer
Thermoskin
    T. arthritic knee wrap
    T. arthritic wrap-around glove
    T. back wrap
    T. brace
    T. heat retainer
Thermos pacemaker
Thermo-STAT rewarming system
thermotherapy
    laser-induced t. (LITT)
    TransUrethral Microwave T.
      (TUMT)
Thermovac tissue pulverizer
ThermoVent heat/moisture exchanger
Thero-Skin gel padding
TherOx
    T. infusion guide wire
    T. infusion guidewire
Theurig sterilizer forceps
THI
    Texas Heart Institute
    THI needle
thick-walled Dacron-backed implant
Thiersch
    T. graft
    T. implant
    T. prosthesis
    T. skin graft knife
    T. suture
    T. wire

thigh
    t. balloon
    t. tourniquet
thigh-high antiembolic stocking
Thillaye
    T. bandage
    T. dressing
thin acupuncture needle
thin-layer chromatograph
**ThinLine EZ bipolar cardiac pacing
  lead**
Thinline uncovered orthotic
Thinlith II pacemaker
ThinPrep 2000 processor
thin-shaft nasal scissors
ThinSite
    T. border hydrogel dressing
    T. topical wound dressing
thin-walled
    t.-w. catheter
    t.-w. introducer catheter
    t.-w. needle
thin-wire Ilizarov fixator
third generation lithotripter
Thole
    T. goniometer
    T. pelvimeter
Thoma
    T. clamp
    T. tissue retractor
Thomas
    T. brush
    T. bur
    T. calipers
    T. cervical collar
    T. cervical collar orthosis
    T. cryoextractor
    T. cryoprobe
    T. cryoptor
    T. cryoretractor
    T. endotracheal tube holder
    T. extrapolated bar graft
    T. femoral shunt
    T. fixation forceps
    T. fixator
    T. full-ring splint
    T. heel
    T. heel orthosis
    T. I&A cannula
    T. Kapsule instrument
    T. keratome
    T. knee splint
    T. Kodel sling
    T. leg splint
    T. magnet
    T. needle
    T. pelvimeter
    T. pessary
    T. posterior splint

T. retractor
T. scissors
T. shot compression forceps
T. shunt
T. spatula
T. splint with Pearson attachment
T. suspension splint
T. uterine curette
T. vascular access shunt
T. walking brace
T. wrench
Thomas-type cervical collar brace
Thompson
T. adenoid curette
T. bronchial catheter
T. carotid artery clamp
T. cervical transilluminator
T. chin support
T. direct full-vision resectoscope
T. dowel
T. drape
T. evacuator
T. femoral head prosthesis
T. femoral neck prosthesis
T. frontal sinus rasp
T. hemiarthroplasty hip prosthesis
T. hip endoprosthesis system
T. hip prosthesis forceps
T. hyperextension fracture frame
T. modification of Denis Browne
splint
T. punch
T. retractor
T. rib shears
T. stem rasp
T. XL endoprosthesis
Thompson-Farley
T.-F. spinal retractor
T.-F. spinal retractor system
Thoms
T. pelvimeter
T. tenaculum
Thoms-Allis
T.-A. intestinal forceps
T.-A. tissue forceps
T.-A. vulsellum forceps
Thomsen rib shears
Thoms-Gaylor uterine biopsy forceps
Thomson
T. adenoid curette
T. lung clamp

Thomson-Walker
T.-W. scissors
T.-W. urethrotome
ThoraCath catheter
thoracentesis needle
thoracic
t. artery forceps
t. cage
t. clamp
t. drain
t. drainage system
t. forceps
t. pedicle screw
t. scissors
t. tissue forceps
t. trocar
thoracoabdominal (TA)
t. stapler
thoracolumbar
t. pedicle screw
t. spinal orthosis (TLSO)
t. standing orthosis
thoracolumbosacral
t. plate
t. spinal orthosis
thoracolumbosacroiliac implant system
Thoracoport
Auto Suture Soft T.
Soft T.
T. trocar
thoracoscope
Boutin t.
Coryllos t.
Cutler forceps t.
Jacobaeus t.
Jacobaeus-Unverricht t.
Moore t.
Sarot t.
Storz t.
thoracostomy tube
thoracotome
Thora-Drain III chest drainage system
Thora-Klex
T.-K. chest drainage system
T.-K. chest tube
Thoralon
T. biomaterial
T. biomaterial TransCyte skin
substitute
T. implant material

T

NOTES

Thora-Port
> T.-P. cannula
> T.-P. obturator

Thoraseal chest tube drainage system

Thoratec
> T. biventricular assist device
> T. mechanical circulatory support system
> T. pump
> T. right ventricular assist device

Thoravision system

Thoreau filter

Thorek
> T. gallbladder aspirator
> T. gallbladder forceps
> T. gallbladder scissors
> T. thoracic scissors

Thorek-Feldman gallbladder scissors

Thorek-Mixter gallbladder forceps

Thorlakson
> T. deep abdominal retractor
> T. lower/upper occlusive clamp
> T. multipurpose retractor

Thornton
> T. adjustable positioner
> T. arcuate triple-edged blade
> T. corneal marker
> T. corneal press-on ruler
> T. 360-degree arcuate keratotomy marker
> T. double corneal ruler
> T. episcleral forceps
> T. fixation forceps
> T. fixation ring
> T. intraocular forceps
> T. iris retractor
> T. low-profile radial marker
> T. malleable spatula
> T. nail
> T. open-wire lid speculum
> T. ophthalmic triple micrometer knife
> T. plate
> T. retrobulbar needle
> T. T-incision diamond knife
> T. tri-square blade

Thornton-Fine ring

Thornwald
> T. antral drill
> T. antral irrigator
> T. antral perforator
> T. antral trephine

THORP
> titanium hollow screw reconstruction plate
>> THORP mandibular reconstruction plate

Thorpe
> T. calipers

> T. conjunctival forceps
> T. corneal forceps
> T. corneoscleral forceps
> T. curette
> T. foreign body forceps
> T. gonioprism lens
> T. 4-mirror goniolaser
> T. 4-mirror goniolaser lens
> T. 4-mirror goniolens
> T. 4-mirror vitreous-fundus lens
> T. pupillary membrane scissors
> T. slit lamp
> T. surgical gonioscope

Thorpe-Castroviejo
> T.-C. calipers
> T.-C. cataract scissors
> T.-C. corneal forceps
> T.-C. fixation forceps

Thorpe-Westcott cataract scissors

Thrasher
> T. intraocular forceps
> T. lens implant forceps

thread
> BioCare t.
> BioHorizon t.
> polyene t.
> SMIC nylon t.
> t. suture
> Wi-Last-Ic t.

threaded
> t. cortical dowel
> t. eye needle
> t. guide pin
> t. interbody fusion cage
> t. rod
> t. titanium acetabular prosthesis

threader
> Allen wire t.
> Borchard wire t.
> Frackelton wire t.
> Hamby wire t.
> t. rod holder pliers
> wire t.

ThreadLoc
> T. implant
> T. non-cast-to abutment
> T. retaining screw

thread-locking device

Three-D worker's back support

Threshold
> T. IMT device
> T. PEP device

Thriftcast alloy

throat
> ears, nose, t. (ENT)
> t. forceps

Throat-E-Vac suction device

thrombectomy
　　t. catheter
　　t. system
Thrombex PMT clot removal system
thrombin-soaked Gelfoam
thromboembolic
　　t. disease (TED)
　　t. disease hose
　　t. disease stocking
Thrombogen absorbable hemostat
thrombolizer
　　Angiocor rotational t.
thrombolytic brush
ThromboScan MRI
thrombosis
　　deep vein t. (DVT)
thrombosuction catheter
thrombus stripper
through-and-through reabsorbable suture
through-cutting forceps tip
through-the-balloon ultrasound
through-the-scope (TTS)
　　t.-t.-s. balloon
　　t.-t.-s. balloon dilator
　　t.-t.-s. bougie
　　t.-t.-s. catheter
　　t.-t.-s. injection needle
throw-away manual dermatome blade
Thruflex
　　T. balloon
　　T. PTCA balloon catheter
Thrust femoral prosthesis
Thudichum
　　T. nasal speculum
　　T. self-retaining ear speculum
thulium-holmium-chromium:yttrium-aluminum-garnet laser
thulium-holmium:YAG laser
thumb
　　t. retractor
　　t. spica cast
　　t. spica splint
　　t. tissue forceps
thumb-dressing forceps
Thumbfit splint
Thumbkeeper
　　Freedom T.
thumb-ring needle holder
Thumb-Saver introducer clamp
Thumper CPR system
ThumSling
　　Action T.

ThumZ'Up functional thumb splint
Thurmond
　　T. iris retractor
　　T. nucleus-irrigating cannula
　　T. pachymeter marker
Thurston-Holland fragment forceps
Thymapad stimulus electrode
thymus retractor
thyroid
　　t. forceps
　　t. retractor
　　t. tenaculum
Ti
　　T. alloy screw
　　T. rotor
Ti-Bac
　　T.-B. acetabular component
　　T.-B. II hip prosthesis
　　T.-B. I, II acetabular cup
Tibbs
　　T. arterial cannula
　　T. semi-automatic suturing device
tibial
　　t. aligner
　　t. augmentation block
　　t. bolt
　　t. broach
　　t. calipers
　　t. collet
　　t. cutter guide
　　t. cutting block
　　t. driver
　　t. endoprosthesis
　　t. fracture brace
　　t. guide
　　t. guide pin
　　t. plate
　　t. plateau prosthesis
　　t. retractor
　　t. stylus
　　t. torsion system
Tibon anterior cervical fusion implant
Tib-Transformer orthosis
Tickner tissue forceps
Ti/CoCr hip prosthesis
Ticonium splint
Ti-Cron suture
Ticsay transpubic needle
Tidal
　　T. Wave handheld capnograph
　　T. Wave Sp capnometer/pulse oximeter

T

NOTES

tie
    cable t.
    gauze neck t.
Tieck-Halle infant nasal speculum
Tieck nasal speculum
Tielle
    T. absorptive dressing
    T. hydropolymer dressing
    T. Plus dressing
Tiemann
    T. bullet forceps
    T. coudé catheter
    T. nail
    T. Neoflex catheter
Tiemann-Foley catheter
Tiemann-Meals tenolysis knife
tie-on needle
tie-over bolster
tier
    knot t.
tiered-therapy
    t.-t. antiarrhythmic device
    t.-t. implantable cardioverter-
      defibrillator
Ti-Fit total hip system
Ti-Frame posterior fixation system
tiger
    T. blade
    t. gut suture
    T. Shark forceps
tightener
    Bowen wire t.
    Harris wire t.
    Kirschner wire t.
    Loute wire t.
    Shiffrin bone wire t.
    Sklar wire t.
    Verner-Joseph wire t.
    wire t.
TiGold clip applier
Tiko
    T. pliable iris retractor
    T. rake retractor
    T. zonule sweeper
Tilastin hip prosthesis
Tilderquist needle holder
Tillary double-ended retractor
Tilley dressing forceps
Tilley-Henckel forceps
Tilley-Lichwitz trocar
Tillyer bifocal lens
tilt
    t. table
    T. and Turn Paragon bed
Tilt-Board
    G5 Vari-Tilt Adjustable T.-B.
tilting-disc
    t.-d. aortic valve prosthesis
    t.-d. heart valve

Tilt-In-Space wheelchair conversion
Timberlake
    T. catheter
    T. electrode
    T. evacuator
    T. irrigating tip
    T. obturator
    T. obturator electrotome
time-based counter
time domain reflectometry instrument
time-gain compensator
time-of-flight
    t.-o.-f. PET imaging system
    t.-o.-f. positron emission
      tomographic camera
timer
    Apgar t.
    Bili-Timer t.
    Medela Apgar t.
    Medtronic automated coagulation t.
TiMesh
    T. bone-plate
    T. burrhole cover
    T. cranial mesh
    T. cranial plating system
    T. craniofacial system
    T. craniomaxillofacial plating
      system
    T. mandibular crib
    T. orbital mesh
    T. orthognathic strap plate
    T. patient-configured titanium
      craniomaxillofacial implant
    T. rigid fixation bone plating
      system
    T. screw
    T. titanium bone plating system
    T. titanium mesh
    T. titanium tray
Timeter pocket spirometer
time-to-pulse height converter
Timoptic Ocumeter
TiMX comprehensive low-back system
TINA monitor
tin-bullet probe
T-incision marker
Tindall scissors
tined
    t. lead pacemaker
    t. ventricular electrode
Tinel
    T. suture
    T. tapered reamer
    T. tourniquet
Tinnant gauge
tinted spectacles
TiOblast dental implant
tip
    Adson brain suction t.

aerosol-barrier pipette t.
Air-Shield-Vickers syringe t.
Andrews-Pynchon suction t.
Andrews suction t.
Batt t.
Beacon radiopaque t.
Becker round dissector t.
Becker twist dissector t.
Bruening biting t.
Colorado electrocautery t.
Combitip Plus pipette t.
conical t.
Cope-Saddekni catheter t.
Cordes punch forceps t.
Corometrics spiral electrode t.
CUSA laparoscopic t.
double-articulated forceps t.
Ducor t.
eel cobra t.
t. electrode
electrode t.
EZ Clean cautery t.
flared ABS t.
Flexoreamer Batt t.
Fournier t.
Fragmatome t.
Frazier suction t.
Gess cannula t.
Girard irrigating t.
grasping forceps t.
t. guard
guillotine cutting t.
Hetter pyramid t.
Illouz modified t.
Illouz standard t.
Implantech SE-100 smoke
  aspiration t.
irrigating t.
Jackson square punch t.
Japanese suction t.
Kahler double-action t.
Keeler lancet t.
Keeler micro spear t.
Keeler puncture t.
Keeler razor t.
Keeler round t.
Keeler triple-facet t.
Kelman t.
K-Flexofile Batt t.
Killian cutting forceps t.
Killian double-articulated forceps t.
Klein cannula t.

Klein 1-hole infiltrator t.
Klein multihole infiltrator t.
Krause oval punch t.
Krause punch forceps t.
Krause square-basket t.
Leasure round punch t.
Leon cobra t.
Marlow Primus t.
Mayo coronary perfusion t.
MegaDyne E-Z clean cautery t.
Mercedes t.
MicroTip phaco t.
Mitchell viscoelastic removal
  I&A t.
Myerson biting t.
OtoClear disposable t.
Pinto dissector t.
plumbeous zirconate titanate t.
Polaris Mansfield/Webster
  deflectable t.
pyramid Toomey t.
Quad cutting t.
Roane bullet t.
Rosenberg dissector t.
rubber acorn t.
Saverburger I&A t.
Scheinmann biting t.
Schuknecht suction t.
Sensor PTFE-nitinol guidewire with
  hydrophilic t.
SE-100 smoke aspiration t.
Simcoe cannula t.
Simcoe interchangeable t.
Sims suction t.
Site guillotine cutting t.
Skimmer laryngeal blade t.
Slip-Coat t.
spatula cannula t.
Spencer oval t.
Struyken angular punch t.
sucker t.
suction t.
Surgi-Fine reusable cannula t.
synthetic sapphire t.
Texas Goodstein sharp t.
through-cutting forceps t.
Timberlake irrigating t.
Tischler-Morgan t.
Toledo flap dissector t.
Toledo standard dissector t.
Toledo V-dissector t.
Toomey pyramid t.

T

NOTES

tip *(continued)*
    Trevisani cannula t.
    Tricut laryngeal blade t.
    TriEye t.
    TULIP t.
    tungsten t.
    TurboSonic t.
    Ultrafyn cautery t.
    Unitri t.
    Universal adenoid punch t.
    V. Mueller cystoscopy t.
    weighted t.
    Yankauer tonsil suction t.
tip-deflecting
    t.-d. catheter
    t.-d. guidewire
    t.-d. wire guide
TIPS
    transjugular intrahepatic portosystemic shunt
    TIPS shunt
TIPSS
    transjugular intrahepatic portosystemic shunt
    TIPSS shunt
Tip-Trol handle
tire
    t. eye implant
    silicone t.
    Watzke t.
tire-grooved silicone
Tischler
    T. cervical biopsy punch
    T. cervical biopsy punch forceps
Tischler-Morgan
    T.-M. biopsy punch
    T.-M. tip
    T.-M. uterine biopsy forceps
Ti-Spacer
    Cohort T.-S.
Tisseel
    T. biologic fibrogen adhesive
    T. fibrin glue
    T. surgical glue
    T. VH fibrin sealant
    T. VH kit
Tissomat device
Tissot spirometer
Tissucol fibrin adhesive material
tissue
    t. adhesive
    t. anchor guide
    t. anchor guide system
    t. culture flask
    Cymetra t.
    t. desiccation needle
    t. desiccation needle electrode
    t. expander
    t. expander template

    t. forceps
    t. glue
    human allograft t.
    t. lifter
    t. morcellator
    t. occlusion clamp
    Ogura t.
    t. press
    t. protector
    t. reflectance oximeter
    t. retractor
    t. scissors
    t. solder
    T. Specific imaging
    T. Tak arthroscopic implant
    T. Tek-II cryostat
    Tutoplast t.
tissue-engineered construct
tissue-grasping forceps
tissue-holding forceps
TissueLink
    T. BPS5.0 bipolar sealer
    T. DS3.0 dissecting sealer
    T. monopolar floating ball
TissueMend fiber membrane
tissue-spreading forceps
Tissue-Tek OCT compound
Tis-U-Trap
    T.-U.-T. endometrial suction
    T.-U.-T. endometrial suction catheter
    T.-U.-T. tissue retrieval device
Titan
    T. Apollo electric flexion distraction table
    T. balloon catheter
    T. endoprosthesis
    T. intramedullary nail system
    T. penile implant
    T. scaler
    T. slow-speed handpiece
    T. stent
titanate ceramic
titanium
    t. alloy implant
    t. alloy Metallograft
    t. alloy needle
    t. aneurysm clip
    t. AO plate
    t. ball-cage heart valve
    t. cable
    t. cage
    t. construct
    t. elastic nail
    t. fixation device
    t. foil
    t. half pin
    t. hollow osseointegrating reconstruction plate

t. hollow screw osseointegrating reconstruction plate
t. hollow screw-plate system
t. hollow screw reconstruction plate (THORP)
t. implant material
t. mandibular staple
t. mesh
t. microconnector
t. microsurgical bipolar forceps
t. miniplate
t. plasma-sprayed dental implant
t. plate
t. prosthesis
t. retinal tack
t. screw
t. spiked washer
t. staple
t. urethral stent
t. vascular clamp
T. VasPort port
t. wire
t. wound retractor
Titmus stereofly
Titus
T. forearm splint
T. tongue depressor
T. venoclysis needle
T. wrist splint
TiUnite dental implant
tivanium
t. alloy
t. hip prosthesis
Tivnen tonsillar forceps
TLC-II portable VAD driver
TLC retractor
T-lens therapeutic contact lens
TLS
TLS suction drain
TLS surgical marker
TLSO
thoracolumbar spinal orthosis
TMJ
temporomandibular joint
TMJ acrylic splint
TMJ Concepts patient-fitted TMJ prosthesis system
TMJ Fossa-Eminence prosthesis
TMJ halter
TMJ head positioner
TMJ reconstruction prosthesis
TMS-2 videokeratoscope

TMS 3-dimensional radiation therapy treatment planning system
Toad finger splint
Tobald syringe
Tobey
T. ear rongeur
T. forceps
Tobin anatomical malar prosthetic implant
Tobold
T. laryngeal forceps
T. laryngeal knife
T. laryngoscopic apparatus
T. tongue depressor
Tobold-Fauvel grasping forceps
Tobolsky elevator
tobramycin-impregnated PMMA implant
Tobruk splint
Tocantins bone marrow biopsy needle
tocodynamometer
guard-ring t.
Nihon t.
tocotonometer
Todd
T. eye cautery needle
T. foreign body gouge
T. stereotaxic guide
Todd-Wells
T.-W. stereotactic guide
T.-W. stereotaxic instrument
T.-W. stereotaxis frame
Todt-Heyer cannula guide
ToDyeFor root canal locator
toe
t. alignment splint
t. comb
t. loop
t. plate
t. prosthesis
toedrop brace
Toennis
T. director
T. dissecting scissors
T. dissector
T. dural hook
T. dural knife
T. needle holder
T. tumor-grasping forceps
Toennis-Adson
T.-A. dissecting scissors
T.-A. dissector
T.-A. forceps

T

NOTES

Tofflemire
T. matrix band
T. retainer
toilet
bidet t.
Toitu cardiovascular monitor
Tolantins bone marrow infusion catheter
Toledo
T. dissector
T. flap dissector tip
T. roller
T. standard dissector tip
T. V-dissector cannula
T. V-dissector tip
Tolentino
T. prism lens
T. vitrectomy lens
T. vitreoretinal cutter
Tolman tonometer
TOM
tube observation model
Tracheostomy TOM
Tomac
T. catheter
T. foam rubber traction dressing
T. forceps
T. goniometer
T. knitted rubber elastic dressing
T. vest-style holder
Tomac-Nélaton catheter
Tomas
T. iris hook
T. suture hook
TomCat PTCA guidewire
Tomenius gastroscope
Tomey
T. angled cannula
T. auto refractor
T. autotopographer
T. ConfoScan confocal microscope
Model P4 microscope
T. G-bevel cannula
T. TMS-1 photokeratoscope
T. topographic modeling system
T. trabeculectomy punch
T. Trooper AutoLensmeter
Tommy
T. hip bar
T. trapeze bar
tomographic
t. scanner
t. skull immobilizer
tomography
computed t. (CT)
electron beam t. (EBT)
electron beam computed t. (EBCT)
emission computerized axial t.

peripheral quantitative computer t. (pQCT)
positron emission t. (PET)
single-photon emission computed t. (SPECT)
t. wedge
Tomolex tomographic system
Tomomatic brain scanner
Tomoscan
T. M CT scanner
T. SR 7000 scanner
tomoscanner
Philips T-60 t.
Tompkins aspirator
TomTec
T. cell harvester
T. echo platform
T. imaging system
tone-reducing ankle-foot orthosis (TRAFO)
tongs
adjustable skull traction t.
Barton-Cone t.
Barton skull traction t.
Böhler t.
Cherry traction t.
Crutchfield t.
Crutchfield-Raney skull traction t.
Crutchfield skeletal traction t.
Edmonton extension t.
Gardner-Wells traction t.
Hinz t.
Raney-Crutchfield skull t.
Reynolds skull traction t.
skull traction t.
traction t.
Trippi-Wells t.
University of Virginia skull t.
Vinke t.
tongue
t. blade
t. depressor
t. depressor blade
t. forceps
t. plate
t. retractor
tongue-retaining device
Tonkaflo pump
Tonomat applanation tonometer
tonometer
air-puff t.
Alcon t.
Allen-Schiotz t.
applanation t.
Bailliart t.
Barraquer t.
Barraquer operating room t.
Berens t.
Carl Zeiss t.

Challenger digital applanation t.
Coburn t.
CT-10 computerized t.
Digilab t.
Draeger t.
Gärtner t.
Goldmann applanation t.
Harrington t.
hollow visceral t.
impression t.
indentation t.
Intermedics intraocular t.
Jena-Schiotz t.
Keeler Pulsair noncontact t.
Krakau t.
Linear KGT t.
Lombart t.
Mack t.
MacKay-Marg t.
Maklakoff t.
McLean t.
Meding tonsil enucleator t.
Mueller electronic t.
Musken t.
noncontact t.
Nuvistor electronic t.
Oculab Tono-Pen t.
Pach-Pen XL t.
Perkins applanation t.
pneumatic t.
pressure phosphene t.
ProTon t.
Proview eye pressure t.
Pulsair t.
Recklinghausen t.
Reichert noncontact t.
Rosner t.
Roush t.
Ruedemann t.
Sauer t.
Sauer-Storz t.
Schiötz t.
Sklar t.
Sklar-Schitz jewel t.
Sluder t.
Sluder-Demarest t.
Storz t.
Storz-Schitz t.
Tolman t.
Tonomat applanation t.
Tono-Pen XL t.
tonometric blood pressure monitor

Tono-Pen XL tonometer
tonsil
t. clamp
t. dissector
t. hook
t. knife
t. sponge
tonsillar
t. abscess forceps
t. artery forceps
t. clamp
t. curette
t. forceps
t. grasping forceps
t. guillotine
t. pillar retractor
t. punch
t. punch forceps
t. scissors
t. snare
t. snare wire
t. suction tube
t. syringe
tonsillectome
Ballenger-Sluder t.
Beck-Mueller t.
Beck-Schenck t.
Brown t.
Daniels hemostatic t.
hemostatic t.
LaForce hemostatic t.
Mack lingual tonsillar t.
Meding tonsil enucleator t.
Moltz-Storz t.
Myles guillotine t.
Sauer hemostatic t.
Sauer-Sluder t.
Sauer-Storz t.
Searcy t.
Seiffert t.
Sluder-Ballenger t.
Sluder-Demarest t.
Sluder-Sauer t.
Sluder tonsillar t.
Storz-Moltz t.
Tydings t.
Van Osdel tonsil enucleator t.
Whiting t.
tonsil-seizing forceps
Tooke
T. angled splitter
T. blade

T

NOTES

Tooke *(continued)*
    T. corneal forceps
    T. corneal knife
    T. iris knife
    T. spatula
Tooke-Johnson corneal knife
tool
    Acuforce 7.0 massage therapy t.
    AcuPressor myotherapy t.
    Avenue insertion t.
    Backnobber II massage t.
    Bates-Jensen pressure ulcer status t.
    cement-removal hand t.
    Gore Smoother crucial t.
    Index Knobber II massage t.
    Magnassager massage t.
    Original Backnobber massage t.
    Original Index Knobber II
     massage t.
    Original Jacknobber massage t.
    OsteoStat disposable power t.
    pressure sore status t.
    spud t.
Toomey
    T. bladder evacuator
    T. forceps
    T. pyramid tip
    T. surgical stainless steel
     instrument set
    T. syringe
    T. syringe kit
tooth
    t. band
    t. cement
    t. guard
tooth-borne distraction device
toothbrush
    DexTBrush t.
    PowerProxi Sonic t.
    Sonicare Plus t.
    Water Pik t.
tooth-colored abutment
toothed
    t. pickups
    t. retractor
    t. tenaculum
    t. thumb forceps
    t. tissue forceps
2-toothed forceps
tooth-extracting forceps
toothless forceps
Topaz
    T. CO_2 laser
    T. flexion table
    T. II SSIR pacemaker
TopCat Contamination Assist Tray
Topcon
    T. aspheric lens
    T. automatic chart projector
    T. IMAGEnet digital imaging
     system
    T. keratometer
    T. LM P5 digital lensometer
    T. noncontact specular
     morphometric analysis
    T. RM-A2300 auto refractor
    T. SL-E series slit lamp
    T. SP-series non-contact specular
     microscope
    T. stereoscopic TRC-series fundus
     camera
top-cover
    Spenco t.-c.
Top-Hat supraannular aortic valve
TopiFoam gel-backed self-adhering foam
  pad
Top Notch automated biopsy system
topographic scanning system
toposcopic catheter
Topper
    T. cannula
    T. dressing sponge
    T. mattress overlay
    T. nonadherent gauze
TopSS
    T. scanning laser ophthalmoscope
    T. topographic scanning system
Torbot
    T. bonding cement
    T. Plastic pouch
    T. Rubber pouch
Torchia
    T. capsular forceps
    T. capsular polisher
    T. conjunctival scissors
    T. corneal knife
    T. eye speculum
    T. lens hook
    T. lens implantation forceps
    T. microbipolar forceps
    T. microcorneal scissors
    T. nucleus-aspirating cannula
    T. tissue forceps
    T. tying forceps
    T. vectis loop
Torchia-Colibri forceps
Torchia-Kuglen hook
Torchia-Vannas micro-iris scissors
Torcon
    T. blue catheter
    T. NB selective angiographic
     catheter
TorFlex transseptal guiding sheath
toric
    t. contact lens
    t. intraocular lens
Toriumi
    T. curved rasp

T. osteotome
T. sharp and dull suction elevators
Torkildsen shunt
Torktherm torque control catheter
torlone fixation pin
Tornado coil
Tornier radial head prosthesis
Toronto
T. Medical CPM exerciser
T. parapodium orthosis
T. splint
T. SPV bioprosthesis
T. SPV stentless porcine valve
Toronto-Western Hospital catheter
TORP
total ossicular reconstruction procedure
Proplast TORP
TORP prosthesis
TORP strut
torpedo
T. eye patch
Gelfoam t.
Torpin
T. automatic uterine gauze packer
T. obstetrical lever
T. vectis
T. vectis blade
T. vectis extractor
torque-control balloon catheter
torqued slot bracket
torque-type prosthesis
torque vise
Torre Cryojet
Torres
T. cross-action forceps
T. needle holder
Torrington French spring needle
torsion
t. bar splint
t. forceps
torsional
telescopic and t. (TT)
torso phased-array coil
Torx driver
Toshiba
T. biplane transesophageal
transducer
T. brain scanner
T. echocardiography machine
T. electrocardiography machine
T. helical CT scanner
T. microendoscope

T. MR scanner
T. Sal 38B real-time
ultrasonography
T. Sonolayer SSH-140A ultrasound
T. SSA-340A Doppler sonography
T. TCE-M-series colonoscope
T. TCT-900S helical CT scanner
T. video endoscope
T. Xpress SX helical CT scanner
T. Xvision scanner
Tosic external fixation system
total
t. alloplastic TMJ reconstruction
prosthesis
t. articular replacement arthroplasty
(TARA)
t. artificial heart
t. contact cast
T. Gym
T. Knee 2100 prosthetic knee
T. O_2/Oxylite oxygen system
t. ossicular prosthesis
t. ossicular reconstruction procedure
(TORP)
t. ossicular replacement prosthesis
t. parenteral nutrition (TPN)
t. parenteral nutrition catheter
T. Recall digital imaging system
T. Synchrony system
t. top implant
total-body compression suit
Totco
T. Autoclip
T. clip
Tote-A-Neb nebulizer
Tothonator orthotic
Toti
T. trephine
T. trephine drill
TouchAmerica BodyTable
Touchlite zoom lens
Touch-Test sensory evaluator
Touma
T. dissector
T. T-type grommet ventilation tube
Tourguide guiding catheter
Tournikwik tourniquet
tourniquet
Adams modification of Bethune t.
automatic t.
t. band
Bethune lobectomy t.

T

NOTES

tourniquet *(continued)*
Bethune lung t.
Bodenstab t.
Campbell-Boyd t.
Campbell-Boyd pneumatic t.
Carr lobectomy t.
closed loop t.
Conn pneumatic t.
Conn Universal t.
cotton-covered t.
t. cuff
Digikit finger t.
Drake t.
Dupuytren t.
Esmarch t.
field t.
forearm t.
Gill renal t.
Grafco t.
Holcombe gastric t.
horseshoe t.
Ideal t.
Johnson & Johnson t.
Kidde t.
Kidde-Robbins t.
Linton t.
Medi-Quet t.
Momberg t.
nonpneumatic t.
Pac-Kit Army-type t.
Petit t.
pneumatic t.
pneumatic ankle t.
Profex arthroscopic t.
Quicket t.
ratchet t.
Robbins automatic t.
Roberts-Nelson lobectomy t.
Roper-Rumel t.
Rumel t.
Rumel-Belmont t.
Rumel ratchet t.
Samway t.
Sebra arm t.
Shenstone t.
Signorini t.
single-loop t.
SMIC auricular t.
t. strap
Sure-Snare t.
Surgikit Velcro t.
thigh t.
Tinel t.
Tournikwik t.
Trussdale t.
Uniquet disposable intravenous t.
Universal t.
U.S. Army t.
Velcro t.

Velket Velcro t.
Weiner t.
Wright pneumatic t.
tourniquet-eyed
t.-e. obturator
t.-e. ratchet stylet
Tovell tube
towel
Charnley t.
t. clamp
t. clip
DisCide disinfecting t.
t. drape
fat t.
t. forceps
Kaycel t.
wound t.
tower
Concept traction t.
T. interchangeable retractor
Linvatec wrist arthroscopy
traction t.
T. muscle forceps
T. rib retractor
T. spinal retractor
T. stent
traction t.
Townley
T. bone graft screw
T. calipers
T. implant
T. TARA prosthesis
T. tissue forceps
T. total knee prosthesis
Townsend
T. biopsy punch
T. endocervical biopsy curette
T. knee brace
Townsend-Gilfillan
T.-G. plate
T.-G. screw
toxemia curette
Toynbee
T. curette
T. diagnostic tube
T. ear speculum
T. otoscope
TPE
thermoplastic elastomer
TPE ankle-foot orthosis
TPE biomechanical foot orthosis
T-pin handle
TPL-6 hip system
TPN
total parenteral nutrition
TPN catheter
TPS-coated
TPS-c. cylinder
TPS-c. screw

TR-28 hip prosthesis
trabeculotome
    Allen-Burian t.
    Harms t.
    McPherson t.
trabeculotomy probe
Trabucco double balloon catheter
TraceHybrid wire guide
Trace hydraulic vein stripper
tracer
    T. Blood Glucose monitor
    T. hybrid wire guide
    radiofrequency t.
    T. ST wire
TrachCare multi-access catheter
tracheal
    t. button
    t. cannula
    t. catheter
    t. dilating forceps
    t. dilator
    t. hook
    t. retractor
    t. safety stitch
    t. scalpel
    t. stent
    t. tenaculum
    t. tube
    t. tube brush
    t. tube changer
    t. tube cuff
tracheobronchoesophagoscope
    Haslinger t.
tracheoesophageal
    t. puncture dilator
    t. shunt
Tracheolife HME oxygen port nebulizer
tracheopharyngeal shunt
tracheoscope
    Haslinger t.
    Jackson t.
    Storz t.
    Storz-Shapshay t.
    Tucker t.
TracheoSoft XLT tracheostomy tube
tracheostoma valve
tracheostomy
    t. button
    t. cannula
    t. hook
    Low Profile PMV 2001 purple t.
    Montgomery t.

    Pitt talking t.
    t. plate
    T. TOM
    t. tube
    t. tube holder
tracheotome
    Salvatore-Maloney t.
    Sierra-Sheldon t.
tracheotomy
    t. cannula
    t. hook
    t. retractor
    t. sponge
Trach-Eze closed suction catheter
Trachguard
    B&B T.
Trachlight lighted intubating stylet
Trach-Mist aerosol drainage bag
Tracho-Foam adhesive disc
trachoma forceps
Trach-Talk
    T.-T. device
    T.-T. tracheostomy tube
Tracker-18
    T. Soft Stream catheter
    T. Unibody catheter
tracker
    Ascension Bird position t.
    T. knee brace
    miniBIRD position t.
    Palumbo patella t.
    patella t.
    Purkinje image t.
Tracker-10 microcatheter
tracker-assisted PRK laser
Trackmaster treadmill
Trac knee system
TRACOEflex tracheostomy tube
Trac Plus catheter
traction
    t. anchor
    t. apparatus
    t. bar
    t. belt
    t. bow
    Bremer halo cervical t.
    Bryant t.
    Buck t.
    cervical AOA halo t.
    C-Flex II cervical t.
    C-Flex supine cervical t.
    Cotrel t.

T

NOTES

traction *(continued)*
- Crutchfield cervical t.
- Crutchfield skeletal t.
- t. device
- Dunlop t.
- Exo-Bed t.
- Exo-Static overhead t.
- t. forceps
- Freiberg t.
- Frejka t.
- Georgiade visor cervical t.
- halo t.
- t. handle
- head halter cervical t.
- Homestretch lumbar t.
- HomeTrac cervical t.
- Houston halo cervical t.
- Jones suspension t.
- Kirschner skeletal t.
- Kirschner wire t.
- t. legging
- lumbosacral support pelvic t.
- McBride tripod pin t.
- Miami Acute Care cervical t.
- Miami J collar cervical t.
- Neufeld t.
- Perkins t.
- Philadelphia collar cervical t.
- Pronex cervical t.
- Quantum 400 true intersegmental t.
- Russell skeletal t.
- Saunders cervical HomeTrac t.
- Sayre suspension t.
- split Russell skeletal t.
- Steinmann t.
- t. suture
- Syms t.
- t. table
- t. tongs
- t. tower
- transfer t.
- Watson-Jones t.

Tracto-Halter gait trainer

tractor
- axial t.
- banjo t.
- Blackburn skull traction t.
- Böhler t.
- Bryant t.
- Buck t.
- Dunlop t.
- Exo-Static overhead t.
- Freiberg t.
- Hamilton pelvic traction screw t.
- Handy-Buck extension t.
- Hoke-Martin t.
- Kestler ambulatory head t.
- Kirschner wire t.
- Lowsley prostatic t.

- Lowsley suprapubic t.
- Lyman-Smith t.
- Muirhead-Little pelvic rest t.
- Neufeld t.
- Orr-Buck extension t.
- Perkins split-weight t.
- prostatic t.
- Rankin prostatic t.
- Russell-Beck extension t.
- Steinmann traction t.
- Syms t.
- Trimline mobile t.
- Tupper t.
- Vinke skull t.
- Watson-Jones t.
- Wells t.
- Young prostatic t.
- Zim-Trac traction splint t.

TRAFO
- tone-reducing ankle-foot orthosis
- TRAFO orthosis

Trailblazer wire

trainer
- AcuTrainer bladder t.
- Bosu balance t.
- impulse inertial exercise t.
- Monark Rehab T.
- positional feedback stimulation t.
- Shuttle Balance balance t.
- Tracto-Halter gait t.

training
- Computer-Aided Fluency Establishment T. (CAFET)
- inspiratory muscle t. (IMT)

Trak Back II digital pullback device

TRAKE-fit
- TRAKE-f. endotracheal tube
- TRAKE-f. tracheostomy tube holder

Trakstar balloon catheter

Tramscope 12 monitor

Tranquility
- T. Auto CPAP system
- T. bilevel CPAP unit
- T. bilevel system
- T. Quest CPAP
- T. Quest CPAP device
- T. Quest CPAP system

transabdominal transducer

transarticular screw

transaxillary needle

transbuccal trocar

transcatheter
- t. patch
- t. umbrella
- t. umbrella implant material

Transcend microguidewire

transcervical tubal access catheter

transconjunctival retractor

transcranial
  t. Doppler probe
  t. Doppler ultrasound
transcutaneous
  t. bilirubinometer
  t. carbon dioxide monitor
  t. cranial electrical stimulator
  t. electrical nerve stimulation
    (TENS)
  t. electrical nerve stimulation
    machine
  t. electrical nerve stimulator
  t. electrical neuromuscular
    stimulator
  t. extraction catheter
  t. lead
  t. monitor
  t. oxygen monitor
  t. pacemaker
TransCyte temporary skin substitute
transducer
  AccuScan t.
  Acuson V510B biplane TEE t.
  Acuson V5M ultrasound t.
  Acuson 128XP t.
  Aloka SSD1700 t.
  anular-array t.
  array ultrasound t.
  Bentley t.
  bifocal multiplane t.
  bite force t.
  Bruel & Kjaer axial t.
  bur hole t.
  Camino catheter-tip t.
  Combitrans monitoring set
    pressure t.
  Cordis Sentron t.
  curved array t.
  Deltran disposable t.
  Diasonics t.
  Dräger MTC t.
  electromagnetic flow t.
  end-fire t.
  endovaginal t.
  epicardial Doppler flow sector t.
  Gaeltec catheter-tip pressure t.
  Gould Statham pressure t.
  Hall-effect strain t.
  high-resolution linear array t.
  HP OmniPlane TEE imaging t.
  ion-specific field effect t.
  linear t.

  linear array t.
  linear 35-MHz t.
  LSC 7000 curved array t.
  magnetic motion t.
  magnetic resonance imaging-guided
    focused ultrasound sector t.
  Medex t.
  microtip pressure t.
  Millar catheter tip pressure t.
  Millar Mikro-Tip catheter
    pressure t.
  M-mode sector t.
  multiplanar t.
  Nellcor Durasensor adult oxygen t.
  Ocuscan 400 t.
  OmniPlane TEE t.
  Oxisensor II adult oxygen t.
  phased-array sector t.
  piezoelectric ultrasound t.
  piezoresistive t.
  pressure t.
  pulsed-wave Doppler t.
  puncture t.
  quartz t.
  range-gated t.
  rotatory-variable-differential t.
  sector t.
  Sentron t.
  Siemens Endo-P endorectal t.
  Sleepscan airflow pressure t.
  Spectramed t.
  Statham external t.
  Therasound t.
  Toshiba biplane transesophageal t.
  transabdominal t.
  transrectal multiplane 3-
    dimensional t.
  TruWave disposable pressure t.
  ultrasound t.
  V510B biplane TEE t.
  V5M multiplane TEE t.
  Voluson sector t.
  wideband sector t.
transducer-tipped catheter
Transeal
  T. dressing
  T. transparent adhesive film
    dressing
Transelast surgical drape
transendoscopic ultrasound
transesophageal
  t. color flow Doppler imaging

T

NOTES

transesophageal *(continued)*
  t. echocardiography probe
  t. pacing system
transfemoral
  t. catheter
  t. endoaortic occlusion catheter
transfer
  t. forceps
  t. traction
TransFix
  T. ACL system
  T. pin
transfixing screw
transfixion
  t. bolt
  t. screw
  t. suture
Transform cardiomyostimulator
transformer
  Coolidge t.
  doughnut t.
  filament t.
  high-voltage t.
  step-down t.
  step-up t.
TransFx external fixation system
transhepatic
  t. biliary stent
  t. portacaval shunt
TransiGel
  T. hydrogel-impregnated gauze
  T. woven gauze dressing
transilluminating telescope
transilluminator
  Briggs t.
  Coldite t.
  Finnoff sinus t.
  Hildreth t.
  Jako t.
  Lancaster ocular t.
  National all-metric t.
  National opal glass t.
  O'Malley-Skia t.
  Tatum ureteral t.
  Thompson cervical t.
  UV t.
  Welch Allyn t.
  Widner t.
transistor
  field-effect t.
  insulated gate field-effect t.
  ion-sensitive field-effect t.
  junction field-effect t. (JFET)
  unijunction t. (UJT)
Transit microcatheter
transit-time flowmeter

transjugular
  t. intrahepatic portosystemic shunt
    (TIPS, TIPSS)
  t. needle
translocation needle
translucent
  t. drain tube
  t. silicone tube
translumbar inferior vena caval
  catheter
transluminal
  t. angioplasty catheter
  t. balloon
  t. endarterectomy catheter
  t. extraction catheter (TEC)
  t. lysing system
transmandibular implant
transmission
  t. electron microscope
  t. line resonator
transmit-receive coil
transmitter
transmitter-receiver
  Itrel programmed t.-r.
transmural
  t. antitachycardia pacemaker
  t. electrical stimulator
transmyocardial pacing stylet
transnasal pancreaticobiliary drain
Transonic
  T. flowmeter
  T. flow probe
  T. laser Doppler perfusion monitor
transoral
  t. catheter
  t. retractor
Transorbent hydrogel topical wound
  dressing
Transorb wound dressing
transosseous
  t. implant
  t. post
  t. suture
transosteal pin implant
transpapillary
  t. drain
  t. endoprosthesis
  t. endoscope
  t. pancreatic stent
transparent
  t. adhesive film dressing
  t. drape
transpedicular screw
transpericardial pacemaker
Transpire wrist orthosis
transplant trephine
Transpore
  T. clear tape
  T. surgical tape dressing

transport catheter
transpubic needle
transpupillary laser
transpyloric feeding tube
TransQFlex iontophoresis electrode
transrectal
    t. multiplane 3-dimensional
       transducer
    t. probe
TransScan
    T. 200 breast imaging system
    T. TS2000 electrical impedance
       breast scanning system
transscleral suture
transseptal
    t. cannula
    t. catheter
    t. sheath
transsphenoidal
    t. bipolar forceps
    t. curette
    t. dissector
    t. speculum
transtelephonic
    t. ambulatory monitoring system
    t. exercise monitor
transthoracic
    t. catheter
    t. pacemaker
    t. pacing stylet
transthoracically implanted ICD
transtracheal oxygen catheter
transurethral
    t. catheter
    t. needle ablation (TUNA)
    t. needle ablation system
    t. ultrasound-guided laser-induced
       prostatectomy (TULIP)
TransUrethral Microwave
   Thermotherapy (TUMT)
transvaginal ultrasound
Transvene
    T. nonthoracotomy implantable
       cardioverter-defibrillator
    T. tripolar electrode
Transvene-RV lead
transvenous
    t. coil
    t. defibrillator lead
    t. electrode
    t. implantable defibrillator
    t. pacemaker catheter

    t. snare
    t. ventricular demand pacemaker
transventricular dilator
transverse
    t. connector
    t. gradient coil
trap
    Allen finger t.
    Burkard spore t.
    collection t.
    Concept digit t.
    DeLee t.
    EndoDynamics suction polyp t.
    extraction t.
    filtered specimen t.
    Hirst spore t.
    in-line t.
    Kramer-Collins Spore t.
    Lukens t.
    Nakao QuickTrap t.
    osseous coagulum t.
    Rusch mucous t.
    sterile specimen t.
TrapEase permanent vena caval filter
trapeze
    t. bar
    overhead frame t.
trapeziometacarpal joint replacement
   prosthesis
trapezium implant
Trapper exchange device
Traquair periosteal elevator
Trattner urethrographic catheter
Traube neurological hammer
TraumaJet wound debridement system
TraumaSeal topical wound closure
   device
traumatic grasping forceps
Travel Bath
Travenol
    T. heart bag
    T. infuser
    T. infusion pump
    T. Tru-Cut biopsy needle
Travert needle
TraxIt continuous-reading precision
   phase-change thermometer
tray
    Bard catheter sterile insertion t.
    Bardex Lubricath sterile Foley t.
    Bard sterile infection control t.
    Bucky view t.

T

NOTES

tray *(continued)*
    Denis Browne t.
    E-Z-EM PercuSet amniocentesis t.
    MetriTray system soaking t.
    orthodontic impression t.
    Papanicolaou smear t.
    PFC offset tibial t.
    Russell gastrostomy t.
    TiMesh titanium t.
    TopCat Contamination Assist T.
    Unimar HSG t.
    Weck microsurgical t.
Treace stapes drill
treadmill
    Aquaciser underwater t.
    AquaGaiter t.
    Cateye T-220 t.
    exercise t.
    Hydrotrack underwater t.
    Jaeger LE3000 t.
    Lifestride t.
    Marquette t.
    Orbiter t.
    Q-Stress t.
    Schwinn light commercial t.
    Trackmaster t.
    Tunturi Jogger-2 self-powered t.
    Universal Tredex t.
treatment
    t. port
    t. table
Tredex bicycle
tree
    BTE Assembly T.
    pinch t.
    pipe t.
trefoil balloon catheter
Trelat
    T. palate raspatory
    T. vaginal speculum
Trelex natural mesh
Trelles metal scleral shield
Trellis infusion catheter
Tremble sphenoid cannula
Trendelenburg
    T. cannula
    T. tampon
Trendelenburg-Craafoord coarctation clamp
Trent
    T. eye retractor
    T. pick
Treon ENT image guidance system
trephine
    Arroyo t.
    Arruga eye t.
    Arruga lacrimal t.
    automated t.
    Bard-Parker t.

    Barraquer corneal t.
    Barron epikeratophakia t.
    Barron-Hessburg corneal t.
    Barron radial vacuum t.
    Barron vacuum t.
    Becker skull t.
    Blackburn t.
    t. blade
    Blakesley lacrimal t.
    Boiler septal t.
    Bonaccolto t.
    Boston t.
    Brown-Pusey corneal t.
    Cardona corneal prosthesis t.
    Castroviejo corneal transplant t.
    chalazion t.
    corneal t.
    Damshek sternal t.
    Davis t.
    DeMartel t.
    D'Errico skull t.
    DeVilbiss skull t.
    DiaPhine t.
    Dimitry chalazion t.
    Dimitry dacryocystorhinostomy t.
    disposable t.
    t. drill
    Elliot corneal t.
    Elschnig t.
    Franceschetti corneal t.
    Galt skull t.
    Garty diamond t.
    Gradle corneal t.
    Green automatic corneal t.
    Greenwood spinal t.
    Grieshaber calibrated corneal t.
    Guyton corneal transplant t.
    hand t.
    handheld t.
    Hanna t.
    Harris t.
    Hessburg-Barron vacuum t.
    Hessburg vacuum t.
    Hippel t.
    Horsley t.
    Iliff lacrimal t.
    Jentzer t.
    Katena t.
    Katena-Barron t.
    Katzin t.
    Keyes cutaneous t.
    King corneal t.
    lacrimal t.
    Lahey Clinic skull t.
    Leksell t.
    Lichtenberg corneal t.
    Londermann corneal t.
    Lorie antral t.
    t. marker

Martinez disposable corneal t.
M-brace corneal t.
Michele t.
Moria t.
Mueller electric corneal t.
Paton see-through corneal t.
pattern t.
Paufique corneal t.
Pharmacia corneal t.
Phemister biopsy t.
Polley-Bickel t.
punch t.
razor blade t.
Robertson corneal t.
Rochester bone t.
Sacker t.
Schanz t.
Scheie t.
Schuknecht temporal t.
scleral t.
Scoville skull t.
Searcy chalazion t.
Sidney Stephenson corneal t.
sinus t.
Sisler lacrimal t.
skull t.
Stille t.
Stock eye t.
Storz chalazion t.
Storz corneal t.
Storz hair transplant t.
Storz-Lieberman DiaPhine t.
Surgistar corneal t.
Terry t.
Thornwald antral t.
Toti t.
transplant t.
Troutman tenotomy t.
Turkel t.
von Hippel mechanical t.
walker corneal t.
Wilder t.
Wilkins t.
Williams & Nicholson t.
Trestle transurethral prostatic catheter
Treves intestinal clamp
Trevisani
T. cannula
T. cannula tip
Trex digital mammography system
Triad
T. defibrillator system

T. facet screw
T. hydrophilic wound dressing
T. lumbar interbody allograft
T. PET balloon
T. prosthesis
T. SPECT imaging system
TriaDyne
T. bed
T. II therapy system
Triage cardiac system
Tria handheld Doppler ultrasound stethoscope
trial
t. component
t. implant
t. prosthesis
triangle
T. gelatin-sealed sling material
t. shoulder abduction brace
triangular
t. ankle fusion frame
t. arm sling
t. bandage
t. dressing
t. forceps
t. jaw forceps
t. rasp
triangulated pedicle screw
triaxial
t. accelerometer
t. Helmholtz coil
t. semiconstrained elbow prosthesis
Tri-Beeled trapezoidal keratome
Tricep hooked-prong grasping forceps
Trichodemolus epilator
Tricodur
T. Epi compression support bandage
T. Omos compression support bandage
T. Talus compression support bandage
tricomponent coaxial system
Tri-Con component
Tricon-M
T.-M cruciate-sparing prosthesis
T.-M patellar prosthesis
Tri-Core cervical support pillow
tricuspid valve strut
Tricut
T. blade
T. laryngeal blade tip

NOTES

Trident resection arthroscopic ablator
Tri-Ex triple-lumen extraction balloon
TriEye
    T. cannula
    T. tip
trifacet knife
Trifecta multipurpose balloon catheter
TriFix spinal instrumentation system
Tri-Flex auxiliary suspension belt
TriFloat Plus pressure-reduction
  mattress
Tri-flow incentive spirometer
trifocal glasses
trigeminal
    t. electrode
    t. knife
    t. scissors
    t. self-retaining retractor
trigeminus cannula
TriGen intramedullary nail
trigger
    t. cannula
    T. Switch
TriggerWheel
    T. device
    T. Wand
Triguide catheter
trilaminate cushion
trileaflet prosthesis
Trilicon external breast prosthesis
Tri-Lock
    T.-L. femoral component
    T.-L. total hip prosthesis with
      Porocoat
Trilogy
    T. acetabular cup
    T. DC, DR, SR pulse generator
    T. DC+ pacemaker
    T. I hearing aid
    T. low-profile balloon dilatation
      catheter
    T. SR+ single-chamber pacemaker
Trilucent breast implant
Trima automated blood collection
  system
Trimble suture stent
Trimedyne
    T. holmium laser
    T. Optilase 1000 device
Trimensional augmentation 3-D shape
Tri-Met apnea monitor
Trimline
    T. knee immobilizer
    T. mobile tractor
trimmer
    calcar t.
    Mallory-Head Interlok calcar t.
    Nordent margin t.
Tri-Motion knee system

Trinica
    T. anterior cervical plate system
    T. System
Trinkle
    T. bone drill
    T. brace
    T. chuck
    T. chuck adapter
    T. screwdriver
    T. socket wrench
    T. Super-Cut twist drill
triode
    t. tube
    t. tube amplifier
Trionix
    T. camera
    T. scanner
Trios M pacemaker
Trio-Temp X Biofil
triphasic spiral CT
Triphasix generator
triplane construct
triple-balloon perfusion catheter
triple-branched stent graft
triple-edge diamond-blade knife
triple-head gamma camera
triple hook
triple-lumen
    t.-l. Arrow catheter
    t.-l. biliary manometry catheter
    t.-l. catheter
    t.-l. central catheter
    t.-l. implant
    t.-l. manometry catheter
    t.-l. needle knife
    t.-l. perfused catheter system
    t.-l. sump drain
triple-thermistor coronary sinus catheter
tripod
    t. grasping forceps
    t. intraocular lens
tripolar
    t. coil defibrillation electrode
    t. Damato curve catheter
    t. electrode catheter
    t. lead
Tri-Port
    T.-P. hemostasis introducer sheath
     kit
    T.-P. sub-Tenon anesthesia cannula
Trippi-Wells tongs
tri-pronged loop
tri-radial resector blade
trisector
    Alfonso nucleus ophthalmic t.
TriStar trocar
TriStim TENS unit
Tri-Tome sphincterotome

Triton
    T. pin collet
    T. power surgical instrument
        system
TriTrac accelerometer
Triumph VR pacemaker
Tri-Wedge total hip system
Trizol RNA extractor
TroCam endoscopic camera
**Trocan disposable CO$_2$ trocar and
    cannula**
trocar
    abdominal t.
    Abelson cricothyrotomy t.
    Allen cecostomy t.
    American Heyer-Schulte-Robertson
        suprapubic t.
    AMS disposable t.
    antral t.
    Apple t.
    Arbuckle-Shea t.
    Argyle t.
    Axiom thoracic t.
    Babcock empyema t.
    BD Potain thoracic t.
    Beardsley cecostomy t.
    Birch t.
    blunt t.
    Bluntport t.
    Boettcher antral t.
    Boettcher-Schnidt antral t.
    brain t.
    Bueleau empyema t.
    Bülau t.
    Cabot t.
    Campbell suprapubic t.
    Castens ascites t.
    Castens hydrocele t.
    Charlton antral t.
    Circon ACMI t.
    Coakley antrum t.
    Cook t.
    Core Dynamics audible t.
    Core Dynamics disposable t.
    Cross needle t.
    Curschmann t.
    Davidson t.
    Dean antral t.
    Denker t.
    Dexide laparoscopic t.
    Dexide locking t.
    Diamond-Flex t.

    disposable t.
    Douglas antrum t.
    Douglas nasal t.
    Dr. White t.
    Duchenne t.
    Duke t.
    Durham tracheotomy t.
    Emmet ovarian t.
    Endopath bladeless t.
    Endopath disposable surgical t.
    Endopath laparoscopic t.
    Endopath surgical t.
    Endopath TriStar t.
    Endo Tip Storz t.
    Entree Plus t.
    Ethicon disposable t.
    Faulkner t.
    Fein antral t.
    Fleurant bladder t.
    Frazier brain-exploring t.
    Gallagher t.
    Haeggstrom antral t.
    Hargin antral t.
    Hasson laparoscopic t.
    Havlicek t.
    Hunt angiographic t.
    Hurwitz thoracic t.
    Ingram t.
    InnerDyne t.
    intercostal t.
    intestinal decompression t.
    Iotec t.
    Jako laser t.
    Jarit disposable t.
    Johannson-Stille cystotomy t.
    Judd t.
    Kido suprapubic t.
    Kolb t.
    Krause antral t.
    Kreutzmann t.
    Landau t.
    LaparoSAC t.
    laparoscopic t.
    laryngeal t.
    Lichtwicz abdominal t.
    Lichtwicz antral t.
    Lillie antral t.
    Livermore t.
    Marlow disposable t.
    Mayo-Ochsner t.
    Monoscopy locking t.
    Morson t.

T

NOTES

trocar *(continued)*
    Myerson antral t.
    Nagashima antroscope t.
    t. needle
    needle t.
    Nelson empyema t.
    Nelson-Patterson empyema t.
    Nelson thoracic t.
    nested t.
    Ochsner gallbladder t.
    Ochsner thoracic t.
    Olympus disposable t.
    Optiview t.
    Origin t.
    PassPort t.
    Patterson empyema t.
    Patterson-Nelson empyema t.
    Pierce antral t.
    Pierce-Kyle t.
    Poole t.
    Potain aspirating t.
    rectal t.
    Reddick-Saye t.
    Rica Universal t.
    Richard Wolf laparoscopic t.
    Roberts abdominal t.
    Ruskin antral t.
    Saber BT blunt-tip surgical t.
    Schwartz t.
    Sewall antral t.
    sharp t.
    Singleton empyema t.
    sinoscopy t.
    Snyder Urevac t.
    Southey anasarca t.
    Southey-Leech t.
    Step laparoscopic t.
    Stiwer t.
    Storz t.
    subcostal t.
    suprapubic t.
    Surgiport disposable t.
    Sweet antral t.
    Synthes transbuccal t.
    thoracic t.
    Thoracoport t.
    Tilley-Lichwitz t.
    transbuccal t.
    TriStar t.
    Ueckermann-Denker t.
    Uni-Shunt split t.
    Universal abdominal t.
    Van Alyea antral t.
    Veirs t.
    Visiport optical t.
    Walther aspirating bladder t.
    Wangensteen internal
      decompression t.
    Weck disposable t.
    Wiener-Pierce antral t.
    Wilson amniotic t.
    Wilson-Baylor amniotic t.
    Wisap disposable t.
    Wolf-Cottle t.
    Wolf needle t.
    Wright-Harloe empyema t.
    Ximed disposable t.
    Yankauer antral t.
trocar-cannula system
trocar-point Kirschner wire
Trocath peritoneal dialysis catheter
trochanter holder
trochanter-holding clamp
trochanteric
    t. awl
    t. bolt
    t. pin
    t. plate
    t. router
    t. wire
Troeltsch
    T. dressing forceps
    T. ear forceps
    T. ear speculum
    T. eustachian catheter
**TroGARD Finesse dilating trocar
system**
Troilius capsulotomy knife
Trokel
    T. hyperopia conformer
    T. lens
Trokel-Peyman laser lens
trolley
    Bolero lift bath t.
Tromner percussion hammer
Troncoso
    T. gonioscope
    T. gonioscopic lens implant
    T. tubular lens
Tronzo
    T. elevator
    T. prosthesis
troposcope
Trotter forceps
Trough gouge
trousers
    Dyna Med anti-shock t.
    MAST t.
    military antishock t. (MAST)
Trousseau
    T. dilating forceps
    T. esophageal bougie
    T. mouthgag
    T. tracheal dilator
Trousseau-Jackson
    T.-J. esophageal dilator
    T.-J. tracheal dilator

Troutman
T. alpha-chymotrypsin cannula
T. blade
T. blade breaker
T. cataract extractor
T. corneal dissector
T. corneal forceps
T. corneal knife
T. corneal splitter
T. eye implant
T. lens loupe
T. lens spatula
T. mastoid chisel
T. microsurgery forceps
T. microsurgical scissors
T. needle
T. needle holder
T. nonincisional lamellar dissector
T. punch
T. superior rectus forceps
T. suture scissors
T. tenotomy trephine
T. tying forceps
T. wave-edge corneal dissector
Troutman-Barraquer
T.-B. corneal fixation forceps
T.-B. iris forceps
T.-B. iris spatula
T.-B. mini blade breaker
T.-B. needle holder
Troutman-Barraquer-Colibri forceps
Troutman-Castroviejo
T.-C. conjunctival scissors
T.-C. corneal section scissors
Troutman-Katzin corneal transplant scissors
Troutman-Llobera fixation forceps
Troutman-Llobera-Flieringa forceps
Troutman-Tooke corneal knife
Trowbridge
T. TerraRound foot
T. triple-speed drill
Trowbridge-Campau
T.-C. bone drill
T.-C. eye magnet
Tru-Arc blood vessel ring
Truarch wire
Trubyte Alma gauge system
Tru-Chrome band material
Tru-clip clip
Tru-Close wound drainage system

Tru-Cut
T.-C. biopsy needle
T.-C. biopsy needle holder
True
T. Blue exercise band
T. Form support stocking
T. Sheathless catheter
True/Fit femoral intramedullary rod system
True/Flex
T./F. intramedullary nail
T./F. intramedullary rod system
True/Lok external fixator
TrueMax 2400 metabolic system
TrueTorque wireguide
TrueVision transvaginal probe
Trufill n-BCA liquid embolic system
Tru-Fit custom-molded shoe
Tru-Incise valvulotome
Trujillo LASIK enhancement wedge
Trulife silicone breast form
TruLine forceps
Tru-Mold shoe
trumpet
Iowa t.
modified nasal t.
nasal t.
t. needle guide
t. valve cannula
t. valve hydrodissector
truncated NMR probe
truncus clamp
trunnion-bearing hip prosthesis
Trupower aspherical lens
Trupp ventricular needle
TruPro cannula
TruPulse
T. CO_2 laser
T. CO_2 laser system
Trush grasping forceps
Trusler-Dean scissors
Trusler infant vascular clamp
truss
Hood t.
inguinal t.
Kansas City band t.
Nu-Form t.
scrotal t.
Trussdale tourniquet
TruStep foot prosthesis

NOTES

Tru-Support
    T.-S. EW bandage
    T.-S. SA bandage
Truszkowski dural dissector
Tru Taper Ethalloy needle
Tru-Trac high-pressure PTA balloon
TruTrak data sampling system
TruWave disposable pressure transducer
TruZone
    T. peak flowmeter
    T. PFM
Trylon hemostatic forceps
TS2000 breast imaging system
T-Scan 2000 breast imaging device
TSH-01 transdermal tape
T-shaped
    T-s. AO plate
    T-s. Edwards-Barbaro syringo-
      peritoneal shunt
T-Span tissue expander
T-spatula
    serrated T-s.
T-Spica bandage
TSRH
    Texas Scottish Rite Hospital
    TSRH buttressed laminar hook
    TSRH circular laminar hook
    TSRH double-rod construct
    TSRH hook-rod
    TSRH pedicle hook
    TSRH pedicle screw-laminar claw
    construct
T-Stick adhesive
TT
    telescopic and torsional
    TT pylon
T-TAC
    T-TAC catheter
    T-TAC system
TTS
    through-the-scope
    Rigiflex esophageal TTS
T-tube
    American Heyer-Schulte T-t.
    bar T-t.
    T-t. catheter
    cul-de-sac irrigation T-t.
    Deaver T-t.
    T-t. drain
    French T-t.
    Houser silicone T-t.
    Kehr T-t.
    Kelly inflatable T-t.
    lacrimal duct T-t.
    Montgomery tracheal T-t.
    polyethylene T-t.
    Pyrex T-t.
    T-t. round suction drain
    T-t. shunt

    silicone T-t.
    T-t. stent
T-type
    T-t. dental implant
    T-t. myringotomy tube
tub
    hydrotherapy t.
tubal
    t. hook
    t. insufflation cannula
    t. scissors
Tubbs
    T. aortic dilator
    T. mitral valve dilator
    T. two-bladed dilator
    T. valvulotome
Tubby tenotomy knife
tube
    Abbott t.
    Abbott-Rawson gastrointestinal
      double-lumen t.
    AccuMark calibrated infant
      feeding t.
    Activent ear t.
    Adson aspirating t.
    Adson brain suction t.
    Adson neurosurgical suction t.
    Aire-Cuf endotracheal t.
    Aire-Cuf tracheostomy t.
    Air-Lon laryngectomy t.
    Air-Lon tracheal t.
    Alesen t.
    American circle nephrostomy t.
    Amersham J t.
    Andersen mercury-weighted t.
    Anderson flexible suction t.
    Andrews-Pynchon suction t.
    anode t.
    Anthony aspirating t.
    Anthony mastoid suction t.
    Anthony suction t.
    antifog t.
    aortic sump t.
    Argyle chest t.
    Argyle-Dennis t.
    Argyle endotracheal t.
    Argyle feeding t.
    Argyle Salem sump t.
    Argyle Sentinel Seal chest t.
    Argyle sump t.
    Armstrong beveled grommet
      drain t.
    Armstrong beveled grommet
      myringotomy t.
    Armstrong beveled grommet
      ventilation t.
    Armstrong V-Vent t.
    Arrow t.
    Asepto suction t.

aspirating t.
aspiration t.
Aspisafe nasogastric t.
Atkins-Cannard tracheotomy t.
Atkinson t.
Ayre t.
Baerveldt glaucoma implant t.
Baerveldt shunt t.
Baker jejunostomy t.
Baker self-sumping t.
Baldwin butterfly ventilation t.
Bard button feeding t.
Bard gastrostomy feeding t.
Bardic t.
Bard PEG t.
Barnes suction t.
Baron ear t.
Baron-Frazier suction t.
Baron suction t.
Baylor intracardiac sump t.
Beall-Feldman-Cooley sump t.
Beardsley empyema t.
Bellocq t.
Bellucci suction t.
Bel-O-Pak suction t.
Benjamin t.
Ben-Jet t.
Bettman empyema t.
bicanalicular silicone t.
Bilbao-Dotter hypotonic
 duodenography t.
Billroth t.
Biolite ventilation t.
Biosystems feeding t.
Bivona Fome-Cuf tracheostomy t.
Bivona Medical Technologies
 customized tracheostomy t.
Bivona sleep apnea tracheostomy t.
Bivona TTS tracheostomy t.
bladder flap t.
Blakemore esophageal t.
Blakemore nasogastric t.
Blakemore-Sengstaken t.
Blue Line cuffed endotracheal t.
bobbin myringotomy t.
Bonney uterine t.
Bouchut laryngeal t.
Bourdon t.
Bower PEG t.
Bowman t.
Brawley nasal suction t.
bronchial t.

Broncho-Cath double-lumen
 endotracheal t.
bronchoscopic disposable suction t.
Bruecke t.
Bucy-Frazier suction t.
Bucy suction t.
Buie rectal suction t.
Butler tonsillar suction t.
calibrated grasping t.
Caluso PEG gastrostomy t.
Cantor intestinal t.
capillary t.
Carabelli endobronchial t.
Carden bronchoscopy t.
Carden laryngoscopy t.
Carlens double-lumen
 endotracheal t.
Carl Zeiss myringotomy t.
Carman rectal t.
Carrel t.
carrier t.
Casselberry sphenoid t.
Castelli-Paparella collar button t.
cathode ray t.
Cattell forked-type T- t.
Cattell gallbladder t.
Celestin endoesophageal t.
Celestin latex rubber t.
Chaoul voltage x-ray t.
Charnley drain t.
Chauffin-Pratt t.
Chaussier t.
chest t.
Chevalier Jackson tracheal t.
coagulation suction t.
Coakley wash t.
Cole endotracheal t.
Cole orotracheal t.
Cole pediatric t.
Cole uncuffed endotracheal t.
collar-button t.
collecting t.
Colton empyema t.
Combitube endotracheal t.
Comfit endotracheal t.
Compat surgical feeding t.
Compat surgical
 gastrojejunostomy t.
Cone-Bucy suction t.
Cone suction t.
conical centrifuge t.
Connell breathing t.

NOTES

T

tube *(continued)*

Connell ether vapor t.
Contigen t.
continuous suction t.
Cooely left ventricular sump t.
Cook County Hospital tracheal
    suction t.
Cooley-Anthony suction t.
Cooley aortic sump t.
Cooley cardiovascular suction t.
Cooley graft suction t.
Cooley intracardiac suction t.
Cooley sump suction t.
Cooley vascular suction t.
Coolidge x-ray t.
corneal t.
Corpak feeding t.
Corpak weighted-tip, self-
    lubricating t.
Costen suction t.
Cottle suction t.
Coupland suction t.
Crawford t.
cricothyrotomy trocar t.
Crookes-Hittorf t.
cuffed endotracheal t.
cuffed tracheostomy t.
CUI myringotomy t.
Dakin t.
Dandy suction t.
David pharyngolaryngectomy t.
Davol t.
Dawson-Yuhl suction t.
Deane t.
Dean wash t.
Deaver t.
DeBakey-Adson suction t.
DeBakey suction t.
Denker t.
Dennis t.
DePaul t.
DeVilbiss suction t.
diagnostic t.
dialysis t.
Diatube-H Vacutainer t.
DIC tracheostomy t.
disposable Yankauer aspirating t.
disposable Yankauer suction t.
Dobbhoff gastrectomy feeding t.
Dobbhoff gastric decompression t.
Dobbhoff nasogastric feeding t.
Dobbhoff PEG t.
Doesel-Huzly bronchoscopic t.
Donaldson drain t.
Donaldson eustachian t.
Donaldson myringotomy t.
Donaldson ventilation t.
double-cannula tracheostomy t.
double-focus t.

double-lumen endobronchial t.
double-lumen endotracheal t.
doughnut tip suction t.
drain-to-wall suction t.
Dr. Bruecke aspirating t.
Dr. Twiss duodenal t.
dual-lumen nasogastric t.
Duke t.
Dundas-Grant t.
Duralite t.
Durham t.
Durham tracheostomy t.
dynamic digit extensor t.
Eastman suction t.
E. Benson Hood Laboratories
    esophageal t.
E. Benson Hood Laboratories
    salivary bypass t.
EDTA Vacutainer blood
    collection t.
Einhorn t.
electron multiplier t.
endobronchial t.
endoesophageal t.
endotracheal t.
Endotrol endotracheal t.
Endo-Tube nasal jejunal feeding t.
enteroclysis t.
EntriStar percutaneous endoscopic
    gastrostomy t.
Eppendorf t.
ET t.
Ethox rectal t.
eustachian t.
Ewald t.
extension t.
Fay suction t.
feeding t.
fenestrated t.
fenestrated tracheostomy t.
Ferguson-Frazier suction t.
Feuerstein drainage t.
Feuerstein split ventilation t.
fiberoptic suction t.
field emission t.
Finsterer myringotomy split t.
Finsterer suction t.
flanged Teflon t.
Flexiflo enteral feeding t.
Flexiflo Inverta-PEG t.
Flexiflo Sacks-Vine t.
Flexiflo Stomate low-profile
    gastrostomy t.
Flexiflo suction feeding t.
Flexiflo tap-fill enteral t.
Flexiflo Taptainer t.
Flexiflo tungsten-weighted
    feeding t.
Flexiflo Versa-PEG t.

flow-regulated suction t.
t. foam
Fome-Cuf endotracheal t.
Fome-Cuf pediatric tracheostomy t.
Franco triflange ventilation t.
Frazier aspirating t.
Frazier brain suction t.
Frazier Britetrac nasal suction t.
Frazier-Ferguson aspirating t.
Frazier-Ferguson ear suction t.
Frazier fiberoptic suction t.
Frazier mastoid suction t.
Frazier modified suction t.
Frazier nasal suction t.
Frazier suction t.
Frederick-Miller t.
Fuller bivalve trach t.
Gabriel Tucker t.
gastric t.
gastrojejunostomy t.
Gastro-Port II feeding t.
gastrostomy t.
gastrostomy feeding t.
Gavriliu gastric t.
Geiger-Müller t.
Gillquist suction t.
Glover suction t.
glutaraldehyde-tanned bovine
  collagen t.
Gomco suction t.
Goode Trim t.
Goode T-tube ventilating t.
Goodhill-Pynchon tonsillar
  suction t.
Gott t.
Gowen decompression t.
Grafco Martin laryngectomy t.
t. graft
graft suction t.
Great Ormond Street pediatric
  tracheostomy t.
grommet drain t.
grommet myringotomy t.
grommet ventilating t.
Guibor Silastic t.
Guilford-Wright suction t.
Guisez t.
Gwathmey suction t.
Haering t.
Hagan surface suction t.
Hakim t.
Haldane t.

Haldane-Priestley t.
Hardy suction t.
Har-el pharyngeal t.
Heimlich t.
Heimlich-Gavrilu gastric t.
Helsper tracheostomy vent t.
Hemagard collection t.
Hemochron P214 glass-activated
  ACT t.
Hemovac suction t.
heparin-bonded Bott-type t.
Herring t.
high heat capacity x-ray t.
Hi-Lo Evac endotracheal t.
Hi-Lo Jet tracheal t.
Holinger open-end aspirating t.
Hossli suction t.
hot cathode x-ray t.
Hotchkiss ear suction t.
Hough-Cadogan suction t.
House-Baron suction t.
House-Radpour suction t.
Houser cul-de-sac irrigator t.
House-Stevenson suction t.
House suction t.
House-Urban t.
Hubbard airplane vent t.
Hugly aspirating t.
Humphrey coronary sinus-sucker
  suction t.
Hunsaker jet ventilation t.
Hymlek portable chest t.
Hyperflex tracheostomy t.
image intensifier t.
image Orthicon t.
Immergut suction t.
Immergut suction-coagulation t.
infusion t.
intracardiac suction t.
intracardiac sump t.
Isolator lysis-centrifugation t.
Israel suction t.
Jackson aspirating t.
Jackson cane-shaped tracheal t.
Jackson laryngectomy t.
Jackson open-end aspirating t.
Jackson-Pratt suction t.
Jackson-Rees endotracheal t.
Jackson silver tracheostomy t.
Jackson tracheal t.
Jackson velvet-eye aspirating t.
Jackson warning stop t.

T

NOTES

tube *(continued)*

Jacques gastric t.
Jako laryngeal suction t.
Jako laser aspirating t.
Jako suction t.
Jarit-Poole abdominal suction t.
Jarit-Yankauer suction t.
Javid bypass t.
jejunal feeding t.
jejunostomy t.
Jesberg aspirating t.
Jiffy t.
Johnson coagulation suction t.
Johnson intestinal t.
Jones Pyrex t.
Jones tear duct t.
J-shaped t.
Jutte t.
Kangaroo silicone gastrostomy
  feeding t.
Kaslow gastrointestinal t.
Kay-Cross suction tip suction t.
Kehr gallbladder t.
Kelly t.
Keofeed t.
Keofeed feeding t.
KeyMed esophageal t.
Kidd U-tube t.
Killian t.
Kistner plastic tracheostomy t.
Klein ventilation t.
Knoche t.
Kos ear suction t.
Kuhn endotracheal t.
Kurz t.
Kurze suction t.
Lacor t.
Lahey Y-tube t.
Lanz low-pressure cuff
  endotracheal t.
Lanz tracheostomy t.
Lar-A-Jext laryngectomy t.
large-bore chest t.
large-caliber chest t.
LaRocca nasolacrimal t.
Laryngoflex reinforced
  tracheostomy t.
Laser-Trach endotracheal t.
Lasertubus endotracheal t.
Leiter t.
Lell tracheal t.
Lenard ray t.
Lennarson t.
Lepley-Ernst tracheal t.
Lester Jones t.
Levin-Davol t.
Levin duodenal t.
Lewis laryngectomy t.
Lezius suction t.

LifePort endotracheal t.
lifesaving t.
Lindemann-Silverstein Arrow
  ventilation t.
Lindholm tracheal t.
Linton esophageal t.
Linton-Nachlas t.
Lonnecken t.
Lo-Por tracheal t.
Lo-Profile tracheostomy t.
Lord-Blakemore t.
Lore-Lawrence tracheotomy t.
Lore suction t.
L.T. Jones tear duct t.
Luer speaking t.
Luer tracheal t.
Lukens collecting t.
Lyon t.
MacKenty laryngectomy t.
Mackler intraluminal t.
Mackray short-cuffed
  endobronchial t.
Madoff suction t.
Magill Safety Clear endotracheal t.
Maingot gallbladder t.
Malecot nephrostomy t.
Malis-Frazier suction t.
malleable multipore suction t.
Mallinckrodt endotracheal t.
Mallinckrodt Laser-Flex t.
Martin laryngectomy t.
Martin tracheostomy t.
Mason suction t.
Massie sliding nail t.
mastoid suction t.
McGowan-Keeley t.
McMurtry-Schlesinger shunt t.
Mead Johnson t.
mediastinal t.
Medina t.
Medoc-Celestin t.
mesh myringotomy t.
Mett t.
MIC bolus gastrostomy t.
MIC gastroenteric t.
MIC jejunal t.
MIC jejunostomy t.
Mic-Key G gastrostomy t.
Mic-Key J gastrostomy t.
Microfuge t.
Microgel surface-enhanced
  ventilation t.
microlaryngeal endotracheal t.
Micron bobbin ventilation t.
Miller-Abbott double-lumen
  intestinal t.
Miller endotracheal t.
Millin suction t.
Mill-Rose t.

Milroy-Piper suction t.
Minnesota t.
Mixter t.
modified suction t.
Molteno shunt t.
molybdenum rotating-anode x-ray t.
molybdenum target t.
Monarch transshaping
  gastrostomy t.
Montando t.
Montefiore tracheal t.
Montgomery esophageal t.
Montgomery-Lofgren tapered Safe-
  T-Tube t.
Montgomery salivary bypass t.
Montgomery tracheal t.
Moore t.
Morch swivel tracheostomy t.
Moretz Tiny Tytan ventilation t.
Moretz Tytan ventilation t.
Morse-Andrews suction t.
Morse-Ferguson suction t.
Morse suction t.
Mosher intubation t.
Mosher life-saving tracheal
  suction t.
Moss balloon triple-lumen
  gastrostomy t.
Moss feeding t.
Moss gastric decompression t.
Moss gastrostomy t.
Moss Mark IV t.
Moss nasal t.
Moulton lacrimal duct t.
Mousseau-Barbin esophageal t.
Mueller-Frazier suction t.
Mueller-Poole suction t.
Mueller-Pynchon suction t.
Mueller suction t.
Mueller-Yankauer suction t.
Muldoon t.
Myerson wash t.
myringotomy drain t.
Nachlas gastrointestinal t.
Nachlas-Linton t.
nasal suction t.
nasobiliary t.
nasocystic drainage t.
nasoendotracheal t.
nasoenteric feeding t.
nasogastric feeding t.
nasojejunal feeding t.

NCC Hi-Lo Jet endotracheal t.
nephrostomy t.
Neuber bone t.
New Luer-type speaking t.
New speaking t.
Newvicon camera t.
Newvicon vacuum chamber
  pickup t.
New York glass suction t.
NG feeding t.
Nilsson-Stille abortion suction t.
Nilsson suction t.
Nishizaki-Wakabayashi suction t.
Norton endotracheal t.
Nunez ventricular ventilation t.
Nuport PEG t.
Nyhus-Nelson gastric
  decompression t.
Nyhus-Nelson jejunal feeding t.
Nystroem abdominal suction t.
O'Beirne sphincter t.
t. observation model (TOM)
obstructed shunt t.
Ochsner gallbladder t.
O'Dwyer t.
O'Hanlon-Poole suction t.
Olshevsky t.
Olympus One-Step Button
  gastrostomy t.
oral endotracheal t.
oral esophageal t.
orgastic t.
oroendotracheal t.
orogastric Ewald t.
orotracheal t.
Ossoff-Karlan laser suction t.
overcouch t.
Oxford nonkinking cuffed t.
Panda gastrostomy t.
Panda nasoenteric feeding t.
Panje t.
Paparella-Frazier suction t.
Paparella myringotomy t.
Paparella type II ventilation t.
Parker t.
Paul intestinal drainage t.
Paul-Mixter t.
pear-shaped extension t.
Pedia-Trake t.
pediatric t.
Pedi PEG t.
Pee Wee low-profile gastrostomy t.

T

NOTES

tube *(continued)*
PEG t.
Penrose t.
percutaneous nephrostomy t.
Per-Lee equalizing t.
Per-Lee myringotomy t.
Per-Lee ventilation t.
Perspex t.
Pertrach percutaneous
  tracheostomy t.
pharyngotympanic t.
photoelectric multiplier t.
photomultiplier t.
Pierce antrum wash t.
pigtail nephrostomy t.
Pilling duralite t.
Pitot t.
Pitt talking tracheostomy t.
plastic-cuffed tracheostomy t.
pleural t.
Pleur-evac suction t.
Plumicon camera t.
Polisar-Lyons adapted tracheal t.
Polisar-Lyons tracheal t.
polyethylene t.
polyvinyl chloride endotracheal t.
Ponsky-Gauderer PEG t.
Ponsky PEG t.
Poole abdominal suction t.
Poppen suction t.
Portex Blue Line tracheostomy t.
Portex Perfit tracheostomy t.
Portex preformed blue line
  tracheal t.
Porto-Vac suction t.
postpyloric feeding t.
preformed polyvinyl chloride
  endotracheal t.
pressure equalization t.
pressure equalizing t.
Pribram suction t.
primordial catheter t.
Proctor suction t.
Pudenz t.
Puestow-Olander gastrointestinal t.
pull-type gastrostomy t.
Pynchon suction t.
Questek laser t.
Quincke t.
Quinton t.
Radius enteral feeding t.
Radpour-House suction t.
RAE endotracheal t.
RAE-Flex tracheal t.
Rand-House suction t.
Rand-Radpour suction t.
rectal t.
rectifier t.
Redivac suction t.

red rubber endotracheal t.
Rehfuss duodenal t.
Rehfuss stomach t.
Reinecke-Carroll lacrimal t.
Replogle t.
Reuter bobbin ventilation t.
Rhoton-Merz suction t.
Rica mastoid suction t.
Ring-McLean sump t.
Ritter suprapubic suction t.
Robertshaw t.
Robinson equalizing t.
Rochester suction t.
Rochester tracheal t.
roentgen t.
Roller pump suction t.
Rosen suction t.
rotating anode x-ray t.
Ruschelit endotracheal t.
Rusch laryngectomy reinforced
  tracheostomy t.
Rusch red rubber rectal t.
Russell suction t.
Ryle duodenal t.
Sachs suction t.
Sacks-Vine PEG t.
SafeCrit microhematocrit t.
Safety Clear Plus endotracheal t.
Salem sump nasogastric t.
salivary bypass t.
Samco t.
Samson-Davis infant suction t.
Sandoz balloon replacement t.
Sandoz Caluso PEG gastrostomy t.
Sandoz feeding/suction t.
Sandoz nasogastric feeding t.
Sandoz suction t.
Sapporo shunt t.
Sarns intracardiac suction t.
Saticon pickup t.
scavenging t.
Schall laryngectomy t.
Schmiedt t.
Schuknecht suction t.
Schuler aspiration/irrigation t.
Scott-Harden t.
Scott nasal suction t.
Securat suction t.
Sengstaken-Blakemore
  esophagogastric tamponade t.
Sengstaken nasogastric t.
Sensiv endotracheal t.
separator t.
Shah myringotomy t.
Shah permanent ventilation t.
Shea-type parasol myringotomy t.
Sheehy collar-button ventilating t.
Sheehy Tytan ventilation t.
Shepard drain t.

Shepard grommet ventilation t.
Sheridan endotracheal t.
Sherman suction t.
Shiley cuffless fenestrated
tracheostomy t.
Shiley disposable cannula low-
pressure cuffed tracheostomy t.
Shiley fenestrated low-pressure
cuffed tracheostomy t.
Shiley French sump t.
Shiley laryngectomy t.
Shiley neonatal tracheostomy t.
Shiley pediatric tracheostomy t.
Shiley single-cannula cuffed
tracheostomy t.
Shiley TracheoSoft XLT
tracheostomy t.
Shiley tracheostomy t.
shunt t.
Silastic eustachian t.
Silastic intestinal t.
Silastic sucker suction t.
Silastic tracheostomy t.
silicone t.
silicone-lubricated endotracheal t.
Silverstein permanent aeration t.
Singer-Blom t.
siphon suction t.
t. site dressing
SMIC mastoid suction t.
Smith t.
Smokeeter t.
smoke evacuator suction t.
smoke removal t.
Snyder Hemovac suction t.
Snyder Surgivac suction t.
Snyder Urevac suction t.
Softech endotracheal t.
SoftForm t.
Soileau Tytan ventilation t.
solid-phase extraction t.
Southey capillary drainage t.
Souttar t.
speaking t.
spiral-wound endotracheal t.
SS bobbin drain t.
SS bobbin myringotomy t.
Stamm gastrostomy t.
Stedman continuous suction t.
stomach t.
Stomate decompression t.
Stomate extension t.

straight chest t.
Stroud-Baron ear suction t.
suction t.
suction-coagulation t.
suction/irrigation t.
Suh ventilation t.
sump t.
Sustagen nasogastric t.
Swenson cholangiography t.
T t.
tear duct t.
T-grommet ventilation t.
Thal-Quick chest t.
thoracostomy t.
Thora-Klex chest t.
tonsillar suction t.
Touma T-type grommet
ventilation t.
Tovell t.
Toynbee diagnostic t.
tracheal t.
TracheoSoft XLT tracheostomy t.
tracheostomy t.
Trach-Talk tracheostomy t.
TRACOEflex tracheostomy t.
TRAKE-fit endotracheal t.
translucent drain t.
translucent silicone t.
transpyloric feeding t.
triode t.
T self-retaining drainage t.
T-type myringotomy t.
Tucker flexible-tip t.
Tucker suction t.
Turkel t.
Turner-Warwick fiberoptic suction t.
Turner-Warwick illuminating
suction t.
twist-in drain t.
twist-in myringotomy t.
tympanostomy t.
Tytan grommet ventilation t.
Tytan ventilation t.
uncuffed endotracheal t.
underwater-seal suction t.
Univent endotracheal t.
urinary drainage t.
uterine t.
U-tube t.
Vacutainer vacuum t.
Valentine irrigation t.
Van Alyea antral wash t.

T

NOTES

tube *(continued)*
    vascular suction t.
    velvet-eye aspirating t.
    Venturi bobbin myringotomy t.
    Venturi collar-button
      myringotomy t.
    Venturi grommet myringotomy t.
    Venturi pediatric myringotomy t.
    Vernon antral wash t.
    Vidicon camera t.
    Vidicon vacuum chamber pickup t.
    Vinyon-N cloth t.
    Vivonex gastrostomy t.
    V. Mueller-Frazier suction t.
    V. Mueller-Poole suction t.
    Voltolini ear t.
    von Eichen antral wash t.
    Vortex tracheostomy t.
    Wangensteen duodenal t.
    Wannagat suction t.
    water-seal chest t.
    Webster infusion t.
    Weck coagulating suction t.
    Weck suction t.
    Welch Allyn suction t.
    Wendl t.
    Wepsic suction t.
    Williams esophageal t.
    Wilson-Cook nasobiliary t.
    Wilson-Cook NJFT-series feeding t.
    Winsburg-White bladder t.
    Wolf suction t.
    Woodbridge t.
    Wullstein microsuction t.
    Xertube t.
    Xomed endotracheal t.
    Xomed Treace ventilation t.
    Xomed Tytan ventilation t.
    x-ray image intensifier t.
    Y t.
    Yankauer aspirating t.
    Yankauer suction t.
    Yasargil suction t.
    Yeder suction t.
    Zollner suction t.
    Zyler t.
**TubeChek esophageal intubation
  detector**
Tubegauz
    T. elastic net
    T. seamless tubular knitted cotton
      bandage
tubeless lithotripter
Tube-Lok tracheotomy dressing
tube-occluding
    t.-o. clamp
    t.-o. forceps
tuberculin syringe
Tubestat lighted stylet

Tubex
    T. gauze dressing
    T. injector
    T. metal syringe
TubiFast bandage
Tubigrip
    T. dressing
    T. elastic support bandage
tubing
    t. adapter
    Argyle Penrose t.
    Bard extension t.
    t. clamp
    t. compressor
    connecting t.
    dialysate t.
    dialysis t.
    Dorsey irrigation t.
    foam t.
    gel t.
    t. hand roller
    Hi Vac t.
    Intramedic PE-50 polyethylene t.
    t. introducer forceps
    Lifemed blood t.
    Ott insufflator filter t.
    Perry latex Penrose drainage t.
    polyethylene t.
    polyvinyl t.
    PVC t.
    ReDeuce pump t.
    shunt t.
    Silastic t.
    Silipos mesh t.
    Simcoe connecting t.
    smoke evacuator t.
    Sub-Lite-Wall t.
    Sur-Fit night drainage container t.
    Surgin insufflation t.
    Teflon t.
    Thera-Band t.
    Tygon t.
    Wolf insufflation t.
    Y-connecting t.
Tubinger
    T. gall stone forceps
    T. self-retaining retractor
Tubipad bandage
Tubiton bandage
Tubsider kneeling seat
tubular
    t. dressing
    t. forceps
    t. magnet
    t. plate
    t. slotted stent
    t. stent
Tubulitec cavity liner
Tuckables underpad

tucker
    T. anterior commissure laryngoscope
    T. appendix clamp
    T. aspirating valve
    T. bead forceps
    Bishop-Black tendon t.
    Bishop-DeWitt tendon t.
    Bishop-Peter tendon t.
    Bishop tendon t.
    T. bronchoscope
    Burch-Greenwood tendon t.
    Burch tendon t.
    T. cardiospasm dilator
    Cooley cardiac t.
    Crafoord-Cooley t.
    T. direct-vision telescope
    T. esophagoscope
    Fink tendon t.
    T. flexible-tip tube
    Green muscle t.
    Green strabismus t.
    T. hallux forceps
    Harrison t.
    T. hemorrhoidal ligator
    ligature t.
    McGuire tendon t.
    T. mid-lighted optic slide laryngoscope
    T. reach-and-pin forceps
    T. retrograde bougie
    Ruedemann-Todd tendon t.
    T. slotted laryngoscope
    Smith-Petersen t.
    Smuckler t.
    T. staple forceps
    T. suction tube
    tendon t.
    T. tracheoscope
    Twirlon ligature t.
    Wayne t.
Tucker-Holinger laryngoscope
Tucker-Jako laryngoscope
Tucker-Levine vocal cord retractor
Tucker-Luikart blade
Tucker-McLane
    T.-M. axis-traction forceps
    T.-M. obstetrical forceps
Tudor-Edwards
    T.-E. bone-cutting forceps
    T.-E. costotome

    T.-E. rib shears
    T.-E. rib spreader
Tufcote epilation probe
Tuffier
    T. abdominal retractor
    T. abdominal spatula
    T. arterial forceps
    T. rib retractor
    T. rib spreader
Tuffier-Raney laminectomy retractor
Tuffnell bandage
TuffSat handheld oximeter
Tuf Nex neck exerciser
Tuf-Skin tape adherent
Tuke bone saw
Tulevech lacrimal cannula
TuliGel heel cup
Tuli heel cup
TULIP
    transurethral ultrasound-guided laser-induced prostatectomy
    TULIP aspiration device
    TULIP probe
    TULIP sheath
    TULIP syringe system
    TULIP tip
    TULIP vena caval MReye filter
tulip-headed pedicle screw
tulle gras dressing
Tumble
    T. Forms feeder
    T. Forms Jettmobile
    T. Forms roll
    T. Forms Tortoise Shell therapy system
    T. Forms Vestibulator
tumbling E cube
Tum-E-Vac gastric lavage
tumor
    t. forceps
    t. probe
    t. screw
tumor-grasping forceps
tumor-replacement endoprosthesis
TUMT
    TransUrethral Microwave Thermotherapy
TUNA
    transurethral needle ablation
tunable
    t. notch filter
    t. pulsed dye laser

T

NOTES

tungsten
    t. anode
    t. carbide bur
    t. eye shield
    t. microdissection needle
    t. microelectrode
    T. syringe shield
    t. tip
tungsten-halogen lamp
tuning fork
Tun-L-Kath epidural catheter
tunnel
    t. drill guide
    t. graft
tunnelable ventricular ICP catheter
tunneled
    t. catheter
    t. eye implant
tunneler
    Cooley cardiac t.
    CPI t.
    Crafoord t.
    Crawford-Cooley t.
    Davol t.
    DeBakey t.
    DeBakey vascular t.
    Dosick t.
    Hallman t.
    Jackson t.
    Kelly-Wick vascular t.
    Noon AV fistular t.
    Noon modified vascular access t.
    Oregon t.
    Scanlan vascular t.
    vascular t.
    vascular access t.
tunnel-type implant material
Tunturi
    T. EL400 bicycle ergometer
    T. hand exerciser
    T. Jogger-2 self-powered treadmill
Tuohy
    T. catheter
    T. lumbar aortography needle
    T. spinal needle
Tuohy-Borst
    T.-B. connector
    T.-B. introducer
    T.-B. sideport adapter
Tuohy-Schliff needle
Tupman osteotomy plate
Tupper tractor
turbinate
    t. electrode
    t. forceps
    t. scissors
turbinectomy scissors
Turbo-Jet dental bur
TurboSonic tip

TurboStaltic pump
TurboVac 90 vacuum
Turbuhaler inhaler
TUR-Cue photometer
Turek spinous process spreader
Turkel
    T. bone biopsy trephine set
    T. liver biopsy needle
    T. prostatic punch
    T. sternal needle
    T. trephine
    T. tube
turkey-claw clamp
TurnAide therapeutic system
turnbuckle
    t. ankle brace
    t. distractor
    t. elbow splint
    t. functional position splint
    t. knee brace
    t. wrist orthosis
Turnbull
    T. adhesion forceps
    T. applicator
    T. cannula
    T. nail nipper
Turn-Easy transfer aid
2-turn epicardial lead
3-turn epicardial lead
Turner
    T. biopsy needle
    T. cord elevator
    T. periosteal elevator
Turner-Babcock tissue forceps
Turner-Doyen retractor
Turner-Warwick
    T.-W. bladder neck spreader
    T.-W. blade
    T.-W. diathermy scissors
    T.-W. fiberoptic suction tube
    T.-W. illuminating suction tube
    T.-W. malleable spoon
    T.-W. needle holder
    T.-W. pediatric perineal retractor ring
    T.-W. posterior urethral retractor
    T.-W. post-urethroplasty review speculum
    T.-W. prostate retractor
    T.-W. stone forceps
    T.-W. urethroplasty needle
Turner-Warwick-Adson forceps
Turning Board exercise system
Turnsoft automatic turning system
turnstile casting stand (TCS)
Turrell
    T. biopsy forceps
    T. sigmoidoscope
    T. specimen forceps

Turrell-Wittner rectal biopsy forceps
Turtle chart
Turvy internal screw fixation
tutoFix cortical pin
Tutoplast
    T. anterior tibialis tendon
    T. auditory ossicle
    T. bone
    T. dura mater
    T. fascia lata
    T. processed allograft
    T. tissue
Tuttle
    T. dressing forceps
    T. obstetrical forceps
    T. proctoscope
    T. sigmoidoscope
    T. thoracic thumb forceps
    T. tissue forceps
Tuttle-Singley thoracic forceps
Tuwave galvanic stimulator/TENS unit
Twardon grommet
Twee alternating cut-off compressor
  stocking
Tweedy canaliculus knife
tweezers
    Arti-holder t.
    Dumont t.
    jeweler's t.
    Kaprelian easy-access t. (KEAT)
    Laser T.
    soldering t.
twill dressing
Twin
    T. Flash scanner
    T. Jet nebulizer
twin-beam CT
twin-coil dialyzer
TwinFix AB absorbable suture anchor
twin knife
TwinMic hearing system
twin-pattern chisel
Twirlon ligature tucker
Twisk
    T. forceps
    T. microscissors
    T. needle holder
    T. scissors
twist
    CamStar rotary t.
    t. drill

    t. drill catheter
    t. fixation hook
twisted
    t. cotton nonabsorbable surgical
    suture material
    t. cotton suture
    t. dermal suture
    t. linen suture
    t. silk suture
    t. virgin silk suture
twister
    Batzdorf cervical wire t.
    Baumgarten wire t.
    cerclage wire t.
    Cooley-Baumgarten wire t.
    Corwin auto wire t.
    Miltex wire t.
    Ochsner wire t.
    orthotic coiled spring t.
    Richards wire t.
    Vital-Cooley-Baumgarten wire t.
    Vital-Cooley wire t.
    Vital wire t.
    wire t.
twist-in
    t.-i. drain tube
    t.-i. myringotomy tube
Twist-Lock drill guard
Twist-Mate ligator
Twist MTX implant
Tworek
    T. bone marrow-aspirating needle
    T. screw guide
    T. transorbital leukotome
    T. Universal gouge
Tycos
    T. gauge
    T. manometer
    T. pressure infuser
Tycron suture
Tydings
    T. automatic ratchet snare
    T. tonsillar clamp
    T. tonsillar knife
    T. tonsillectome
    T. tonsil-seizing forceps
    T. tonsil snare
Tydings-Lakeside tonsillar forceps
Tygon
    T. catheter
    T. endoesophageal prosthesis

T

NOTES

Tygon *(continued)*
    T. tubing
    T. tubing circuit
tying forceps
Tyler-Gigli saw
Tyler spiral Gigli saw
Tylok
    T. cerclage
    T. high-tension cerclage cabling
      system
tympanic membrane thermometer
tympanomastoid suture
tympanometer
    diagnostic t.
    handheld diagnostic t.
    MicroTymp2 handheld t.
    MI34 diagnostic t.
    Welch Allyn MicroTymp
      impedance t.
tympanoplasty
    t. forceps
    t. knife
tympanoscope
    Hopkins t.

tympanostomy tube
tympanum
    t. perforator
    t. perforator handle
Typhoon
    T. cutter blade
    T. microdebrider blade
Tyrer nerve root retractor
Tyrrell
    T. clamp
    T. foreign body forceps
    T. hook
    T. hook retractor
    T. skin hook
Tyrrell-Gray suture
Tyshak
    T. balloon
    T. balloon valvuloplasty catheter
TY stent
Tytan
    T. grommet ventilation tube
    T. tube inserter
    T. ventilation tube

U

U suture
U X-Acto gouge

U-1100 UV-Vis spectrophotometer

UBC

University of British Columbia
Upper Body Cycle
UBC brace

UBIS 5000 ultrasound bone sonometer

UC

UC strip
UC strip catheter tubing fastener

UCBL

University of California Berkeley
Laboratory
UCBL orthosis

U-channel stripping dural substitute

UCI prosthesis

Uckermann cotton applicator

UCLA

University of California Los Angeles
UCLA CAPP TD hook
UCLA functional long leg brace

U-clip

Duane U-c.
nitinol U-c.

U-Clip anastomotic device

UCOheal orthotic

UCOlite orthotic

U-Control training device

Uebe applicator

Ueckermann-Denker trocar

Uffenorde bone curette

UGI

upper gastrointestinal
UGI endoscope

UHMWPe

ultra-high molecular weight polyethylene
UHMWPe ball liner

UJT

unijunction transistor

Ulanday double cannula

Ulbrich wart curette

UlcerJet system

Uldall

U. subclavian hemodialysis cannula
U. subclavian hemodialysis catheter

Ullrich

U. bone-holding forceps
U. dressing forceps
U. fistula knife
U. tubing clamp
U. uterine knife
U. vaginal speculum

Ullrich-Aesculap forceps

Ullrich-St.

U.-St. Gallen forceps
U.-St. Gallen self-retaining retractor

ulnar rasp

Ulrich bone-holding forceps

Ulson fixator system

Ultec Pro alginate hydrocolloid dressing

Ultex

U. lens
U. lens implant
U. thin extra thin hydrocolloid
dressing

Ultigard underpad

Ultima

U. Bloc bite block
U. femoral component
U. hip replacement system
U. OPCAB system
U. 2000 photocoagulator
U. total hip prosthesis

UltiMA mammography system

Ultimate

U. knee
U. nasal mask
U. quilted comply underpad

Ultimax

U. distal femoral intramedullary
rod system
U. Haig II nail system

Ultra

U. Cover transducer cover
U. Dream Ride infant car bed
U. Duet colostomy
U. Duet colostomy irrigating sleeve
U. Duet urostomy
U. 8 intraaortic balloon catheter
U. Lite II headlight
U. low-resistance voice prosthesis
U. pacemaker
U. Twin bag system
U. ultrasonic aspirator
U. view SP slit lamp lens
U. Voice speech aid
U. Y-set system

UltraBag system

Ultrabrace

U. brace
U. orthosis

Ultra-Care heel/elbow protector

Ultracast alloy

ultracentrifuge

Sorvall Discovery SE u.

UltraCision

U. harmonic scalpel
U. ultrasonic knife

U

UltraCon
U. RGP contact lens
U. rigid gas permeable contact
lens
Ultra-Core biopsy needle
Ultracor prosthetic valve
UltraCross catheter
Ultra-Cut
U.-C. Cobb curette
U.-C. Cobb spinal gouge
U.-C. Hibbs gouge
U.-C. Hoke osteotome
U.-C. Smith-Petersen osteotome
**Ultra-Drive bone cement removal
system**
UltraEase ultrasound pad
UltraEdge keratome blade
UltraEnergy orthotic
Ultrafast
U. CT scanner
U. magnetic resonance imaging
U. MRI
Ultrafera wound dressing
ultrafiltration membrane
UltraFine erbium laser
Ultra-Fit brief
UltraFix
U. anchor
U. MicroMite anchor suture
U. rotator cuff suture anchor
system
Ultraflex
U. dynamic splint system
U. esophageal stent system
U. Microvasive stent
U. nitinol expandable esophageal
stent
U. self-adhering male external
catheter
U. self-expanding stent
U. stent delivery system
**Ultra-Flow double-lumen high-flow
catheter**
UltraFoam seating cushion
UltraForm
U. mattress overlay
U. therapeutic mattress
Ultrafuse catheter
Ultrafyn
U. cautery tip
U. thermal cautery
Ultra-Guard hip orthosis system
**ultra-high molecular weight polyethylene
(UHMWPe)**
Ultra-Image A-scan scanner
Ultraject
U. contrast media syringe
U. prefilled syringe

UltraLine
U. laser
U. Nd:YAG laser fiber
UltraLite
U. flow-directed microcatheter
U. one-piece convex disposable
system
Ultramark-series ultrasound
Ultramark ultrasound system
**Ultramatic Rx Master Phoroptor
refractor**
Ultramer catheter
Ultra-Neb 99 ultrasonic nebulizer
UltraPACS diagnostic imaging system
UltraPak enteral closed feeding system
UltraPower
U. bur guard
U. drill system
UltraPulse
U. 5000C CO_2 laser
U. surgical laser
Ultrascan digital B system
Ultrascope obstetrical Doppler
**Ultraseed ultrasound-guided
brachytherapy system**
Ultra-Select nitinol PTCA guidewire
**UltraShaper Automate durable keratome
system**
Ultra-Sil cannula
UltraSling glenohumeral joint sling
UltraSom NT polysomnography system
ultrasonic
u. biomicroscope
u. bone-cutting instrument
u. cleaner basket
u. dissector
u. electrode
u. fiberendoscope
u. flow director
u. harmonic scalpel
u. inhaler
u. irrigating needle
u. lithotripter
u. micrometer
u. nebulizer
u. scaler
u. stone crusher
u. tactile sensor
ultrasonically activated scalpel
ultrasonogram
A-scan u.
B-scan u.
endoscopic u.
gray-scale u.
ultrasonography
endoscopic color Doppler u.
intraportal endovascular u.
Toshiba Sal 38B real-time u.

ultrasonometer
   Achilles+ u.
   QUS-2 calcaneal u.
ultrasonoscope
   Bronson u.
UltraSorb suture anchor
ultrasound
   u. ablation catheter
   Acuson u.
   Acuson 128XP/10 Doppler u.
   ADR Ultramark 4 u.
   Advantage u.
   AI 5200 diagnostic u.
   Alcon Digital B 2000 u.
   Aloka 650CL u.
   Aloka linear u.
   Aloka OB/GYN u.
   Aloka sector u.
   Ansaldo AU560 u.
   Aspen digital u.
   ATL Ultramark-series real-time u.
   BladderManager u.
   BladderScan BVI2500 diagnostic u.
   u. bone analyzer
   u. catheter probe
   catheter probe u.
   color flow Doppler u.
   continuous-wave Doppler u.
   CooperVision u.
   Diasonics u.
   Doppler u.
   Doptone u.
   duplex u.
   Dynatron 150 u.
   EchoEye u.
   Elscint ESI-3000 u.
   endoanal u.
   EndoSound endoscopic u.
   EUB-series portable u.
   GE RT 3200 Advantage II u.
   HDI-series color Doppler
      imaging u.
   Hitachi EUB-series diagnostic u.
   HP Sonos 2500 cardiac/vascular
      diagnostic u.
   Interspec Apogee CX 100 u.
   Interspec XL u.
   Intertherapy intravascular u.
   intracoronary vascular u. (IVUS)
   intraductal u.
   intraluminal u. (ILUS)
   Intrascan u.
   Irex Exemplar u.
   LeFort urethral u.
   Medison 3D/4D u.
   u. monitor
   Netra intravascular u.
   Ophthascan S u.
   Performa u.
   Photopic u.
   Pie Medical u.
   PowerVision u.
   u. probe
   ProSound SSD-5500 u.
   pulsed Doppler u.
   real-time u.
   Rich-Mar 510 external u.
   RT 3200 Advantage u.
   Shimadzu cardiac u.
   Shimadzu IIQ u.
   Shimadzu SDU-400 u.
   Siemens SI 400 u.
   Siemens Sonoline Elegra u.
   Siemens Sonoline Prima u.
   SieScape u.
   Sonicator portable u.
   Sonicator therapeutic u.
   Sonolayer SSA-270A-30 u.
   Sonoline Prima u.
   SonoSite digital u.
   Spectra-Diasonics u.
   u. stethoscope
   through-the-balloon u.
   Toshiba Sonolayer SSH-140A u.
   transcranial Doppler u.
   u. transducer
   transendoscopic u.
   transvaginal u.
   Ultramark-series u.
   Vingmed CFM-series u.
   Vingmed System Five u.
ultrasound-tipped catheter
UltraStep orthotic
ultra-stiff wire
UltraStim electrode
Ultrata capsulorrhexis forceps
Ultrathane Amplatz ureteral stent
ultra-thin
   u.-t. balloon
   u.-t. pancreatoscope
   u.-t. surgical blade
Ultrathin Diamond balloon
ultratome
   Microvasive u.

U

NOTES

Ultratome XL triple-lumen sphincterotome
ultraviolet (UV)
u. detector
u. lamp
u. laser
u. light
u. radiation (UVR)
ultraviolet-blocking intraocular lens
ultraviolet-light-polymerized resin
Ultra-vue amniocentesis needle
Ultra-X external fixation system
Ultrex
U. cylinder
U. Plus penile prosthesis
Ultroid coagulator
ULT-Svi calibrated end-tidal gas analyzer
UM
Universal modular
umbilical
u. artery catheter
u. clip
u. cord clamp
u. scissors
u. tape
u. vein catheter
u. venous catheter
umbiliclamp
SurgiMed u.
Umbili Clip
Umbilicup umbilical cord blood collection device
Umbilicutter umbilical cord cutter and clamp
umbrella
ASDOS double u.
atrial septal defect occluder system u.
Bard clamshell septal u.
Bard PDA u.
clamshell septal u.
u. filter
PDA u.
U. punctum plug
Rashkind u.
transcatheter u.
umbrella-type prosthesis
UMI
UMI amniocentesis kit
UMI Cath-Seal catheter
UMI Cath-Seal sheath
UMI transseptal Cath-Seal catheter introducer
U-Mid-O$_2$ Jet set
unabsorbable suture
uncoated mesh stent
unconstrained prosthesis
uncuffed endotracheal tube

undergarment
Attends beltless u.
First Quality belted u.
MaxiCare adult disposable u.
Protection Plus belted u.
Safe & Dry u.
underglove
Biogel Indicator u.
underpad
Attends u.
Birdseye quilted u.
Breathables air-permeable u.
Canadian Ibex quilted u.
chamois u.
Comfort Quilt u.
Dignity Plus u.
Dri-flo u.
Excel Plus u.
Excel quilted u.
Harmonie u.
Macima reusable u.
MaxiFlo breathable u.
Med-I-Pad u.
Night Preservers u.
PatientGuard u.
Pinnacle reusable u.
Polylite quilted u.
PrimeTime disposable u.
Sahara super absorbent reusable u.
Senepads u.
Sofnit Birdseye reusable u.
Spectra quilted u.
SureCare/Medical disposable u.
Tuckables u.
Ultigard u.
Ultimate quilted comply u.
underwater
u. diathermy
u. electrode
u. seal drainage system
underwater-seal suction tube
undyed suture
unfilled resin
Unfolder
U. intraocular lens implantation system
U. Silver implantation instrument
UNI
UNI reservoir
UNI shunt catheter
uniaxial
u. accelerometer
u. accelerometer unit
u. strain gauge
unibevel chisel
Unica CO$_2$ laser system
Unicare breast pump
Unicath all-purpose catheter
Unicat knife

unicompartmental knee implant
unicondylar prosthesis
Uni-Flate 1000 penile prosthesis
Uniflex
    U. calibrated step drill
    U. distal targeting awl
    U. drill bushing
    U. intramedullary nail
    U. nailing system
    U. polyurethane adhesive surgical
      dressing
Uni-frame patient immobilization system
UniFuse infusion catheter
Uni-Gard
    U.-G. piggyback connector
    U.-G. Quik Cath
Unigraft
    U. bone graft material
    U. knife
UniHeart nebulizer
unijunction transistor (UJT)
Unilab
    U. Surgibone
    U. Surgibone collagen hemostatic
      material
    U. Surgibone surgical implant
unilateral
    u. removable partial denture
Uni-Lead ECG electrode system
Unilink
    U. anastomotic device
    U. hand surgery system
Unilith pacemaker
Unimar
    U. Cervex brush
    U. HSG tray
    U. J needle
    U. J-needle
    U. Pipelle
    U. Pipelle curette
UniMax 2000 laser micromanipulator
Unipass endocardial pacing lead
uniplanar intraocular lens
Uniplane rocker
UniPlast Imaging and Archiving system
unipolar
    u. atrial pacemaker
    u. atrioventricular pacemaker
    u. cautery
    u. cutting loop
    u. electrode
    u. glass electrode

    u. pacemaker
    u. sequential pacemaker
UniPort
    U. hemostasis introducer sheath kit
    U. Plus vein harvesting system
    VasoView U.
Uniquet disposable intravenous
    tourniquet
Uni-Sem intrauterine catheter
Unisensor unitip pressure sensor
    catheter
UniShaper single-use keratome
Uni-Shunt
    U.-S. abdominal slip clip
    U.-S. catheter passer
    U.-S. cranial anchoring clip
    U.-S. hydrocephalus shunt
    U.-S. split trocar
Unison bone plate system
UniSpacer knee system
Unistat bilirubinometer
unit
    Accucare TENS u.
    Accu-o-Matic TENS u.
    Acu-Ray x-ray u.
    AdvanTeq II TENS u.
    Alcon cryosurgical u.
    Alcon Phaco-Emulsifier
      phacoemulsification u.
    Amoils cryosurgical u.
    Amoils-Keeler cryo u.
    Apex MiniTENS TS-1701 TENS u.
    Arrow-Trerotola PTD rotator
      drive u.
    Aspen Excaliber electrosurgical u.
    Atmolit suction u.
    AtriCure ablation and sensing u.
    Autocon electrosurgical u.
    Autoflex II continuous passive
      motion u.
    Back Bubble gravity traction u.
    Baird Electric System 5000 Power
      Plus electrosurgical u.
    Bart abdominoperipheral
      angiography u.
    BCD Plus cardioplegic u.
    BICAP u.
    BiliBed phototherapy u.
    BioMed TENS u.
    Biosound 2000 II ultrasound u.
    BiPAP u.
    bipolar electrosurgical u.

U

NOTES

unit (*continued*)

Birtcher Hyfrecator electrosurgical u.
Bovie electrocautery u.
Buck Universal convoluted traction u.
Burdick microwave diathermy electrosurgical u.
Burton Electricator electrosurgical u.
Cadwell 5200A somatosensory evoked potential u.
CardioNet mobile outpatient cardiac telemetry u.
C-arm portable x-ray u.
cautery u.
Cavitron cautery u.
Cavitron phacoemulsification u.
Celay milling u.
Century bicarbonate dialysis control u.
Cilco ultrasound u.
Collins Eagle I spirometry u.
ConMed Excalibur-Plus electrosurgical u.
CoolPac hands-free u.
CooperVision I&A u.
cryosurgical u.
CSV Bovie electrosurgical u.
Cybex trunk extension/flexion u.
DeVilbiss I&A u.
Diasonics DRF ultrasound u.
Discover Cryo-Therapy u.
DualStim TENS u.
DynaLator ultrasound u.
Dynasplint knee extension u.
ECG trigger u.
Eclipse TENS u.
EEA disposable loading u.
Efica CC dynamic air therapy u.
EIE MiniEndo piezoelectric ultrasonic u.
Elan electrosurgical u.
ElastaTrac home lumbar traction u.
electrosurgical u.
enhanced external counterpulsation u.
Exakt cutting/grinding u.
Exo-Overhead traction u.
Flexicair eclipse low air loss therapy u.
Flowtron DVT prophylactic deep venous thrombosis u.
Fox I&A u.
FracSure u.
Freedom dental u.
FreeDop portable Doppler u.
Frigitronics cryosurgical u.

Galileo computerized measurement u.
Gass I&A u.
Gaymar Thermacare warming u.
G5 Fleximatic massage/percussion u.
GIA II loading u.
Gibson I&A u.
Giotto Image mammography u.
Girard ultrasonic u.
Hampton electrosurgical u.
HeatProbe u.
Heliodent dental x-ray u.
Hercules 7000 mobile x-ray u.
HomeTrac cervical traction u.
Hounsfield u.
Hyde irrigator & aspirator u.
Hydrocollator heating u.
I&A u.
Iceman continuous cold therapy u.
image processing u.
inhalation breath u.
InjecTx u.
Intermedics phaco I&A u.
intrapleural sealed drainage u.
Irvine I&A u.
Jace hand continuous passive motion u.
JACE-Stim electrotherapy u.
Keeler cryophake u.
Keeler cryosurgical u.
Kelman-Cavitron I&A u.
Kelman cryosurgical u.
Kelman I&A u.
Kinetic Dual-Channel ultrasound u.
Kreiselman resuscitation u.
KryMed cryopexy u.
Laerdal compact suction u.
laminar air flow u.
Leksell stereotactic gamma u.
L-F Uniflex diathermy electrosurgical u.
linear accelerator u.
Lithostar lithotripsy u.
Living Air XL-15 u.
Lumix dental x-ray u.
Magnatherm pulsed therapy high-frequency u.
Magnatherm SSP electromagnetic therapy u.
Magnetrode cervical u.
Malis electrocoagulation u.
Maxima II TENS u.
Mayfield radiolucent base u.
McKesson suction bottle u.
Mettler Dia-Sonic electrosurgical u.
Micro-Pulsar TENS u.
MiniStim TENS u.
Moblvac suction u.

molecular recognition u. (MRU)
Mr. PainAway Health-Up TENS u.
Myotrace Plus electromyography u.
Neosonic piezo ultrasonic u.
Neuromod TENS u.
Neuro-Pulse TENS u.
NeuroStim TENS u.
N_2O cryosurgical u.
Ocoee scalp cleansing u.
Ocutome vitrectomy u.
One-Touch electrolysis u.
Orbix x-ray u.
Orthoceph x-ray u.
Orthotic Research and Locomotor
    Assessment U. (ORLAU)
Ortho Trac motorized traction u.
Osada Beaver-XL handpiece u.
Osmo reverse-osmosis u.
Oti Vac lighted suction u.
over-the-door traction u.
Peyman vitrectomy u.
Peyman vitreophage u.
Poly-Mesam 7-channel ambulatory
    recording u.
Portaray dental x-ray u.
Premier I&A u.
ProMax maxillofacial x-ray u.
Pulmonex dynamic air therapy u.
Pulsar obstetrical 2-channel
    TENS u.
Radionics bipolar coagulation u.
Resuscitaire neonatal
    resuscitation u.
Rollet I&A u.
Sensimatic electrosurgical u.
Sheffield gamma u.
Siemens MRI u.
Siemens Somatom DRH CT
    analyzer u.
Signa 1.5 Tesla u.
Skylark TENS u.
Solfy ZX ultrasonic u.
Solitens TENS u.
Solitens transcutaneous electrical
    nerve stimulation u.
Sonicator Plus 930 therapy u.
sonography u.
Sophie mammography u.
Soprano cryotherapy u.
S-Scort new-Duet suction u.
Stayoden 9000F TENS u.
Storz-Walker retinal detachment u.

Strobex Mark II electrosurgical u.
Surgitron portable radiosurgical u.
Surgitron radiofrequency u.
Sylva I&A u.
TA II loading u.
Ten-O-Matic TENS u.
TENS u.
Tensmax TENS u.
Tesla superconductive magnet u.
Thermalator heating u.
ThermoFlex thermotherapy u.
Tranquility bilevel CPAP u.
TriStim TENS u.
Tuwave galvanic
    stimulator/TENS u.
uniaxial accelerometer u.
Vari-Stim u.
Visitec aspiration u.
Visitec vitrectomy u.
V-Vac suction u.
Wangensteen suction u.
Windmill suction evacuation u.
X-Cel dental x-ray u.
Yoshida dental x-ray u.
Zamorano-Dujovny localizing u.

Unitech
    U. instrument
    U. Toomey cannula
United
    U. Sonics J shock phaco
        fragmentor system
    U. States Catheter & Instruments
        (USCI)
    U. States Surgical circular stapler
Unitek
    U. appliance
    U. I decubitus mattress
    U. II convoluted innerspring
        mattress system
Unitome knife
Unitrax
    U. modular endoprosthesis
    U. unipolar system
Unitri
    U. cannula
    U. tip
Unitron Esteem CIC hearing aid
Unity-C
    U.-C cardiac pacemaker
    U.-C pacemaker
Unity VDDR pacemaker

NOTES

U

Uni-Vent
  U.-V. Eagle portable ventilation system
  U.-V. ventilator
Univent endotracheal tube
Universal
  U. abdominal trocar
  U. acetabular graft impactor
  U. adenoid punch tip
  U. Aerobicycle
  U. aspirator
  U. bone plate
  U. cannula
  U. catheter access port
  U. chuck handle
  U. clip remover
  U. conformer
  U. connector
  U. drainage catheter
  U. drill point
  U. esophagoscope
  U. eye shield
  U. F breathing system
  U. Fitstep exerciser
  U. fixation driver
  U. fixation screw
  U. forceps
  U. gastroscope
  U. gauge
  U. goniometer
  U. head holder
  U. hex screwdriver
  U. joint device
  U. Kerrison rongeur
  U. Mack lamp
  U. malleable valvulotome
  U. modular (UM)
  U. nasal saw
  U. nasal saw blade
  U. phaco manipulator
  U. Plus instrument system
  U. prosthesis
  U. radial component
  U. reducer cap
  U. retractor
  U. screwdriver
  U. sheath
  U. slit lamp
  U. speculum
  U. speculum holder
  U. stent
  U. support splint
  U. swivel
  U. T-adapter
  U. tourniquet
  U. Tredex treadmill
  U. two-speed hand drill
  U. vaginal probe
  U. ventilation meter (UVM)

  U. wire clamp
  U. wire scissors
Uni-Versatil sling
University
  U. of Akron artificial heart
  U. of British Columbia (UBC)
  U. of British Columbia brace
  U. of California Berkeley Laboratory (UCBL)
  U. of California Biomechanics Laboratory heel cup
  U. of California Los Angeles (UCLA)
  U. of Florida linear accelerator
  U. of Illinois biopsy needle
  U. of Illinois marrow needle
  U. of Illinois sternal puncture needle
  U. of Iowa cotton applicator
  U. of Kansas corneal forceps
  U. of Kansas hook
  U. of Kansas spatula
  U. of Michigan gonioscope
  U. of Michigan Mixter thoracic forceps
  U. of Virginia skull tongs
Univision low-vision microscopic lens
Uniweave catheter
Uni-Yeast-Tek system
Unloader
  U. Bi-ComPF brace
  U. Express knee brace
Unna
  U. boot
  U. comedo extractor
  U. paste boot
  U. zinc boot
Unna-Flex
  U.-F. compression wrap
  U.-F. elastic Unna boot
  U.-F. paste bandage
  U.-F. Plus compression dressing
  U.-F. Plus venous ulcer convenience pack
  U.-F. Plus venous ulcer kit
Unna-Pak compression dressing and wrap
Unopette
  U. capillary pipette
  U. system
unstented pulmonary homograft heart valve
unsutured Dacron prosthesis
unzipper
  Katzen flap u.
Up and About system
uPACS picture archiving system
up-angled hook

upbiting
- u. bean forceps
- u. cup forceps
- u. forceps

upcupped forceps

upcurved basket forceps

Updegraff
- U. cleft palate needle
- U. staphylorrhaphy needle

updraft nebulizer

Uplift
- Carter-Thomason U.

UPO-16 stapler

upper
- U. Body Cycle (UBC)
- u. cervical spine anterior/posterior construct
- u. extremity myoelectric prosthesis
- u. gastrointestinal (UGI)
- U. Hands self-retaining retractor
- u. lateral scissors
- u. lid elevator
- U. 7 model head halter
- u. occlusive clamp

upper-lateral exposing retractor

Uppsala gall duct forceps

upright foot pedal cycloergometer

UPS 2020 ambulatory manometry system

upturned forceps

upward-bent forceps

upward-cutting triangular knife

Urban
- U. microscope
- U. retractor
- U. Walkers

Urbanski strut guide

Urbantschitsch
- U. eustachian bougie
- U. nasal forceps

Urchin heart positioner

Ureflex ureteral catheter

UreSil
- U. biliary catheter
- U. embolectomy/thrombectomy catheter
- U. irrigation catheter
- U. occlusion balloon catheter
- U. radiopaque silicone-band vessel loop
- U. Tru-Incise valvulotome
- U. Vascu-Flo carotid shunt

ureteral
- u. basket stone dislodger
- u. catheter obturator
- u. clamp
- u. dilatation catheter
- u. implant
- u. meatotomy electrode
- u. occlusion balloon catheter
- u. stent
- u. stone basket
- u. stone extractor
- u. stone forceps
- u. stone retriever
- u. stylet

ureteric retrieval net

ureteropyeloscope
- Karl Storz flexible u.

ureteroscope
- Applied Medical mini u.
- Circon ACMI MR-series u.
- flexible u.
- Micro-6 u.
- PanoView rod-lens u.
- stiletto u.
- Storz 27022 SK u.
- Wolf rigid u.

ureterotome
- Campbell u.
- Korth u.
- optical u.
- Otis u.

Uretex pubourethral sling

urethane
- Poron cellular u.

urethra cup pessary

urethral
- u. catheter
- u. female dilator
- u. forceps
- u. instillation cannula
- u. male dilator
- u. meatal dilator
- u. sound

UrethraMax urethral catheter

urethrographic
- u. cannula
- u. cannula clamp
- u. catheter

urethroplasty needle

urethroscope
- Albarran u.
- Judd u.

U

NOTES

urethroscope *(continued)*
    Lowsley u.
    Microlens u.
urethrotome
    u. blade
    bougie u.
    Hertel bougie u.
    Huffman-Huber infant u.
    infant u.
    Keitzer infant u.
    Kirkheim-Storz u.
    Maisonneuve u.
    Otis u.
    Riba u.
    Sachs u.
    Storz u.
    Storz-Kirkheim u.
    Thomson-Walker u.
urethrotomy
    optical internal u. (OIU)
Urias pressure splint
Uribe orbital implant
Uri-Cath set
Uridome catheter
Uri-Drain
    U.-D. leg bag
    U.-D. male incontinence device
Uridrop catheter
Urihesive
    U. expandable adhesive
    U. moldable adhesive strip
urinal
    condom u.
    Feminal female u.
    male u.
    Millie female u.
urinary
    u. catheter
    u. control urethral insert
    u. drainage bag
    u. drainage tube
    u. incontinence clamp
    u. incontinence prosthesis
    u. leg bag
    u. night drainage bottle
Urisheath
    Conveen Security+ Conveen self-
      sealing U.
    Conveen self-sealing U.
    Security+ Self-Sealing U.
Urisys 2400 urine analyzer
Uri-Two petri dish
Uro-Bond II brush-on silicone adhesive
Urocam video camera
Urocare
    U. Foley catheter
    U. latex reusable leg bag
Uro-Cath external catheter
UroCoil self-expanding stent

Uro-Con Texas style male external catheter
Uro-Cup female vaginal urinary collection system
Urocyte diagnostic cytometry system
urodynamic catheter
urodynamics chair
Uroflo cystometer
uroflowmeter
    Dantec Urodyn u.
    Drake u.
    Etude cystometer u.
    Synectics-Dantec Flo-Lab II u.
Urofoam-1, -2 adhesive foam strip
Uro-Guide stent
Urolase
    U. CO_2 laser
    U. neodymium:YAG laser fiber
urological
    u. catheter
    u. soaking basin
Uroloop vaporizing cutting electrode
UroLume
    U. endourethral Wallstent prosthesis
    U. urethral stent
    U. Wallstent
UroMax II high-pressure balloon catheter
Uro-Safe vinyl disposable leg bag
Uro-San Plus external catheter
Urosheath incontinence device
UROS infuser
UroSnare cystoscopic tumor snare
Urosoft stent
Urospiral urethral stent
urostomy
    Ultra Duet u.
Urovac bladder evacuator
UroVive system
Urowave microwave thermotherapy system
Urquhart periosteal elevator
Urrets-Zavalia
    U.-Z. depressor
    U.-Z. probe
    U.-Z. retinal surgical lens
    U.-Z. scleral depressor
Urschel-Leksell rongeur
Urschel rongeur
URYS 800 nerve stimulator
U.S.
    U.S. Army bone chisel
    U.S. Army double-ended retractor
    U.S. Army gauze scissors
    U.S. Army gouge
    U.S. Army osteotome
    U.S. Army tourniquet
    U.S. Army umbilical scissors

USA
    USA Elite System rotating continuous-flow resectoscope
    USA plaster spreader
    USA Series Distortion-Free Hydro laparoscope
USCI
    United States Catheter & Instruments
    USCI Bard catheter
    USCI bifurcated Vasculour II prosthesis
    USCI cannula
    USCI Finesse guiding catheter
    USCI Goetz bipolar electrode
    USCI Hyperflex guidewire
    USCI introducer
    USCI Mini-Profile PTCA balloon dilatation catheter
    USCI NBIH bipolar electrode
    USCI pacing electrode
    USCI Positrol coronary catheter
    USCI probe
    USCI Probe balloon-on-a-wire dilatation system
    USCI Sauvage EXS side-limb prosthesis
    USCI shunt
    USCI Vario permanent pacemaker
USCI-DeBakey vascular prosthesis
U-shaped
    U-s. cannula
    U-s. forceps
    U-s. retractor
U-sheet sheet
Usher
    U. Marlex mesh dressing
    U. Marlex mesh implant
    U. Marlex mesh prosthesis
U-splint splint
Ussing chamber
U-sutures
    Cooley U-s.
Utah
    U. arm electronic prosthesis
    U. artificial arm
    U. total artificial heart
UT bag system
uterine
    u. activity monitor
    u. artery forceps
    u. aspirator

    u. biopsy curette
    u. biopsy punch
    u. biopsy punch forceps
    u. cannula
    u. clamp
    u. cornual access catheter
    u. curette
    u. dilator
    u. elevator
    u. evacuator
    U. Explora Curette endometrial sampling device
    u. injector
    u. irrigating curette
    u. manipulator
    u. needle
    u. ostial access catheter
    u. polyp forceps
    u. probe
    u. scissors
    u. scoop
    u. self-retaining cannula
    u. sound
    u. specimen forceps
    u. suction curette
    u. tenaculum
    u. tenaculum forceps
    u. tube
    u. vacuum aspirating curette
    u. vacuum cannula
    u. vulsellum forceps
uterine-dressing forceps
uterine-elevating forceps
uterine-grasping forceps
uterine-holding forceps
uterine-manipulating forceps
uterine-packing forceps
Uterobrush endometrial sample collector
utility
    u. bandage scissors
    u. forceps
    u. shears
Utrata
    U. capsulorrhexis forceps
    U. foldable lens cutter
    U. foldable lens retriever
U-tube
    U-t. drain
    U-t. stent
    U-t. tube
U-type dental implant

U

NOTES

UV
    ultraviolet
        UV transilluminator
UV-blocking filter
uvea-fixated intraocular lens
uvea-supported intraocular lens
Uvex lens
UV-Flash ultraviolet germicidal
    exchange device

Uviolite lamp
UVM
    Universal ventilation meter
UVR
    ultraviolet radiation
UVR-absorbing intraocular lens
uvular retractor

V.

V. Mueller amputating saw
V. Mueller aortic clamp
V. Mueller auricular appendage clamp
V. Mueller-Balfour abdominal retractor
V. Mueller biopsy forceps
V. Mueller blunt hook
V. Mueller bone-cutting forceps
V. Mueller bulldog clamp
V. Mueller cross-action bulldog clamp
V. Mueller curved operating scissors
V. Mueller cystoscopy tip
V. Mueller diamond rasp
V. Mueller embolectomy catheter
V. Mueller fiberoptic retractor
V. Mueller-Frazier suction tube
V. Mueller-Gigli saw
V. Mueller-LaForce adenotome
V. Mueller laser Allis forceps
V. Mueller laser Backhaus towel forceps
V. Mueller laser Crile micro-arterial forceps
V. Mueller laser Rhoton microforceps
V. Mueller laser Rhoton microneedle holder
V. Mueller laser Rhoton microscissors
V. Mueller laser Rhoton microtying forceps
V. Mueller laser Singley tissue forceps
V. Mueller laser tubal scissors
V. Mueller mastoid curette
V. Mueller myringotomy blade
V. Mueller nonperforating towel forceps
V. Mueller operating scissors
V. Mueller paracervical nerve block needle
V. Mueller-Poole suction tube
V. Mueller pudendal nerve block needle
V. Mueller ruler
V. Mueller ruler calipers
V. Mueller screwdriver
V. Mueller Tip-Trol handle
V. Mueller TUR drape
V. Mueller tying forceps
V. Mueller Universal handle
V. Mueller vascular loop
V. Mueller vena caval clamp
V. Mueller-Vital laser Babcock forceps
V. Mueller-Vital laser Heaney needle holder
V. Mueller-Vital laser Julian needle holder
V. Mueller-Vital laser Mayo dissecting scissors
V. Mueller-Vital laser Potts-Smith forceps

V1 halo ring
V33W high-density endocavity probe
VA

VA magnetic orbital implant
VA shunt

Vabra

V. aspirator
V. assembly
V. cannula
V. catheter
V. cervical aspirator
V. suction curette

V.A.C.

Vacuum Assisted Closure
V.A.C. dressing
V.A.C. Therapy wound healing system

Vac

Sani V.

Vacher self-retaining retractor
Vac-Lok

V.-L. immobilization cushion
V.-L. patient immobilization system

Vac-Pac positioner
Vac-Pak pad
Vactro perilimbal suction apparatus
Vacuconstrictor erection device
Vacu-Irrigator

Vozzle V.-I.

Vaculance

Microlet V.

Vacupac portable vacuum system
Vac-U-Port

Bemis V.-U.-P.

Vacurette

Berkeley V.
V. catheter
V. suction curette

Vacutainer

V. drain
V. holder
V. needle
V. Safety-Gard needle

V

Vacutainer *(continued)*
 V. specimen tube system
 V. vacuum tube
Vacu-tome knife
Vacutron suction regulator
vacuum
 v. apparatus
 v. aspiration catheter
 v. aspirator
 V. Assisted Closure (V.A.C.)
 v. cannula
 v. constriction device
 v. controller
 v. cup catheter
 v. curette
 v. entrapment device
 v. erection device
 v. extraction device
 v. extractor
 v. fixation ring
 v. intrauterine cannula
 v. intrauterine probe
 MultiVac v.
 v. pillow
 Quiet-Vac v.
 Rainbow v.
 v. retractor
 v. tube voltmeter
 TurboVac 90 v.
vacuuming needle
vacuum-operated viscous restraint
VAD
 vascular access device
 venous access device
 ventricular assist device
 DeBakey VAD
 HeartSaver VAD
Vaduz hand
vaginal
 v. aluminum electrode
 v. bag
 v. candle
 v. contraceptive film
 v. cuff clamp
 v. cylinder
 v. dilator
 v. hysterectomy forceps
 v. laser measuring rod
 v. mold
 v. probe ultrasound wand
 v. prolapse prosthesis
 v. retractor
 v. spatula
 v. speculum
 v. speculum loop
 v. stent
Vaginard metal speculum
vaginometer

vaginoscope
 Huffman-Huber infant v.
 Huffman infant v.
VagiTrac vaginal retractor
vagotometer
 Burge v.
vagotomy
 v. retractor
 v. stripper
Vail
 V. lid everter
 V. lid retractor
Vairox
 V. high-compression vascular
 stocking
 V. support stocking
Vaiser-Cibis muscle retractor
Vaiser sponge
Vakutage
 V. curette
 V. suction system
Valchev uterine manipulator
Valdoni clamp
Valentine
 V. irrigation tube
 V. irrigator
 V. splint
valgus bar
Validyne manometer
Valin
 V. forceps
 V. hemilaminectomy self-retaining
 retractor
Valle hysteroscope
Valleylab
 V. ball electrode
 V. cautery
 V. CUSA CEM system
 V. electrocautery
 V. Force 1C electrosurgical
 generator
 V. laparoscopic instrument
 V. loop electrode
 V. pencil
 V. REM system
Valley Vac smoke evacuation system
Valliex uterine probe
Valls prosthesis
Valtrac
 V. absorbable biofragmentable
 anastomosis ring
 V. BAR
ValueWalker brace
valve
 Accu-Flo pressure v.
 Ahmed glaucoma v.
 Ambu-E v.
 Angell-Shiley bioprosthetic heart v.

Angell-Shiley xenograft prosthetic v.
Angestat introducer with hemostasis v.
Angiocor prosthetic v.
antisiphon v.
aortic bioprosthetic v.
apicoaortic conduit heart v.
apicoaortic shunt heart v.
Argyle anti-reflux v.
Argyle-Salem sump anti-reflux v.
ATS Open Pivot bileaflet heart v.
ball-occluder v.
Baxter mechanical v.
Beall disc heart v.
Beall mitral v.
Beall-Surgitool disc prosthetic v.
Benchekroun ileal v.
Beverly referential v.
Bianchi v.
Bicer-val prosthetic v.
bileaflet tilting-disc prosthetic v.
Biocor porcine stented mitral v.
Biocor prosthetic v.
Biocor stentless porcine aortic v.
bioprosthetic heart v.
Bio-Vascular prosthetic v.
Björk-Shiley mitral v.
Blom-Singer v.
bovine pericardial v.
Braunwald-Cutter ball prosthetic v.
Braunwald heart v.
bulb and thumb screw v.
caged-ball heart v.
Capetown aortic prosthetic v.
CarboMedics bileaflet prosthetic heart v.
CarboMedics Orbis prosthetic heart v.
CarboMedics Top Hat supraannular v.
Carpentier-Edwards bioprosthetic v.
Carpentier-Edwards mitral annuloplasty v.
Carpentier-Edwards pericardial v.
Carpentier-Edwards Perimount mitral v.
Carpentier-Edwards porcine supraannular v.
Carpentier pericardial v.
Carpentier ring heart v.
cerebral spinal fluid v.

Codman Hakim programmable v.
Codman-Medos programmable v.
convexoconcave heart v.
Cooley-Bloodwell-Cutter v.
Cooley-Cutter disc prosthetic v.
Coratomic prosthetic v.
Cordis-Hakim v.
CPHV OptiForm mitral v.
Cross-Jones aortic v.
Cross-Jones caged mitral v.
CRx v.
CryoLife-O'Brien stentless heart v.
cryopreserved homograft v.
CryoValve SG allograft heart v.
CSF v.
Cutter-Smeloff mitral v.
DeBakey prosthetic heart v.
DeBakey-Surgitool prosthetic v.
Delrin disc heart v.
Delta v.
Denver v.
Diamond v.
diastolic fluttering aortic v.
v. dilator
Dua antireflux v.
dual-chamber flushing v.
Duostat rotating hemostatic v.
Duraflow heart v.
Duromedics bileaflet mitral v.
eccentric monocuspid tilting-disc prosthetic v.
Edwards-Duromedics bileaflet heart v.
Edwards Prima Plus v.
Edwards seamless heart v.
Emiks heart v.
expiratory v.
Fink v.
flexible cardiac v.
floating disc heart v.
flushing v.
Freestyle stentless v.
glutaraldehyde-tanned bovine heart v.
glutaraldehyde-tanned porcine heart v.
Gott butterfly heart v.
Hakim high-pressure v.
Hakim precision v.
Hakim programmable v.
Hall v.
Hall-Kaster heart v.

V

NOTES

valve *(continued)*
Hall prosthetic heart v.
Hancock bioprosthetic heart v.
Hancock heterograft heart v.
Hancock II tissue v.
Hancock modified orifice v.
Hancock porcine v.
Hans Rudolph 3-way v.
Harken ball heart v.
Harken prosthetic v.
Harken-Starr v.
Hasner v.
heart v.
Heidbrink expiratory spill v.
Heimlich chest drainage v.
Heimlich heart v.
Heimlich Vygon pneumothorax v.
Hemex prosthetic v.
Heyer-Pudenz v.
Heyer-Schulte v.
v. holding chamber (VHC)
hollow Silastic disc heart v.
Holter elliptical v.
Holter-Hausner v.
Holter high-pressure v.
Holter medium-pressure v.
Holter mini-elliptical v.
Holter straight v.
Hufnagel-Kay heart v.
Hufnagel prosthetic v.
impedance threshold v.
Intact bioprosthetic v.
Intact xenograft v.
Ionescu-Shiley artificial cardiac v.
Ionescu-Shiley pericardial v.
Ionescu tri-leaflet v.
I-S artificial cardiac v.
Jatene arterial switch v.
Jatene-Macchi prosthetic v.
Kay-Shiley heart v.
Kay-Suzuki heart v.
Kock nipple v.
Krupin-Denver eye v.
Labcor Synergy v.
Lanz pressure regulating v.
v. leaflet excision scissors
3-legged cage heart v.
lens mitral heart v.
LeVeen v.
Lewis-Leigh positive-pressure
  nonrebreathing v.
Lifemed heterologous heart v.
Liks Russian disc rotation heart v.
Lillehei-Kaster pivoting-disc
  prosthetic mitral v.
Liotta-BioImplant LPB prosthetic v.
Lopez enteral v.
low-profile mitral heart v.

Magovern-Cromie ball-cage
  prosthetic v.
Magovern heart v.
Malteno v.
Medos v.
Medos-Hakim v.
Medtronic Freestyle stentless v.
Medtronic-Hall monocuspid tilting-
  disc v.
Medtronic-Hall prosthetic heart v.
Medtronic Hancock II tissue v.
Medtronic Intact bioprosthetic v.
Medtronic Mosaic heart v.
Medtronic prosthetic v.
Mishler dual-chamber v.
Mishler flushing v.
Mitamura fine ceramic heart v.
Mitroflow pericardial prosthetic v.
Mitroflow Synergy PC aortic
  heart v.
Molteno v.
Montgomery speaking v.
Mosaic porcine bioprosthetic
  heart v.
Nezhat-Dorsey trumpet v.
nonrebreathing v.
Novus hydrocephalic v.
Omnicarbon prosthetic heart v.
Omniscience tilting-disc v.
On-X bileaflet prosthetic heart v.
Open Pivot heart v.
OptiForm mitral v.
Orbis prosthetic heart v.
Orbis-Sigma v.
v. outflow strut
Passy-Muir v. (PMV)
Passy-Muir speaking v.
Passy-Muir tracheostomy
  speaking v.
Peep v.
Pemco prosthetic v.
Perimount mitral v.
Phoenix ancillary v.
Phoenix cruciform v.
PlegiaGuard pressure relief v.
PMV-series tracheostomy and
  ventilator speaking v.
polyethylene seat heart v.
pop-off v.
porcine heart v.
pressure-activated safety v.
programmable v.
v. prosthesis
prosthetic heart v.
Provox tracheoesophageal
  speaking v.
PS Medical Flow Control v.
Pudenz flushing v.

Puig Massana-Shiley annuloplasty v.
pulmonary autograft v.
Pyrolyte ball-cage heart v.
quadricusp stentless mitral bioprosthetic v.
Quattro mitral v.
Quick Drain v.
v. retractor
Ross pulmonary porcine v.
rotating hemostatic v.
Rudolph 1-way respiratory v.
Safsite v.
Sanders v.
v. scissors
Shiley convexoconcave heart v.
Shiley monostrut heart v.
Shiley Phonate speaking v.
v. shunt
silicone ball heart v.
silicone disc heart v.
Singer-Blom v.
SJM Masters series v.
SJM Quattro mitral v.
SJM Regent v.
Smeloff-Cutter ball-cage prosthetic v.
Smeloff heart v.
SmokEvac trumpet v.
Sophy programmable v.
speaking v.
Spitz-Holter v.
Spivack v.
spring ball v.
Starr-Edwards cloth-covered metallic ball heart v.
Starr-Edwards prosthetic aortic v.
Starr-Edwards prosthetic mitral v.
Starr-Edwards Silastic v.
Starr-Edwards silicone rubber ball v.
Stellite ball-cage heart v.
Stellite ring material of prosthetic v.
stented bioprosthetic v.
stentless porcine aortic v.
stent-mounted allograft v.
stent-mounted heterograft v.
Stephen-Slater v.
St. Jude Medical bileaflet tilting-disc aortic v.
St. Jude Medical Biocor v.

St. Jude Medical BioImplant v.
St. Jude Medical Masters series v.
St. Jude Medical Quattro mitral v.
St. Jude Medical Regent v.
SynerGraft heart v.
Tascon prosthetic v.
Tekna mechanical heart v.
tilting-disc heart v.
titanium ball-cage heart v.
Top-Hat supraannular aortic v.
Toronto SPV stentless porcine v.
tracheostoma v.
Tucker aspirating v.
Ultracor prosthetic v.
unstented pulmonary homograft heart v.
Vascor porcine prosthetic v.
ventilator speaking v.
Wada-Cutter heart v.
Wessex prosthetic v.
X-Cell v.
Xenomedica prosthetic v.
Xenotech prosthetic v.

valved
v. holding chamber
v. voice prosthesis
valve-ended catheter
valvotome
expanding v.
spade-shaped v.
valvuloplasty balloon catheter
valvulotome
angioscopic v.
antegrade v.
Bakst v.
bread knife v.
Brock v.
Carmody v.
Chalnot v.
Derra v.
expandable LeMaitre v.
Gerbode mitral v.
Gohrbrand v.
Gore EZE-Sit v.
Hall v.
Harken v.
Himmelstein pulmonary v.
Intramed angioscopic v.
Leather antegrade v.
Leather retrograde v.
Longmire v.
Longmire-Mueller curved v.

NOTES

V

valvulotome *(continued)*
    Malm-Himmelstein pulmonary v.
    Mills v.
    Neider v.
    Potts expansile v.
    Potts-Riker v.
    retrograde v.
    Samuels v.
    Sellor v.
    Tru-Incise v.
    Tubbs v.
    Universal malleable v.
    UreSil Tru-Incise v.
VAMOS
    Variable Anesthesia Monitoring System
      VAMOS anesthetic gas monitor
VAMP
    venous arterial blood management
      protection system
van
    V. Alyea antral cannula
    V. Alyea antral trocar
    V. Alyea antral wash tube
    V. Alyea frontal sinus cannula
    V. Alyea sphenoid cannula
    V. Aman pigtail catheter
    V. Aman pulmonary pigtail
      catheter
    V. Andel dilation catheter
    V. Beek nerve approximator clamp
    V. Buren bone-holding forceps
    V. Buren canvas roll sound
    V. Buren catheter
    V. Buren catheter guide
    V. Buren dilating sound
    V. Buren dilator
    V. Buren sequestrum forceps
    V. Buren urethral sound
    v. de Graaf generator
    V. Der Pas hysteroscope
    V. Doren uterine biopsy punch
      forceps
    V. Hove bag
    V. Loenen operating keratoscope
    V. Osdel guillotine
    V. Osdel irrigating cannula
    V. Osdel tonsil enucleator
      tonsillectome
    V. Ruben forceps
    v. Slyke apparatus
    v. Sonnenberg gallbladder catheter
    v. Sonnenberg sump catheter
    v. Sonnenberg sump drain
    v. Sonnenberg-Wittich catheter
    V. Struyken nasal forceps
    V. Struyken nasal punch
    V. Tassel pigtail catheter
Vanadium arch bar cutter
Vancaillie uterine cannula

Vancare shower/commode transfer chair
Vance
    V. percutaneous Malecot
      nephrostomy catheter
    V. prostatic aspiration cannula
Vance-Kish urethral illuminated catheter
Vanderbilt
    V. arterial forceps
    V. deep-vessel forceps
    V. University hemostatic forceps
    V. University vessel forceps
    V. vessel clamp
Vander-Lift lift
Vander Pool sterilizer forceps
Vanghetti limb prosthesis
Vanguard endograft
VanishPoint syringe
Vannas
    V. abscess knife
    V. capsulotomy scissors
    V. corneal scissors
    V. fixation forceps
    V. iridocapsulotomy scissors
Vantage
    V. graft
    V. indirect ophthalmoscope
    V. Performance monitor
    V. tube-occluding forceps
Vantec
    V. dilator
    V. grasping forceps
    V. loop retriever
    V. occlusion balloon catheter
    V. stone basket
    V. ureteral balloon dilatation
      catheter
    V. urinary stent
Vantex central venous catheter
Vantos vacuum extractor
VAPC dorsiflexion assist orthosis
VAPORbar instrument
vaporizer
    cool mist v.
    Cool-vapor v.
    Dench v.
    draw-over v.
    flow-over v.
    Fluotec v.
    Goldman v.
    Israel Benzedrine v.
    Maxi-Myst v.
    Muraco v.
    Ohmeda Sevotec 5 v.
    Penlon v.
VAPORloop instrument
vapor-permeable dressing
VaporTome resection electrode
VaporTrode roller electrode

Vapotherm 2000i respiratory therapy device
Vapr
  V. arthroscopic system
  V. coagulation and cautery device
Vapro Vapor pressure osmometer
Var-A-Pulse wound debridement system
Varco
  V. dissecting clamp
  V. forceps
  V. gallbladder clamp
  V. gallbladder forceps
variable
  V. Anesthesia Monitoring System (VAMOS)
  v. positive airway pressure (VPAP)
  v. rate pacemaker
  v. screw placement system
  v. spinal plating
  V. Spot DermaStat
  v. stiffness endoscope
  v. stiffness guidewire
variable-angle gamma camera
variable-axis knee
variable-flow insufflator
variable-focus scope
Varian
  V. brachytherapy system
  V. Cary-118C spectrophotometer
  V. CT scanner
  V. LINAC
  V. linear INAC accelerator
  V. MLC system
  V. model 3600 gas chromatograph
  V. NMR spectrometer
Vari-Angle
  V.-A. clip
  V.-A. McFadden clip applier
  V.-A. temporary clip approximator
Vari bladebreaker
VariCare system
Varick elastic dressing
Varicoscreen contact thermography
Vari-Duct hip and knee orthosis
Varidyne drain
Variflex catheter
Vari-Flex prosthetic foot
Varigray
  V. implant
  V. lens
Varigrip spine fixation system
Variject needle

VariLift spinal cage
Varilux
  V. Infinity lens
  V. lens implant
  V. Plus lens
Varimic 900 microscope
Vari-Mix II amalgamator
Vari/Moist wound dressing
Varioligator kit
Varisource remote afterloading catheter
Varis radiation oncology system
Vari-Stim
  V.-S. III handheld nerve stimulator
  V.-S. unit
Varivas
  V. loop graft
  V. vein graft
Vari-Zone variable density convoluted mattress overlay
vas
  v. clamp
  v. hook
  v. isolation forceps
Vasamedics PR-434 implantable prism laser probe
Vasa Trainer exercise machine
Vas-Cath
  V.-C. dialysis catheter
  V.-C. Opti-Plast peripheral angioplasty catheter
  V.-C. Soft-Cell catheter
Vasceze vascular access/flush device
Vasconcelos-Barretto clamp
Vasco-Posada orbital retractor
Vascor
  V. porcine prosthetic valve
  V. sterile retraction tape
VascuClamp vascular clamp
VascuCoil peripheral vascular stent
Vascufil suture
Vascu-Guard
  V.-G. bovine pericardial surgical patch
  V.-G. peripheral vascular patch
vascular
  v. access catheter
  v. access device (VAD)
  v. access needle
  v. access tunneler
  v. clamp
  v. clip
  v. clip applier

V

NOTES

vascular *(continued)*
 v. dilator
 v. dissector
 v. graft clamp
 v. graft prosthesis
 v. hemostatic device
 v. loop
 v. needle holder
 v. scissors
 v. sealing device
 v. sheath
 v. silk suture
 v. spring retractor
 v. stent
 v. suction tube
 v. tape
 v. tissue forceps
 v. tunneler
VascuLink
 V. vascular access graft
 V. vascular access guidewire
Vasculour-II vascular prosthesis
VascuPatch
 Shelhigh No React V.
Vascu-Sheath catheter
Vascushunt carotid balloon shunt
Vascutech circular blade
Vascutek
 V. Gelseal vascular graft
 V. knitted vascular graft
 V. vascular prosthesis
 V. woven vascular graft
vasectomy forceps
Vaseline
 V. gauze dressing
 V. wick dressing
Vaso-Cath peritoneal dialysis catheter
vasocillator
 v. fracture appliance
 v. fracture frame
VasoExtor lead extraction system
VasoSeal
 V. ES arterial sealing device
 V. VHD extravascular sealing device
Vasotrac blood pressure monitoring system
Vasotrax
 V. BP monitor
 V. handheld monitoring device
vasovasostomy clamp
VasoView
 V. balloon
 V. balloon dissection system
 V. Uniport
 V. Uniport Plus endoscopic vein harvesting system
Vasport access port
Vastack needle

VAT pacemaker
Vauban speculum
Vaughan
 V. abscess knife
 V. periosteotome
Vaughn sterilizer forceps
Vaxcel
 V. Mini-Stick
 V. Mini-Stick vascular entry kit
 V. peripherally inserted central catheter
VAX-D therapy table
V510B biplane TEE transducer
Vbeam laser
VBH
 Vogel-Bale-Hohner
 VBH head holder
V-blade
 Blount V.-b.
 V.-b. plate
V-Cath catheter
V-clip
 McKenzie V.-c.
VDD
 VDD pacemaker
 VDD pacing lead
V-dissector
 Coleman V.-d.
vectis
 Anis irrigating v.
 anterior chamber irrigating v.
 v. blade
 v. cesarean forceps
 cul-de-sac irrigating v.
 Drews irrigating v.
 Drews-Knolle reverse irrigating v.
 irrigating-aspirating v.
 Knolle-Pearce v.
 Look irrigating v.
 v. loop
 Peczon I&A v.
 Pierce I&A v.
 Pierce irrigating v.
 plastic disposable irrigating v.
 Sheets irrigating v.
 Snellen v.
 Torpin v.
Vector
 V. intertrochanteric nail
 V. large-lumen guiding catheter
 V. low back analysis system
VectorVision neuronavigation system
Vectra vascular access graft
Vedder loop
Veeder tip snare
Veenema-Gusberg
 V.-G. prostatic biopsy cup
 V.-G. prostatic biopsy needle
 V.-G. prostatic punch

Veenema retropubic self-retaining retractor
Vehmehren costotome
Veidenheimer resection clamp
veil
    Conformant 2 wound v.
vein
    v. dilator
    v. graft cannula
    v. graft ring marker
    v. graft stent
    v. hook retractor
    v. retractor
    v. stripper
Veingard dressing
Veinlase captured-pulse laser
Veirs
    V. canaliculus rod
    V. cannula
    V. dacryocystorhinostomy set
    V. needle
    V. trocar
Velcro
    V. extenders splint
    V. fastener
    V. restraint
    V. tourniquet
Veley headrest
Velket Velcro tourniquet
velocimeter
    Doppler laser v.
    FloMap v.
    laser Doppler v.
    optical Doppler v.
Velocity stent
velolaryngeal endoscope
velour collar graft
Velpeau
    V. bandage
    V. cast
    V. shoulder immobilizer
    V. sling
    V. sling dressing
    V. snare
    V. stockinette
    V. wrap
velum
    Baker v.
velvet-eye aspirating tube
vena
    v. caval cannula
    v. caval clamp
    v. caval clip
    v. caval filter
    v. caval forceps
    V. Tech dual vena caval filter
    V. Tech LGM vena caval filter
    V. Tech LP vena caval filter
Venable
    V. bone plate
    V. screw
Venable-Stuck
    V.-S. fracture pin
    V.-S. nail
Venaflo needle
VenaFlow
    V. compression system
    V. vascular graft
Venaport guiding catheter
veneer retention wire
Venflon cannula
Veni-Gard stabilization dressing
venipuncture needle
Vennes pancreatic dilation set
venoclysis cannula
Venodyne
    V. boot
    V. pneumatic compression device
    V. venous compression system
Venofit medical compression stocking
Venoflex medical compression stocking
venoscope
    Landry vein light v.
venous
    v. access device (VAD)
    v. access port
    v. arterial blood management protection system (VAMP)
    v. cannula
    v. catheter
    v. flow controller (VFC)
    v. irrigation catheter
    v. needle
    v. occlusion plethysmograph
    v. pressure gradient support stocking
    v. thrombectomy catheter
    v. Y adapter
    v. Y connector
VentAire bottle system
Ventak
    V. AICD
    V. AICD pacemaker

V

NOTES

Ventak *(continued)*
    V. AV III DR automatic
      implantable cardioverter-defibrillator
    V. ECD pacemaker
    V. Mini II, III defibrillator
    V. Mini IV AICD
    V. P AICD
    V. Prizm 2 automatic implantable
      cardioverter-defibrillator
    V. PRx implantable cardioverter-
      defibrillator
Ventana 320 automated immunostainer
VentCheck handheld respiratory
  monitor
vented-electric HeartMate LVAD
Ventex dressing
Ventifoam traction dressing
ventilated mask
ventilation
    v. adapter
    v. bronchoscope
ventilator
    Achieva portable v.
    Adult Star 2000 v.
    Aequitron v.
    Amadeus v.
    Amsterdam v.
    Avea v.
    Avian transport v.
    Babybird II v.
    Babyflex v.
    Bear 1, 2, 3 adult-volume v.
    Bear Cub infant v.
    Bennett MA-1 v.
    Bennett PR-2 v.
    Bennett pressure-cycled v.
    Bio-Med MVP-10 neotal/pediatric
      transport v.
    Bird MK VIII pressure-cycled v.
    Bird pressure-cycled v.
    Bird 8400STi v.
    blow-by v.
    Bourns-Bear v.
    Bourns infant pressure v.
    Breeze E150 v.
    Breeze infant v.
    CPAP v.
    Critical Care v.
    cuirass v.
    Dräger v.
    Emerson postoperative v.
    Esprit critical care v.
    extrathoracic v.
    Galileo v.
    Hamilton v.
    Healthdyne v.
    high-frequency jet v.
    HVF v.
    ICV-10 v.

Infant Star high-frequency v.
Infrasonics v.
IVAC v.
KnightStar 330 bi-level v.
Lifecare v.
LTV800 v.
Max v.
mechanical v.
MicroVent v.
Monaghan 300 v.
Morch v.
MVV v.
Neovent v.
Newport E100M v.
Newport HT50 v.
Newport Wave VM200 v.
Ohio critical care v.
Peep v.
Pneumotron v.
pneumo-wrap v.
pneuPAC v.
portable volume v.
Porta-Lung noninvasive
  extrathoracic v.
PR-2 v.
pressure v.
pressure-cycled v.
v. pressure manometer
pressure-preset v.
Pulmo-Aide v.
Puritan Bennett v.
Quantum PSV pressure support v.
Respironics BiPAP bilevel v.
Searle volume v.
Sechrist Millenium
  infant/pediatric v.
Servo-series v.
Siemens-Elema Servo-series
  900C v.
Siemens Servo-series v.
Smart Trigger Bear 1000 v.
v. speaking valve
Star v.
TBird v.
Uni-Vent v.
Venturi v.
Veolar v.
Vickers Neovent v.
Vip Bird neonatal v.
Vix infant v.
volume v.
volume-cycled v.
volume-limited v.
Wave VM200 v.
Yung percutaneous mastoid v.
Ventimask
venting catheter
VentNet remote monitoring system
Vent-O-Vac aspirator

Ventra catheter
Ventricor pacemaker
ventricular
    v. arrhythmia monitor
    v. assist device (VAD)
    v. asynchronous pacemaker
    v. cannula
    v. catheter
    v. catheter introducer
    v. demand-inhibited pacemaker
    v. demand pacemaker
    v. demand pulse generator
    v. demand-triggered pacemaker
    left v. (LV)
    v. needle
    v. sump
ventricular-suppressed pacemaker
ventricular-triggered pacemaker
ventriculoatrial shunt
ventriculogram retractor
ventriculography catheter
ventriculoperitoneal (VP)
    v. shunt
ventriculoscope
    4-channel Aesculap v.
    rigid v.
ventriculosubarachnoid
Ventritex
    V. Angstrom MD implantable
    cardioverter-defibrillator
    V. Cadence device
    V. Cadence ICD
    V. Cadence implantable
    cardioverter-defibrillator
    V. Contour cardioverter-defibrillator
    V. Contour pulse generator
    V. TVL system
Ventrix
    V. fiberoptic intracranial monitor
    V. True Tech ICP catheter
    V. tunnelable ventricular intracranial
    pressure monitoring system
ventroposterolateral
VentTrak monitoring system
Ventura spreader
Venture
    V. demand oxygen delivery device
    V. II HomeFill complete home
    oxygen system
    V. sponge
Ventureyra ventricular catheter

Venturi
    V. apparatus
    V. bobbin myringotomy tube
    V. collar-button myringotomy tube
    V. grommet myringotomy tube
    V. insufflator
    V. mask
    V. meter
    V. pediatric myringotomy tube
    V. spirometer
    V. ventilation adapter
    V. ventilator
Venturi-Flo valve system
Veolar ventilator
Vera bond alloy
Vera-Lift back belt
Veratex cotton roll
Verbatim balloon catheter
Verbrugge
    V. bone clamp
    V. bone-holding forceps
    V. needle
    V. retractor
Verbrugge-Souttar craniotome
Veress
    V. laparoscopic cannula
    V. peritoneum cannula
    V. pneumoperitoneum needle
    V. spring-loaded laparoscopic
    needle
Veress-Frangenheim needle
Vergs phaco chopper
Verhoeff
    V. capsular forceps
    V. cataract forceps
    V. dissecting scissors
    V. suture
Veridian umbilical clamp
Veriflex guidewire
Verifuse ambulatory infusion pump
Veripath peripheral guiding catheter
VeriSoft steerable guidewire
Verity ADx pacemaker
Verlow brace
Vermont spinal fixator
Verner
    V. speculum
    V. stripper
Verner-Joel cutter
Verner-Joseph
    V.-J. scissors
    V.-J. wire tightener

V

NOTES

Verner-Kalinowski speculum
Verner-Smith monitor
Vernier calipers
Vernon
    V. antral wash tube
    V. David sigmoidoscope
    V. wire cutter
    V. wire-cutting scissors
Verruca-Freeze clinical freezing system
Versaback Safe Station back system
Versa bath seat
VersaBond
    V. cement
    V. structural adhesive
VersaClamp flex clamp
VersaClimber exercise machine
VersaDerm dressing
VersaDoc Model 5000 imaging system
Versadopp Doppler probe
Versaflex steerable catheter
Versaflow pump
Versa-Fracture femoral fixation system
Versa-Fx femoral device
VersaLap lapping fixture
VersaLight
    V. laser
    V. photodynamic therapy
Versalok
    V. low-back fixation device
    V. low-back fixation system
Versalon all purpose sponge
VersaLoop curette
Versa-PEG gastrostomy kit
VersaPoint system
Versaport trocar system
VersaPulse
    V. cosmetic holmium laser
    V. Select laser
VersaTack
    V. stapler
    V. stapling device
VersaTool eye sponge
Versatrac lumbar retractor system
Versatrax
    V. cardiac pacemaker
    V. II pacemaker
Verse-Webster clamp
Versi-Splint carry bag
VerSys hip system
VertaBrace brace
VertAlign spinal support system
vertebral
    v. body impactor
    v. spacer
    v. spreader
vertebrated
    v. catheter
    v. probe
Vertetrac ambulatory traction system

Vertex
    V. camera
    V. Plus MCD/AC gamma camera
    V. reconstruction system
vertical
    v. forceps
    v. ring curette
VertiGraft
    V. extured allograft bone guidewire
    V. textured allograft bone graft
Vertis PNT system
vertometer
Vesely nail
Vesely-Street nail
vesical retractor
Vesica percutaneous bladder neck
    suspension kit
vesicoamniotic shunt
vesicular transport system
Vess chair
vessel
    v. band
    v. clamp
    v. clip
    v. dilator
    v. forceps
    v. knife
    v. loop
    v. occluder
    v. occlusion system
    v. punch
vessel-occluding clamp
vessel-sizing catheter
vest
    V. airway clearance system
    Bremer AirFlo thoracic
      stabilization v.
    Bremer halo v.
    Circumpress gynecomastia v.
    V. direct forward-vision telescope
    EZ-On v.
    halo v.
    Little cargo v.
    Mark VII cooling v.
    Orthotrac pneumatic v.
    ThAIRapy v.
    weighted v.
VestaBlate balloon system
VEST ambulatory ventricular function
    monitor
vestibular clamp
Vestibulator
    Tumble Forms V.
Vet-Co vacuum system
Vezien abdominal scissors
VFC
    venous flow controller
    Actis VFC
V-Flex Plus PTX stent

VG slit lamp
VHC
    valve holding chamber
    AeroChamber VHC
    AeroPEP Plus VHC
Viabahn
    V. endoprosthesis
    V. graft
vial
    Nickerson Biggy v.
Viasorb absorbent dressing
Viatorr endoprosthesis
Viatronix V3D virtual colonoscopy
  system
Viba-Brush
    V.-B. endocervical brush
    Rovers V.-B.
Viboch iliac graft retractor
Vibracare massager
Vibram
    V. rockerbottom shoe
    V. walking base
Vibrasonic hearing instrument
vibrating-reed electrometer
vibrating scissors
vibrator
    Magic Wand v.
Vibrodilator probe
Vibro-Graver
    Burgess V.-G.
vibrometer
Vic
    V. hair transplant knife
    V. Vallis running hair knife
Vicat needle
Vick-Blanchard hemorrhoidal forceps
Vickerall round ringed forceps
Vickers
    V. isolator
    V. M85a microdensitometer
    V. needle holder
    V. Neovent ventilator
    V. ring-tip forceps
    V. Treonic hemoheater
Vico angled manipulator
Vicor pacemaker
Vicryl
    V. pop-off suture
    V. Rapide suture
    V. SH suture
Victor-Bonney forceps
Victoreen dosimeter

Victorian collar dressing
Victory alloy
Vidal-Hoffman fixator frame
VidaMed TUNA system
Vidar scanner
Vidas automated immunoassay system
Vidaurri
    V. cannula
    V. LASIK flap irrigator
video
    v. display camera
    v. duodenoscope
    v. monitor
    v. otoscope
    v. processor
    v. push enteroscope
    v. recorder
    v. specular microscope
    V. ZoomScope
videobronchoscope
videoduodenoscope
    Fujinon ED7-XU2 v.
    Fujinon 310XU v.
videoelectroscope
    Fujinon CEG-FP-series v.
    Fujinon EG7-series v.
videoendoscope
    double-channel v.
    fiberoptic v.
    Olympus GIF-T-series v.
videohydrolaparoscope
videohydrothorascope
videokeratoscope
    computer-assisted v.
    EyeSys v.
    PAR-C-Scan v.
    TechnoMed C-Scan v.
    TMS-2 v.
videolaparoscope
videoscope
    SlimSIGHT ultraslim GI v.
videosigmoidoscope
videostrobe
Vidicon
    V. camera tube
    V. vacuum chamber pickup tube
Vi-Drape
    V.-D. bowel bag
    V.-D. incise drape
    V.-D. wound protector
Vi-drape
    3M V.-d.

V

NOTES

Vienna
    V. Britetrac nasal speculum
    V. nasal speculum
    V. wire suture
Viers
    V. erysiphake
    V. needle
Vieth-Mueller horopter
viewer
    Mammoviewer v.
Viewing
    V. Wand
    V. Wand system
ViewSite video monitor
Vigger-5 eye forceps
VigiFOAM dressing
Vigilance monitoring system
Vigilon primary wound dressing
Vigor
    V. DDDR pacemaker
    V. DR pacemaker
Vigorimeter
    Martin V.
Viking
    V. cannula
    V. IV nerve monitoring device
    V. needle
    V. Optima guiding catheter
Vilex cannulated screw
Villalta retractor
Villard button
Villasenor-Navarro fixation ring
Villasensor ultrasonic pachymeter
Vilmann-Hancke biopsy handle instrument
vimentin filament
Vim needle
Vim-Silverman biopsy needle
Vimule pessary
Vinciguerra
    V. LASEK protector
    V. PRK/LASEK spatula
Vinciguerra-Carones LASEK spatula
Vingmed
    V. CFM-series ultrasound
    V. System Five ultrasound
Vinke
    V. retractor
    V. skull tractor
    V. tongs
vinyl glove
Vinyon-N cloth tube
Vioform gauze dressing
Viomedex surgical marking pen
Vip
    V. Bird infant/pediatric volume monitor
    V. Bird neonatal ventilator
Viper PTA catheter

Virag injector
ViraGuard viral-blocking transducer protector
ViraType probe
Virchow
    V. brain knife
    V. cartilage knife
    V. chisel
    V. skin graft knife
Virden rectal catheter
Viresolve ultrafiltration membrane
virgin
    V. hip screw
    v. silk suture
Virginia needle
Viridis laser
Virilis I, II penile implant
Viro-Tec suture
virtual
    v. biopsy system
    v. labor monitor
    v. reality head-mounted display
    v. reality simulator
    v. retinal display
Virtuoso
    V. LX Smart CPAP system
    V. portable three-dimensional imaging system
    V. shape camera
Virtus
    V. splinter clamp
    V. splinter forceps
Visa II PTCA catheter
viscera-holding forceps
visceral forceps
viscera retainer
Viscoat viscoelastic
viscoelastic
    Cilco v.
    CooperVision v.
    sodium hyaluronate v.
    Viscoat v.
Viscoflow angled cannula
Viscoheel
    V. K, N orthosis
    V. SofSpot orthosis
Viscolens lens
viscometer
    Brookfield v.
Viscopaste PB7 gauze dressing
Viscoped insole
viscosimeter
    capillary tube plasma v.
ViscoSpot heel cushion
vise
    allograft bone v.
    AlloGrip bone v.
    Benda finger v.
    v. forceps

Gam-Mer v.
pin v.
torque v.
vise-grip pliers
Visi-Black surgical needle
Visica
    V. cryoablation system
    V. treatment system
Visicath
    V. endoscope
    V. viewing catheter
Visidex II blood glucose testing strip
Visidrape
    V. Mini Aperture drape
    V. Mini Incise drape
    V. ophthalmic drape
Visiflex drape
Visi-Flow
    V.-F. irrigation starter set
    V.-F. stoma cone
Visijet hydrokeratome
Visilex mesh
Visiline disposable sigmoidoscope
Visio-Gem color system
Vision
    V. camera
    V. Epic wheelchair
    Hydra V.
    V. Magnetom 1.5-tesla system
    V. MRI scanner
    V. PTCA catheter
    V. Sciences bronchoscope EndoSheath system
    V. Sciences VSI 2000 flexible sigmoidoscope system
    V. Ten V-scan scanner
Visiontech lens
Visiport
    V. optical trocar
    V. port
Visi-Spear eye sponge
Visitec
    V. angled lens hook
    V. anterior chamber cannula
    V. aspiration unit
    V. capsule polisher curette
    V. circular knife
    V. corneal shield
    V. corneal suture manipulating hook
    V. cortex extractor
    V. crescent knife

    V. double-cutting cystotome
    V. double iris hook
    V. EdgeAhead phaco slit knife
    V. I&A cannula
    V. intraocular lens dialer
    V. iris retractor
    V. lens
    V. lens pusher
    V. nucleus removal loop
    V. retrobulbar needle
    V. RK zone marker
    V. stiletto knife
    V. straight lens hook
    V. surgical vitrectomy system
    V. syringe
    V. Vico manipulator
    V. vitrectomy unit
Visi-Tube catheter
Vismark surgical skin marker
Vista
    V. Brite Tip guiding catheter
    V. Brite tip IG introducer guide
    V. disposable skin stapler
    V. pacemaker
    V. Tesla MRI scanner
Vistech wall chart
Vistec x-ray detectable sponge
Vistnes
    V. applier bar
    V. rubber band
visual
    v. obturator
Visual-Tech machine
Visuflo wand
Visulab system
Visulas
    V. argon laser
    V. Nd:YAG laser
    V. YAG laser
visuscope ophthalmoscope
Visx
    V. 2020 excimer laser
    V. STAR S3 ActiveTrak eyetracker
    V. Star S2 excimer laser
    V. Star S2 excimer laser system
    V. Twenty/Twenty system
    V. Wavefront system
    V. WaveScan wavefront system
Vitacrilic dental acrylic
VitaCuff
    V. antimicrobial cuff
    V. dressing

NOTES

V

VitaCuff *(continued)*
- V. infection control device
- V. tissue-interface barrier

Vita-Gel acrylic

Vitagraft
- V. arteriovenous shunt
- V. vascular graft

Vital
- V. French eye-needle holder
- V. general tissue forceps
- V. intestinal forceps
- V. lung-grasping forceps
- V. microsurgery needle holder
- V. microvascular needle holder
- V. needle holder forceps
- V. neurosurgical needle holder
- V. operating scissors
- V. skin stapler
- V. wire-cutting scissors
- V. wire twister

Vitalab
- V. Flexor clinical chemistry analyzer
- V. ViVa clinical chemistry analyzer

Vital-Adson tissue forceps
Vital-Babcock tissue forceps
Vital-Baumgartner needle holder
Vital-Castroviejo eye needle holder
Vital-Cooley
- V.-C. French-eye needle holder
- V.-C. general tissue holder
- V.-C. intracardiac needle holder
- V.-C. microvascular needle holder
- V.-C. neurosurgical needle holder
- V.-C. operating scissors
- V.-C. wire-cutting scissors
- V.-C. wire twister

Vital-Cooley-Baumgarten wire twister
Vitalcor
- V. cardioplegia infusion cannula
- V. venous return catheter

Vital-Cottle dorsal angled scissors
Vital-Crile-Wood needle holder
Vital-Cushing tissue forceps
Vital-DeBakey cardiovascular needle holder
Vital-Derf eye needle holder
Vital-Duval intestinal forceps
Vital-Evans pelvic tissue forceps
Vital-Finochietto needle holder
Vital-Fomon angular scissors
Vital-Halsey eye-needle holder
Vital-Heaney needle holder
Vital-Jacobson spring-handled needle holder
Vital-Julian needle holder
Vital-Kalt eye needle holder

Vital-Knapp
- V.-K. iris scissors
- V.-K. strabismus scissors

Vitallium
- V. alloy
- V. clip
- V. cobalt-chrome alloy prosthesis
- V. cup
- V. device
- V. drill
- V. Elliott knee plate
- V. eye implant
- V. Hicks radius plate
- V. implant material
- V. mesh component
- V. miniplate
- V. Moore self-locking prosthesis
- V. nail
- V. screw
- V. Wainwright blade plate
- V. Walldius mechanical knee plate

Vital-Masson needle holder
Vital-Mayo dissecting scissors
Vital-Mayo-Hegar needle holder
Vital-Metzenbaum dissecting scissors
Vital-Mills vascular needle holder
Vital-Neivert needle holder
Vital-Nelson dissecting scissors
Vital-New Orleans needle holder
Vitalock
- V. cluster acetabular component
- V. solid-back acetabular component
- V. talon acetabular component

Vitalograph
- V. aerosol inhalation monitor
- V. bacterial/viral filter
- V. BreathCO monitor
- V. Escort spirometer

Vital-Olsen-Hegar needle holder
Vital-Potts-Smith forceps
Vital-Rochester needle holder
Vital-Ryder needle holder
Vital-Sarot needle holder
VitalSAT pulse oximeter
Vital-Stratte needle holder
Vital-Wangensteen
- V.-W. needle holder
- V.-W. tissue forceps

Vital-Webster needle holder
Vita-Stat automatic device
Vitatron
- V. catheter electrode
- V. Diamond ICD
- V. Diamond II pacemaker
- V. E catheter

Vitax female catheter
Vit Commander vitreous cutter

Vitesse
    V. Cos laser catheter
    V. E-II coronary catheter
Vitoss synthetic bone
Vitox femoral head
Vitrasert intraocular ganciclovir implant
Vitrathene jacket
Vitrea 3D system
vitrectomy sponge
vitrector
    Alcon v.
    catheter v.
    Cilco v.
    CooperVision v.
    Frigitronics v.
    Kaufman v.
    Kaufman II v.
    Machemer VISC v.
    mechanical v.
    Microvit v.
    ocutome v.
    O'Malley v.
    Peeler-Cutter v.
    Peyman v.
    v. probe
    Storz Premiere Microvit v.
vitreophage
    Kaufman v.
vitreoretinal infusion cutter
vitreous
    v. aspirating cannula
    v. aspirating needle
    v. infusion suction cutter
    v. pencil
    v. scissors
    v. sweep spatula
    v. transplant needle
vitreous-grasping forceps
Vivalith-10 pacemaker
Vivalith II pulse generator
Vivant ultrasonic scaler
Vivatron pacemaker
Vivonex
    V. gastrostomy tube
    V. jejunostomy catheter
Vivosil
    V. implant
    V. prosthesis
Vix infant ventilator
VixOne nebulizer
ViziLite disposable light

V-lance
    V.-l. blade
    V.-l. knife
    V.-l. Sharpoint
V-Lok disposable blood pressure cuff
V5M
    V5M multiplane TEE transducer
    V5M transesophageal
    echocardiographic monitor
V-medullary nail
Vnus
    V. Closure catheter
    V. Closure vein reflux system
    V. Restore catheter
Vocare bladder system
VoCoM thyroplasty implant
Voda catheter
Vogel-Bale-Hohner (VBH)
Vogel-Bale-Hohner head holder
Vogelfanger-Beattie stapler
Vogelfanger blood vessel stapler
Vogel infant adenoid curette
Vogler hysterectomy forceps
Vogt-Barraquer corneal needle
Vogt toothed capsular forceps
voice
    v. button
    v. intensity controller
    v. prosthesis sizer
Void-Ease urine collection bag
Volk
    V. conoid implant
    V. conoid lens
    V. high-resolution aspherical lens
    V. Minus power noncontact adapter
    V. panretinal lens
    V. Plus power noncontact adapter
    V. QuadrAspheric fundus lens
    V. retinal scale adapter
    V. SuperField NC lens
    V. SuperPupil XL lens
    V. Super Quad 160 lens
    V. UltraField contact lens adapter
    V. yellow filter adapter
Volkmann
    V. bone curette
    V. bone hook
    V. finger retractor
    V. hand retractor
    V. pocket retractor
    V. rake retractor
    V. scoop

V

NOTES

Volkmann *(continued)*
    V. splint
    V. spoon
    V. vas hook
Voller curette
voltage amplifier
voltmeter
    digital v.
    electronic v.
    vacuum tube v.
Voltolini
    V. ear tube
    V. nasal speculum
Voltz wrist joint prosthesis
volume
    v. controller
    v. displacement spirometer
    v. ventilator
volume-cycled ventilator
volume-limited ventilator
volumeter
    Dräger v.
    foot v.
    hand v.
volumetric
    v. diffusive respirator
    v. infusion pump
Volurex incentive spirometer
Voluson
    V. sector transducer
    V. ultrasound system
Volutrol control apparatus
vomerine gouge
vomer septal forceps
von
    v. Andel biliary dilation catheter
    v. Eichen antral cannula
    v. Eichen antral wash tube
    v. Graefe cautery
    v. Graefe cystotome
    v. Graefe electrocautery
    v. Graefe fixation forceps
    v. Graefe iris forceps
    v. Graefe knife
    v. Graefe muscle hook
    v. Graefe strabismus hook
    v. Graefe tissue forceps
    v. Hippel mechanical trephine
    V. Lackum transection shift jacket
    v. Langenbeck periosteal elevator
    V. Mandach capsule fragment forceps
    V. Mandach clot forceps
    v. Petz apparatus
    v. Petz clip
    v. Petz forceps
    v. Petz intestinal clamp
    v. Rosen splint
    v. Saal medullary pin

    v. Seemen rongeur
    v. Szulec hook
vonSonnenberg-Wittich catheter
Voorhees
    V. bag
    V. needle
Voris intervertebral disc rongeur
Voris-Oldberg intervertebral disc forceps
Vorse
    V. tube-occluding clamp
    V. tube-occluding forceps
Vorse-Webster
    V.-W. forceps
    V.-W. tube-occluding clamp
Vortex
    V. Clear-Flow port
    V. router
    V. stabilization system
    V. tracheostomy tube
Vortx coil
Voxel system
VoxelView system
Voxgram digital holography system
Voyager Aortic IntraClusion device
Vozzle Vacu-Irrigator
VP
    ventriculoperitoneal
VPAP
    variable positive airway pressure
        VPAP II ST-A ventilatory assistance system
VPI
    VPI nonadhesive colostomy system
    VPI nonadhesive condom catheter
    VPI nonadhesive ileostomy system
    VPI nonadhesive urostomy system
    VPI stone basket
    VPI urinary leg bag
VPI-Ambrose resectoscope forceps
VPI-Jacobellis microhematuria catheter set
VP shunt
VS
    VS femoral stem
    VS shunt
VSI 2000 sigmoidoscope
V-slit lamp
V-Star laser
V-suture
    Marshall V-s.
V-type intertrochanteric plate
VueCath spinal endoscopic system
VueLock anterior cervical plate system
Vueport balloon occlusion guiding catheter
Vulcan
    V. ablator probe

V. EAS ElectroThermal
Arthorscopy System
vulcanite
v. bur
v. chisel
vulsellum
Bland v.
cervical v.
v. clamp
Donald v.
Fenton bulldog v.
v. forceps
Henrotin v.
Jacobs v.
Kelly v.
MGH v.
Seyand v.
Skene v.
Teale v.

Vu-Max vaginal speculum
Vuport balloon-occlusion catheter
V-Vac
V-V. suction device
V-V. suction unit
VVD mode pacemaker
VVI
VVI bipolar Programalith
pacemaker
VVI single-chamber pacemaker
VVI/AAI pacemaker
**VVIR single-chamber rate-adaptive
pacemaker**
VVT pacemaker
Vygantas-Wilder retinal drainage probe
Vygon Nutricath S catheter
Vynacron resin
Vynagel dental resin

NOTES

V

Wachenfeldt
  W. clip-applying forceps
  W. suture clip forceps
Wachsberger bur
WACH shoe
Wachtenfeldt
  W. butterfly clip
  W. wound clip
Wachtenfeldt-Stille retractor
Wackenheim clivus canal line
Wacker Sil-Gel 604 silicone cement
Wada-Cutter heart valve
Wada hingeless heart valve prosthesis
Wadia elevator
Wadsworth
  W. lid clamp
  W. lid forceps
  W. scissors
Wadsworth-Todd
  W.-T. cautery
  W.-T. electrocautery
wafer
  BCNU-impregnated polymer w.
  carmustine w.
  Coloplast w.
  Curagel w.
  Gliadel w.
  polyanhydride biodegradable
    polymer w.
  Stomahesive sterile w.
  Sur-Fit w.
  wax bite w.
Waffle
  W. mattress replacement system
  W. seating cushion
Wagener hook
Wagner
  W. antral punch
  W. apparatus
  W. bone lever
  W. distraction device
  W. knife
  W. laryngeal brush
  W. leg-lengthening distraction
    device
  W. resurfaced prosthesis
  W. revision hip system
  W. rongeur
Wainstock eye suturing forceps
waist belt
Wakeling fetal heart monitor
Walb knife
Waldeau fixation forceps
Walden-Aufricht nasal retractor
Waldenberg apparatus

Waldenstrom laryngeal forceps
Walden telescope
Waldeyer
  W. forceps
  W. ring
Waldmar link
Wales
  W. rectal bougie
  W. rectal dilator
WALK
  weight-activated locking knee
Walkabout oxygen conserver
walker
  AmbulMate w.
  W. articulator
  w. aspirator
  Body Armor w.
  Body Armor short leg w.
  CAM W.
  Castaway II fixed ankle w.
  Castaway leg w.
  w. cautery
  W. coagulating electrode
  W. coagulator
  Comfy w.
  w. corneal scissors
  w. corneal trephine
  Darco Body Armor w.
  Delta w.
  DH pressure relief w.
  EasyStep w.
  Equalizer air w.
  w. forceps
  front-wheeled w.
  W. gallbladder retractor
  Guardian w.
  hemiambulator w.
  W. hollow quill pin
  w. lid everter
  W. lid retractor
  Low Profile w.
  Lumex w.
  Maddacrawler prone support w.
  w. magnet
  Merry W.
  Moon W.
  Nextep Contour lower-leg w.
  Nextep Silhouette lower-leg w.
  obese w.
  ORLAU swivel w.
  pneumatic w.
  ProROM w.
  W. ring curette
  Rollator Nova w.
  W. ruptured-disc curette

W

walker *(continued)*
Sabel cast w.
W. scleral ruler
short leg w.
Steady Step w.
w. submucous elevator
w. suction tonsillar dissector
Sure-Gait folding w.
W. tonsillar needle
Urban W.'s
W. ureteral meatotomy electrode
3-wheel w.
Walker-Apple scissors
Walker-Atkinson scissors
Walker-Lee sclerotome
walking
w. brace
w. heel
w. heel cast
w. pole
Walk-'n-tone exerciser
Walk-Rite orthotic
Wallaby II phototherapy system
Wallace
W. cesarean forceps
W. Flexihub central venous
pressure cannula
W. pipette
Wallace-Maloney knife
Wallach
W. Bio-Tool sterilizer
W. cryosurgical pain blocker
W. cryosurgical pencil
W. Endocell endometrial cell
sampler
W. LL100 cryosurgical system
W. minifreezer cryosurgical
instrument
W. ZoomScope colposcope
W. ZoomStar colposcope
**Wallach-Papette disposable cervical cell
collector**
**Walldius Vitallium mechanical knee
prosthesis**
Wallgraft
W. endoprosthesis
W. endoprosthesis stent-graft
Wallich
W. abortion scoop
W. bone curette
W. placental scoop
Wallner interstitial prostate implanter
Wallstent
W. biliary endoprosthesis
W. delivery device
W. esophageal prosthesis
W. iliac endoprosthesis
Schneider esophageal W.
Schneider Magic W.

self-expanding Easy W.
W. self-expanding stent
W. spring-loaded stent
UroLume W.
Wal-Pil-O neck pillow
Walrus
W. Advancit catheter
W. Angioflus catheter
Walser
W. corneoscleral punch
W. matrix
Walsh
W. dermal curette
W. footplate chisel
W. hook
W. hook-type dermal curette
W. pressure ring
W. tissue forceps
Walsham
W. nasal septal forceps
W. septal straightener
W. septum-straightening forceps
Walter
W. corneal spud
W. nasal retractor
W. Reed implant
W. splinter forceps
Walter-Deaver retractor
Waltham-Street bougie
Walther
W. aspirating bladder trocar
W. female catheter
W. kidney pedicle clamp
W. pedicle clamp
W. tissue forceps
W. urethral dilator
W. urethral sound
Walther-Crenshaw meatal clamp
Walton
W. comedone extractor
W. curette
W. ear knife
W. foreign body gouge
W. meniscal clamp
W. meniscal forceps
W. rib shears
W. rongeur
W. round gauge spud
W. scissors
Walton-Allis tissue forceps
Walton-Liston forceps
Walton-Ruskin rongeur
Walton-Schubert
W.-S. punch
W.-S. uterine biopsy forceps
waltzing areolar lifter
Walzl hysterectomy forceps
wand
AccESS w.

ArthroCare plasma scalpel w.
Bevel w.
CollagENT w.
Connor straight nonirrigating w.
CoVac w.
Dome w.
Elekta viewing w.
ENTec Plasma W.'s
EVac Plasma w.
flexible w.
Hummingbird w.
irrigating Connor w.
Powell w.
programmer w.
ReFlex w.
straight Connor irrigating w.
Thera Cane massager w.
TriggerWheel w.
vaginal probe ultrasound w.
Viewing W.
Visuflo w.

wandering atrial pacemaker
Wang
W. applicator
W. lens
W. needle
Wang-Binford edge detector
Wangensteen
W. anastomosis clamp
W. apparatus
W. awl
W. deep ligature carrier
W. dissector
W. drain
W. dressing
W. duodenal tube
W. gastric-crushing anastomotic clamp
W. internal decompression trocar
W. intestinal forceps
W. intestinal needle
W. needle holder
W. patent ductus clamp
W. retractor
W. suction
W. suction unit
W. tissue forceps
Wangensteen-Vital needle holder
Wannagat
W. injection needle
W. suction tube
Wan sideport nucleus manipulator

Wappler
W. bridge
W. cold cautery
W. cystoscope with microlens optics
W. electrode
W. microlens cystourethroscope
W. pneumotome
W. polypectomy snare
W. resectoscope with microlens optics
Warburg apparatus
Ward
W. French-eye needle
W. French needle
W. nasal chisel
W. nasal osteotome
W. periosteal elevator
Ward-Lempert lens loop
Ware cancer cell collector
Warm
W. 'n Form lumbosacral back support
W. Springs brace
W. Springs crutch
warmer
Alton and Dean blood/fluid w.
Bair Hugger forced-air w.
Fenwal blood w.
fluid w.
gel w.
high-capacity fluid w.
hypothermia oxygen w.
Kreiselman infant w.
Maxone I.V. fluid/blood w.
Ohio w.
Omni infant heel w.
radiant heat w.
Thermasonic gel w.
Warm'N'Form insert
WarmTouch patient warming system
Warm-Up active wound therapy system
Warne penile sheath
Warren-Mack rotating drill
Warren splenorenal shunt
Warren-Wilder retriever
Warsaw hip prosthesis
Wartenberg
W. neurological hammer
W. pinwheel
Warthen
W. forceps

NOTES

W

Warthen *(continued)*
    W. spur crusher
    W. spur-crushing clamp
Wart Stick wart remover
Warwick-James dental elevator
Was-Catheter catheter
washer
    biconcave w.
    BioCuff w.
    w. crimper
    female w.
    Gravlee jet w.
    w. holder
    male w.
    Microwell w.
    Olympus Europe ETD automated
      endoscope w.
    plate-spacer w.
    rotation-stop w.
    Salzburg biconcave w.
    spiked w.
    Synthes ligament w.
    titanium spiked w.
WasherLoc
    W. implant
    W. tibial graft fixation device
washing catheter
washout cannula
Wasko common duct probe
wasp-waist laryngoscope
Watanabe
    W. apparatus
    W. arthroscope
    W. catheter
    W. pin
    W. pin holder
watchmaker forceps
Watco 2001 knee immobilizer
water
    w. bed
    W. Bike aquatic therapy machine
    w. cushion lithotripter
    w. dressing
    w. gauge
    W. Pik irrigator
    W. Pik toothbrush
    w. probe
    w. scalpel
Waterfield needle
water-filled balloon sheath
water-infusion esophageal manometry catheter
Waterlase Millennium laser
Waterman
    W. folding bronchoscope
    W. rib contractor
    W. sump drain
water-perfused catheter

Waterpillow
    Mediflow W.
Waters
    W. M-440 fixed wavelength
      detector
    W. muscle stimulator
    W. positioner
water-seal
    w.-s. chest tube
    w.-s. drain
water-sealed spirometer
Waterston-Cooley shunt
Waterston shunt
water-trap drain
Watson
    W. capsule
    W. duckbill forceps
    W. heart value holder
    W. skin graft knife
    W. speculum
    W. tonsil-seizing forceps
Watson-Cheyne dry dissector
Watson-Jones
    W.-J. bandage
    W.-J. bone gouge
    W.-J. bone lever
    W.-J. elevator
    W.-J. frame
    W.-J. guide pin
    W.-J. nail
    W.-J. traction
    W.-J. tractor
Watson-Williams
    W.-W. conchotome
    W.-W. ethmoidal punch
    W.-W. ethmoid-biting forceps
    W.-W. intervertebral disc rongeur
    W.-W. nasal polyp forceps
    W.-W. needle
    W.-W. sinus rasp
Watts
    W. locking clamp
    W. tenaculum
Watzke
    W. band
    W. cuff
    W. forceps
    W. silicone sleeve
    W. tire
Waugh
    W. dissecting diathermy forceps
    W. dressing forceps
    W. prosthesis
    W. tissue forceps
Waugh-Brophy forceps
wave-edge knife
waveform generator
waveguide catheter
2-wavelength near-infrared spectroscope

**WaveMap intracoronary pressure
system**
WaveScan wavefront system
wave-tooth forceps
Wave VM200 ventilator
WaveWire
W. guidewire
W. guidewireXact graft-fixation
system
W. pressure guidewire
W. wire
wax
Aluwax bite and impression w.
w. bite wafer
Bite wafer denture bite w.
bone w.
w. bougie
w. carver
Carver dental w.
w. curette
dental w.
Flex-E-Z w.
Flexo w.
Godiva w.
Horsley bone w.
Kwik w.
Parafil w.
PD dental w.
Peck inlay w.
Plastodent w.
Swissedent w.
Sylver-Wax dental w.
wax-removing spatula
3-way
3-w. bridge
3-w. Foley catheter
3-w. irrigating catheter
2-way catheter
Wayfarer prosthesis
Wayne tucker
W. D. Johnson epicardial retractor
wearable
w. cardioverter-defibrillator device
w. speech processor
Weary
W. brain spatula
W. nerve hook
W. nerve root retractor
Weaveknit
W. vascular graft
W. vascular prosthesis

Weaver
W. chalazion clamp
W. chalazion curette
W. chalazion forceps
W. sinus probe
W. trocar introducer
Webb
W. bolt
W. cannula
W. interchangable vein stripper
W. pin
W. retractor
W. stove bolt
**Webb-Balfour self-retaining abdominal
retractor**
Weber
W. aortic clamp
W. canaliculus knife
W. colonic insufflator
W. hip implant
W. iris knife
W. lens loop
W. lens scoop
W. Permalock
W. rectal catheter
W. tissue scissors
W. winged catheter
Weber-Elschnig
W.-E. lens
W.-E. lens loop
Web needle holder
Webril
W. bandage
W. dressing
web-spacer
C-bar w.-s.
Webster
W. abdominal retractor
W. coronary sinus catheter
W. infusion cannula
W. infusion tube
W. needle holder
W. orthogonal electrode catheter
W. ruler
W. skin graft knife
Webster-Halsey needle holder
Webster-Kleinert needle holder
Webster-Vital needle holder
Weck
W. astigmatism ruler
W. clamp
W. clip applier

W

NOTES

Weck *(continued)*
- W. coagulating suction tube
- W. dermatome
- W. disposable cannula
- W. disposable trocar
- W. electrosurgery pencil
- W. endoscopic suture punch
- W. eye shield
- W. Hemoclip ligating clip
- W. high-flow laparator
- W. hysterectomy forceps
- W. iris scissors
- W. knife
- W. microscope
- W. microsurgical tray
- W. Prep blade
- W. rectal biopsy forceps
- W. shears
- W. sponge
- W. suction tube
- W. suture-removal scissors
- W. suture scissors
- W. towel forceps
- W. uterine biopsy forceps
- W. wire-cutting scissors

Weck-Cel
- W.-C. dressing
- W.-C. implant
- W.-C. microsponge
- W.-C. sponge

Weck-Cell surgical spear
Weck-Edna nonperforating towel clamp
Weck-Harms forceps
Weck-Prep orderly razor
Weck-Spencer suture scissors
Wedeen wire passer
Weder
- W. dissector
- W. retractor

Weder-Solenberger
- W.-S. pillar retractor
- W.-S. tonsillar retractor

wedge
- w. adjustable cushioned heel
- w. adjustable cushioned heel shoe
- ball w.
- bumper w.
- C. B. T. bumper w.
- 45-degree spinal w.
- 55-degree tomography w.
- DePuy VertiGraft bone w.
- disconnect w.
- Duo-Cline contoured bed w.
- W. electrosurgical resection device
- w. filter
- Good 'N Bed w.
- inner heel w.
- Kaltenborn-Evjenth Concept Wedge mobilization w.

- knee w.
- Livingston peribulbar w.
- medial heel w.
- medial heel-and-sole w.
- medial sole w.
- Medline w.
- Medpor biomaterial w.
- membrane delamination w.
- Najo head w.
- Positex knee w.
- w. pressure balloon catheter
- w. resection clamp
- roof w.
- Saunders mobilization w.
- w. spirometer
- W. TAG suture anchor system
- Tempur PC seat w.
- Tepperwedge w.
- The W.
- tomography w.
- Trujillo LASIK enhancement w.

wedge-line needle
wedge-shaped support
Weeks
- W. eye forceps
- W. eye speculum
- W. needle

Weerda
- W. endoscope
- W. laparoscope
- W. laryngoscope

Wegenke stent exchange accessory
Wehbe arm holder
Wehmer
- W. cephalometer
- W. cephalostat

Wehrs incus prosthesis
Weider tongue depressor
Weidmann Spirette mouthpiece
Weiger-Zollner forceps
weight
- ankle w.
- w. boot
- EyeClose external eyelid w.
- Femina vaginal w.
- FemTone vaginal w.
- gold w.
- SutureGroove gold eyelid w.

weight-activated locking knee (WALK)
weightbearing brace
weighted
- w. glove
- w. posterior retractor
- w. tip
- w. vaginal speculum
- w. vest

weight-relieving orthosis
Weil
- W. ethmoidal forceps

W. implant
W. lacrimal cannula
W. pelvic sling
W. pelvic snare
Weil-Blakesley
    W.-B. conchotome
    W.-B. ear forceps
    W.-B. ethmoidal forceps
    W.-B. pituitary rongeur
Weil-modified Swanson implant
Weimert epistaxis packing
Weinberg
    W. rib spreader
    W. vagotomy retractor
Weiner
    W. cannula
    W. speculum
    W. tourniquet
    W. uterine biopsy forceps
Weingartner
    W. ear forceps
    W. rongeur
Weinmann SomnoMask mask
Weinstein
    W. horizontal retractor
    W. intestinal retractor
Weis chalazion forceps
Weise jack screw
Weisenbach sterile forceps holder
Weisman
    W. cannula
    W. ear curette
    W. forceps
    W. tenaculum
Weisman-Graves open-sided vaginal speculum
Weiss
    W. fixed wing epidural needle
    W. forceps
    W. gold dilator
    W. needle
    W. speculum
    W. spring
Weissbarth vaginal speculum
Weitlaner
    W. brain retractor
    W. hinged retractor
    W. microsurgery retractor
    W. retractor
    W. self-retaining retractor
Welch
    W. Allyn anal biopsy forceps
W. Allyn anoscope
W. Allyn dual-purpose otoscope
W. Allyn fiberoptic sigmoidoscope
W. Allyn flexible sigmoidoscope
W. Allyn halogen penlight
W. Allyn illuminated speculum
W. Allyn KleenSpec fiberoptic disposable sigmoidoscope
W. Allyn KleenSpec vaginal speculum
W. Allyn laryngoscope
W. Allyn laryngoscope blade
W. Allyn MicroTymp impedance tympanometer
W. Allyn operating otoscope
W. Allyn ophthalmoscope
W. Allyn PneumoCheck spirometer
W. Allyn pocket scope
W. Allyn proctoscope
W. Allyn rectal hook
W. Allyn rectal probe
W. Allyn Schiller AT-1, AT-2 electrocardiograph
W. Allyn Schiller SP-series spirometer
W. Allyn single fiber illumination headlight
W. Allyn standard retinoscope
W. Allyn streak retinoscope
W. Allyn suction tube
W. Allyn transilluminator
W. Allyn video colonoscope
W. Allyn video endoscope
Weldon miniature bulldog clamp
Wellaminski antral perforator
Weller
    W. cartilage forceps
    W. cartilage scissors
    W. meniscal forceps
    W. total hip joint prosthesis
Wellington
    W. Hospital vaginal retractor
    W. Hospital vaginal speculum
well-leg
    w.-l. holder
    w.-l. support
Wells
    W. enucleation scoop
    W. enucleation spoon
    W. forceps
    W. irrigator
    W. Johnson cannula

W

NOTES

Wells (*continued*)
  W. pedicle clamp
  W. scleral suture pick
  W. stereotaxic apparatus
  W. tractor
96-well scanning fluorometer
Wellwood-Ferguson introducer
Welsh
  W. cortex extractor
  W. cortex-stripper cannula
  W. flat olive-tipped
  W. flat olive-tipped double cannula
  W. iris retractor
  W. olive-tipped needle
  W. ophthalmic forceps
  W. pupil-spreader forceps
  W. rubber bulb erysiphake
  W. Silastic erysiphake
Wendl tube
Wenger slotted plate
Wepsic
  W. fiberoptic cautery
  W. suction tube
Werb
  W. angled stricturotome
  W. right-angle probe
  W. scissors
Wergeland
  W. double cannula
  W. double needle
Wertheim
  W. deep surgery scissors
  W. hysterectomy forceps
  W. kidney pedicle clamp
  W. needle holder
  W. splint
  W. uterine forceps
  W. vaginal forceps
Wertheim-Cullen
  W.-C. compression forceps
  W.-C. hysterectomy forceps
  W.-C. kidney pedicle clamp
  W.-C. kidney pedicle forceps
Wertheim-Navratil
  W.-N. forceps
  W.-N. needle
Wertheim-Reverdin pedicle clamp
Weser dental hinge
Wesley-Jessen lens
Wesolowski
  W. bypass graft
  W. Teflon graft
  W. vascular prosthesis
Wessex prosthetic valve
Wesson
  W. mouthgag
  W. perineal self-retaining retractor
  W. vaginal retractor

West
  W. blunt dissector
  W. blunt elevator
  W. hand dissector
  W. lacrimal cannula
  W. lacrimal chisel
  W. nasal bone gouge
  W. nasal chisel
  W. nasal dressing forceps
  W. plastic dissector
  W. Shur cartilage clamp
Westaby stent
West-Beck
  W.-B. periosteotome
  W.-B. spoon curette
Westcott
  W. biopsy needle
  W. conjunctival scissors
  W. curved tenotomy scissors
  W. double-end scissors
  W. micro scissors
  W. needle
  W. spring-action scissors
  W. stitch scissors
  W. tenotomy scissors
  W. utility scissors
Westcott-Scheie scissors
Wester
  W. meniscal clamp
  W. meniscectomy scissors
Westerman-Jensen needle
Westermark-Stille forceps
Westermark uterine dressing forceps
Western external urinary catheter
Westfield-style
  W.-s. acromioclavicular immobilizer
  W.-s. envelope sling
Westmacott dressing forceps
Weston rectal snare
Westphal
  W. gall duct forceps
  W. hemostatic forceps
wet
  w. bandage
  w. cup
  w. dressing
wet-field
  w.-f. cautery
  w.-f. coagulator
  w.-f. electrocautery
Wet-Stop enuresis alarm
wet-to-dry dressing
Weve electrode
Wexler
  W. catheter
  W. self-retaining abdominal
    retractor
  W. Universal joint abdominal
    retractor

W. vaginal retractor
W. X-P large abdominal retractor
Wexler-Balfour retractor
Wexler-Bantam retractor
Wextran sponge
whalebone
    w. eustachian probe
    w. filiform bougie
    w. filiform catheter
Wheaton
    W. brace
    W. bunion splint
    W. Pavlik harness
    W. tissue homogenizer
wheel
    w. bur
    Carborundum grinding w.
    Excell polishing w.
    pin w.
    shoulder w.
wheelchair
    Action Jr pediatric w.
    Action 4XP tilt system w.
    Amigo mechanical w.
    Applause Super-Hemi w.
    A-6S w.
    W. Buddy bag
    w. cushion
    Epic w.
    HiRider motorized lift w.
    Hoveround HVR 100 w.
    iBOT w.
    Invacare w.
    Jay J2 w.
    Kid-Kart w.
    Kusch'kin Ace w.
    Lumex lightweight w.
    Lumex Tilt-in-Space reclining w.
    Nitro w.
    w. pad
    power w.
    Pride Jazzy 1103 Mini electric w.
    Quickie Carbon w.
    Quickie EX w.
    Quickie GPS w.
    Quickie GP Swing-Away w.
    Quickie GPV w.
    Quickie Kidz Pediatric w.
    Quickie Recliner w.
    Quickie Ti w.
    Regency XLC power w.
    Rx Rocker w.

    self-propelling w.
    Skil-Care reclining w.
    Slam'r w.
    Spirea adjustable foldable w.
    Vision Epic w.
    Zippie 2 w.
    Zippie P500 w.
Wheeler
    W. blade
    W. cyclodialysis spatula
    W. cyclodialysis system
    W. cystotome
    W. discission knife
    W. graft
    W. iris knife
    W. iris spatula
    W. malleable-shape knife
    W. plaque forceps
    W. prosthesis
    W. spherical eye implant
    W. vessel forceps
3-wheel walker
whip
    W. appliance
    w. bougie
Whip-Mix articulator
whirlpool
whirlybird
    Hough w.
    w. needle
    w. probe
    w. stapes excavator
whisker
    slotted w.
whisk-packets dressing
Whisper
    W. guidewire
    W. Mist cool mist humidifier
whistle
    Bárány noise apparatus w.
    coaching w.
    Galton ear w.
    peak flow w.
    w. stent
Whistler bougie
Whistle-Stop wireless aversive stimulator
whistle-tip
    w.-t. drain
    w.-t. Foley catheter
    w.-t. ureteral catheter
Whitacre spinal needle

W

NOTES

Whitcomb-Kerrison
- W.-K. laminectomy punch
- W.-K. rongeur

white
- W. bone chisel
- w. braided silk suture
- W. clamp
- W. foam pessary
- W. glaucoma pump shunt
- W. mallet
- w. nylon suture
- W. Plume absorbent gauze
- W. scissors
- W. screwdriver
- W. tenaculum
- W. tonsillar forceps
- w. twisted suture

Whitehall Glacier pack
Whitehead-Jennings mouthgag
Whitehead mouthgag
White-Lillie
- W.-L. retractor
- W.-L. tonsillar forceps

White-Oslay prostatic forceps
White-Proud uvular retractor
Whiteside prosthesis
White-Smith forceps
WhiteStar power modulation technology
Whiting
- W. mastoid curette
- W. mastoid rongeur
- W. tonsillectome

Whitman
- W. arch support
- W. fracture appliance
- W. fracture frame
- W. plate

Whitmore bag
Whitmyer headrest
Whitney
- W. single-use plastic curette
- W. superior rectus forceps

Whitten fixation ring
Whittle spud
Whitver penile clamp
whole blood aggregometer
whole-body
- w.-b. counter
- w.-b. digital scanner
- w.-b. MR imaging system

Wholey
- W. balloon occlusion catheter
- W. Hi-Torque floppy guidewire
- W. Hi-Torque modified J guidewire
- W. wire

Wholey-Edwards catheter
Whylie uterine dilator

Wiberg
- W. fracture staple
- W. fracture stapler
- W. raspatory

Wichman retractor
wick
- Bone-Dri femoral surgical w.
- w. catheter
- w. dressing
- gauze w.
- glaucoma w.
- Pope w.
- Silastic w.
- Staar glaucoma w.

wicking glue patch
Wickman uterine forceps
wideband
- w. sector transducer
- W. urinary catheter

wide-base quad cane
wide-field eyepiece
wide-seal diaphragm
wide-tray bite relator
Widex hearing aid
Widner transilluminator
Wiechel scissors
Wiechel-Stille bile duct scissors
Wieder
- W. dental retractor
- W. pillar retractor
- W. tonsillar dissector

Wieder-Solenberger pillar retractor
Wiegerinck culdocentesis puncture set
Wiener
- W. antral nasal rasp
- W. corneal hook
- W. eye needle
- W. eye speculum
- W. hysterectomy forceps
- W. keratome
- W. MRI filter
- W. scleral hook
- W. suture hook
- W. Universal frontal sinus rasp

Wiener-Pierce
- W.-P. antral rasp
- W.-P. antral trocar

Wies chalazion forceps
Wiet
- W. graft measuring instrument
- W. otologic cup forceps
- W. otologic scissors
- W. retractor

Wigand endoscopic instrument
Wigderson ribbon retractor
Wiggle coronary guidewire
Wigmore plaster saw
Wikco ankle machine

Wikström
W. arterial forceps
W. gallbladder clamp
Wikström-Stilgust clamp
Wiktor GX Hepamed coated coronary artery stent system
Wi-Last-Ic thread
Wild
W. laser
W. lens
W. M 690 operating microscope
Wildcat wire
Wilde
W. ear forceps
W. ear polyp snare
W. ethmoidal forceps
W. ethmoidal punch
W. laminectomy forceps
W. nasal-cutting forceps
W. nasal-dressing forceps
W. nasal punch
W. nasal snare
W. septal forceps
Wilde-Blakesley
W.-B. ethmoidal forceps
W.-B. scissors
Wilde-Bruening
W.-B. ear snare
W.-B. nasal snare
Wilder
W. band spreader
W. cystotome
W. cystotome knife
W. dilating forceps
W. foreign body hook
W. lacrimal dilator
W. lens hook
W. lens loop
W. lens scoop
W. loupe
W. pick
W. scleral depressor
W. scleral self-retaining retractor
W. trephine
Wilde-Troeltsch forceps
Wildgen-Reck metal locator magnet
Wildhirt laparoscope
Wiles prosthesis
Wilgnath alloy
Wilkadium alloy
Wilke
W. boot

W. boot brace
W. boot prosthesis
Wilkerson
W. choanal bur
W. intraocular lens-insertion forceps
Wilkes self-retaining retractor
Wilkinson
W. ring-frame abdominal retractor
W. self-retaining abdominal retractor
Wilkinson-Deaver blade
Wilkins trephine
Wilkoro alloy
Willauer
W. intrathoracic forceps
W. raspatory
W. scissors
Willauer-Deaver retractor
Willauer-Gibbon periosteal elevator
Willett
W. clamp
W. placental forceps
W. placenta previa forceps
W. scalp flap forceps
William
W. Dixon Cratex point
W. Harvey arterial blood filter
W. Harvey cardiotomy reservoir
William-House suction-irrigator
Williams
W. back brace
W. cardiac device
W. cartilage knife
W. clamp
W. craniotome
W. cystoscopic needle
W. discectomy forceps
W. esophageal tube
W. eye speculum
W. gastrointestinal forceps
W. interlocking Y nail
W. internal pelvimeter
W. intestinal forceps
W. lacrimal dilator
W. lacrimal probe
W. L-R guiding catheter
W. microclip
W. microlumbar retractor
W. & Nicholson trephine
W. orthosis
W. perforator
W. rod

W

NOTES

Williams *(continued)*
- W. rod self-retaining retractor
- W. screwdriver
- W. splinter forceps
- W. tissue forceps
- W. tonsillar electrode
- W. Uni-Quad leg holder
- W. uterine forceps
- W. varices injection overtube
- W. vessel-holding forceps

Williamsburg forceps
Williamson biopsy needle
Williamson-Noble scissors
Williams-Watson ethmoidal punch
Williger
- W. bone curette
- W. ear curette
- W. elevator
- W. hammer
- W. raspatory

Willock respiratory jacket
Wills
- W. Eye Hospital cautery
- W. Eye Hospital ophthalmic forceps
- W. Eye lacrimal retractor
- W. spoon with spatula

Wilman clamp
Wilmer
- W. chisel
- W. conjunctival scissors
- W. iris forceps
- W. iris retractor
- W. iris scissors
- W. refractor

Wilmer-Bagley
- W.-B. iris expressor
- W.-B. lens expressor
- W.-B. retractor

Wilmer-Converse conjunctival scissors
Wilmington plastic jacket
Wilson
- W. amniotic trocar
- W. awl
- W. bimetric distalizing arch
- W. clamp
- W. foreign body forceps
- W. fracture appliance
- W. intraocular scissors
- W. retractor
- W. rib spreader
- W. spinal frame
- W. spinal fusion plate
- W. vein stripper

Wilson-Baylor amniotic trocar
Wilson-Cook
- W.-C. bronchoscope biopsy forceps
- W.-C. coagulation electrode
- W.-C. colonoscopy biopsy forceps

- W.-C. cytology brush
- W.-C. dilating balloon
- W.-C. double-channel sphincterotome
- W.-C. eight-wire basket stone extractor
- W.-C. endoprosthesis
- W.-C. esophageal prosthesis
- W.-C. esophageal Z-stent
- W.-C. feeding tube kit
- W.-C. fine-needle aspiration catheter
- W.-C. gastric balloon
- W.-C. gastroscopy biopsy forceps
- W.-C. grasping forceps
- W.-C. hot biopsy forceps
- W.-C. mini stent retriever
- W.-C. nasobiliary tube
- W.-C. needle electrode
- W.-C. NJFT-series feeding tube
- W.-C. papillotome
- W.-C. polypectomy snare
- W.-C. prosthesis repositioner
- W.-C. Protector wire guide
- W.-C. retrieval forceps
- W.-C. stent
- W.-C. stone basket
- W.-C. Tracer wire guide
- W.-C. tripod grasping forceps
- W.-C. wire-guided sphincterotome

Wilson-Kirbe speculum
Wilson-Mayo stand
Wiltberger spinous process spreader
Wiltek papillotome
Wil-Tex alloy
Wilton-Webster
- W.-W. coronary sinus thermodilution catheter
- W.-W. thermodilution pacing catheter

Wiltse
- W. cross-bracing spinal fixation system
- W. iliac retractor
- W. pedicle screw fixation system
- W. system H construct
- W. system single-rod construct
- W. system spinal rod

Wiltse-Bankart retractor
Wiltse-Gelpi self-retaining retractor
WinABP ambulatory blood pressure monitor
Wincor enucleation scissors
Windmill suction evacuation unit
window
- W. cervical plate system
- w. clip
- w. rasp
- w. rasp marker

windowed esophageal balloon
Winer catheter
wing
    w. clip
    suture w.
4-wing
    4-w. Malecot drain
    4-w. Malecot retention catheter
winged
    w. catheter
    w. retractor blade
    w. steel needle
Wingfield fracture frame
2-wing Malecot drain
Winkelmann circumcision clamp
Winquest tibial/femoral extraction
    system
Winsburg-White
    W.-W. bladder tube
    W.-W. retractor
Winston
    W. cervical clamp
    W. SD catheter
Winter
    W. elevator
    W. facial fracture appliance
    W. Helping Hand
    W. ovum forceps
    W. placental forceps
    W. splint
Winter-Nassauer placental forceps
Winternitz sound
wipe
    Alkare adhesive remover w.
    AllKare protective barrier w.
    Kimwipes absorbent w.'s
    Remove adhesive remover w.
    Sani-Cloth HB disposable w.
    Sani-Cloth Plus germicidal
      disposable w.
wire
    Amplatz torque w.
    Amplex guide w.
    Ancrofil clasp w.
    w. appliance
    atrial pacing w.
    auger w.
    Australian orthodontic w.
    Australian Special Plus w.
    Babcock stainless steel suture w.
    Baron suction tube-cleaning w.
    beaded cerclage w.

    Birtcher Hyfrecator cautery w.
    w. bivalve vaginal speculum
    bone fixation w.
    braided w.
    brass w.
    Brooker w.
    Bunnell pull-out w.
    cerclage w.
    Charnley trochanter w.
    circumdential w.
    Coffin transpalatal w.
    coiled spiral pusher w.
    Commander PTCA w.
    Compere fixation w.
    Conceptus Robust guide w.
    control w.
    Cope w.
    Cordis Stabilizer marker w.
    core w.
    coronary w.
    Cragg Convertible w.
    Cragg FX w.
    Cragg infusion w.
    crenulated tantalum w.
    w. crimper
    Crozat orthodontic w.
    w. cutter
    Dall-Miles cerclage w.
    delivery w.
    Dentaflex w.
    diathermy w.
    w. drill
    w. driver
    Drummond w.
    ear snare w.
    eel w.
    endocardial w.
    E Wildcat orthodontic w.
    extra-flexible w.
    extra stiff Amplatz w.
    w. fixation bolt
    flow w.
    FloWire Doppler w.
    Force w.
    Gigli spiral saw w.
    Gilmer w.
    Glidewire Gold surgical guide w.
    w. guide
    Hahnenkratt orthodontic w.
    Hancock temporary cardiac
      pacing w.
    high-torque w.

W

NOTES

wire *(continued)*
House piston w.
hydrophilic-coated guide w.
intermaxillary w.
interosseous w.
intracoronary Doppler flow w.
Isola w.
Isotac pilot w.
Ivy w.
Jarabak arch w.
J exchange w.
Johnson canaliculus w.
J retention w.
Katzen infusion w.
Killip w.
Kirschner w.
Kirschner boring w.
w. lid speculum
ligature tie w.
lingual w.
Linx extension w.
w. loop
w. loop stapes dilator
Lunderquist coat hanger w.
Luque cerclage w.
Luque sublaminar w.
magnet w.
Magnum w.
Markley orthodontic w.
Medi-Tech w.
w. mesh eye implant
w. mesh self-expandable stent
w. mesh stent
monofilament snare w.
Monorail guide w.
Mullan w.
nasal snare w.
needle-knife w.
Neivert-Eves tonsillar w.
nitinol shape-memory alloy w.
olive w.
outrigger w.
over-tying w.
pacing w.
w. passer
Pathfinder w.
PD orthodontic w.
platinum w.
platinum-iridium electrode w.
Prima FX laser w.
w. probe
protector plus w.
pusher w.
Quadcat w.
RadiMedical fiberoptic pressure-
  monitoring w.
rectangular w.
Remaloy w.

Remanium w.
Respond w.
RingMASTER guide w.
Roadrunner w.
Rotablator w.
Rotafloppy w.
round chuck-end Kirschner w.
Sadowsky hook w.
Sage w.
w. saw
Scimed-Choice floppy w.
w. scissors
Seldinger retrograde w.
w. side blade
Simcoe anterior chamber
  retaining w.
Sippy esophageal dilator pusher w.
w. snare
space-age w.
spinous process w.
w. splint
square w.
stainless steel w.
w. stapes prosthesis
Sterling-Spring orthodontic w.
Stertzer-Myler extension w.
stiffening w.
w. stylet
sublaminar w.
suture w.
tantalum w.
TherOx infusion guide w.
Thiersch w.
w. threader
w. tightener
titanium w.
tonsillar snare w.
Tracer ST w.
Trailblazer w.
trocar-point Kirschner w.
trochanteric w.
Truarch w.
w. twister
ultra-stiff w.
veneer retention w.
WaveWire w.
Wholey w.
Wildcat w.
Wironit clasp w.
Wirotom clasp w.
Wizdom guide w.
Zimaloy beaded suture w.
w. Zytor suture
wire-closure forceps
wire-crimping forceps
wire-cutting suture scissors
wire-fat ear prosthesis
wire-fixation buckle

wireguide
TFE-coated w.
TrueTorque w.
wire-guided
w.-g. hydrostatic balloon
w.-g. metal spiral retrieval device
w.-g. oval intracostal dilator
w.-g. papillotome
w.-g. polyvinyl bougie
w.-g. sphincterotome
wire-holding forceps
wire-loop
w.-l. keratoscope
w.-l. strut
wire-passing awl
wire-pulling forceps
6-wire spiral-tip Segura basket
wire-tightening clamp
wire-twisting forceps
wiring retractor
Wironit clasp wire
Wirosol investment material
Wirotom clasp wire
Wirovest investment material
Wirthlin splenorenal shunt clamp
Wisap
W. diagnostic/operating laparoscope
W. disposable cannula
W. disposable trocar
W. insufflator
Wisconsin
W. laryngoscope
W. laryngoscope blade
Wise
W. dilator
W. iridotomy laser lens
W. orbital retractor
W. sphincterotomy laser lens
Wis-Foregger laryngoscope
Wishard
W. catheter
W. ureteral catheter
Wis-Hipple
W.-H. laryngoscope
W.-H. laryngoscope blade
Wisorb
W. malleolar screw
W. spinal fusion system
Wissinger
W. rod
W. set

Wister
W. forceps holder
W. nipper
W. vascular clamp
Withers tendon passer
Wit portable TENS system
Witt dental light
Wittmoser optical arm
Wittner
W. cervical biopsy punch
W. uterine biopsy forceps
Witzel
W. enterostomy catheter
W. gastrostomy
Wixson hip positioner
Wizard
W. cardiac device
W. gamma counter
W. microdebrider
Wizdom guide wire
Woakes nasal saw
Wolf
W. antral needle
W. arthroscope
W. aspiration/injection system
W. biopsy forceps
W. biting-basket forceps
W. cataract delivery forceps
W. curved-basket forceps
W. delivery system
W. dermal curette
W. disposable cannula
W. drain
W. drainage cannula
W. endoscope
W. eye forceps
W. graft
W. hemostatic bag
W. implant
W. insufflation tubing
W. lithotrite
W. Loktite mouthgag
W. meniscal retractor
W. needle trocar
W. nephrostomy catheter
W. photolaparoscope
W. Piezolith 2300 lithotripsy device
W. prosthesis
W. resectoscope
W. return-flow cannula
W. rigid panendoscope

NOTES

W

Wolf *(continued)*
  W. rigid ureteroscope
  W. suction tube
  W. uterine cuff forceps
Wolf-Castroviejo needle holder
Wolf-Cottle trocar
Wölfe-Böhler
  W.-B. cast breaker
  Wölfe-Böhler cast remover
  Wölfe-Böhler plaster cast spreader
Wölfe-Krause graft
Wolfe loop electrode
Wolferman drill
wolffian drain
Wolff standup cheiroscope
Wolf-Henning gastroscope
Wolf-Knittlingen gastroscope
Wolf-Post rhinoscope
Wolfram needle electrode
Wolf-Schindler gastroscope
Wolfson
  W. forceps
  W. gallbladder retractor
  W. intestinal clamp
  W. spur crusher
  W. spur-crushing clamp
Wolf-Yoon
  W.-Y. applicator
  W.-Y. ring
Wollaston doublet
Wolvek
  W. fixation device
  W. sternal approximation fixation
  W. sternal approximator
Women's Tradition brace
WonderBrace Convertible
Wong-Staal scissors
wood
  W. aortography needle
  W. bulldog clamp
  W. colonic kit
  W. glasses
  W. lamp
  W. light
  w. roll dressing
  W. screw
  w. tongue blade
  w. tongue depressor
Woodbridge tube
Wooden
  W. Uniplane rocker
  W. Wobble balance board
Woodruff
  W. screw
  W. screwdriver
  W. spatula knife
  W. ureteropyelographic catheter
Woodson
  W. dental periosteal elevator

  W. double-ended dissector
  W. dural separator
  W. obstetrical spoon
  W. packer
  W. plug
  W. probe
  W. spatula
Woods Surgitek bra
Woodward
  W. antral rasp
  W. forceps
  W. retractor
  W. sound
  W. thoracic artery forceps
Woodward-Potts intestinal forceps
Woolley tibia punch
Wool'n Gel seating cushion
Wooten eye needle
Worcester
  W. City Hospital speculum
  W. instrument holder
Word Bartholin gland catheter
Work-Bruening diagnostic head
Workhorse percutaneous transuluminal angioplasty balloon catheter
workstation
  AquariusBLUE 2D/3D imaging w.
  Dimaq integrated ultrasound w.
  EnSite 3000 electrophysiology w.
  LEEP system 1000 w.
  Mayfield/Acciss stereotactic w.
  OB-View w.
  RAMS w.
  robot-assisted microsurgery w.
world standard Olsen bipolar cable
Worm curving suture passer
Worrall
  W. deep retractor
  W. headband
Worst
  W. corneal bur
  W. corneal contact glasses
  W. double-ended pigtail probe
  W. gonioprism contact lens
  W. iris claw lens
  W. lobster-claw lens
  W. Medallion lens
  W. needle
Wort antral retractor
Worth
  W. advancement forceps
  W. amblyoscope
  W. chisel
  W. cystotome
  W. muscle forceps
  W. strabismus forceps
wound
  w. clip
  w. closure forceps

w. drain
w. drainage collector
w. drainage reservoir
w. dressing
w. spreader
W. Stick Photo Facts Card
w. towel
wound-clip forceps
Wound-Evac kit
Woun'Dres collagen hydrogel wound dressing
WoundSpan Bridge II dressing
woven
w. cotton gauze
w. Dacron catheter
w. Dacron fabric graft
w. Dacron tube graft
w. elastic bandage
w. silk catheter
woven-tube vascular graft prosthesis
Wozniak Sur-Lok chuck
wrap
Ace w.
Action elbow w.
Action wrist w.
ArtAssist w.
bias w.
Biocell w.
BodyIce cold pack w.
braceRAP w.
CircPlus w.
Circulon w.
Coban self-adherent w.
Coflex w.
digit w.
DK 201 cryotherapy w.
Dura-Kold reusable compression ice w.
Dura-Soft soft-compression reusable ice or heat w.
Elasto-Gel hot and cold therapy cervical neck w.
Elasto-Gel shoulder therapy w.
Electro-Link joint w.
Flex-Wrap self-adherent w.
Ice Wedge hot/cold therapy w.
iodophor-impregnated adhesive w.
kastRAP w.
Kerlix w.
KneeRAP compressive w.
Kold W.
magnetic w.

3M Coban LF self-adherent w.
Nylatex w.
Ocu-Guard ophthalmic w.
Primer compression w.
shoulderRAP w.
Stimprene w.
super w.
SurePress compression w.
Tecnol ankle w.
thermal plastic w.
Thermoskin arthritic knee w.
Thermoskin back w.
Unna-Flex compression w.
Unna-Pak compression dressing and w.
Velpeau w.
wraparound
w. dressing
w. inactive electrode
Wratten 6B filter
wrench
Barton w.
beaded pin w.
Canakis w.
Cloward spanner w.
DynaTorq w.
Hagie w.
Halifax w.
Harrington flat w.
hexagonal w.
hex socket w.
Kurlander orthopaedic w.
Richmond subarachnoid w.
Santa Casa w.
slotted w.
socket w.
spanner w.
spinal slip w.
Stader w.
Stille w.
T-handle w.
T-handle nut w.
Thomas w.
Trinkle socket w.
Wright
W. Care-TENS device
W. fascia needle
W. knee plate
W. knee prosthesis
W. nasal snare
W. ophthalmic needle
W. peak flow meter

W

NOTES

1065

Wright *(continued)*
    W. peak flowmeter
    W. pneumatic tourniquet
    W. respirometer
    W. spirometer
    W. tonsillar snare
    W. Universal brace
Wright-Crawford needle
Wright-Guilford
    W.-G. curette
    W.-G. cutting block
    W.-G. double-edged knife
    W.-G. drum elevator
    W.-G. elevator knife
    W.-G. fenestrometer
    W.-G. flap knife
    W.-G. footplate pick
    W.-G. incudostapedial knife
    W.-G. middle ear instrument
    W.-G. roller knife
    W.-G. stapes pick
    W.-G. wire cutter
Wright-Harloe empyema trocar
Wrightlock spinal fusion system
Wright-Rubin
    W.-R. forceps
    W.-R. forceps guard
Wrigley forceps
wrist
    w. bandage
    Wrist Restore brace
Wristaleve support
wristband
    SeaBands acupressure w.
wrist-driven prehension orthosis
Wristlet
    Freedom USA W.
Writer
    STA-Pen W.
W-shaped
    W-s. forceps
    W-s. ileoneobladder
Wullen stone dislodger
Wullstein
    W. chuck adapter
    W. diamond bur

    W. double-edged knife
    W. drill
    W. ear forceps
    W. ear scissors
    W. endaural retractor
    W. high-speed bur
    W. microsuction tube
    W. ototympanoscope otoscope
    W. ring curette
    W. self-retaining ear retractor
    W. transplant spatula
    W. tympanoplasty forceps
Wullstein-House forceps
Wullstein-Paparella forceps
Wullstein-Weitlaner self-retaining retractor
Wunderer modification activator
Wurd catheter
Wurmuth spatula
Wurth
    W. spur crusher
    W. vein stripper
Würzburg
    W. maxillofacial plating system
    W. plate
Wurzelheber dental elevator
WuScope system
Wutzler scissors
Wyler subdural strip electrode
Wylie
    W. drain
    W. endarterectomy set
    W. endarterectomy stripper
    W. hypogastric clamp
    W. J vascular clamp
    W. lumbar bulldog clamp
    W. renal vein retractor
    W. spatula
    W. splanchnic retractor
    W. stem pessary
    W. tenaculum forceps
    W. uterine dilator
    W. uterine forceps
    W. uterine tenaculum
Wylie-Post rhinoscope
Wynne-Evans tonsillar dissector

Xact
    X. cushion
    X. graft-fixation system
X-Acto utility knife
Xanar
    X. 20 Ambulase CO_2 laser
    X. laser adapter
    X. laser bronchoscope
Xcalibur otologic drill
X-Cel dental x-ray unit
X-Cell valve
Xcelon nylon balloon material
XeCl excimer laser
Xemex pulmonary artery catheter
Xenaderm ointment
XenoDerm graft
xenograft
    Angell-Shiley porcine x.
    bovine x.
    bovine pericardial heart valve x.
    Carpentier-Edwards x.
    Ionescu-Shiley x.
    Ionescu-Shiley pericardial x.
Xenomedica prosthetic valve
xenon
    x. arc
    x. arc coagulator
    x. arc lamp
    x. arc photocoagulator
    x. cold light fountain
    x. flash lamp
    x. light source
xenon-chloride excimer laser
Xenophor femoral prosthesis
Xenotech prosthetic valve
Xercise
    X. band
    X. Tube resistive device
Xeroflo dressing
Xeroform
    X. dressing
    X. gauze
Xertube
    X. resistance band
    X. tube
XFix DynaFix system
Xia spinal system
Xillix
    X. LIFE-GI fluorescence endoscopy
      system
    X. LIFE-Lung system
Ximatron simulator
Ximed
    X. disposable cannula
    X. disposable trocar

Xi-scan fluoroscope
XKnife
    X. knife
    X. software for stereotactic
      radiation therapy
    X. stereotactic radiosurgery system
XL
    extra large
    XL illuminator
    Jung Autostainer XL
XL-11 Ranfac percutaneous
    cholangiographic catheter
X-long cement forceps
Xltek
    X. EEG
    X. electroencephalogram
Xoman drill
Xomed
    X. Audiant bone conductor
    X. Doyle nasal airway splint
    X. dual-chamber pacemaker
    X. endotracheal tube
    X. intraoral artificial larynx
    X. Kartush tympanic membrane
      patcher
    X. rectal probe
    X. Silastic splint
    X. sinus irrigation kit
    X. sinus secretion collector
    X. Skimmer shaver
    X. Treace ventilation tube
    X. Tytan ventilation tube
Xomed-Treace nerve integrity monitor
XO-soft-sole orthotic
Xpeedior series catheter
Xplorer 1000 digital imaging system
XP peritympanic hearing instrument
Xpress/SW helical CT scanner
Xpress/SX helical CT scanner
X-Press vascular closure system
XPS
    XPS Sculpture system
    XPS Straightshot micro tissue
      resector system
    XPS Striaghtshot micro tissue
      resector
XQ video instrument
x-ray
    x.-r. calipers
    x.-r. detectable laparotomy sponge
    x.-r. generator
    x.-r. image intensifier tube
    x.-r. overlay
    x.-r. spectrometer
    x.-r. tomographic microscope

X

Xsensor Pressure Mapping system
X-Sizer catheter
XT
    XT cardiac device
    InSound XT
    XT radiopaque coronary stent
X-Tend back protector
X-Tend-O knee flexer

Xtrac
    X. excimer laser
    X. laser system
X-Trel spinal cord stimulation system
X-Trode electrode catheter
XXL balloon dilatation catheter
Xyrel pacemaker

Y

Y adapter
Y B Sore cushion
Y connector
Y drain
Y hook
Y jaws
Y stent
Y tube

YAG

yttrium-aluminum-garnet
YAG laser

Yaghouti LASIK polisher
YagLazr system
Yale

Y. brace
Y. Luer-Lok needle
Y. Luer-Lok syringe

Yalon intraocular lens
Yamagishi

Y. stapler
Y. viscocanalostomy cannula

Yamanda knife
Yang needle
Yankauer

Y. antral punch
Y. antral trocar
Y. aspirating tube
Y. bronchoscope
Y. ear curette
Y. esophagoscope
Y. ethmoidal forceps
Y. eustachian catheter
Y. hook
Y. laryngoscope
Y. ligature passer
Y. middle meatus cannula
Y. nasopharyngeal speculum
Y. salpingeal curette
Y. salpingeal probe
Y. scissors
Y. septal needle
Y. suction tube
Y. suture needle
Y. tonsil suction tip

Yankauer-Little forceps
Yannuzzi fundus laser lens
Yarmo morcellizer
Yasargil

Y. Aesculap scissors
Y. aneurysm clip applier
Y. applying forceps
Y. arachnoid knife
Y. arterial forceps
Y. bayonet needle holder

Y. bayonet scissors
Y. bipolar forceps
Y. carotid clamp
Y. clip-applying forceps
Y. cross-legged clip
Y. curette
Y. dissector
Y. flat serrated ring forceps
Y. ligature carrier
Y. microclip
Y. microdissector
Y. microforceps
Y. microneedle holder
Y. microraspatory
Y. microscissors
Y. microvascular bayonet scissors
Y. microvessel clip-applying forceps
Y. neurosurgical bipolar forceps
Y. raspatory
Y. scalp flap retractor
Y. scoop
Y. spring hook
Y. suction tube
Y. tissue lifter

Yasargil-Aesculap aneurysm clip
Yasargil-Leyla brain retractor
Yashica Dental Eye II camera
Yazujian cataract bur
Y-bandage dressing
Y-bone plate
Y-connecting tubing
Yeates drain
Yeder suction tube
Yellen circumcision clamp
yellow-eyed dilating bougie
Yellow Springs probe
yellow-tip aspirator
Yeoman

Y. biopsy punch
Y. probe
Y. proctoscope
Y. sigmoidoscope
Y. uterine biopsy forceps
Y. uterine forceps

Yeoman-Wittner rectal forceps
Yield nonadherent gauze dressing
Y-Knot device
Yoon

Y. tubal sterilization ring

Yoon-ring applicator
Yoshida

Y. dental x-ray unit
Y. tonsillar dissector

You-Bend hemodialysis catheterization kit

Y

Youens lens
Youlten nasal inspiratory peak flow meter
Young
Y. anterior prostatic retractor
Y. bifid retractor
Y. bladder retractor
Y. boomerang needle holder
Y. bulb retractor
Y. cystoscope
Y. cystoscopic rongeur
Y. intestinal forceps
Y. lateral prostatic retractor
Y. ligature carrier
Y. lobe forceps
Y. needle holder
Y. pediatric rectal dilator
Y. prostatectomy forceps
Y. prostatic enucleator
Y. prostatic forceps
Y. prostatic retractor
Y. prostatic tractor
Y. renal pedicle clamp
Y. rubber dam fracture frame
Y. tongue forceps
Y. urological dissector
Y. uterine forceps
Y. vaginal dilator
Younge
Y. endocervical curette
Y. endometrial curette
Y. irrigator
Y. uterine forceps
Younge-Kevorkian forceps
Young-Hryntschak boomerang needle holder
Young-Millin boomerang needle holder
Younken double-lumen drain
Yours Truly asymmetrical external breast form
Y-port connector
YSI
YSI Foley probe
YSI neonatal temperature probe
YSI telethermometer
Y-trough catheter
yttrium-aluminum-garnet (YAG)
y.-a.-g. laser
Yuan screw
Yucca wood splint
Yueh centesis disposable catheter needle
Yu-Holtgrewe
Y.-H. blade
Y.-H. prostatic retractor
Yumiko-Lita catheter
Yund
Y. acetabular skid
Y. ligamentum teres knife
Yung percutaneous mastoid ventilator

Z

Z retractor
Z stent
Z Strong blood pressure device

ZAAG

Zest Anchor Advanced Generation
ZAAG dental implant system

Zachary-Cope clamp
Zachary-Cope-DeMartel colon clamp
Zaldivar

Z. anterior procedure (ZAP)
Z. degree gauge
Z. iridectomy forceps
Z. iridectomy scissors
Z. limbal relaxing incision marker
Z. reverse capsulorrhexis forceps

Zalkind-Balfour

Z.-B. blade
Z.-B. self-retaining retractor

Zalkind lung retractor
Zamorano-Dujovny localizing unit
Zander apparatus
Zang metatarsal cap
ZAP

Zaldivar anterior procedure
ZAP diamond knife

Zarski gallstone scoop
Za-Stent

Z.-S. biliary stent

ZA-Stent endoscopic biliary stent system
Zaufal bone rongeur
Zaufel-Jansen

Z.-J. bone rongeur
Z.-J. ear hook

Zavala lung biopsy needle
Zavod

Z. aneroid pneumothorax apparatus
Z. bronchospirometry catheter

Zawadzki
Z-Clamp hysterectomy forceps
Zebra exchange guidewire
Zeeifel angiotribe forceps
Zeichner implant
Zein loop
Zeiss

Z. aspheric lens
Z. Axioskop microscope
Z. binocular prism telescope
Z. carbon arc slit lamp
Z. cine adapter
Z. coagulator
Z. colposcope
Z. Endolive endoscope

Z. FF450 fundus camera
Z. goniolens
Z. gonioscope
Z. H laser
Z. IDO3 phase-contrast microscope
Z. lens loupe
Z. MD binocular
Z. operating camera
Z. operating field loupe
Z. operating microscope
Z. ophthalmoscope
Z. OPMI CS-NC2 surgical microscope system
Z. OPMI drape
Z. Opmilas surgical laser
Z. OPMI Mdo ophthalmic surgical microscope
Z. OPMI Pro magis microscope
Z. small beam splitter
Z. Super Lux 40 light source
Z. vertex refractometer
Z. Visulas 690s laser
Z. xenon arc photocoagulator

Zeiss-Barraquer cine microscope
Zeiss-Contraves operating microscope
Zeiss-Gullstrand loupe
Zeiss-Jena surgical microscope
Zeiss-Nordenson fundus camera
Zeiss-Scheimpflug camera
Zeitels

Z. UM glottiscope
Z. universal modular glottiscope

Zelicof orthopaedic awl
Zell pad
Zelsmyr Cytobrush
Zener diode
Zenith AAA endovascular graft
Zenker

Z. forceps
Z. raspatory
Z. retractor

Zenoderm dural implant
Zenotech

Z. graft
Z. synthetic ligament

Zephir anterior cervical plate system
Zephyr rubber elastic dressing
Zeppelin

Z. clamp
Z. obstetrical forceps

ZeroG pressure relief pad
ZeroRad body scan
ZeroTip nitinol stone retrieval basket
Zerowet Splashfield shield

Z

Zest
  Z. Anchor Advanced Generation
    (ZAAG)
  Z. Anchor Advanced Generation
    implant system
  Z. dental bone anchor
  Z. subperiosteal implant
Zeta
  Z. coronary stent
  Z. probe nylon filter
Zetafuge centrifuge instrument
Zeus
  Z. computer-controlled robotic
    system
  Z. surgical system
  Z. voice-controlled robotic system
Z-fixation nail
Zickel
  Z. II subtrochanteric rod
  Z. nail
  Z. supracondylar rod
Ziegler
  Z. blade
  Z. cautery
  Z. cautery electrode
  Z. ciliary forceps
  Z. electrocautery
  Z. eye speculum
  Z. iris knife
  Z. iris needle
  Z. lacrimal dilator
  Z. lacrimal probe
  Z. needle probe
  Z. wash bottle
Ziegler-Furness clamp
Zielke
  Z. bifid hook
  Z. curette
  Z. derotator bar
  Z. pedicular instrumentation
  Z. rod
  Z. scoliosis gouge
  Z. screw
zigzag stent
Zilver biliary stent
Zimalate twist drill
Zimaloy
  Z. beaded suture wire
  Z. cobalt-chromium-molybdenum
    alloy
  Z. epiphyseal staple
  Z. femoral head prosthesis
Zimberg esophageal hiatal retractor
Zimcode traction frame
Zim-Flux dressing
Zimfoam
  Z. finger splint
  Z. head halter

  Z. pad
  Z. pin
Zimmer
  Z. airplane splint
  Z. anatomic hip prosthesis system
  Z. antiembolism stocking
  Z. arthroscope
  Z. bone cement
  Z. bone-holding clamp
  Z. bur
  Z. cartilage clamp
  Z. Centralign Precoat hip prosthesis
  Z. clavicular cross splint
  Z. clip
  Z. CPT hip system
  Z. dermatome
  Z. extractor
  Z. fracture frame
  Z. goniometer
  Z. hand drill
  Z. low-viscosity adhesive
  Z. Orthair reamer
  Z. pin
  Z. Pulsavac wound debridement
    system
  Z. saw
  Z. saw blade
  Z. screwdriver
  Z. shoulder prosthesis
  Z. skin graft mesher
  Z. snare
  Z. suction irrigator
  Z. tibial locking screw
  Z. tibial nail cap
  Z. tibial prosthesis
  Z. Universal drill
Zimmer-Hall drive system
Zimmer-Hoen forceps
Zimmer-Hudson shank
Zimmer-Kirschner hand drill
Zimmer-Schlesinger forceps
Zimmon
  Z. biliary stent
  Z. catheter
  Z. endoscopic biliary stent set
  Z. endoscopic pancreatic stent set
  Z. esophagogastric balloon
    tamponade set
  Z. papillotome
  Z. sphincterotome
Zimocel dressing
Zim-Trac
  Z.-T. traction splint
  Z.-T. traction splint tractor
Zim-Zip rib belt splint
Zinco
  Z. Gunslinger II shoulder
    immobilizer
  Z. Hyperex thoracolumbar brace

zinc oxide bandage
Zinnanti
- Z. uterine manipulator (ZUMI)
- Z. uterine manipulator-injector catheter
- Z. Z-clamp clamp

Zinn endoillumination infusion cannula
zipper
- Z. antidisconnect device
- Z. Medical hypoallergenic tracheostomy tube neck band
- z. ring

Zippie
- Z. P500 wheelchair
- Z. 2 wheelchair

Zipser
- Z. meatal clamp
- Z. meatal dilator

Zipster rib guillotine
Zipzoc
- Z. medicated stocking
- Z. stocking compression dressing

Ziramic
- Z. femoral head
- Z. femoral head prosthesis

zirconia
- z. orthopaedic prosthesis
- z. orthopaedic prosthetic head

Ziskie operating laparoscope
Ziski iris clip intraocular lens
Zitron pacemaker
ZM-1 colonoscope
Z-Med balloon catheter
ZMR hip system
ZMS intramedullary fixation system
Zmurkiewicz
- Z. brain clip
- Z. clip applier

Zobec sponge dressing
Zoeffle soft intraocular lens
Zoellner
- Z. hook
- Z. needle
- Z. raspatory
- Z. scissors

Zoladex implant
Zoll
- Z. NTP noninvasive pacemaker
- Z. PD1200 external defibrillator

Zollinger
- Z. leg holder
- Z. multipurpose tissue forceps
- Z. splint

Zollinger-Gilmore vein stripper
Zollner suction tube
Zonas
- Z. porous adhesive tape dressing
- Z. porous tape

zone
- large loop excision of transformation z. (LLETZ)
- large loop excision of transition z. (LLETZ)

Zone Specific II meniscal repair system
zonule
- z. separator
- z. stripper

zoom
- Somatom Volume Z.

ZoomScope
- Z. colposcope
- Video Z.

Zoroc resin plaster dressing
Zower speculum
Zplate-ATL anterior spinal fixation system
Z-plate plate
Z-Sampler endometrial suction curette
Z-Scissors hysterectomy scissors
Z-stent
- Colonic Z-s.
- esophageal Z-s.
- Gianturco Z-s.
- modified Z-s.
- polyethylene-covered Z-s.
- Wilson-Cook esophageal Z-s.

ZTT acetabular cup
Zucker
- Z. multipurpose bipolar catheter
- Z. splint

Zucker-Myler cardiac device
Zuelzer
- Z. awl
- Z. hook plate

Zuker bipolar pacing electrode
Zuma
- Z. coronary guiding catheter
- Z. guiding catheter

ZUMI
- Zinnanti uterine manipulator
- ZUMI catheter

Zund-Burguet apparatus

NOTES

Z

Zuni
- Z. exercise system
- Z. gym
- Z. harness

Zurich
- Z. dilatation catheter
- Z. pediatric maxillary distractor

Zutt clamp
Zwanck radium pessary
Zweifel
- Z. angiotribe
- Z. appendectomy clamp
- Z. needle holder
- Z. pressure clamp

Zweifel-DeLee cranioclast
Zweymuller-Alloclassic prosthesis
Zweymuller hip prosthesis
Zyclast collagen hemostatic material
Zyderm
- Z. I or II collagen hemostatic material
- Z. I or II collagen implant

zygoma
- z. elevator
- z. hook

Zyler
- Z. head halter
- Z. tube

Zylik
- Z. cannula
- Z. microclip
- Z. ophthalmoendoscope

Zylik-Joseph hook
Zylik-Michaels
- Z.-M. retractor
- Z.-M. scissors
- Z.-M. speculum

Zyoptix laser
Zyplast injectable collagen implant
Zyranox femoral head
Zywiec electrode

Appendix 1
Illustrations

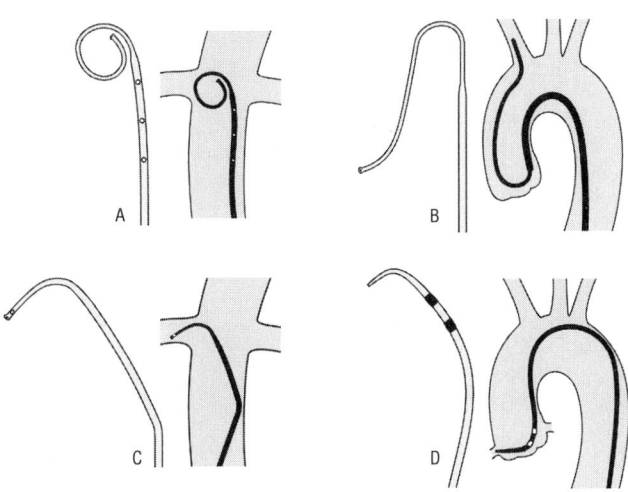

Figure 1. Angiographic catheters: (A) Aortic catheter with side holes; (B) Side-bending cerebral catheter (sidewinder); (C) Side-bending catheter for selective viewing of visceral vessels; (D) Judkins coronary catheter.

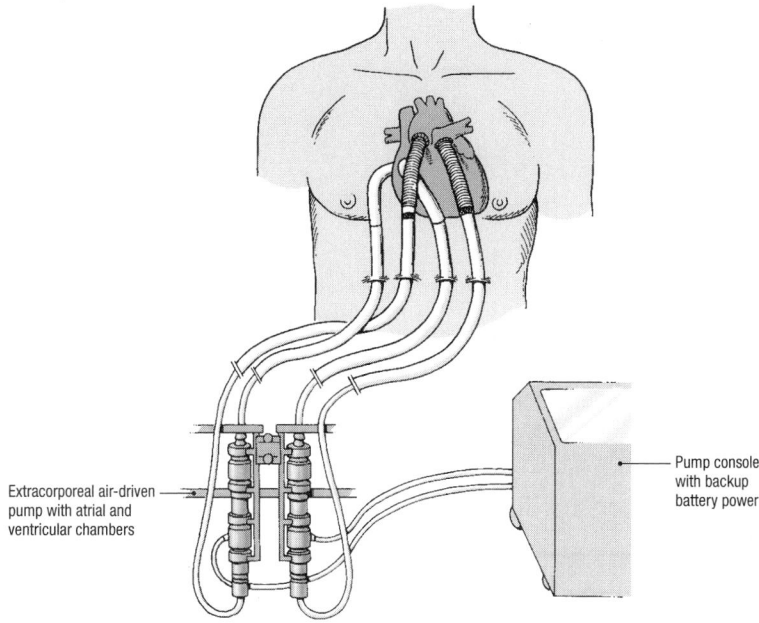

Pump console
with backup
battery power

Extracorporeal air-driven
pump with atrial and
ventricular chambers

Figure 2. Abiomed BVS-5000 biventricular support system.

Appendix 1

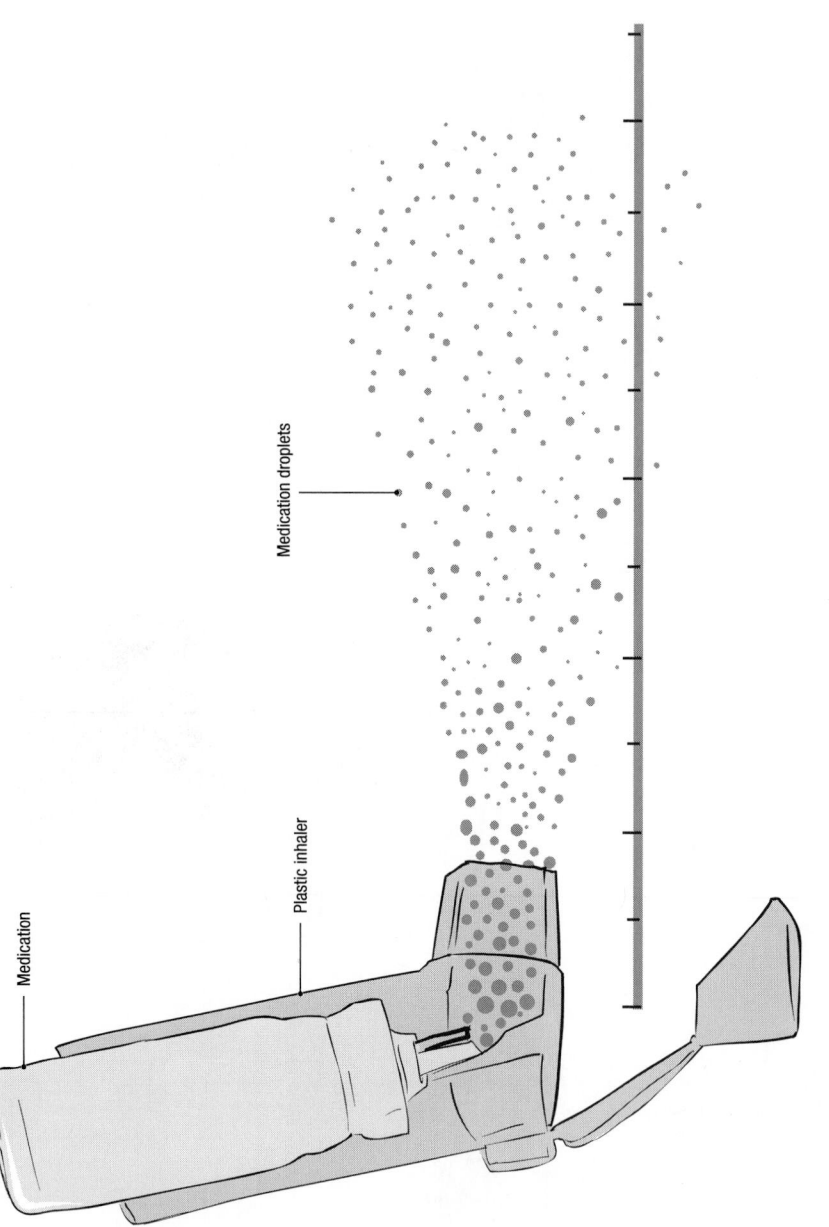

Figure 3. Metered dose inhaler (MDI).

A2

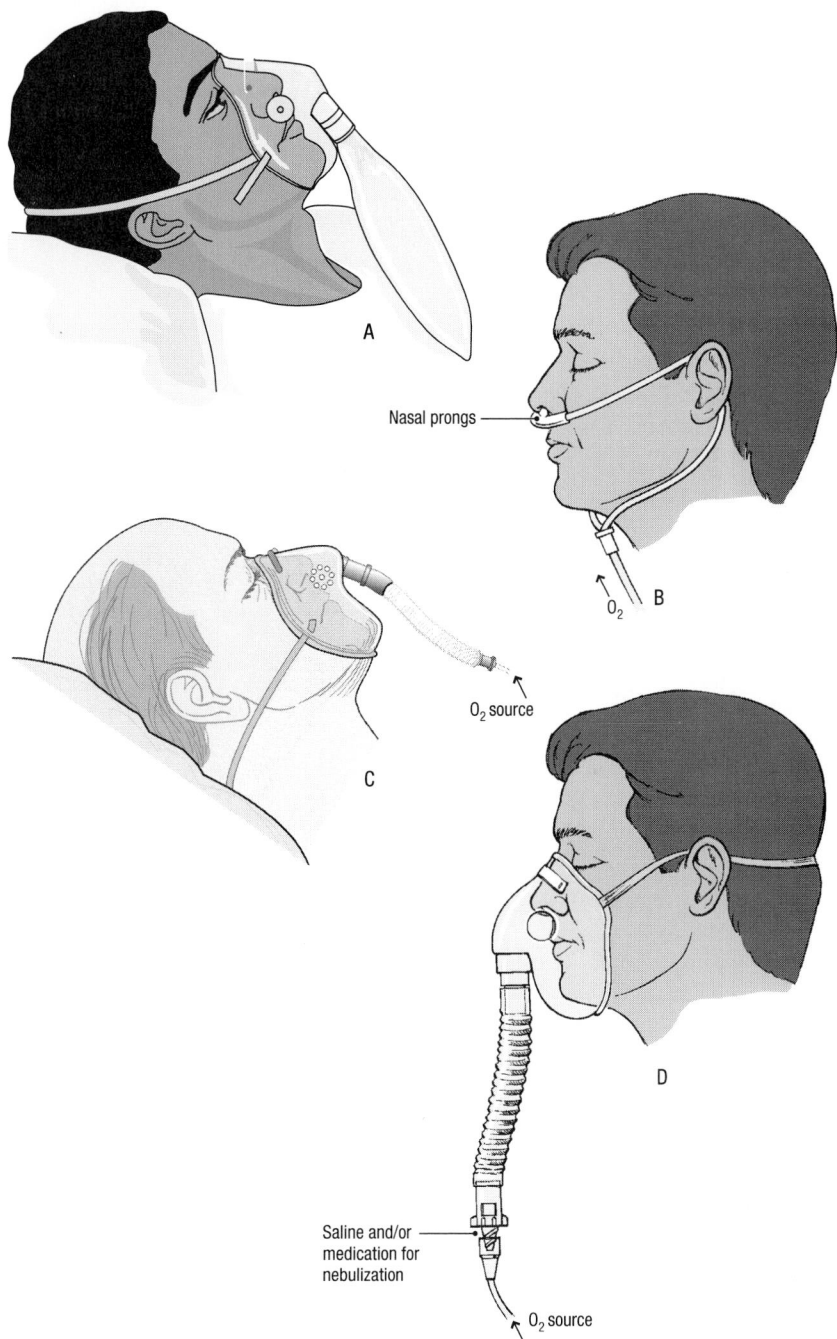

Figure 4. (A) Nonrebreathing mask; (B) Nasal oxygen cannula; (C) Ventimask; (D) Venturi mask with nebulizer.

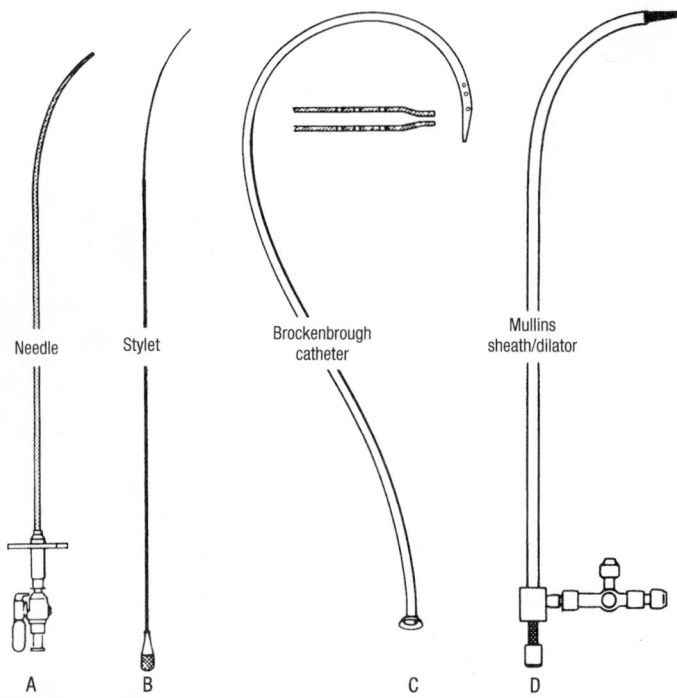

Figure 5. (A) Brockenbrough needle; (B) Bing stylet used in conjunction with the following: (C) Brockenbrough catheter; (D) Mullins sheath/dilator system.

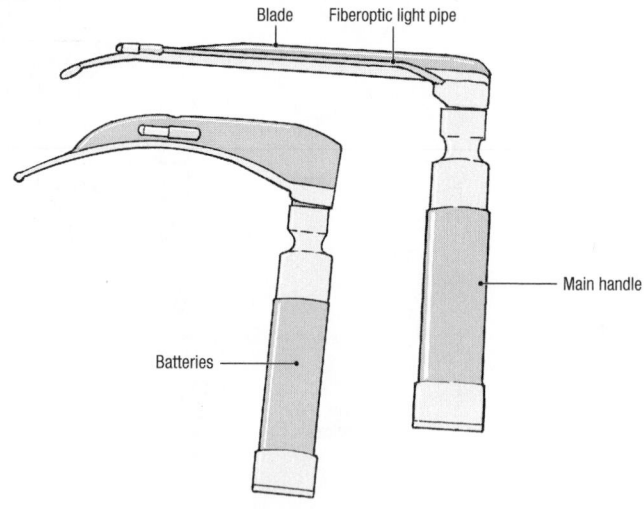

Figure 6. MacIntosh laryngoscope.

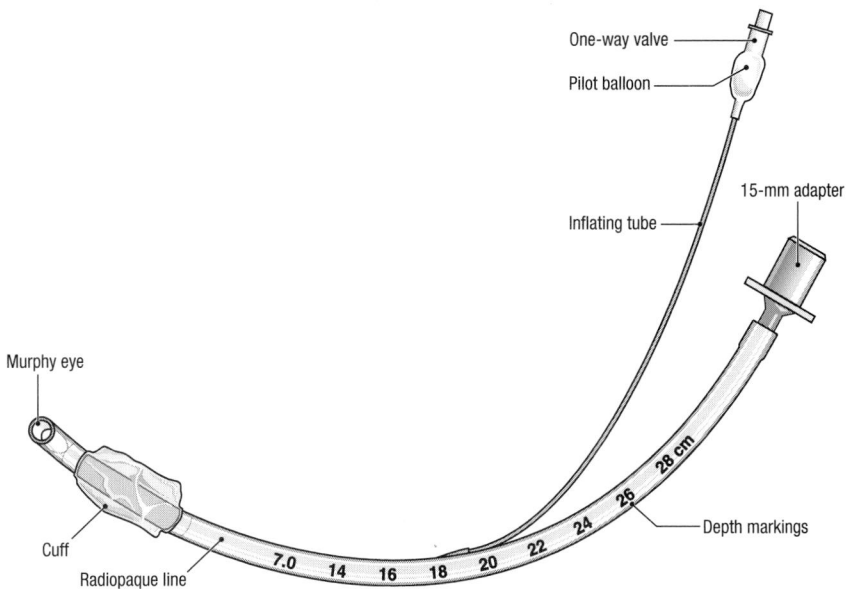

One-way valve

Pilot balloon

15-mm adapter

Inflating tube

Murphy eye

Depth markings

Cuff

7.0   14   16   18   20   22   24   26   28 cm

Radiopaque line

Figure 7. Parts of an endotracheal tube.

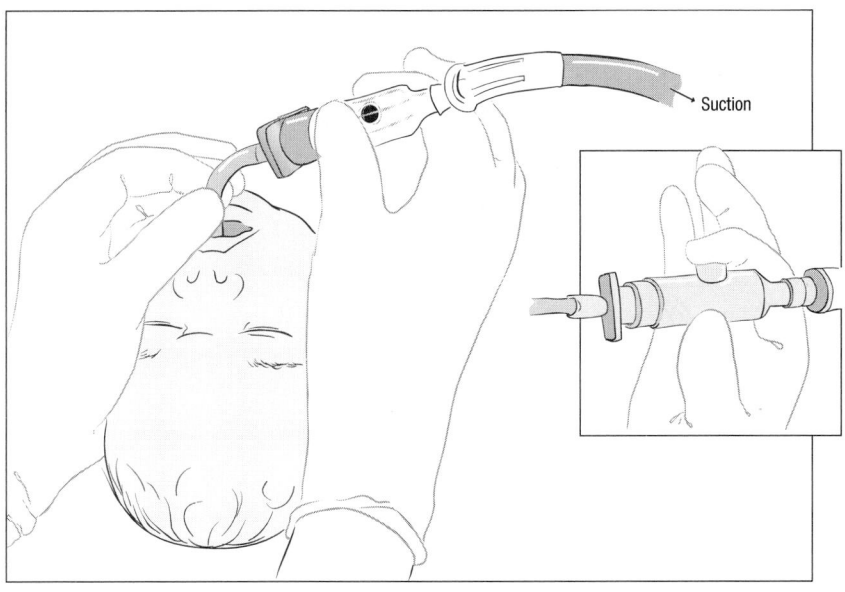

Suction

Figure 8. Meconium aspirator.

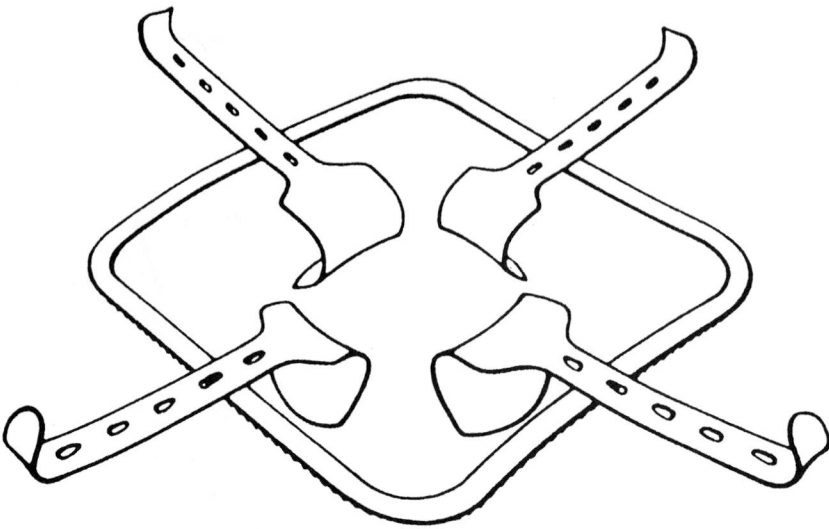

Figure 9. Kirschner abdominal retractor.

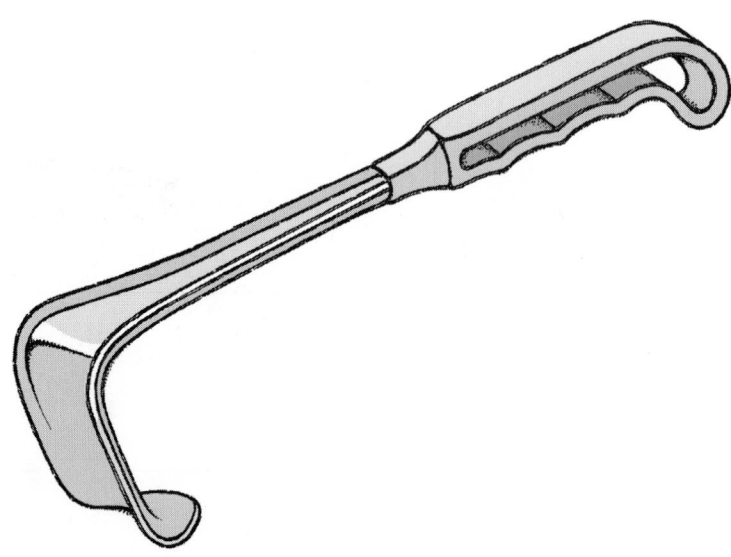

Figure 10. Abdominal retractor.

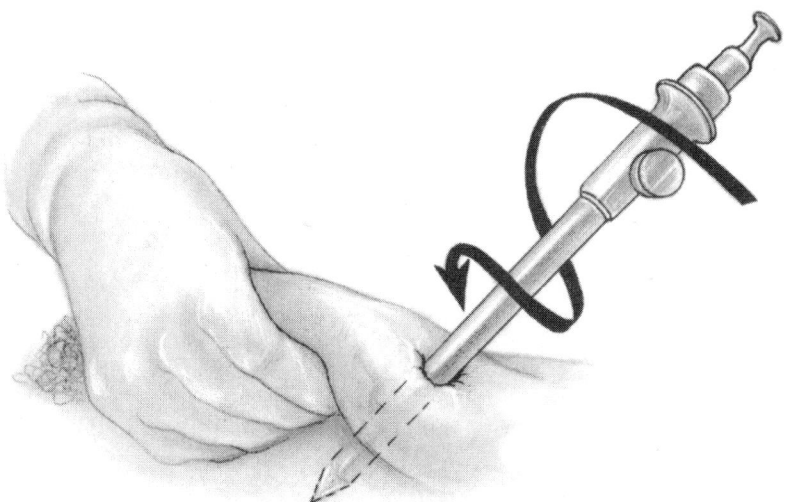

Figure 11. Trocar.

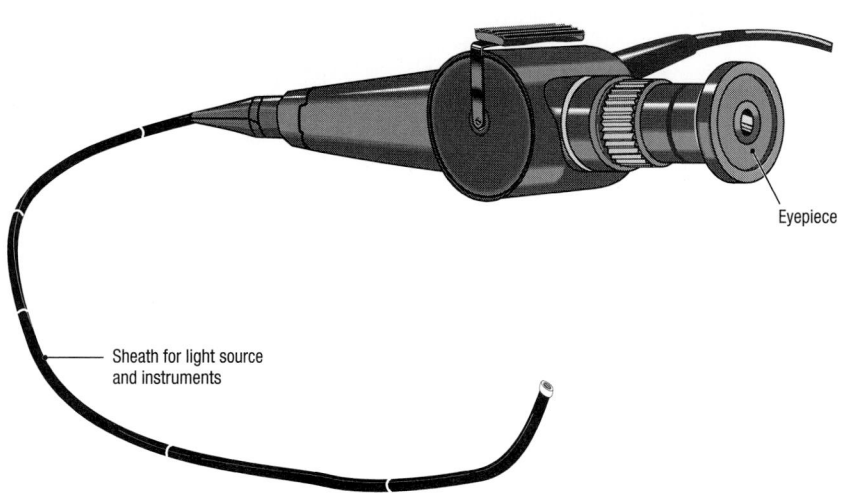

Figure 12. Endoscope.

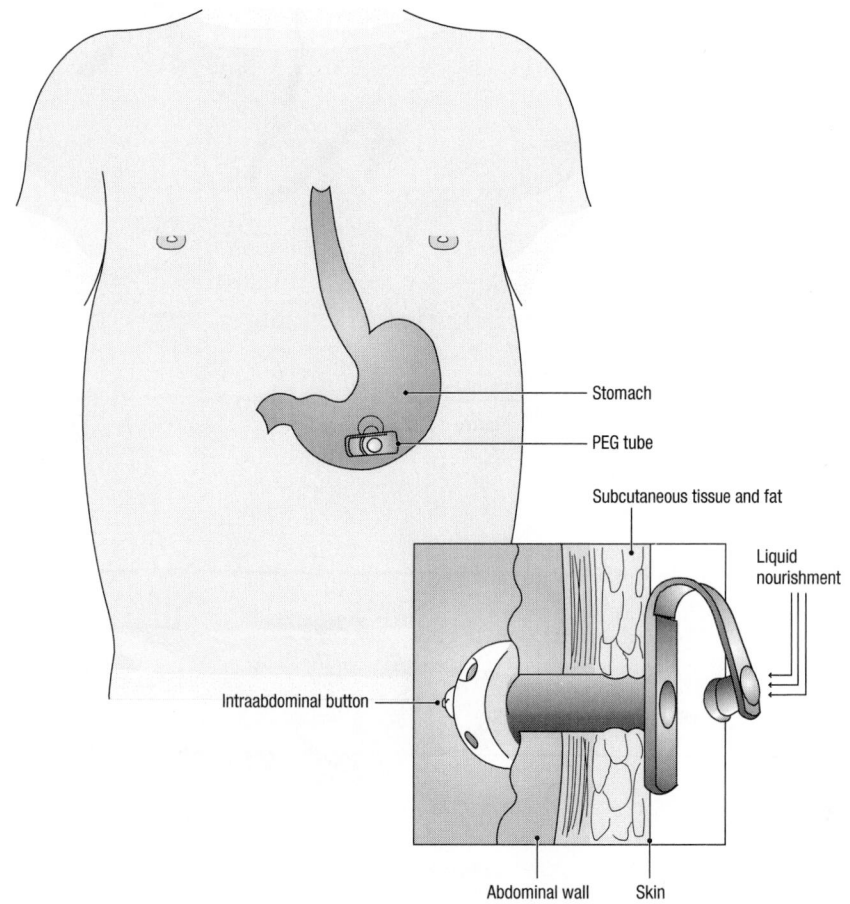

Figure 13. Percutaneous endoscopic gastrostomy (PEG) tube and button.

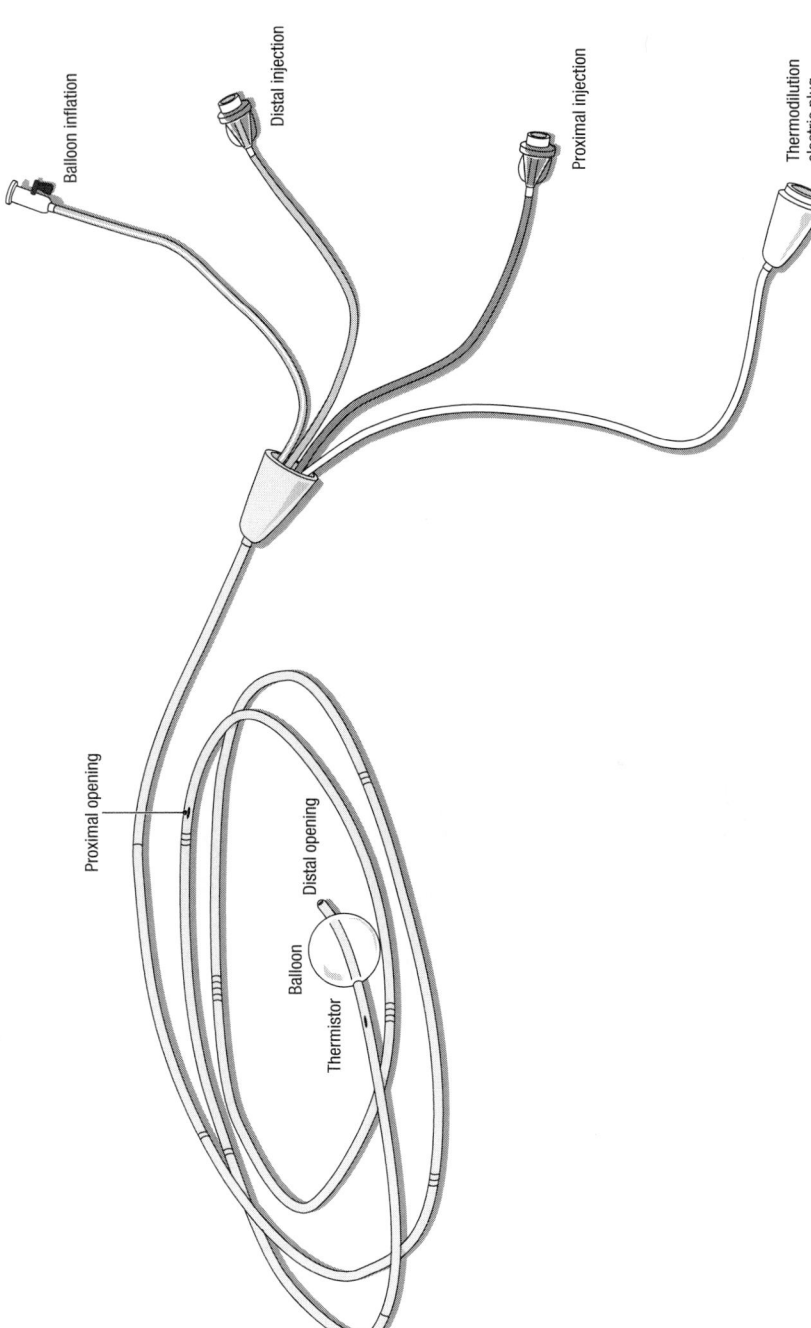

Balloon inflation

Distal injection

Proximal injection

Thermodilution electric plug

Proximal opening

Distal opening

Balloon

Thermistor

Figure 14. Swan-Ganz thermodilution catheter.

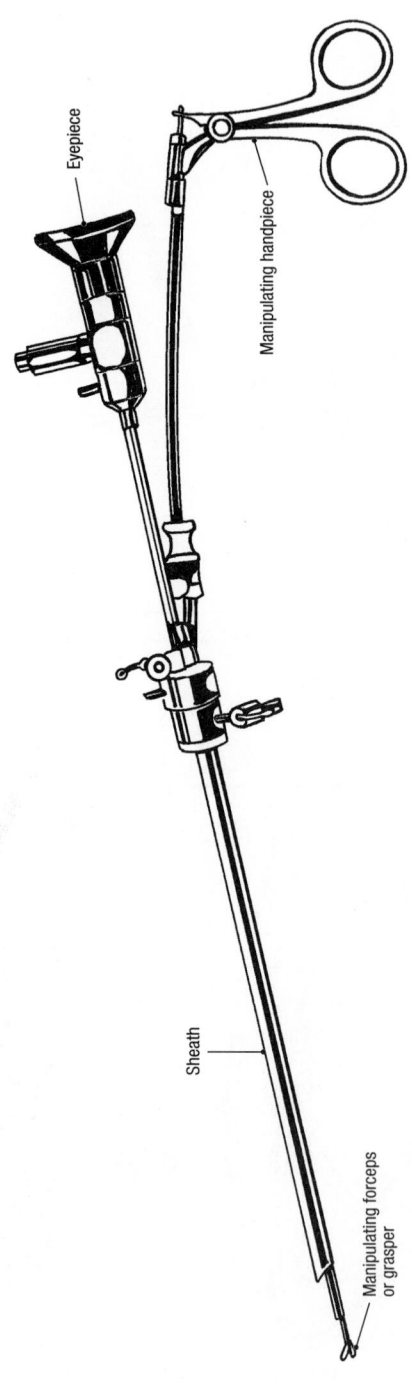

Eyepiece

Manipulating handpiece

Sheath

Manipulating forceps or grasper

Figure 15. Hysteroscope.

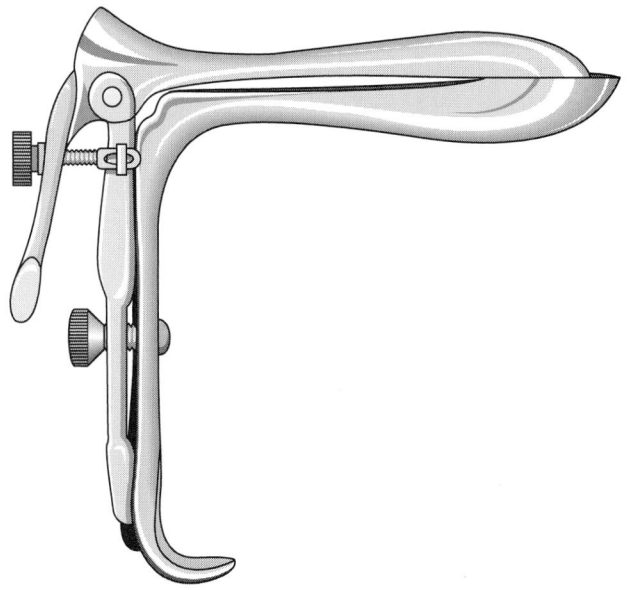

Figure 16. Vaginal bivalve speculum.

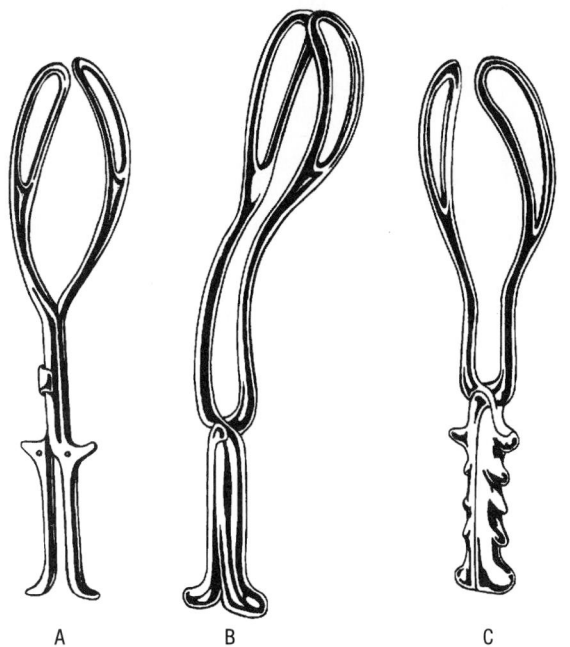

A   B   C

Figure 17. Obstetrical forceps: (A) Kjelland; (B) Piper; (C) Simpson.

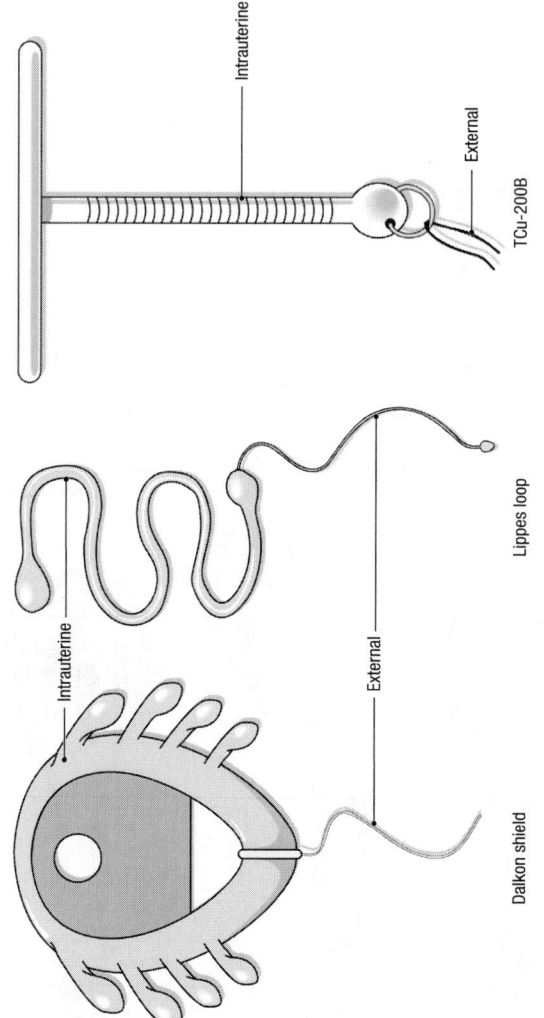

Figure 18. Intrauterine devices.

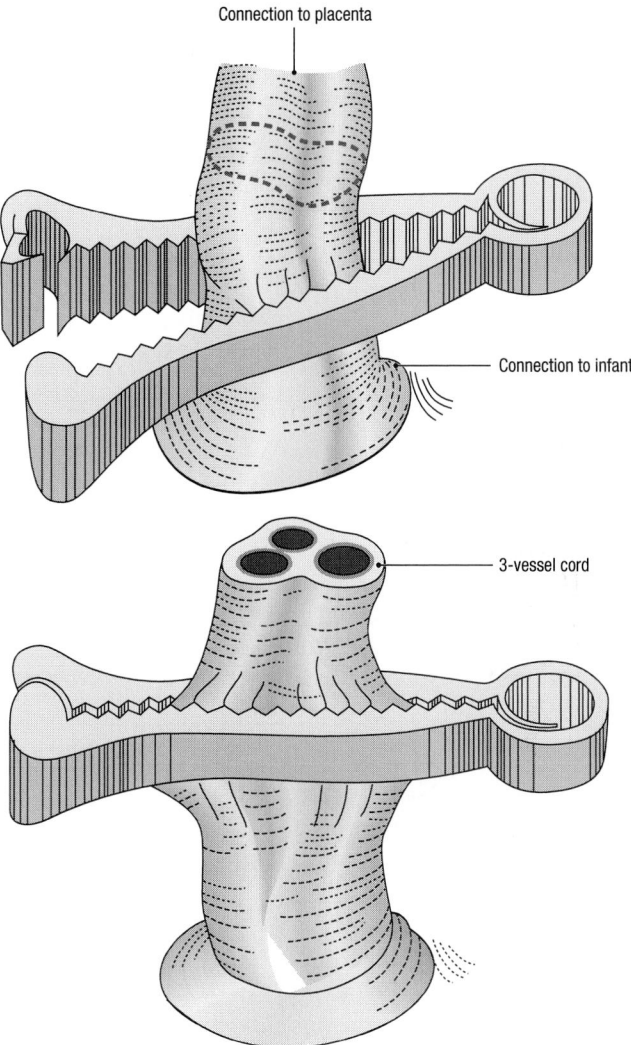

Figure 19. Umbilical cord clamp.

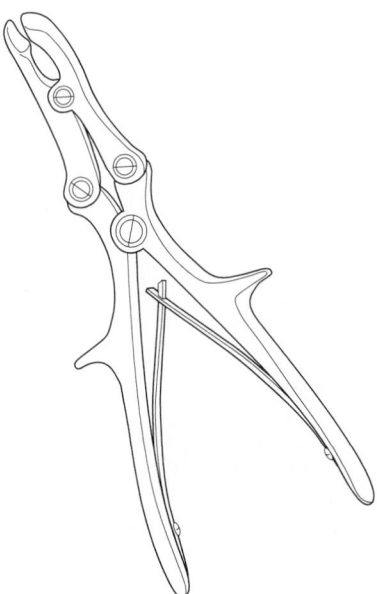

Figure 20. Rongeur.

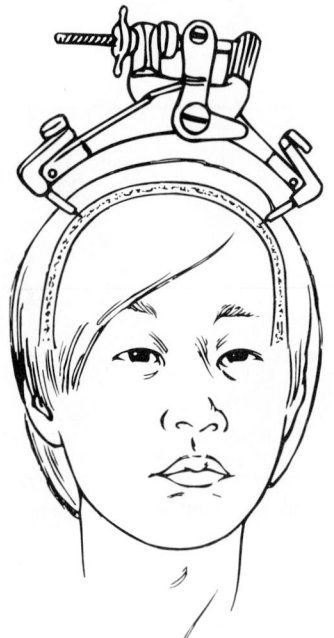

Figure 21. Raney-Crutchfield skull tongs.

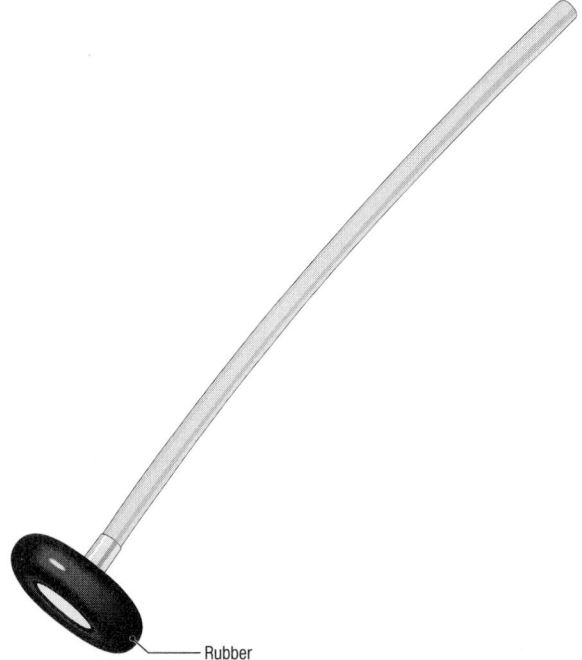

Rubber

Figure 22. Babinski percussion hammer.

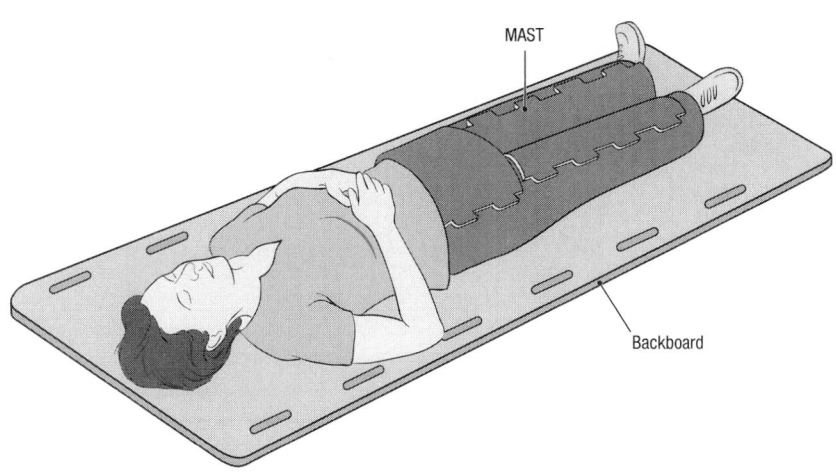

MAST

Backboard

Figure 23. Medical antishock trousers (MAST).

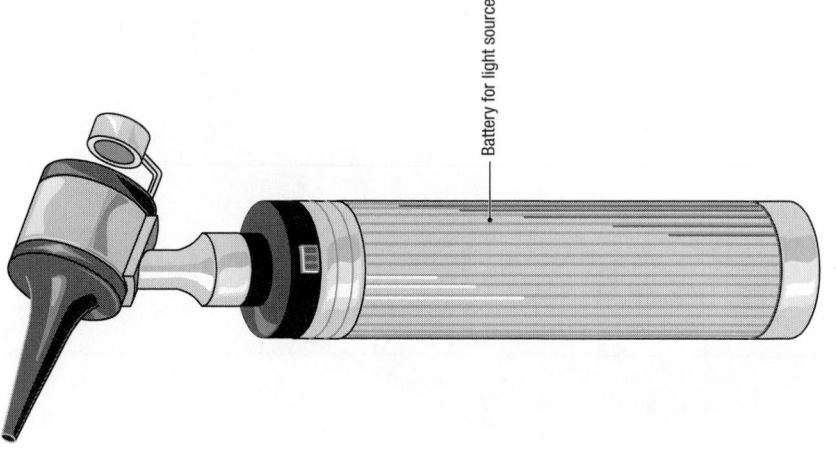

Battery for light source

Figure 25. Ophthalmoscope.

Battery for light source

Figure 24. Otoscope.

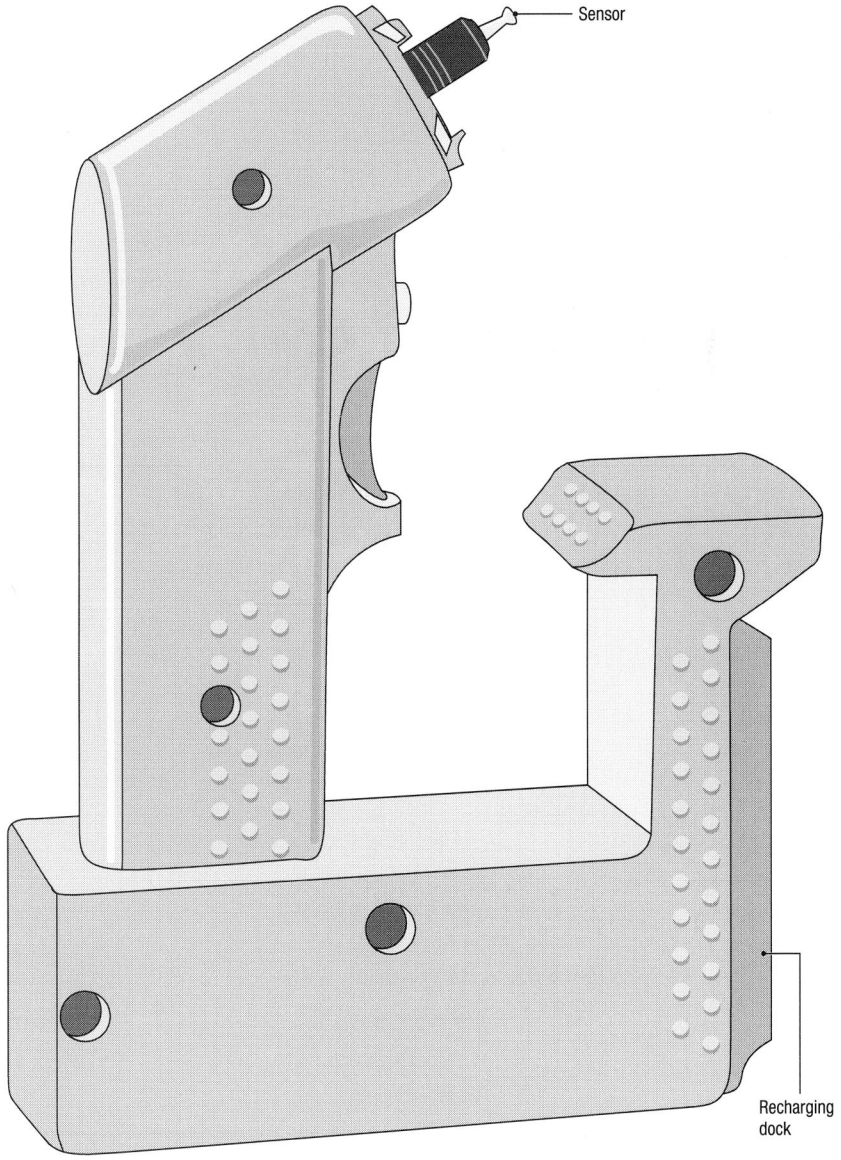

Sensor

Recharging dock

Figure 26. Tympanic membrane thermometer.

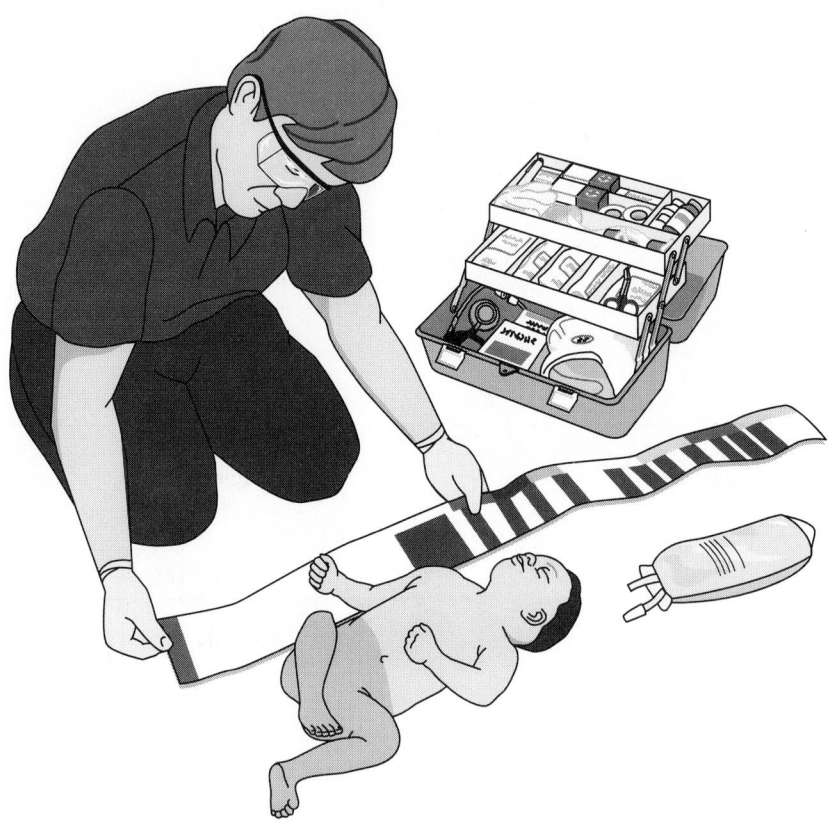

Figure 27. Broselow tape. Used to estimate body weight and tracheal tube size based on body length in small children.

Sample Reports and Dictation

CORONARY ARTERY BYPASS GRAFTING

PREOPERATIVE DIAGNOSIS: Coronary artery disease.

POSTOPERATIVE DIAGNOSIS: Coronary artery disease.

PROCEDURE PERFORMED: Coronary artery bypass grafting.

INDICATIONS: The patient was seen in preoperative consultation. The risks, benefits, and options were identified. The risks include damage to other organ systems, bleeding, infection, transfusion, anesthesia, and death. The patient elected to proceed with coronary artery bypass grafting.

DETAILS OF PROCEDURE: The patient was taken to the operating room, placed in the supine position. Radial artery catheter and Swan-Ganz catheter were placed. He underwent general endotracheal anesthesia. A Foley catheter was placed, and he was prepped and draped.

A saphenous vein was harvested from the leg. Multiple small skip incisions were made over the saphenous vein. Branch points were controlled with clips and ties. After the vein was excised, the wound was irrigated with antibiotic and closed with running Vicryl and a running, subcuticular Vicryl.

A vertical midline skin incision was made. This was carried down to the sternum. The sternum was divided with a saw. The mammary artery was harvested with clip and cautery technique. Prior to dividing the mammary artery distally, the patient was systemically heparinized. The mammary artery was divided, sprayed externally with a papaverine solution and then stored in papaverine-soaked sponge. The pericardium was incised. Pericardial stay sutures were placed. Deep pericardial sutures were placed. The octopus retractor was used. Distal vessels were controlled with silastic tapes.

By coronary angiography the PDA had a 50% proximal lesion; however, on visual inspection of this artery, it was much more heavily diseased. The saphenous vein was anastomosed to it with a running 7–0 Prolene suture in an end-to-side fashion. A side-to-side anastomosis was then performed to the posterior lateral branch of the right coronary artery with a 7–0 Prolene in a side-to-side fashion. Following this, a side-to-side anastomosis was performed of the obtuse marginal with a 7–0 Prolene suture. A partial occlusion clamp was placed. Two holes were created. The proximal anastomosis was created with 6–0 Prolene suture in an end-to-side fashion. A free segment of reverse saphenous vein was anastomosed to the aorta with 6–0 Prolene suture in an end-to-side fashion. The partial occlusion clamp was removed and the vein grafts de-aired. A side-to-side anastomosis was then performed to the lower 2 diagonals with a 7–0 Prolene in a side-to-side manner. Following this, an end-to-side anastomosis was performed with the higher of the 2 diagonals in an end-to-side manner to perform a sequential vein graft. The left internal mammary artery was then anastomosed to the LAD with a 7–0 Prolene suture in an end-to-side fashion.

We radiographed the LAD out distally, and the mammary artery was taken beyond its bifurcation. The mammary artery was slightly smaller beyond its bifurcation, however it was a usable conduit. This was noted. In the event the patient was to have coronary angiography, we may notice some tapering of the mammary artery itself right before the LAD anastomosis.

Then protamine was given. Blake drains were placed. Once we were satisfied with hemostasis, the sternum was reapproximated with stainless steel wires. The subcutaneous tissues were irrigated with antibiotic and closed with running Vicryl and the skin was closed with running subcuticular Vicryl.

EXTRACAPSULAR CATARACT EXTRACTION WITH INSERTION OF INTRAOCULAR LENS

PREOPERATIVE DIAGNOSIS: Visually significant cataract.

POSTOPERATIVE DIAGNOSIS: Visually significant cataract.

PROCEDURE PERFORMED: Extracapsular cataract extraction with insertion of an intraocular lens, left eye.

DETAILS OF PROCEDURE: Prior to surgery, a Honan intraocular pressure reducer balloon was placed over the left eye. The balloon pressure was then inflated to 30 mmHg and allowed to remain in place prior to surgery. The patient was taken to the operating room where local anesthesia was administered with lidocaine 2% with epinephrine for a Nadbath lid block. Retrobulbar anesthesia and akinesia were achieved with an equal mixture of Marcaine 0.75% with epinephrine and lidocaine 4% along with Wydase. The patient was then prepped and draped in the usual sterile ophthalmic manner and attention was directed to the left eye.

A lid speculum was inserted between the lids, and the intraocular pressure was measured with a Schiotz tonometer. The remainder of the procedure was conducted through the use of the Weck ophthalmic microscope.

The eye was stabilized with a 4–0 black silk superior rectus traction suture and was subsequently deflected downward. A limbal peritomy was performed with Westcott scissors from 10 o'clock around to 2 o'clock. Eraser bipolar cautery was utilized to affect hemostasis. A scleral incision was made 2 mm superior to the superior limbus with a 6610 Beaver blade to one-half the depth of the sclera for 12 mm in length. The dissection was then carried posteriorly from the base of the incision into clear cornea. A #75 Beaver blade was utilized to create a stab wound into clear cornea at 2 o'clock to provide an access port. A keratome was utilized to enter the anterior chamber through the base of the corneoscleral wound at 10 o'clock.

Healon was injected into the anterior chamber through a cystitome needle. The needle was subsequently used to affect an anterior capsulotomy, and capsular forceps were utilized to affect a circular tear capsulorrhexis capsulotomy. Balanced salt solution was injected underneath the capsule to dissect the nucleus free from the capsule.

The 10 o'clock incision was then enlarged with right and left cutting corneoscleral scissors to 12 mm in length. Through the use of a lens loop and Colibri forceps, the nucleus was expressed through the wound. Two interrupted 10–0 nylon sutures were then inserted through the corneoscleral wound, dividing the wound into equal thirds.

A Cavitron irrigation and aspiration tip was inserted through the wound, and lens cortical material was irrigated and aspirated. Following this, the posterior capsule was noted to be intact, and Healon was injected into the anterior chamber.

An Iolab posterior chamber intraocular lens, Model G-708G of 22-diopter power had previously been soaked in balanced salt solution. The lens was flushed with fresh balanced salt solution and coated with Healon. Angled McPherson tying forceps were then used to insert the lens through the scleral incision with the inferior foot of the haptic passing beneath the anterior capsule at 6 o'clock. Long-angled McPherson tying forceps were then used to place the superior foot of the haptic through the pupil behind the anterior capsule at 12 o'clock. A Sinskey hook was utilized to rotate the lens and ensure its stability. Miochol-E was injected into the anterior chamber to constrict the pupil.

Balanced salt solution was then utilized to deepen the chamber and firm up the eye. Additional 10–0 nylon interrupted sutures were utilized to close the corneoscleral wound. At the completion of the maneuver, the wound was watertight. The eye evidenced normal pressure, and the pupil was round, central, and lay immediately over the haptic of the posterior chamber lens. The conjunctival wound was coapted with bipolar cautery. Gentamicin and Celestone, 0.5 mL each, were separately injected through the inferior conjunctival cul-de-sac into the sub-Tenon space. The Barraquer lid speculum was removed, Maxitrol ointment instilled, and a patch and Fox shield placed over the eye.

HEMICOLECTOMY AND PANCREATICODUODENECTOMY (WHIPPLE PROCEDURE)

PREOPERATIVE DIAGNOSIS: Suspected pancreatic neoplasm.

POSTOPERATIVE DIAGNOSIS: Suspected pancreatic neoplasm, pathology pending.

PROCEDURES PERFORMED
1. Partial colectomy with anastomosis (right hemicolectomy).
2. Pancreaticoduodenectomy (Whipple procedure).

DETAILS OF PROCEDURE: The patient was brought to the operating suite and was administered a general intubation anesthetic. Foley catheter was placed to gravity drainage. The abdomen was prepped with Betadine and sterilely draped.

A midline incision was made with a scalpel and electrocautery through the subcutaneous fat and then through the rectus fascia. The peritoneal cavity was entered above the level of the umbilicus. The lower abdomen and pelvis were obliterated, with adhesions involving the omentum. These omental adhesions involved the entire lower abdomen and pelvis. Dissection was carried out with electrocautery and Metzenbaum scissors to free up the omentum and to free up multiple loops of small bowel which were adherent to each other. There were noted to be sutures from a previous surgery in what appeared to be the sigmoid colon. The patient also had sutures in the distal small bowel, about 6 to 8 cm from the ileocecal valve, also consistent with what appeared to be some type of small bowel resection.

The ascending colon was mobilized with sharp dissection, and palpation revealed a soft mass within the proximal ascending colon. Dissection was carried around the hepatic flexure, incising the peritoneum, separating it into pedicles, which were clipped and then divided. Dissection was carried around and through the gastrocolic tissue. Again this tissue was either divided between large Weck clips or between clamps, and the tissue was tied with 2–0 silk. It was at this point that a mass was noted in the head of the pancreas that measured about 3 × 4 cm. The remainder of the pancreas was smooth with only 1 or 2 other areas of slight induration, one in the body and one in the tail.

There were enlarged lymph nodes around the common bile duct. These were soft. One of these was removed and sent for frozen section. Meanwhile, dissection was carried out to complete mobilization of the terminal small bowel and the ascending colon over to the midtransverse colon. The omentum was divided up to the midpoint of the transverse colon. The vessels along the right side of the middle colic artery and vein were sacrificed after the bowel had been divided between a bowel clamp and a Kocher clamp. The dissection extended to the origin of the right colic and ileocolic vessels, and these vessels were divided between clamps and tied with 0 silk. There were small palpable nodes evident in the proximal mesocolon. These nodes were included as much as possible. The duodenum was dissected away from the mesocolon to allow for proximal ligation of the respective vessels. The distal small bowel was divided between a Kocher clamp and a bowel clamp. This was just proximal to the area of the previous anastomosis. The remaining mesentery of the terminal ileum and cecum was divided between clamps and tied with 2–0 silk.

The bowel was then prepared for an end-to-end anastomosis. This was carried out in 2 layers with the outer layer of interrupted seromuscular 3–0 silk and an inner layer of continuous interlocking 3–0 chromic. The mesenteric defect was closed with interrupted 3–0 silk. By this time word was received that the lymph node removed from the common bile duct area did not show any evidence of malignancy. Both right and left lobes of the liver were unremarkable to palpation. The gallbladder was moderately distended. The stomach was unremarkable. There was no evidence of any tumor studding the peritoneum. There was no free fluid within the peritoneal cavity. At this point, the patient's family was informed of the situation involving the pancreas. After discussion, it was decided to proceed at this time with the pancreaticoduodenectomy for the suspected neoplasm at the head of the pancreas.

The midline incision was extended up to the xiphoid. The self-retaining Bookwalter retractor was used, and the mobilization of the duodenum was completed to the inferior vena cava. The ligament of Treitz was mobilized by incising the peritoneum there. Gastroepiploic vessels were divided near their origin at the region of the head of the pancreas, and the head of the pancreas and duodenum were mobilized. The dissection was carried along the middle colic vein to the identified superior mesenteric vein, which then led into the identification of the portal vein. Blunt dissection was carried out easily over the portal vein behind the neck of the pancreas. The neck of the pancreas was totally normal. Dissection was then carried out in the lesser curvature area of the stomach over the duodenum to identify the gastroduodenal vessel. This was identified as being separate from the hepatic artery. The gastroduodenal vessel was encircled with a vessel loop. The opening was made in the lesser sac, and dissection was carried out over the superior aspect of the pancreas to allow for passage of a large Kelly clamp behind the neck of the pancreas. Again, a vessel loop was wrapped around the neck of the pancreas. Dissection was then carried out over the common bile duct, separated from the hepatic artery and the portal vein. The common bile duct appeared to be about 8 to 9 mm in diameter. It was encircled again with a vessel loop. At this point another enlarged node was located just above the neck of the pancreas near the celiac access. This lymph node was not hard, but it was enlarged and appeared to be slightly discolored. At this point there was no evidence of any extension of the tumor beyond the region of the head of the pancreas. It was elected then to proceed with the pancreaticoduodenectomy.

The pancreas was divided over its neck, with the TA-55 stapler applied across the proximal portion. The severed neck of the pancreas had bleeding, which was controlled easily with several 3–0 silk sutures. The pancreatic duct was found to lie in the posterior portion of the gland, and it measured perhaps 3 mm to 4 mm. Dissection was carried along the lateral aspect, right along the portal vein. The pancreaticoduodenal arteries were divided between clamps. The tissue along here was separated into small pedicles, and these were divided between clamps and tied with 2–0 silk. In this fashion, the head of the pancreas and the uncinate process were removed and dissection carried up towards the gastroduodenal vessel, which was then divided between clamps and tied with 2–0 silk. The distal common bile duct was also subsequently divided, and this allowed resection of the head of the pancreas along with the uncinate process.

The duodenum was divided between clamps just distal to the pylorus, and the small bowel at the duodenojejunal junction was divided as well, with a TA-55 stapler being applied distally and then the bowel transected. The resected specimen then was the head of the pancreas, duodenum and distal common bile duct. Later inspection revealed that the preserved pylorus and 3 cm of duodenum appeared a bit dusky, and so I elected to resect the distal half of the stomach as well. The antrectomy was carried out by dividing the gastric vessels and ligating them with 0 silk.

The pancreaticojejunostomy anastomosis was carried out. This was an end-to-side fashion. The outer layer of the pancreaticojejunostomy was interrupted 3–0 silk. The inner layer was mucosa to mucosa with interrupted 4–0 silk, and the anterior outer layer was interrupted 3–0 silk in 2 layers. Approximately 8 cm distal to this anastomosis, the site was selected for the choledochojejunostomy. Before this was accomplished, the gallbladder was resected. The gallbladder was taken down from the fundus to the cystic duct in the usual fashion with electrocautery and also in some areas tissue divided between clamps, tied, and divided with 2–0 silk. Weck clips were also used in these areas. The dissection was carried down to identify the cystic artery, which was ligated with 2–0 silk and divided. The cystic duct was dissected down and then divided and ligated with 2–0 silk. The choledochojejunostomy was an end-to-side anastomosis. This was carried out in essentially 1 layer with interrupted 3–0 Vicryl, although 3–0 silk was used on either side of the anastomosis. The loop of jejunum was then brought around so that a gastrojejunostomy could be performed. This again was an end-to-side anastomosis. The midpoint of the stomach was divided between a ball clamp, which was applied along the greater curvature for about 4 cm, and then the medial half of the stomach was closed with a TA-90 stapler, 4.8 staple height. Again the anastomosis was carried out in 2 layers. An outer layer was interrupted 3–0 seromuscular silk, and the inner layer was continuous interlocking 3–0 chromic. All 3 anastomoses were accomplished with excellent blood supply to the respective organs and without any tension.

Irrigation of the abdominal cavity was carried out. Inspection revealed good hemostasis. Some of the omentum over the transverse colon appeared to be dusky, so this was resected. Next, 2 Jackson-Pratt drains were brought through the abdominal wall, 1 on the right side and 1 on the left side. One was placed near the area of the choledochojejunostomy, and the other 1 was located near the pancreaticojejunostomy. These were secured to the skin using 2–0 nylon. After an accurate sponge, instrument, and needle count was conducted, the abdomen was closed with continuous 1–0 Panacryl. The skin was approximated with skin staples. The patient was subsequently transferred to a cart and taken to recovery in good condition.

IMPLANTATION OF IMPLANTABLE CARDIOVERTER-DEFIBRILLATOR (ICD)

PROCEDURES PERFORMED
1. Dual-chamber implantable cardioverter-defibrillator implantation.
2. Interrogation of reprogramming.
3. Fluoroscopy.
4. Superior vena cava leads ×2.
5. Intracardiac atrial and ventricular pacing and recording.
6. Defibrillation threshold testing.
7. Echocardiogram ×4.

COMPLICATIONS: None.

ANESTHESIA: ASA classification class III. Deep conscious sedation provided by the anesthesia service.

MEDICATIONS: Ancef 1 g IV given prior to the implantation.

DETAILS OF PROCEDURE: The patient was taken to the clinical laboratory in the fasting state. He has had documented clinical ventricular tachycardia as well as coronary artery disease and left ventricular dysfunction. During electrophysiological study, he was found to have inducible ventricular tachycardia and no reversible cause for his arrhythmia was present. He also has significant sinus node dysfunction with symptomatic bradycardia.

The left upper chest was prepared in the usual sterile fashion. Local anesthetic was applied to the skin. A 3-cm incision was performed inferior and parallel to the clavicle. Two separate punctures of the left axillary vein were performed, and the guidewire was left in place. Pocket was manufactured through a combination of sharp and blunt dissection. Good hemostasis was present.

Through the guidewire in the left axillary vein, 2 separate sheaths were placed toward the SVC. The atrial and ventricular leads were advanced through each of these sheaths and placed primarily into the right atrium.

The right ventricular lead was then advanced into the right ventricular apex. After documenting satisfactory pacing parameters, the lead position was secure. The right atrial lead was then placed in the right atrial appendage. After documenting satisfactory pacing parameters, the lead position was secured with silk sutures.

Of note, after removing the sheath for the right ventricular lead, air within the pulmonary artery was noted on the fluoroscopy. The patient developed desaturation and cough. Immediately, a Swan-Ganz catheter was advanced into the pulmonary artery and the air within the pulmonary artery was aspirated. This led to complete resolution of the cough and immediate improvement in desaturations. The Swan-Ganz catheter was removed.

Good hemostasis was present in the pocket. Intracardiac atrial and ventricular pacing and recording was performed. A dual-chamber generator from St. Jude was then connected to the leads and placed in the pocket. The pocket was irrigated copiously with antibiotic solution before and after placement of the generator in the pocket. The pocket was closed in layers with 2–0 and 3–0 Vicryl. Dermabond was applied to the skin.

Defibrillation testing threshold was performed. Two separate episodes of ventricular fibrillation were induced 5 minutes apart. During the first episode, a 20-J shock was delivered, successfully restoring sinus rhythm. Charge time was 3.9 seconds with a defibrillation impedance of 42 ohms and 100% sensing when programmed to a sensitivity of 1.0 mV. For the second episode, a 15-J shock successfully restored sinus rhythm after a charge time of 2.7 seconds. Impedance was 42 ohms and again there was 100% sensing when programmed to a sensitivity of 0.3 mV. At the end of the procedure, no complications were noted and the patient recovered from the sedation well.

FINDINGS
1. Successful implantation of a dual-chamber Epic DR, model #V235, dual-chamber pulse generator from St. Jude Medical, serial #17060.
2. Implantation of a St. Jude 1688TC, 52-cm lead in the right atrial appendage, serial #DN14249. The measured R wave was 3.1 mV with a pacing impedance of 504 ohms and an acute pacing threshold of 0.9 V at 0.5 msec.
3. Successful implantation of St. Jude 1580, 65-cm lead in the right ventricular apex, and an acute pacing threshold of 0.8 V at 0.5 msec.
4. Defibrillation threshold equal to or less than 15 J.

IMPRESSION: Successful implantation of a dual-chamber implantable cardioverter-defibrillator.

RECOMMENDATIONS
1. Maximize beta blockade for the treatment of his coronary artery disease and congestive heart failure and minimize the possibility of sinus tachycardia being detected as ventricular tachycardia. His clinical tachycardia had a relatively low ventricular rate; therefore, his ventricular tachycardia detection is set at 140 beats per minute.
2. Chest x-ray, antibiotics, electrocardiogram, and observation.

LAPAROSCOPIC-ASSISTED HYSTERECTOMY AND BILATERAL SALPINGO-OOPHORECTOMY

PREOPERATIVE DIAGNOSIS: Endometriosis and spasmodic dysmenorrhea, refractory to conservative treatment.

POSTOPERATIVE DIAGNOSIS: Endometriosis and spasmodic dysmenorrhea, refractory to conservative treatment.

PROCEDURE PERFORMED: Laparoscopic-assisted hysterectomy and bilateral salpingo-oophorectomy.

DETAILS OF PROCEDURE: After informed consent was obtained, the patient was taken to the operating room where she underwent general endotracheal anesthesia. The patient was then prepped and draped in normal sterile fashion in the dorsal supine position in Allen stirrups. A Foley catheter was placed, and a Rubin cannula was placed in the cervix. The infraumbilical area was injected with Xylocaine. A 1-cm incision was then made. The Veress needle was then placed. Two towel clips were then placed on the skin to elevate the abdomen. The Veress needle was placed through this incision with proper placement verified by saline drop test and an opening pressure of 3 mmHg. The abdomen was then insufflated. The pelvis was examined and noted to be grossly normal. Two additional 10-mm trocars were placed in the left and right lower quadrants under direct visualization. Each area was injected with lidocaine first. The pelvis was fully examined.

The uterus was grossly normal and retroverted. There were normal bilateral tubes and ovaries. There was a small amount of endometriosis along the posterior uterosacral ligaments which was ablated. Next, the left infundibulopelvic ligament was clamped and cut using the Endostapler. Prior to this being transected, care was taken to verify that the ureter was not in the clamp. The remainder of the broad ligament was then serially transected using the stapling device. Once again, prior to transection and stapling, each pedicle was checked to ensure that there was no ureter noted in the clamp. In a similar fashion, the right infundibulopelvic ligament was clamped and transected using the stapler. Once again, the ureter was identified prior to any transection. The remainder of the broad ligament was transected in a similar fashion. The bladder was elevated, and the peritoneum above the bladder was incised with the Endoshears. The space was developed using the Endoshears. All areas appeared to be dry.

Attention was then turned to the vagina. The patient was converted to high stirrups using the Allen stirrups. A weighted speculum was placed in the most posterior vagina with a Deaver retractor in the anterior vagina. The cervix was grasped with 2 thyroid Lahey clamps. The mucosa of the cervix was circumscribed with Bovie cautery.

The bladder was bluntly dissected off of the lower uterine segment, and the peritoneum was then entered. The posterior cul-de-sac was grasped with a Kocher clamp and elevated. Curved Mayo scissors were used to enter the posterior cul-de-sac. A speculum was then placed. A Heaney clamp was then used on the right side to clamp across the uterosacral complex. This was then transected and suture ligated with 0 Vicryl. In a similar fashion, the left uterosacral was transected, cut, and suture ligated with 0 Vicryl. The small amount of remaining broad ligament was then clamped with Heaney clamps on each side, transected, and suture ligated with 0 Vicryl. The uterus was then easily delivered through the vagina.

The vaginal cuff and perineum were closed together using a 2–0 Vicryl from 12 o'clock to 6 o'clock, being tied in the midline. The uterosacral ligament pedicles had been tagged, and these were tied in the midline and reattached to the vaginal cuff. The vaginal cuff, once it was sewn, was noted to be hemostatic. The Foley catheter drained clear urine.

The patient was taken out of stirrups, awakened, extubated, and transferred to the recovery room in stable condition. The patient tolerated the procedure well. All counts were correct ×3. The patient received Ancef for antibiotic prophylaxis.

LE FORT OSTEOTOMY AND GENIOPLASTY

PREOPERATIVE DIAGNOSES: Maxillary hypoplasia, mandibular hypoplasia, and mandibular retrogenia.

POSTOPERATIVE DIAGNOSES: Maxillary hypoplasia, mandibular hypoplasia, and mandibular retrogenia.

PROCEDURES PERFORMED: A 3-piece Le Fort I osteotomy with internal rigid fixation, bilateral sagittal split mandibular advancement osteotomy with internal rigid fixation, and advancement genioplasty with internal rigid fixation.

INDICATIONS: The patient is an otherwise healthy female who presents with masticatory dysfunction secondary to her maxillary hypoplasia in the transverse dimension and mandibular hypoplasia in the sagittal dimension, creating an anterior open bite of approximately 2 mm and an overjet of approximately 6 mm. She had been in an orthognathic treatment plan for the past 18 months and is currently at the surgical component stage. All of the risks were reviewed with the patient and her mother. A decision was made for advancement of the chin as well as the mandible in a 3-piece Le Fort I osteotomy. There were no contraindications based on her history and physical provided by her primary care physician.

DETAILS OF PROCEDURE: The patient was taken to the operating room and placed in a supine position on the operating table. Monitors for general anesthesia were placed and verified. She was induced to sleep with IV propofol, and a nasal endotracheal tube was passed without difficulty. The eyes were lubricated, taped, and the head turban was placed. The nasal endotracheal tube was secured to the head turban. The patient was prepped and draped in a usual fashion for an intraoral procedure. A throat pack was placed. Using a wire driver, a K wire was placed through the nasal bridge area. Measurements from the nasal pin to the central incisor brackets were recorded. A total of 10 mL of 0.5% Sensorcaine and 1:200,000 epinephrine was injected in an infiltrative fashion into the maxillary vestibule bilaterally. A 1-mm crosscut Fischer bur was used to section the maxillary arch wire between teeth numbers 6 and 7, 10, and 11. Utilizing a Bovie, a circumvestibular incision was created from the second premolar on the right extending to the second premolar on the left.

The elevators were used to expose the anterior and lateral aspects of the maxilla. Care was taken to protect the infraorbital nerves bilaterally. Subperiosteal dissection was created in a tunnel-like fashion to the pterygoid plates bilaterally with a Freer elevator. The nasal mucosa was elevated from the lateral nasal walls and the floor of the nose with a Woodson elevator and a curved Freer elevator. A reciprocating saw was used to create a standard Le Fort I osteotomy cut bilaterally. The curved reciprocating saw was used to osteotomize the posterior lateral aspects of the maxilla bilaterally. A 1-mm crosscut Fischer bur was used to make vertical cuts from the Le Fort I cut extending inferiorly between the cuspid and lateral bilaterally. A large curved osteotome was used to osteotomize the pterygoid plates bilaterally. The nasal septum was released with the nasal septal osteotome. The curved lateral nasal osteotomes were used to osteotomize the lateral nasal walls.

Next, the maxilla was down-fractured. The greater palatine vessels remained intact. A large round bur was used to remove the maxillary nasal crest as well as the portion of the nasal walls bilaterally. With the maxilla down-fractured, a reciprocating saw was used to make paramidline cuts from the posterior aspect of the hard palate extending to the premaxilla bilaterally. These cuts were then jointed to the vertical cuts between the cuspid and laterals using the 1.6 crosscut Fischer bur. The Smith spreader was used to segment the osteotomy into 3 segments, as well as the lone standing hard palate in the middle. An interim splint was then placed into the maxillary dentition and held in place with 26-gauge stainless steel wires. The mandible was then rotated into the splint and intermaxillary fixation was achieved with 26-gauge stainless steel wire loops. The maxillary-mandibular complex was then rotated into the correct vertical position based on the measurements taken from the nasal pin. Once this was achieved, the maxilla was fixated with 1.5-mm titanium plates and screws. The intermaxillary fixation was released, and there was reproducible occlusion into the splint. The interim splint was then released, and the final splint was placed against the maxillary dentition and secured with 26-gauge stainless steel wires. A total of 10 mL of 0.5% Sensorcaine and 1:200,000 epinephrine was injected in infiltrative fashion into the posterior mandible bilaterally.

Next, the maxillary wound was closed in a V-to-Y fashion utilizing 4–0 Monocryl sutures. The 15 blade was used to make a mucoperiosteal incision in the left posterior mandible approximately 1 cm in length from the mid portion of the vertical ramus extending toward the second molar on the buccal aspect. The periosteal elevator was used to expose the lateral aspect of the body of the mandible, as well as the medial aspect of the vertical ramus, with care taken to protect the neurovascular bundle. A Lindemann bur was used to create the medial osteotomy cut and a 1.5 crosscut Fischer bur was used to extend this cut along the anterior ramus then through the body of the mandible and into the inferior border. Wooden handle osteotomes were used to split the proximal and distal segments, and the neurovascular bundle remained within the distal segment throughout. The segments separated, packing was placed, and attention was turned to the right posterior mandible and identical incision, dissection, and osteotomy cuts were performed. The segments were split and the neurovascular bundle was within the distal segment. Next, the distal segment was rotated into the final splint and secured with 26-gauge stainless steel wire loops creating intermaxillary fixation. Attention turned back to the right posterior mandible and a Jeter clamp was used to secure the proximal and distal segment. An 11 blade was used to make a stab incision on the cheek and the trocar was passed through this incision. The proximal and distal segments were rigidly fixated with 2-mm bicortical titanium screws ×3. The trocar and Jeter clamp were removed, and an identical procedure was used to fixate the left proximal and distal segment. With the segments fixated, the intermaxillary fixation was released and there was reproducible occlusion into the splint.

Next, the mandible was rotated back into the splint and secured with two 26-gauge wire loops. Next, a standard genioplasty incision was created with a 15 blade and care was taken to dissect out the middle nerves. A reciprocating saw was used to create an inferior border osteotomy of the anterior mandible. The inferior border was then advanced 5 mm and secured with a 5-mm titanium plate and screws using 8 screws in total. Next, the mandibular posterior wounds were closed with 4–0 Monocryl sutures in a running fashion. The genioplasty incision was closed in layer fashion first by fixating the muscle bilaterally. The mucosa was secured with 4–0 Vicryl sutures in a running fashion. The oral cavity was irrigated and the maxillary fixation was released and the oral cavity was suctioned. The throat pack was removed. A nasogastric tube was passed into the stomach, and the stomach was decompressed and the tube was removed. Elastics were placed on the surgical lugs. The cheek wounds were closed with 5–0 nylon sutures ×1 each and Steri-Strips were placed. A Jobst fascioplasty was applied. The nasal pin was removed. The patient was then turned over to the anesthesia service having tolerated the procedure well. She was taken to the recovery room in stable condition.

LIVER TRANSPLANT AND BROVIAC CATHETER PLACEMENT

PREOPERATIVE DIAGNOSIS: Biliary atresia.

POSTOPERATIVE DIAGNOSIS: Biliary atresia.

PROCEDURES PERFORMED
1. Liver transplant.
2. Broviac catheter placement.

INDICATIONS: The child has biliary atresia. She was evaluated by our multidisciplinary transplant committee and a liver transplant was recommended. The parents gave informed written consent to proceed.

DETAILS OF PROCEDURE: The patient was brought to the operating room and general anesthesia was induced. A urinary catheter was subsequently placed in the bladder, and anesthesiology placed monitoring devices and infusion lines. The abdomen, neck, and chest were prepped with Betadine and draped in sterile styles. An incision over the right neck was made and carried down until the external jugular vein was identified. It was divided proximally, and then a 7-French double-lumen Broviac catheter was placed in the subcutaneous tunnel exiting in the anterior chest and guided down through the external jugular vein and into the central venous system. Fluoroscopy revealed the catheter to be in satisfactory position. The wound was closed with 2 layers of absorbable suture after securing the catheter to the vein with a silk suture. The catheter was affixed to the skin at the exit site with nylon suture.

The bilateral subcostal incision was made at the site of the portoenterostomy. When the peritoneal cavity was entered, it was apparent there was a dense amount of adhesions throughout the abdomen. These were painstakingly dissected free, exposing the liver. During the course of the dissection, a colotomy occurred at the splenic flexure on the transverse colon. This was closed with a single layer of silk suture. Attention was turned to the portal, which was skeletonized. The previous Roux-en-Y limb was identified and dissected free. It was divided as close as possible to the liver. The hepatic artery was identified, and we divided the right and left hepatic arteries individually. There were numerous large lymph nodes present, which were carefully dissected free and resected. The lymphatics were ligated with silk sutures. The portal limb was identified and was noted to be extremely diminutive. This had been expected based on the MRA. It was carefully dissected free up to the bifurcation and divided. It was noted that there was very little flow in the portal vein.

The attachments of the liver to retroperitoneum were then divided medially and laterally. It was apparent that the caudate lobe encircled the vena cava, and it was not possible to remove the liver with the cava in situ. Therefore, clamps were placed on the cava above and below the liver, and the liver was resected. It was apparent that the portal vein would not be satisfactory for portal inflow, but the inferior vena cava appeared satisfactory in position and size. Therefore, the decision was made to use the vena cava as portal inflow.

The new liver was then sutured into place using a 5–0 Prolene running suture for the suprahepatic anastomosis and a 7–0 Prolene suture for the hepatic artery anastomosis, which was from an aortic patch of the donor to a branch going to the right and left hepatic arteries on the recipient. The portal vein of the donor was then anastomosed to the inferior vena cava of the recipient using running 6–0 sutures. The clamps were released, and the liver flushed nicely. Prior to releasing the clamps, the infrahepatic cava of the donor was oversewn with 4–0 Prolene suture. The liver achieved satisfactory color and texture and began to make bile. There was a strong pulse palpable in the hepatic artery, and the portal vein anastomosis appeared satisfactory. The previous Roux-en-Y limb was then used to fashion a hepaticojejunostomy using interrupted 5–0 PDS sutures. This was fashioned over a 5-French biliary stent that had been placed on the back table through the donor cystic duct and guided up the gallbladder fossa, where the peritoneum had been oversewn. Some silk sutures were used to suture the Roux-en-Y limb up to the porta and some connective tissue to relieve any tension that might occur at a later time. There was no tension on the anastomosis at this time. It was checked by infusion of the biliary catheter with saline, and there was no evidence of a leakage. The catheter was then brought out the right flank and secured with nylon suture to the skin.

The abdomen was irrigated with warm saline and, after a final check for hemostasis, was closed with running 2–0 Prolene suture in the fascia and running subcuticular stitch in the skin. The patient tolerated the procedure well.

LOW TRANSVERSE CESAREAN SECTION

PREOPERATIVE DIAGNOSIS: Intrauterine pregnancy at 38 weeks.

POSTOPERATIVE DIAGNOSIS: Intrauterine pregnancy at 38 weeks.

PROCEDURE PERFORMED: Repeat low transverse cesarean section with upper midline vertical uterine extension.

DETAILS OF PROCEDURE: The patient was taken to the operating room after successful epidural anesthesia had been placed in labor and delivery. She was placed in the supine position on the operating room table with her right side elevated and supported with a bag. The patient's abdomen was then prepared and draped in a sterile manner. An Allis clamp was used to check for an appropriate level of anesthesia, and the patient's breathing was noted to be unlabored.

A scalpel was used to make a Pfannenstiel incision through the old scar, which was excised and removed. The incision was extended through the subcutaneous tissue with the scalpel, and the bleeding was controlled with an electrocautery device. The fascia of the abdominis muscle was identified and nicked transversely with the Mayo scissors. Kocher clamps were placed on the proximal fascial flap, which was bluntly and sharply dissected from the rectus abdominis muscle. Kocher clamps were then placed on the lower fascial flap, which was bluntly and sharply dissected free from the rectus abdominis muscle. The median raphe was then bluntly and sharply dissected in a careful manner. The parietal peritoneum was visualized, grasped with hemostats using a 3-point technique and nicked with a scalpel, and the incision extended both cephalad and caudad.

There were omental adhesions present to the anterior abdominal wall, presumed due to the previous cesarean section. These were carefully lysed with electrocautery. A bladder blade was positioned, and the peritoneal serosa was grasped with pickups and nicked with the Metzenbaum scissors, and the incision extended transversely with the Metzenbaum scissors.

A scalpel was used to score a low transverse uterine incision, which was then extended utilizing blunt dissection. The surgeon's hand was placed into the uterus to remove the fetal head, but it was necessary to extend the incision through the rectus muscles, the fascia, and the skin to remove the fetal head safely. There was a nuchal cord $\times 2$, which was reduced and the nares and oropharynx bulb suctioned prior to removing the remainder of the fetus. The infant cried spontaneously. The cord was clamped and cut, and the neonate was handed off the field to the waiting neonatologist in attendance. The infant weighed 8 pounds 3 ounces and had Apgar scores of 9 at 1 minute and 10 at 5 minutes. Cord gases were obtained, as was cord blood.

At this time, the uterus was exteriorized and wrapped in a moist towel. The vertical upper midline extension in the uterus was reapproximated using #1 chromic sutures in a running locked fashion. The second layer was reapproximated using #1 chromic sutures in a simple fashion. Hemostasis was excellent. The peritoneal serosa was reapproximated with 3–0 Vicryl in a running fashion. The low transverse uterine incision was closed in 2 layers, the first was a #1 chromic running locked stitch, and the second a #1 chromic running imbricating stitch. Cautery was used to assure complete hemostasis. After copious irrigation with normal saline, the bladder flap was reapproximated with 3–0 Vicryl in a running fashion.

The cul-de-sac was wiped free of all blood and clots, and the uterus was returned to the abdominal cavity. An Interceed barrier was placed over the upper vertical uterine incision, and the pelvic gutters were freed of all blood and clots. Once again, the uterine incision was inspected and found to have excellent hemostasis.

The parietal peritoneum was reapproximated with 3–0 Vicryl in a running fashion. The rectus muscles were reapproximated with 2–0 chromic sutures in a running fashion. The area was irrigated once again with normal saline, and hemostasis was noted to be excellent. The rectus muscles were reapproximated using 3–0 Vicryl in a running fashion, and the skin was reapproximated utilizing metallic skin staples. A sterile, mildly compressive dressing was applied.

The Foley catheter was noted at this time to be draining clear urine. The sponge, needle, instrument, and lap counts were reported as being correct ×2 prior to the final closure.

The patient was taken to the recovery room in stable condition with an estimated blood loss of 700 mL. She tolerated the procedure well. The neonate was sent to the newborn nursery in excellent condition.

MYRINGOTOMY WITH TONSILLECTOMY AND ADENOIDECTOMY

PREOPERATIVE DIAGNOSES: Recurrent otitis media, adenotonsillar hypertrophy.

POSTOPERATIVE DIAGNOSES: Recurrent otitis media, adenotonsillar hypertrophy.

PROCEDURES PERFORMED: Bilateral myringotomy with tubes and tonsillectomy and adenoidectomy.

DETAILS OF PROCEDURE: With the patient in the supine position, general endotracheal anesthesia was established. The patient was prepped and draped in the routine fashion for tubes and tonsillectomy and adenoidectomy. The operating microscope was used. A large wax plug was removed from the left ear and then an anterior-inferior myringotomy was made. Scant amount of serous fluid was aspirated from the middle ear space and a Paparella-type tube was placed. Cortisporin drops were then placed in the middle ear and ear canal. The patient was repositioned and the right ear canal was cleaned and then an anterior-inferior myringotomy was made. Again, scant fluid was obtained and a Paparella tube was placed. Again, Cortisporin drops were placed in the ear canal.

The patient was repositioned. A Crowe-Davis mouth gag was inserted, and the patient placed in the Rose position. The soft palate was retracted with a red rubber catheter and the adenoids were examined with the mirror. The nasopharynx was completely filled with adenoid tissue, blocking the posterior choanae. Then using adenoid curettes, the adenoid pad was removed sharply and then the nasopharynx was packed with cotton balls. The left tonsil was then grasped with a retractor. The midline incision was made along the anterior tonsillar pillar and then carried posteriorly to the posterior pillar using a Harmonic scalpel. Then using the Harmonic scalpel, the tonsil was dissected from the tonsillar fossa. The right tonsil was then removed in a similar fashion. Several bleeding points were then cauterized with the suction cautery. The nasopharyngeal packs were then removed and the nasal cavity was irrigated with saline solution. Bleeding points were controlled with suction cautery. The nose was again irrigated. There was no active bleeding. The patient was then extubated and taken to the recovery room in satisfactory condition.

OPEN DONOR NEPHRECTOMY

PREOPERATIVE DIAGNOSIS: The patient is acting as a living, related kidney donor to her brother.

POSTOPERATIVE DIAGNOSIS: The patient is acting as a living, related kidney donor to her brother.

PROCEDURE PERFORMED: Open left donor nephrectomy.

INDICATIONS: The patient has volunteered to be a living, related kidney donor to her brother, who suffers from end-stage renal disease. The patient was referred for evaluation as a prospective live kidney donor, and she was deemed to be a suitable candidate.

DETAILS OF PROCEDURE: After informed consent was obtained from the patient, she was brought to the operating room and placed supine on the operative table.

After successful induction of general endotracheal anesthesia, a Foley catheter as well as an IV line were placed. An orogastric tube was also placed. The patient was then placed in the left lateral decubitus position, at which time her entire left side was placed perpendicular to the operating table. A kidney rest was then applied to an area superior to the iliac crest to make the skin tense by the left-sided kidney. Her left shoulder was also placed over on top of her, and so she was essentially perpendicular to the operating table. After we were content with how she was placed on the operating table, we next prepped in the usual sterile fashion for a donor nephrectomy. We identified the twelfth rib, and approximately 1 fingerbreadth below the twelfth rib an incision was made for an approximate length of about 18 cm. The incision ended close to the lateral border of the rectus muscle. Electrocautery was then used to cut the skin and the subcutaneous fat. The latissimus dorsi, as well as the 3 layers of the abdominal wall, was then excised in its entirety. This was done with cautery. Once this was done, we were able to gently palpate the kidney, which was superior and lateral, and using careful blunt as well as cautery dissection, we were able to find the peritoneum. We were able to reflect this medially while keeping the kidney in the retroperitoneal space.

Once this was done, a Bookwalter retractor was placed into the operative field for retraction both cephalad and caudad, and laterally and medially. Using careful dissection, we were able to open up Gerota fascia, the plane on top of the kidney. This was extended with electrocautery superiorly, and we were able to use the cautery to excise all of the attachments this had in adventitia to the superior pole of the kidney.

We next identified the adrenal gland, which was noted in its entirety. We found the adrenal vein. This was divided between silk sutures. We were able to essentially dissect out the entire kidney circumferentially, first at the superior pole, then extending medially and inferiorly, and then finally the inferior pole. We next found a large ovarian vein, and this was divided between silk ties. In addition, a posterior-lying lumbar vein was identified and also divided between silk sutures. We reflected the kidney, observing its inferior side, and we found the ureter. We dissected this on top of the psoas, and we left a large amount of adventitious tissue around the entire circumference of the ureter.

Once the veins were identified, we were able to manipulate the kidney and find both renal arteries. The superior pole, which was the main renal artery, had a diameter of approximately 4 to 5 mm. We dissected this with some difficulty to its entrance into the aorta. The lower pole artery, which was approximately 3 mm, was also found and dissected along its entire length to the aorta. The dissection was a little bit difficult, based upon the size of the kidney which was large and the fact that the patient was relatively big herself and the kidney lay relatively deep. We then carefully inspected the hilum of the kidney, and it was noted to be intact.

Once this major dissection was completed, we placed a right-angle clamp quite distally on the ureter. We did not trace it on top of the iliac, and we divided it and we tied off the distal end with a 3–0 silk tie. A very minimal amount of urine was noted to emanate from the ureter. Once this was done, we had vessel loops placed around all the major vessels. We clamped off the inferior artery with a right-angle clamp right on top of the aorta; the vessel was cut. We placed a right-angle clamp on top of the main artery, which was the more superior one; this was cut. Finally, we placed a Satinsky clamp on the renal vein, and we cut on top of this. Once this was done, the kidney was removed.

On the back table, both renal arteries, the major one and the lower pole one, were irrigated with approximately 200 to 300 mL of urecholine. We placed 200 mL through the main renal artery and approximately 100 mL through the inferior artery. The kidney was noted to blanch well, and there was good emanation of the effluent through the renal vein. The kidney was then packaged in 3 sterile bags and taken to the operating room for implantation.

We next turned our attention back to the donor. We tied off both renal arteries with double suture of 2–0 silk. Our attention was then directed towards the cut renal vein. The renal vein orifice was oversewn using a 5–0 Prolene suture, which was sutured in a double-row fashion. When we removed the Satinsky, there was excellent hemostasis.

The operative field was then flooded with antibiotic saline, and hemostasis was really quite excellent. We next turned our attention to closing the wound. The wound was closed in two running layers of 1–0 Novafil. The transversalis muscle was closed first with a buried stitch of running Novafil, and once this was closed the external and internal oblique muscles were closed in a single layer of running Novafil. The fascia was noted to coapt together very well. Prior to closing the fascia, we brought down the kidney rest and repositioned the table. Finally, the skin was closed using a subcuticular stitch of 4–0 Monocryl. The skin was noted to coapt together very well. Once this was done, the skin was washed off of all preparatory Betadine, and Steri-Strips were placed on top of the wound. Finally, sterile gauze was placed on top of this.

OPEN REDUCTION AND INTERNAL FIXATION OF HIP FRACTURE

PREOPERATIVE DIAGNOSIS: Intertrochanteric fracture, left hip.

POSTOPERATIVE DIAGNOSIS: Intertrochanteric fracture, left hip.

PROCEDURES PERFORMED: Open reduction and internal fixation of intertrochanteric fracture, left hip, with DHS hip screw and 4-hole sideplate.

INDICATIONS: This elderly female fell at the boarding home where she lives on the day of admission and sustained an intertrochanteric fracture of her left hip.

DETAILS OF PROCEDURE: Under satisfactory spinal anesthesia, the patient was placed on the Telos table, and I was able to do some traction with some manipulation and reduction. This was checked in the AP and lateral position. She was then prepped and draped in this position.

A 6-inch incision was made, beginning at the tip of the greater trochanter and going distally along the lateral thigh. Sharp dissection was used to go through the subcutaneous fat. Hemostasis was achieved with electrocoagulation. The fascia was incised in line with the incision, and the vastus lateralis muscle was split by sharp dissection down to the underlying femur, and a Bennett retractor placed. Under C-arm control, a guidewire was placed up into the neck. The greater trochanter had fractured right at the place where the guidewire went, so this made placement rather easy. This was checked on the AP and lateral, and the 135-degree angle guide was used. It was then measured and determined that a 90-mm compression hip screw was needed. The wire was then driven in a little further, and the drill for the hip screw and sideplate barrel was run over the screw under x-ray control. This was then removed, and the 90-mm compression hip screw was placed over the guidewire and again checked in the AP and lateral. It was found to be in good position, and had very good purchase in the head.

The 135-degree angle, 4-hole sideplate was placed, the barrel of which was slipped over the shaft of the screw and fixed to the femoral shaft. It was held in place with a Jackson bone clamp. A total of 4 screws were put in place by drilling, measuring, and putting in 4 tap screws. The 4 tap screws consisted of one 40-mm, two 38-mm, and one 6-mm screw. Finally, all of them were tightened down. The Jackson clamp was removed, and the wound was irrigated. The vastus lateralis muscle was allowed to fall back together.

The fascia was closed with #1 Vicryl interrupted sutures. The subcutaneous fat was closed with 0 Vicryl interrupted inverted sutures, and the skin was closed with skin staples. A Betadine dressing was applied. The patient left the operating room in satisfactory condition with no drains and no complications. Prior to the procedure, the patient received 1 g IV Ancef.

PLATE AND SCREW HARDWARE REMOVAL

PREOPERATIVE DIAGNOSIS: Metatarsalgia, left foot.

POSTOPERATIVE DIAGNOSES
1. Metatarsalgia, left foot.
2. Stable nonunion, left first metatarsophalangeal joint.

PROCEDURES PERFORMED
1. Removal of hardware, left foot.
2. Bone biopsy, left first metatarsal bone.
3. Shortening osteotomies, left second and third metatarsals.

DETAILS OF PROCEDURE: The patient was brought to the operating room and placed on the operating table in a supine position. Following the administration of intravenous sedation, an infiltrative block of 0.5% Marcaine plain was administered to the left foot in ankle block fashion. The left foot was then prepped and draped in the usual sterile manner. A well-padded pneumatic tourniquet was placed on the left ankle and the limb exsanguinated via gravity. Upon adequate exsanguination of the limb, the cuff was inflated to 250 mmHg. Attention was now directed to the left foot where a surgical scar was noted over the dorsal aspect of the first metatarsophalangeal joint.

In the first metatarsophalangeal joint area, a dorsal incision was performed over the previous surgical scar. This incision was deepened in the same plane, taking care to clamp, cauterize, or ligate any superficial bleeders as necessary. Blunt and sharp dissection was utilized to penetrate the soft tissue layers, with care being taken to preserve and retract all vital structures. Moderate scar tissue was noted in the surgical area, consistent with multiple previous surgeries.

Blunt and sharp dissection was utilized to penetrate the soft tissue layers until reaching the level of the internal fixation plate and screws. The hardware was exposed via sharp dissection. Bony growth was noted around the metallic plate overlying the dorsal aspect of the fusion site. The internal fixation screws were removed utilizing the AO screwdriver in the standard AO technique. The periosteal elevator was then utilized to free the plate and remove it from the surgical field in toto. There, overlying the plate and screws, was abnormal-appearing fibrous tissue which was sent for pathology. There was no evidence of abscess formation in the area. Inspection of the plate and screws did not demonstrate any evidence of biocorrosion or infection.

Upon removal of the hardware, the first metatarsophalangeal joint area was manipulated. Inspection demonstrated fibrous tissue at the fusion site at the interface of the proximal phalanx and first metatarsal. The interface of the metatarsal and graft proximally appeared solid and well healed. Motion was noted across the fusion site with manipulation of the area distally.

Wound cultures were also taken in this area due for aerobic and anaerobic bacterial cultures. In addition, a deep bone biopsy was taken for pathology to rule out pseudoarthrosis versus osteomyelitis. The surgical site was flushed copiously with normal saline and closed in a layered fashion utilizing 2–0 and 3–0 Vicryl to reapproximate the deep tissues, 4–0 Vicryl to reapproximate the subcutaneous tissues, and 4–0 nylon to reapproximate the skin margins.

Attention was now directed to the lesser metatarsals where a dorsal incision was performed between the second and third metatarsal bones. This incision was deepened in the same plane, taking care to clamp, cauterize, or ligate any superficial bleeders as necessary. Blunt and sharp dissection was utilized to penetrate soft tissue layers with care being taken to preserve and retract all vital structures.

Attention was first directed towards the second metatarsal bone, where the extensor tendon and neurovascular structures were retracted from the surgical site. Upon reaching the level of the periosteum and joint capsule, this tissue layer was incised in a linear fashion to provide exposure to the distal aspect of the second metatarsal bone and second metatarsal head. The periosteum was reflected from its underlying bony attachments to facilitate exposure. A 0.045 K-wire was then driven from dorsal to plantar through the metatarsal neck, slightly medial to center point to serve as an axis guide. The power bone saw was then utilized to perform a V-shaped osteotomy with the apex oriented distally and long medial arm through the metatarsal bone. Upon completion of the osteotomy, the axis guide was removed. An approximate 3-mm wedge of bone was then removed from the shorter lateral arm of the osteotomy to provide for shortening of the second metatarsal bone. Temporary fixation was achieved via K wire and bone clamp fixation.

Attention was then directed to the third metatarsal bone, where a similar V-shaped osteotomy with long medial arm was performed. A 3-mm wedge of bone was removed from the shorter lateral arm of the osteotomy to also provide for shortening of the metatarsal bone. Temporary fixation was achieved via bone clamps, and intraoperative radiographs were taken. The radiographs demonstrated shortening of the metatarsal bones and rebalancing of the forefoot.

Permanent fixation of the osteotomies was achieved utilizing 2-mm cortical screws inserted parallel from medial to lateral across the metatarsal bone in standard AO fashion. Upon permanent fixation, a second set of intraoperative radiographs was taken. They demonstrated preservation of the metatarsal parabola through the shortening osteotomies of the second and third metatarsal bones. It was not deemed necessary to perform an additional osteotomy beneath the fourth metatarsal bone at this time as this area remained clinically asymptomatic for him.

The surgical site was flushed copiously with normal saline, and the wound was closed in a layered fashion utilizing 3–0 Vicryl to reapproximate the periosteal and capsular tissues, 4–0 Vicryl to reapproximate the subcutaneous tissues and 5–0 Vicryl to reapproximate the skin margins in continuous subcuticular fashion.

The patient left the operating room in good condition with all digits warm and viable. The left lower extremity was immobilized in a well-padded fiberglass posterior splint beneath compressive dressings.

PORT-A-CATH PLACEMENT

PREOPERATIVE DIAGNOSES: Need for IV access for chemotherapy. Carcinoma of the colon.

POSTOPERATIVE DIAGNOSES: Need for IV access for chemotherapy. Carcinoma of the colon.

PROCEDURE PERFORMED: Insertion of left subclavian Port-A-Cath.

ANESTHESIA: IV sedation plus local 1% Xylocaine and 0.5% Marcaine.

INDICATIONS: This woman has need for IV access for chemotherapy.

DETAILS OF PROCEDURE: The patient was placed in the Trendelenburg position on the operating table. A rolled sheet was placed between the shoulder blades. The neck and chest wall were prepped and draped in a sterile fashion. Infiltration of local anesthesia carried out. A needle was inserted beneath the mid aspect of the left clavicle and the subclavian vein with ease. Free flow of blood was obtained and the syringe was removed. A guidewire was passed through the needle confirming good position in the right atrium and the left subclavian vein. Following this a 6-cm incision was made including the puncture site for the pocket. The pocket was created with blunt dissection inferiorly on the chest wall musculature. The wound was defatted for easier access for the Port-A-Cath. The Port-A-Cath, which was heparinized, was then sutured to the fascia with interrupted 3–0 silk sutures. It was then cut to size. Following, a dilator was partially passed over the guidewire and the dilator removed and the dilator and peel-away sheath were fed over the guidewire. The guidewire was removed. The peel-away sheath was advanced as the dilator was withdrawn, and the Port-A-Cath was easily threaded through the peel-away sheath, and the peel-away sheath was removed. It was confirmed in good position in the right atrium. There was no evidence of arrhythmia. The catheter was easily was irrigated and aspirated. The wound was irrigated and was cleaned and dry. The wound was then closed in layers with 3–0 and 4–0 Vicryl and Steri-Strips. Sterile dressings were applied. Final sponge, needle and instrument counts were correct. The patient tolerated the procedure well and transferred to the recovery room for observation.

PUBOVAGINAL SLING

PREOPERATIVE DIAGNOSIS: Urinary incontinence.

POSTOPERATIVE DIAGNOSIS: Urinary incontinence.

PROCEDURE PERFORMED: Pubovaginal sling.

DETAILS OF PROCEDURE: In lithotomy position, the patient was prepped and draped in sterile fashion. A 16-French Foley catheter was placed initially into the bladder. An Allis clamp was placed on the vaginal mucosa. The bladder neck was then identified and marked using a sterile marking pencil. The vaginal mucosa was then infiltrated using 1% Xylocaine with epinephrine to help aid in hydrodissection. Following this, Malis scissors were then used to dissect the vaginal flap, which was in the shape of an inverted U. Dissection was performed laterally to the pelvic side-walls and in the retropubic space bilaterally. Following this, a transverse incision was made in the suprapubic region down to the level of the rectus fascia. Stamey needles were then placed on either side of the bladder neck.

Following this, the fascia lata graft was then prepared using a mattress suture of 0 Prolene on either side. Having marked the midline, the 0 Prolene suture was then placed through either eye of the Stamey needles, and the sutures were brought out through the abdominal wall. Cystoscopy was then performed, which was within normal limits. A 4-French open-ended catheter was placed up each ureteral orifice and easily passed, and normal efflux of urine could be seen from each ureteral orifice. The midline of the fascia lata flap was then attached to the underlying vaginal wall in the midline using 4–0 Vicryl. A running suture of 2–0 chromic was used to approximate the vaginal incisions. The sutures of 0 Prolene were then tied across each other along the anterior rectus fascia and allowed good suspension of the bladder neck. The subcutaneous tissue in the abdominal incision was then approximated using interrupted sutures of 3–0 chromic. The skin edges were approximated using a running suture of 4–0 Vicryl. The patient tolerated the procedure well.

RETROPUBIC PROSTATECTOMY AND PELVIC LYMPH NODE DISSECTION WITH NERVE SPARING

PREOPERATIVE DIAGNOSIS: T2C, NX, M0 prostate cancer.

POSTOPERATIVE DIAGNOSIS: T2C, NX, M0 prostate cancer.

PROCEDURES PERFORMED
1. Radical retropubic prostatectomy.
2. Bilateral pelvic lymph node dissection.

INDICATIONS: The patient is a 60-year-old male who was noted to have an elevated PSA of 13.7 on routine screening. He underwent a transrectal ultrasound and biopsy which revealed approximately 9 out of 10 cores positive for adenocarcinoma of the prostate. Gleason score was 7/10. He was then treated with 3 months of neoadjuvant hormonal therapy. His PSA preoperatively had decreased to 0.1 on androgen blockade.

DETAILS OF PROCEDURE: The patient was brought back to the operating room and a general anesthetic was administered. He was placed on the table in the supine position with it flexed 20 degrees. He had pneumatic compression stockings placed on his lower extremities. He was then prepped and draped in the usual sterile fashion. A midline incision was made, starting just left of the umbilicus and carried down to the pubic bone. The fascia was split in the midline as well as the rectus muscle, and the retropubic space was then entered. Each obturator fossa was delineated using blunt dissection. A fixed Balfour retractor was then placed.

A left pelvic lymph node dissection was then performed in the usual fashion. Care was taken to avoid the obturator nerve. There were no grossly enlarged nodes in the area. Clips were used to control bleeding and lymph drainage.

Attention was then directed to the right-hand side where a similar dissection was performed. Once again there was no damage to the obturator nerve, and there were no grossly enlarged lymph nodes.

Each of the specimens was then passed off the operative field, and frozen section analysis did not reveal any adenocarcinoma.

The endopelvic fascia was then identified and defatted. It was split along its lateral borders from the puboprostatic ligaments and down to the bladder neck. The dorsal vein complex and endopelvic fascia were then gathered using a curved Babcock clamp. Two 0 Vicryl suture ligatures were placed at the bladder neck to control back-bleeding.

A Goldwasser clamp was then passed between the anterior urethra and dorsal vein complex, and a 0 Vicryl suture was then tied around this complex. A second 0 Vicryl suture ligature was also placed in the most distal portion. The dorsal vein complex was then divided using electrocautery, and excellent hemostasis was noted. The prostatic apex was then identified with further sharp and blunt dissection.

When adequate urethral length was determined to have been obtained, the anterior half of the urethra was then divided sharply using the #15 blade. The Foley catheter was then passed into the wound and divided. The posterior urethra was then sharply transected in a similar fashion. The catheter was then used to provide some subtle traction of the prostate. The rectourethralis was taken down using a right-angle clamp and electrocautery. Each neurovascular bundle was also tied and ligated.

The prostate was noted to be small, at approximately 15 g, and adherent to the rectum. A plane was established, and the prostate was able to be mobilized up to the bladder neck.

The lateral pedicles were controlled using 2–0 Vicryl sutures and divided. A small horizontal incision was then made over the seminal vesicles and ampulla of the vas. Each of these structures was then dissected out using sharp and blunt dissection. Clips were used to control bleeding. The seminal vesicles were able to be removed in their entirety. Each vas was clipped and ligated.

An anatomic bladder neck-preserving dissection was then performed, and the prostate was sharply transected off the bladder neck. The bladder mucosa was everted using a running 4–0 Monocryl suture. Two 0 Vicryl sutures were placed at the 6 o'clock position to tighten the bladder neck to 20 French.

Four 2–0 Monocryl sutures were placed in this bladder neck at equally spaced distances. A Greenwald sound was then placed into the distal urethral stump, and the corresponding bladder neck sutures were then placed into the urethral stump under direct visualization.

The bladder neck was then brought down to the urethral stump using a curved Babcock clamp. The wound had been inspected for any bleeding and all bleeding was confirmed to be controlled. The wound was also irrigated with large amounts of normal saline. The anastomosis was then tied down and, upon testing, was shown to be watertight.

Two #10 round Jackson-Pratt drains were then brought out through each lower abdominal quadrant in a separate stab wound incision. They were used to drain each obturator fossa and around the anastomosis. The fascia was reapproximated using interrupted #1 figure-of-8 Vicryl sutures. The subcutaneous tissue was closed with a running 2–0 chromic suture. The skin was reapproximated using staples. Each drain was sutured in with a 2–0 silk suture. The patient tolerated the procedure well. He was then discharged to the postanesthesia care unit in stable condition.

ROUX-EN-Y GASTRIC BYPASS SURGERY

PREOPERATIVE DIAGNOSIS: Morbid obesity.

POSTOPERATIVE DIAGNOSIS: Morbid obesity.

PROCEDURE PERFORMED: Antecolic laparoscopic gastric bypass, 150 cm, with enteroscopy.

ANESTHESIA: General endotracheal.

BLOOD LOSS: 25 mL.

SPECIMENS: None.

INDICATIONS: A 33-year-old woman with a BMI of 58 who has failed physician-directed weight loss. She suffers from depression, sleep apnea, and urinary stress incontinence. She is, therefore, taken for a 150-cm bypass because of her BMI.

OPERATIVE FINDINGS: Both the liver and the omentum were reasonable.

DETAILS OF PROCEDURE: In the supine position on the operating table, the patient was appropriately padded. General endotracheal anesthesia was undertaken. Foley catheter was sterilely placed. The footboard was placed onto the bed. There was a slight bend to the knees using pillows. The patient was strapped in at the waist, and the abdomen was prepped in the usual sterile fashion with sterile drape to follow.

The 10-mm Optiview trocar was placed in the left upper abdomen under direct visualization into the abdomen. Insufflation was undertaken with 15 mmHg of carbon dioxide. Laparoscopy confirmed good trocar placement and no injury to abdominal organs with trocar placement. Four additional ports were placed in the upper abdomen under direct visualization. Adhesions to the anterior surface of the abdomen were divided where needed using the Harmonic shears, and the omentum was retracted up over the colon.

The ligament of Treitz was positively identified, and the bowel was measured to the end of the biliopancreatic limb. The small bowel was divided using the Endo GIA with the 3.5-mm staples and a Seamguard. The mesentery was divided using the Harmonic shears, and clips were needed until we had a 15-cm mobility on the Roux-en-Y limb. We took great care to preserve the arcades to both the Roux-en-Y and the biliopancreatic limb. We measured distally to the appropriate distance in the mid small bowel and performed a side-to-side anastomosis by making 2 small kissing enterotomies and passing the Endo GIA with the 2.5-mm staples into both limbs, firing the stapler, and removing properly. The enterotomy was approximated by securing both staple lines with 2–0 Monocryl and running the 2 sutures to the middle with a full-thickness inverting suture line and tying in the middle. The suture line and staple line both appeared intact and hemostatic.

The mesenteric defect was approximated with 2–0 silk running suture and the Petersen defect was approximated with 2–0 silk running suture. We split the omentum using the Harmonic shears to create a trough for the Roux-en-Y to go into the upper abdomen.

The stomach was divided 4 cm below the angle of His using the Endo GIA with 3.5-mm staples. A Hurst dilator, 34 French, was carefully passed by the anesthesiologist down into the pouch parallel to the lesser curvature. The Endo GIA with the 3.5-mm staples was then fired for 1 fire parallel to the lesser curvature, creating a pouch the diameter of the 34-French Hurst dilator. We then completed the stomach division with the Endo GIA using 4.1-mm staples with the Seamguard up to the angle of His. The patient tolerated this quite well. Hemostasis was excellent and assured with clips, where needed.

The anastomosis between the apex of the small gastric pouch and the side of the small bowel was performed by running 2–0 silk posterior layer from the staple line on the stomach to the antimesenteric surface of the small bowel, running this down from the antimesenteric surface of the small bowel to the posterior edge of the stomach and then back to the staple line at the apex of the small gastric pouch. We then removed the apex of the staple line for 1.5 cm and made a small enterotomy in the side of the small bowel. The inner layer of 2–0 Vicryl was placed with the knot on the outside and full-thickness bites of small bowel and stomach. The Hurst dilator was then passed down into the small bowel, and we completed the anterior layer with another Vicryl 2–0 running and then tied the 2 Vicryl sutures together. The anterior layer of silk was then placed starting at the upper edge of the silk and tying down to the lower edge of the silk so that the 2 anterior and posterior sutures were tied together. This was performed over the 34-French Hurst dilator. The Hurst dilator was then removed and the abdomen was irrigated and dried. There was no tension on the anastomosis.

A clamp was placed across the small bowel. I went to the head of the bed and passed the gastroscope per oral under direct visualization down to the anastomosis through the stomach. It appeared as a small stomach. Hemostasis was excellent. I passed through the anastomosis, which was airtight, watertight, and hemostatic. We filled the upper abdomen with saline and made sure there were no bubbles, insufflating inside the stomach. The scope was withdrawn under direct visualization.

I went down to the lower abdomen and I changed my gown and gloves and removed the clamp off the bowel. We aspirated the fluid.

Hemostasis was found to be excellent throughout the abdomen. The trocars were removed under direct visualization, the abdomen desufflated, the skin edges approximated with 4–0 Monocryl, and sterile dressings applied. The patient tolerated the procedure extremely well and was taken from the operating room in stable condition.

SPINAL FUSION WITH BAK CAGES AND ROD INSTRUMENTATION

PREOPERATIVE DIAGNOSIS: Degenerative disc disease, L4–5 and L5–S1.

POSTOPERATIVE DIAGNOSIS: Degenerative disc disease, L4–5 and L5–S1.

PROCEDURES PERFORMED: Posterior lumbar interbody fusion, L4–5, and L5–S1 using BAK threaded fusion cages and Danek pedicle screws with local autogenous bone graft under fluoroscopy.

ANESTHESIA: General.

DETAILS OF PROCEDURE: The patient was identified and taken to the operating room, where he was given general anesthesia. He was given antibiotics, and the Foley catheter was placed as well as sequential compression stockings applied. He was transferred onto the surgical table in the prone position on the spinal frame. The back was prepped and draped in the usual sterile fashion. The initial approach to the spine as well as the decompression at the L4–5 and L5–S1 levels were done by the cosurgeon and will be dictated separately.

The fusion was done using the posterior lumbar interbody technique. BAK instrumentation was used. The L4–5 level was addressed first. The alignment guide was placed over the L4–5 disc space and the disc incised with a knife. The initial drill was used to make a hole into the disc space and then spacers were put in sequentially up to a size #12. The x-ray image intensifier was brought into the operating room and draped in a sterile fashion and introduced over the patient to provide a crosstable lateral x-ray of the lumbar spine. An x-ray was taken at every step of the way to provide optimal positioning of all instruments and implants.

The C-ring retractor was placed over the spacer on the left side, and the locking tube sleeve was inserted into the body of L4 and L5. The hole was then drilled with the hand drill and tapped with the hand tap. Loose fragments were removed with the straight pituitary. The assistant held retraction and protection on the nerve roots and dura at all times. At no time were these structures injured.

The cage was then selected and packed with bone graft. There was an abundant quantity of high-quality cancellous bone from the laminectomy, so no bone graft was needed from the iliac crest. This bone graft was packed into the cage at the distal end and then the cage was inserted. The proximal end of the cage was then packed with bone as well. The same technique was then done on the right-hand side and the same technique was done at the L5–S1 level for a total of 4 cages.

Because this was a 2-level cage procedure, the pedicle screw instrumentation was used to augment the stabilization. The pedicle screw was put into the L4 vertebral body by making a bur hole at the junction of the facet joint and transverse process on the left. The assistant held visual and palpable protection of the pedicle and then the curette was used to make an entry hole into the pedicle. This hole was then replaced with the screw. The same technique was done on the contralateral side and at the S1 level bilaterally. The screw from L4 to S1 was connected to the other S1 screw with a rod on both sides, and then the rods were locked into place with the locking nuts. The rods were then connected with a transverse connector piece. A rigid construct was obtained. Final x-rays were taken, and the wound was then closed in anatomic layers using interrupted Vicryl suture for the deep layer and staples for the skin. Sterile dressing was applied and the patient was taken to the recovery room in stable condition.

TOTAL HIP ARTHROPLASTY WITH SALZER APR II PROSTHESIS

PREOPERATIVE DIAGNOSIS: Osteoarthritis, left hip.

POSTOPERATIVE DIAGNOSIS: Osteoarthritis, left hip.

PROCEDURE PERFORMED: Left total hip arthroplasty with Salzer APR II prosthesis.

DETAILS OF PROCEDURE: Under epidural anesthesia supplemented by general anesthesia, the patient was placed in the left lateral decubitus position. The left hip was prepped and draped in the usual fashion. A 10-inch incision was made, centering over the greater trochanter. The incision was deepened and small bleeders were cauterized. The short external rotator was divided close to bone, together with the posterior capsule. The hip was dislocated posteriorly. Severe osteoarthritis was noted. The femoral neck was cut at the appropriate level and angle. The acetabulum was exposed. Osteophytes were excised. The floor was cleared of soft tissue. The acetabulum was reamed progressively to 53 mm in diameter. This was under-reamed by 2 mm. A trial with a 54-mm trial acetabular component was done. Fit and alignment were excellent. The trial component was removed. The 55-mm, porous-coated acetabular component was press-fit into place. Excellent alignment and fixation were noted. The liner was inserted with the overhang posteriorly and inferiorly. The femoral canal was then prepared by reaming and broaching to 13.5-mm stem size. A trial was made with the neutral neck 32-mm head component. The hip was reduced, and a stable range of movement was noted. An AP view taken showed good position and length.

The hip was again dislocated, and the trial femoral component was removed. The femoral canal was prepared for cementing by brushing and washing. The canal was plugged with the Universal cement restrictor plug. The canal was lavaged with pulsatile lavage and dried thoroughly. Two bags of cement were mixed in the vacuum mixer, and using the cement syringe, a 13.5-mm, nonporous stem with a 14-mm centralizer was cemented in place. On setting of the cement, excellent alignment and fixation were noted. The 4-mm neck, 32-mm head component was tapped onto the femoral stem, and the hip was reduced. A stable range of movement was noted. Hemostasis was checked. The hip was drained with one Hemovac drain.

Closure was done using #1 Vicryl to reattach the short external rotators and the posterior capsule. The fascial layer was closed with #1 Vicryl, the subcutaneous layer with 2–0 and 3–0 Vicryl, and the skin with staples. The incision was dressed with Xeroform gauze, 4 × 4 gauze, and a Cover-Roll dressing.

The patient tolerated the procedure well and left for the recovery room in stable condition.

Appendix 3
Common Terms by Procedure

Coronary Artery Bypass Grafting

anastomosed
bifurcation
Blake drain
branch point
clip and cautery technique
coronary angiography
coronary artery bypass grafting
coronary artery disease
de-aired
deep pericardial suture
end-to-side anastomosis
end-to-side fashion
end-to-side manner
Foley catheter
free segment
general endotracheal anesthesia
internal mammary artery
left anterior descending (LAD)
obtuse marginal
octopus retractor
papaverine-soaked sponge
papaverine solution
partial occlusion clamp
pericardial stay suture
pericardium
posterior descending artery (PDA)
posterior lateral branch
prepped and draped
7–0 Prolene suture
protamine
proximal anastomosis
proximal lesion
radial artery catheter
reapproximated
reverse saphenous vein
right coronary artery
risks, benefits, and options

running Vicryl
saphenous vein
sequential vein graft
side-to-side anastomosis
side-to-side fashion
side-to-side manner
silastic tape
skip incision
stainless steel wire
subcutaneous tissue
subcuticular Vicryl
supine position
Swan-Ganz catheter
systemically heparinized
vein graft
vertical midline skin incision
visual inspection

Extracapsular Cataract Extraction with Insertion of Intraocular Lens

access port
akinesia
anterior capsulotomy
anterior chamber
aspiration tip
balanced salt solution
Barraquer lid speculum
Beaver blade
bipolar cautery
4–0 black silk superior rectus traction
    suture
capsular forceps
Cavitron irrigation
Celestone
circular tear capsulorrhexis
    capsulotomy
clear cornea
coapted

Colibri forceps
corneoscleral scissors
corneoscleral wound
cul-de-sac
cystitome needle
deepen the chamber
epinephrine
equal mixture
eraser bipolar cautery
expressed
extracapsular cataract extraction
foot of the haptic
Fox shield
gentamicin
Healon
Honan intraocular pressure reducer
   balloon
intraocular lens
intraocular pressure
Iolab posterior chamber intraocular
   lens
irrigated and aspirated
keratome
lens cortical material
lens loop
lidocaine 2% with epinephrine
lid speculum
limbal peritomy
local anesthesia
Maxitrol ointment
Marcaine 0.75% with epinephrine
McPherson tying forceps
Miochol-E
Nadbath lid block
nucleus
10–0 nylon suture
patch and Fox shield
posterior capsule
retrobulbar anesthesia
Schiotz tonometer
scleral incision
Sinskey hook
stab wound

sub-Tenon space
superior limbus
usual sterile ophthalmic manner
Weck ophthalmic microscope
Westcott scissors
Wydase

Hemicolectomy and Pancreaticoduodenectomy (Whipple Procedure)

abdominal wall
adhesion
anastomosis
ascending colon
ball clamp
Betadine
blunt dissection
Bookwalter retractor
bowel clamp
choledochojejunostomy
clipped and divided
colic vessel
common bile duct
cystic duct
divided between clamps and tied
duodenum
electrocautery
end-to-end anastomosis
end-to-side fashion
enlarged lymph node
Foley catheter
free fluid
frozen section
fundus
gallbladder
gastrocolic tissue
gastroduodenal vessel
gastroepiploic vessel
gastrojejunostomy
general intubation anesthetic
gravity drainage
greater curvature
head of the pancreas

Appendix 3

hemostasis
hepatic flexure
ileocecal valve
ileocolic vessel
induration
inferior vena cava
Jackson-Pratt drain
jejunum
Kelly clamp
Kocher clamp
lesser curvature area of the stomach
level of the umbilicus
ligament of Treitz
loop of jejunum
loop of small bowel
lower abdomen and pelvis
mesenteric defect
mesentery of the terminal ileum and
    cecum
mesocolon
Metzenbaum scissors
middle colic artery and vein
midline incision
midtransverse colon
mucosa to mucosa
neck of the pancreas
neoplasm
obliterated
omental adhesion
omentum
outer layer
palpable node
palpation
1–0 Panacryl
pancreatic neoplasm
pancreaticoduodenal artery
pancreaticoduodenectomy
pancreaticojejunostomy anastomosis
partial colectomy with anastomosis
pathology pending
pedicle
peritoneal cavity
peritoneum

portal vein
proximal ascending colon
proximal ligation
proximal mesocolon
rectus fascia
right and left lobes of the liver
right hemicolectomy
scalpel
self-retaining Bookwalter retractor
3–0 seromuscular silk
sharp dissection
2–0 silk
sigmoid colon
skin staple
skin was approximated
small bowel resection
sponge, instrument, and needle count
staple height
sterilely draped
subcutaneous fat
superior mesenteric vein
suspected neoplasm
suspected pancreatic neoplasm
TA-55 stapler
terminal small bowel
transverse colon
tumor studding
uncinate process
vessel loop
3–0 Vicryl
Weck clip
Whipple procedure
xiphoid

Implantation of Implantable Cardioverter-Defibrillator (ICD)
Ancef 1 g IV
arrhythmia
ASA classification class III
beta blockade
bradycardia

clinical laboratory
congestive heart failure
coronary artery disease
deep conscious sedation
defibrillation impedance
defibrillation testing threshold
defibrillation threshold testing
Dermabond
desaturation
dual-chamber implantable cardioverter-
    defibrillator implantation
dual-chamber pulse generator
echocardiogram
electrophysiological study
fasting state
fluoroscopy
guidewire
hemostasis
implantation
inducible ventricular tachycardia
interrogation of reprogramming
intracardiac atrial and ventricular
    pacing and recording
joule (J)
20-J shock
lead position
left axillary vein
left ventricular dysfunction
local anesthetic
microvolt (mV)
ohm
pacing impedance
pacing parameter
prepared in the usual sterile fashion
pulmonary artery
right atrial appendage
right atrial lead
right atrium
right ventricular apex
right ventricular lead
sharp and blunt dissection
sinus node dysfunction
sinus rhythm

sinus tachycardia
St. Jude Medical
superior vena cava (SVC)
superior vena cava lead
Swan-Ganz catheter
usual sterile fashion
ventricular fibrillation
ventricular tachycardia

Laparoscopic-Assisted Hysterectomy and Bilateral Salpingo-Oophorectomy

Allen stirrups
Ancef
anterior vagina
antibiotic prophylaxis
bilateral salpingo-oophorectomy
bilateral tubes and ovaries
Bovie cautery
broad ligament
curved Mayo scissors
Deaver retractor
direct visualization
dorsal supine position in Allen stirrups
endometriosis
Endostapler
Foley catheter
general endotracheal anesthesia
grossly normal and retroverted
Heaney clamp
high stirrups
informed consent was obtained
infraumbilical area
infundibulopelvic ligament
insufflated
Kocher clamp
Lahey clamp
laparoscopic-assisted hysterectomy and
    bilateral salpingo-oophorectomy
left lower quadrant
lower uterine segment
mucosa of the cervix

opening pressure
peritoneum
posterior cul-de-sac
prepped and draped in normal sterile
    fashion
refractory to conservative treatment
right lower quadrant
saline drop test
serially transected
spasmodic dysmenorrhea
stapling device
suture ligated
towel clip
transected, cut, and suture ligated
ureter
uterosacral complex
uterosacral ligament pedicle
vaginal cuff
Veress needle
0 Vicryl
weighted speculum
Xylocaine

Le Fort Osteotomy and Genioplasty

advancement genioplasty
anterior ramus
bicortical titanium screws
bilateral sagittal split mandibular
    advancement osteotomy
buccal aspect
central incisor bracket
circumvestibular incision
crosscut Fischer bur
curved osteotome
curved reciprocating saw
cuspid
down-fractured
elevator
Fischer bur
floor of the nose
Freer elevator
genioplasty incision

greater palatine vessel
hard palate
head turban
inferior border
infiltrative fashion
infraorbital nerve
intermaxillary fixation
internal rigid fixation
Jeter clamp
Jobst fascioplasty
K wire
large curved osteotome
lateral nasal wall
Le Fort I osteotomy
Lindemann bur
mandibular hypoplasia
mandibular retrogenia
masticatory dysfunction
maxillary arch wire
maxillary dentition
maxillary fixation
maxillary hypoplasia
maxillary nasal crest
maxillary vestibule
medial osteotomy
4–0 Monocryl suture
mucoperiosteal incision
nasal bridge
nasal endotracheal tube
nasal mucosa
nasal pin
nasogastric tube
neurovascular bundle
occlusion
open bite
oral cavity
orthognathic treatment plan
osteotomize
osteotomy cut
overjet
3-piece Le Fort I osteotomy
posterior mandible
propofol

proximal and distal segments
pterygoid plate
reciprocating saw
round bur
0.5% Sensorcaine and 1:200,000
  epinephrine
Smith spreader
splint
stainless steel wire
stainless steel wire loop
Steri-Strips
subperiosteal dissection
supine position
surgical lug
throat pack
titanium plate and screw
vertical ramus
V-to-Y fashion
wire driver
wooden handle osteotome
Woodson elevator

Liver Transplant and Broviac Catheter Placement

absorbable suture
aortic patch
bifurcation
bilateral subcostal incision
biliary atresia
biliary catheter
Broviac catheter placement
caudate lobe
central venous system
colotomy
connective tissue
dissected free
donor cystic duct
double-lumen Broviac catheter
exit site
external jugular vein
fluoroscopy
5-French biliary stent

7-French double-lumen Broviac
  catheter
gallbladder fossa
general anesthesia was induced
hepatic artery anastomosis
hepaticojejunostomy
inferior vena cava
informed written consent
infusion line
in situ
liver transplant
lymphatics
lymph node
magnetic resonance angiography
  (MRA)
monitoring device
multidisciplinary transplant committee
nylon suture
oversewn
peritoneal cavity
portal inflow
portal limb
portoenterostomy
5–0 Prolene running suture
retroperitoneum
Roux-en-Y limb
satisfactory position
silk suture
single layer of silk suture
skeletonized
splenic flexure
subcostal incision
subcutaneous tunnel
subcuticular stitch
suprahepatic anastomosis
transverse colon
urinary catheter
vena cava

Low Transverse Cesarean Section

abdominal cavity
abdominis muscle

Allis clamp
anterior abdominal wall
Apgar score
bladder blade
bladder flap
bluntly and sharply dissected
bulb suctioned
cautery
cephalad and caudad
#1 chromic suture
clear urine
compressive dressing
copious irrigation
cord blood
cord gas
cord was clamped and cut
cul-de-sac
electrocautery
epidural anesthesia
estimated blood loss
exteriorized and wrapped in a moist
    towel
fascial flap
fetal head
final closure
Foley catheter
hemostasis
hemostat
Interceed barrier
intrauterine pregnancy
Kocher clamp
labor and delivery
low transverse cesarean section
lysed
Mayo scissors
median raphe
Metzenbaum scissors
neonate
neonatologist
nicked
normal saline
nuchal cord ×2
omental adhesion

operating room table
oropharynx
parietal peritoneum
pelvic gutter
peritoneal serosa
Pfannenstiel incision
pickup
3-point technique
reapproximated
rectus abdominis muscle
repeat low transverse cesarean section
running imbricating stitch
running locked fashion
running locked stitch
scalpel
simple fashion
sponge, needle, instrument, and lap
    counts were reported as being correct
    ×2
subcutaneous tissue
supine position
upper midline extension
uterine extension
3–0 Vicryl

Myringotomy with Tonsillectomy and Adenoidectomy

adenoid curette
adenoid pad
adenoid tissue
adenotonsillar hypertrophy
anterior tonsillar pillar
aspirated
bilateral myringotomy with tubes
bleeding point
Cortisporin drop
Crowe-Davis mouth gag
ear canal
general endotracheal anesthesia
Harmonic scalpel
middle ear space

midline incision
nasopharyngeal pack
nasopharynx
operating microscope
Paparella tube
posterior choanae
recurrent otitis media
red rubber catheter
retractor
Rose position
serous fluid
soft palate
suction cautery
tonsillar fossa
tonsillectomy and adenoidectomy
wax plug

Open Donor Nephrectomy
adrenal gland
adrenal vein
adventitia
adventitious tissue
antibiotic saline
Betadine
Bookwalter retractor
buried stitch
cautery dissection
cephalad and caudad
coapt
donor nephrectomy
double-row fashion
effluent
electrocautery
end-stage renal disease
external oblique muscle
Foley catheter
general endotracheal anesthesia
Gerota fascia
hemostasis
hilum of the kidney
iliac crest
inferior pole
internal oblique muscle

IV line
kidney rest
latissimus dorsi
left lateral decubitus position
living, related kidney donor
4–0 Monocryl
1–0 Novafil
open left donor nephrectomy
orogastric tube
ovarian vein
peritoneum
posterior-lying lumbar vein
5–0 Prolene suture
psoas
renal artery
retroperitoneal space
right-angle clamp
Satinsky clamp
silk suture
silk tie
Steri-Strips
subcuticular stitch
suitable candidate
transversalis muscle
urecholine
ureter

Open Reduction and Internal Fixation of Hip Fracture
Ancef
angle guide
AP and lateral position
Bennett retractor
Betadine dressing
C-arm control
compression hip screw
DHS hip screw
electrocoagulation
fascia
good purchase
guidewire
4-hole sideplate
greater trochanter

Appendix 3

hemostasis
intertrochanteric fracture
Jackson bone clamp
manipulation
open reduction and internal fixation
prepped and draped
reduction
satisfactory condition
satisfactory spinal anesthesia
sharp dissection
sideplate barrel
skin staple
subcutaneous fat
tap screw
Telos table
traction
vastus lateralis muscle
0 Vicryl interrupted inverted suture
#1 Vicryl interrupted suture
x-ray control

Plate and Screw Hardware Removal

abscess formation
administration of intravenous sedation
aerobic and anaerobic bacterial culture
ankle block fashion
AO screwdriver
apex oriented distally
axis guide
biocorrosion
blunt and sharp dissection
bone biopsy
bone clamp
bony attachment
bony growth
capsular tissue
clamp, cauterize, or ligate
clinically asymptomatic
closed in a layered fashion
compressive dressing
continuous subcuticular fashion

cortical screw
deep tissue
dorsal incision
exsanguinated via gravity
exsanguination
fibrous tissue
first metatarsophalangeal joint
flushed copiously
fusion site
hardware
infiltrative block
internal fixation plate and screw
in toto
intraoperative radiograph
joint capsule
0.045 K-wire
lesser metatarsal
0.5% Marcaine plain
metatarsal bone
metatarsal parabola
metatarsalgia
normal saline
osteomyelitis
periosteal elevator
periosteum
permanent fixation
placed on the operating table in a supine
    position
power bone saw
prepped and draped in the usual sterile
    manner
pseudoarthrosis
reapproximate the deep tissue
removal of hardware
scar tissue
shortening osteotomy
skin margin
soft tissue layer
standard AO technique
subcutaneous tissue
superficial bleeder
surgical area
surgical scar

A58

temporary fixation
3–0 Vicryl
vital structure
V-shaped osteotomy
wedge of bone
well-padded fiberglass posterior splint
well-padded pneumatic tourniquet
wound culture

Port-A-Cath Placement
arrhythmia
carcinoma of the colon
chest wall musculature
defatted
dilator
final sponge, needle and instrument
    counts were correct
free flow of blood
guidewire
heparinized
infiltration of local anesthesia
interrupted 3–0 silk suture
intravenous (IV)
irrigated and aspirated
IV access for chemotherapy
IV sedation plus local
left subclavian Port-A-Cath
0.5% Marcaine
need for IV access for chemotherapy
patient tolerated the procedure well
peel-away sheath
Port-A-Cath
prepped and draped in a sterile fashion
puncture site
right atrium
rolled sheet
sterile dressing
Steri-Strips
subclavian vein
transferred to the recovery room
Trendelenburg position
1% Xylocaine

Pubovaginal Sling
Allis clamp
bladder neck
2–0 chromic
cystoscopy
efflux of urine
fascia lata graft
Foley catheter
hydrodissection
interrupted sutures
inverted U
lithotomy position
Malis scissors
mattress suture
open-ended catheter
pelvic sidewall
prepped and draped in sterile fashion
0 Prolene suture
pubovaginal sling
retropubic space
rectus fascia
running suture
skin edge
Stamey needle
sterile marking pencil
subcutaneous tissue
suprapubic region
suspension of the bladder neck
transverse incision
ureteral orifice
urinary incontinence
vaginal flap
vaginal mucosa
4–0 Vicryl
within normal limits
1% Xylocaine with epinephrine

Retropubic Prostatectomy and Pelvic Lymph Node Dissection with Nerve Sparing
adenocarcinoma
ampulla of the vas

anastomosis
androgen blockade
anterior urethra
backbleeding
Balfour retractor
bilateral pelvic lymph node dissection
bladder mucosa
blunt dissection
clipped and ligated
core positive for adenocarcinoma
curved Babcock clamp
defatted
dorsal vein complex
electrocautery
elevated PSA
endopelvic fascia
Foley catheter
frozen section analysis
general anesthetic was administered
Goldwasser clamp
Gleason score
Greenwald sound
grossly enlarged lymph node
hemostasis
horizontal incision
Jackson-Pratt drain
lateral pedicle
lymph drainage
midline incision
4–0 Monocryl suture
neoadjuvant hormonal therapy
neurovascular bundle
normal saline
obturator fossa
obturator nerve
6 o'clock position
pneumatic compression stockings
postanesthesia care unit
posterior urethra
prepped and draped in the usual sterile
    fashion
prostate cancer
prostatic specific antigen (PSA)

pubic bone
puboprostatic ligament
radical retropubic prostatectomy
rectourethralis
retropubic space
rectus muscle
right-angle clamp
seminal vesicle
sharp and blunt dissection
split in the midline
supine position
transected
transrectal ultrasound
umbilicus
urethral length
urethral stump
0 Vicryl suture ligature
watertight

Roux-en-Y Gastric Bypass Surgery

anastomosis
angle of His
antecolic laparoscopic gastric bypass
anterior surface of the abdomen
antimesenteric surface
biliopancreatic limb
body mass index (BMI)
direct visualization
Endo GIA
enteroscopy
enterotomy
Foley catheter
footboard
full-thickness inverting suture line
gastric pouch
general endotracheal anesthesia
Harmonic shears
hemostasis
Hurst dilator
insufflation
laparoscopy
lesser curvature

ligament of Treitz
mesenteric defect
2–0 Monocryl
morbid obesity
omentum
Optiview trocar
Petersen defect
physician-directed weight loss
prepped in the usual sterile fashion
Roux-en-Y limb
Seamguard
side-to-side anastomosis
2–0 silk running suture
sleep apnea
staple line
sterile drape
sterile dressing
suture line
trocar placement
urinary stress incontinence
Vicryl suture

Spinal Fusion with BAK Cages and Rod Instrumentation

alignment guide
augment
autogenous bone graft
BAK instrumentation
BAK threaded fusion cage
bur hole
cancellous bone
connector piece
C-ring retractor
crosstable lateral x-ray
curette
Danek pedicle screws
degenerative disc disease
dura
entry hole
facet joint
fluoroscopy
Foley catheter
general anesthesia

hand drill
hand tap
iliac crest
interrupted Vicryl suture
laminectomy
2-level cage procedure
L4–5 level
locking nut
locking tube sleeve
L5–S1 level
L4 vertebral body
nerve root
optimal positioning
pedicle screw instrumentation
posterior lumbar interbody fusion
posterior lumbar interbody technique
prepped and draped in the usual sterile
 fashion
prone position
rigid construct
sequential compression stockings
spinal frame
straight pituitary
surgical table
transverse process
x-ray image intensifier

Total Hip Arthroplasty with Salzer APR II Prosthesis

acetabular component
acetabulum
alignment and fixation
anteroposterior (AP)
AP view
broaching
cauterized
cement syringe
centralizer
Cover-Roll dressing
epidural anesthesia
fascial layer
femoral canal
femoral neck

4 × 4 gauze
greater trochanter
Hemovac drain
left lateral decubitus position
neutral neck
nonporous stem
osteoarthritis
osteophyte
porous-coated acetabular component
posterior capsule
prepped and draped in the usual fashion
pulsatile lavage
range of movement

reaming and broaching
Salzer APR II prosthesis
short external rotator
small bleeder
soft tissue
subcutaneous layer
total hip arthroplasty
trial femoral component
under-reamed
Universal cement restrictor plug
vacuum mixer
3–0 Vicryl
Xeroform gauze

Appendix 4
Common Manufacturers and Websites

Editor's Note: Mergers, acquisitions, and new entrants in the medical and scientific equipment industry contribute to this collection.

Manufacturer	Website
Abbott Laboratories	www.abbott.com
Accurate Surgical & Scientific Instrument Corp.(ASSI)	www.accuratesurgical.com
Accuscope	www.accuscope.com
Accutome	www.accutome.com
Achilles USA	www.achillesusa.com
ACI Medical	www.acimedical.com
Ackrad Laboratories, Inc.	www.ackrad.com
Acme United Corp., Medical Division	www.acmeunited.com
ACMI Circon	www.circon.com
Acromed Corp.	www.johnsonandjohnson.com
ACS (Applied Cardiac Systems)	www.acsholter.com
Action Products, Inc.	www.actionproducts.com
Acuson, Inc.	www.acuson.com
Adenna, Inc.	www.adenna.com
Advanced Bionics	www.bionicear.com
Advanced Neuromodulation Systems	www.ans-medical.com
Advanced Orthopedic Systems, Inc.	www.advancedortho.qpg.com
AdvantaJet	www.advantajet.com
Aesculap, Inc.	www.aesculap.de
Alcon Surgical, Inc.	www.alconlabs.com
Aldrich Chemical Co.	www.sigma-aldrich.com/aldrich/
Alimed, Inc.	www.alimed.com
Allen Surgical Co. Ltd.	www.allensfuture.com
Allergan Inc.	www.allergan.com
Allied Healthcare	www.alliedhpi.com
Alltech Associates, Inc.	www.alltechweb.com
Aloka Co., LTD.	www.aloka.co.jp
American Endoscopy/Amersham Corp.	www.amersham.com
American Type Culture Collection	www.atcc.org
Amersham Corp.	www.amersham.com
Angeion Corp.	www.angeion.com
Apple Medical Corp.	www.applemed.com
Applied Cardiac Systems, Inc. (ACS)	www.acsholter.com
Applied Imaging Corp.	www.cytovision.com
Arrow International, Inc.	www.arrowintl.com

Atlas Surgical	www.sahaj.com
Auto Suture	www.autosuture.com
Bausch & Lomb Surgical, Inc.	www.blsurgical.com
Baxter Healthcare Corp.	www.baxter.com
Bayer Diagnostics	www.bayerdiag.com
BBL Microbiology Systems/ Becton Dickinson	www.bd.com
Beckman Coulter, Inc. (Beckman Instruments)	www.beckman.com
Becton Dickinson and Co.	www.bd.com
Beere Precision Medical Instruments, Inc.	www.beeremedical.com
Beltone Electronics Corp.	www.beltone.com
Benson Medical Instruments	www.bensonmedical.com
Biodex Medical Systems, Inc.	www.biodex.com
Bioject, Inc.	www.bioject.com
Bio-Logic Systems, Corp.	www.blsc.com
Bio-Lok International, Inc.	www.biolok.com
Bio-Med Devices, Inc.	www.biomeddevices.com
Bio-Medicus, Inc.	www.medtronic.com
Biomet, Inc.	www.biomet.com
Bio-Rad Laboratories Ltd.	www.bio-rad.com
Biosound Esaote	www.biosound.com
Bird & Cronin Medical	www.birdcronin.com
Bivona Medical Technologies	www.bivona.com
Bledsoe Brace Systems	www.bledsoebrace.com
Boehringer Mannheim Corporation	www.boehringer-mannheim.com
Boekel Scientific	www.boekelsci.com
Boston Scientific Corporation	www.bsci.com
Braintree Scientific, Inc.	www.braintreesci.com
Brasseler USA/Komer Medical	www.brasselerusa.com
Braun Medical, Inc.	www.bbraunusa.com
Breas	www.breas.com
Bristol-Myers Co./Mead Johnson & Company	www.bms.com www.meadjohnson.com
Bristol-Myers Squibb Pharmaceutical	www.bms.com
Bruel & Kjaer Instruments, Inc.	www.bk.dk
Bruker Instruments	www.bruker.com
C.B. Fleet Co., Inc.	www.cbfleet.com
Canon USA, Inc.	www.usa.canon.com
Carbomedics, Inc.	www.carbomedics.com
Cardinal Health	www.cardinal.com
Cardiovascular Innovations, Inc.	www.cvico.com
Cardiovascular Systems/3M Health Care	www.3m.com

Carl Zeiss, Inc.	www.zeiss.com
Carolina Medical, Inc.	www.caromed.com
Carrington Laboratories, Inc.	www.carringtonlabs.com
Cavitron Surgical Systems, Inc./ Valleylab, Inc.	www.valleylab.com
Cavitron/Syntel Division/Alcon Surgical	www.alconlabs.com
Cell Robotics	www.cellrobotics.com
Cetylite Industries, Inc.	www.cetylite.com
Chiron Corporation	www.chiron.com
Cho-Pat, Inc.	www.cho-pat.com
Chughtai	www.chughtaidental.com
Ciba Vision Corporation	www.cibavision.com
Cincinnati Surgical Company	www.cincinnatisurgical.com
Circon Corporation	www.circoncorp.com
Circon ACMI	www.acmicorp.com
Clarus Medical Systems, Inc.	www.clarus-medical.com
CliniMed Systems, Inc.	www.clinimed.com
COBE Laboratories, Inc. (Gambro BCT)	www.cobebct.com
Codman & Shurtleff, Inc.	www.codmanjnj.com
Coherent, Inc.	www.cohr.com
Conmed	www.conmed.com
Cook Incorporated	www.cookincorporated.com/ products/
Cook Urological, Inc.	www.cookurological.com
CooperSurgical, Inc.	www.coopercos.com
CooperVision, Inc.	www.coopervision.com
Cordis Corporation (Johnson & Johnson ultimate parent)	www.cordis.lu
Corometrics Medical System, Inc.	www.gemedicalsystems.com
Corpak USA	www.corpakgroupusa.com
Coulter Corporation	www.coulter.com
Craft de Pak	http://users.erols.com/craftdepak
C. R. Bard, Inc.	www.crbard.com
Critikon, Inc.	www.gemedicalsystems.com
Cryomedics, Inc./Cabot Medical Corp.	www.circoncorp.com
Custom Ultrasonics, Inc.	www.customultrasonics.com
Cypress Bioscience, Inc.	www.cypressbio.com
DaKoCytomation	www.dakousa.com
Datascope Corp	www.datascope.com
Datex-Ohmeda	www.datex-ohmed.com
Davol, Inc.	www.davol.com
Denison Orthopedic Appliance Corp.	www.cddenison.com
Dentsply International, Inc.	www.dentsply.com

Denver Biomedical	www.denverbio.com
DePuy Orthopaedics, Inc.	www.depuy.com
DeRoyal Industries, Inc.	www.deroyal.com
Diasonics	www.diasonics.com
Dicon	www.dicon.com
Doran Instruments, Inc.	www.diagnosysllc.com
Dornier MedTech	www.dornier.com
Dow Medical	www.dow.com
Draeger, Inc. Critical Care Systems	www.draeger.com
Du Pont Company	www.dupont.com
Dynamed Biomedical	www.dynamed.com
Dyonics, Inc/Smith & Nephew Dyonics, Inc.	www.smith-nephew.com
E-Z-EM, Inc.	www.ezem.com
EBI Medical Systems, Inc./Biomet, Inc.	www.biomet.com
	www.ebimedical.com
Eli Lilly	www.lilly.com
Elmed, Inc.	www.elmed.com
Erie Scientific Co.	www.eriesci.com
Ethicon Endo-Surgery	www.eesonline.com
Everest Medical Corp.	www.everestmedical.com
Fenwal Electronics, Inc.	http://content.honeywall.com/sensing/ hss/SensorSystems/sencoa.asp
Fillauer, Inc.	www.fillauer.com
Fischer Imaging Corporation	www.fischerimaging.com
Fisher Scientific Co.	www.fisher.co.uk
Flowtronics, Inc.	www.flowtronics.net
Frank Stubbs Co., Inc.	www.fstubbs.com
Freeman Manufacturing Company	www.freemanmfg.com
Fresenius USA, Inc.	www.fmcna.com
Fujinon, Inc.	www.fuginon.com
Gambro BCT	www.cobebct.com
Gaymar Industries, Inc.	www.gaymar.com
GE Medical Systems	www.gemedicals.com
General Electric CGR USA	www.ge.com
Genzyme Corporation	www.genzyme.com
Glaxo, Inc.	www.glaxowellcome.com
Gomco/Allied Health Care Products, Inc.	www.alliedhpi.com
Gore & Associates, Inc., W. L. (Gore-Tex)	www.gore.com
Gould Instrument Systems, Inc.	www.gould.co.uk
Graham-Field, Inc.	www.grahamfield.com
Grass-Telefactor	www.grass-telefactor.com
Greenwald Surgical Co., Inc.	www.greenwaldsurgical.com
Guidant Corp.	www.guidant.com

Hemocue, Inc.	www.hemocue.com
HemoTec, Inc.	www.braunbiosystems.com
Hewlett-Packard Co.	www.hp.com
Hitachi Denshi America, Ltd.	www.hdal.com
Hitachi Instruments, Inc.	www.hii.hitachi.com
Hoffman-La Roche, Ltd./	www.roche.com
Roche Diagnostic Systems, Inc.	
Hollister, Inc.	www.hollister.com
Hologic, Inc.	www.hologic.com
Horizon Medical Products, Inc.	www.ingenstudio.com/HMP/
Hu-Friedy Manufacturing Co., Inc.	www.hu-friedy.com
Hyclone Laboratories, Inc.	www.hyclone.com
Hydro-Med, Inc.	www.hydromed.com
Inamed Corp.	www.inamed.com
Incstar Corp.	www.diasorin.com
Infimed, Inc.	www.infimed.com
International Biomedical, Inc.	www.int-bio.com
Invacare Corporation	www.invacare.com
Jarit Instruments	www.jarit.com
Johnson & Johnson	www.jnj.com
Kapp Surgical Instrument, Inc.	www.kappsurgical.com
Karl Storz	www.karlstorz.com
Katena Products, Inc.	www.katena.com
Kendall Co.	www.kendallhq.com
Kerr Dentistry	www.kerrdental.com
Keymed, Inc.	www.keymedinc.com
Kinamed, Inc.	www.kinamed.com
Kirwan Surgical Products, Inc.	www.kirwans.com
Kodak Company	www.kodak.com
Kontron Instruments, Inc.	www.kontronmedical.com
KT Medical, Inc.	www.ktmedical.com
Kurzweil Applied Intelligence, Inc.	www.kurzweiltech.com
Labconco Corp.	www.labconco.com
Laser Diagnostic Technologies, Inc.	www.laserdiagnostic.com
Laserscope	www.laserscope.com
Lawton USA Surgical Instruments	www.instruman.com.au
Leica Microsystems, Inc.	www.leica-microsystems.com
Life Medical Technologies, Inc.	www.lifemedicalequipment.com
(Life Medical Equipment)	
Life-Tech, Inc.	www.life-tech.com
Linvatec Corporation	www.linvatec.com
LKC Technologies, Inc.	www.lkc.com
Lone Star Medical Products	www.lsmp.com

Lumex	www.lumex.com
Lumiscope Company, Inc.	www.lumiscope.net
Luxtec Corp.	www.luxtec.com
Machida, Inc.	www.machidascope.com
Mallinckrodt Medical, Inc.	www.mallinckrodt.com
Maramed Orthopedic Systems	www.maramed.com
Marco Ophthalmic, Inc.	www.marcooph.com
Maxxim Medical	www.maxximmedical.com
Medical Graphics Corporation	www.medgraphics.com
Medical Devices International	www.cprmicroshield.com
Medstone International, Inc.	www.medstone.com
Meditron Devices, Inc.	www.meditronmedical.com
Medline Industries, Inc.	www.medline.com
Medrad, Inc.	www.medrad.com
Medtronic, Inc.	www.medtronic.com
Medtronic Ophthalmics	www.medtronicophthalmics.com
MegaDyne Medical Products, Inc.	www.megadyne.net
Mennen Medical Corp.	www.mennenmedical.com
Mentor Corp.	www.mentorcorp.com
Merck & Co., Inc.	www.merck.com
Merlyn Pharmaceuticals	www.merlynp.homestead.com
Micro-Aire Surgical Instruments, Inc.	www.microaire.com
MicroBiologics, Inc.	www.microbiologics.com
Micromedics, Inc.	www.micromedics-usa.com
Microtek Medical, Inc.	www.microtekmed.com
Microvasive/Boston Scientific Corp.	www.bsci.com
Midas Rex Pneumatic Tools	www.medtronic.com/neuro/midasrex
Midmark Corporation	www.midmark.com
Milex Products, Inc.	www.milexproducts.com
Mill-Rose Laboratories, Inc.	www.mrlabsinc.com
Millar Instruments, Inc.	www.millarinstruments.com
Miltex Instrument Co., Inc.	www.miltex.com
Minntech Corporation	www.minntech.com
Mityvac/Neward Enterprises, Inc.	www.lincolnindustrial.com
Moss Tubes, Inc.	www.mosstubesinc.com
Nautilus	www.nautilus.com
NDL Products	www.ndlproducts.com
Nellcor, Inc.	www.nellcor.com
New Life Systems, Inc.	www.newlifesystems.com
New World Medical, Inc.	www.ahmedvalve.com
Ney Company, J. M.	www.deringerney.com
Nichols Institute Diagnostics	www.nicholsdiag.com
Nihon Kohden (America), Inc.	www.nkusa.com

Nikon Inc., Instrument Group	www.nikonusa.com
Nomos Corporation	www.nomos.com
Nordic Track	www.nordictrak.com
Nova Biomedical Corporation	www.nova.ch
Nova Ortho-Med, Inc.	www.novaortho-med.com
Novartis AG	www.novartis.com
Novo Industries A/S	www.novo.dk
Nuaire, Inc.	www.nuaire.com
Nalge Nunc International	www.nalgenunc.com
Oculus of America/Insight Instruments, Inc.	www.insightinstruments.com
Ohio Medical Instrument Co., Inc.	www.schaerermayfieldusa.com/index.html
Ohmeda (Datex-Ohmeda)	www.datex-ohmeda.com
Olympus America, Inc.	www.olympus.com
Onyx Medical Corp.	www.onyxmedical.com
Optimed Technologies, Inc.	www.optimed.com
Orion Medical Products, Inc.	www.orimed.com
Ormco Orthodontics	www.ormco.com
Orthoband Company, Inc.	www.orthoband.com/orthoband/intro.htm
Ortho-Care, Inc.	www.ortho-care.com
Ortho Med, Inc.	www.novaortho-med.com
Osada Electric Co., Inc.	www.osadausa.com
Osteotech, Inc.	www.osteotech.com
Otomed, Inc.	www.otomed.com
Padgett Instruments, Inc.	www.padgettinst.com
Palco Laboratories	www.palcolabs.com
Pall Corporation	www.pall.com
Pascal Company, Inc.	www.pascaldental.com
Passy-Muir, Inc.	www.passy-muir.com
Pentax Precision Instrument Corp.	www.pentaxmedical.com
Perma-Type Co., Inc.	www.perma-type.com
Perkin-Elmer Corp., Nelson Analytical	www.perkin-elmer.com
Philips Medical Systems North America	www.medical.philips.com
Physitemp Instruments, Inc.	www.physitemp.com
Pilling Weck, Inc.	www.pillingweck.com
Pioneer Medical Systems, Inc.	www.pioneermed.com
PLC Medical Systems	www.plcmed.com
PML Microbiologicals	www.pmlmicro.com
PMT Corp.	www.pmtcorp.com
Polaroid Corp. Medical Products	www.polaroid-oem.com/medical.htm
Poly Scientific R&D Corp.	www.polyrnd.com
Poly Vac, Inc.	www.polyvac.com

Popper & Sons, Inc.	www.popperandsons.com
Possis Medical, Inc.	www.possis.com
Pozzi Dental Products	www.americantooth.com/pozzi.htm
Precision Medical, Inc.	www.pmp.net
Premier Dental Products Co.	www.premusa.com
Proctor & Gamble	www.pg.com
Propper Manufacturing Co., Inc.	www.proppermfg.com
Puritan Bennett Corp.	www.puritanbennett.com
(Nellcor Puritan Bennett)	
Quest Medical, Inc.	www.questmedical.com
Quinton Instrument Co.	www.quinton.com
Ramvac Corporation	www.ramvac.com
Ranfac Corporation	www.ranfac.com
Rayfield Technology, Inc.	www.rayglobe.com
Redfield Corporation	www.redfieldcorp.com
Rehab Designs, Inc.	www.rehabdesigns.com
Rehabilicare	www.complextechnologies.com
Respironics	www.respironics.com
Ricca Chemical Company	www.riccachemical.com
Richard Wolf Medical Instruments	www.richard-wolf.com
RJL Systems, Inc.	www.rjlsystems.com
Roche Diagnostic Systems, Inc.	http://us.diagnostics.roche.com
Rocky Mountain Orthodontics	www.rmortho.com
Roho, Inc.	www.rohoinc.com
Ross Laboratories/Ross Products Division	www.rosslaboratories.com
	www.ross.com
Rumex International Co.	www.rumex-international.com
Rusch, Inc.	www.rusch.com
Rush-Berivon, Inc.	www.netdoor.com/com/berivon
Sammons Preston Roylan, Inc.	www.sammonspreston.com
Sanderson-Macleod, Inc.	www.sandersonmacleod.com
Sandhill Scientific, Inc.	www.sandhillsci.com
Sargent-Welch Scientific Co.	www.sargentwelch.com
Scanlan International, Inc.	www.scanlangroup.com
Schering-Plough Corporation	www.schering-plough.com
Schneider (USA), Inc.	http://www.bsci.com
(Boston Scientific subsidiary)	
Schott Fibre Optics, Inc.	www.schott.co.uk
Schuco International	www.schuco.co.uk
SciMed Life Systems (Boston Scientific)	www.bsci.com
Searle & Co., G.D./Buchler Instruments	www.searle.com
(Labconco)	www.labconco.com
Sechrist Industries, Inc.	www.sechristind.com

Seitz Corporation	www.seitzcorp.com
SensorMedics Corp	www.sensormedics.com
SensoMotorie Instruments	www.smi.de
Shandon Lipshaw, Inc.	www.shandon.com
Sharpoint/Surgical Specialties Corp.	www.sharpoint.com
Shimadzu Corporation	www.shimadzu.com
Shippert Medical Technologies Corp.	www.shippertmedical.com
Siemens Corporation	www.siemens.com
Sigma Diagnostics	www.sigma-aldrich.com
Silipos	www.silipos.com
Sklar Instrument Company	www.sklarcorp.com
Smith and Nephew DonJoy, Inc.	www.donjoy.com
Smith & Nephew Dyonics, Inc.	www.smith-nephew.com
Smith and Nephew Richards, Inc.	www.smith-nephew.com
Smith and Nephew Roylan, Inc.	www.roylan.com
SmithKline Beecham	www.sb.com
Snowden-Pencer	www.snowdenpencer.com
Sodem Systems	www.sodemsystems.com
Sofamor Danek Group	www.sofamordanek.com
Sola Optical USA Inc./Sola Ophthalmics	www.sola.com
Sontec Instruments, Inc.	www.sontecinstruments.com
Sony Electronics, Inc., Medical Systems	www.sony.com
SpaceLabs Medical, Inc.	www.spacelabs.com
Sparta Surgical Corp.	www.pillingweck.com/sparta.html
Spectrum Surgical Instruments Co.	www.spectrumsurgical.com
Spencer Technologies	www.spencertechnologies.com
STAAR Surgical Co.	www.staar.com
Stephens Instruments, Inc.	www.stephensinst.com
Sterion, Inc.	www.sterion.com
St. Jude Medical Co.	www.sjm.com
Stryker Corporation, Medical Division	www.strykercorp.com
Stryker Howmedica Osteonics	www.howost.com
Sulzer Carbomedics, Inc.	www.carbomedics.com
Sumitomo Electric U.S.A.	www.sumitomoelectric.com
Sun-Med, Inc.	www.sunmedica.com
Sutter Corp.	www.sutter.com
Synectic Engineering, Inc.	www.synectic.net
Tartan Orthopedics, Ltd.	www.tartanortho.com
Taut, Inc.	www.taut.com
Terumo Medical Corp.	www.terumomedical.com
Thomas Scientific	www.thomassci.com
Thoratec Corp.	www.thoratec.com
Toolmex Corp.	www.toolmex-polmach.co.uk

TomTec Imaging Systems	www.tomtec.de
Topcon America Corp.	www.topcon.com
Toshiba America Medical Systems	www.toshiba.com
Trimedyne, Inc.	www.trimedyne.com
Truform Orthotics & Prosthetics	www.surgicalappliance.com/truform.html
Tulip Products, Inc.	www.tulipmedical.com
Tyco International	www.tycoint.com
United States Catheter & Instrument Co./ Bard Inc. (USCI)	www.crbard.com
Urocare Products, Inc.	www.urocare.com
U.S. Endoscopy Group	www.usendoscopy.com
U.S. Orthotics, Inc.	www.usorthotics.com
U.S. Surgical	www.ussurgical.com
Vacumed	www.vacumed.com
Valley Forge Scientific Corp.	www.vfsc.com
Valleylab, Inc.	www.valleylab.com
Vance Products, Inc.	www.cookuro.com
Varian	www.varian.com
Vasamedics	www.vasamedics.com
Viasys Healthcare, Inc.	www.viasyshealthcare.com
Vicon Industries, Inc.	www.vicon-cctv.com
Vingmed U.S.A.	www.vingmed.se
Vision Science	www.visionscience.com
Visx, Inc.	www.visx.com
Vital Signs, Inc.	www.vital-signs.com
Volk Optical	www.volk.com
Vygon Corp.	www.vygonusa.com
Walter Lorenz Surgical, Inc.	www.lorenzsurgical.com
Wampole Laboratories	www.wampolelabs.com
Weck Closure Systems	www.weckclosure.com
Weck Instruments	www.teleflex.com/medicalgr.htm
Weidmann Plastics Technology	www.weidmann-plastics.com/medical.htm
Welch Allyn, Inc.	www.welchallyn.com
Wells Johnson Co.	www.wellsgrp.com
Whittaker Bioproducts, Inc./ BioWhittaker, Inc.	www.cambrex.com
Wilson Cook Medical, Inc.	www.cookgroup.com/wilson_cook/
Wisap USA	www.wisap.com
Wright Medical Technologies	www.wmt.com
Wyeth-Ayerst Laboratories, Inc.	www.ahp.com/wyeth_labs.htm
Ximed Medical Systems	www.ximedgroup.com

Xomed Surgical Products	www.xomed.com
Zeiss Humphrey Systems	www.humphrey.com
Zimmer, Inc.	www.zimmer.com
Zoll Medical Corp.	www.zoll.com